MW01526225

The Adult and Pediatric Spine

Third Edition

The Adult and Pediatric Spine

Third Edition

Volume 2

Editors-in-Chief

John W. Frymoyer, M.D., M.S.
Professor Emeritus of Orthopaedics and Rehabilitation
Department of Orthopaedics and Rehabilitation
Former Dean, University of Vermont College of Medicine
Burlington, Vermont

Sam W. Wiesel, M.D.
Professor and Chair
Department of Orthopaedics
Georgetown University Medical Center
Washington, D.C.

Associate Editors

Howard S. An, M.D.
The Morton International Professor
Department of Orthopedic Surgery
Rush Medical College of Rush University
Director of Spine Surgery
Rush-Presbyterian-St. Luke's Medical Center
Chicago, Illinois

Scott D. Boden, M.D.
Professor of Orthopaedics
Emory University School of Medicine
Atlanta, Georgia
Director
The Emory Spine Center
Decatur, Georgia

William C. Lauerman, M.D.
Professor
Department of Orthopaedic Surgery
Georgetown University School of Medicine
Georgetown University Medical Center
Washington, D.C.

Lawrence G. Lenke, M.D.
The Jerome J. Gilden Professor of Orthopaedic Surgery
Department of Orthopaedic Surgery
Washington University School of Medicine
St. Louis, Missouri

Robert F. McLain, M.D.
Member, Surgical Staff
Director, Spine Fellowship Program
Cleveland Clinic Spine Institute and the Department of Orthopaedic Surgery
The Cleveland Clinic Foundation
Cleveland, Ohio

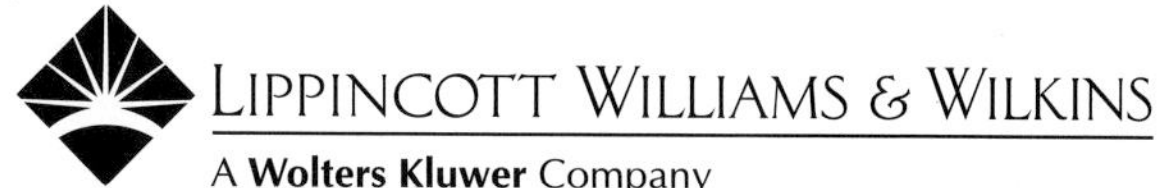

Philadelphia • Baltimore • New York • London
Buenos Aires • Hong Kong • Sydney • Tokyo

Acquisitions Editor: Robert Hurley
Developmental Editor: Julia Seto
Supervising Editor: Patrick Carr
Production Editor: Erica Broennle Nelson, Silverchair Science + Communications
Manufacturing Manager: Colin Warnock
Cover Designer: Marsha Cohen
Compositor: Silverchair Science + Communications
Printer: Courier Westford

530 Walnut Street
Philadelphia, PA 19106 USA
LWW.com

Printed in the USA

Library of Congress Cataloging-in-Publication Data

The adult and pediatric spine / editors-in-chief, John W. Frymoyer, Sam W. Wiesel ; associate editors, Howard S. An ... [et al.].-- 3rd ed.
p. ; cm.
Rev. ed. of: The adult spine. 2nd ed. c1997.
Includes bibliographical references and index.
ISBN 0-7817-3549-1
1. Spine--Abnormalities. 2. Spine--Wounds and injuries. 3. Spine--Diseases--Treatment. 4. Spine--Surgery. 5. Pediatric orthopedics. 6. Pediatric neurology. I. Frymoyer, John W. II. Wiesel, Sam W. III. Adult spine.
[DNLM: 1. Spinal Diseases. 2. Orthopedic Procedures--methods.. 3. Spinal Injuries. 4. Spine. WE 725 A2435 2003]
RD768.A32 2003
616.7'3--dc22

2003060573

---

10 9 8 7 6 5 4 3 2 1

To my wife, Nan P. Frymoyer, a patient educator who has suffered through three editions of *The Adult Spine* with infinite patience, good humor, and love, while constantly reminding, "It is the patient who is number one!"

—J.W.F.

For Anneliese Holland Wiesel—Barbara's and my first grandchild, who represents the future.

—S.W.W.

Contents

II. PEDIATRIC SPINE

Editor: Lawrence G. Lenke

Adult Deformity

Editor: William C. Lauerman

Operative Techniques for Pediatric and Adult Spinal Deformity

Editor: William C. Lauerman

VOLUME 2

III. CERVICAL SPINE

Editor: Howard S. An

Operative Techniques

Editor: William C. Lauerman

Contributing Authors

Kamran Aflatoon, D.O.
Instructor
Department of Orthopaedic Surgery
Johns Hopkins University School of Medicine
Baltimore, Maryland

Nicholas U. Ahn, M.D.
Assistant Professor of Orthopaedic Surgery
University of Missouri—Kansas City School of Medicine
Truman Medical Center
Kansas City, Missouri
Attending Spine Surgeon
Heartland Spine & Specialty Hospital
Overland Park, Kansas

Uri M. Ahn, M.D.
Attending Orthopaedic Surgeon
New Hampshire Spine Institute
Bedford, New Hampshire

Todd J. Albert, M.D.
Professor and Vice Chairman
Department of Orthopaedic Surgery
Jefferson Medical College of Thomas Jefferson University
Philadelphia, Pennsylvania

Glenn M. Amundson, M.D.
Heartland Spine & Specialty Hospital
Overland Park, Kansas

Howard S. An, M.D.
The Morton International Professor
Department of Orthopedic Surgery
Rush Medical College of Rush University
Director of Spine Surgery
Rush-Presbyterian-St. Luke's Medical Center
Chicago, Illinois

Paul A. Anderson, M.D.
Associate Professor
Department of Orthopedics and Rehabilitation
University of Wisconsin Hospital and Clinics
Madison, Wisconsin

Gunnar B. J. Andersson, M.D., Ph.D.
Professor and Chairman
Department of Orthopedic Surgery
Rush Medical College of Rush University
Rush-Presbyterian-St. Luke's Medical Center
Chicago, Illinois

Paul J. Apostolides, M.D.
Associate Attending Physician
Department of Neurosurgery
Greenwich Hospital
Greenwich, Connecticut

Hyun W. Bae, M.D.
Research Director
The Spine Institute at St. John's Health Center
Santa Monica, California

Jonathan J. Baskin, M.D.
Division of Neurological Surgery
Barrow Neurological Institute
St. Joseph's Hospital and Medical Center
Phoenix, Arizona

Drew A. Bednar, M.D.C.M., F.R.C.S.(C)
Associate Clinical Professor of Orthopedic Surgery
Department of Surgery
McMaster University Undergraduate Medical Programme School of Medicine
Hamilton, Ontario
Canada

John M. Beiner, M.D.
Clinical Instructor
Department of Orthopaedics
Yale-New Haven Hospital
New Haven, Connecticut

Theodore A. Belanger, M.D.
Miller Orthopaedic Clinic
Charlotte, North Carolina

Gordon R. Bell, M.D.
Vice Chairman, Department of Orthopaedic Surgery
Vice Chairman, Cleveland Clinic Spine Institute
The Cleveland Clinic Foundation
Cleveland, Ohio

Edward C. Benzel, M.D.
Chairman, Cleveland Clinic Spine Institute
Department of Neurosurgery
The Cleveland Clinic Foundation
Cleveland, Ohio

Philip Michael Bernini, M.D.
Department of Orthopaedic Surgery
Dartmouth Medical School
Dartmouth-Hitchcock Medical Center
Lebanon, New Hampshire

Sigurd H. Berven, M.D.
Assistant Professor in Residence
Department of Orthopaedic Surgery
University of California, San Francisco, School of Medicine
San Francisco, California

Randal R. Betz, M.D.
Professor
Department of Orthopaedic Surgery
Temple University School of Medicine
Shriners Hospital for Children, Philadelphia
Philadelphia, Pennsylvania

Stanley J. Bigos, M.D.
Professor Emeritus
Departments of Orthopedic Surgery and Environmental Health
University of Washington School of Medicine
Seattle, Washington

Ashok Biyani, M.D.
Assistant Professor
Department of Orthopedic Surgery
Medical College of Ohio
Toledo, Ohio

Oheneba Boachie-Adjei, M.D.
Associate Clinical Professor of Orthopaedics
Department of Orthopaedic Surgery
Joan and Sanford I. Weill Medical College and Graduate School of Medical Sciences of Cornell University
Hospital for Special Surgery
New York, New York

Scott D. Boden, M.D.
Professor of Orthopaedics
Emory University School of Medicine
Atlanta, Georgia
Director
The Emory Spine Center
Decatur, Georgia

David S. Bradford, M.D.
Professor and Chairman
Department of Orthopaedic Surgery
University of California, San Francisco, School of Medicine
San Francisco, California

Gregory T. Brebach, M.D.
Attending Orthopedic Spine Surgeon
Department of Orthopedic Surgery
Good Shepherd Hospital
Barrington, Illinois

J. Kenneth Burkus, M.D.
Staff Physician
The Hughston Clinic
Columbus, Georgia

James E. Cain, Jr., M.D.
Orthopaedic Associates of Milwaukee
Milwaukee, Wisconsin

Marco A. Campello, Ph.D.
Associate Clinical Director
Occupational and Industrial Orthopaedic Center
New York University Medical Center
Hospital for Joint Diseases
New York, New York

John J. Carbone, M.D.
Assistant Professor
Department of Orthopaedic Surgery
Johns Hopkins University School of Medicine
Johns Hopkins Bayview Medical Center
Baltimore, Maryland

Eugene J. Carragee, M.D.
Professor of Orthopaedic Surgery
Orthopaedic Surgery Department
Director, Spinal Surgery Section
Stanford University School of Medicine
Stanford, California

Adrian T. H. Casey, M.B., B.S., F.R.C.S., S.N.
Consultant Spinal Neurosurgeon
Victor Horsley Department of Neurosurgery
National Hospital for Neurology and Neurosurgery
London, United Kingdom

Ezequiel H. Cassinelli, M.D.
Clinical Instructor
Department of Orthopaedic Surgery
University of Pittsburgh School of Medicine
University of Pittsburgh Medical Center
Pittsburgh, Pennsylvania

Daniel J. Clauw, M.D.
Professor of Medicine
Department of Internal Medicine
Division of Rheumatology
University of Michigan Medical School
Ann Arbor, Michigan

David H. Clements, M.D.
Associate Professor
Department of Orthopaedic Surgery
Cooper University Hospital
Camden, New Jersey

Jean-Valery C. E. Coumans, M.D.
Instructor in Surgery
Department of Neurosurgery
Harvard Medical School
Massachusetts General Hospital
Boston, Massachusetts

Renn Crichlow, M.D.
Resident
Department of Orthopaedic Surgery
Massachusetts General Hospital
Boston, Massachusetts

H. Alan Crockard, D.Sc., M.B., F.R.C.S., F.D.S.R.C.S, F.R.C.P
Professor
Victor Horsley Department of Neurosurgery
National Hospital for Neurology and Neurosurgery
London, United Kingdom

Scott D. Daffner, M.D.
Department of Orthopaedic Surgery
Thomas Jefferson University Hospital
Philadelphia, Pennsylvania

Mark B. Dekutoski, M.D.
Assistant Professor
Department of Orthopedic Surgery
Mayo Clinic
Saint Mary's Hospital
Rochester Methodist Hospital
Rochester, Minnesota

Rick B. Delamarter, M.D.
Associate Clinical Professor
Department of Orthopaedic Surgery
University of California, Los Angeles, UCLA School of Medicine
Los Angeles, California
St. John's Health Center
Santa Monica, California

Richard A. Deyo, M.D., M.P.H.
Professor
Departments of Medicine and Health Services
University of Washington School of Medicine
Seattle, Washington

Curtis A. Dickman, M.D.
Director of Spinal Research
Division of Neurological Surgery
Barrow Neurological Institute
Phoenix, Arizona

Matthew B. Dobbs, M.D.
Assistant Professor
Department of Orthopaedic Surgery
Washington University School of Medicine
St. Louis Children's Hospital
St. Louis, Missouri

William F. Donaldson III, M.D.
Associate Professor of Orthopaedic Surgery
Associate Professor of Neurologic Surgery
Chief of Spine Service
Department of Orthopaedic Surgery
University of Pittsburgh School of Medicine
University of Pittsburgh Medical Center
Pittsburgh, Pennsylvania

Daryll C. Dykes, M.D., Ph.D.
Staff Surgeon
Twin Cities Spine Center
Minneapolis, Minnesota

Thomas A. Einhorn, M.D.
Professor and Chairman
Department of Orthopaedic Surgery
Boston University School of Medicine
Boston University Medical Center
Boston, Massachusetts

Sanford E. Emery, M.D., M.B.A.
Professor and Chairman
Department of Orthopaedics
Robert C. Byrd Health Sciences Center
West Virginia University School of Medicine
Morgantown, West Virginia

Kevin Farmer, M.D.
Department of Orthopaedic Surgery
Johns Hopkins University School of Medicine
Baltimore, Maryland

Richard G. Fessler, M.D., Ph.D.
John Harper Seeley Professor and Chief
Department of Neurosurgery
University of Chicago Division of Biological Sciences
Pritzker School of Medicine
Chicago, Illinois

Jeffrey S. Fischgrund, M.D.
Department of Orthopaedic Surgery
William Beaumont Hospital
Royal Oak, Michigan

Mitchell K. Freedman, D.O.
Clinical Instructor
Department of Physical Medicine and Rehabilitation
Jefferson Medical College of Thomas Jefferson University
The Rothman Institute
Philadelphia, Pennsylvania

David M. Fribourg, M.D.
Spine Surgeon
The Spine Institute
St. John's Health Center
Santa Monica, California

Guy Fried, M.D.
Assistant Professor
Department of Physical Medicine and Rehabilitation
Jefferson Medical College of Thomas Jefferson University
Magee Rehabilitation Hospital
Philadelphia, PA

John W. Frymoyer, M.D., M.S.
Professor Emeritus of Orthopaedics and Rehabilitation
Department of Orthopaedics and Rehabilitation
Former Dean, University of Vermont College of Medicine
Burlington, Vermont

Timothy A. Garvey, M.D.
Associate Professor
Department of Orthopaedic Surgery
University of Minnesota Medical School—Minneapolis
Twin Cities Spine Center
Minneapolis, Minnesota

Robert J. Gatchel, Ph.D., A.B.P.P.
Professor of Psychiatry
Department of Psychiatry
University of Texas Southwestern Medical Center at Dallas Southwestern Medical School
Dallas, Texas

Alexander J. Ghanayem, M.D.
Associate Professor and Chief
Department of Orthopaedic Surgery and Rehabilitation
Division of Spine Surgery
Loyola University Chicago Stritch School of Medicine
Maywood, Illinois

Sanjitpal S. Gill, M.D.
Fellow
Department of Orthopaedic Surgery
Emory University School of Medicine
Atlanta, Georgia
The Emory Spine Center
Decatur, Georgia

John A. Glaser, M.D.
Professor of Orthopaedic Surgery
Department of Orthopaedic Surgery
Medical University of South Carolina College of Medicine
Charleston, South Carolina

Michael E. Goldsmith, M.D.
Clinical Associate Professor
Department of Orthopaedic Surgery
Georgetown University School of Medicine
Georgetown University Medical Center
Washington, D.C.

Eric J. Graham, M.D.
Spine Fellow
Department of Orthopaedic Surgery
University of Pittsburgh School of Medicine
University of Pittsburgh Medical Center
Pittsburgh, Pennsylvania

Jonathan N. Grauer, M.D.
Assistant Professor
Department of Orthopaedics and Rehabilitation
Yale University School of Medicine
New Haven, Connecticut

Richard D. Guyer, M.D.
Associate Clinical Professor and Co-Director of Texas Back Institute Spine Fellowship
Department of Orthopaedic Surgery
University of Texas Southwestern Medical Center at Dallas Southwestern Medical School
Dallas, Texas
Presbyterian Hospital of Plano
Plano, Texas

Scott Haldeman, D.C., M.D., Ph.D., F.R.C.P.(C)
Adjunct Professor
Department of Epidemiology
School of Public Health
University of California, Los Angeles, David Geffen School of Medicine at UCLA
Los Angeles, California
Clinical Professor
Department of Neurology
University of California, Irvine, College of Medicine
Irvine, California
Adjunct Professor
Research Department
Southern California University of Health Sciences
Whittier, California

Manny Halpern, Ph.D.
Assistant Research Professor
Departments of Environmental Health Science and Ergonomics and Biomechanics
Occupational and Industrial Orthopaedic Center
New York University School of Medicine
New York, New York

James S. Harrop, M.D.
Assistant Professor
Department of Neurosurgery
Jefferson Medical College of Thomas Jefferson University
Thomas Jefferson University Hospital
Philadelphia, Pennsylvania

Andrew C. Hecht, M.D.
Assistant Professor of Orthopaedic Surgery
Chief, Spine Surgery
Mount Sinai School of Medicine of New York University
Mount Sinai Medical Center
New York, New York

John Gaylord Heller, M.D.
Professor of Orthopaedic Surgery
Department of Orthopaedic Surgery
Emory University School of Medicine
Atlanta, Georgia
Spine Fellowship Director
The Emory Spine Center
Decatur, Georgia

Fraser C. Henderson, M.D.
Associate Professor
Department of Neurosurgery
Georgetown University School of Medicine
Georgetown University Medical Center
Washington, D.C.

Shawn M. Henry, D.O.
Associate Clinical Professor
University of North Texas
Orthopedic Spine Surgeon
Texas Back Institute
Fort Worth, Texas

Francis J. Hornicek, M.D., Ph.D.
Associate Professor of Orthopaedic Surgery
Department of Orthopaedic Surgery
Harvard Medical School
Chief, Orthopaedic Oncology
Massachusetts General Hospital
Boston, Massachusetts

Serena S. Hu, M.D.
Associate Professor
Department of Orthopaedic Surgery
University of California, San Francisco, School of Medicine
San Francisco, California

Jeffrey G. Jarvik, M.D., M.P.H.
Associate Professor
Departments of Radiology and Neurosurgery
Adjunct Associate Professor
Department of Health Services
University of Washington School of Medicine
Seattle, Washington

Paul Jeffords, M.D.
Resident
Department of Orthopaedics
Emory University School of Medicine
Atlanta, Georgia

Louis G. Jenis, M.D.
Clinical Assistant Professor of Orthopaedic Surgery
Department of Orthopaedic Surgery
Tufts University School of Medicine
New England Baptist Hospital
Boston, Massachusetts

Safdar N. Khan, M.D.
Research Fellow
Spinal Surgical Service
Joan and Sanford I. Weill Medical College and Graduate School of Medical Sciences of Cornell University
Hospital for Special Surgery
New York, New York

Bong-Soo Kim, M.D.
Department of Surgery
Division of Neurosurgery
University of Chicago Division of Biological Sciences Pritzker School of Medicine
Chicago, Illinois

David H. Kim, M.D.
Attending Spine Surgeon
Department of Orthopaedic Surgery
The Boston Spine Group
Boston, Massachusetts

John S. Kirkpatrick, M.D.
Associate Professor
Division of Orthopaedic Surgery
University of Alabama School of Medicine
Birmingham, Alabama

John P. Kostuik, M.D., F.R.C.S.(C)
Professor
Department of Orthopaedics
Johns Hopkins University School of Medicine
The Johns Hopkins Outpatient Center
Baltimore, Maryland

Timothy R. Kuklo, M.D., J.D.
Assistant Professor of Surgery
Department of Orthopaedic Surgery and Rehabilitation
Walter Reed Army Medical Center
Washington, D.C.

William C. Lauerman, M.D.
Professor
Department of Orthopaedic Surgery
Georgetown University School of Medicine
Georgetown University Medical Center
Washington, D.C.

Daniel D. Lee, M.D.
Department of Orthopaedic Surgery
Johns Hopkins University School of Medicine
Baltimore, Maryland

Ronald A. Lehman, Jr., M.D.
Major, Medical Corps
Senior Resident
Department of Orthopaedic Surgery and Rehabilitation
Walter Reed Army Medical Center
Washington, D.C.

Mesfin A. Lemma, M.D.
Assistant Professor
Department of Orthopaedic Surgery
Johns Hopkins University School of Medicine
Baltimore, Maryland

Lawrence G. Lenke, M.D.
The Jerome J. Gilden Professor of Orthopaedic Surgery
Department of Orthopaedic Surgery
Washington University School of Medicine
St. Louis, Missouri

Peter J. Lennarson, M.D.
Assistant Professor of Surgery
Uniformed Services University of the Health Sciences F. Edward Hébert School of Medicine
Bethesda, Maryland
Clinical Instructor
Department of Surgery
Wright State University School of Medicine
Dayton, Ohio

Kai-Uwe Lewandrowski, M.D.
Fellow in Spine Surgery
Cleveland Clinic Spine Institute
The Cleveland Clinic Foundation
Cleveland, Ohio

Isador H. Lieberman, M.D., M.B.A., F.R.C.S.(C)
Orthopaedic and Spinal Surgeon
Department of Orthopaedics
The Cleveland Clinic Foundation
Cleveland, Ohio

Angela M. Lis, P.T., M.A., C.I.E.
Instructor
Program of Ergonomics and Biomechanics
New York University School of Medicine
Occupational and Industrial Orthopaedic Clinic
Orthopaedic Department
Hospital for Joint Diseases
New York, New York

Randall T. Loder, M.D.
Professor of Orthopaedic Surgery
Department of Orthopaedic Surgery
Indiana University School of Medicine
Riley Hospital for Children
Indianapolis, Indiana

John E. Lonstein, M.D.
Clinical Professor
Department of Orthopaedic Surgery
University of Minnesota Medical School—Minneapolis
Twin Cities Spine Center
Minneapolis, Minnesota

Roger M. Lyon, M.D.
Department of Pediatric Orthopaedic Surgery
Medical College of Wisconsin
Orthopaedic Surgery Clinic
Milwaukee, Wisconsin

Alexandre Marinho, M.D.
University of Iowa Roy J. and Lucille A. Carver College of Medicine
Iowa City, Iowa

Tom G. Mayer, M.D
Clinical Professor of Orthopedic Surgery
Department of Orthopaedic Surgery
University of Texas Southwestern Medical Center at Dallas Southwestern Medical School
Dallas, Texas

Daniel Mazanec, M.D.
Director, Cleveland Clinic Spine Institute
The Cleveland Clinic Foundation
Cleveland, Ohio

Brian R. McCall, M.D.
Assistant Instructor of Orthopaedics
Department of Orthopaedics
Georgetown University School of Medicine
Georgetown University Medical Center
Washington, D.C.

Don McGeary, Ph.D. candidate
Productive Rehabilitation Institute of Dallas for Ergonomics (PRIDE)
Dallas, Texas

Robert F. McLain, M.D.
Member, Surgical Staff
Director, Spine Fellowship Program
Cleveland Clinic Spine Institute and the Department of Orthopaedic Surgery
The Cleveland Clinic Foundation
Cleveland, Ohio

Robert W. Molinari, M.D.
Assistant Professor of Surgery
Uniformed Services University of the Health Sciences F. Edward Hèbert School of Medicine
Chief, Spinal Surgery Service
Madigan Army Medical Center
Tacoma, Washington

Gerd Mueller, M.D.
Director, Rueckenzentrum
Hamburg, Germany

Peter O. Newton, M.D.
Pediatric Orthopedic and Scoliosis Center
Children's Hospital of San Diego
San Diego, California

Margareta Nordin, Dr.Sci.
Professor
Departments of Orthopaedic and Environmental Medicine
New York University School of Medicine
Hospital for Joint Diseases
New York, New York

James W. Ogilvie, M.D.
Professor
Departments of Orthopaedic Surgery and Pediatrics
University of Minnesota Medical School—Minneapolis
Minneapolis, Minnesota

Joseph Orchowski, M.D.
Spine Fellow
Department of Orthopaedic Surgery
Washington University School of Medicine
St. Louis, Missouri

Frank X. Pedlow, M.D.
Chief, Spine Surgery
Department of Orthopaedic Surgery
Massachusetts General Hospital
Boston, Massachusetts

David W. Polly, Jr., M.D.
Professor of Orthopaedic Surgery
Department of Orthopaedic Surgery
Chief, Spine Service
University of Minnesota Medical School—Minneapolis
Minneapolis, Minnesota

Christopher S. Raffo, M.D.
Assistant Instructor of Orthopaedics
Department of Orthopaedics
Georgetown University School of Medicine
Georgetown University Medical Center
Washington, D.C.

Raj D. Rao, M.D.
Associate Professor of Orthopaedic Surgery
Director of Spine Surgery
Department of Orthopaedic Surgery
Medical College of Wisconsin
Milwaukee, Wisconsin

Daniel Refai, M.D.
Department of Neurosurgery
Washington University School of Medicine
St. Louis, Missouri

John M. Rhee, M.D
Assistant Professor
Department of Orthopaedic Surgery
Emory University School of Medicine
Atlanta, Georgia
The Emory Spine Center
Decatur, Georgia

K. Daniel Riew, M.D.
Associate Professor
Department of Orthopaedic Surgery
Washington University School of Medicine
Chief, Cervical Spine Surgery
Barnes-Jewish Hospital
St. Louis, Missouri

Jeffrey S. Ross, M.D.
Head, Division Research
Department of Radiology
The Cleveland Clinic Foundation
Cleveland, Ohio

Andrew A. Sama, M.D.
Instructor of Orthopaedic Surgery
Department of Orthopaedic Surgery
Joan and Sanford I. Weill Medical College and Graduate School of Medical Sciences of Cornell University
Hospital for Special Surgery
New York, New York

Faheem Sandhu, M.D., Ph.D.
Department of Surgery
Division of Neurosurgery
University of Chicago Division of Biological Sciences Pritzker School of Medicine
Chicago, Illinois

Harvinder S. Sandhu, M.D., M.B.A.
Associate Professor
Department of Orthopaedic Surgery
Joan and Sanford I. Weill Medical College and Graduate School of Medical Sciences of Cornell University
Hospital for Special Surgery
New York, New York

Steven C. Scherping, Jr., M.D.
Assistant Professor of Orthopaedic Surgery
Department of Orthopaedic Surgery
Georgetown University School of Medicine
Georgetown University Medical Center
Washington, D.C.

Brian M. Scholl, M.D.
Spine Surgery Fellow
Department of Orthopaedics
University of Tennessee, Heath Science Center, College of Medicine
Campbell Clinic
Memphis, Tennessee

David L. Scott, M.D.
Assistant Orthopaedic Surgeon
Department of Orthopaedic Surgery
Massachusetts General Hospital
Boston, Massachusetts

Saeed A. Shaikh, M.D., F.R.C.P.(C)
Department of Rheumatology
St. Catherine's General Hospital
Ontario, Canada

Mudit Sharma, M.D.
Neurosurgery Resident
Department of Neurosurgery
Georgetown University School of Medicine
Georgetown University Medical Center
Washington, D.C.

Harry L. Shufflebarger, M.D.
Head, Division of Spinal Surgery
Department of Orthopedic Surgery
Miami Children's Hospital
Miami, Florida

Brian G. Smith, M.D.
Associate Professor
Department of Orthopaedics
Connecticut Children's Medical Center
Hartford, Connecticut

Volker K. H. Sonntag, M.D., F.A.C.S.
Clinical Professor of Surgery
University of Arizona College of Medicine
Tucson, Arizona
Vice Chairman, Division of Neurological Surgery
Director, Residency Program
Chairman, Spine Section
Barrow Neurological Institute
Phoenix, Arizona

Paul D. Sponseller, M.D., M.B.A.
Professor of Orthopaedic Surgery
Department of Orthopaedic Surgery
Johns Hopkins University School of Medicine
Baltimore, Maryland

Daniel J. Sucato, M.D., M.S.
Assistant Professor
Department of Orthopaedic Surgery
University of Texas Southwestern Medical Center at Dallas Southwestern Medical School
Texas Scottish Rite Hospital
Dallas, Texas

Brett A. Taylor, M.D
Assistant Professor
Department of Orthopaedic Surgery
Washington University School of Medicine
St. Louis, Missouri

Kerry J. Thompson, M.D.
Department of Interventional Neuroradiology
Anne Arundel Medical Center
Annapolis, Maryland

P. Justin Tortolani, M.D.
Scoliosis and Spine Center
St. Joseph's Hospital
Baltimore, Maryland

Ensor E. Transfeldt, M.D.
Associate Professor
Department of Orthopaedic Surgery
University of Minnesota Medical School—Minneapolis
Department of Orthopaedics
Abbott Northwestern Hospital
Twin Cities Spine Center
Minneapolis, Minnesota

Vincent C. Traynelis, M.D.
Professor of Neurosurgery
Department of Neurosurgery
University of Iowa Roy J. and Lucille A. Carver College of Medicine
Iowa City, Iowa

Eeric Truumees, M.D.
Adjunct Faculty
Bioengineering Center
Orthopaedic Director
Gehry Biomechanics Laboratory
Wayne State University School of Medicine
Detroit, Michigan
Attending Spine Surgeon
Department of Orthopaedic Surgery
William Beaumont Hospital
Royal Oak, Michigan

Alexander R. Vaccaro, M.D.
Professor
Department of Orthopaedic Surgery
Jefferson Medical College of Thomas Jefferson University
The Rothman Institute
Philadelphia, Pennsylvania

Vance E. Watson, M.D.
Assistant Professor of Radiology and Neurosurgery
Departments of Radiology and Neurosurgery
Georgetown University School of Medicine
Georgetown University Medical Center
Washington, D.C.

Mark Weidenbaum, M.D.
Associate Professor, Clinical
Department of Orthopedic Surgery
Columbia University College of Physicians and Surgeons
New York, New York

Sherri R. Weiser, Ph.D.
Research Assistant Professor
Departments of Orthopaedics and Environmental Medicine
New York University School of Medicine
Hospital for Joint Diseases
New York, New York

Sam W. Wiesel, M.D.
Professor and Chair
Department of Orthopaedics
Georgetown University Medical Center
Washington, D.C.

David A. Wong, M.D., M.Sc., F.R.C.S.(C)
Assistant Clinical Professor
University of Colorado School of Medicine
Director, Advanced Center for Spinal Microsurgery
Presbyterian/St. Luke's Medical Center
Denver, Colorado

Kirkham B. Wood, M.D.
Clinical Associate Professor
Department of Orthopaedic Surgery
University of Minnesota Medical School—Minneapolis
Fairview-University Medical Center
Minneapolis, Minnesota

S. Tim Yoon, M.D., Ph.D.
Assistant Professor
Department of Orthopaedic Surgery
Emory University School of Medicine
Atlanta, Georgia

Thomas A. Zdeblick, M.D.
Professor and Chairman
Department of Orthopedics and Rehabilitation
University of Wisconsin Medical School
University of Wisconsin Hospital and Clinics
Madison, Wisconsin

Reinhard D. Zeller, M.D.
Hospital St. Vincent de Pau, Ortho
Paris, France

Preface to the First Edition

Two decades ago a small handful of books and no journals were available to physicians and surgeons who daily encountered spinal disorders. Today, multiple journals and texts are devoted to this topic; yet a comprehensive text has been unavailable to bring together the epidemiology and socioeconomic consequences of spinal disease, its causation and diagnosis, its prevention, and the myriad of nonoperative and operative approaches that are used with varying degrees of success.

The editors and publisher of *The Adult Spine* identified this important need two years ago. Our overall goal was simple: create a book that would serve as *the* reference text for every physician treating adult spine disorders. Our approach was somewhat more complex: Identify all of the important topics in spinal disorders from the foramen magnum to the coccyx, and get the recognized authorities to produce chapters that give the reader the most up-to-date information on those topics. Write chapters that can stand alone so that the reader can find the needed information, illustrated with original drawings and radiographs, and supported by a complete bibliography. At the same time, our editorial group was charged with the important task of making the individual chapters form a comprehensive whole.

The task has been complex. The effort has been monumental to produce a two-volume text comprising 104 chapters, over 400 original illustrations and 2,000 images, and a bibliography of nearly 9,000 references. To complete such a project in two years and thus keep the text at the "cutting edge" has required remarkable devotion from the editors, publisher, illustrators, and librarians.

All of us associated with this project are proud of the final product. We hope you, who read this text, will find it contains all of the important, timely information you need to understand and treat your patients with spinal disorders. If you and they benefit, then our efforts will have been well worth it.

John W. Frymoyer
Thomas B. Ducker
Nortin M. Hadler
John P. Kostuik
James N. Weinstein
Thomas S. Whitecloud III

Preface

The third edition of *The Adult and Pediatric Spine* builds on two previous editions of *The Adult Spine*. While creating a new face for this text, this edition adheres to the goal for the first edition, which was to "create a book that would serve as the reference text for every physician treating adult spine disorders." It was the editors' and publisher's aspiration that the text contain all the important, timely information needed to understand and treat patients with spinal disorders. The basic mission and challenge was to intertwine the science of the spine, the art of medical care, and the complex social and economic climate in which the illness is experienced and care is provided. Published and anecdotal reviews indicated, to a very real measure, that these aspirations were met in both the first and second editions. That is a tribute to the associate editors—Thomas B. Ducker, Norton M. Hadler, John P. Kostuik, James N. Weinstein, and Thomas S. Whitecloud III—to the 108 contributors, to the publisher—Raven Press—and to Kathy Alexander, who shepherded the first edition from an embryonic idea to a two-volume text. The second edition, published by Lippincott–Raven, maintained the basic format of the first edition and presented the most current information.

This third edition, *The Adult and Pediatric Spine*, attempts to respond to the rapidly changing environment, knowledge, and technology surrounding the diagnosis, treatment, and prevention of spinal disorders in the twenty-first century. Editor-in-chief John Frymoyer and the publisher, Lippincott Williams & Wilkins, determined that an entirely "new look" was required. Co-editor-in-chief Sam Wiesel brings his extensive editing experience in the spinal literature along with his commitment and leadership in the area of "best practice." Five new associate editors, Howard An, Scott Boden, William Lauerman, Lawrence Lenke, and Robert McLain, bring their scientific knowledge, clinical expertise, and enthusiasm to this project. The majority of the authors also are new and are current or emerging experts in many of the new scientific and clinical breakthroughs that are occurring. Readers familiar with the previous editions will recognize major changes in this edition.

The title reflects the addition of a new section devoted to the issues of pediatric spinal disorders. Although the growing spine creates distinct issues in diagnosis and particularly, treatment, many of the basic approaches and technologies are applicable to both pediatric and adult patients. This section also responds to the readers of the first two editions, who opined the inclusion of pediatrics would be an important addition.

The pace of new technology and new diagnostic and therapeutic approaches in the past decade is breathtaking and is reflected in many new chapters. The diagnostic tools available to the practitioner abound. Far more detailed information is now available from computed tomography scans and magnetic resonance imaging. Newer technologies, such as positron emission tomography, hold promise for the earlier diagnosis of spinal infections. New knowledge about human genetics and genetic engineering is transforming the face of treatment and will probably allow for prevention in the future. Today, stimulation of osteogenic induction and transduction is a reality. Tomorrow, it is quite possible that induced growth factors will allow the formation of new and functional discs. Pharmacologic advances abound. In many ways, the prevention and treatment of osteoporosis was, at best, crude just 10 years ago. Today, not only is there effective prevention, but also effective treatment for those who have suffered significant bone loss. There also has been major growth in instrumentation systems and implants that allow the surgeon to address the most complex spinal deformities and diseases.

At the same time that all of these advances are occurring, the environment in which health care is rendered continues to be uncertain. The costs of medical care continue to grow at a pace far greater than either the U.S. or world economy. Significant parts of the population are without or have suboptimal health care. The aging population creates its own special challenges, particularly in the affordability of medications and, therefore, access to optimum health care. Numerous reports raise significant questions about the quality of health care, particularly as it is delivered in the hospital environment. All of these issues surround the delivery of care to patients with spinal disorders. In addition, spinal disorders have an unusual place in health care. Spinal disorders are ubiquitous in society. Although most are benign and many are self-limited, the attendant costs are astronomical, particularly in the context of the workplace environment. Thus, the practicing physician and surgeon must understand the environment in which the spinal disorder occurs and the many psychosocial factors that can positively or negatively affect outcomes. The combination of these socioeconomic issues and continued major scientific advances create far more complexity for the practitioners who are ordering and interpreting diagnostic information and attempting to formulate an optimum, hopefully cost-effective, therapeutic approach.

We are proud of the edition's "new face." In the first edition, we stated that, "We hope you, who read this text, will find it contains all of the important, timely information you need to understand and treat your patients with spinal disorders. If you and they benefit, then our efforts will have been well worth it." That continues to be our aspiration for *The Adult and Pediatric Spine*.

J.W.F.

It is both an honor and a personal pleasure to join John Frymoyer as a co-editor-in-chief in this edition of *The Adult and Pediatric Spine*. The first two editions of this text with Dr. Frymoyer as the sole editor-in-chief have truly set a standard for excellence in a specialty text. These books have been used as both a sole source and as a definitive reference. They have also had appeal to a multidisciplinary audience. The future, I think, is bright. As Dr. Frymoyer mentioned above, we have a new set of editors who represent the next generation. They have brought enthusiasm and vigor. This book also features an excellent group of authors, each an expert in his or her specific area. It has been a very exciting and stimulating experience to work with all of the editors and authors. I am truly appreciative of each contribution. Dr. Frymoyer and I are both extremely proud of the final text.

S.W.W.

III

Cervical Spine

Editor

Howard S. An

CHAPTER 31

Congenital Anomalies of the Cervical Spine

Randall T. Loder

Congenital anomalies of the pediatric cervical spine reflect aberrant growth and developmental processes. A knowledge of the normal embryology, growth, and development of the pediatric cervical spine is necessary to understand these conditions.

NORMAL EMBRYOLOGY, GROWTH, AND DEVELOPMENT

Embryology

Embryology of the Occiput-Axis-Atlas Complex

The occiput is formed from four or five somites. All definitive vertebrae develop from the caudal sclerotome half of one segment and the cranial sclerotome half of the next succeeding segment (1). These areas of primitive mesenchyme separate from each other during fetal growth, chondrify, and then subsequently ossify. This chondrification and ossification is a passive process, following the blueprint laid down by the mesenchymal anlage. Due to this sequencing, the cranial half of the first cervical sclerotome remains as a half segment between the occipital and atlantal rudiments and is known as the *proatlas*. The primitive centrum of this proatlas becomes the tip of the odontoid process, whereas its arch rudiments assist in the formation of the occipital condyles (2). The vertebral arch of the atlas separates from its respective centrum, becoming the ring of C-1; the separated centrum fuses with the proatlas above and the centrum of C-2 below to become the odontoid process and body of C-2. The axis forms from the second definitive cervical vertebral mesenchymal segment. The odontoid process is the fusion of the primitive centrum of the atlas and the proatlas half segment. The posterior arches of C-2 form from only the second definitive cervical segment.

Thus, the atlas is made up of three main components: the body and two neural arches. The axis is made up of four main components: the body, two neural arches, and the odontoid (or five components, if the proatlas rudiment is considered).

Embryology of Vertebrae C-3 to C-7

These vertebrae follow the normal formation schema of all vertebrae (3). A portion of the mesenchyme from the sclerotomal centrum creates two neural arches that migrate posteriorly and around the neural tube. This forms the pedicles, laminae, spinous processes, and a very small portion of the body. The majority of the body is formed by the centrum. An ossification center develops in each of the two neural arches and one in the vertebral center, with a synchondrosis formed by the cartilage between the ossification centers.

Normal Growth and Development

Atlas

Ossification exists only in the two neural arches at birth (4). These ossification centers extend posteriorly toward the rudimentary spinous process to form the posterior synchondrosis and anteriorly to form the facets. Anteromedial to each facet the neurocentral synchondroses form, joining the neural arches and the body; this occurs on each side of the expanding anterior ossification center. The body starts to ossify between 6 months and 2 years of age, usually in a single center. By 4 to 6 years of age, the posterior synchondrosis fuses, followed by the anterior ones. The final internal diameter of the pediatric C-1 spinal canal is determined by 6 to 7 years of age. Periosteal appositional growth on the external surface leads to thickening and an increased height but does not change the internal size of the spinal canal.

Axis

The odontoid develops two primary ossification centers that typically coalesce within the first 3 months of life and are separated from the C-2 centrum by the dentocentral synchondrosis (5,6). This synchondrosis is below the level of the C-1 to C-2 facets. It contributes to the overall height of the odontoid as well as the body of C-2. It is continuous throughout the vertebral body and facets and coalesces with the anterior neurocentral synchondroses. These synchondroses progressively close, starting first in the regions of the facets, next at the neurocentral synchondroses, and finally at the dentocentral synchondrosis. This closure occurs between 3 and 6 years of age. The tip of the dens is comprised of a cartilaginous region similar to an epiphysis, the chondrum terminale. When it develops an ossification center between 5 and 8 years of age, it becomes the ossiculum terminale, which fuses to the remainder of the odontoid between 10 and 13 years of age.

The posterior neural arches are partially ossified at birth, joined by the posterior synchondrosis. By 3 months of age, the posterior growth of these arches forms the rudimentary spinous process, which at 1 year of age becomes ossified. By 3 years of age, the posterior synchondrosis has fused. Similar to the axis, the posterior and anterior atlantal synchondroses close by age 6, and there is again no further increase in spinal canal size after this age.

C-3 through C-7

At birth, all three ossification centers are present (7,8). The anterior synchondrosis (neurocentral synchondrosis) is slightly anterior to the base of the pedicle; it typically closes between 3 and 6 years of age. The posterior synchondrosis is at the junction of the two neural arches and usually closes by 2 to 4 years of age. In the neonate and young child, the articular facets are quite horizontal but become more vertically oriented as the child ages. They are also more horizontal in the upper cervical spine than in the lower cervical spine. The vertebral bodies enlarge circumferentially by periosteal appositional growth, whereas they grow vertically by endochondral ossification. Secondary ossification centers develop at the tips of the spinous processes and the cartilaginous ring apophyses of the bodies around the time of puberty. These ring apophyses are involved in the vertical growth of the body. These secondary ossification centers fuse with the vertebral body at approximately age 25 years.

Normal Radiographic Parameters

There are certain normal radiographic parameters that indicate pathology of the cervical spine in adults but in children represent normal developmental processes. These parameters are the atlanto-occipital and atlantodens interval (ADI), pseudosubluxation and pseudoinstability, and normal cervical spine motion in children. ADI and atlanto-occipital motion are determined on lateral flexion-extension views that should be conducted voluntarily with the patient awake. The ADI is the space between the anterior aspect of the dens and the posterior aspect of the anterior ring of the atlas. An ADI of more than 5 mm on flexion-extension lateral radiographs indicates instability (9,10). This is more than the 3-mm adult value limit. This difference is due to the increased cartilage content of the odontoid and ring of the atlas in children, as well as increased ligamentous laxity in children. In extension, overriding of the anterior arch of the atlas on top of the odontoid can also be seen in up to 20% of children (11).

A mild increase in this interval may indicate a subtle disruption of the transverse atlantal ligament. In adults, this ligament ruptures approximately at an interval of 5 mm (12). In chronic atlantoaxial conditions (e.g., rheumatoid arthritis, Down syndrome, congenital anomalies), the ADI is less useful. In these children, who are frequently hypermobile but do not have a ruptured transverse atlantal ligament, the ADI is increased beyond the 3- to 5-mm range. It is here that the complement of the ADI, or the space available for the cord (SAC), is useful (Fig. 1). This space is the distance between the posterior aspect of the dens and the anterior aspect of the posterior ring of the atlas or the foramen magnum. A decrease in the SAC to 13 mm or less may be associated with neurologic problems (13).

In patients in whom there is attenuation of the transverse atlantal ligament but without rupture, the alar ligament does provide some stability. It acts like a checkrein (14), first tightening up in rotation and then becoming completely taut as the odontoid process continues to move posteriorly a distance equivalent to its full transverse diameter. This safety zone between the anterior wall of the spinal canal of the atlas and axis and the neural structures is an anatomic constant equal to the transverse diameter of the odontoid. This constant defines Steel's rule of thirds: one-third cord, one-third odontoid, and one-third space. The cord can move into this space (safe zone) when the odontoid moves posteriorly due to an attenuated transverse atlantal ligament. It is here that the alar

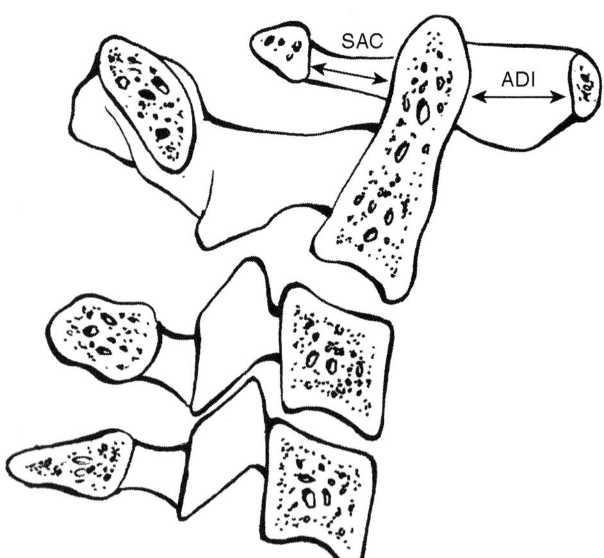

FIG. 1. Atlantoaxial instability. The atlantodens interval (ADI) increases as the space available for the spinal cord (SAC) decreases. SAC less than 13 mm is significant.

ligament becomes taut, acting as a checkrein and secondary restraint, preventing further movement of the odontoid into the cord. In the chronic situation, it is important to recognize when this safe zone has been exceeded and the child enters the region of impending spinal cord compression. In the case of trauma, the alar ligament is insufficient to prevent a fatal cord injury in the event of another neck injury similar to the one that caused the initial interruption of the transverse atlantal ligament.

Normal ranges of motion at the atlanto-occipital interval are not well defined. In a series of 40 healthy college freshmen, the tip of the odontoid remained directly below the basion of the skull in both flexion and extension (15). Thus, the joint should not allow any horizontal translation during flexion and extension. Tredwell et al. (16) feel that a posterior subluxation of the atlanto-occipital relationship in extension of 4 mm indicates instability. This can be measured as the distance between the anterior margin of the condyles at the base of the skull and the sharp contour of the anterior aspect of the concave joint of the atlas anteriorly, or as the distance between the occipital protuberance and the superior arch of the atlas posteriorly. Another method to measure this posterior subluxation of the atlanto-occipital joint uses the technique of Wiesel and Rothman (17). With this technique, occiput to C-1 translation from maximum flexion to maximum extension should be no more than 1 mm in normal adults. Norms for children have not been established for either of these techniques, however.

Pseudosubluxation

It is known that the C2-3 and to a lesser extent the C3-4 interspaces in children have a normal physiologic displacement (18). In a study of 161 children (11), marked anterior displacement of C-2 on C-3 was observed in 9% of children between 1 and 7 years of age. In some children, the anterior physiologic displacement of C-2 on C-3 was so pronounced that it appeared pathologic (pseudosubluxation). To differentiate this from pathologic subluxation, Swischuk has used the posterior cervical line drawn from the anterior cortex of the posterior arch of C-1 to the anterior cortex of the posterior arch of C-3 (Fig. 2) (19). In physiologic displacement of C-2 on C-3, the posterior cervical line may (a) pass through the cortex of the posterior arch of C-2, (b) touch the anterior aspect of the cortex of the posterior arch of C-2, or (c) come within 1 mm of the anterior cortex of the posterior arch of C-2. In pathologic dislocation of C-2 on C-3, the posterior cervical line misses the posterior arch of C-2 by 2 mm or more.

The causes of pseudosubluxation relates to the change in the planes of the articular facets that occurs with growth. The lower cervical spine facets change from 55 to 70 degrees, whereas the upper facets (i.e., C-2 to C-4) may have initial angles as low as 30 degrees that gradually change to 60 to 70 degrees. This variation in facet angulation, along with normal looseness of the soft tissues and intervertebral discs, and the relative increase in size and weight of the skull compared to the trunk, are the major factors responsible for this pseudosubluxation. Because this pseudosubluxation is a normal physiologic condition, no treatment is needed.

Normal Lower Cervical Spine Motion

Generally, the interspinous distances increase with increasing age, with the smallest at C4-5 and the largest at C6-7, until 15 years of age, when it is the largest at C5-6 (10). The anteroposterior displacement from hyperflexion to hyperextension decreases from C2-3 to C6-7. The angular displacement is highest at C3-4 and C4-5 (15 degrees) for those children 3 to 8 years of age, C4-5 (17 degrees) for those aged 9 to 11 years of age, and C5-6 (15 degrees) for those aged 12 to 15 years of age.

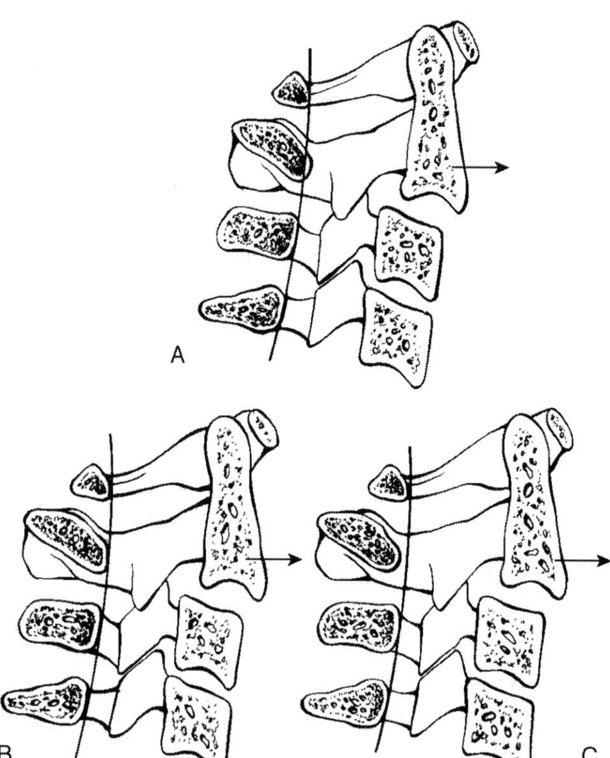

FIG. 2. The posterior line of Swischuk, showing the normal limits. **A:** Passing through or just behind the anterior cortex of C-2. **B:** Touching the anterior aspect of the cortex of C-2. **C:** Coming within 1 mm of the anterior aspect of the cortex of C-2.

CONGENITAL PROBLEMS

Torticollis

Torticollis is a combined rotatory and head tilt deformity and indicates a problem at C1-2 (because 50% of the cervical spine rotation occurs at this joint). A head tilt alone indicates a more generalized problem in the cervical spine. The differential diagnosis of torticollis is large (20) and can be either osseous (e.g., basilar impression) or nonosseous (e.g., congenital muscular torticollis). This chapter discusses only those that have a congenital basis.

Congenital Muscular Torticollis (Congenital Wryneck)

Congenital muscular torticollis is the most common cause of torticollis in the infant and young child, presenting at a median age of 2 months (21). A disproportionate number of these children have a history of a primiparous birth, or the mothers had a breech or difficult delivery. It has, however, been reported in children with normal births and even in children born by cesarean section (21–23). Rarely is there a familial tendency (24,25).

The exact etiology is unknown, but there are several theories. Because of the birth history, one theory is that of a compartment syndrome occurring from soft-tissue compression of the neck at the time of delivery (26). Surgical histopathologic sections suggest occlusion of the veins supplying the sternocleidomastoid muscle (27). This occlusion may result in a compartment syndrome as manifested by edema, degeneration of muscle fibers, and muscle fibrosis. This fibrosis is variable, ranging from small amounts to the entire muscle. MRI studies demonstrate abnormal signals in the sternocleidomastoid muscle but no discrete masses within the muscle (26). The muscle diameter is increased two to four times that of the contralateral muscle. In older patients, the signals are consistent with atrophy and fibrosis, similar to the pathologic changes encountered in compartment syndromes of the leg and forearm. It has been suggested that the clinical deformity is related to the ratio of fibrosis to remaining functional muscle. If ample muscle remains, the sternocleidomastoid will probably stretch with growth, and the child will not develop torticollis; if fibrosis predominates, there is little elastic potential, and torticollis will develop. Another theory is *in utero* crowding, because three of four children have the lesion on the right side (22), and up to 20% have developmental hip dysplasia (28). The fact that it can occur in children with normal birth histories or in children born by cesarean section challenges the perinatal compartment syndrome theory and supports the *in utero* crowding theory. The fact that it can occur in families (24,29) (supporting a genetic predisposition) also questions the compartment syndrome theory. A third theory is primarily a neurogenic causation (30), supported by histopathologic evidence of denervation and reinnervation. The primary myopathy initially may be due to trauma or ischemia, or both, and involves the two heads of the sternocleidomastoid muscle unequally. With continuing fibrosis of the sternal head, the branch of the spinal accessory nerve to the clavicular head of the muscle can be entrapped, leading to a later progressive deformity (30).

The final theory concerns mesenchymal cells remaining in the sternocleidomastoid from fetal embryogenesis. Recent histopathologic studies have demonstrated the presence of both myoblasts and fibroblasts in the sternocleidomastoid tumor in varying stages of differentiation and degeneration (31). The source of these myoblasts and fibroblasts is unknown. After birth, environmental changes stimulate these cells to differentiate, and the sternocleidomastoid tumor develops. Hemorrhagic and inflammatory reactions would be expected if the tumor was a result of perinatal birth trauma or intrauterine positioning, yet these cells were not seen in the sternocleidomastoid histopathologic studies. The occurrence of torticollis depends on the fate of the myoblasts in the mass. If the myoblasts undergo normal development and differentiation, then no persistent torticollis will occur, and conservative treatment will likely succeed. If the myoblasts mainly undergo degeneration, then the remaining fibroblasts produce large amounts of collagen with a scar-like contraction of the sternocleidomastoid muscle and the typical torticollis.

Contracture of the sternocleidomastoid muscle tilts the head toward the involved side and rotates the chin toward the opposite shoulder. There are three clinical subgroups: (a) sternocleidomastoid tumor (43% of cases), (b) muscular torticollis (31% of cases), and (c) postural torticollis (22% of cases) (32). The clinical features of congenital muscular torticollis depend on the time at which the physician evaluates the child. It is often discovered in the first 6 to 8 weeks of life, because the neck was not examined previously (33). If the child is examined during the first 4 weeks of life, a mass or tumor may be palpable in the neck (22,34). It is characteristically a nontender, soft enlargement beneath the skin and located within the sternocleidomastoid muscle belly. This tumor reaches its maximum size within the first 4 weeks of life and then gradually regresses. After 4 to 6 months of life, the contracture and torticollis are the only clinical findings. In some children, the deformity is not noticed until after 1 year of age; this calls into question the congenital part of the name as well as the perinatal compartment syndrome theory. Recent studies (35) indicate that the rate of associated hip dysplasia in children with congenital muscular torticollis is 8%, lower than the previously cited 20% (28). Regardless of the exact prevalence of hip dysplasia in children with congenital muscular torticollis (28,33,36), a hip examination should be performed. The sternocleidomastoid tumor subgroup, the most severe group, presents at an earlier age and is associated with a higher prevalence of breech presentation (19%), difficult labor (56%), and hip dysplasia (6.8%) (32).

If the deformity is progressive, skull and face deformity can develop (plagiocephaly), often within the first year of life. The facial flattening occurs on the side of the contracted muscle and is probably due to the sleeping position of the child (37). Children in the United States usually sleep prone, and in this position, it is more comfortable for them to lie with the affected side down. The face therefore remodels to conform to the bed. If the child sleeps supine, reverse modeling of the contralateral skull occurs. In the child untreated for many years, the level of the eyes and ears becomes unequal and can result in considerable cosmetic deformity.

Cervical spine radiographs should be obtained to differentiate a muscular torticollis from congenital vertebral malformations. Plain radiographs of the cervical spine in children with muscular torticollis are always normal, aside from the head tilt and rotation. If any suspicion exists about the status of the hips, appropriate imaging should be done (ultrasound or radiographs), depending on the age of the child and expertise of the ultrasonographer.

As the deficit in cervical rotation increases, the relative risk for a previous sternocleidomastoid tumor, hip dysplasia, and likelihood of needing surgery increases (38,39). Treatment initially consists of conservative measures (23,34,40–42). Good results can be expected with stretching exercises alone, with one clinical study reporting 90% success (40) and another reporting 95% (39). Those children with a sternocleidomastoid tumor respond less favorably to conservative stretching exercises than those with a simple muscle torticollis; none of the children with postural torticollis need surgery (39). The extent of sternocleidomastoid fibrosis on ultrasound examination is also predictive of the need for surgery (43,44). In those cases in which only the lower one-third of the muscle was involved with fibrosis, all responded to conservative therapy, whereas in those cases where the entire length of the muscle was involved with fibrosis, surgery was needed in 35% of the children (45).

The exercises are performed by the caregivers and guided by the physiotherapist. The ear opposite the contracted muscle should be positioned to the shoulder, and the chin should be positioned to touch the shoulder on the same side as the contracted muscle. When adequate stretching has occurred in the neutral position, the exercises should be graduated up to the extended position, which achieves maximum stretching and prevents residual contractures. Treatment measures to be used along with stretching consist of modifying the child's toys and crib so that the neck is stretched when the infant is reaching for or looking at objects of interest. The exact role of the efficacy of these stretching measures versus a natural history of spontaneous resolution is not known.

Stretching measures usually fail when the deformity persists after 1 year of age (39,41,46,47), and surgery is recommended. The child's neck and anatomic structures are larger, making surgery easier. Established facial deformity or a limitation of more than 30 degrees of motion usually precludes a good result, and surgery is required to prevent further facial flattening and further cosmetic deterioration (41). Asymmetry of the face and skull can improve as long as adequate growth potential remains after the deforming pull of the sternocleidomastoid is removed; good (but not perfect) results can be obtained as late as 12 years of age (42,48). The best time for surgical release is between the ages of 1 and 4 years (34,49); for those treated before the age of 3 years, excellent results can be expected in nearly all cases (48).

Surgical treatments include a unipolar release either at the sternoclavicular or mastoid poles, a bipolar release, a middle one-third transection, and even complete resection. Although these surgical procedures are usually done open, an endoscopic approach has been recently described (50). The bipolar release combined with a Z-plasty of the sternal attachment yielded 92% satisfactory results in one series, whereas only 15% satisfactory results were obtained with other procedures (46). The middle one-third transection has also been reported to give 90% satisfactory results (51). The Z-plasty lengthening maintains the V-contour of the neck and cosmesis, which the middle one-third transection does not. Structures that can be injured from surgery are the spinal accessory nerve, the anterior and external jugular veins, the carotid vessels and sheath, and the facial nerve. Skin incisions should never be located directly over the clavicle because of cosmetically unacceptable scar spreading but rather should be made one finger breadth proximal to the medial end of the clavicle and sternal notch and in line with the cervical skin creases. The postoperative protocol can vary from simple stretching exercises to cast immobilization. An orthosis to maintain alignment of the head and neck is probably a desirable part of the initial postoperative protocol.

Atlanto-Occipital Anomalies

Occipitocervical synostosis, basilar impression, and odontoid anomalies are the most common malformations of the occipitovertebral junction, with an occurrence of 1.4 to 2.5 per 100 children (52). Both genders are equally affected. These lesions arise from a malformation of the mesenchymal anlages at the occipitovertebral junction.

These children resemble those with the Klippel-Feil syndrome—short, broad necks, restricted neck movements, low hairline, high scapula, and torticollis (53,54). The skull may be deformed and shaped like a "tower skull." Other associated anomalies include dwarfism, funnel chest, jaw anomalies, cleft palate, congenital ear deformities, hypospadias, genitourinary tract defects, and syndactyly. Neurologic symptoms may occur during childhood, but more often present during later adulthood, around the age of 40 to 50 years. They progress slowly and relentlessly and can be initiated by traumatic or inflammatory processes. Rarely do they present suddenly or dramatically, although they have been reported as a cause of sudden death. The most common signs and symptoms are neck and occipital pain, vertigo, ataxia, limb paresis, paresthesias, speech disturbances, hoarseness, diplopia, syncope, auditory malfunction, and dysphagia (55,56).

Standard radiographs are difficult to obtain due to fixed bony deformities; overlapping shadows from the mandible, occiput, and foramen magnum; and the patient's difficulty in cooperating. An x-ray beam directed 90 degrees perpendicular to the skull, rather than the cervical spine, usually gives a satisfactory view of the occipitocervical junction. Further studies [computed tomography (CT) scans] are usually needed. The anterior arch of C-1 is commonly assimilated to the occiput, often with a hypoplastic posterior ring. The height of C-1 is also variably decreased, allowing the odontoid to project upward into the foramen magnum (primary basilar impression). The position of the odontoid relative to the opening of the foramen magnum has been described by McRae by measuring the distance from the posterior aspect of the odontoid to the posterior ring of C-1 or the posterior lip of the foramen magnum, whichever is closer (54,57). This should be determined in flexion because this position maximizes the reduction in the SAC. If this distance is less than 19 mm, a neurologic deficit is usually present. Lateral flexion-extension views of the upper cervical spine often show up to 12 mm of space between the odontoid and the C-1 ring anteriorly (54); associated C1-2 instability eventually develops in 50% of these patients (56). The odontoid may also be misshapen or misdirected posteriorly. Up to 70% of these children have a congenital fusion between C2-3. Occipital vertebrae and condylar hypoplasia can also occur.

The MRI is used to image the neural structures. Posterior encroachment on the upper spinal cord or medulla often occurs by a dural constricting band, with resultant neurologic findings. Compression from the posterior lip of the foramen magnum or dural constricting band can disturb the posterior columns with a loss of proprioception, vibration, and tactile senses. Nystagmus also commonly occurs, due to posterior cerebellar compression. Vascular disturbances from vertebral artery involvement can result in brainstem ischemia, manifested by syncope, seizures, vertigo, and unsteady gait. Cerebellar tonsil herniation can also occur (53). The altered mechanics of the cervical spine may result in a dull, aching pain in the posterior occiput and neck with intermittent stiffness and torticollis. Irritation of the greater occipital nerve may cause tenderness in the posterior scalp.

The posteriorly projecting odontoid can cause anterior compression of the brainstem or upper cervical cord. This produces a range of findings and symptoms, depending on the location and degree of compression. Pyramidal tract signs and symptoms (spasticity, hyperreflexia, muscle weakness, gait disturbances) are most common, although sometimes cranial nerve involvement is manifested by diplopia, tinnitus, dysphagia, or auditory disturbances.

Treatment is difficult, because surgical intervention carries a much higher morbidity and mortality risk than with anomalies of the odontoid (53,56,58). For this reason, nonoperative methods should be attempted initially. Cervical collars, braces, and traction often help for persistent complaints of head and neck pain, especially when the complaints follow minor trauma or infection. Immobilization may only achieve temporary relief if neurologic deficits are present. Those with evidence of a compromised upper cervical area should take precautions not to expose themselves to undue trauma.

When symptoms or signs of an unstable C1-2 complex are present, a posterior C1-2 fusion is indicated. Preliminary traction to attempt reduction is used if necessary. If a reduction is possible, and there are no neurologic signs, surgery has a better prognosis (53,56). Posterior signs or symptoms may be an indication for posterior decompression, depending on the evidence of dural or osseous compression. Results vary from complete resolution to increased neurologic deficits and even death (53,58). The role of concomitant posterior fusion has not yet been determined, but if the decompression (either anterior or posterior) could potentially destabilize the spine, then concomitant posterior fusion should be strongly considered.

Basilar Impression

Basilar impression occurs when the skull floor is indented by the upper cervical spine. The tip of the dens is more cephalad and sometimes protrudes into the opening of the foramen magnum. This may encroach on the brainstem, risking neurologic damage from direct injury, vascular compromise, or cerebrospinal fluid flow alteration (59,60).

There are two types of basilar impression: primary and secondary. Primary basilar impression is a congenital abnormality often associated with other vertebral defects (Klippel-Feil syndrome, odontoid abnormalities, atlanto-occipital fusion, and atlas hypoplasia). The prevalence of primary basilar impression in the general population is 1% (61).

Secondary basilar impression, the less common type, is a developmental condition attributed to softening of the osseus structures at the skull base, which can be produced by any disorder of osseous softening that can lead to secondary basilar impression (62). These include metabolic bone diseases [e.g., Paget's disease (63,64)], renal osteodystrophy, rickets and osteomalacia (65), bone dysplasias and mesenchymal syndromes [osteogenesis imperfecta (66–70)], achondroplasia (71), and hypochondroplasia (72), neurofibromatosis (73), and rheumatologic disorders (e.g., rheumatoid arthritis), and ankylosing spondylitis (74,75). The softening allows the odontoid to migrate cephalad and into the foramen magnum.

These patients typically present with a short neck (78% in one series) (62), which is an apparent, rather than real, deformity because of the basilar impression. They also show asymmetry of the skull or face (68%), painful cervical motion (53%), and torticollis (15%). Neurologic signs and symptoms are often present (76). Many children have acute onset of symptoms precipitated by minor trauma (77). In cases of isolated basilar impression, the neurologic involvement is basically a pyramidal syndrome associated with proprioceptive sensory disturbances [motor weakness (85%), limb paresthesias (85%)]. In cases of basilar impression associated with Arnold-Chiari malformations, the neurologic involvement is usually cerebellar (motor in coordination with ataxia, dizziness, and nystagmus). In both types, the patients may complain of neck pain and headache in the distribution of the greater occipital nerve and cranial nerve involvement, particularly those which emerge from the medulla oblongata [trigeminal (V), glossopharyngeal (IX), vagus (X), and hypoglossal (XII)]. Ataxia is a very common

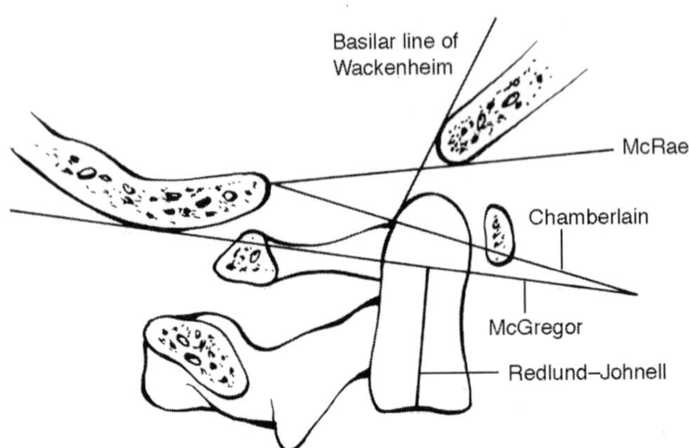

FIG. 3. Lines for assessing basilar invagination. The basilar line of Wackenheim is along the clivus into the cervical canal. The odontoid transects the line in basilar invagination. The McRae line (basion to opisthion), which demonstrates the amount of odontoid protrusion into the foramen magnum, is abnormal whenever the odontoid tip protrudes beyond and into the foramen magnum. The Chamberlain line runs from the posterior lip of the foramen magnum to the dorsal margin of the hard palate. The odontoid bisects this line in early basilar invagination. The McGregor line runs from the upper surface of the posterior edge of the hard palate to the most caudad point of the skull (>4.5 mm is abnormal). The Redlund-Johnell line is the distance between the C-2 inferior vertebra to the McGregor line. Values less than 35 mm (men) or 30 mm (women) indicate basilar invagination.

finding in children (77). Hydrocephalus may develop due to obstruction of the cerebrospinal fluid flow by obstruction of the foramen magnum from the odontoid.

Basilar impression is difficult to assess radiographically (Fig. 3). The most commonly used reference lines are Chamberlain's (59), McRae's (78), and McGregor's (79) measured from the lateral radiograph. McGregor's line is a line from the posterosuperior aspect of the hard palate to the lowermost point on the midline occipital curve. It is the best method for screening, because the landmarks can be clearly defined at all ages on a routine lateral radiograph. Any odontoid tip greater than 4.5 mm above the line is concerning for basilar invagination. McRae's line is helpful in assessing the clinical significance of basilar impression because it defines the opening of the foramen magnum; in those who are symptomatic, the odontoid projects above this line. Chamberlain's line is drawn from the posterior lip of the foramen magnum to the dorsal margin of the hard palate. No more than one-third of the odontoid should project above this line. CT with sagittal plane reconstructions can show the osseous relationships at the occipitocervical junction more clearly, and magnetic resonance imaging shows the neural anatomy (Fig. 4). Occasionally, vertebral angiography is needed (80).

Treatment of basilar impression is difficult and requires a multidisciplinary approach (orthopedic and neurosurgery, neuroradiology) (69,70,81,82). The symptoms can rarely be improved by custom-made orthoses (83). The primary treatment is surgical. If the symptoms are due to a hypermobile odontoid, then surgical stabilization in extension at the occipitocervical junction is needed. Anterior excision of the odontoid is needed if it cannot be reduced (81,84,85) but should be preceded by posterior stabilization and fusion. If the symptoms are from posterior impingement or suboc-

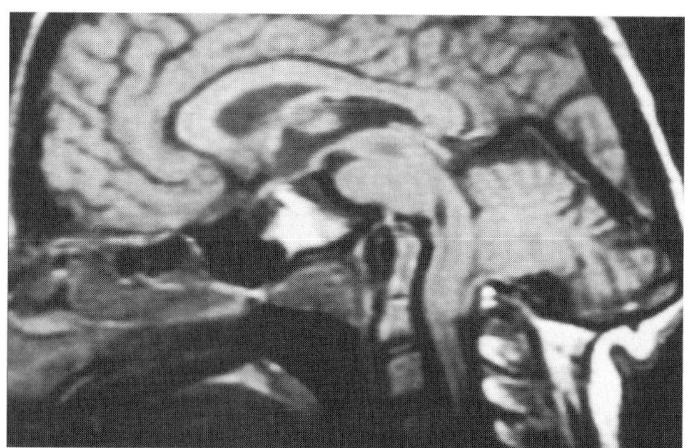

FIG. 4. Sagittal magnetic resonance image of the brain and upper cervical spine shows the odontoid process beyond the margins of the foramen magnum indenting the brainstem. This patient had osteogenesis imperfecta and had posterior occipitocervical fusion. (Courtesy of Howard S. An, M.D.)

cipital decompression, often an upper cervical laminectomy is required. The dura often needs to be opened to look for a tight posterior band (53,54). Posterior stabilization should also be performed. In a recent series of 190 cases, those without an isolated Arnold-Chiari malformation were appropriately treated by decompression of the foramen magnum; transoral anterior decompression was reserved for those without an associated Arnold-Chiari malformation (86). These are general statements, and each case should be individually considered. Secondary basilar impression tends to progress despite arthrodesis (70).

Unilateral Absence of C-1

Unilateral absence of C-1 is a congenital malformation of the first cervical vertebrae and is, in essence a hemiatlas, or a congenital scoliosis of C-1. It was first described by Doubousset (87) in 17 children. The problem is often associated with other anomalies common to children with congenital spine deformities.

Two-thirds of the children present at birth, whereas the others develop a torticollis and are noticed later. A lateral translation of the head on the trunk with variable degrees of lateral tilt and rotation is a typical finding, best appreciated from the back. There may also be severe tilting of the eye line. The sternocleidomastoid muscle is not tight, although regional aplasia of the muscles in the nuchal concavity of the tilted side is noted. Neck flexibility is variable and decreases with age. The condition is not painful. Plagiocephaly can occur and increases as the deformity increases. Neurologic signs (headaches, vertigo, and myelopathy) are present in approximately one-fourth of the patients. The natural history is unknown because this anomaly has only recently been described.

Standard anteroposterior and lateral radiographs rarely give the diagnosis, although the open-mouth odontoid view may suggest it. Tomograms or CT scans are usually needed to see the anomaly. The defect can range from a hypoplasia of the lateral mass to a complete hemiatlas with rotational instability and basilar impression. Occasionally, the atlas is occipitalized. There are three types of this disorder. Type I is an isolated hemiatlas. Type II is a partial or complete aplasia of one hemiatlas, with other associated anomalies of the cervical spine (e.g., fusions of the third and fourth vertebrae, or congenital bars in the lower cervical vertebrae. Type III is a partial or complete atlanto-occipital fusion and symmetric or asymmetric hemiatlas aplasia with or without anomalies of the odontoid or lower cervical vertebrae.

Once this condition is diagnosed, radiographs of the entire spine are needed to rule out other congenital vertebral anomalies. Vertebral angiography and MRI are needed if operative intervention is planned. Arterial anomalies are often found on the aplastic side (e.g., multiple loops, vessels smaller than normal, and abnormal routes between C-1 and C-2), and many of these children have stenosis of the foramen magnum or an Arnold-Chiari malformation.

The initial management is to observe the deformity and document the presence or absence of progression. This observation is primarily clinical because radiographic measurements are difficult to obtain. If the deformity is progressive, bracing does not halt progression. Surgery is recommended for severe deformities. Preoperative gradual correction with a halo is used. An ambulatory method of gradual cervical spine deformity correction has been recently described using the halo-Ilizarov technique (88). A posterior fusion from the occiput to C-2 or C-3 is then performed. Decompression of the spinal canal is necessary when the canal size is not ample, either at the time or if it is projected not to be able to fully accommodate the developed spinal cord. The ideal age for posterior fusion is between 5 and 8 years, when the canal reaches adult size.

Familial Cervical Dysplasia

Familial cervical dysplasia, a recently described atlas deformity (89), has an autosomal-dominant genetic pattern with complete penetrance and variable expressivity. Clinical presentation varies from an incidental finding, a passively correctable head tilt, suboccipital pain, or decreased cervical motion, to a clunking of the upper cervical spine.

Plain radiographs are difficult to interpret. Various anomalies of C-1, most commonly a partial absence of the posterior ring of C-1, are typically seen. Various anomalies of C-2 also coexist, commonly a shallow hypoplastic left facet. Other dysplasias of the lateral masses, of the facets and posterior elements, and occasionally spondylolisthesis are seen. Occiput to C-1 instability is frequently observed, and C1-2 instability is rarely seen. The delineation of this complex anatomy is often best seen with a CT scan and three-dimensional reconstructions. When symptoms of instability are present, an MRI in flexion and extension is recommended to assess the presence and magnitude of neural compression. Neural compression at the occipitocervical junction is created by instability from the malformation(s).

Frequent observation (every 6 to 12 months) is recommended to ensure that instability does not develop either clinically (e.g., progressive weakness and fatigue or objective signs of myelopathy) or radiographically (lateral flexion-extension views). Surgery is recommended for persistent pain, torticollis, and especially neurologic symptoms. A posterior fusion from the occiput to C-2 is usually required, with gradual preoperative reduction using an adjustable halo cast (88).

Klippel-Feil Syndrome

The Klippel-Feil syndrome is a triad of a low posterior hairline, short neck, and limited neck motion (90–93) resulting from congenital fusions of the cervical vertebrae. Other anomalies in the musculoskeletal and other organ systems frequently occur. The congenital fusions result from abnormal embryologic formation of the cervical vertebral mesenchymal anlages. This embryologic insult, although yet unknown, is not limited to the cervical vertebrae, explaining the other associated anomalies with Klippel-Feil syndrome. The annual incidence of congenital cervical fusion is approximately 0.7% (94). In some instances, Klippel-Feil syndrome is familial, indicating a genetic transmission (95–97).

Limited neck motion of varying degrees is seen. Approximately one-third of patients have an associated Sprengel's deformity. The other anomalies associated with the syndrome are scoliosis (both congenital and idiopathic) (90), congenital limb deficiency (98), renal anomalies (99–103), deafness (104–107), synkinesis (mirror movements) (108,109), pulmonary dysfunction (110–112), and congenital heart disease (113,114). Varying degrees of vertebral fusion, ranging from simple block vertebrae to multiple and bizarre anomalies, are observed radiographically (Fig. 5). Klippel-Feil syndrome can be divided into three types depending on the extent of vertebral involvement; type I involves the cervical and upper thoracic vertebrae, type II involves the cervical vertebra alone, and type III involves the cervical vertebra as well as lower thoracic or upper lumbar vertebrae (115). Flexion and extension lateral radiographs are useful to assess for cervical instability. Any segment adjacent to unfused segments may result in hypermobility and neurologic symptoms (116–119). A common pattern is fusion of C1-2 and C3-4, leading to a high risk of instability at the unfused C2-3 level (120).

A thorough evaluation should be undertaken to ensure that no congenital cardiac or other neurologic abnormalities exist (33,121,122). Renal imaging should be done on all children; a simple renal ultrasound is usually quite adequate for initial evaluation (123,124). The neural axis is most easily visualized with an MRI. An MRI should be obtained whenever any concern for neurologic involvement exists on a clinical basis, as well as before any orthopedic spinal procedure (125,126). Flexion-extension lateral radiographs should also be obtained before any general anesthetic to rule out any occult instability of the cervical spine. When flexion-extension radiographs are difficult to interpret (which is not uncommon due to the multiple anomalous vertebrae), a flexion-extension CT scan can be quite useful, especially at the C1-2 level.

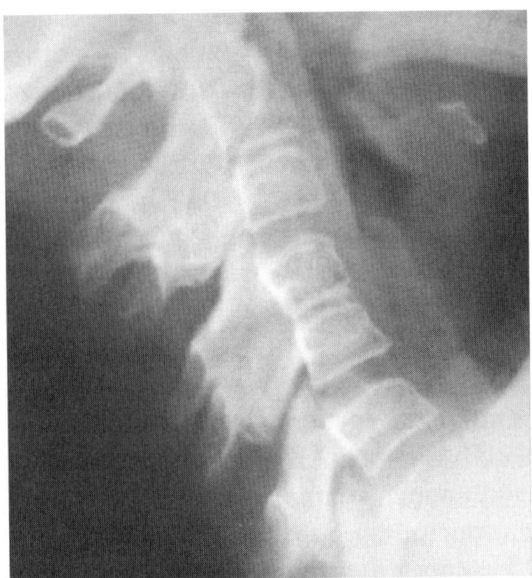

FIG. 5. Lateral radiograph shows block vertebrae (C-2 to C-3 and C-4 to C-5) with slight instability at C-3 to C-4 in a patient with Klippel-Feil syndrome.

The natural history of these children primarily depends on the occurrence of severe renal or cardiac problems, which may limit life expectancy. Instability of the cervical spine (127) can develop with neurologic involvement, especially in the upper segments or in those with iniencephaly (127,128). The more numerous the occipitoatlantal anomalies, the higher the neurologic risk (129). Later in life, degenerative joint and disc disease develops in those with lower segment instabilities. Because children with large fusion areas are at high risk for developing instabilities, strenuous activities should be avoided, especially contact sports. Beyond observation and restricted activities, other nonsurgical methods of treatment are cervical traction, collars, and analgesics when mechanical symptoms appear, which is usually in the adolescent or adult patient. Surgical fusion is needed when neurologic symptoms arise from instability. The real dilemma is whether prophylactic stabilization should be undertaken for asymptomatic hypermobile segments. To date, there are no guidelines on this topic. If stabilization is necessary, the need for accompanying decompression depends on the exact anatomic circumstance, as does the need for combined anterior-posterior versus simple posterior fusions alone. Surgery solely for cosmesis is unwarranted and quite risky (130,131).

Sandifer's Syndrome

Sandifer's syndrome is a syndrome of gastroesophageal reflux (often from a hiatal hernia) resulting in abnormal posturing of the neck and trunk, usually resulting in torticollis (132,133). It is commonly seen in infants or in children with cerebral palsy. The torticollis is believed to be an attempt on the part of the child to decrease the esophagitis pain secondary to the reflux. The majority present in infancy. On occasion, the diagnosis may be delayed and not discovered until childhood. The abnormal posturing may also present as opisthotonos or neural tics and often mimics central nervous system (CNS) disorders. The diagnosis of symptom-causing gastroesophageal reflux is frequently overlooked (134). The associated risk of gastroesophageal reflux is high (up to 40% of infants) (135) with the principal symptoms being vomiting, failure to thrive, recurrent respiratory disease, dysphagia, various neural signs, torticollis, and even respiratory arrest. On careful examination of these infants, the tight and short sternocleidomastoid muscle or its tumor is not seen, eliminating congenital muscular torticollis. Further evaluation excludes skeletal dysplasias, congenital anomalies of the cervical spine, postinfectious causes, and CNS disorders (e.g., extraocular muscle or vestibular apparatus disorders and CNS neoplasms). In these situations, the physician should consider Sandifer's syndrome in the differential diagnosis.

Plain radiographs of the cervical spine are needed to rule out congenital anomalies or skeletal dysplasias. Contrast studies of the upper gastrointestinal tract usually demonstrate hiatal hernia or gastroesophageal reflux (136). Esophageal pH studies may be necessary; many children (both asymptomatic and symptomatic) show evidence of gastroesophageal reflux (137). Medical therapy of the reflux and esophagitis is the first treatment used. When this fails, fundoplication can be considered. In otherwise healthy children, this procedure is usually curative (136).

Other Syndromes

Fetal Alcohol Syndrome

The teratogenic fetal alcohol syndrome is characterized by CNS dysfunctions, growth deficiencies, facial anomalies, and variable major and minor malformations. The children present with developmental delay, especially in motor milestones; failure to thrive; mild to moderate retardation; mild microcephaly; distinct facies (hypoplasia of the facial bones and circumoral tissues); and congenital cardiovascular anomalies. Abnormal necks are not uncommon and are similar to Klippel-Feil syndrome. Fusion of two or more cervical vertebrae occurs in approximately one-half of the children, resembling Klippel-Feil syndrome (138–140). However, fetal alcohol syndrome is distinctly different than Klippel-Feil syndrome, because the major visceral anomaly in Klippel-Feil syndrome is the genitourinary system, whereas in fetal alcohol syndrome, it is the cardiovascular system (140). Radiographic imaging and treatment recommendations regarding the cervical spine are the same as for Klippel-Feil syndrome.

Craniofacial Syndromes

Cleft lip or palate is the most common craniofacial anomaly. It can be a solitary finding or, more often, it is associated with other syndromes and anomalies. Children with cleft anomalies have a 13% associated risk of cervical spinal anomalies, compared to the 0.8% risk in children undergoing orthodontic care for other reasons (noncleft) (141). The incidence is highest in those with soft-palate and submucous clefts (45%). These anomalies are predominantly in the upper cervical spine and are usually spina bifida or vertebral body hypoplasia. The potential for instability is not known, nor is the natural history. No documented information regarding treatment is available; however, the clinician should be aware of this association and make sound clinical judgments as needed.

Craniosynostosis Syndromes (Crouzon's Syndrome, Pfeiffer's Syndrome, Apert's Syndrome, Goldenhaar's Syndrome)

Craniosynostosis syndromes exhibit cervical spine fusions (neural arch, facet fusions, and block vertebrae), occipitoatlantal fusions, and butterfly vertebrae (142–147). Fusions are more common in Apert's syndrome (affecting 71%) than in Crouzon's syndrome, in which 38% are affected (142). Upper cervical fusions are most common in Crouzon's and Pfeiffer's syndromes (144), whereas in Apert's syndrome, the fusions are more likely to be complex and involve C-5 to C-6 (142). However, this syndromal variation is not accurate enough for syndromic differentiation. Congenital cervicothoracic scoliosis is frequently seen in Goldenhaar's syndrome, usually from hemivertebrae (144).

The cervical fusions are progressive with aging; in younger children, the vertebrae appear to be separated by intervertebral discs, but as the child ages, the vertebrae fuse together. Recommendations for treatment are not specifically known; the same principles as in Klippel-Feil syndrome should be followed. One major problem is the potential difficulty with intubation in these children. Odontoid anomalies are rare; however, if any question exists regarding the stability of the cervical spine, lateral flexion-extension radiographs should be obtained.

Dysplasias

Skeletal Dysplasias

Spondyloepiphyseal dysplasia, Morquio syndrome and other mucopolysaccharidoses, achondroplasia, pseudoachondroplasia, chondrodysplasia punctata, and multiple epiphyseal dysplasia have their own unique parameters regarding epidemiology, etiology, and clinical features. The cervical spine is frequently involved (148,149). Overall, 48% of individuals with skeletal dysplasias show upper cervical anomalies (150).

The clinical features of upper cervical instability are often quite subtle and difficult to differentiate in children with skeletal dysplasias from preexisting mechanical problems in the lower limbs associated with joint laxity and epiphyseal malformation (e.g., genu valgum, loss of endurance, tiredness). Later, sleep apnea and loss of hand-motor coordination can occur, with eventual paraparesis or quadriparesis and loss of urinary or bowel sphincter control.

Odontoid hypoplasia with instability on lateral flexion-extension views is the most frequently seen problem. Varying degrees of vertebral body dysplasia are also present. The overall proportion of children with upper cervical anomalies and skeletal dysplasias is 100% for those with Morquio's syndrome, 75% for those with other mucopolysacchandoses, 83% for those with spondyloepiphyseal dysplasia congenita, and 57% for those with pseudoachondroplasia. Children with Hurler's syndrome often show correction of odontoid dysplasia after successful bone marrow transplantation (151).

Flexion-extension CT scans or MRI are often needed to better delineate the neuroanatomy. The vertebral body and odontoid hypoplasia, as well as ligamentous laxity, leads to instability and myelopathy. The relative risk and natural history for irreversible neurologic damage is unknown in most of these dysplasias; however, children with Morquio's syndrome are at a very high risk.

All children with skeletal dysplasias should be screened for upper cervical instability prior to any surgical procedure. Those with Morquio's syndrome should be routinely screened as early as possible, regardless of whether surgery and general anesthesia are planned in the near future, due to their very high risk for instability. When instability develops, upper cervical fusion, often from the occiput to C-3 to C-4 is needed. Halo-cast immobilization is often required; instrumentation, except for interspinous wiring, is rarely indicated.

Combined Soft-Tissue and Skeletal Dysplasias

Neurofibromatosis

Neurofibromatosis is the most common single gene disorder in humans. The proportion of patients with neurofibromatosis and cervical spine involvement is difficult to assess [30% in the series of Yong-Hing et al. (152)]; 44% of those with scoliosis or kyphosis had cervical spine lesions. The children are often asymptomatic (152). Symptoms, when they do occur, are diminished and manifest as painful neck motion, torticollis, dysphagia, deformity, and neurologic signs ranging from mild pain and weakness to paraparesis or quadriparesis (73,153). Neck masses constituted 20% of presenting symptoms in one study of neurofibromatosis patients (154).

Radiographic features of neurofibromatosis in the cervical spine are vertebral body deficiencies and dysplasia or scalloping (152,155). This is often associated with kyphosis (lordosis being less common) and foraminal enlargement. A dystrophic cervicothoracic scoliosis can also develop (156). Lateral flexion-extension radiographs are recommended for all neurofibromatosis patients before general anesthesia or surgery. MRI is quite helpful for assessing the involvement of neural structures and dural ectasia. CT scans are useful for evaluating the upper cervical spine complex and bony definition of the neural foramen. The natural history regarding the cervical spine is unknown, but those with severe kyphosis often develop neurologic deterioration.

Surgical indications are cord or nerve root compression, C-1 to C-2 rotary subluxation, pain, and neurofibroma removal (153,152). Laminectomy alone without accompanying arthrodesis is contraindicated (157). Halo-cast/vests are usually needed after fusions, with or without internal fixation, which is usually simple interspinous wiring. Kyphosis usually requires anterior and posterior fusions. If there are no indications for surgical treatment, then the patient should be closely followed. Pseudarthroses are frequent when isolated posterior fusions are performed.

Marfan Syndrome

Marfan syndrome affects ligamentous laxity and bone morphology. It is due to a mutation in the gene coding for the glycoprotein fibrillin, which has been mapped to the long arm of chromosome 15. Abnormalities regarding the cervical spine in this syndrome are primarily identified radiographically rather than by clinical examination (158,159). Focal cervical kyphosis involving at least three consecutive vertebra occurs in 16%, with an average kyphosis of 22 degrees. The normal cervical lordosis is absent in 35%. Atlantoaxial hypermobility is common (54%). There is also an increased risk of radiographic basilar impression (36%). Unlike Down syndrome, there is no increased association with cervical skeletal anomalies such as persistent synchondrosis and spina bifida occulta of C-1. In spite of these radiographic abnormalities observed in patients with Marfan syndrome, symptoms or neurologic compromise are rare. Neck pain is not increased compared to the general population. Patients with Marfan syndrome should be advised to avoid sports with high-impact loading on the cervical spine; it does not appear necessary to routinely perform cervical radiographs for those undergoing general anesthesia. Atlantoaxial rotatory subluxation may be increased in those with Marfan syndrome, and this should be specially noted during surgical positioning.

Os Odontoideum

Os odontoideum is an anomaly where the tip of the odontoid process is divided by a wide transverse gap, leaving the apical segment without its basilar support (160,161). It is quite rare; the exact incidence is unknown. It most likely represents an unrecognized fracture at the base of the odontoid or damage to the epiphyseal plate during the first few years of life (160,162). Either of these can compromise the blood supply to the developing odontoid, resulting in the os odontoideum. MRI scans have further documented the presence of nuchal cord changes consistent with trauma (163). Some authors believe that it may represent a congenital anomaly instead of occult trauma (164), and it is for this reason that it is included in this chapter on congenital anomalies.

These children usually present with local neck pain, and occasionally transitory episodes of paresis, myelopathy, or cerebral-brainstem ischemia due to vertebral artery compression from the upper cervical instability. Sudden death can also occur, but it is rare.

Radiographically, an os odontoideum is seen as an oval or round ossicle with a smooth sclerotic border, is of variable size, and is located in the position of the normal odontoid tip. On occasion, it can be located near the basioccipital area of the foramen magnum. There are three radiographic types of os odontoideum; round, cone, and blunt tooth (165). The base of the dens is usually hypoplastic. It is often difficult to differentiate an os odontoideum from nonunion following a fracture. The gap between the os and the hypoplastic dens is wider than in a fracture and usually well above the level of the facets. Tomograms and CT scans are useful to further delineate the bony anatomy, and flexion-extension lateral radiographs are useful to assess instability (Fig. 6). The instability index and sagittal plane rotation angle can be measured (166). The presence of myelopathy is highly correlated with a sagittal plane rotation angle 20 degrees and an instability index 40%; it is also most common in the round type of os odontoideum (165).

The neurologic symptoms are due to cord compression from posterior translation of the os into the cord in extension, or the odontoid into the cord in flexion. Increased motion at the C-1 to C-2 level can lead to vertebral artery occlusion ischemia of the

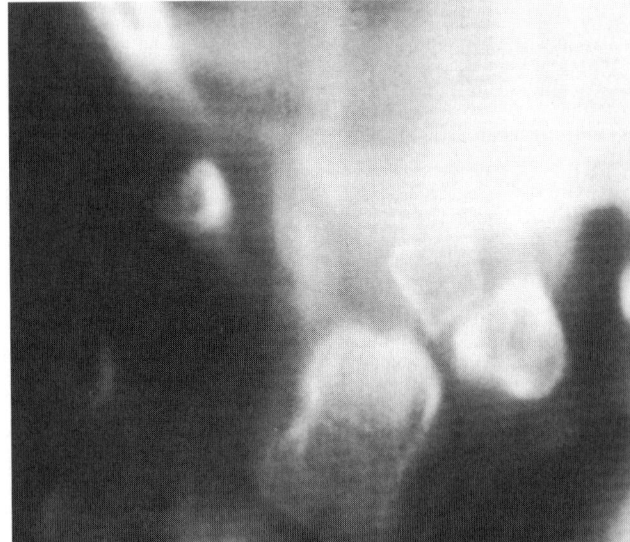

FIG. 6. Lateral radiograph shows os odontoideum. Atlantodens interval and space available for the spinal cord are within normal limits.

brainstem and posterior fossa structures, resulting in seizures, syncope, vertigo, and visual disturbances. The long-term natural history is unknown.

Those with local pain or transient myelopathies can expect recovery with cervical traction or immobilization. Subsequently, only nonathletic activities should be allowed, but the curtailment of activities in the pediatric age group can be difficult. One must weigh the risk of a small insult leading to catastrophic quadriplegia or death in determining an appropriate level of activity.

Surgery is indicated when there is 10 mm or more of instability (ADI) or a SAC of 13 mm or less (13), neurologic involvement, progressive instability, or persistent neck pain. A Gallie-type fusion is recommended. The surgeon must be careful when tightening the wire so that the os is not pulled back posteriorly into the canal and cord, with disastrous consequences. In small children, the wire may be eliminated. In all children, a Minverva or halo cast or vest is also used in the postoperative period. C-1 to C-2 screw fixation has been reported in pediatric atlantoaxial instability (167) for those children older than 4 years of age.

REFERENCES

1. O'Rahilly R, Meyer DB. The timing and sequence of events in the development of the human vertebral column during the embryonic period proper. *Anat Embryol* 1979;57:167–176.
2. Sensenig EC. The development of the occipital and cervical segments and their associated structures in human embryos. *Contrib Embryol Carnegie Inst* 1957;36:141–156.
3. O'Rahilly R, Muller F, Meyer DB. The human vertebral column at the end of the embryonic period proper. 1. The column as a whole. *J Anat* 1980;131:565–575.
4. Ogden JA. Radiology of postnatal skeletal development. XI. The first cervical vertebrae. *Skeletal Radiol* 1984;12:12–20.
5. Ogden JA. Radiology of postnatal skeletal development. XII. The second cervical vertebra. *Skeletal Radiol* 1984;12:169–177.
6. Ogden JA, Murphy MJ, Southwick WO, et al. Radiology of postnatal skeletal development. XIII. C1-2 interrelationships. *Skeletal Radiol* 1986;15:433–438.
7. Fesmire FM, Luten RC. The pediatric cervical spine: developmental anatomy and clinical aspects. *Emer Med* 1989;7:133–142.
8. Ogden JA. *Skeletal injury in the child*, 2nd ed. Philadelphia: WB Saunders, 1990.
9. Locke GR, Gardner II, van Epps EF. Atlas-dens interval (ADI) in children. A survey based on 200 normal cervical spines. *AJR Am J Roentgenol* 1966;97:135–140.
10. Pennecot GF, Gouraud D, Hardy JR, et al. Roentgenographical study of the stability of the cervical spine in children. *J Pediatr Orthop* 1984;4:346–352.
11. Cattell HS, Filtzer DL. Pseudosubluxation and other normal variations in the cervical spine in children. *J Bone Joint Surg Am* 1965;47-A:1295–1309.
12. Fielding JW, Cochran GVB, Lawsing JF III, et al. Tears of the transverse ligament of the atlas. A clinical and biomechanical study. *J Bone Joint Surg Am* 1974;56-A:1683–1691.
13. Spierings ELH, Braakman R. The management of os odontoideum. *J Bone Joint Surg Br* 1982;64-B:422–428.
14. Steel HR. Anatomical and mechanical considerations of the atlantoaxial articulations. *J Bone Joint Surg Am* 1968;50-A:1481–1482.
15. El-Khoury GY, Clark CR, Dietz FR, et al. Posterior atlantooccipital subluxation in Down syndrome. *Radiology* 1986;159:507–509.
16. Tredwell SJ, Newman DE, Lockitch G. Instability of the upper cervical spine in Down syndrome. *J Pediatr Orthop* 1990;10:602–606.
17. Wiesel SW, Rothman RH. Occipitoatlantal hypermobility. *Spine* 1979;4:187–191.
18. Bailey DK. The normal cervical spine in infants and children. *Radiology* 1952;59:712–719.
19. Swischuk LE. Anterior displacement of C2 in children: physiologic or pathologic. A helpful differentiating line. *Radiology* 1977;122:759–763.
20. Armstrong D, Pckrell K, Fetter B, et al. Torticollis: an analysis of 271 cases. *Plast Reconstr Surg* 1965;35:14–25.
21. Ho BCS, Lee EH, Singh K. Epidemiololgy, presentation, and management of congenital muscular torticollis. *Sing Med J* 1999;40:675–679.
22. Lin CM, Low YS. Stemomastoid tumor and muscular torticollis. *Clin Orthop* 1972;86:144–150.
23. MacDonald D. Stemomastoid tumor and muscular torticollis. *J Bone Joint Surg Br* 1969;51-B:432–443.
24. Thompson F, McManus S, Colville J. Familial congenital muscular torticollis. *Gun Orthop* 1986;202:193–196.
25. Engin C, Yavuz SS, Sahm Fl. Congenital muscular torticollis: is heredity a possible factor in a family with five torticollis patients in three generations? *Plast Reconstr Surg* 1997;99:1147–1150.
26. Davids JR, Wenger DR, Mubarak SJ. Congenital muscular torticollis: sequela of intrauterine or perinatal compartment syndrome. *J Pediatr Orthop* 1993;13:141–147.
27. Whyte AM, Lufkin RB, Bredenkamp J, et al. Sternocleidomastoid fibrosis in congenital muscular torticollis: MR appearance. *J Comput Assist Tomogr* 1989;13:163–166.
28. Weiner DS. Congenital dislocation of the hip associated with congenital muscular torticollis. *Clin Orthop* 1976;121:163–165.
29. Hosalkar H, Gill IS, Gujar P, et al. Familial torticollis with polydactyly: manifestations in three generations. *Am J Orthop* 2001;30:656–658.
30. Sarnat HB, Morrissy RT. Idiopathic torticollis: sternocleidomastoid myopathy and accessory neuropathy. *Muscle Nerve* 1981;4:374–380.
31. Tang S, Liu Z, Quan X, et al. Sternocleidomastoid pseudotumor of infants and congenital muscular torticollis: fine structure research. *J Pediatr Orthop* 1998;18:214–218.
32. Cheng JCY, Tang SP, Chen TMK, et al. The clinical presentation and outcome of treatment of congenital muscular torticollis in infants—a study of 1086 cases. *J Pediatr Surg* 2000;35:1091–1096.
33. Morrison DL, MacEwen GD. Congenital muscular torticollis: observations regarding clinical findings, associated conditions, and results of treatment. *J Pediatr Orthop* 1982;2:500–505.
34. Ling CM. The influence of age on the results of open stemomastoid tenotomy in muscular torticollis. *Clin Orthop* 1976;116:142–148.
35. Walsh JJ, Morrissy RT. Torticollis and hip dislocation. *J Pediatr Orthop* 1998;18:219–221.
36. Hunmier CD Jr, MacEwen GD. The coexistence of torticollis and congential dysplasia of the hip. *J Bone Joint Surg Am* 1972;54-A:1255–1256.
37. Brackbill Y, Douthitt IC, West H. Psychophysiologic effects in the neonate of prone versus supine placement. *J Pediatr* 1973;81:82–84.
38. Cheng JCY, Au AWY. Infantile torticollis: a review of 624 cases. *J Pediatr Orthop* 1994;14:802–808.
39. Cheng JCY, Wong MWN, Tang SP, et al. Clinical determinants of the outcome of manual stretching in the treatment of congenital muscular torticollis in infants. *J Bone Joint Surg Am* 2001;83-A:679–687.
40. Binder H, Eng GD, Gaiser IF, et al. Congenital muscular torticollis: results of conservative management with long-term follow-up in 85 cases. *Arch Phys Med Rehabil* 1987;68:222–225.
41. Canale ST, Griffin DW, Hubbard CN. Congenital muscular torticollis. A long-term follow-up. *J Bone Joint Surg Am* 1982;64-A:810–816.
42. Coventry MB, Harris LE. Congenital muscular torticollis in infancy. *J Bone Joint Surg Am* 1959;41-A:815–822.
43. Cheng JC-Y, Metrewell C, Chen TM-K, et al. Correlation of ultrasonographic imaging of congenital muscular torticollis with clinical assessment in infants. *Ultra Med Biol* 2000;26:1237–1241.
44. Hsu TC, Wang C-L, Wong M-K, et al. Correlation of clinical and ultrasonographic features in congenital muscular torticollis. *Arch Phys Med Rehabil* 1999;80:637–641.
45. Lm J-N, Chou M-L. Ultrasonographic study of the sternocleidomastoid muscle in the management of congenital muscular torticollis. *J Fed Surg* 1997;32:1648–1651.
46. Ferkel RD, Westin GW, Dawson EG, et al. Muscular torticollis. A modified surgical approach. *J Bone Joint Surg Am* 1983;65-A:894–900.
47. Wei JL, Schwartz KM, Weaver AL, et al. Pseudotumor of infancy and congenital muscular torticollis: 170 cases. *Laryngoscope* 2001; 1-11:688–695.
48. Cheng JCY, Tang SP. Outcome of surgical treatment of congenital muscular torticollis. *Gun Orthop* 1999;362:190–200.
49. Tse P, Cheng J, Chow Y, et al. Surgery for neglected congenital torticollis. *Acta Orthop Scand* 1987;58:270–272.

50. Burstein FD, Cohen SR. Endoscopic surgical treatment for congenital muscular torticollis. *Plast Reconstr Surg* 1998;101:25–26.
51. Gurpinar A, Kiristioglu I, Balkan E, et al. Surgical correction of muscular torticollis in older children with Peter G. Jones technique. *J Pediatr Orthop* 1998;18:598–601.
52. MacAlister A. Notes on the development and variations of the atlas. *J Anat Physiol* 1983;27:519–542.
53. Bharucha EP, Dastur HM. Craniovertebral anomalies (a report on 40 cases). *Brain* 1964;87:469–480.
54. McRae DL, Barnum AS. Occipitalization of the atlas. *AJR Am J Roentgenol* 1953;70:23–46.
55. Greenberg AD. Atlantoaxial dislocation. *Brain* 1968;91:655–684.
56. Wadia NH. Myelopathy complicating congenital atlantoaxial dislocation (a study of 28 cases). *Brain* 1967;90:449–472.
57. McRae DL. The significance of abnormalities of the cervical spine. *AJR Am J Roentgenol* 1960;84:3–25.
58. Nicholson JT, Sherk HH. Anomalies of the occipitocervical articulation. *J Bone Joint Surg Am* 1968;50-A:295–304.
59. Chamberlain WE. Basilar impression (platybasia): bizarre developmental anomaly of occipital bone and upper cervical spine with striking and misleading neurologic manifestations. *Yale J Biol Med* 1939;11:487–496.
60. Taylor AR, Chakravorty BC. Clinical syndromes associated with basilar impression. *Arch Neurol* 1964;10:475–484.
61. Burwood RJ, Watt I. Assimilation of the atlas and basilar impression. *Gun Radiol* 1974;25:327–333.
62. de Barros MC, Farias W, Ataide L, et al. Basilar impression and Arnold-Chiari malformation. *J Neurol Neurosurg Psychiatr* 1968;31: 596–605.
63. Epstein BS, Epstein JA. The association of cerebellar tonsillar herniation with basilar impression incident to Paget's disease. *AJR Am J Roentgenol* 1969;107:535–542.
64. Poppel MH, Jacobson HG, Duff BK, et al. Basilar impression and platybasia in Paget's disease. *Radiology* 1953;61:639–644.
65. Hurwitz U, Shepherd WHY. Basilar impression and disordered metabolism of bone. *Brain* 1966;89:223–234.
66. Harkey HL, Crockard HA, Stevens JM, et al. The operative management of basilar impression in osteogenesis imperfecta. *Neurosurg* 1990;27:782–786.
67. Pozo JL, Crockard HA, Ransford AO. Basilar impression in osteogenesis imperfecta. *J Bone Joint Surg Br* 1984;66-B:233–238.
68. Rush PJ, Berbrayer D, Ieilly BJ. Basilar impression and osteogenesis imperfecta in a three-year-old girl: CT and MRI. *Pediatr Radiol* 1989;19:142–143.
69. Hayes M, Parker G, Ell J, et al. Basilar impression complicating osteogenesis imperfecta type IV: the clinical and neuroradiological findings in four cases. *J Neurol Neurosurg Psychiatry* 1999;66:357–364.
70. Sawin PD, Menezes AH. Basilar invagination in osteogenesis imperfecta and related osteochondrodysplasias: medical and surgical management. *J Neurosurg* 1997;86:950–960.
71. Yamada H, Nakamura S, Tajima M, et al. Neurological manifestations of pediatric achondroplasias. *J Neurosurg* 1981;54:49–57.
72. Wong VCN, Fung CF. Basilar impression in a child with hypochondroplasia. *Pediatr Neurol* 1991;7:62–64.
73. Isu T, Miyasaka K, Abe H, et al. Atlantoaxial dislocation associated with neurofibromatosis. *J Neurosurg* 1983;58:451–453.
74. Hallah JT, Fallahi S, Hardin JG. Nonreducible rotational head tilt and atlantoaxial lateral mass collapse. Clinical and roentgenographic features in patients with juvenile rheumatoid arthritis and ankylosing spondylitis. *Arch Intern Med* 1983;143:471–474.
75. Martel W, Holt JF, Cassidy JT. Roentgenologic manifestations of juvenile rheumatoid arthritis. *AJR Am J Roentgenol* 1962;88:400–423.
76. Michie I, Clark M. Neurological syndromes associated with cervical and craniocervical anomalies. *Arch Neurol* 1968;18:241–247.
77. Teodori JB, Painter MJ. Basilar impression in children. *Pediatrics* 1984;74:1097–1099.
78. McRae DL. Bony abnormalities in the region of the foramen magnum: correlation of the anatomic and neurologic findings. *Acta Radiol* 1960;40:335–354.
79. McGregor M. Significance of certain measurements of skull in diagnosis of basilar impression. *Br J Radiol* 1948;21:171–181.
80. Pasztor E, Vajda I, Piffko P, et al. Transoral surgery for basilar impression. *Surg Neurol* 1980;14:473–476.
81. Menezes AR, van Gilder JC, Graf CJ, et al. Craniocervical abnormalities: a comprehensive surgical approach. *J Neurosurg* 1980;53:444–454.
82. Wood DE, Good TL, Hahn J, et al. Decompression of the brain stem and superior cervical spine for congenital/acquired craniovertebral invagination: an interdisciplinary approach. *Laryngoscope* 1990;100: 926–931.
83. Hunt TE, Dekaban AS. Modified head-neck support for basilar impression with brain-stem compression. *Can Med Assoc J* 1982; 126:947–948.
84. Menezes AR, van Gilder JC. Transoral-transpharyngeal approach to the anterior craniocervical junction. *J Neurosurg* 1988;69:895–903.
85. Sakou I, Morizono Y, Morimoto N. Transoral atlantoaxial anterior decompression and fusion. *Clin Orthop* 1984;187:134–138.
86. God A, Bhatjiwale M, Desai K. Basilar invagination: a study based on 190 surgically treated patients. *J Neurosurg* 1998;88:962–968.
87. Doubousset J. Torticollis in children caused by congenital anomalies of the axis. *J Bone Joint Surg Am* 1986;68-A:178–188.
88. Graziano GP, Herzenbeig JE, Hensinger RN. The halo-Ilizarov distraction cast for correction of cervical deformity. *J Bone Joint Surg Am* 1993;75-A:996–1003.
89. Saltzman CL, Hensinger RN, Blane CE, et al. Familial cervical dysplasia. *J Bone Joint Surg Am* 1991;73-A:163–171.
90. Hensinger RN, Lang JE, MacEwen GD. Klippel-Feil syndrome. A constellation of associated anomalies. *J Bone Joint Surg Am* 1974; 56-A:1246–1253.
91. Klippel M, Feil A. Un cas dabsence des vertebres cercvicales. *Nouvell Iconographie de la Salpétrière* 1912;25:223–250.
92. Morrison SG, Perry LW, Scott LP III. Congenital brevicollis (Klippel-Feil syndrome). *Am J Dis Child* 1968;1-15:614–620.
93. Shooul MI, Ritvo M. Clinical and roentgenological manifestations of the Klippel-Feil syndrome (congenital fusion of the cervical vertebrae, brevicollis). Report of eight additional cases and review of the literature. *AJR Am J Roentgenol* 1952;68:369–385.
94. Brown MW, Templeton AW, Hodges FJ III. The incidence of acquired and congenital fusions in the cervical spine. *AJR Am J Roentgenol* 1964;92:1255–1259.
95. Thompson E, Haan E, Sheffield L. Autosomal-dominant Klippel-Feil anomaly with cleft palate. *Clin Dysmorphol* 1998;7:11–15.
96. Clarke RA, Kearsley JH, Walsh DA. Patterned expression in familial Klippel-Feil syndrome. *Teratology* 1996;53:152–157.
97. Clarke RA, Catalan G, Diwan AD, et al. Heterogeneity in Klippel-Feil syndrome: a new classification. *Pediatr Radiol* 1998;28:967–974.
98. Thomsen M, Krober M, Schneider U, et al. Congenital limb deficiencies associated with Klippel-Feil syndrome. A survey of 57 subjects. *Ada Orthop Scand* 2000;71:461–464.
99. Duncan PA. Embryologic pathogenesis of renal agenesis associated with cervical vertebral anomalies (Klippel-Feil phenotype). *Birth Defects* 1977;13:91–101.
100. Gehring GG, Shenasky JH II. Crossed fusion of renal pelves and Klippel-Feil syndrome. *J Urol* 1976;1-16:103–104.
101. Mecklenburg RS, Krueger PM. Extensive genitourinary anomalies associated with Klippel-Feil syndrome. *Am J Dis Child* 1974; 128:92–93.
102. Moore WB, Matthews TI, Rabinowitz R. Genitourinary anomalies associated with Klippel-Feil syndrome. *J Bone Joint Surg Am* 1975; 57-A:355–357.
103. Ramsey J, Bliznak J. Klippel-Feil syndrome with renal agenesis and other anomalies. *AJR Am J Roentgenol* 1971;113:460–463.
104. McLay K, Maran AGD. Deafness and the Klippel-Feil syndrome. *J Laryngol Otol* 1969;83:175–184.
105. Palant DI, Carter BL. Klippel-Feil syndrome and deafness. A study with polytomography. *Am J Dis Child* 1972;123:218–221.
106. Stark EW, Borton TE. Hearing loss and the Klippel-Feil syndrome. *Am J Dis Child* 1972;123:233–235.
107. Stark EW, Borton I. Klippel-Feil syndrome and associated hearing loss. *Arch Otolaryngol* 1973;97:415–419.
108. Baird PA, Robinson GC, Buckler WSJ. Klippel-Feil syndrome. A study of mirror movement detected by electromyography. *Am J Dis Child* 1967;113:546–551.
109. Gunderson CH, Solitare GB. Mirror movements in patients with the Klippel-Feil syndrome. *Arch Neurol* 1968;18:675–679.
110. Baga N, Chusid EL, Miller A. Pulmonary disability in the Klippel-Feil syndrome. *Clin Orthop* 1969;67:105–110.

111. Chaurasia BD, Singh MP. Ectopic lungs in a human fetus with Klippel-Feil syndrome. *Anat Anz* 1977;142:205–208.
112. Krieger AJ, Rosomoff HL, Kuperman AS, et al. Occult respiratory dysfunction in a craniovertebral anomaly. *J Neurosurg* 1969;31:15–20.
113. Falk RH, Mackinnon J. Klippel-Feil syndrome associated with aortic coarctation. *Br Heart J* 1976;38:1220–1221.
114. Nora JJ, Cohen M, Maxwell GM. Klippel-Feil syndrome with congenital heart disease. *Am J Dis Child* 1961;102:110–116.
115. Thomsen MN, Schneider U, Weber M, et al. Scoliosis and congenital anomalies associated with Klippel-Feil syndrome types I–III. *Spine* 1997;21:396–401.
116. de Graaff R. Congenital block vertebrae C2-C3 in patients with cervical myelopathy. *Acta Neurochir* 1982;61:111–126.
117. Hall JE, Simmons ED, Danylchuk K, et al. Instability of the cervical spine and neurological involvement in Klippel-Feil syndrome. *J Bone Joint Surg Am* 1990;72-A:460–462.
118. Lee CK, Weiss AB. Isolated congenital cervical block vertebrae below the axis with neurological symptoms. *Spine* 1981;6:118–124.
119. Strax TE, Baran E. Traumatic quadriplegia associated with Klippel-Feil syndrome: discussion and case reports. *Arch Phys Med Rehabil* 1975;56:363–365.
120. Epstein NE, Epstein JA, Zilkha A. Traumatic myelopathy in a seventeen-year-old child with cervical spinal stenosis (without fracture or dislocation) and a C2-3 Klippel-Feil fusion. *Spine* 1984;9:344–347.
121. Illingsworth RS. Attacks of unconsciousness in association with fused cervical vertebrae. *Arch Dis Child* 1956;31:8–11.
122. Mosberg WH Jr. The Klippel-Feil syndrome. Etiology and treatment of neurologic signs. *J Nerv Ment Dis* 1953;117:479–491.
123. Drvaric DM, Ruderrnan RJ, Conrad RW, et al. Congenital scoliosis and urinary tract abnormalities: are intravenous pyelograms necessary? *J Pediatr Orthop* 1987;7:441–443.
124. MacEwen GD, Winter RB, Hardy JH. Evaluation of kidney anomalies in congenital scoliosis. *J Bone Joint Surg Am* 1972;54-A:1451–1454.
125. Ritterbusch IF, McGinty LD, Spar J, et al. Magnetic resonance imaging for stenosis and subluxation in Klippel-Feil syndrome. *Spine* 1991;16:539–541.
126. Ulmer JL, Elster AD, Ginsburg LE, et al. Klippel-Feil syndrome: CT and MR of acquired and congenital abnormalities of cervical spine and cord. *J Comp Assist Tomogr* 1993;17:215–224.
127. Pizzutillo PD, Woods M, Nicholson L, et al. Risk factors in Klippel-Feil syndrome. *Spine* 1994;19:2110–2116.
128. Sherk HH, Shut L, Chung S. Iniencephalic deformity of the cervical spine with Klippel-Feil anomalies and congenital evaluation of the scapula. *J Bone Joint Surg Am* 1974;56-A:1254–1259.
129. Rouvreau P, Glorion C, Langlais J, et al. Assessment and neurologic involvement of patients with cervical spine congenital synostosis as in Klippel-Feil syndrome: study of 19 cases. *J Pediatr Orthop Br* 1998;7:179–185.
130. Bonola A. Surgical treatment of the Klippel-Feil syndrome. *J Bone Joint Surg Br* 1956;38-B:440–449.
131. Deburge A, Briard J-L. Cervical hemivertebra excision. *J Bone Joint Surg Am* 1981;63-A:1335–1338.
132. Murphy WJ Jr, Gellis SS. Torticollis with hiatus hernia in infancy. *Am J Dis Child* 1977;131:564–565.
133. Ramenofsky ML, Buyse M, Goldberg MJ, et al. Gastroesophageal reflux and torticollis. *J Bone Joint Surg Am* 1978;60-A:1140–1141.
134. Bray PF, Herbst JJ, Johnson DG, et al. Childhood gastroesophageal reflux. Neurologic and psychiatric syndromes mimicked. *JAMA* 1977;327:1342–1345.
135. Darling DB, Fisher JH, Gellis SS. Hiatal hernia and gastroesophageal reflux in infants and children: analysis of the incidence in North American children. *Pediatrics* 1974;54:450–455.
136. Johnson DG, Herbst JJ, Oliveros MA, et al. Evaluation of gastroesophageal reflux surgery in children. *Pediatrics* 1977;59:62–68.
137. Jolley SG, Johnson DG, Herbst JJ, et al. An assessment of gastroesophageal reflux in children by extended pH monitoring of the distal esophagus. *Surgery* 1978;84:16–24.
138. Lowry RB. The Klippel-Feil anomalad as part of the fetal alcohol syndrome. *Teratolgy* 1977;16:53–56.
139. Neidengard L, Carter TE. Klippel-Feil malformation complex in fetal alcohol syndrome. *Am J Dis Child* 1978;1-32:929–930.
140. Tredwell SJ, Smith DF, Macleod PJ, et al. Cervical spine anomalies in fetal alcohol syndrome. *Spine* 1982;7:331–334.
141. Sandham A. Cervical vertebral anomalies in cleft lip and palate. *Cleft Palate J* 1986;23:206–214.
142. Hemmer KM, McAlister WH, Marsh JL. Cervical spine anomalies in the craniosynostosis syndromes. *Cleft Palate J* 1987;24:328–333.
143. Louis DS, Argenta LC. The orthopaedic manifestations of Goldenhaar's syndrome. *Surg Round Orthop* 1987;7:43–46.
144. Sherk HH, Whitaker LA, Pasquariello PS. Facial malformations and spinal anomalies. A predictable relationship. *Spine* 1982;7:526–531.
145. Anderson PJ, Hall CM, Evans RD, et al. Cervical spine in Pfeiffer's syndrome. *J Craniofac Surg* 1996;7:275–279.
146. Moore MH, Lodge ML, Clark BE. Spinal anomalies in Pfeiffer syndrome. *Cleft Palate Craniofac J* 1995;32:251–254.
147. Anderson PJ, Hall CM, Evans RD, et al. The cervical spine in Saethre-Chotzen syndrome. *Cleft Palate Craniofac J* 1997;34:79–82.
148. Lachrnan RS. Neurologic abnormalities in the skeletal dysplasias: a clinical and radiological perspective. *Am J Med Genet* 1997;69:33–43.
149. Lachman RS. The cervical spine in the skeletal dysplasias and associated disorders. *Pediatr Radiol* 1997;27:402S–408S.
150. Skeletal Dysplasia Group. Instability of the upper cervical spine. *Arch Dis Child* 1989;64:283–288.
151. Hite SH, Peters C, Krivit W. Correction of odontoid dysplasia following bone-marrow transplantation and engraftment (in Hurler MPS 1H). *Pediatr Radiol* 2000;30:464–470.
152. Craig JB, Govender S. Neurofibromatosis of the cervical spine. *J Bone Joint Surg Br* 1992;74-B:575–578.
153. Adkins JC, Ravitch MM. The operative management of von Recklinghausen's neurofibromatosis in children, with special reference to lesions of the head and neck. *Surgery* 1977;82:342–348.
154. Crawford AR Jr. Osseous manifestations of neurofibromatosis in childhood. *J Pediatr Orthop* 1986;6:72–78.
155. Yong-Hing K, Kalamchi A, MacEwen GD. Cervical spine abnormalities in neurofibromatosis. *J Bone Joint Surg Am* 1979;61-A:695–699.
156. Nijiand EA, van den Berg MP, Wuisman PIJM, et al. Correction of a dystrophic cervicothoracic spine deformity in Recklinghausen's disease. *Clin Orthop* 1998;349:149–155.
157. Giaia G, Mandelli D, Capaccioni B, et al. Postlaminectomy cervical dislocation in von Recklinghausen's disease. *Spine* 1998;23:273–276.
158. Hobbs WR, Sponseller PD, Weiss A-PC, et al. The cervical spine in Marfan syndrome. *Spine* 1997;22:983–989.
159. Herzka A, Sponseller PD, Pyeritz RE. Atlantoaxial rotatory subluxation in patients with Marfan syndrome. *Spine* 2000;25:524–526.
160. Fielding JW, Hesninger RN, Hawkins RJ. Os odontoideum. *J Bone Joint Surg Am* 1980;62-A:376–383.
161. Wollin DG. The os odontoideum. *J Bone Joint Surg Am* 1963;45-A:1459–1471.
162. Verska JM, Anderson PA. Os odontoideum. A case report of one identical twin. *Spine* 1997;22:706–709.
163. Kuhns LR, Loder RT, Parley FA, et al. Nuchal cord changes in children with os odontoideum: evidence for associated trauma. *J Pediatr Orthop* 1998;18:815–819.
164. Sakaida H, Waga S, Kojima T, et al. Os odontoideum associated with hypertrophic ossiculum terminale. *J Neurosurg* 2001;94:140–144.
165. Matsui H, Imada K, Tsuji H. Radiographic classification of os odontoideum and its clinical significance. *Spine* 1997;22:1706–1709.
166. Watanabe M, Toyama Y, Fujimura Y. Atlantoaxial instability in os odontoideum with myelopathy. *Spine* 1996;21:1435–1439.
167. Wang J, Vokshoor A, Kim S, et al. Pediatric atlantoaxial instability: management with screw fixation. *Pediatr Neurosurg* 1999;30:70–78.

CHAPTER 32

Rehabilitation of the Patient with Tetraplegia and Paraplegia

Mitchell K. Freedman, Alexander R. Vaccaro, Scott D. Daffner, and Guy Fried

The medical community and the general lay community are oriented toward the "cure of spinal cord injuries." The practice of rehabilitation management is dedicated toward this end as well. However, the rehabilitation team is also oriented toward minimizing progression of injury; preventing and limiting secondary medical problems that result from spinal cord injury (SCI); and maximizing functional abilities to enable the patient to achieve the maximal quality of life in their home, workplace, and community. Rehabilitation of the patient with SCI begins at the time of injury and continues through their acute stay in the hospital, and into the rehabilitative stage of their acute injury. This is a life-long project, however, and a comprehensive rehabilitation program should address the needs of the spinal cord–injured patient on a lifetime basis.

EPIDEMIOLOGY

There are approximately 180,000 to 230,000 patients with spinal cord injuries in the United States. Based on patients hospitalized with spinal cord injuries, the incidence rate in the United States appears to be 30 to 40 new injuries per 1 million population per year. There may be another 10 to 20 fatal injuries per 1 million population per year in which the patient expires before reaching the hospital. Nearly one-half of all injuries occur in patients who are between 16 and 30 years of age. The age of the patient with SCI is slowly increasing, however. The average age of a patient injured between 1973 and 1977 was 28.5 years old. Between 1994 and 1998, the average age of a patient with a SCI had increased to 36 years old. Men experience 81% of spinal cord injuries, with black and Hispanic men at higher risk. Demographic data indicates patients with SCI have fewer years of education, are more likely to be unemployed, and are single (1–5).

Motor vehicle accidents account for 43% of spinal cord injuries. Intentional violence accounts for 18.9% of injuries; the vast majority of these injuries are gunshot wounds. Falls (18.8%) and sports (11.1%) are the other major causes of spinal cord injuries. The majority of sports-related injuries are related to diving accidents. The majority of intentional violence and motor vehicle injuries occurs in patients younger than 30 years of age, whereas patients who experience SCI related to falls generally are elderly (1,3).

A high index of suspicion is required to identify SCI in patients with multiple trauma. Similarly, patients with overt SCI must be examined carefully for other injuries. SCI in and of itself can blunt signs and symptoms related to other visceral injuries, as well as pain responses to other injuries in a multitrauma patient. The most frequent associated injuries are fractures (29%) and head injury (12%). Pneumothorax and hemothorax are also frequently associated injuries (3,5).

MORTALITY

The mortality after SCI is greatest during the year after the injury. In patients who survive more than 24 hours, the most common cause of death is pneumonia, followed by nonischemic heart disease and pulmonary embolism. Other common etiologies of death in the first year postinjury include pulmonary embolism and sepsis (6).

Overall, life expectancy in patients with SCI has increased in recent decades. The life expectancy decreases with severity of injury, however. The leading cause of death in patients who survive for more than 5 years is pneumonia, followed by nonischemic heart disease and unintentional injury (6).

PATHOPHYSIOLOGY OF SPINAL CORD INJURY

Neurologic dysfunction secondary to traumatic SCI is a dynamic process initiated by a mechanical injury that disrupts the neuronal and glial architecture. Excessive external forces result in distraction, compression, or translation of the spinal cord. The degree of injury is dependent on the amount of energy applied to the cord and the mechanism and level of injury to the cord, and the individual patient issues range from their spinal cord dimensions to concurrent medical issues (7). The mechanical injury may include vertebral fracture or dislocation, ligamentous damage, and vascular injury. The damage to the spinal cord initiates a secondary cascade of events that exacerbates the neurologic injury (8). Vascular damage occurs within 15 minutes of injury; punctate hemorrhage is seen in the gray and white matter. Bleeding progresses centrifugally, with hemorrhagic lesions found first in the gray matter, but also in the white matter by 3 to 5 days postinjury (9). Subsequent edema and hemorrhage resulting from endothelial inflammation and leakage progress peripherally, as well as posteriorly and caudally (10). Small intramedullary and pial arteries and veins are occluded,

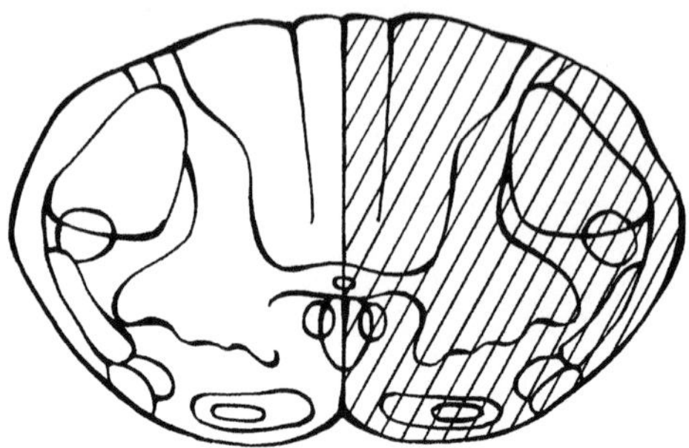

FIG. 2. Brown-Séquard syndrome. A hemisection of the spinal cord resulting in ipsilateral loss of strength and proprioception and contralateral loss of pain and temperature.

which results in further ischemia (10). Cellular injury and death with axonal disruption, cell fragmentation, and myelin breakdown occur within several hours of injury (11). Demyelination and wallerian degeneration may be seen in long fiber tracts distal to the zone of injury (11).

Acute changes in the spinal cord occur from 48 hours to 1 week postinjury. Interstitial edema and resorption of cellular debris and hemorrhage occurs. Cavitation occurs as injured tissue is absorbed. Over time, cystic areas may coalesce to form a syrinx (12). Scar tissue replaces degenerated gray and white matter.

CLINICAL MANIFESTATIONS OF SPINAL CORD INJURY

A lesion is defined as *complete* when there is no evidence of sensory or motor function in the sacral segments 48 to 72 hours postinjury. Lack of sensation at the anal mucocutaneous junction or inability of the external anal sphincter to voluntarily contract can be identified by physical examination.

An *incomplete* injury is defined as preservation of at least partial sensory or motor function below the neurologic level, or both, and including the sacral segments. The sacral segments are at the more peripheral edges of the major tracts in the spinal cord (Fig. 1). Because injury is initiated in the center of the cord and progresses peripherally, any tissue that is spared is most likely to be peripheral. Degree and presentation of injury vary greatly (13).

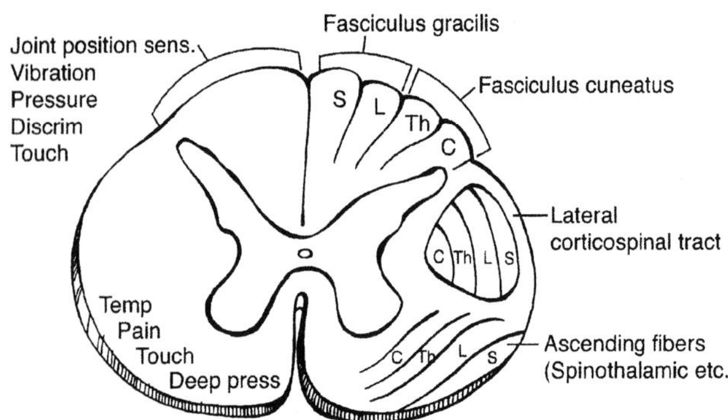

FIG. 1. Cross section of the spinal cord demonstrating the major tracts of the spinal cord.

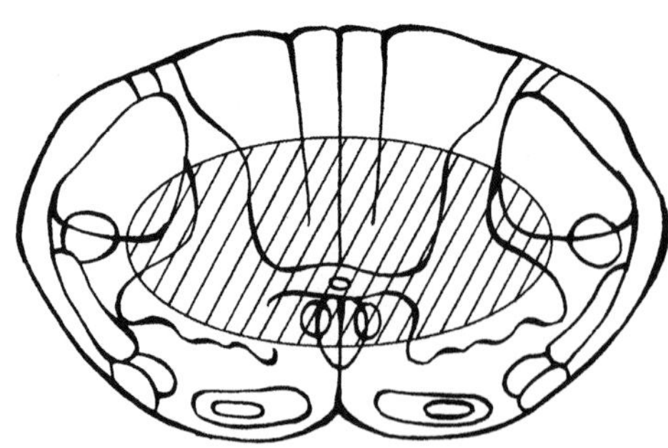

FIG. 3. Central cord syndrome. Injury results in sacral sparing and preferentially upper- more than lower-extremity weakness.

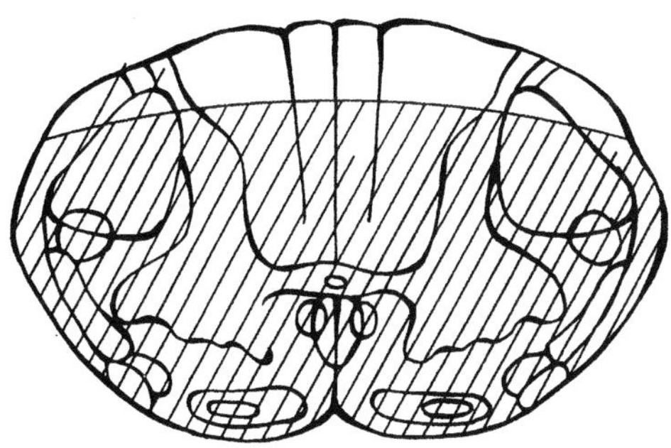

FIG. 4. Anterior cord syndrome. Injury results in variable loss of motor function as well as pain and temperature. Proprioception is preserved.

Brown-Séquard syndrome (Fig. 2) is the result of a hemisection of the spinal cord. It is rarely seen as a pure syndrome because physiologic hemisection of the cord rarely occurs in clinical practice. Elements of Brown-Séquard injury are frequently seen with incomplete injury, however, and in particular, with knife and gunshot wounds. Injury to the posterior column results in the loss of ipsilateral proprioception. The motor function also is lost ipsilaterally because the motor fibers in the corticospinal tract run ipsilaterally after crossing in the lower medulla. There is contralateral loss of pain and temperature sensation secondary to injury to the lateral spinothalamic tract (14).

The central cord syndrome (Fig. 3) is characterized by sacral sparing and greater motor deficits in the upper limbs than in the lower limbs due to damage to the central cord (15). It frequently occurs in hyperextension injuries and is commonly seen in elderly patients after a fall.

Anterior spinal cord syndrome (Fig. 4) occurs due to direct damage to the anterior spinal cord secondary to a mechanical lesion, such as a bone fragment or herniated disc, or because of vascular insufficiency produced by injury to the anterior spinal artery. In a severe injury, there is complete loss of motor function as well as sensitivity to pain and temperature, but gross touch and proprioception are preserved (16).

Posterior cord syndrome (Fig. 5) is infrequently seen. Posterior column injury impairs position and vibratory sensation, with relative preservation of anterior and lateral column function (13).

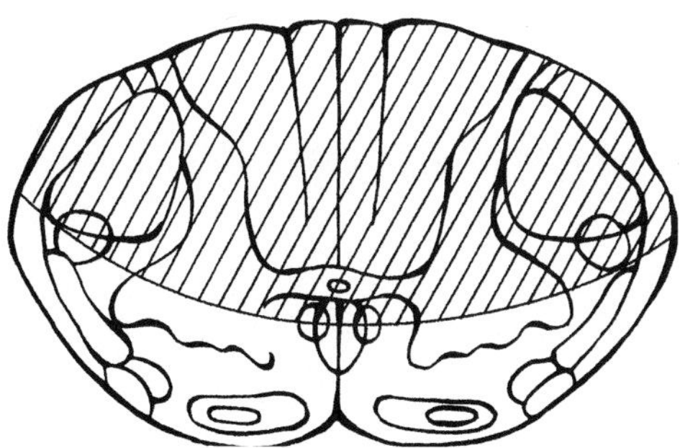

FIG. 5. Posterior cord syndrome. Injury results in loss of proprioception and variable preservation of motor function and pain and temperature sensation.

REHABILITATION

The rehabilitation team consists of multiple disciplines. The *physiatrist* is a physician who specializes in physical medicine and rehabilitation. The physiatrist should be in charge of the patient's overall medical care and take charge of the organization of the rest of the rehabilitation team, which includes the following: other physicians involved in the patient's care, nursing, physical therapy, occupational therapy, social services, psychology, recreational therapy, and vocational services. The patient is a vital member of the team as well.

The physical therapist addresses upper- and lower-extremity range of motion and strengthening, as well as all types of functional mobility. The occupational therapist also addresses upper-extremity range of motion and strengthening as well as activities of daily living, homemaking, and recreational and vocational activities. The nursing staff assists the physiatrist in caring for basic medical problems as well as in helping to manage bowel, bladder, and skin problems. Psychology and social services work with the patient and his or her family to help with the adjustment to disability and life planning.

Impairment is defined as "any loss or abnormality of psychological, physiologic or anatomic structure or function" (17). The patient with SCI may have an impairment consisting of a fracture or a bony injury and the subsequent injury to the spinal cord. *Disability* is "any restriction or lack resulting from an impairment of ability to perform an activity in the manner within the range considered normal for a human being" (17). The disability in a patient with SCI varies depending on the degree of injury and subsequent neurologic damage. Disability may involve the patient's ability to turn in bed, transfer, walk, or use a wheelchair. Other examples of disabilities involve activities of daily living as well as recreational, homemaking, and vocational activities.

A *handicap* is a "disadvantage for a given individual resulting from an impairment or disability that limits or prevents the fulfillment of a role that is normal for that individual" (17). SCI patients may have difficulty functioning in a previous job because of accessibility or the setup of their workstation. The issue of "being handicapped" refers to the limitations of the external environment or society in accommodating a patient with a disability so that they may continue to function. It is the job of the rehabilitation team to address all of the aforementioned issues.

Acute Stage

The initial stage of rehabilitation is an evaluation and stabilization phase. It begins with the immediate immobilization of the patient's spine. Patients with acute quadriplegia may have difficulty with breathing. The ABCs of airway, breathing, and circulation must be addressed immediately to prevent the patient's death, as well as to maximize oxygenation of the spinal cord. Control of the airway must be accomplished while limiting further damage to the spinal cord. All of the other issues in the care of acute trauma may be present, including hypovolemic shock and pulmonary dysfunction, as well as the concomitant management of fractures and visceral injuries.

When the patient is seen within 8 hours of injury, they generally receive 30 mg per kg of methylprednisolone over a 15-

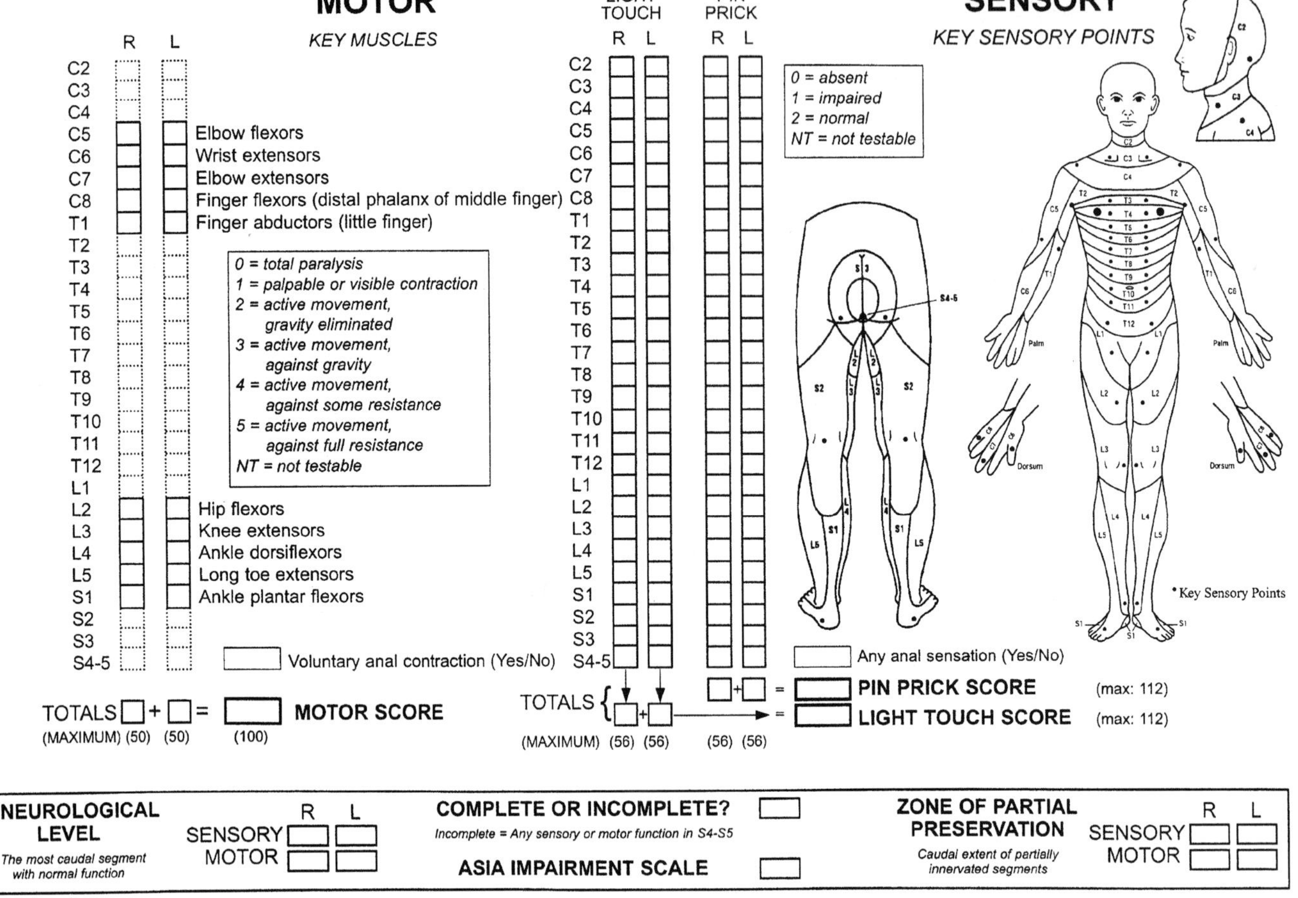

ASIA
STANDARD NEUROLOGICAL CLASSIFICATION OF SPINAL CORD INJURY
MOTOR
KEY MUSCLES
R L
C2
C3
C4
C5 Elbow flexors
C6 Wrist extensors
C7 Elbow extensors
C8 Finger flexors (distal phalanx of middle finger)
T1 Finger abductors (little finger)
T2
T3
T4
T5
T6
T7
T8
T9
T10
T11
T12
L1
L2 Hip flexors
L3 Knee extensors
L4 Ankle dorsiflexors
L5 Long toe extensors
S1 Ankle plantar flexors
S2
S3
S4-5
0 = total paralysis
1 = palpable or visible contraction
2 = active movement, gravity eliminated
3 = active movement, against gravity
4 = active movement, against some resistance
5 = active movement, against full resistance
NT = not testable
Voluntary anal contraction (Yes/No)
TOTALS + = MOTOR SCORE
(MAXIMUM) (50) (50) (100)
LIGHT TOUCH
PIN PRICK
R L
R L
SENSORY
KEY SENSORY POINTS
0 = absent
1 = impaired
2 = normal
NT = not testable
Any anal sensation (Yes/No)
TOTALS
(MAXIMUM) (56) (56) (56) (56)
PIN PRICK SCORE (max: 112)
LIGHT TOUCH SCORE (max: 112)
Palm
Dorsum
* Key Sensory Points
NEUROLOGICAL LEVEL
The most caudal segment with normal function
R L
SENSORY
MOTOR
COMPLETE OR INCOMPLETE?
Incomplete = Any sensory or motor function in S4-S5
ASIA IMPAIRMENT SCALE
ZONE OF PARTIAL PRESERVATION
Caudal extent of partially innervated segments
R L
SENSORY
MOTOR

FIG. 6. Summary sheet of international Standards for Neurological and Functional Classification of Spinal Cord Injury. (From the American Spinal Injury Association. *International standards for neurological and functional classification of spinal cord injury.* Chicago: American Spinal Injury Association, 1996, with permission.)

minute period. After 45 minutes, they then receive 5.4 mg per kg per hour for 23 hours (18).

Classification of Injury

It is important to identify residual function objectively. If there is a decrement in neurologic function, acute surgical treatment may be necessary. Furthermore, the process of prognostication and plan for postrehabilitation phase can be initiated.

During the initial phase of injury, the level and degree of neurologic injury is established. The criteria for diagnosing the level of SCI has been established by the American Spinal Injury Association (ASIA) (Fig. 6) (19,20). The key muscles are evaluated to establish the motor level of injury. The level is named for the segment above the most cephalad abnormal segment. A muscle that is rated as 3 or 4 is considered normal, provided the next rostral muscle is a 5. Key sensory points are evaluated to establish the sensory level of the injury. The sensory level is the dermatome that is intact to pinprick and touch above the highest abnormal level. Hyperesthesia or hypesthesia to pinprick is graded as a 1. Inability to detect pinprick is a 0.

A neurologic level is determined for each side of the body. The examination identifies whether the patient is complete or incomplete. The patient who is incomplete has evidence of some residual sensory or motor function (or both) in the sacral segments. Based on all the physical findings, the ASIA Impairment Scale is then used to classify the degree of completeness of injury (Table 1).

Subacute Stage

The second phase in a rehabilitation program is the period immediately after the stabilization of the spinal injury. During that phase, there are multiple issues. The patient is often medically unstable. With a cervical spine injury, the patient may be in a halo or a cervical collar. There may be concurrent skeletal injuries,

TABLE 1. *ASIA Impairment Scale*

- ❑ A = Complete: No motor or sensory function is preserved in the sacral segments S4-5.
- ❑ B = Incomplete: Sensory but not motor function is preserved below the neurologic level and includes the sacral segments S4-5.
- ❑ C = Incomplete: Motor function is preserved below the neurologic level, and more than one-half of key muscles below the neurologic level have a muscle grade <3.
- ❑ D = Incomplete: Motor function is preserved below the neurologic level, and at least one-half of key muscles below the neurologic level have a muscle grade ≥3.
- ❑ E = Normal: Motor and sensory function are normal.

which limit progress as well. The patient and the family are often in the acute throes of trying to come to grips with their injury. Prognostication is discussed with the patient and the family members. Initial teaching about medical problems is instituted. Interim and long-term discharge and planning begins immediately.

Therapy begins at the bedside and progresses to the gym as rapidly as possible. The patients may receive splints for their hands or to keep tension on their heel cords. Range-of-motion exercises are instituted. Nutritional support is critical in this stage to prevent decubitus ulcers, as is the use of an appropriate mattress and wheelchair padding. Once the patient is medically stable, they are transferred to the rehabilitation center.

Neurologic Recovery

The prognosis after an acute traumatic injury may be more accurate at 72 hours after the acute injury than in the emergency room. Patients who suffer an ASIA A injury (complete) rarely become incomplete after 72 hours (21). Even if patients with an ASIA A injury become incomplete (B), rarely is there progression to an ASIA C or D classification (22).

Patients with an ASIA B injury often progress to a grade C or D level of incompleteness, however. Careful sensory examination is essential, because the patient with an ASIA B injury who has preservation of pinprick sensation has an excellent chance to progress of an ASIA D or E level (23). The patient who has an ASIA B level without preservation of pinprick is less likely to progress to an ASIA C or D classification (24).

The patient with a complete tetraplegia often gains one motor level in the first 1 to 2 years, but the neurologic level generally does not change between acute admission and discharge. The overall recovery rate of one root level of function has been reported to occur in up to 90% of patients (25). A patient who has at least 2/5 strength in their zone of injury generally gains one neurologic level within 3 to 6 months of their injury. Patients who have 0/5 strength at the level caudal to the neurologic level of injury gain a level in the first 3 to 6 months in up to 40% of patients. Patients who have a C-4 injury are less likely to progress by one motor level (22,26).

Patients recover at the level of injury by various mechanisms. There may be some recovery of partially damaged neurons. Peripheral sprouting of spared neurons occurs and allows further recovery over months to years. Incomplete lesions recover by receptor upregulation and by expanse of synaptic fields, which allows an increase in the influence of spared pathways (27,28).

Magnetic resonance imaging of the spinal cord may also prognosticate future recovery. When there is hemorrhaging in the spinal cord, there is a suggestion of a poor prognosis, whereas a contusion followed by edema dictates a better prognosis. Obviously, the best prognosis occurs when the spinal cord has a normal appearance (27,29).

Functional Recovery

The average level of function in a patient directly depends on the severity of their neurologic injury (5,30). It is difficult to prognosticate about patients with incomplete injuries because of the variability in the timing of return of function, as well as the variability in recovery of neurologic function and the severity of spasticity. The variability in levels of function for patients with similar injuries also varies to a certain degree with the patient's motivation, age, body habitus, and general state of health.

C2-4 Tetraplegia

The patient who experiences a C2-4 lesion is a high tetraplegic. These patients are dependent for nearly all of their activities of daily living, including bed mobility and transfers. They may be independent with the use of a power wheelchair or may require a pneumatic or chin control–driven power wheelchair. A power recliner allows them to independently shift weights.

C-5 Tetraplegia

The most common injury level at the time of admission of a tetraplegic patient is the C-5 level. The patient with a C-5 tetraplegia has intact biceps function and may be able to use a manual wheelchair for short distances and equipment for the wheels. They are dependent for weight shifts and longer distance wheelchair propulsion. Mobility is most functional with a power wheelchair. In general, they require assistance with most of their activities of daily living. Feeding and grooming with assistive devices is feasible.

C-6 Tetraplegia

Patients with a C-6 tetraplegia have intact wrist extension. In general, the musculature in their shoulders is stronger as well. Because they have wrist extension, a tenodesis may improve their hand function. These patients are able to use a manual wheelchair for moderate distances with plastic rims or lugs. Certain transfers may be feasible in an athletic patient as well. Upper-extremity dressing and bathing are manageable, but the patient generally needs assistance with their lower extremities.

C-7 Tetraplegia

A patient with C-7 tetraplegia has intact triceps muscles. Transfers are often feasible even without a transfer board. This capability can vary, however, depending on the size of the patient and the degree of their spasticity. Wheelchair propulsion should be independent indoors and often is independent outdoors. The patient should be independent with all grooming and feeding. They have the potential for independence with washing and dressing the upper and lower extremities with equipment.

C-8 to T-1 Tetraplegia

The patient with C-8 to T-1 tetraplegia should be independent with all transfers indoors and outdoors. All of their activities of daily living can be performed without equipment, unless the degree of spasticity or the patient's body habitus makes assistive devices for these activities necessary.

Ambulation

Patients with complete tetraplegia generally are not capable of functional ambulation. Patients with a complete high paraplegia can occasionally walk, but this is rare. In the patient who is a superb athlete, ambulation may be feasible with a bilateral knee-ankle orthosis and bilateral assistive devices. Ambulation is quite laborious and has a high energy consumption. The gait is a swing-to, as opposed to a reciprocal pattern, with a slow velocity. These patients are much more functional out of a wheelchair (30).

The tetraplegic with an incomplete lesion at 72 hours may have a good prognosis to walk at 1 year. Maynard and colleagues reported that 47% of sensory incomplete patients and 87% of motor incomplete patients at 72 hours were walking at 1 year (31). Crozier reported that patients who have 3/5 quadriceps strength by 2 months have a good prognosis for ambulation at 1 year (23).

There is a difference between therapeutic ambulation and functional ambulation. *Therapeutic ambulation* describes the patient who walks for exercise only. This patient may need assistance to don and doff their orthosis or to arise from the floor or sitting position to a standing position so they can walk. All of these activities are extremely laborious. *Indoor functional ambulation* implies that the patient is able to walk on a full- or part-time basis within the home. They are able to don and doff their orthosis. They can transfer from the floor or sitting position to a standing position. They can use their ambulation to perform activities around the house, but they may prefer to use the wheelchair outdoors or for longer distance ambulation. The *community ambulator* is the patient who is independent with ambulation and generally does not use the wheelchair for mobility outside the house.

The incomplete patient has a good prognosis to ambulate in some capacity (28,30). However, there is a great degree of variation in how functional the ambulation is based on their age, body habitus, degree of spasticity, residual function, and motivation. Furthermore, what the rehabilitation team defines as "successful ambulation" may not match up with the patient's expectations as to what constitutes "walking." Patients are often not happy with ambulation if they need to use an assistive device or a brace.

Upper-Extremity Reconstructive Surgery

Moberg estimated that 60% of patients with tetraplegia can benefit from upper-extremity procedures (32). Such procedures must have focused functional goals. Patients must be at least 1 year postinjury and have demonstrated neurologic stability for a minimum of 6 months. Patients must be committed to postoperative recovery and rehabilitation. Range of motion, strength, and sensation must be carefully evaluated throughout the entire upper extremity to assure the highest possibility that the surgery will be successful. A muscle that is considered for transfer must have at least 4/5 strength (33). Severe spasticity of a muscle group may be a contraindication.

In general, upper-extremity reconstructive surgery involves the transfer of a tendon of a nonessential but functioning muscle to a position where it can provide a new function for the patient. For example, the patient with a C-5 injury has functional use of the deltoid, elbow flexors, and brachioradialis. These patients therefore have the ability to flex their elbows. If the patient has 4/5 strength in the deltoid, then a posterior deltoid to triceps transfer can be performed so that the patient can have active elbow extension. Another surgical option might include a brachioradialis to extensor carpi radialis transfer, with the goal being to provide active wrist extension.

There are a variety of other reconstructive procedures. Moberg's key-pinch procedure is used in the C-6 tetraplegic to allow functional pinch between the thumb and the side of the index finger. The flexor hallucis longus tendon is secured proximally to the distal radius to create a flexor pollicis longus tenodesis. An intramedullary screw is inserted through the distal thumb and across the interphalangeal joint to prevent interphalangeal joint flexion, and promote fusion of that joint. The extensor pollicis longus and brevis tendons are secured proximally to the metacarpophalangeal joint to prevent excessive flexion. Other procedures are available to assist with active grasp and improve hand control in patients with a C-7 level injury. For example, some flexion can be restored by transferring the brachioradialis to the flexor pollicis longus. Finger flexion may be restored by the transfer of the extensor carpi radialis longus, flexor carpi ulnaris, or pronator teres to the flexor digitorum profundus.

Functional Neuromuscular Stimulation

Patients with upper-motor neuron dysfunction have intact peripheral nerves. These nerves can be stimulated electrically to provide muscular contraction (34), whereas in the case of a lower-motor neuron lesion, external electrical stimulation cannot be effective because of axonotmesis and subsequent wallerian degeneration. Overzealous electrical stimulation can actually impair recovery in lower-motor neuron injury and should be avoided in muscles affected by nerve root injury (23).

Electrical stimulation may be initiated by transcutaneous, percutaneous, or implanted electrodes. The goal is to stimulate weak muscles, which may help the patient to coordinate remaining muscular contraction more efficiently, but there is no proof that electrical stimulation expedites neurologic recovery. Neuromuscular stimulation is also used for a stationary bicycle program that provides cardiovascular conditioning and helps retard the progression of osteoporosis and lessens spasticity. Patients also use electrical stimulation to assist with standing and ambulation, although it is less commonly used for routine functional purposes.

Adjustment to Disability

Patients who have experienced an SCI respond in a variety of fashions to the injury based on their social, economic, and educational background. Significant depression often is the initial, and normal, response to a catastrophic injury. Supportive counseling is appropriate, and the patient's support system should be encouraged to provide support. Additional measures include antidepressant medication and group psychological treatment. Patients who are newly injured often support one another. Patients who are removed from their initial SCI and have successfully adjusted to life postinjury also can serve as role models and "sounding boards" to patients with acute and subacute injury.

Suicide after Spinal Cord Injury

Six percent of deaths after SCI are related to suicide. SCI patients are at higher risk of committing suicide in the years immediately after injury, but by 10 years, the suicide rate mirrors that of the general population (35,36).

Discharge Planning in Spinal Cord Injury

More than 90% of individuals who experience SCI are discharged to a private residence in the community. The average length of stay in acute rehabilitation is approximately 60 days. Nursing homes account for 4% of discharges. This depends in part on the patient's support system, as well as the severity of their medical issues and accessibility of their dwelling (36,37).

Marriage after Spinal Cord Injury

Separation and divorce after SCI is a frequent occurrence. However, patients who remain married for 1 year after SCI are often still married at 5 years postinjury. Ninety percent of patients who are single at the time of SCI are single at the fifth anniversary of the injury (36).

Education and Employment

Approximately 59% of patients who experience SCI are employed at the time of the injury. After the injury, the rate of employment declines, but then increases to a peak of 30% approximately 10 years later. There are multiple factors that determine whether or not a patient is able to return to work. Severity of injury correlates inversely with chances of returning to gainful employment. White race, younger age at the time of injury, and the number of years of education correlate with a higher chance of employment.

In the years immediately after SCI, the average education level is below that of the general population. At 15 years postinjury, the educational level of SCI patients exceeds that of the average national level (36,38).

MEDICAL PROBLEMS AFTER SPINAL CORD INJURY

Cardiovascular Complications

Deep Vein Thrombophlebitis

SCI greatly increases the risk of deep vein thrombophlebitis (DVT) and subsequent pulmonary embolism in the acute phase of the injury. Venous stasis and hypercoagulability result from bed rest and paralysis. Prospective studies indicate that 47 to 100% of acute SCIs develop DVT (39). Approximately 62% of patients demonstrate a positive venogram study by postinjury day 8 (40). DVT is at lower risk to occur in patients with chronic injury.

DVT is difficult to diagnose on physical examination in the patient with SCI. Patients often have lower-extremity edema secondary to poor venous return and variations in fluid volume in the body. Tenderness in the calves often cannot be detected because of neurologic injury. Pulmonary embolism occurs in approximately 4% of SCI patients during their initial hospitalization (41). Symptoms of pulmonary embolism, such as shortness of breath, may be masked by shortness of breath secondary to other pulmonary problems, such as atelectasis and pneumonia, or the level of paralysis. It may also present as a fever of unknown origin. Pulmonary embolism may present with sudden death.

Prophylactic strategies must be used to screen for DVT. The patient must be examined daily. In the first several weeks, weekly venous imaging via ultrasonography is a sound strategy. The physician must have a low threshold to order subsequent ultrasonographic tests to detect DVT or chest x-rays and ventilation perfusion studies to rule out pulmonary embolism.

Pneumatic compression devices and compression hose should be used during the first 2 weeks after the injury. If DVT is detected, then the pneumatic compression device must be discontinued. Low-molecular-weight heparin, such as enoxaparin, 30 mg, or heparin, 5,000 U subcutaneously every 12 hours, should be instituted 72 hours postinjury and continued for 2 to 3 months. Vena cava filters are indicated if anticoagulation is contraindicated, such as in patients with recent cerebral hemorrhages or upper gastrointestinal bleeding. Vena cava filters are also indicated in patients with multiple risk factors for DVTs, such as cancer, leg fractures, congestive heart failure, obesity, or age older than 70 years (42,43).

Cardiac Function

Patients with high thoracic and cervical SCI experience significant injury to their sympathetic nervous system. The sympathetic fibers that originate in the lower thoracic spine and in the lumbar spine become disinhibited, and there is a loss of supraspinal control. Parasympathetic fibers that originate in the brainstem are spared. Thus, the potential exists for an unopposed parasympathetic response in patients with complete or incomplete SCI above T-6. Sympathetic activity after an injury is low, whereas in the subacute and chronic phase there is often an exaggerated sympathetic response. Heart rate and oxygen uptake may not increase normally with exercise in a patient with a higher SCI. Stroke volume is diminished because of poor venous return. Cardiac output may be diminished because of the diminished heart rate and stroke volume. Impaired autonomic response also limits positive cardiac chronotropy and inotropy (9,44,45).

Orthostatic Hypotension

Orthostatic hypotension is a frequent phenomenon in a patient with tetraplegia. It is most often seen when the patient transfers from the supine position to a sitting position. The patient may present with dizziness, lightheadedness, or syncope. Orthostatic hypotension is most likely the result of diminished venous return to the heart secondary to fluid pooling in the lower extremities, because muscle contraction is limited and there is ineffective vasoconstriction secondary to the impaired autonomic response. However, there is some evidence of an altered cerebral blood flow provoking these symptoms, as opposed to a decrease in the absolute value of the blood pressure (2). Other medications that the patient may be taking can exacerbate symptoms as well, such as antidepressants and alpha-adrenergic blockers for bladder management.

Patients with orthostasis can be managed conservatively. Pressure garments to the lower extremities and abdominal binders can be used to assist venous return. Elevated leg rests may limit venous pooling. Patients should be progressed in a very slow manner from a supine to an upright position. Caregivers must be sensitive to hypotensive symptoms, and the patient should immediately be placed in a reclined position with their legs above their heart when symptoms occur. Medication options may include sodium chloride tablets, ephedrine, and fludrocortisone.

Bradycardia

Bradycardia may occur shortly after SCI. The parasympathetic influence on the heart may provoke cardiac arrhythmias, a particular risk in the patient with high tetraplegia. Tracheal suction can provoke bradycardia and even asystole. Cardiac arrest has been reported (46–48). Atropine is the treatment for acute episodes, but recurrent significant brachycardia may require pacemaker insertion.

Autonomic Dysreflexia

Autonomic dysreflexia results from an extreme sympathetic response from below the level of the lesion. It is associated with injuries at T-7 and above. Noxious stimulation results in an excessive sympathetic outflow in the absence of a parasympathetic response. Presenting symptoms include headache, anxiety, nasal congestion, flushing, bradycardia or tachycardia, and hypertension. It may be provoked by any nociceptive problem below the level of the injury, in particular, a distended bladder from urinary retention or a blocked catheter. Other factors reported to provoke autonomic dysreflexia include fecal impaction, urinary calculi, decubiti, and ingrown toenails (49,50).

Initial management includes sitting the patient up. Whenever possible, the inciting problem should be treated. Topical nitroglycerine may be used to help decrease blood pressure expeditiously. If hypotension occurs, the nitrate can be cleaned off. Other options may include an alpha-adrenergic blocking agent, such as terazosin or oral nifedipine, but these should be reserved as the last choice as the patient may well become hypotensive shortly after the dysreflexia has resolved (51).

Altered Thermoregulation

SCI patients frequently are hyperthermic or hypothermic. The hypothalamus controls body temperature. When core body temperatures are low, shivering occurs and vasoconstriction reduces blood flow to the extremities. When the core body temperature is elevated, sweating occurs and peripheral vasodilation shunts blood to the extremities. These mechanisms are lost or impaired in patients with SCI. Treatment involves climate control and addition or subtraction of blankets (57). Infection, medication, DVT, and heterotopic ossification are a few of the possibilities to consider. If a fever occurs, it cannot be assumed altered regulation is causative. The patient with a fever from poikilothermia is often not tachycardic, whereas the patient with sepsis generally does have a rapid heart rate.

Pulmonary Complications

Pulmonary disease and, in particular, pneumonia are frequent reasons for death in patients with SCI (6). Atelectasis, pneumonia, and restrictive lung disease are commonly seen (52).

Patients with high tetraplegia may have impaired diaphragmatic function secondary to involvement of the spinal cord above the C3-5 levels or secondary to peripheral root injury, impairing phrenic nerve function. Even in patients with lower tetraplegia, the chest wall and abdominal musculature function is impaired. Thus, even when the diaphragm is spared, the patient's ability to cough is reduced. Patients demonstrate paradoxical breathing. The abdomen elevates during inspiration and, as the diaphragm descends, there is a retraction of the chest wall secondary to negative intrathoracic pressure. In the neurologically intact patient, this retraction is opposed by the muscles of the chest wall. When the chest wall musculature is impaired, the chest muscles cannot oppose this movement and the cough mechanism is impaired. The accessory neck muscles of respiration may assist breathing. Patients with high tetraplegia may use oral musculature to assist their breathing, a phenomenon termed *glossopharyngeal breathing* (6,29).

Immediately after injury, patients develop atelectasis and are particularly at risk for pneumonia. Patients have difficulty clearing secretions because of impaired cough. Respiratory failure can occur rapidly. Mechanical ventilation may be necessary shortly after the initial injury. Vital capacity is generally diminished in high tetraplegia. This parameter is monitored carefully, and is a good indication of overall pulmonary function (53).

The baseline treatment is a pulmonary toilet, including chest PT and postural drainage. A "Quad cough" involves manual splinting of the abdominal musculature to help improve the patient's cough. The optimal position for this maneuver is in a supine position, in which the weight of the abdominal viscera can descend on the diaphragm and reset it at a higher level, allowing greater inspiration. A mini-nebulizer is used to dispense bronchodilators and mucolytic therapy. Guaifenesin may be used to reduce the viscosity of pulmonary secretions. Pneumococcal vaccination should be dispensed to patients. Infections must be treated aggressively (53).

Patients with C-4 injuries can generally be weaned off the ventilator, but this varies in elderly patients or if other pulmonary problems coexist. Up to 50% of patients with C-3 tetraplegia stand a chance of ultimately being weaned off of the ventilator as well (54).

Gastrointestinal Problems

In patients with SCI, abdominal pathology is difficult to diagnose early. With sustained fevers or autonomic dysreflexia, one must be concerned about an intraabdominal problem as the precipitating factor. Often, the patient cannot give reliable localization of an abdominal problem. They may perceive an abnormal vague sensation or even pain in the abdomen. On physical examination, there may be a change in the abdominal tone or an overall increase in spasticity. Abdominal sounds may be lost as well (55).

Prophylactic medications are frequently given to prevent gastrointestinal bleeding. This may occur as the result of unimposed parasympathetic action secondary to impaired sympathetic innervation, with an increased acid secretion. An H_2-blocker is often given to the patient for the first 2 to 3 months' postinjury (55,56).

Neurogenic Bowel

Neurogenic bowel dysfunction results from an upper-motor neuron injury to the bowel. Patients become incontinent of stool secondary to impaired colonic transit and stool retention secondary to spasticity of the anal sphincter. Volitional control of defecation is lost secondary to impaired sensation and motor control. The reflexes allowing defecation are present, however, and these reflexes are used to establish a bowel routine.

A bowel routine is an attempt to invoke continence on a patient who is incontinent, with a goal to limit incontinence and promote regular defecation. This often involves a stool softener, such as Colace, 100 mg t.i.d. A cathartic, such as Senokot or possibly Dulcolax, is given 8 to 10 hours before the desired time of the patient's defecation. The patient is given a fleet bisacodyl enema or a rectal suppository 12 hours later. A digital stimulation may replace or complement the application of the enema. Rectal stimulation activates the rectocolic reflex and stimulates evacuation. The patient should be upright when possible. The patient's normal timing of evacuation is used to promote maximal elimination. A bowel routine is generally performed daily or every other day. Fluid intake, degree of rectal and colonic tone, and other medications may affect the success of a bowel routine. The bowel routine is timed to be after a meal to take advantage of the gastrocolic reflex. Some prefer an evening routine, whereas others prefer a morning routine. The doses may be altered depending on the success of the program. Fiber supplements, such as Metamucil, may add bulk if the stool is loose.

Antibiotics may cause diarrhea or secondary infection with *Clostridia difficile*. Impaction is a frequent occurrence, even in the face of a regular bowel routine. Sometimes immobilization hypercalcemia may contribute toward constipation as well. An abdominal x-ray may help to establish whether the patient is evacuating well.

Neurogenic Bladder

Patients with tetraplegia have impaired bladder function secondary to upper-motor neuron injury. Immediately after the injury, there is a period of spinal shock and the bladder is flaccid. Over time, the detrusor becomes spastic and there are uninhibited contractions. The sphincter also becomes spastic. Detrusor-sphincter dyssynergia occurs as the patient loses the ability to relax the sphincter when the detrusor contracts. This results in urinary retention and high bladder pressures; hydronephrosis, ureteral reflux, and recurrent infection may also occur (Fig. 7). In the past, renal complications secondary to bladder dysfunction was the leading cause of death in SCI patients. This is no longer the case, however. Patients are also at higher risk for urinary calculi and bladder cancer (42).

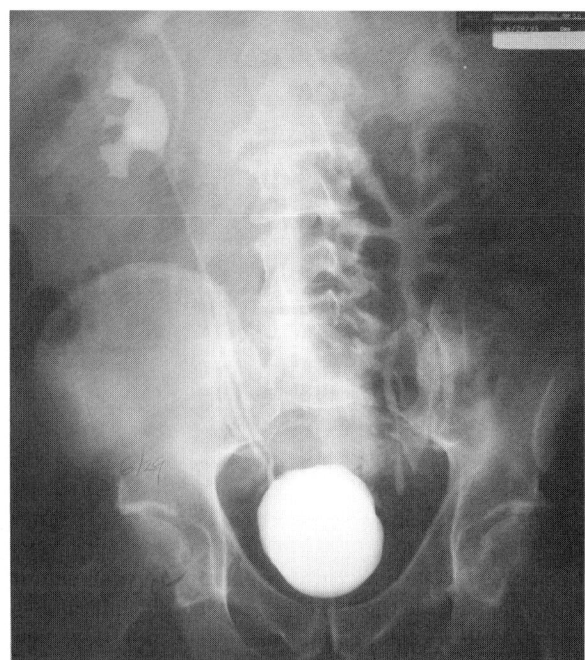

FIG. 7. Cystogram in a spinal cord injury patient demonstrating vesicoureteral reflux secondary to neurogenic bladder.

After acute SCI, an indwelling catheter is put into place. The patient must be allowed adequate hydration, and intermittent catheterization is not practical. In the long run, removal of the indwelling catheter is a major goal. Asymptomatic bacteriuria is frequently seen in the patient with a Foley catheter, as well as in patients on intermittent catheterization. Asymptomatic colonization of the bladder should not be treated with antibiotics but instead be reserved for symptomatic urinary tract infections.

The long-term goal of bladder management is to promote low pressure voiding and to provide a storage site for urine. The intravesicular pressure should be under 40 to 60 cm H_2O. Bladder contraction may be inhibited by oxybutynin or tolterodine. The patient who has a skilled attendant or has good hand function is placed on fluid restriction below 1,800 cc per day, and intermittent catheterization is performed every 4 to 6 hours. Acceptable residual volumes are 400 to 500 cc.

In men, reflex voiding into a condom catheter may be an option. The individual's anatomy must be such that a condom catheter is feasible. The sphincter needs to be defeated by an alpha-adrenergic blocking agent, such as terazosin, doxazosin, or tamsulosin. The other option is a surgical procedure, such as sphincterotomy. Women do not have the option of voiding into a condom catheter, but a suprapubic catheter or ureteral diversion can be considered. A Foley catheter is less desirable because of local soft tissue problems and increased risk of cancer and infection. Bladder management by electrical stimulation may be an option in the future (57).

Spasticity

The patient with tetraplegia is prone to have spasticity. *Spasticity* is a velocity-dependent increase in resistance to a passive stretch, characterized by increased deep tendon reflexes, clonus,

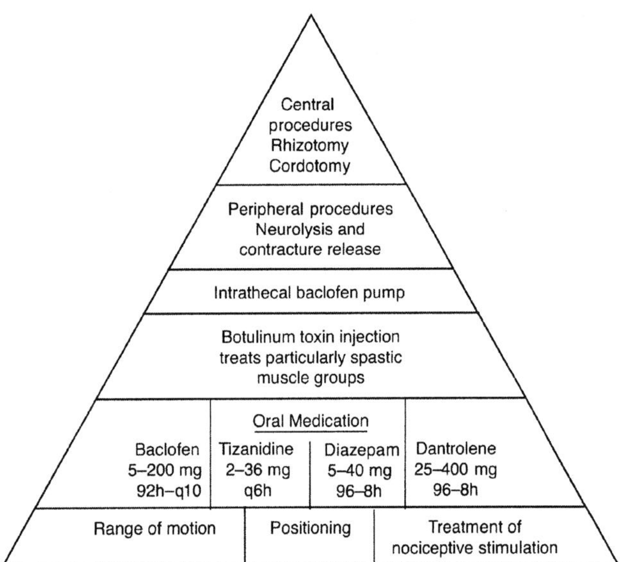

FIG. 8. Treatment of spasticity in tetraplegia.

and involuntary muscle contraction, and it creates a number of significant problems. Spasticity may be painful. Positioning in the bed or in the wheelchair may be altered. Uncontrolled limb movements may drag the skin across surfaces and predispose patients to decubiti. Transfers and ambulation may be impaired. On the other hand, spasticity may provide muscle contraction, which may assist with mobility. Muscle contractions decrease the chances of DVT and retard the progression of osteoporosis.

The treatment of spasticity must target specific goals. It is treated only if it interferes with function, promotes decubiti or poor hygiene, or induces pain. The baseline treatment involves a regular range of motion program (Fig. 8). Removal of nociceptors that exacerbate the spasticity is critical. Strategies may include optimal bowel and bladder routines, treatment of ingrown toenails, elimination of decubiti, and so forth. Medications to diminish spasticity include baclofen, clonidine, tizanidine, diazepam, and Dantrium. Motor-point blocks with phenol or botulinum toxin may be helpful in reducing the spasticity of a particularly troublesome muscle group. Neurolytic blocks of peripheral nerves are used also. Intrathecal baclofen pump may be effective in patients with uncontrolled spasticity. Other procedures such as rhizotomy and cordotomy are rarely performed (58).

Decubitus Ulcers

The pressure ulcer is the most common cause of morbidity in SCI patients in the United States. It occurs in 15% of patients during the first year postinjury, whereas patients with chronic SCI have an annual incidence of 25% (44,59,60).

Excessive pressure is the leading factor in the causation of decubiti. The type and intensity of pressure lead to greater skin breakdown. Sustained pressure above capillary pressure is all that is required to cause tissue damage. Shearing stresses occur secondary to spasticity. Maceration with sweat, urine, or feces also predisposes patients to the problem. Common sites for injury include areas over bony prominences including occiput, scapula, sacrum, ischium, greater trochanter, and heel. Poor nutrition, impaired circulation, and infection can promote skin breakdown as well. Impaired sensation, alteration of consciousness, and substance abuse impede the prevention of decubiti (61).

The best treatment for a decubitus ulcer is prevention. Patients must be turned in bed every 2 hours, and positioned to minimize pressure over bony surfaces. Patients at particularly high risk may benefit from special mattresses. Seating in the wheelchair must be optimal. Regular pressure relief every 15 minutes must be used when the patient is in the wheelchair. The patient's skin must be monitored multiple times throughout the day. Other factors that should be managed include optimal nutrition, reduction of spasticity, optimal bowel and bladder hygiene, and discontinuation of smoking.

When the decubitus does occur, pressure to the involved area must be eliminated. For instance, the patient with an ischial ulcer must go to bed rest. The necrotic tissue must be débrided surgically or with topical enzymatic débridement. The wound is cleansed on a regular basis with saline, and some prefer alternating wet to dry dressings. If the decubitus is infected, intravenous antibiotics may be required, particularly when an underlying osteomyelitis is suspected. Bone biopsy is the most effective tool for diagnosis, as well as for ascertaining the offending bacteria and determining the most appropriate antibiotic for treatment. Deep ulcers may require surgical débridement and reconstruction with a myocutaneous flap, usually accompanied by débridement of any underlying bony prominence.

Pain in Spinal Cord Injury

Pain is a significant issue in the majority of patients with SCI. It may be so severe that many patients would trade pain relief for the loss of bowel, bladder, or sexual function. Forty-four percent of patients with chronic SCI claim the pain interferes with their daily activities. It generally presents within 6 months of injury (62–64).

SCI pain is generally classified as musculoskeletal, neuropathic (which may be central or peripheral), or visceral discomfort. Other sources of pain may include complex regional pain syndromes, headaches, and pain from posttraumatic syrinx (65,66).

Central or diffuse pain is generally referred to as *spinal pain* and is quite common. It is perceived to be caudal to the level of the injury, or it may be in a saddle distribution. It is described as cutting, burning, piercing, radiating, tight, cool, or nagging. Acute onset of spinal pain must raise the question as to whether or not there is an underlying problem, such as a syrinx or a new peripheral problem. Conservative management includes patient education, biofeedback and relaxation techniques, hypnosis, and cognitive strategies for pain management. Medication options include tricyclic antidepressants; membrane stabilizers, such as gabapentin or carbamazepine; and Tramadol. Narcotic usage in central pain syndromes is controversial. Intrathecal baclofen also has been used with some success in central pain syndromes.

Neuropathic pain can also emanate from the zone of injury. This pain may be segmental in nature and characterized as sharp, electric, paresthesia-like, or burning. It is often worse with inactivity. The patient may suffer from local allodynia, which is pain from a nonpainful stimulus, or hyperalgesia, which is excessive pain from a painful stimulation.

Treatment options for radicular pain are similar to that of central pain, but the area involved may be more localized. In these instances desensitization, TENS unit, Lidoderm patches, or topical capsaicin may be useful. Medications used are similar to those used for central pain syndromes. A dorsal root entry-zone ablation may also be considered for these patients (67).

Visceral pain from the abdomen or chest often presents as a vague, nondescript discomfort in the chest, abdomen, and pelvic area. Its projection is probably mediated via the autonomic nervous system, which emanates from cephalad to the injury. Central pain symptomatology or spasticity may worsen. There may be changes in local abdominal tone. Treatment must be directed toward the individual visceral etiology, for example, cholecystatony in a patient with symptomatic gallstones.

Musculoskeletal discomfort is a frequent occurrence after SCI. Patients rely heavily on upper extremities for mobility. Muscles may be used in a novel manner, and muscle function may become unbalanced secondary to joint contractures and injuries to other muscles in the extremities. Spasticity also causes muscle imbalances, which may make certain muscles work harder to overcome spastic muscle groups.

Shoulder discomfort is quite frequent. C-5 and C-6 tetraplegics have impaired muscle activity, which predisposes them toward rotator cuff dysfunction secondary to biomechanical instability of the shoulder. Similarly, lateral epicondylitis is a frequent occurrence because the wrist extensors are weak and those muscle groups are constantly being used (68–70).

Treatment of musculoskeletal injuries is directed toward maximizing range of motion and strengthening individual muscle groups within a pain-free zone. Equipment should be used to decrease the stress on muscle groups. Wheelchairs should appropriately fit the patient. There may be times when it is appropriate to place a patient in a power wheelchair to put the impaired joint to rest. Nonsteroidal antiinflammatories, joint injections, and modalities including ultrasonography, ice, and electrical stimulation may be helpful. Heat must be used with great care because sensation is impaired. The SCI patient should generally not receive heat treatment in an area with impaired sensation. If hot packs are used, they must be monitored carefully.

Heterotopic Ossification

Heterotopic ossification occurs in 16 to 53% of patients after SCI (71) and is defined as the deposition of new bone around the joint (Fig. 9). Heterotopic ossification may be recognized within the first 2 months after injury. The most prominent joint involved is the hip, followed by the knee. It occurs below the level of the SCI unless there is a concomitant head injury or burn.

Heterotopic ossification may present only with limitation of range of motion in the affected joint, or the presentation may be swelling, local heat, and a fever. In these instances, differential diagnoses includes hematoma, infection, fracture, tumor, and DVT.

During the active phase, the sedimentation rate and alkaline phosphatase level are elevated, and plain radiographs may be normal. Later x-rays reveal the process after sufficient ossification has taken place. The third phase of the bone scan becomes abnormal 7 to 10 days before plain x-rays (72,73).

Baseline treatment includes aggressive range of motion to maintain joint mobility. Contractures of the hip can be disastrous, as this may alter seating and promote decubiti. Functional activities, including transfers, ambulation, and activities of daily living, may be impaired as well by metatrophic bone formation.

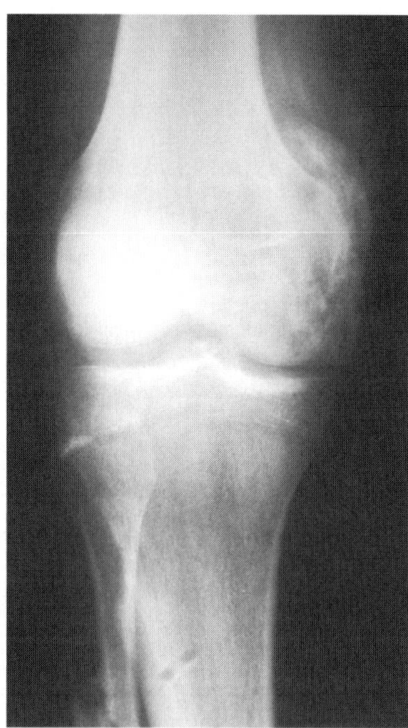

FIG. 9. Heterotopic ossification of the knee in a tetraplegic patient.

Medication options may include disodium etidronate, given 20 mg per kg per day for 2 weeks. The patient is then given 10 mg per kg per day for at least an additional 10 weeks. Nonsteroidal antiinflammatories, particularly indomethacin (Indocin), can be used because of their interference with bone formation. Low-dose irradiation can also be given to prevent worsening of heterotopic ossification (74–76).

Surgical resection of heterotopic ossification is performed in patients when restriction of motion has caused significant functional compromise. Surgery cannot take place until the bone has fully matured, as determined by serial x-ray films, bone scans, and alkaline phosphatase levels. Surgical complications may include excessive bleeding, fracture, infection, and recurrent heterotopic ossification (77).

Osteoporosis and Pathologic Fractures

Bone mineral loss is greatest within the first 4 months after SCI, with the greatest loss in the pelvis and proximal femur. Maximal bone loss occurs at 18 months, and then metabolic equilibrium is established. The greatest loss occurs in areas rich with trabecular bone, such as the upper tibia, which may suffer a total loss of 50% of bone by 18 months (78).

Fractures occur in approximately 4% of patients with chronic SCI. This figure probably underestimates the true frequency of fracture, because many fractures go undiagnosed. Patients are at risk for a fracture secondary to osteoporosis especially in the setting of repetitive passive range of motion exercises. Additionally, patients with an SCI are at higher risk for falls. The majority of fractures are in the distal femur and proximal tibia (Fig. 10) (79,80).

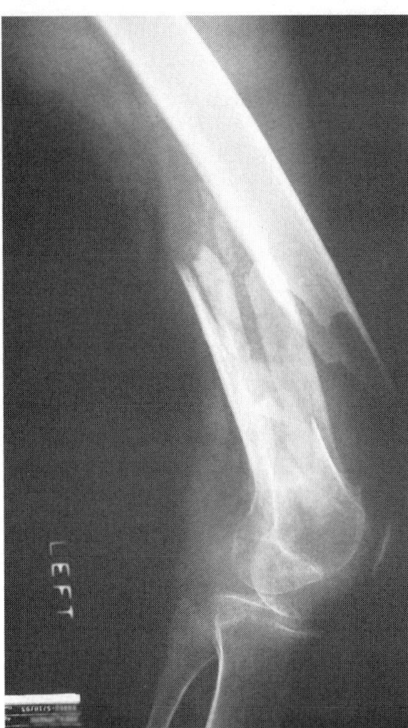

FIG. 10. Pathologic fracture of the femur in a patient with osteoporosis secondary to spinal cord injury.

The treatment of osteoporosis includes mobilization out of bed and standing. Tiludronate, which is a bisphosphonate, may be effective in reducing bone resorption (81). Electrical stimulation to promote muscle activity may also be beneficial.

Patients with chronic SCI generally are treated with conservative, closed treatment of long bone fractures. The fractures generally heal within 3 to 4 weeks. Soft splints are used when possible, because plaster casts may promote skin breakdown. Shortening, angulation, and even nonunion is acceptable in the lower extremities of patients who are nonambulatory. Problematic fractures include those in the femoral neck and subtrochanteric regions. In contrast, patients who are ambulatory often require a surgical stabilization. Open reduction and internal fixation is generally used for lower-extremity fractures presenting with the acute SCI. The indications for open reduction and internal fixation in ambulatory SCI patients are similar to the indications for the general population (82,83).

SUMMARY

SCIs are devastating, and their effects are manifest long after the initial injury. Patients with these injuries are commonly at risk for numerous medical complications. The physical injuries and disabilities associated with SCI are frequently accompanied by psychosocial issues.

Rehabilitation of patients with SCI begins almost immediately after the injury and is carried out by a multidisciplinary team of physicians, nurses, therapists, and social workers, headed by a physiatrist. The specific aims of therapy depend on the neurologic level and severity (complete or incomplete) of the injury, with the ultimate goal of optimizing function and achieving maximal neurologic recovery.

REFERENCES

1. Chiles BW III, Cooper P. Acute spinal cord injury. *N Engl J Med* 1996;334:514–520.
2. Gonzalez F, Chang JY, Banovac K, et al. Autoregulation of cerebral blood flow in patients with orthostatic hypotension after spinal cord injury. *Paraplegia* 1991;29:1–7.
3. Meyers AR. The epidemiology of traumatic spinal cord injury in the United States. In: Nesathurai S, ed. *The rehabilitation of people with spinal cord injury*, 2nd ed. Malden, MA: Blackwell Science Inc., 2001:9–13.
4. Nobunaga AI, Go BK, Karunas RB. Recent demographic and injury trends in people served by the model spinal cord injury care system. *Arch Phys Med Rehabil* 1999;80:1372–1382.
5. Staas WE, Formal CS, Freedman MK, et al. Spinal cord injury and spinal cord injury medicine. In: DeLisa JA, Gans BM, eds. *Rehabilitation medicine: principles and practice*, 3rd ed. Philadelphia: Lippincott–Raven Publishers, 1998:1259–1291.
6. DeVivo MJ, Stover SL. Long-term survival and causes of death. In: Stover SL, DeLisa JA, Whiteneck GG, eds. *Spinal cord injury*. Gaithersburg, MD: Aspen, 1995:289–316.
7. Amar AP, Levy MC. Pathogenesis and pharmacological strategies for mitigating secondary damage in acute spinal cord injury. *Neurosurg* 1999;44:1027–1040.
8. Allen AR. Surgery of experimental lesion of spinal cord equivalent to crush injury of fracture dislocation of spinal column: a preliminary report. *JAMA* 1911;57:878–880.
9. Teasell RW, Arnold JMO, Krassioukov A, et al. Cardiovascular consequences of loss of supraspinal control of sympathetic nervous system after spinal cord injury. *Arch Phys Med Rehabil* 2000;81:506–516.
10. Tator CH, Koyanagi I. Vascular mechanisms in the pathophysiology of human spinal cord injury. *J Neurosurg* 1997;86:483–492.
11. Bresnahan JC, King JS, Martin GF, et al. A neuroanatomical analysis of spinal injury in the rhesus monkey. *J Neurol Sci* 1976;28:521–542.
12. Curat WL, Kingsley DP, Kendall BE, et al. MRI in chronic spinal cord trauma. *Neuroradiol* 1992;35:30–35.
13. Bosch A, Stauffer S, Nickel MD. Incomplete traumatic quadriplegia, a ten year review. *JAMA* 1971;216:473–478.
14. Brown-Séquard CE. Lectures on the physiology and pathology of the central nervous system and on the treatment of organic nervous affectations. *Lancet* 1868;2:593–596, 659–662, 755–757, 821–823.
15. Schneider RC, Cherry G, Pantek H. The syndrome of acute central cervical spinal cord injury. *J Neurosurg* 1954;11:546–577.
16. Schneider RC. The syndrome of acute anterior spinal cord injury. *J Neurosurg* 1955;12:95–122.
17. World Health Organization. International classification of impairments, disabilities, and handicaps: a manual of classification relating to the consequences of disease. Geneva: World Health Organization, 1980.
18. Bracken MB, Shepard MJ, Collins WF Jr, et al. A randomized, controlled trial of methylprednisolone or naloxone in the treatment of acute spinal cord injury: results of the second National Acute Spinal Cord Injury Study. *N Eng J Med* 1990;322:1405–1411.
19. American Spinal Injury Association. International standards for neurological classification of spinal cord injury. Chicago: American Spinal Injury Association, 1996.
20. Ditunno JF Jr, Young W, Donovan WH, et al. The international standards booklet for neurological and functional classification of spinal cord injury. *Paraplegia* 1994;32:70–80.
21. Brown PJ, Marino RJ, Herbison GJ, et al. The 72 hour examination as a predictor of recovery in motor complete quadriplegia. *Arch Phys Med Rehabil* 1991;72:546–548.
22. Ditunno JF Jr, Cohen ME, Formal C, et al. Functional outcomes. In: Stover SL, DeLisa JA, Whiteneck GG, eds. *Spinal cord injury*. Gaithersburg, MD: Aspen, 1985:170–184.
23. Crozier KS, Graziani V, Ditunno JF Jr, et al. Spinal cord injury: prognosis for ambulation based on sensory examination in patients who are initially motor complete. *Arch Phys Med Rehabil* 1991; 72:119–121.
24. Katoh S, El Masry WS. Motor recovery of patients presenting with

motor paralysis and sensory sparing following cervical spinal cord injury. *Paraplegia* 1995;33:506–509.
25. Stauffer ES. Neurologic recovery following injuries to the cervical spinal cord and nerve roots. *Spine* 1984;9:532–534.
26. Ditunno JF, Stover SL, Freed MM, et al. Motor recovery of the upper extremities in traumatic quadriplegia: a multicenter study. *Arch Phys Med Rehabil* 1992;73:431–436.
27. Kirshblum SC, O'Connor KC. Predicting neurologic recovery in traumatic cervical spinal cord injury. *Arch Phys Med Rehabil* 1998; 79:1456–1466.
28. Little JW, Ditunno JF Jr, Stiens SA, et al. Incomplete spinal cord injury: neuronal mechanisms of motor recovery and hyperreflexia. *Arch Phys Med Rehabil* 1999;80:587–599.
29. Clough P. Glossopharyngeal breathing: its application with a traumatic quadriplegic patient. *Arch Phys Med Rehabil* 1983;64:384–385.
30. Consortium for Spinal Cord Medicine. Outcomes following traumatic spinal cord injury: clinical practice guideline for health-care professionals. Washington, DC: Paralyzed Veterans of America, 1999.
31. Maynard FM, Reynolds GG, Fountain S, et al. Neurological prognosis after traumatic quadriplegia: three-year experiences of California regional spinal cord injury care system. *J Neurosurg* 1979; 50:611–616.
32. Moberg EA. The present state of surgical rehabilitation for the upper limb in tetraplegia. *Paraplegia* 1987;25:351–356.
33. Waters RL, Sie IH, Gellman H, et al. Functional hand surgery following tetraplegia. *Arch Phys Med Rehabil* 1996;77:86–94.
34. Chae J, Triolo RJ, Kilgore K, et al. Functional neuromuscular stimulation. In: DeLisa JA, Gans BM, eds. *Rehabilitation medicine: principles and practice*, 3rd ed. Philadelphia: Lippincott–Raven, 1998:611–631.
35. Consortium for Spinal Cord Medicine. Depression following spinal cord injury: a clinical practice guideline for primary care physicians. Washington, DC: Paralyzed Veterans of America, 1998.
36. Dijkers MP, Abela MB, Gans B, et al. The aftermath of spinal cord injury. In: Stover SL, DeLisa JA, Whiteneck GG, eds. *Spinal cord injury*. Gaithersburg, MD: Aspen, 1995:185–212.
37. Eastwood EA, Hagglund KJ, Ragnarsson KT, et al. Medical rehabilitation length of stay and outcomes for persons with traumatic spinal cord injury 1990–1997. *Arch Phys Med Rehabil* 1999;80:1457–1463.
38. Krause JS, Kewman DK, DeVivo MJ, et al. Employment after spinal cord injury: an analysis of cases from the model spinal cord injury systems. *Arch Phys Med Rehabil* 1999;80:1492–1500.
39. Merli GJ, Herbison GJ, Ditunno JF. Deep vein thrombophlebitis in acute spinal cord injured patients. *Arch Phys Med Rehabil* 1988; 69:661–664.
40. Rossi EC, Green D, Rosen JS, et al. Sequential changes in factor VIII and platelets preceding deep vein thrombosis in patients with spinal cord injury. *Br J Haematol* 1980;45:143–151.
41. Clinical outcomes from the model systems. In: Stover SL, DeLisa JA, Whiteneck GG, eds. *Spinal cord injury.* Gaithersburg, MD: Aspen, 1995:302–305.
42. Consortium for Spinal Cord Medicine. Clinical practice guideline—spinal cord medicine: prevention of thromboembolism in spinal cord injury. Washington, DC: Paralyzed Veterans of America, 1997.
43. McKinley WO, Jackson AB, Cardenas DD, et al. Long-term medical complications after traumatic spinal cord injury: a regional model system analysis. *Arch Phys Med Rehabil* 1999;80:1402–1409.
44. Drory Y, Ohry A, Brooks ME, et al. Arm crank ergometry in chronic spinal cord injured patients. *Arch Phys Med Rehabil* 1990;71:389–392.
45. Figoni SF. Exercise responses and quadriplegia. *Med Sci Sports Exerc* 1993;25:433–441.
46. Frankel HL, Mathias CJ, Spalding JMK. Mechanism of reflex cardiac arrest in tetraplegic patients. *Lancet* 1975;2:1183–1185.
47. Gilgoff IS, Davidson-Ward SL, Hohn AR. Cardiac pacemaker in high spinal cord injury. *Arch Phys Med Rehabil* 1991;72:601–603.
48. Mathias CJ. Bradycardia and cardiac arrest during tracheal suction mechanisms in tetraplegic patients. *Eur J Intens Care Med* 1976;2: 147–156.
49. Colachis SC III. Autonomic hyperreflexia with spinal cord injury. *J Spinal Cord Med* 1992;15:171–196.
50. Erickson RP. Autonomic hyperreflexia: pathophysiology and medical management. *Arch Phys Med Rehabil* 1980;61:431–440.
51. DeSantis N. Autonomic dysfunction. In: Nesathurai S, ed. *The rehabilitation of people with spinal cord injury*, 2nd ed. Malden, MA: Blackwell Science, Inc., 2001:71–74.
52. Fishburn MJ, Marino RJ, Ditunno JF Jr. Atelectasis and pneumonia in acute spinal cord injury. *Arch Phys Med Rehabil* 1991;71:197–200.
53. Cohn JR. Pulmonary management of the patient with spinal cord injury. *Trauma Q* 1993;9:65–71.
54. Wicks AB, Mentar RR. Long-term outlook in quadriplegic patients with initial ventilator dependency. *Chest* 1986;90:406–410.
55. Juler GI, Eltorai IM. The acute abdomen in spinal cord injury patients. *Paraplegia* 1985;23:118–123.
56. Kewalramani LS. Neurogenic gastroduodenal ulceration and bleeding associated with spinal cord injuries. *J Trauma* 1979;19:259–265.
57. Nygaard IE, Kreder KJ. Urologic management in patients with spinal cord injuries. *Spine* 1996;21:128–132.
58. Stein AB, Pomerantz F, Schectman J. Evaluation and management of spasticity in spinal cord injury. *Topics in Spinal Cord Rehabil* 1997;2:70–83.
59. Carlson CE, King RB, Kirk PM, et al. Incidence and correlates of pressure ulcers development after spinal cord injury. *Rehab Nursing Res* 1992;1:34–40.
60. Whiteneck GG, Charlifue SW, Frankel HC, et al. Mortality, morbidity and psychosocial outcomes of persons spinal cord injured more than twenty years ago. *Paraplegia* 1992;30:617–630.
61. Koziak M. Etiology and pathology of ischemic ulcers. *Arch Phys Med Rehabil* 1959;40:62–69.
62. Ankle AG, Staughelle JK. Pain and life quality within two years of spinal cord injury. *Paraplegia* 1995;33:555–559.
63. Beric A, Dimitrijevic M, Lindblom V. Central dysthesia syndrome in spinal cord injury patients. *Pain* 1988;34:109–116.
64. Nepomuceno C, Fine PR, Richards JS, et al. Pain in patients with spinal cord injury. *Arch Phys Med Rehabil* 1979;60:605–609.
65. Donovan WH, Dimitrijevic MR. Neurophysiologic approaches to chronic pain following spinal cord injury. *Paraplegia* 1982;20:135–146.
66. Sidall PJ, Taylor DA, Cousins MJ. Classification of pain following spinal cord injury. *Spinal Cord* 1997;35:69–75.
67. Friedman AH, Nashold BS Jr. DREZ lesions for relief of pain related to spinal cord injury. *J Neurosurg* 1986;65:465–469.
68. Campbell C, Koris M. Etiologies of shoulder pain in cervical spinal cord injury. *Clin Orthop* 1996;322:140–145.
69. Sie IH, Waters RL, Adkins RH, et al. Upper extremity pain in the postrehabilitation spinal cord injured patient. *Arch Phys Med Rehabil* 1992;73:44–48.
70. Silfverskiold J, Waters RL. Shoulder pain and functional disability in spinal cord injury patients. *Clin Orthop* 1991;272:141–145.
71. Venier LH, Ditunno JF Jr. Heterotopic ossification in the paraplegic patient. *Arch Phys Med Rehabil* 1971;52:475–479.
72. Freed JH, Hahn H, Menter R, et al. The use of the three phase bone scan in the early diagnosis of heterotopic ossification and the value of Didronel therapy. *Paraplegia* 1982;13:208–216.
73. Orzel JA, Rudd TG. Heterotopic bone formation: clinical, laboratory, and imaging correlation. *J Nuclear Med* 1985;26:125–132.
74. Ayers DG, Evarts CM, Parkinson TR. The prevention of heterotopic ossification in high risk patients by low dose radiation therapy after total hip arthroplasty. *J Bone Joint Surg (Am)* 1986;68: 1423–1430.
75. Garland DE, Betzabe A, Venos KG, et al. Siphosphonate treatment for heterotopic ossification in spinal cord injury patients. *Clin Orthop* 1983;176:197–200.
76. Schmidt SA, Kjaersgaard-Andersen P, Pedersen NW, et al. The use of indomethacin to prevent the formation of heterotopic bone

after total hip replacement. *J Bone Joint Surg (Am)* 1988;70: 834–838.

77. Stover SL, Niemann Tulloss JR. Experience with surgical resection of heterotopic bone in spinal cord injury patients. *Clin Orthop* 1991;263:71–77.
78. Garland DE, Stewart CA, Adkins RH, et al. Osteoporosis after spinal cord injury. *J Orthop Res* 1992;10:371–378.
79. Freehafer A. Limb fractures in patients with spinal cord injury. *Arch Phys Med Rehabil* 1995;76:823–827.
80. Ragnarsson KT, Sell GH. Lower extremity fractures after spinal cord injury: a retrospective study. *Arch Phys Med Rehabil* 1981; 62:418–423.
81. Chappard D, Minaire P, Privat C, et al. Effects of tiludronate on bone loss in paraplegic patients. *J Bone Miner Res* 1995;10:112–118.
82. Garland DE, Reiser TV, Singer DI. Treatment of femoral shaft fractures associated with acute spinal cord injuries. *Clin Orthop* 1985;197:191–195.
83. McMaster W, Stauffer E. The management of long bone fracture in the spinal cord patient. *Clin Orthop* 1975;112:44–52.

CHAPTER 33

Injuries to the Upper Cervical Spine

Paul A. Anderson

The upper cervical spine has a unique anatomic arrangement, with relatively large bony lateral masses and strong ligaments. It consists of the occipitoatlantal and atlantoaxial articulations, their bony and ligamentous structures, and the neurovascular bundles that course through. Its function is to transition between the skull and spinal column, to protect the spinal cord, and to allow a wide range of motion. Additionally, the movement of this articulation is closely integrated to the visual system. A mobile occipitocervical articulation is essential for wide visual fields. Ocular motion in humans is limited to only 30 degrees, with the remaining view range coming from rotatory motion in the upper cervical spine. Additionally, proprioception in these joints is extensive so that the brain can coordinate vision (1).

The bony structures are strong and relatively spared from osteoporosis until very late in life. Injuries require significant trauma, usually rapid deceleration or direct trauma to the cranium or face. Only in the elderly, in whom the odontoid fractures secondary to falls, are less severe injuries observed. Concomitant spinal trauma at other levels occurs in 10 to 20% of cases. Craniofacial and closed-head injuries are common and make the diagnosis and treatment of upper cervical injuries more difficult. Neurologic injuries are rare because of the relative increased cross-sectional area of the spinal canal in this region. When present, however, they may be catastrophic, resulting in respiratory embarrassment and often death. Additionally, cranial nerve and vertebral artery injuries may be present in contrast to other spinal trauma.

This chapter reviews the evaluation of the upper cervical spine, describes common fracture patterns and their mechanism of injury, and presents treatment algorithms. Specifics of surgical treatment, such as fusion and orthotic management, are found in Chapters 32 and 38 through 40.

ANATOMY

Bony Anatomy

Occiput

The *occipitocervical articulation* is a highly complex structure that forms a transition between the skull base and spinal column (Fig. 1). The occipital bone has four components. The squamous

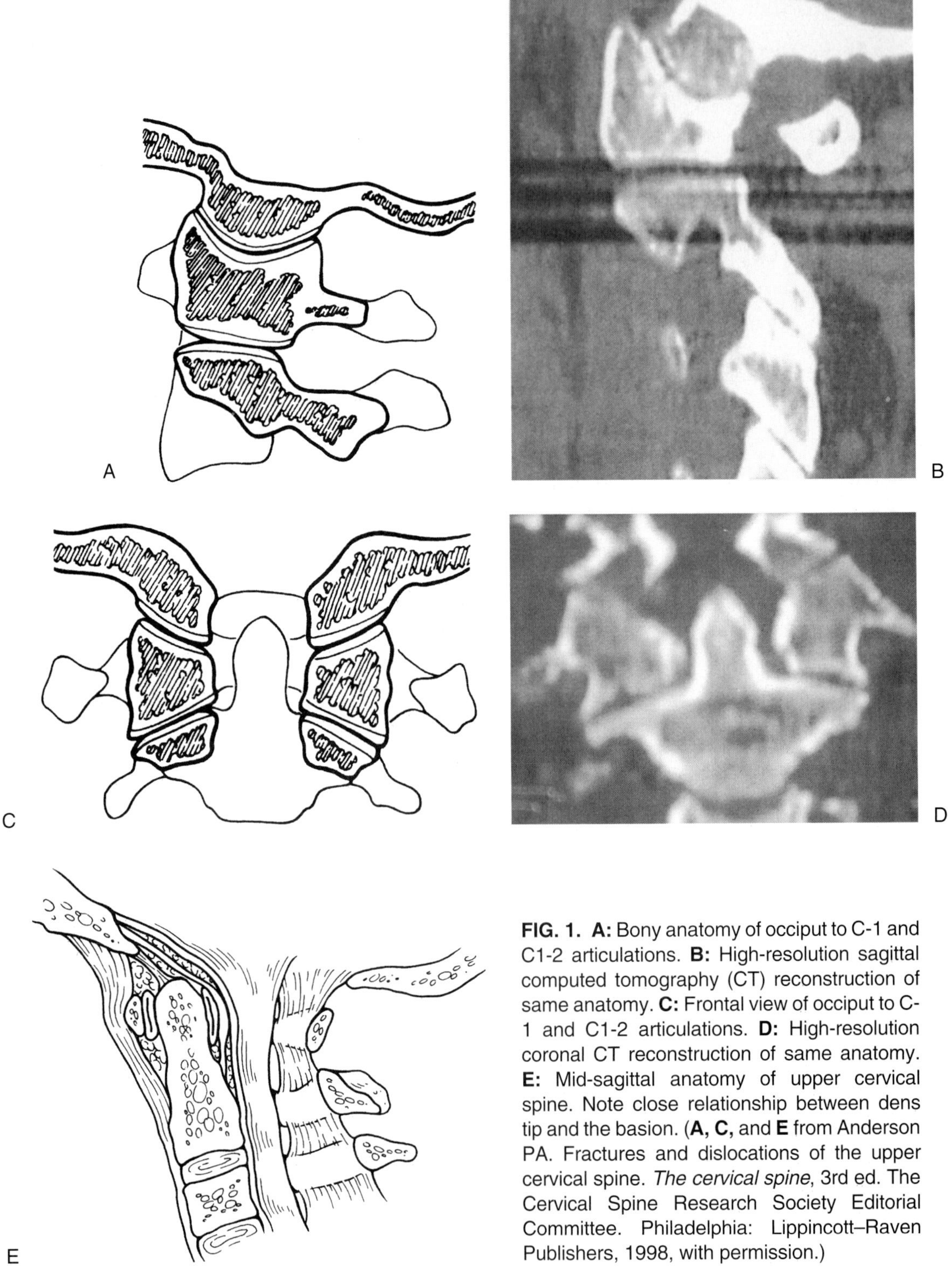

FIG. 1. A: Bony anatomy of occiput to C-1 and C1-2 articulations. **B:** High-resolution sagittal computed tomography (CT) reconstruction of same anatomy. **C:** Frontal view of occiput to C-1 and C1-2 articulations. **D:** High-resolution coronal CT reconstruction of same anatomy. **E:** Mid-sagittal anatomy of upper cervical spine. Note close relationship between dens tip and the basion. (**A, C,** and **E** from Anderson PA. Fractures and dislocations of the upper cervical spine. *The cervical spine*, 3rd ed. The Cervical Spine Research Society Editorial Committee. Philadelphia: Lippincott–Raven Publishers, 1998, with permission.)

part projects posteriorly from foramen magnum and fuses rostrally with the parietal bones at the Lambda suture. The *opisthion* is the posterior midline demarcation of foramen magnum. Two paired lateral parts have downward projects, *occipital condyles*, which form the articulation with the atlas. The occipital condyles are located along the anterolateral aspect of foramen magnum. When viewed from the front, the condyles are wedge shaped, extending caudally more medially than laterally. Viewed laterally, they form a near semicircle. Just anterior to the occipital condyle is the hypoglossal canal, transmitting cranial nerve XII. Further lateral, at the junction of the occipital and petrous bones, is the *jugular foramen*, containing the internal jugular vein and cranial nerves IX, X, and XI. The basilar part of the occiput forms the anterior aspect of foramen magnum, the *basion*, and fuses with the sphenoid. Extending upward from the basion is a bony plate, the *clivus*. This is an important landmark, as it is easily identifiable on radiographs and aids in determining occipitocervical alignment. More rostrally, the clivus forms the posterior aspect of the sella turcica.

Atlas

The *atlas* is a ringed bone with a large central spinal canal. The two large lateral masses are connected by a short anterior and a longer posterior arch. On the anterior surface, a tubercle is present for attachment of the longus colli muscle. Behind the anterior arch is a fovea, for articulation with the odontoid process of the axis. Tubercles are located anteromedially on the inner surface of the lateral masses for attachment of the transverse ligament. The posterior arch has a groove and, occasionally, a foramen on its cranial surface for the vertebral artery and first cervical nerve. When viewed anteriorly, the lateral masses are wedge shaped with articular surfaces that are congruent with those of the occipital condyles. Inferiorly, there is a slightly convex articular surface for contact with the axis. The transverse process extends more widely than all the other cervical vertebrae and lies just behind the internal jugular vein and accessory nerve. Contained in the transverse process are the vertebral artery and a venous plexus.

Axis

The *axis* is the most unique vertebrae, characterized by the odontoid process, or dens, which projects cranially from the body of C-2 into the anterior one-third of the atlas. The dens forms an articulation anteriorly with the atlas and from behind with the transverse ligament. The body of the axis joins to the dens and extends laterally, forming large lateral masses. On the cranial surface of the lateral masses are slightly convex surfaces for articulation with the atlas. The surface contours aid in rotation of C-1 on C-2. The lateral masses are connected posteriorly through short pedicles or a bony isthmus to the posterior facets, which articulate with C-3. The facets are oriented in similar directions to the other cervical vertebrae. The lamina of C-2 is large and overhangs C-3. A large bifid spinous process forms a major attachment of the nuchal ligaments and the short cranial rotator muscles. The transverse process of the axis is small and obliquely oriented. Numerous anomalies exist in its placement and orientation, making the vertebral artery more likely to be injured during surgical procedures and from trauma.

Ligamentous Anatomy

The craniocervical ligaments are essential for survival. They can be categorized into *external craniocervical*, which lie outside the spinal canal, and *internal craniocervical* ligaments.

External Craniocervical Ligaments

The *ligamentum nuchae* is a heavy condensation of collagenous tissue attaching to the external occipital protuberance, to the spinous process of C-2, and to all the remaining cervical spinous processes. A small number of fibers extend to C-1. Redundant capsular ligaments are present in the occipitoatlantal and atlantal-axial articulations. Intervertebral discs and ligamentum flavum are absent in the upper cervical spine.

Thin fibrous elastic bands are located between the anterior aspect of foramen magnum and the anterior arch of C-1, and between the posterior aspect of foramen magnum and posterior arch of C-1. These are termed the *anterior* and *posterior occipitoatlantal membranes*. Similar bands are present between the atlas and axis and are called the *anterior* and *posterior atlantoaxial membranes*. These are redundant tissues, having little structural strength.

Internal Craniocervical Ligaments

The internal craniocervical ligaments are located anterior to the spinal cord in three layers and provide most of the stabilization of the craniocervical region (Fig. 2). The odontoid ligaments lie the most anterior and consist of the apical ligament and the alar ligaments. The apical ligament is a small fibrous band extending between the dens tip and the basion and has a rudimentary function in humans. The alar ligaments are stout horizontal ligaments that extend from the lateral surface of the dens tip to the anteromedial surface of the occipital condyles. Dvorak identified two components of the alar ligaments, upper and lower, which have different biomechanical functions (2). The middle layer of internal craniocervical ligaments is the cruciate ligament. The *transverse ligament* is the horizontal component of this structure and is a strong condensation of fibers extending between the medial aspect of the atlantal lateral masses and behind the dens. A synovial membrane can be present between the transverse ligament and the dens. Triangular fibrous bands extend from the transverse ligament cranially to foramen magnum and caudally to C-2. Posterior to the cruciate ligament is a broad thin ligament, the *tectorial membrane*. This structure is the continuation of the posterior longitudinal ligament and attaches to the anterior rim of foramen magnum.

Neurovascular Anatomy

The *pons* and *medulla oblongata* lie directly posterior to the clivus and pass through foramen magnum to become the spinal cord. The cerebellar tonsils occasionally protrude through foramen magnum posterior to the spinal cord; in normal anatomy, they should not extend more than 5 mm. Behind and contained by the occipital bone is the cerebellum. Cranial nerves IX, X, and XI originate in the medulla and pass downward and ventral, continuing out the jugular foramen, which is located anterior and lateral to the occipital condyles. Cranial nerve XII courses similarly but passes out the hypoglossal foramen, which is located more medial and posterior than the jugular foramen, closer to the occipital condyle.

The vertebral arteries are unique, as they are the only arteries that join together rather than divide. This redundancy presumably allows atlantoaxial rotation such that one artery can be occluded with the contralateral maintaining cerebral blood flow. During life one vertebral artery, usually the left, becomes more dominant. The vertebral artery ascends on each side in the fora-

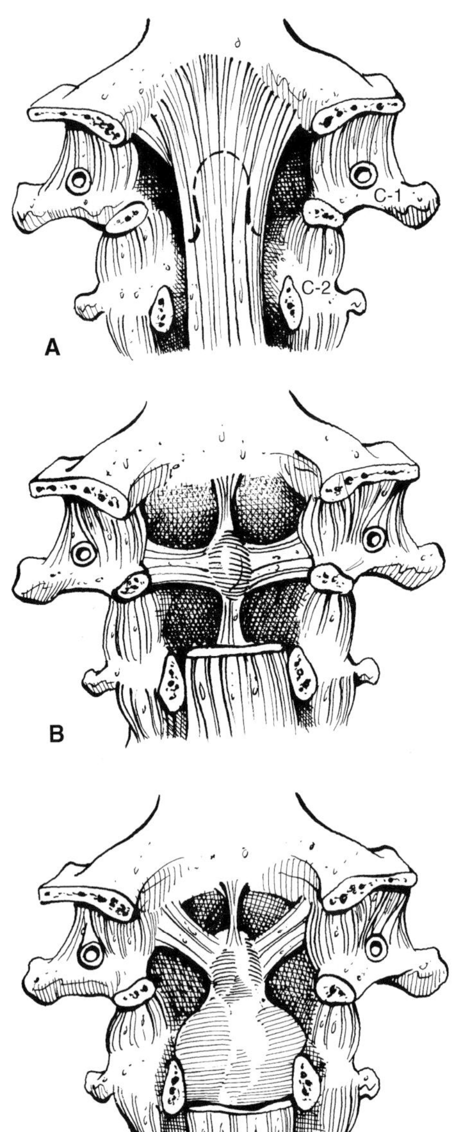

FIG. 2. A: Internal craniocervical ligaments lie in three layers, all anterior to the spinal cord. The most dorsal layer is the tectorial membrane, a continuation of the posterior longitudinal ligament. **B:** The middle layer of the internal craniocervical ligaments is the cruciate ligament. This important stabilizer of C1-2 anterior translation is composed of a horizontal component, the transverse ligament, and triangular vertical bands extending cranially to the basion and caudally to C-2. **C:** The anterior layer of the internal craniocervical ligaments is the odontoid ligaments. These are the rudimentary apical ligament and the essential alar ligaments. The alar ligaments extend from the lateral aspect of the dens tip to the medial aspect of the occipital condyles. A lower portion of the alar ligament attaches to the medial aspect of the atlas lateral masses.

men transversum from C-6 to C-2. In C-2 the artery loops, turning more lateral to ascend in the foramen transversarium of C-1, which lies more lateral. Along the cranial surface of the atlas, the arteries turn medial and cross on top of the atlas in a groove. At the lateral edge of the posterior occipitoatlantal membrane, the arteries perforate the dura and arachnoid and pass into foramen magnum. They then course ventrally on the medulla oblongata, and at the level of the pons, they join together to form the basilar artery.

BIOMECHANICS AND KINEMATICS

The occipital cervical articulation is highly specialized to allow wide range of motion and yet protect its important contents. It lacks inherent bony stability, having several strong ligamentous structures to maintain stability. To facilitate atlantoaxial rotation, the stabilizing ligaments extend from the occiput to the axis and are not joined to the atlas. The atlas thus acts simply as a bushing.

The range of motion of the occiput to C-1 and C1-2 articulation has been summarized by Panjabi (3). Head nodding is created by flexion-extension at occiput to C-1 and ranges 13 to 35 degrees. Flexion-extension at C1-2 is less, 5 to 20 degrees. Flexion at the occiput to C-1 is limited by impaction between the basion and dens tip and, similarly, extension between the occiput and atlantal posterior arch. Flexion occurring at occiput to C-1 results in tightening of the tectorial membrane at C1-2, which becomes a check rein for flexion at C1-2. The same mechanism limits extension at C1-2. Axial rotation at occiput to C-2 and C1-2 is limited by tightening of the contralateral alar ligaments. During this movement, the ipsilateral alar ligament relaxes. Lateral bending is more complex. During left lateral bending at both articulations, the upper portion of the contralateral alar ligament and the lower portion of ipsilateral alar tighten (2,4). Translational movement anteroposteriorly or vertically is less than 2 mm between the occiput and atlas. At C1-2, 2 to 3 mm of anterior translation and up to 3 mm of distraction can be observed.

MECHANISM OF INJURY

The high incidence of fatalities from injuries in the upper cervical spine attests to the importance of its integrity to life. Adams performed forensic evaluation of 155 persons killed in traffic accidents (5–7). Twelve died of occipitoatlantal dislocation with brainstem injury (5). In all cases, the alar ligaments and tectorial membranes were torn. He opined that the mechanism of injury was distraction with combinations of extension, rotation, and posterior translation. Fourteen deaths were attributable to atlantoaxial dislocations (6). Six of these victims had odontoid fractures and one an atlas fracture, all of whom had disruption of the atlantoaxial facet capsules. The mechanism of injury was thought to be head and neck impaction, as all patents had skull base fractures or other craniofacial injuries. In another 21 fatalities, a ligamentous injury to the craniocervical articulation without dislocation of the occipitoatlantal or atlantoaxial joints was observed (7). This has only rarely been reported. Alar ligament avulsion was present in 20 of 25. Eight had laceration of the tectorial membrane, and subaxial cervical trauma was seen in 10. Severe cranial trauma was seen in all patients in this group. These reports were similar to investigations by Alker, Bucholz, and Jonsson indicating that the craniocervical junction is injured by severe trauma, and concomitant head and neck injuries are common (8–10). The two main mechanisms of injury are distraction with avulsion of the alar ligaments and tectorial membranes and craniofacial impaction. These forensic studies confirm the *in vitro* biomechanical studies that demonstrate the importance of the alar ligaments, tectorial membrane, and transverse ligament to the stability of the upper cervical spine (11).

PATIENT ASSESSMENT

All patients with trauma are treated according to Advanced Trauma Life Support guidelines (12). Achieving and maintaining an airway may be difficult in patients with upper cervical trauma secondary to vertebral displacement, retropharyngeal hematoma, facial fractures, or respiratory depression from neurologic injury. In patients with potential upper cervical injuries, intubation, if required, should be performed with an assistant stabilizing the head and as little neck motion as possible. Accompanying craniofacial trauma may warrant tracheostomy. After the primary and secondary assessments, the entire spinal column is assessed. Patients who are awake usually complain of pain, stiffness, crepitation, or neurologic symptoms. Many injuries are purely ligamentous, however, and are not initially associated with significant pain. Obtunded patients are more difficult to evaluate and are largely assessed radiographically.

During the spinal assessment, the patient is log-rolled and the entire spine is inspected. The occiput, all cervical, thoracic, and lumbar spinous processes are palpated for tenderness, hematoma, or gaps. A detailed neurologic exam according to American Spinal Injury Association guidelines is performed and recorded in the medical record (13). In upper cervical injuries, detailed examination of the cranial nerves should be performed. As observed in forensic studies, neurologic injuries in the upper cervical spine are often associated with death. However, with improved on-the-scene care, including cardiopulmonary resuscitation and in-field intubation, more patients are surviving injury and requiring emergency treatment. Neurologic trauma may include various complete and incomplete cord injuries and even brainstem injury. Cranial nerve injuries, especially of VI, VII, IX, XI, and XII, occur with skull-base and occipitocervical trauma. Uncommon neurologic injuries are the cruciate paralysis of Bell and the Wallenberg syndrome (14).

Radiologic Assessment

Radiographic imaging of the upper cervical spine provides the most important screening procedure. Controversy exists as to whether all awake asymptomatic patients should have radiographs. Until evidence is conclusive, however, the author strongly recommends the three-view cervical series. Patients who were undergoing head computed tomography (CT) for closed-head injury or craniofacial trauma should have a cervical-screening CT. Blakemore has shown spiral CT to be more accurate and cost effective than plain radiography in these patients (15,16). Similarly, patients with abnormal or questionable findings on plain radiographs should also undergo CT.

Interpretation of plain radiographs of the upper cervical spine is difficult because of overlying osseous structures, the presence of various tubes, the obliquity of the occipitoatlantal articulation, and artifacts from even slight head rotations from malpositions. Injuries in the upper cervical spine are the most likely missed, especially occipitoatlantal dislocation and odontoid fracture. On the lateral view, the alignment of the occipitoatlantal should be accurately determined. Focal retropharyngeal swelling is common in upper cervical injury. The basion, located at the end of clivus, should lie above the dens tip. The continuity of the spinolaminar line between C-1 and C-3 should be assessed. The location of spinolaminar point of C-2 should lie within 2 mm of the line connecting C-1 and C-3. The anterior atlantodens interval should be measured and is less than 3 mm in adults and 5 mm in children.

Harris has studied radiologic parameters in normals and in patients with occipitoatlantal instability (17,18) (Fig. 3). He has described the Rule of 12: In 95% of normals, the dens tip is located within 12 mm of the basion. Also, the basion is located within 12 mm of a line drawn along the posterior cortical margin of the axis, termed the *posterior axial line*. Other parameters, such as the Powers ratio and Lee's X line, have been described but are less sensitive than the Harris Rule of 12 (18).

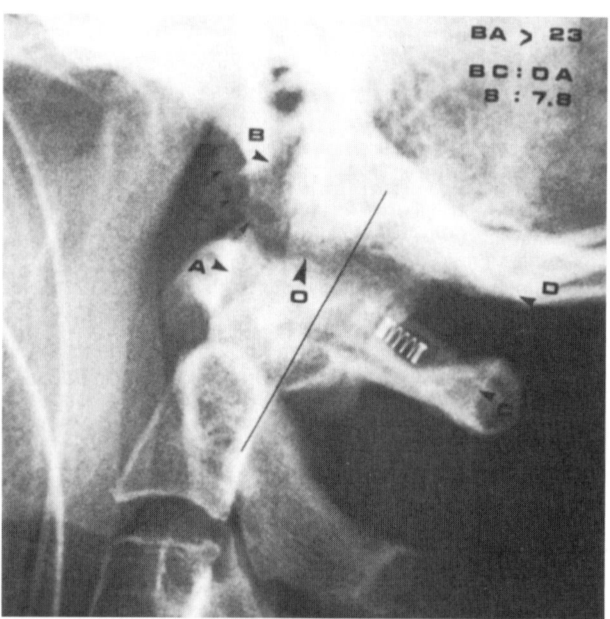

FIG. 3. This lateral cervical spine radiograph demonstrates an occipitocervical dissociation in this 22-year-old patient with respiratory-dependent quadriplegia. *A* identifies the anterior arch of the atlas, *B* the basion, *C* the posterior arch of the atlas, and *D* the opisthion. The tip of the odontoid is labeled *O.* Harris recommended extending a line along the posterior aspect of the axis body, the *posterior axial line.* The distance from the basion to the odontoid tip is the basion dens interval (BDI). The BDI should measure 12 mm or less. In this patient, the BDI was 13 mm. The basion axis interval (BAI) is the distance to the posterior axial line and should measure less than 12 mm. In this patient, the BAI measured 20 mm. Powers ratio is derived from a quotient of the distances of AD to BC and should be greater than 0.9. In this case the quotient was 0.94, despite the patient having an atlanto-occipital dissociation. The patient was treated with occipitocervical fusion and recovered independent ambulatory function 6 months postoperatively.

Anteroposterior visualization of the upper cervical spine requires an open-mouth view and patient cooperation (Fig. 1D). Rarely, congruency of the occipitoatlantal articulation can be seen. The dens waist and body should be inspected for fracture. The atlantal masses should be symmetric in size and in distance from the dens. Asymmetry usually reflects malposition, but may be secondary to ligamentous injury and rotational instability. Spreading of the atlantolateral masses over those of the corresponding axis is suggestive of C-1 ring fracture.

Computed Tomography

Fine-section CT, 1.25- to 2.50-mm slice thickness, with coronal and sagittal reconstruction, is ideally suited to evaluate the upper cervical spine. CT is indicated in patients with suspicious or actual injuries on plain radiographs and in patients with altered consciousness who are undergoing head CT. Analyzing the congruency of the articulation is of prime importance. In all positions, the occipital condyles align congruent to the concavities in the atlas lateral masses and should not be distracted by more than 2 mm (Fig. 1B). Malalignment of the atlantoaxial articulation is suggestive of inadequate patient positioning, rotary subluxation, or transverse ligament injury. Avulsion fractures of the alar ligament or transverse ligaments attachments indicate probable instability.

Magnetic Resonance Imaging

Magnetic resonance imaging (MRI) can be used to identify ligamentous disruptions, especially with T2-weighted or short inversion imaging recovery sequences (19). For logistical reasons, these techniques have rarely been helpful in the evaluation of trauma patients. MRI is useful to demonstrate spinal cord injury, epidural and retropharyngeal hematoma, and occult fracture.

Dynamic Imaging

Flexion-extension radiographs can result in spinal displacement and spinal cord injury, and therefore are not recommended in evaluation of patients with upper cervical spine trauma (20). Rarely, the stability requires immediate determination. In these cases, a supervised traction test or fluoroscopic flexion-extension examination can be performed (21–23).

FACTORS INFLUENCING TREATMENT

A variety of bony and ligamentous injuries occur in the upper cervical spine. Proper management requires identification, correct classification, early stabilization, and, finally, definitive treatment. Important factors that influence treatment are stability, the presence or absence of ligamentous integrity, neurologic function, associated injuries, and demographics, such as age.

Concept of Stability

Stability is a commonly used term but lacks validation and consensus. The author agrees with the definition proposed by White that stability indicates the spine can withstand physiologic loads without the potential for neurologic defects, progressive deformity, or long-term dysfunction from pain and disability. Stability is also temporal and should be considered in the following time frames: immediately, such as on the scene or in the emergency department; during mobilization a short time after injury; and after healing for 2 to 4 months. If at all times the fracture is unstable, such as with occipitocervical dislocation, then obviously surgical treatment is warranted.

Neurologic Injury

The presence of a neurologic injury is often devastating. High spinal cord injuries result in respiratory-dependent quadriplegia and require intubation and ventilation for survival. Cranial nerve injuries may impair gag reflexes and swallowing mechanisms, making aspiration and malnutrition a risk. All patients with cord injuries should have immediate reduction, respiratory support, maintenance of systolic blood pressure to greater than 90 mm Hg, and high-dose methylprednisolone according to the National Acute Spinal Cord Injury III protocol (24). In patients with cord injuries, nonoperative treatment with the halo vest reduces vital capacity by 30 to 40%, which may lead to prolonged ventilation (25). In general, most patients with significant neurologic injuries are treated by rigid internal fixation and bony fusion.

Bony versus Ligamentous Injury

Ligamentous injuries have a poor prognosis for healing in the upper cervical spine; therefore, most patients with documented injury to the important stabilizing ligaments, such as the tectorial membrane, alar ligaments, or transverse ligament, are candidates for surgery. Bony injuries, on the other hand, have an excellent capacity to heal, and most are treated nonoperatively. A notable exception is the type II odontoid fracture. Impingement from displaced fracture is rare in the upper cervical spine, as most bony injuries divide the spinal column and result in widening. Neurologic deficits, if present, are usually secondary to vertebral subluxation or vertebral artery injury.

Demographics

Age has an important influence on treatment and prognosis. Fractures in the elderly are often low energy secondary to a fall but are associated with a high incidence of morbidity and mortality, similar to that of hip fractures (26–28). Neurologic injuries in the age group are usually fatal; this should be discussed with the patient and family. However, children with respiratory-dependent quadriplegia can survive long term and sometimes return to school.

The upper cervical spine is a common site of spinal injury in children. This is thought to be secondary to the high head to trunk size ratio; immature articulations, especially at the occiput lending little or no bony stability; generalized ligamentous laxity; weak musculature; and concentration of force vectors at the craniocervical junction because of the small stature of children. Delays in diagnosis are often seen, with potential catastrophic consequences. Adult immobilization techniques are inadequate for children because of their large head size, which creates cervical hyperflexion when lying supine on a standard backboard (29).

Associated Injuries

Multisystem, skeletal, and other spinal injuries are frequent and attest to the high energy that most patients sustain when injuring the upper cervical spine. The ATLS guidelines for resuscitation, diagnosis, and stabilization should be followed (12). Most patients with multiple injuries and unstable upper cervical spines should have the neck immobilized by a halo vest or tong traction until the patients are medically stable for definitive treatment. In these cases, surgery is usually recommended to allow early mobilization and to avoid prolonged bed rest. Craniofacial trauma may preclude immobilization in cervicothoracic orthosis or placement of tongs or halo devices. Discussion with the maxillofacial team and neurologic surgeons is important to avoid iatrogenic complications.

TREATMENT OF SPECIFIC UPPER CERVICAL INJURIES

In this section, injuries are discussed from rostral to caudal, including occipital condyle fractures, occipitocervical dislocations, axis fractures, atlantoaxial ligamentous injury, odontoid fracture, traumatic spondylolisthesis of the axis, and C-2–body fractures.

Occipital Condyle Fractures

Occipital condyle fractures were once thought to be rare injuries, but they are increasingly being diagnosed due to the widespread use of CT to evaluate closed-head trauma and the craniocervical junction (30). Most injuries are stable unless associated with disruption of the alar ligament.

Mechanism of Injury

The mechanism of injury is direct cranial trauma or rapid head deceleration. Head trauma applied to the skull vertex, through the mandible or when the spinal column pushes up into a fixed head, has been shown to create basilar skull fractures, including the occipital condyles (31). These mechanisms are attested by the fact that the majority of patients present with closed-head injury and up to one-fourth have skull base fractures.

Diagnosis

Occipital condyle fractures are rarely seen on plain radiographs. Hanson reviewed 95 patients with 107 occipital condyle fractures and could retrospectively make the diagnosis in only one case (30). Soft-tissue retropharyngeal swelling was the only common suggestive finding. Similarly, using a cryoplane sectioning technique of the upper cervical spine in fatalities of road accidents, Jonsson identified nine fractures in 22 victims, all of whom had negative plain radiographs (10).

Fine-section CT with coronal and sagittal reconstruction is highly accurate. Continuing the CT to include at least C-4 is used routinely in patients undergoing CT for closed-head trauma. MRI was not found to be particularly useful by Hanson, although increased signal in the occipital condyle or in the articulation was often visualized (30). In assessing occipital condyle fractures, the status of the alar ligaments and tectorial membrane should be determined. Vertical displacement of the occipitoatlantal by 2 mm or atlantoaxial joint by 3 mm indicates ligamentous instability. Patients with occipital condyle fractures and anterior or posterior displacement have occipitocervical instability, which is discussed in a later section.

Clinical Symptoms

Patients, when awake, complain of suboccipital head or neck pain and may have limited motion. Midline tenderness may be lacking. A variety of neurologic syndromes have been repeated, including the cruciate palsy of Bell, Wallenberg syndrome, respiratory-dependent quadriplegia, and incomplete quadriplegia. Associated basilar skull fractures may lead to cranial nerve palsy including nerves IX, X, XI, and XII (32). On occasion, associated skull fractures may require cranial decompression. Injury to the vertebral artery has been reported with associated Wallenberg syndrome (33). Patients may present late with chronic suboccipital pain secondary to missed occipital condyle fracture and posttraumatic arthrosis (34).

Classification

The *Anderson classification* of occipital condyle fractures is based on fracture location, morphology, and presence of associated ligamentous instability (32) (Fig. 4).

Type I

Type I injuries are comminuted fractures secondary to axial loading mechanics. They are stable as long as the contralateral side is intact.

Type II

Type II injuries are occipital condyle associated with skull base fractures (Fig. 5). These can be unilateral or bilateral and have been reported to be associated with ring fractures through the basion. Most type II fractures are stable. However, if sufficient comminution is present or if the condyle is sheared off the occiput and displaced, they may be unstable.

Type III

Type III injuries are avulsion fractures secondary to tensile forces in the alar ligaments (Fig. 5). The stability of this injury is dependent on the displacement of the articulation between occiput and atlas, and the atlas and axis. Deliganis has also pointed out that stability should also be based on whether the injury is unilateral or bilateral (35). Three types of bilateral injuries were observed: bilateral occipital condyle fractures, unilateral occipital condyle fracture with contralateral widening of the occipitoatlantal joint, and unilateral occipital condyle fractures with the contralateral widening of the atlantoaxial joint. Unilat-

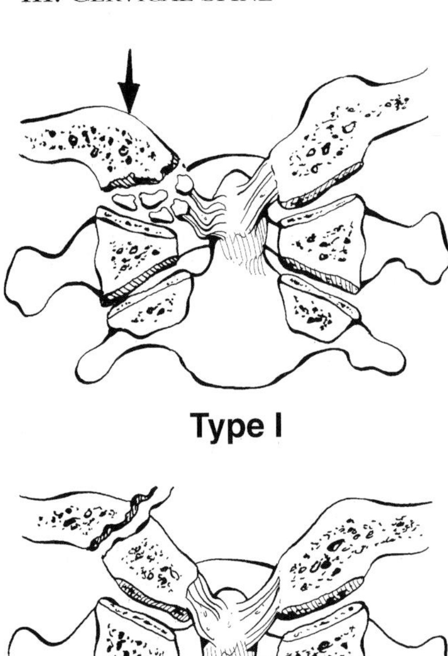

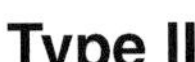

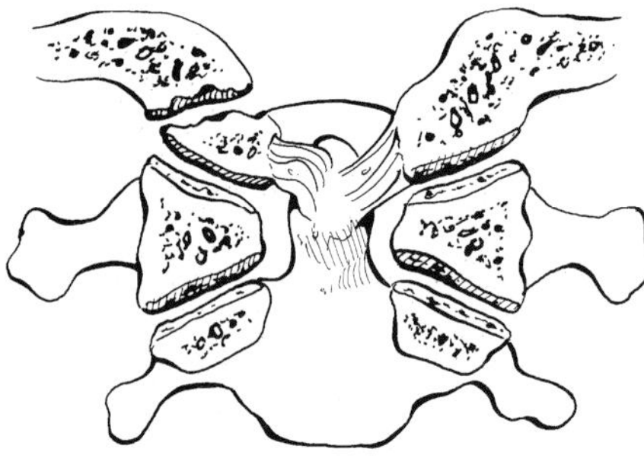

FIG. 4. Anderson and Montesano classification of occipital condyle fractures. Type I is an impaction fracture. Type II is a fracture of the occipital condyle involving the skull base. Type III is an avulsion fracture. This type III injury may represent occipitocervical instability.

eral injuries proved to be stable and were successfully treated nonoperatively in 80% of cases, whereas 67% of bilateral cases had occipitocervical fusion.

Initial Treatment

The emergent treatment of occipital condyle fractures is immobilization in an extraction collar. Associated cranial nerve injuries may require airway, nutritional, and otorhinolaryngologic support. The initial treatment of occipital condyle fractures with occipitoatlantal instability is discussed in a later section.

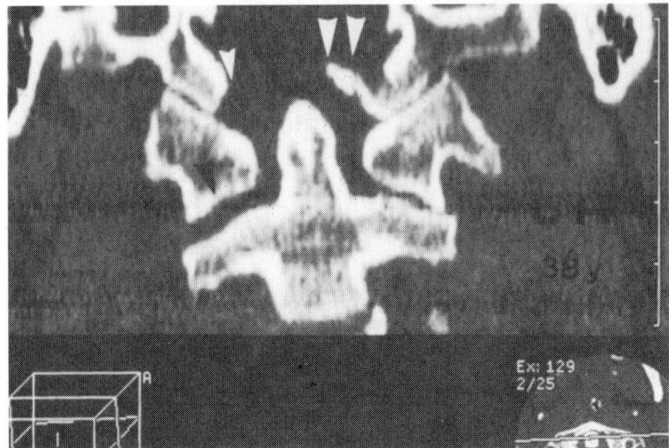

FIG. 5. The computed tomography coronal reformation of the upper cervical spine reveals a type III occipital condyle fracture on the patient's left side (*large arrows*), and a type II avulsion injury on the right side (*small arrow*). The patient was successfully treated in a halo vest.

Definitive Treatment

Type I and stable type II fractures are treated in a soft collar or cervicothoracic brace for 6 to 8 weeks. Unstable type II injuries in which there is collapse creating torticollis or condylar displacement may require traction, halo vest, or occipitocervical fusion.

Unilateral type III and nondisplaced type III injuries are treated by a cervicothoracic brace. Unstable type III injuries are treated similarly to occipitocervical instabilities by occipitocervical fusion using rigid internal fixation.

Occipitoatlantal Dislocation

Occipitoatlantal dislocations are usually the result of violent trauma. There is a higher incidence in the pediatric population. Until recently, survivors of these injures were rare and the diagnosis often delayed with adverse consequences. Attention to airway and proper ventilation at the accident scene is allowing patients to survive until arrival at the emergency department. Improved understanding of the pathoanatomy, biomechanics, and imaging has led to early diagnosis and more effective treatment that prevents further neurologic deterioration.

Mechanism of Injury

Occipitoatlantal instability is caused by the loss of ligamentous integrity of the alar ligaments, their bony attachments, and the tectorial membrane. The most common mechanism is rapid deceleration-acceleration, often from vehicular trauma. Pediatric pedestrians struck by vehicles or children crushed by deployment of airbags are being increasingly reported. Concomitant craniofacial trauma mechanisms are seen, especially in forensic studies. Imaizumi analyzed 11 fatalities with occipitoatlantal dislocations (36). Nine had vertebral artery injury, four had associated basilar skull fractures, four had atlantoaxial dislocation, and all had other facial trauma (36).

Diagnosis

All trauma patients require careful assessment of the craniocervical junction to determine the integrity of craniocervical ligaments and the alignment of the upper cervical articulation. Findings that suggest craniocervical injury are retropharyngeal soft-tissue swelling, displacement to the basion from the dens tip, increased space between the occiput and cervical spine, and increased atlantodens interval. The Harris Rule of 12, as described previously, is abnormal in 95% of patients with occipitocervical instability (18) (Fig. 6). Occipital condyle fracture is present in 30 to 50% of cases. Definitive diagnosis is made from CT with reformations. Alignment is best assessed on sagittal reconstruction in the plane of the articulations. The occiput-atlantal joint should be congruent and have no greater than 2 mm distraction. In 30% of cases, a unilateral occipitoatlantal injury is present with contralateral distraction injury of atlanto-axial articulation (37). Increased atlantodens interval from transverse ligament injury is seen in 30 to 50% of cases (37).

Clinical Symptoms

Patients are often obtunded from head trauma, and the diagnosis is made radiographically. Patient symptoms are similar to those of occipital condyle fractures. Cases with bilateral dislocations

A,B

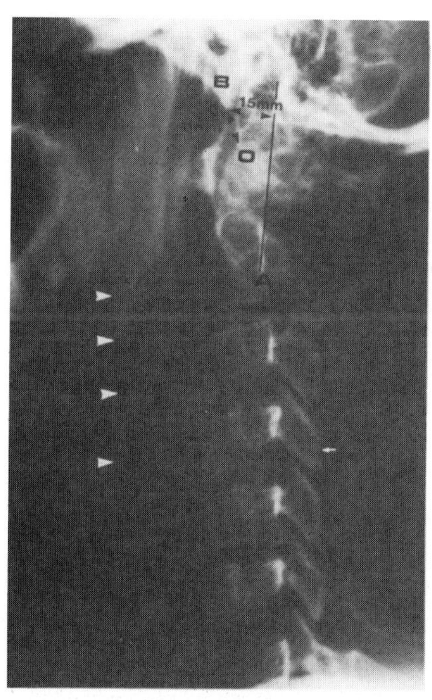

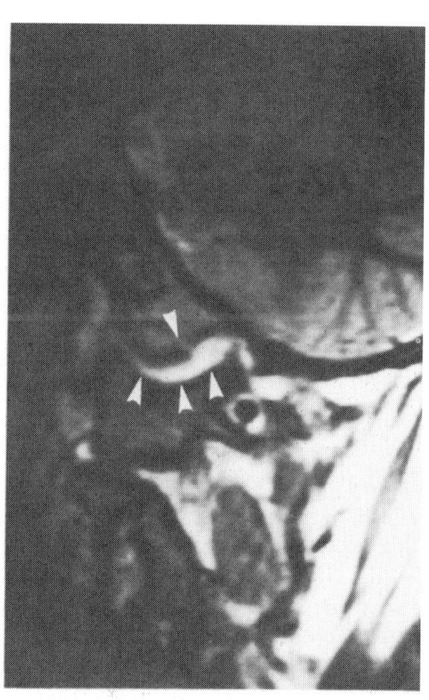

C,D

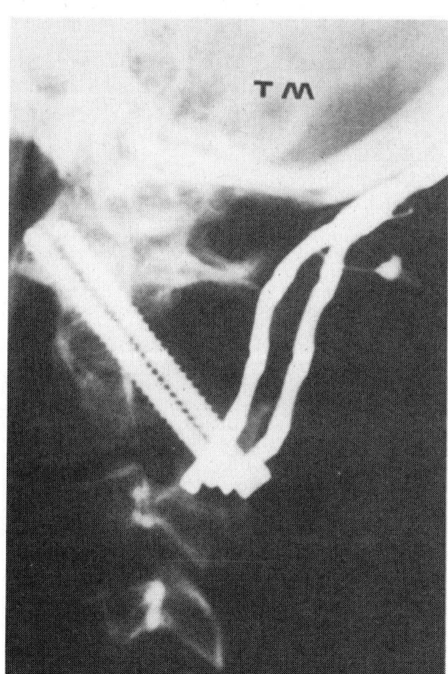

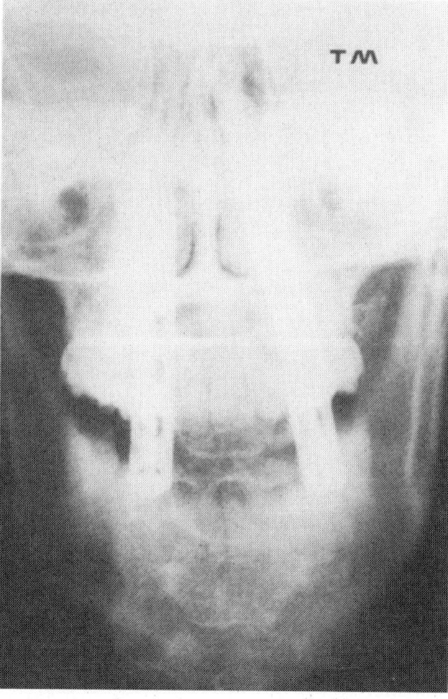

FIG. 6. A: Lateral cervical spine radiograph of a neurologically intact 22-year-old woman involved in a high-speed motor vehicle accident demonstrates prevertebral soft-tissue swelling (*arrows*) and anterior subluxation of the occipital condyles on the lateral masses of the atlas. The basion dens interval measures 11 mm, and the basion axis interval (*B–O*) measures 15 mm. **B:** Increased signal intensity of the occipitocervical and atlantoaxial joints on T2-weighted magnetic resonance imaging correlates with severe ligamentous injuries of the cervicocranial junction. Arrows point to anterior and vertical subluxation of the occipital condyles on the atlas. **C:** The lateral flexion C-spine radiograph taken 3 months postoperatively demonstrates solid occipitocervical fusion achieved with titanium reconstruction plates and atlantoaxial transarticular screw fixation with corticocancellous iliac crest bone graft. The patient remained neurologically normal and is pain free. **D:** Anteroposterior radiograph demonstrates occipitocervical plating.

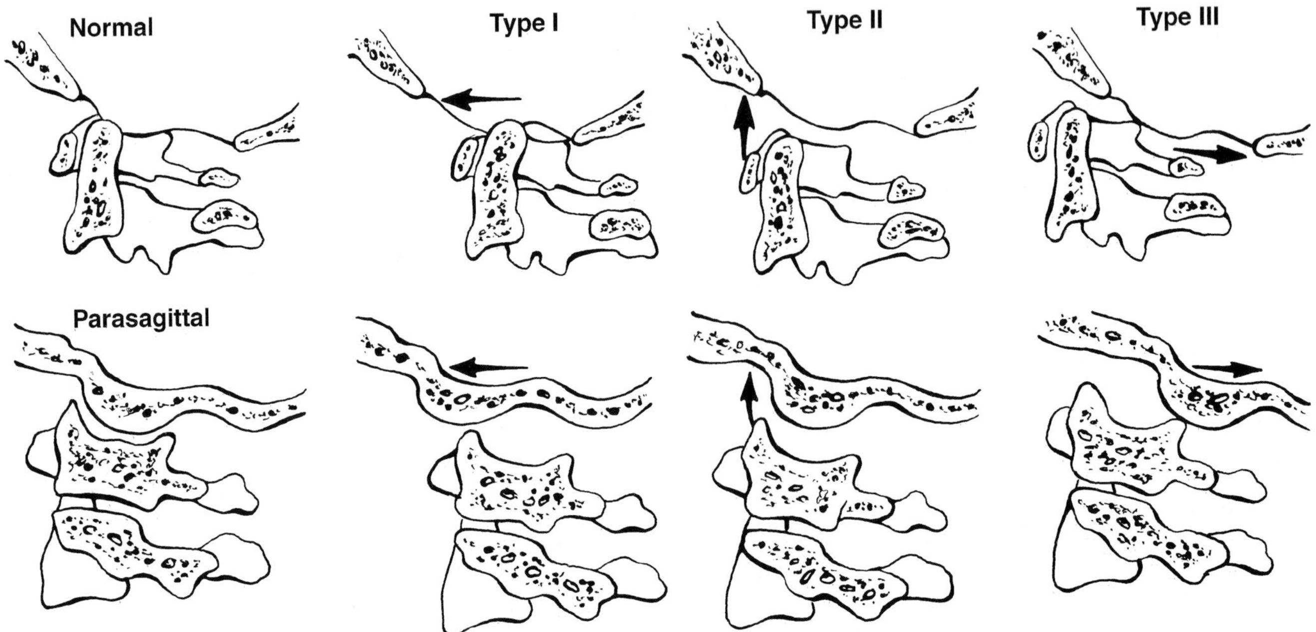

FIG. 7. Classification of occipitocervical instabilities. Normal. Type I—anterior. Type II—vertical. Type III—posterior. (Modified from Traynelis VC, Marano GD, Dunker RO, et al. Traumatic atlanto-occipital dislocation. Case report. *J Neurosurg* 1986;65:863–870.)

or significant distraction are associated with respiratory dependent brainstem injury, cerebral anoxia, and early death.

Classification

Occipitoatlantal dislocation has been classified according to the direction of subluxation, although this is largely dependent on position technique and does little to direct treatment. Traynelis described anterior, posterior, and vertical injuries (38) (Fig. 7). Anderson added vertical distraction injuries at C1-2 as a form of occipitoatlantal dislocation because the primary stabilizer, the alar ligaments, and tectorial membrane span from occiput to C-2 (37). Other considerations of stability are whether injuries are unilateral or bilateral and the severity of ligamentous injury. Similar to knee ligament injuries, there can be a sprain with some residual integrity or complete rupture without any stabilizing properties and a poor prognosis. Injuries that are purely unilateral associated with minimal displacement are generally stable and have a better prognosis.

Initial Treatment

Early diagnosis and immediate treatment are essential to avoid neurologic deterioration or even death. Respiratory compromise must be treated by intubation and ventilation. Intubation may be difficult secondary to retropharyngeal hematoma, fracture displacement, or facial fracture and may require tracheostomy. Initially, the patient should be immobilized by sandbags or tape across the forehead. Traction is contraindicated in occipitoatlantal dislocation. The author therefore recommends placement of the halo vest and reduction as soon as possible. Reduction is achieved by careful positioning of the head relative to thorax. In cases of distraction injuries, use of gravity by having the patient sit partially upright may aid reduction.

Definitive Treatment

The treatment of occipitoatlantal instability is based on the severity of ligamentous injury. Unilateral or bilateral injuries with little initial displacement, especially in children, may have treatment attempted by the halo vest. Careful follow-up is warranted to monitor alignment.

Patients with bilateral subluxation or any dislocation should have posterior occipito–C-2 fusion with rigid internal fixation (Fig. 6). The aggressive approach is warranted to avoid catastrophic loss of reduction and spinal cord injury. Currently, the author recommends a plate and screw or rod-screw construct with autogenous iliac bone graft.

Atlas Fracture

Traumatic injuries to the atlas are common and are associated with other spine fractures in 10 to 20% of cases. The C-1 ring is wide, which accounts for low incidence of neurologic complications. In general, these are relatively benign with satisfactory outcome, although loss of rotation is to be expected.

Mechanism of Injury

Several biomechanical studies to determine the mechanism of atlas fractures have been performed. Teo used a finite element model and found that significant local stress occurred in the anterior and posterior arches during compression loading (39). The

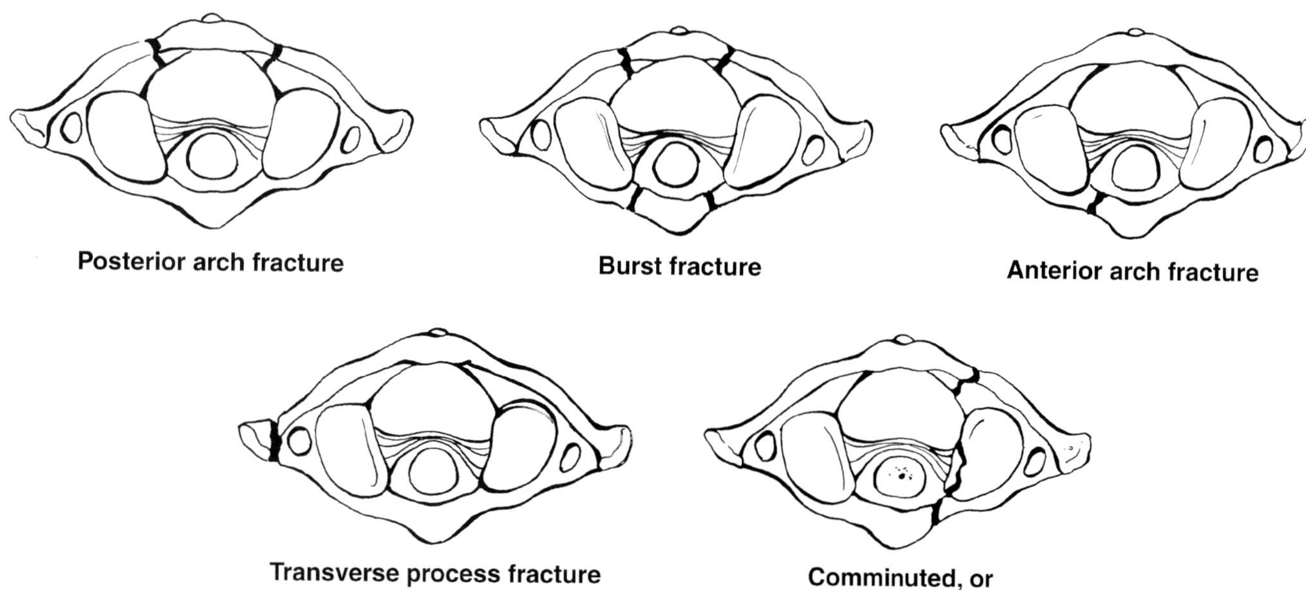

FIG. 8. C-1 ring injuries. (Redrawn from Bronwer, Jupiter, Levine, et al., eds. *Skeletal trauma, fractures, dislocations, ligamentous injuries.* Philadelphia: WB Saunders, 1992.)

groove in the posterior arch for the vertebral artery was subjected to large bending moments, accounting for their high fracture incidence. Panjabi performed compression failure tests and found that atlas fracture occurred at 3,050 N in the neutral position and only 2,000 N when the neck was extended (40). Beckner applied tensile forces to the atlas and measured that only 1.6 mm of radial displacement occurred before failure (41). Thus, biomechanical studies confirm that atlas fractures are likely from axial loading and extension forces.

After the atlas fracture, outward spreading of the lateral masses is resisted by the transverse ligament. Continued loads of up to 2,000 N can result in ligamentous injury. Spence found that this occurred with an average of 6.9 mm of offset of C-1 on C-2 (42). In experimental studies, transverse ligament ruptures occur in midsubstance and from bony avulsion off the medial aspect of the lateral mass. This is similar to clinical observations (40,43).

Diagnosis

Atlas fractures are usually easily visualized on lateral and open-mouth radiographs. Anterior arch fractures are associated with retropharyngeal swelling. Posterior arch fractures must be differentiated from congenital defects. On the open-mouth radiographs, the C-1 lateral masses should lie symmetrically over those of C-2. If they extend wider, a Jefferson-type fracture is present. Rarely, an anterior or posterior atlantoaxial facet dislocation is present. CT is indicated to determine the extent of bony and ligamentous injury. Avulsion fractures of the transverse ligament indicate C1-2 instability. MRI may show disruption of the transverse and alar ligaments (44).

Clinical Symptoms

Patients with atlas fracture complain of suboccipital pain and have local tenderness. Neurologic manifestations are rare other than C-1 or C-2 radiculopathy. A careful assessment of the entire spinal column is required, as other fractures are common.

Classification

Atlas fractures are classified according to location of the fracture and to the integrity of the transverse and alar ligaments (Fig. 8) (45).

Anterior Arch Fracture

Anterior arch fractures can be vertical or transverse secondary to avulsion from the longus colli muscle. Isolated bilateral arch fractures are potentially unstable when associated with potential posterior atlantoaxial dislocation. This has been called the *plow fracture*, in which the dens is forced through the atlantoanterior arch, resulting in the posterior dislocation (46). This rare injury is unstable and often associated with spinal cord injury.

Lateral Mass Fracture

Isolated lateral mass fractures are rare. When the lateral aspect of the ring is intact, they are stable. Rarely, the entire lateral mass is comminuted or separated from the C-1 ring. These are essentially variants of the Jefferson fracture. Transverse process fractures are stable, although they have the potential for vertebral artery injury.

Posterior Arch Fracture

Posterior arch fractures are common and may be confused with incomplete ossification. Cervical CT is required, as many posterior arch fractures are associated with other C-1 or cervical injuries.

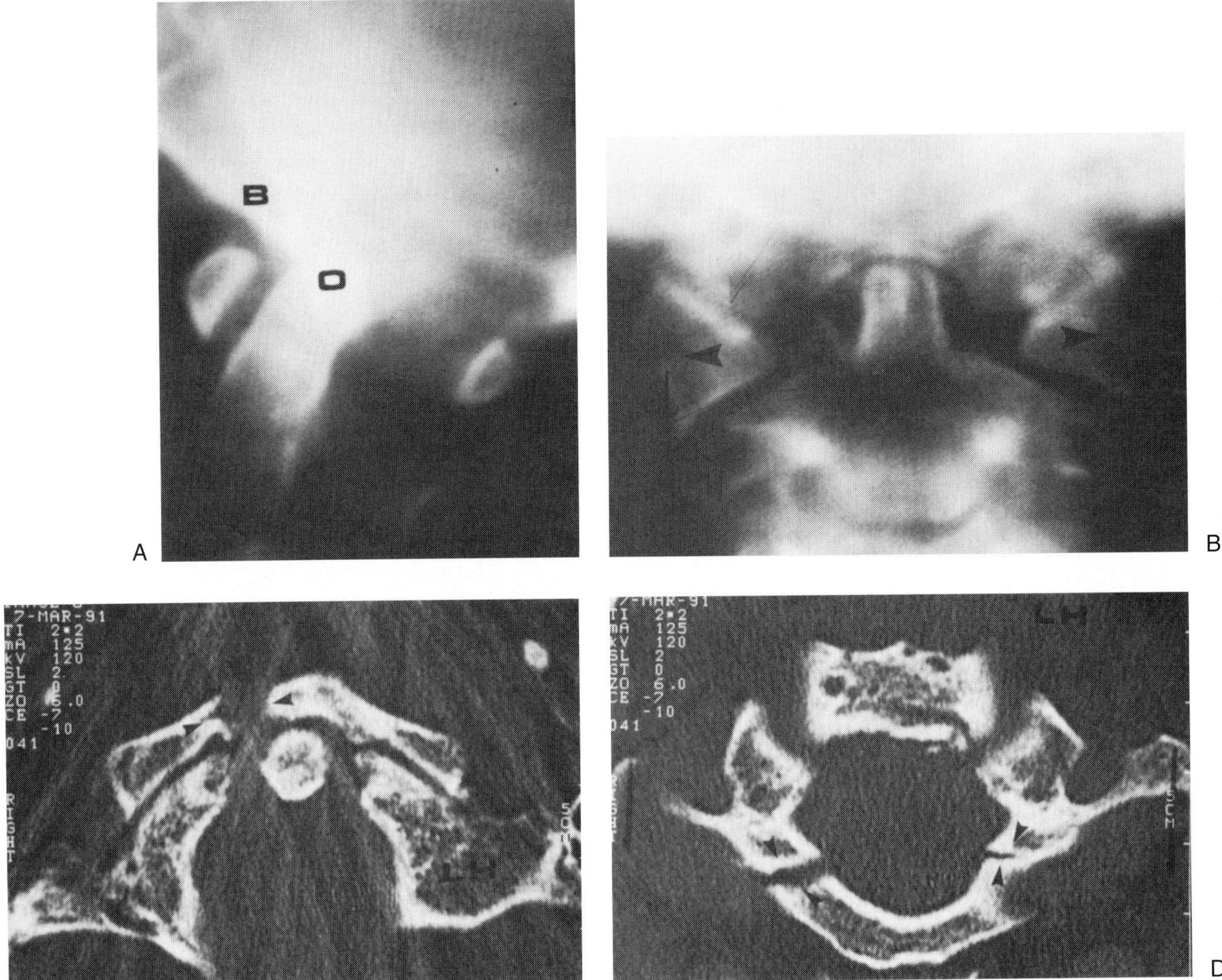

FIG. 9. A: Lateral tomography demonstrates cranial migration of the dens (O) to the foramen magnum (B) due to the unstable burst injury of the atlas and resultant loss of height of the C-1 ring. An increased atlantodens interval of 5 mm is present. After reduction with cranial traction, this 42-year-old patient was successfully treated with a halo vest. **B:** The open-mouth odontoid view demonstrates overhang of 6 mm on the left C-1 lateral mass over the C-2 lateral mass and 8 mm on the right. Arrowheads indicate lateral displacement of the C-1 lateral masses. A combined lateral mass overhang of more than 6.9 mm is suspicious for an unstable axis fracture with transverse ligament disruption. **C:** Axial computed tomography (CT) demonstrates a displaced three-part atlas fracture with avulsion of the transverse ligament. The anterior arch fracture is seen on this CT scan (*arrows*). **D:** The posterior arch fractures are visualized on this CT scan (*arrows*).

Bursting-Type Fracture

The Jefferson fracture is a bursting-type fracture and has a variable pattern. These can consist of two-, three-, or four-part fractures. Displacement occurs radially, thus increasing the spinal canal diameter. Displacement of the lateral masses has the most significant consequences (Fig. 9). As they separate, subluxation of the occipitoatlantal and atlantoaxial articulations occurs. Combined lateral mass displacement relative to C-2 of 6.9 mm indicates disruption of the transverse ligament and potential for C1-2 instability (42). In greater than 50% of cases, an avulsion fracture of the transverse ligament from C-1 is present (43). Jefferson fractures with intact transverse ligaments are stable, whereas those with greater than 6.9 mm displacement are unstable.

Initial Treatment

Patients with unstable atlas fracture are initially treated with cranial tong traction. These include most Jefferson-type fractures, the anterior plow fracture, and unstable lateral mass fracture. Increasing traction weight may be required to reduce the bursting-type fractures. This is best monitored on open-mouth axial views. Other stable fracture types are initially maintained in extraction collars.

Definitive Treatment

Stable atlas fractures including the anterior arch, lateral mass, and posterior arch are treated by a cervical orthosis for 6 to 8 weeks. Few outcome reports are available, although long-term symptoms or disability is not to be expected. The patient should be informed that a loss of range of motion is likely if the fracture involves the articular surfaces.

The anterior plow fracture is treated by reduction and immobilization in a halo vest. In patients with significant neurologic injuries or with multiple injuries, C1-2 fusion may be warranted. The Magerl technique would be most appropriate for these injuries.

The management of the Jefferson fracture is controversial. The stable type with intact transverse ligament is most commonly treated by immobilization in the halo vest for 10 to 12 weeks. Alternatively, patients may be immobilized in a cervicothoracic brace. Lee documented satisfactory outcome in 12 patients with stable Jefferson fracture treated in a cervicothoracic brace (47). Results comparing these methods are lacking.

Unstable Jefferson fractures have the potential for increasing outward displacement of the lateral masses during healing, nonunion, and late C1-2 instability. Outcomes, although retrospective, confirm the relative benign course of these fractures (45,48). The author recommends halo vest management for 10 to 12 weeks for the patient with unstable Jefferson fracture. During healing, displacement of the lateral masses should be assessed on open-mouth radiographs. Traction or even surgery may be warranted if alignment cannot be maintained.

After 12 weeks, patients should have a flexion-extension radiograph to determine if C1-2 instability is present from failure of healing of the transverse ligament injury. Rarely, greater than 3.5 mm of translation occurs, necessitating a posterior C1-2 fusion.

Largely to avoid halo vest immobilization and to maintain anatomic alignment, more aggressive surgical approaches have been proposed. None of these approaches has been systematically studied or compared to the outcomes of halo treatment. McGuire achieved successful healing using a posterior C1-2 arthrodesis with the Magerl C1-2 translational screw (49). This technique could be indicated for patients who fail the halo vest, who are multiply injured, or are elderly. In Europe, several other strategies have been implemented. Ruf recommended anterior osteosynthesis with screw placed transorally into C-1 lateral masses connected by a wire or a custom rod system (50). Another technique is to perform a similar C-1 osteosynthesis from a posterior approach or even combined anterior and posterior instrumentation (51). These aggressive and potential highly morbid techniques require validation that significant patient benefit occurs before they should be used.

Atlantoaxial Instability

Atlantoaxial instability is defined as nonphysiologic motion between C-1 and C-2. Instability at the atlantoaxial articulation can occur from injury to the transverse and alar ligaments, the odontoid process, the anterior arch, or lateral masses of the atlas. The most commonly discussed form of atlantoaxial instability is anterior subluxation secondary to rupture of transverse ligament. Other directions of instability should be considered including vertical, posterior, lateral, and rotation. Descriptions of a comprehensive system are lacking. In this section, the concept of atlantoaxial dislocation is reviewed. Many instabilities are associated with other upper cervical injuries and are reviewed separately.

Mechanism

The intricate arrangement of the anterior arch of C-1, the odontoid process, and the transverse and alar ligaments maintains atlantoaxial stability and provides up to 90-degree rotational movement. Instability can be associated with injury to any of these structures. After odontoid fracture, displacement can occur in any direction, especially anterior or posterior. Other causes of anterior instability are transverse ligament rupture. Fielding found that the transverse ligaments failed at an 84-kilopond force when applied by an anterior-directed force (52). Increasing displacement was prevented by alar ligaments. Another mechanism of injury is by downward forces onto the atlantolateral masses of the occipital condyles, as described in Bursting-Type Fracture. Spence determined that an average 6.9 mm of anterior displacement occurred after rupture of the transverse ligament (42). In severe cases, there is associated alar ligamentous rupture with associated occipitocervical instability. This occurs in 30 to 50% of cases initially recognized as transverse ligament rupture (37). Rotational instability theoretically indicates injury to at least one of the alar ligaments, although this also occurs in children from upper respiratory infections, so-called Grisel's syndrome. A very rare injury is posterior dislocation in which the anterior arch lies posterior to the dens (53). This injury is associated with rupture of the alar and apical ligaments and is caused presumably by an upward or distractive force.

Diagnosis

Plain radiographic findings of atlantoaxial instability include increased anterior atlantodens interval, a change in the spinolaminar line between C-1 and C-2 and C-3, widening between C1-2 lamina, and a change in the parallel contours between the dens and anterior arch (Fig. 10). On the anteroposterior open-mouth view, rotational instabilities are characterized by loss of symmetry in size and shape of the atlantal lateral masses, ipsilateral loss of joint space, and a difference greater than 2 mm of the distance between the dens and lateral masses. However, small amounts of head rotation during positioning can complicate assessment. The diagnosis is best confirmed with CT and reconstructions. The alignment of the atlantoaxial articulation should be symmetric. Fractures of the C-1 ring and avulsion fracture of the transverse ligament are notable. T2-weighted or short inversion imaging recovery MRI may be helpful in identifying ligamentous disruption, occult bony injury, and hemorrhage (44). Clinically, MRI has been logistically difficult and not as useful. Dynamic radiographs may be required to identify atlantoaxial instability. Flexion-extension view can show an increase in the atlantodens interval, confirming transverse ligament injury. With isolated alar ligament rupture, the displacement between the dens and lateral atlantal mass may be different on open-mouth right and left bending. More practical is dynamic CT, performed in neutral, right, and left rotation. Dvorak used this technique and measured the relative rotation between C-1 and C-2 in these positions (54,55). He found that alar ligament transection increased rotation to the opposite side at occiput to C-1 and C1-2.

Classification

The classification of atlantoaxial instability is based on direction and consideration of the osseous and ligamentous struc-

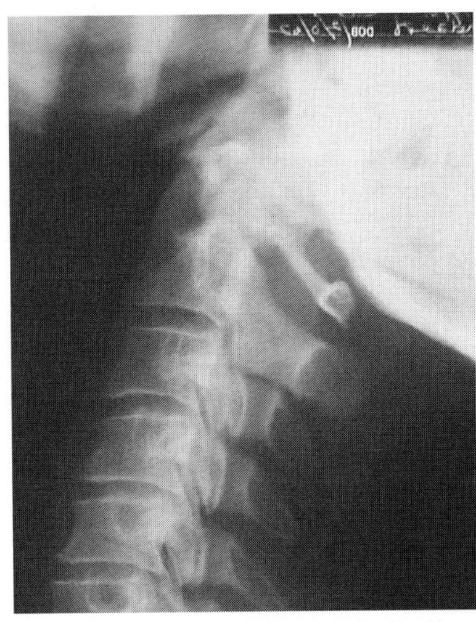

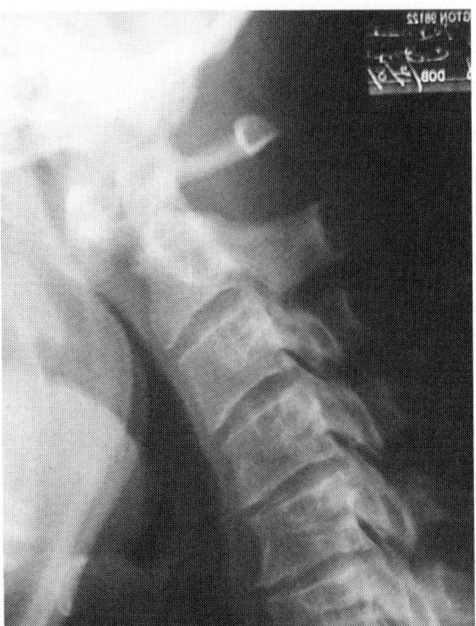

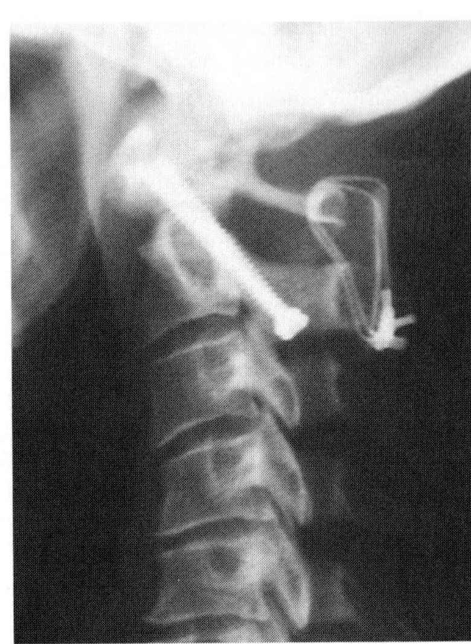

A–C

FIG. 10. A: Extension lateral radiograph of a 35-year-old nurse involved in a motor vehicle accident. She complained of neck pain, but the radiograph was interpreted as normal. Her husband was treated for traumatic spondylolisthesis of the axis with a halo vest. **B:** Flexion radiograph 9 months after injury. An increased anteroatlantodens interval is seen, indicating traumatic rupture of the transverse ligament. She continued to complain of disabling suboccipital pain without neurologic deficit. **C:** Postoperative lateral radiograph after C1-2 transarticular fixation combined with Brooks fusion performed with polyethylene cable and autogenous iliac graft. Her symptoms completely resolved.

tures injured (Table 1). Most, if not all, injuries are unstable, resulting in the potential for displacement between C-1 and C-2. Each direction of displacement may be caused by a purely ligamentous injury, a bony injury, or combination. In particular, odontoid fractures may be associated with atlantoaxial instability in any direction. Associated injuries to the occipitoatlantal region occur frequently because of the interrelationship of all ligaments.

Anterior

Anterior instability can be caused by odontoid fracture with anterior dislocation, transverse ligament injury, transverse ligament combined with alar ligament injury, and unstable Jefferson fracture.

Posterior

Posterior atlantoaxial instability is usually secondary to odontoid fracture with posterior displacement. Rare causes are anterior arch fracture with posterior dislocation, the so-called plow fracture, and posterior dislocation of the anterior arch of C-1 behind the dens. This has been described by Fielding as type IV rotatory instability (53).

Lateral

Lateral instability results from an incompetent odontoid process, especially os odontoideum, alar ligament injury, and from fracturing of the lateral masses of C-1 or C-2.

Vertical

Vertical instability is present when there is greater than 3 mm of distraction between the atlas and axis. This indicates rupture of the alar ligament and tectorial membrane and, therefore, a form

TABLE 1. *Atlantoaxial instability*

Anterior
Transverse ligament rupture
Odontoid fracture
Associated occipitocervical instability (alar ligament rupture)
Unstable Jefferson fracture
Posterior
Odontoid fracture
Posterior dislocation (type IV Fielding)
Lateral
Fracture lateral mass C-1
Fracture lateral mass C-2
Unilateral alar ligament rupture
Rotatory
Facet subluxation (Fielding I)
Transverse ligament rupture (3–5 mm displacement) (Fielding II)
Transverse and alar ligament rupture (>5 mm displacement) (Fielding III)
Vertical
Alar ligament and tectorial membrane rupture

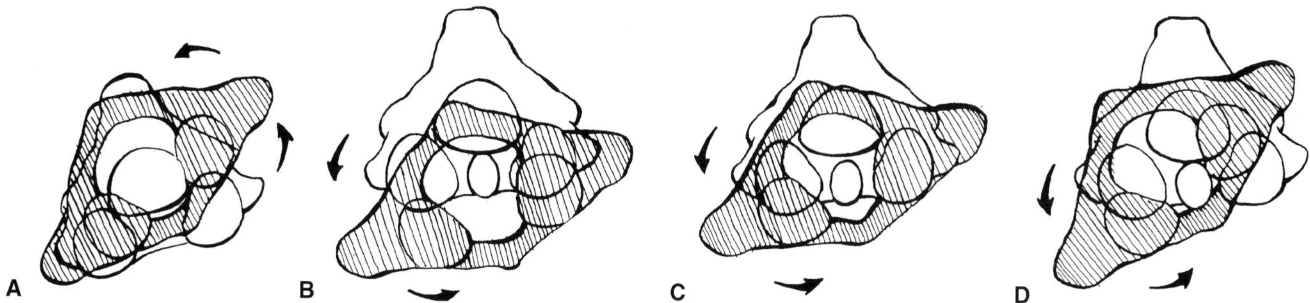

FIG. 11. Fielding classification of rotary subluxation. **A:** Type I: Rotation about the dens without anterior translation. **B:** Type II: Rotation about one lateral mass with anterior translation of 3 to 5 mm. **C:** Type III: Rotation about one lateral mass with anterior translation greater than 5 mm. **D:** Type IV: Posterior displacement of C-1 on C-2. (Redrawn from Bronwer BD, Jupiter JB, Levine AM, et al, eds. *Skeletal trauma, fractures, dislocations, ligamentous injuries.* Philadelphia: WB Saunders, 1992.)

of occipitocervical instability. It is often observed that displacement occurs at C1-2 on one side and between the occiput to C-1 on the contralateral side.

Rotation

Rotatory instability has been classified by Fielding (53) (Fig. 11). Type I is a forward subluxation on one side and posterior subluxation contralaterally. The transverse ligament is theoretically intact, as there is no increase in the atlantodens interval.

Type II is anterior subluxation on one side, pivoting on the contralateral joint. There is an increased atlantodens interval up to 5 mm, indicating injury to the transverse ligament.

Type III is anterior subluxation of both articulations, one greater than the other, and an increased atlantodens interval greater than 5 mm. This injury represents transverse and alar ligament injury.

Type IV is the rare and usually fatal injury of posterior dislocation of the C-1 arch behind the dens.

Initial Treatment

Atlantoaxial fractures are inherently unstable and are initially placed in traction with light amounts of weight. Overdistraction is likely if there is alar ligament injury. Reduction can be achieved by careful head positioning or application of weight. Alternatively, patients can be placed in the halo vest until a decision can be made regarding definitive treatment.

Definitive Treatment

Treatment depends on the osseous and ligamentous injuries. Displaced odontoid fractures are treated as described later. Anterior, lateral, and rotatory subluxation with transverse ligament injury are treated by C1-2 fusion using internal fixation. This aggressive approach is mandated because transverse ligamentous injury has a poor prognosis for healing except when associated with avulsion fractures. Dickman reported that all transverse ligament injuries with avulsion fracture healed without surgery (43).

Vertical instability is simply a variant of occipitocervical instability and is treated by occipitocervical fusion.

Type I rotatory instabilities may be stable and are frequently not associated with trauma. Closed reduction using sedation and head halter or cranial tong traction often results in reduction. Patients are then immobilized in a collar for 4 to 6 weeks. Reoccurrences are usually associated with transverse ligament incompetence and may require posterior C1-2 fusion.

Type II and III injuries are unstable and have a poor prognosis. Posterior C1-2 fusion with internal fixation is recommended.

Odontoid Fracture

Odontoid fractures are common injuries occurring in 8 to 10% of all cervical traumas. Although thought to be relatively benign, 10% of cases are associated with spinal cord injury. In the elderly, this combination is often fatal. Associated cervical trauma is present in 10 to 20% of cases, especially posterior arch fractures of C-1. A well-established classification system accurately predicts prognosis and directs treatment (56).

Mechanism of Injury

Odontoid fractures occur in a bimodal age distribution from corresponding high- and low-energy mechanisms. In younger patients, fractures are caused by forces of rapid acceleration-deceleration or from blows to the cranium or face (Fig. 12). In the elderly, most occur secondary to falls (28). The biomechanical cause of odontoid fractures has been studied (57–59). Anterior and posterior shear forces have been shown to result in odontoid fractures in *in vitro* models. In anterior shear, forces are applied in an anterior direction creating tensioning of the transverse ligament and shearing of the odontoid. This is confirmed clinically, as 10% of patients with odontoid fractures have associated transverse ligament injuries (60). In posterior shear, the opposite occurs with odontoid loading occurring through the anterior arch of C-1. In the elderly, thoracic kyphosis pushes the head forward, which becomes prominent to receive injury during falls. This creates posterior shear forces and odontoid fractures. With sufficient posterior displacement, spinal cord injury can occur. Rotational forces applied by the

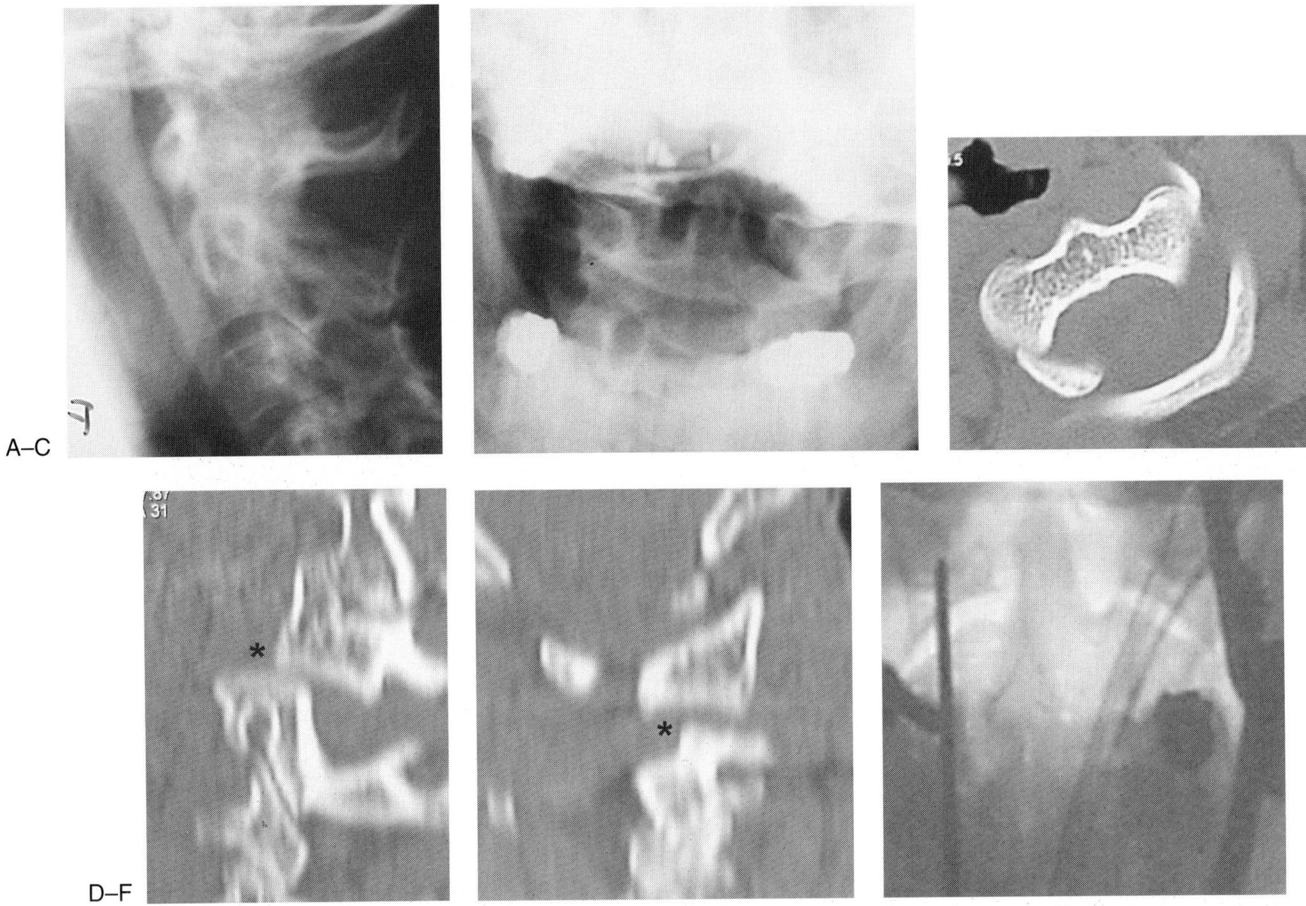

FIG. 12. **A:** A 37-year-old man was struck from behind with a 100-lb box. He complained of occipital pain and torticollis for the next 22 months. He had the typical cock-robin head position of rotary subluxation of C1-2, with the head rotated to the left and tilted to the right. Lateral radiograph is unremarkable. **B:** Open-mouth radiograph shows absence of the right C1-2 joint space, decreased width of the C-1 lateral mass, and increased distance between the dens and right C-1 lateral mass. **C:** On the axial CT, there is a C1-2 facet subluxation anteriorly on the right and posteriorly on the left. **D:** Posterior subluxation of left C1-2 facet (*star*). **E**: Sagittal reformation of right C1-2 facet showing probably physiologic anterior subluxation (*star*). He was treated by posterior C1-2 fusion with the transarticular technique. **F:** Intraoperative open-mouth showing restoration of symmetric lateral masses and joint space. The right guide pin for the transarticular screw is in the proper position.

alar ligaments may be more important in producing fracture than clinically suspected.

Diagnosis

Odontoid fractures are one of the most commonly missed spinal fractures. In retrospect, the fracture lines or other signs, such as retropharyngeal swelling, are present. However, nondisplaced fractures may not be apparent initially. The lateral and open-mouth views should be critically evaluated for odontoid fractures. If the open-mouth view is obscured, then CT should be considered. Harris has described a confluence of bony shadows that create a ring at the base of the odontoid (61). Discontinuity of this ring is indicative of an odontoid fracture. Fine-section CT with reformations is highly accurate, despite worries that transverse fractures may be missed. In patients with fractures on plain radiograph, CT should be obtained to evaluate the entire cervical spine, looking for concomitant injuries.

Clinical Symptoms

In awake patients, odontoid fracture is associated with upper cervical pain. However, nondisplaced fractures may be relatively painless. Painful head rotation and swallowing difficulties from retropharyngeal hematoma may be present. Spinal cord injury occurs in 10% of cases, especially in the elderly.

Classification

The Anderson and d'Alonzo classification is widely accepted and is predictive of prognosis (56) (Fig. 13).

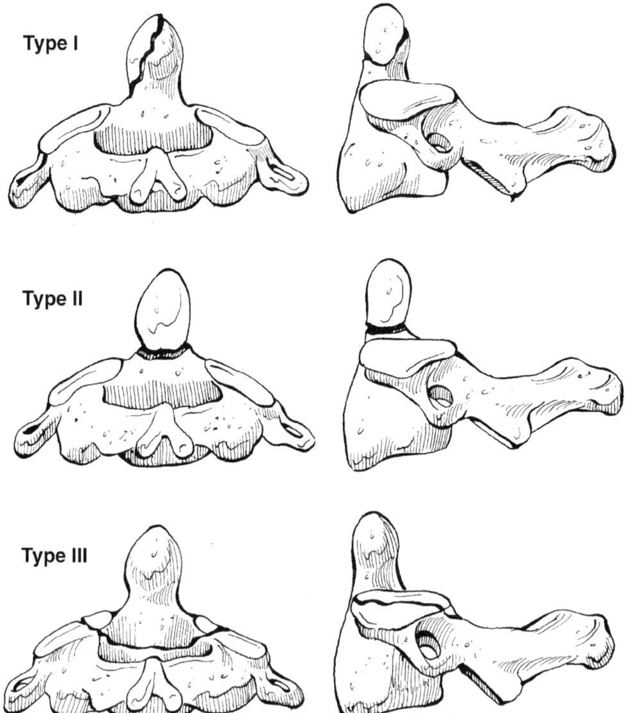

FIG. 13. Anderson and d'Alonzo classification of odontoid fractures.

Type I

Type I injuries are avulsion fractures of the lateral dens tip secondary to the alar ligament. Therefore, they may be associated with occipitocervical instability, as discussed previously.

Type II

Type II injuries are fractures through the waist of the dens. The fracture occurs through cortical bone having a small cross-sectional area. Significant anterior or posterior displacement can occur.

Type III

Type III injuries are fractures that extend into the body of C-2. They have a broad fracture surface of trabecular bone and, therefore, a good prognosis. Displacement, if present, is usually anterior.

Initial Treatment

The initial treatment of patients with odontoid fractures is to immobilize the cervical spine with traction or the halo vest. In patients with displacement, reduction should be obtained by tong traction. Excessive weight should be avoided, as overdistraction may have an adverse effect on healing. Reduction is obtained by relative positioning of the head and thorax or by the halo vest. The two-tong traction technique may be helpful in difficult cases (62).

Definitive Treatment

Type I

Type I injuries, which are rare, should be carefully evaluated for occipitoatlantal instability. If present, then they are treated by occipitocervical fusion. Stable type I injuries are treated by collar immobilization for 6 weeks.

Type II

The treatment of type II injuries is controversial. Nonoperative treatment is associated with a high failure rate, whereas operative care can lead to loss of range of motion or other iatrogenic complications. Type II fractures treated without halo vest immobilization or when missed have a near 100% chance of nonunion (63). Therefore, the majority of patients with type II fractures should at least have treatment by the halo vest. However, nonunion with the use of the halo vest treatment occurs in 15 to 85% of cases (Fig. 14). Numerous factors associated with nonunion have been identified (64). Clark found that displacement of more than 5 mm resulted in nonunion when treated by a halo vest (63). Similarly, Hadley identified displacement of 6 mm as a significant risk of nonunion (65). Hadley also described a variant that is a comminuted type II fracture. This fracture type has a uniformly poor prognosis and should be treated surgically. Aebi has also described an anterior oblique fracture type that is usually anteriorly displaced and is also associated with a high rate of nonunion (66). Odontoid screw fixation is inadequate treatment for this fracture type, as the fracture line runs parallel to the screw trajectory.

The adequacy and stability of reduction are important in healing. Ryan measured the contact between fracture fragments at different displacements (67). Only 20% of malreduction resulted in 40% loss of contact area. Fracture site stability may not be achieved in a halo vest, as described by Anderson (68) (Fig. 15). Also, prolonged traction, especially if fragments are distracted, has been associated with failure. Other risk factors include an older patient population and posterior displaced fractures (69). Additionally, transverse ligament interposition in the fracture site may lead to nonunion. The current recommended treatment for type II fractures is based on the risk of nonunion, the associated injuries, and the patient's age.

Type II fractures that have good progress are those that are transverse without comminution and have less than 4 to 5 mm initial displacement. The recommended treatment is by a halo vest for 10 to 12 weeks. During healing, the reduction should be assessed frequently. Alternatively, direct odontoid screw fixation can be performed. This has the advantage of being a direct fracture repair, thus maintaining atlantoaxial motion. However, Jeanneret reported that patients treated by odontoid screw fixation maintained only 50% of normal C1-2 motion (70).

Patients with fractures at high risk for nonunion—those with greater than 5 mm initial displacement, fracture comminution or angulation, an anterior oblique pattern, associated spinal cord injury, or other pulmonary injuries—are candidates for surgery. Younger patients can be treated with odontoid screw osteosynthesis or posterior C1-2 fusion (Fig. 15). The risks and benefits of

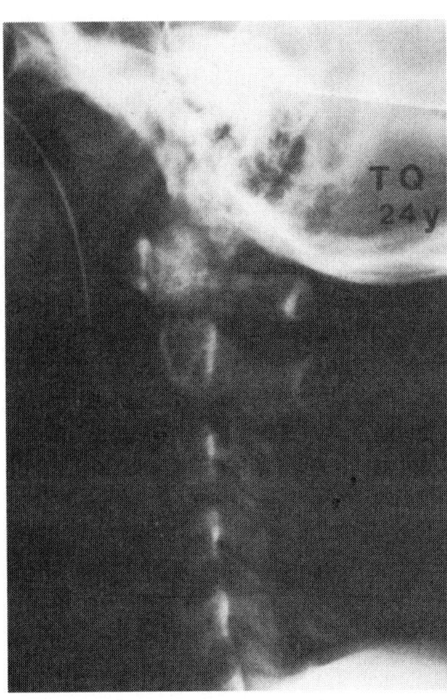

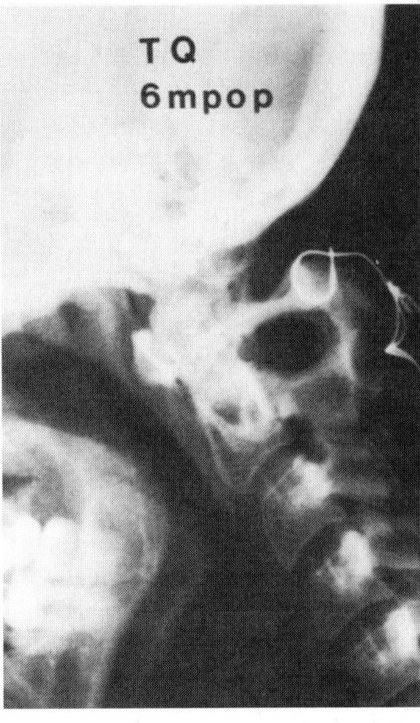

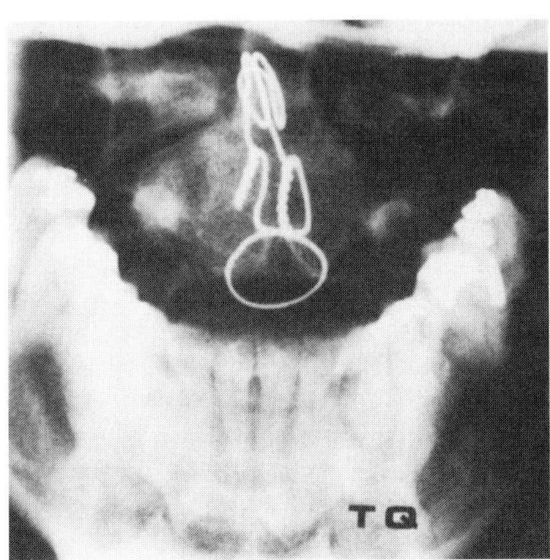

A–C

FIG. 14. A: This type II odontoid fracture in a 24-year-old woman failed to unite despite 4-month treatment in a halo vest. The lateral cervical spine radiograph demonstrates an established nonunion at the base of the odontoid. **B:** Successful fusion was achieved using the Gallie technique. The lateral view demonstrates remodeling of the posterior bone graft and healing of the fracture 6 months postoperatively. **C:** The anteroposterior view demonstrates correct wire placement.

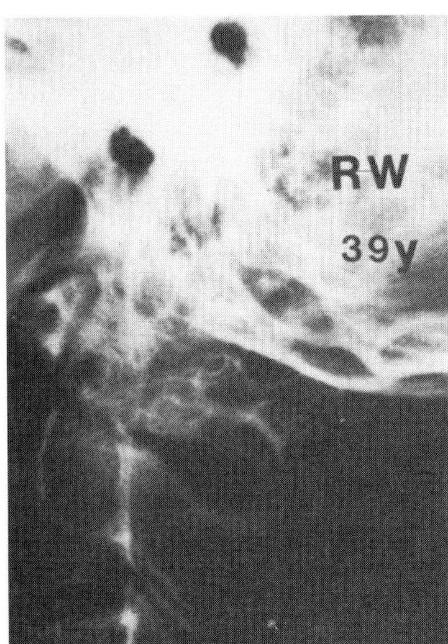

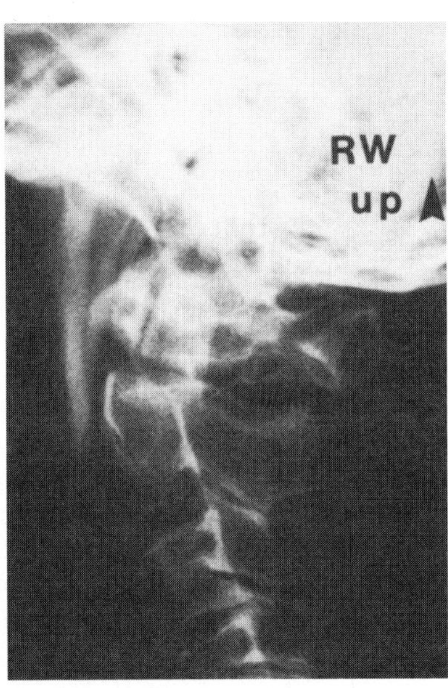

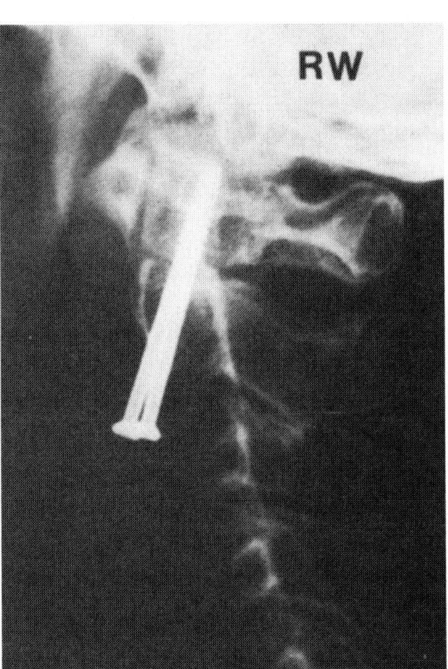

A–C

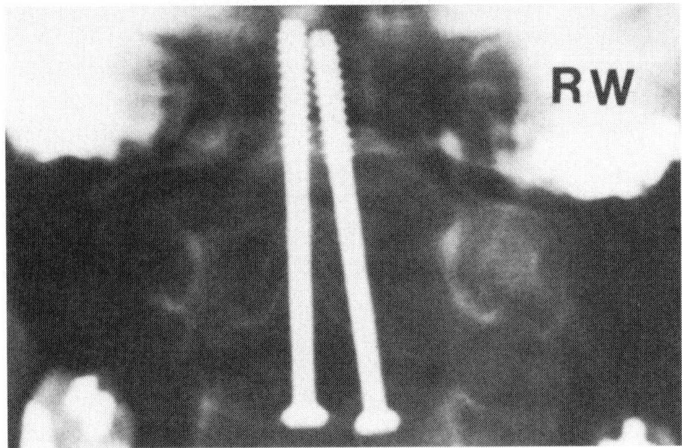

D

FIG. 15. A: The lateral radiograph taken in a recumbent position demonstrates a well reduced type II odontoid fracture in this man. **B:** An upright view taken in the halo vest shows posterior translation of the dens. Despite several repeat reduction attempts carried out in the upright position, a stable reduction could not be maintained. **C:** Surgical stabilization of the odontoid in an anatomically reduced position was carried out with two 3.5-mm cannulated screws, as seen on the postoperative lateral radiographs. **D:** Postoperative anteroposterior radiograph. Note slight convergence of the odontoid screws.

each procedure should be explained to patients and their input allowed in the decision-making process. Disadvantages of odontoid screws are that only partial range of motion is preserved, success is only 90%, swallowing or voice disturbance occurs in 5 to 20% of cases, and there is a small risk of spinal cord injury (71–73). Older patients or those with unfavorable fracture pattern are treated by posterior C1-2 fusion.

The surgical technique for posterior cervical fusion is described elsewhere (Chapter 40C). In patients with odontoid fracture, the author recommends the transarticular screw technique or C1-2 fixation as described by Harms (74,75) (Fig. 15). Adequate reduction must be achieved for safe screw placement. Wire techniques such as Gallie or Brooks provide insufficient stabilization, can result in posterior displacement of C-1 on C-2 during wire tightening, and require postoperative immobilization in the halo vest (76,77).

The anatomy and biomechanics of odontoid screw fixation have been investigated. Heller measured the internal dimensions of the odontoid and found that insufficient cross-sectional diameter (i.e., less than 7 mm) for two 3.5-mm screws can be present in 10% of individuals (78). The use of two screws has the advantage of improved rotational control, although several biomechanical investigations have demonstrated that there is little or no advantage to two screws compared to a single-screw technique (79–81).

Type III

Clark reported that type III fractures heal in 95% of cases when treated by the halo vest (63). Others have demonstrated a small series of patients with successful healing using the cervicothoracic brace (82). Unstable type III fractures or treatment failures are treated by a posterior C1-2 fusion. Type III fractures are a relative contraindication for odontoid screw fixation.

Elderly Patients

Odontoid fractures in the elderly are associated with significant morbidity and mortality similar to that of hip fractures (27,28,83). Halo treatment or even a short period of bed rest in tong traction is poorly tolerated and can be associated with mortality. In healthier geriatric patients, an aggressive surgical approach by early posterior C1-2 fusion with rigid internal fixation is warranted (Fig. 16). In patients with significant dementia or severe medical comorbidities, benign treatment by a soft collar should be considered with the knowledge that a nonunion will occur. Odontoid screw fixation is not recommended in the elderly and can be associated with significant morbidity and mortality (84).

Pediatric Odontoid Fracture

Pediatric odontoid fracture can be difficult to diagnose and to differentiate from the odontoid synchrosis. This growth center is located between the dens and C-2 body and is fused by age 11 years. Displacement at any age is abnormal; therefore, one should be suspicious of a fracture. Pediatric odontoid fractures are treated by reduction and stabilization in a halo vest and rarely require surgery.

A–C

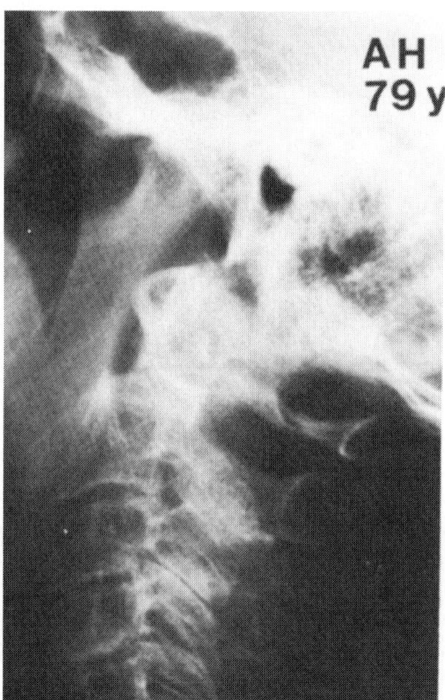

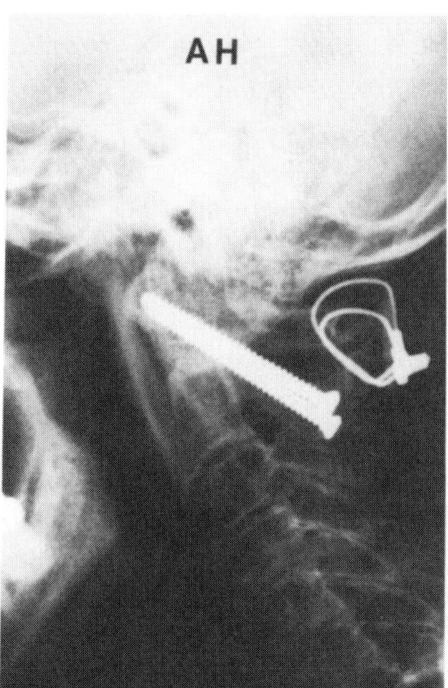

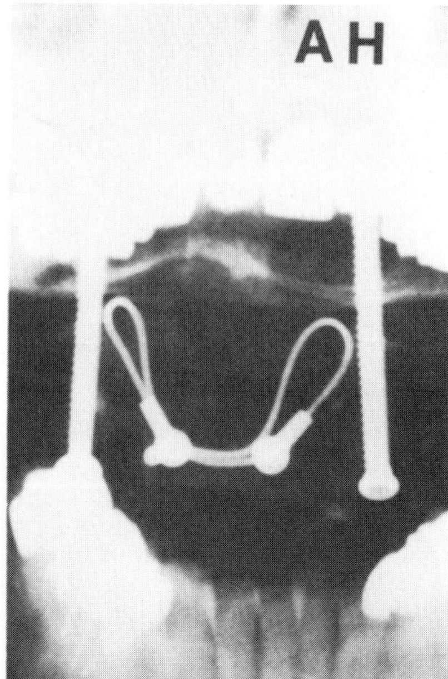

FIG. 16. A: This neurologically intact woman presented with an unstable, posteriorly displaced type II odontoid fracture. Due to the age of the patient and initial fracture displacement, surgical stabilization of the C1-2 segment was performed. **B:** Atlantoaxial fusion was achieved with transarticular facet screws using the technique described by Magerl, and an iliac crest bone graft was performed. The screws properly angle toward the midpoint of the anterior atlantal arch. **C:** Postoperative open-mouth view.

Traumatic Spondylolisthesis of the Axis

This injury pattern is commonly referred to by the moniker *hangman's fractures*, but it is more appropriately called *traumatic spondylolisthesis of the axis*. Although originally described by Schneider as the cause of death in judicial hanging, forensic findings after recent hangings in Washington state have given less credence to the name (85). These studies indicate that traumatic spondylolisthesis of the axis is a rare cause of death in these circumstances and that craniocervical distraction with arterial rupture is the fatal mechanism. In traumatic spondylolisthesis of the axis, the injury is a fracture through the relatively small osseous strut connecting the superior to the inferior facet, the pars interarticularis, sometimes referred to as an *isthmus* or *pedicle* (86).

Mechanism of Injury

The majority of cases of traumatic spondylolisthesis of the axis are caused by hyperextension from head and facial impaction. These extension axial loading forces create bending stress in the pars and ultimately failure. After the pars fracture, the C2-3 disc is placed under tension and, with sufficient force, can fail. Thus, a bony injury occurs in the pars with a variable amount of soft-tissue injury to the C2-3 disc. A flexion component is often apparent. Indication of this is seen because many injuries are anteriorly angulated and associated with anterior translation or, in rare circumstances, are associated with C2-3 facet dislocations. Whether flexion is a primary force or from a rebound is not clear. Variable amounts of rotation and lateral bending are evident as fracture lines in the pars interarticularis are rarely symmetric.

Clinical Symptoms

Patients often have signs of external craniofacial trauma, such as contusion, abrasion, or fractures. The spinal canal enlarges in the majority of cases; therefore, neurologic consequences are rare, although a small percentage of fatalities in forensic studies result from these injuries. Pain and tenderness at the easily palpable C-2 spinous process are to be expected. Vertebral artery injuries have been reported and when bilateral are usually fatal.

Classification

Effendi proposed a classification based on the severity of associated soft tissue injury, especially the C2-3 disc (87). This has been modified by Levine to four types (88) (Fig. 17).

Type I

A *type I* injury is a bilateral pars fracture with less than 3 mm of anterior C2-3 subluxation. This is stable by virtue of the intact C2-3 discoligamentous complex.

Type II

A *type II* injury is associated with a discoligamentous injury at C2-3. There is displacement of the pars fracture and anterior translation of the C-2 body. In the type IIa as described by Levine, there is distraction across the C2-3 disc and flexion angulation of the C-2 body and dens.

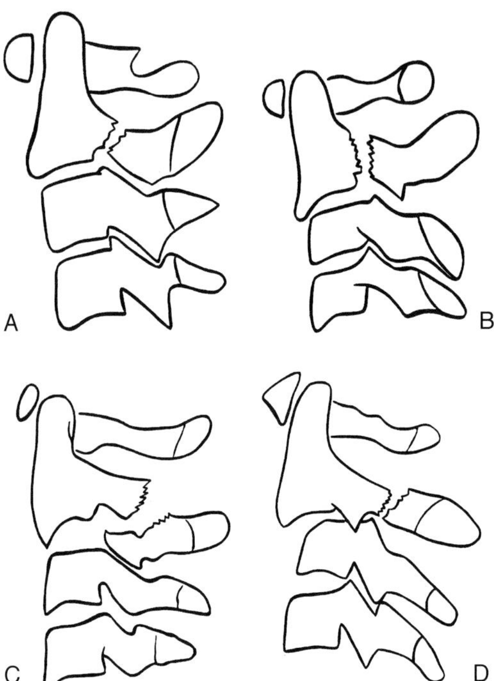

FIG. 17. Levine classification of traumatic spondylolisthesis of the axis. **A:** Type I. **B:** Type II. **C:** Type IIa. **D:** Type III.

Muller subclassifies type II fractures as flexion, extension, and listhesis (89). The flexion and extension types were generally stable and had a good prognosis. The listhesis types were unstable even in the halo vest and were associated with neurologic and other injuries. This analysis is similar to the classification proposed by Francis based on amount of initial displacement (86).

Type III

Type III injuries are fractures of the pars interarticularis with C2-3 facet dislocations. These cannot be reduced by cranial tong traction because of the division between the anterior and posterior segments of C-2.

Diagnosis

Traumatic spondylolisthesis of the axis is usually easy to identify on plain radiographs. Children do not have a synchondrosis in the pars and, therefore, pars defects are likely to be traumatic in origin (20). CT is helpful to see the fracture location, as many extend into the vertebral body. This has been described as an atypical hangman's fracture (90). In type II fractures, Levine recommends flexion-extension radiographs to determine stability. The author cannot agree with this technique due to concerns over possible spinal cord injury (20). In such cases, the author would simply choose to treat more aggressively with the halo vest rather than simple orthosis.

Initial Treatment

Patients with traumatic spondylolisthesis of the axis should be immobilized by tong traction or halo vest. Given that the common name is *hangman's fracture*, only light traction weights should be applied. Alignment may be improved by changing the angle of the applied traction or relative position of head and thorax. Type III injuries are irreducible and should be treated surgically in a timely manner.

Definitive Treatment

Type I injuries are stable and can be treated by immobilization in a cervicothoracic brace. After orthotic application, upright radiographs should be obtained to assess maintenance of alignment.

Type II fractures are unstable and are treated by reduction and halo vest immobilization. Healing is expected to occur uniformly, despite its unstable nature and significant initial displacement.

A controversy exists regarding the treatment of type IIa fractures. If reduction is achieved, they can be treated similarly to type II fractures. If reduction fails, or if it cannot be maintained, then longer periods of bed rest with traction may be required. Once the fracture becomes "sticky," the patient can be managed in a halo vest. Over 95% of these injuries heal with satisfactory outcomes (Fig. 18). Some patients with type II or IIa fracture have been successfully treated by a cervicothoracic orthosis (91). The author has used this in multiply injured patients and the morbidly obese. Other more aggressive approaches for managing type II fractures have been described, including osteosynthesis using C-2 pedicle screws and anterior C2-3 fusion with plate. These techniques are indicated for patients who fail halo treatment or who do not tolerate orthotic management. In a review of 74 patients with hangman's fractures, Greene reported that seven could not be managed in an orthosis and were treated surgically (92). Muller recommends surgery for all type II listhesis fracture types (89).

The surgical treatment of traumatic spondylolisthesis of the axis is by reduction and osteosynthesis, with pedicle screw fixation or by anterior cervical fusion at C2-3 and plate stabilization. In the small series reported, these techniques have had satisfactory outcomes (89,93,94). Biomechanically, the osteosynthesis technique preserves C2-3 motion but is not as stiff as anterior plate stabilization (95).

A
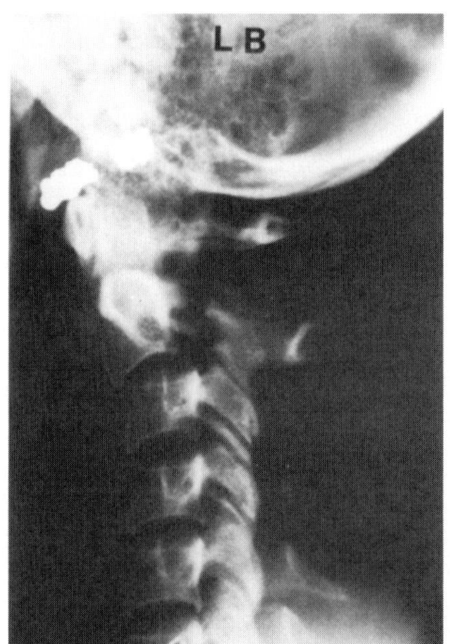

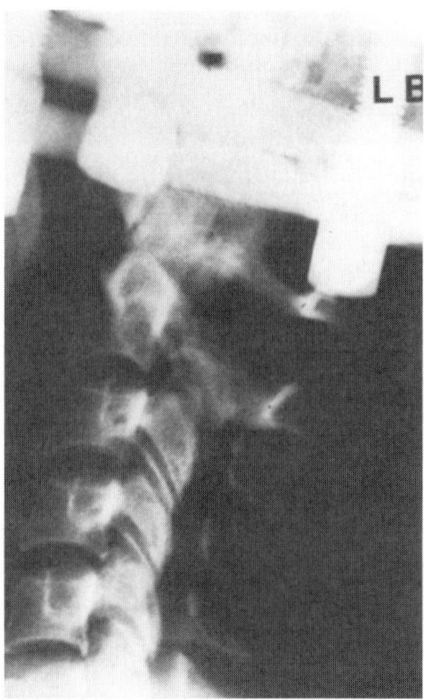

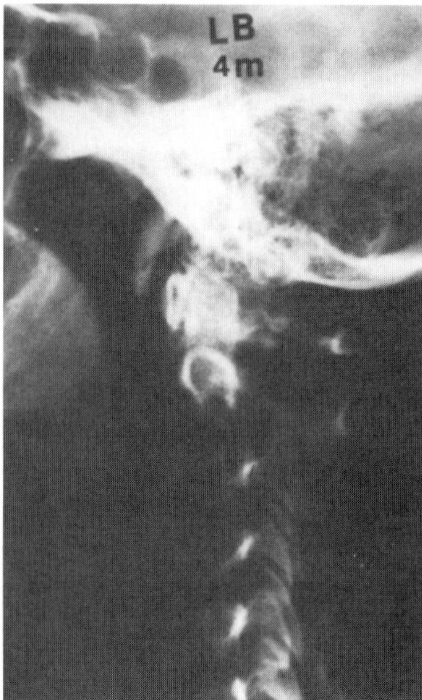

C,D

B
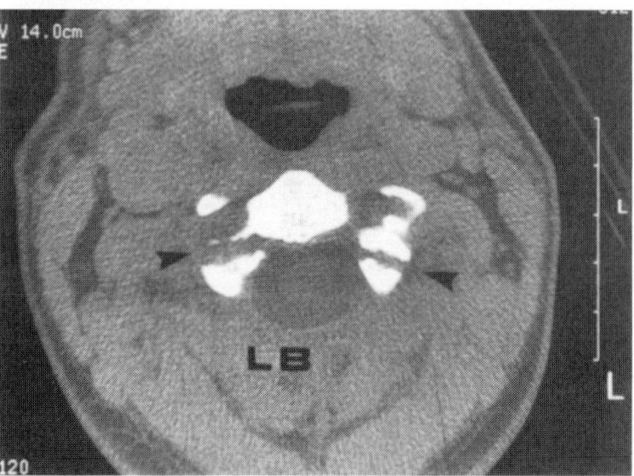

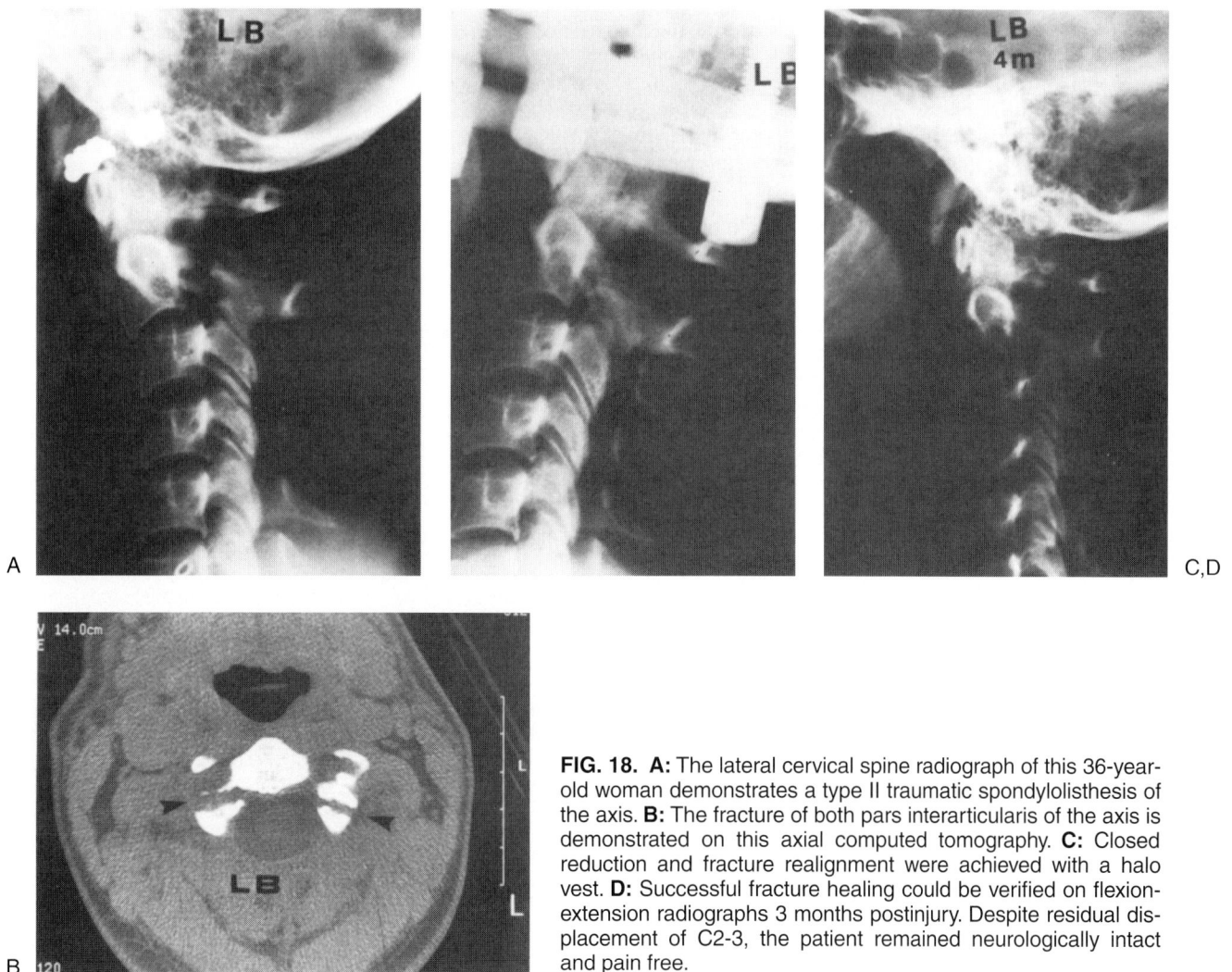

FIG. 18. A: The lateral cervical spine radiograph of this 36-year-old woman demonstrates a type II traumatic spondylolisthesis of the axis. **B:** The fracture of both pars interarticularis of the axis is demonstrated on this axial computed tomography. **C:** Closed reduction and fracture realignment were achieved with a halo vest. **D:** Successful fracture healing could be verified on flexion-extension radiographs 3 months postinjury. Despite residual displacement of C2-3, the patient remained neurologically intact and pain free.

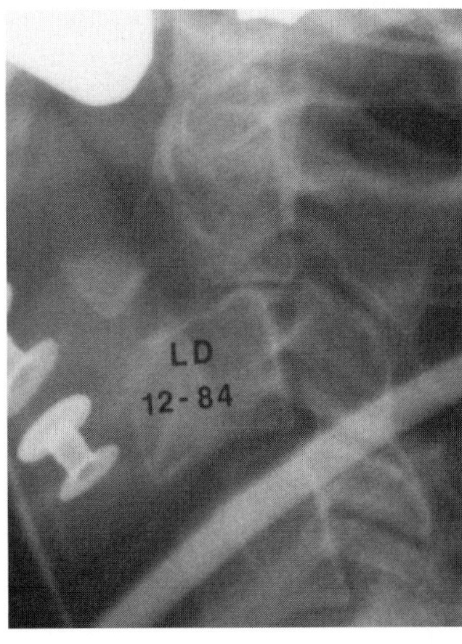

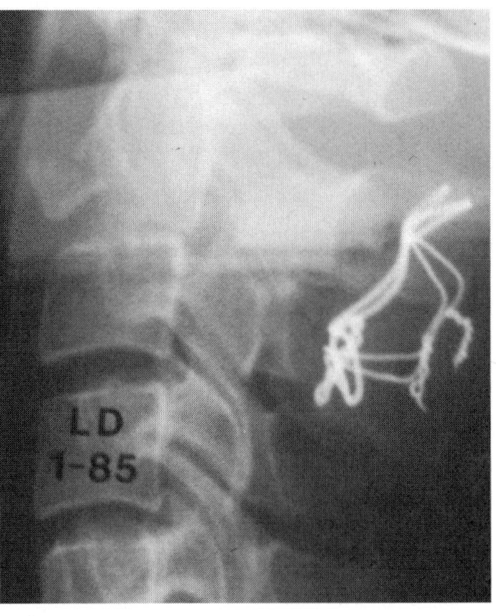

A,B

FIG. 19. A: This 22-year-old man sustained a hyperextension injury resulting in an extension teardrop fracture, type I C-2 body fracture. He had a central cord syndrome, which improved with reduction. Because of the instability despite halo vest, he was treated by posterior cervical fusion. **B:** Postoperative lateral radiograph after C2-3 fusion.

Type III fractures are irreducible and are treated by open reduction and internal fixation. The C2-3 facet dislocation is reduced manually. Machining away a small amount of the superior facet of C-3 may facilitate reduction. Once reduced, stabilization is performed by the interspinous wire technique or plate and screw fixation. The latter technique is more complex and associated with risk of complications, but it has the advantage of combining fixation of the C2-3 facet dislocation with screw stabilization of the C-2 pars fracture. In the wire technique, the pars fracture still requires treatment, usually with halo vest. The prognosis for healing is excellent in the few cases that have been reported; however, patients with type III injury often have severe spinal cord injuries with residual deficits if they survive.

Axis Body Fractures

Axis body fracture has been poorly recognized as a specific entity and is often simply a variant of the odontoid or hangman's fracture or is similar to injuries in the subaxial cervical spine. These fractures are localized below the odontoid process and involve the C-2 vertebral body.

Classification

Fujimira has developed the first classification system of these injuries (96).

Type I

Type I injuries are extension teardrop fractures from the anterior-inferior endplate of C-2. Most injuries are stable unless associated with greater than 4 mm of posterior vertebral displacement.

Type II

Type II injuries are horizontal shear fractures through the body located more caudally than type III odontoid fractures.

Type III

Type III injuries are bursting-type fractures of the C-2 body.

Type IV

Type IV injuries are unstable sagittal cleavage fractures.

Diagnosis

C-2 vertebral body injuries are usually easily visualized on plain radiographs. CT allows assessment of the spinal canal and determination of facet alignment.

Initial Treatment

The initial treatment is to stabilize the neck with extraction collar or tong traction. The patients with displaced injuries should have reduction by traction. Unstable injuries are assessed by CT or MRI before surgical treatment.

Definitive Treatment

The treatment is primarily based on fracture stability and displacement of the atlantoaxial articulation. Stable fracture with minimal displacement can be treated by a cervicothoracic brace. Unstable injuries have a good prognosis because of the large bony surfaces involved, and therefore are best treated in a halo vest. Fractures that cannot be maintained in the halo vest or are associated with ligamentous injury should be treated by posterior C1-2 fusion. The type I extension teardrop fracture, if significantly displaced, is treated by posterior C2-3 fusion (Fig. 19).

COMPLICATIONS

Upper cervical injuries are associated with significant morbidity and mortality. Death usually occurs at the accident scene but can also occur during the early phase of hospitalization. Most often death is secondary to neurologic injury, cerebrovascular insufficiency, or multiple injuries. Mortality rates of elderly patients with odontoid fracture are 23 to 26% (26). Treatment by aggressive stabilization and mobilization has significantly reduced the high mortality rate as reported by Bednar (27). Neurologic injuries may be associated with respiratory failure and require intubation. Vertebral displacement during intubation can be prevented by an assistant holding the head in neutral alignment. Tracheostomy may be required if facial fractures are present. Additionally, protection of the airway may be compromised in patients with cranial nerve injuries, which occur in up to 30% of patients with occipitocondyle fractures or occipitoatlantal dislocations.

Delay in Diagnosis

Delay in diagnosis of upper cervical injuries occurs frequently because of the variable anatomy, importance of ligament integrity, lack of visualization of articulations radiographically, and alterations in consciousness of patients. Most commonly missed patterns with the greatest potential for adverse consequences are occipitoatlantal dislocations and odontoid fracture. Neurologic injury and even death have been reported in these missed injuries (97). Timely diagnosis can be made using proper clinical and radiographic protocols to evaluate all trauma patients. CT with reconstruction is the most reliable method to evaluate questionable or suspected cases. Upper cervical injuries are associated with other cervical trauma in 20 to 30% of cases; therefore, when an injury is identified, a complete assessment of the spine is required.

Neurologic Deterioration

Neurologic deterioration is uncommon except when associated with missed injury. Budshuk reported deterioration in 75% of patients after missed upper cervical injury. Patients who present with neurologic deterioration require prompt assessment of cervical alignment and MRI to determine canal patency. In autopsy studies, epidural hematomas and vascular injuries are frequently noted, which may lead to deterioration in survivors. Treatment requires administration of high-dose methylprednisolone, reduction of malalignment, and possibly urgent decompression and stabilization.

Vascular Injury

Vascular injury, especially to the vertebral arteries, is more common than appreciated (98). The clinical consequences of isolated vascular artery are uncertain, although cases of delayed stroke or death and neurologic deterioration have been observed in patients with vertebral artery injury and subsequent thrombosis of the basilar artery. Distractive injuries such as occipitoatlantal dislocation, atlantoaxial rotary subluxation, and fractures involving the foramen transversarium are most likely associated with arterial injury. The treatment of identified vertebral artery injury is controversial. A reasonable approach is to place patients on a course of acute thrombotic prophylaxis to prevent ascending thrombosis. This may, of course, complicate management of patients with other system trauma.

Nonunion

Nonunion of bony injuries except for type II odontoid fracture is uncommon. Nonunion of atlantal posterior arch fractures is usually insignificant and does not require treatment. Transverse ligament injuries associated with avulsion fracture heal in the majority of cases, whereas midsubstance injuries require surgery. Atlantoaxial rotary subluxations may continue to be unstable and require C1-2 posterior fusion if there is associated transverse ligament injury. The rare patient with nonunion of traumatic spondylolisthesis of the axis is managed by anterior C2-3 fusion with plate fixation. Odontoid fracture nonunions that occur in 5% of type III and up to 80% of type II injuries when treated in a halo vest are treated by posterior C1-2 fusion.

Loss of Reduction

The upper cervical spine has little inherent bony stability and therefore, when injured, may have a high degree of instability. Loss of reduction is not infrequent in occipitoatlantal dislocation, transverse ligament injury, and odontoid and hangman's fractures despite halo vest immobilization. When treated nonoperatively, frequent radiographs should be obtained to assess alignment. Before discharge, an upright radiograph is obtained to assess fracture site mobility. Anderson compared upright and supine radiographs in patients with unstable cervical injuries managed with a halo vest and found that 1.9 mm of fracture site translation and 8 degrees of angulation occurred between the two positions (68).

Chronic Pain and Disability

In the absence of neurologic injury, upper cervical injuries have a good prognosis overall with a minimal amount of disability. However, injury to these highly mobile articulations or from the effects of surgery can lead to joint arthrosis, pain, and loss of range of motion. Even osteosynthesis of odontoid fracture is associated with 50% loss of atlantoaxial rotation (70). Patients with missed fractures or nonunions present with pain, diminished neck motion, and often torticollis. Late diagnosis may be evaluated using bone scan and CT. Painful arthritic joints can be treated successfully by appropriate posterior fusion.

CONCLUSION

The upper cervical spine is a commonly injured region with potential for significant morbidity and mortality. Increasing numbers of patients are surviving these injuries and presenting for treatment. Early attention to maintenance of airway and ventilation and proper techniques of stabilization are essential for survival. Imaging, particularly CT, provides sufficient details to allow proper classification and to determine the extent of injuries. Initial treatment of the spine injury includes reduction of vertebral displacement if malalignment is present. Definitive treatment is determined by injury type; patient demographics, such as age, presence of associated injuries, and neurologic deficits; and whether the injury is bony or ligamentous. The most common complications are delayed or missed injuries and loss of reduction. In the elderly, early mobilization with orthosis or by surgery should be considered.

REFERENCES

1. Rabischong P. Comprehensive anatomy of the upper cervical spine. Read at the XVIII Annual Meeting of the Cervical Spine Research Society. Paris, France: June 14, 2002.
2. Dvorak J, Schneider E, Saldinger P, et al. Biomechanics of the craniocervical region: the alar and transverse ligaments. *J Orthop Res* 1988;6:452–461.
3. Panjabi MM, Dvorak J, Sandler A, et al. Cervical spine kinematics and instability. In Cervical Spine Research Society, ed. *The cervical spine*, 3rd ed. Philadelphia: Lippincott–Raven Publishers, 1998:55–57.
4. Crisco JJD, Panjabi MM, Dvorak J. A model of the alar ligaments of the upper cervical spine in axial rotation. *J Biomech* 1991;24: 607–614.
5. Adams VI. Neck injuries: I. Occipitoatlantal dislocation—a pathologic study of 12 traffic fatalities. *J Forensic Sci* 1992;37:556–564.
6. Adams VI. Neck injuries: II. Atlantoaxial dislocation—a pathologic study of 14 traffic fatalities. *J Forensic Sci* 1992;37:565–573.
7. Adams VI. Neck injuries: III. Ligamentous injuries of the craniocervical articulation without occipito-atlantal or atlanto-axial facet dislocation—a pathologic study of 21 traffic fatalities. *J Forensic Sci* 1993;38:1097–1104.
8. Alker GJ, Oh YS, Leslie EV, et al. Postmortem radiology of head-neck injuries in fatal traffic accidents. *Radiology* 1975;114:611–617.
9. Bucholz RW, Burkhead WZ. The pathological anatomy of fatal atlanto-occipital dislocations. *J Bone Joint Surg* 1979;61:248–250.
10. Jonsson H, Bring G, Rauschning W, et al. Hidden cervical spine injuries in traffic accident victims with skull fractures. *J Spinal Disord* 1991;4:251–256.
11. Werne S. Studies in spontaneous atlas dislocations. *Acta Orthop Scan (Suppl)* 1957;23:1–109.
12. American College of Surgeons. *Advanced trauma life support manual*. Chicago, 1992.
13. American Spinal Injury Association. *Standards for neurological and functional classification of spinal cord injury*. Chicago, 1992.
14. Dickman CA, Hadley MN, Pappas CT, et al. Cruciate paralysis: a clinical and radiographic analysis of injuries to the cervicomedullary junction. *J Neurosurg* 1990;73:850–858.
15. Blackmore CC, Mann FA, Wilson AJ. Helical CT in the primary trauma evaluation of the cervical spine: an evidence-based approach. *Skeletal Radiol* 2000;29:632–639.
16. Hanson JA, Blackmore CC, Mann FA, et al. Cervical spine injury: a clinical decision rule to identify high-risk patients for helical CT screening. *AJR Am J Roentgenol* 2000;174:713–717.
17. Harris JH, Carson GC, Wagner LK. Radiologic diagnosis of traumatic occipitovertebral dissociation: 1. Normal occipitovertebral relationships on lateral radiographs of supine subjects. *AJR Am J Roentgenol* 1994;162:881–886.
18. Harris JH Jr, Carson GC, Wagner LK, et al. Radiologic diagnosis of traumatic occipitovertebral dissociation: 2. Comparison of three methods of detecting occipitovertebral relationships on lateral radiographs of supine subjects. *AJR Am J Roentgenol* 1994;162: 887–892.
19. Bundschuh CV, Alley JB, Ross M, et al. Magnetic resonance imaging of suspected atlanto-occipital dislocation. Two case reports. *Spine* 1992;17:245–248.
20. Budorick TE, Anderson PA, Rivara FP, et al. Flexion-distraction fracture of the cervical spine. A case report. *J Bone Joint Surg* 1991; 88:572–577.
21. Davis JW, Parks SN, Detlefs CL, et al. Clearing the cervical spine in obtunded patients: the use of dynamic fluoroscopy. *J Trauma* 1995; 39:435–438.
22. Harris MB, Kronlage SC, Carboni PA, et al. Evaluation of the cervical spine in the polytrauma patient. *Spine* 2000;25:2884–2891.
23. White AA, Panjabi MM. The problem of clinical instability in the human spine: a systematic approach. In: *Clinical biomechanics of the spine*, 2nd ed. Philadelphia: Lippincott, 1990:277–378.
24. Bracken MB, Shepard MJ, Holford TR, et al. Methylprednisolone or tirilazad mesylate administration after acute spinal cord injury: 1-year follow up. Results of the third National Acute Spinal Cord Injury randomized controlled trial. *J Neurosurg* 1998;89:699–706.
25. Lind B, Bake B, Lundqvist C, et al. Influence of halo vest treatment on vital capacity. *Spine* 1987;12:449–452.
26. Alander DH, Andreychik DA, Stauffer ES. Early outcome in cervical spinal cord injured patients older than 50 years of age. *Spine* 1994;19:2299–2301.
27. Bednar DA, Parikh J, Hummel J. Management of type II odontoid process fractures in geriatric patients; a prospective study of sequential cohorts with attention to survivorship. *J Spinal Disord* 1995;8:166–169.
28. Lieberman IH, Webb JK. Cervical spine injuries in the elderly. *J Bone Joint Surg Br* 1994;76:877–881.
29. Herzenberg JE, Hensinger RN, Dedrick DK, et al. Emergency transport and positioning of young children who have an injury of the cervical spine. The standard backboard may be hazardous. *J Bone Joint Surg* 1989;71:15–22.
30. Hanson JA, Deliganis AV, Baxter AB, et al. Radiologic and clinical spectrum of occipital condyle fractures: retrospective review of 107 consecutive fractures in 95 patients. *AJR Am J Roentgenol* 2002;178:1261–1268.
31. McElhaney JH, Hopper RH, Nightingale RW, et al. Mechanisms of basilar skull fracture. *J Neurotrauma* 1995;12:669–678.
32. Anderson PA, Montesano PX. Morphology and treatment of occipital condyle fractures. *Spine* 1988;13:731–736.
33. Miyazaki C, Katsume M, Yamazaki T, et al. Unusual occipital condyle fracture with multiple nerve palsies and Wallenberg syndrome. *Clin Neurol Neurosurg* 2000;102:255–258.
34. Stroobants J, Fidlers L, Storms JL, et al. High cervical pain and impairment of skull mobility as the only symptoms of an occipital condyle fracture. Case report. *J Neurosurg* 1994;81:137–138.
35. Deliganis AV, Baxter AB, Hanson JA, et al. Radiologic spectrum of craniocervical distraction injuries. *Radiographics* 2000;20 Spec No:S237–S250.
36. Imaizumi T, Sohma T, Hotta H, et al. Associated injuries and mechanism of atlanto-occipital dislocation caused by trauma. *Neurol Med Chir* 1995;35:385–391.
37. Anderson PA. Upper cervical spine trauma. In: Bulstrode C, Buckwalter J, Carr A, et al., eds. *Oxford textbook of orthopaedics and trauma*. Oxford: Oxford University Press, 2002;2082–2101.
38. Traynelis VC, Marano GD, Dunker RO, et al. Traumatic atlanto-occipital dislocation. Case report. *J Neurosurg* 1986;65:863–870.
39. Teo EC, Ng HW. First cervical vertebra (atlas) fracture mechanism studies using finite element method. *J Biomech* 2001;34:13–21.
40. Panjabi MM, Oda T, Crisco JJ, et al. Experimental study of atlas injuries. I. Biomechanical analysis of their mechanisms and fracture patterns. *Spine* 1991;16S:460–465.
41. Beckner MA, Heggeness MH, Doherty BJ. A biomechanical study of Jefferson fractures. *Spine* 1998;23:1832–1836.
42. Spence KF Jr, Decker S, Sell KW. Bursting atlantal fracture associated with rupture of the transverse ligament. *J Bone Joint Surg* 1970;52:543–549.
43. Dickman CA, Greene KA, Sonntag VK. Injuries involving the transverse atlantal ligament: classification and treatment guidelines based upon experience with 39 injuries. *Neurosurgery* 1996;38:44–50.
44. Dickman CA, Mamourian A, Sonntag VK, et al. Magnetic resonance imaging of the transverse atlantal ligament for the evaluation of atlantoaxial instability. *J Neurosurg* 1991;75:221–227.
45. Levine AM, Edwards CC. Fractures of the atlas. *J Bone Joint Surg* 1991;73:680–91.
46. Broom MJ, Krompinger WJ, Bond SD. Fracture of the atlantal arch causing atlanto-axial instability. Report of a case. *J Bone Joint Surg* 1986;68:1289–1291.
47. Lee TT, Green BA, Petrin DR. Treatment of stable burst fracture of the atlas (Jefferson fracture) with rigid cervical collar. *Spine* 1998;23:1963–1967.
48. Hadley MN, Dickman CA, Browner CM, et al. Acute traumatic atlas fractures: management and long-term outcome. *Neurosurgery* 1988;23:31–35.
49. McGuire RA Jr, Harkey HL. Primary treatment of unstable Jefferson's fractures. *J Spinal Disord* 1995;8:233–236.

50. Ruf M, Melcher R, Harms J. Transoral reduction and osteosynthesis of C1 as a function preserving option in the treatment of unstable Jefferson's fractures. Read at the XVIII Annual Meeting Cervical Spine Research Society. Paris, France: June 14, 2002.
51. Kluger PJ. A new method for intra-segmental osteosynthesis of dislocated Jefferson's fractures. Read at the XVIII Annual Meeting Cervical Spine Research Society. Paris, France: June 14, 2002.
52. Fielding JW, Cochran GB, Lawsing JF, et al. Tears of the transverse ligament of the atlas. A clinical and biomechanical study. *J Bone Joint Surg* 1974;56:1683–1691.
53. Fielding JW, Hawkins RJ. Atlanto-axial rotatory fixation. (Fixed rotatory subluxation of the atlanto-axial joint). *J Bone Joint Surg* 1977;59:37–44.
54. Dvorak J, Hayek J, Zehnder R. CT-functional diagnostics of the rotatory instability of the upper cervical spine. Part 2. An evaluation on healthy adults and patients with suspected instability. *Spine* 1987;12:726–731.
55. Dvorak J, Panjabi M, Gerber M, et al. CT-functional diagnostics of the rotatory instability of upper cervical spine. 1. An experimental study on cadavers. *Spine* 1987;12:197–205.
56. Anderson LD, D'Alonzo RT. Fractures of the odontoid process of the axis. *J Bone Joint Surg* 1974;56:1663–1674.
57. Doherty BJ, Heggeness MH, Esses S. A biomechanical study of odontoid fractures and fracture fixation. *Spine* 1993;18:178–184.
58. Graham RS, Oberlander EK, Stewart JE, et al. Validation and use of a finite element model of C-2 for determination of stress and fracture patterns of anterior odontoid loads. *J Neurosurg* 2000;93:117–125.
59. Mouradian WH, Fietti VG, Cochran GV, et al. Fractures of the odontoid: a laboratory and clinical study of mechanisms. *Orthop Clin North Am* 1978;9:985–1001.
60. Greene KA, Dickman CA, Marciano FF, et al. Transverse atlantal ligament disruption associated with odontoid fractures. *Spine* 1994;19:2307–2314.
61. Harris JH, Burke JT, Ray RD, et al. Low (type III) odontoid fracture: a new radiographic sign. *Radiology* 1984;153:353–356.
62. Star AM, Jones AA, Cotler JM, et al. Immediate closed reduction of cervical spine dislocations using traction. *Spine* 1990;15:1068–1072.
63. Clark CR, White AA. Fractures of the dens. A multicenter study. *J Bone Joint Surg* 1985;67:1340–1348.
64. Schatzker J, Rorabeck CH, Waddell JP. Non-union of the odontoid process. An experimental investigation. *Clin Orthop* 1975;108:127–137.
65. Hadley MN, Browner CM, Liu SS, Sonntag VK. New subtype of acute odontoid fractures (type IIA). *Neurosurgery* 1988;22:67–71.
66. Aebi M, Etter C, Coscia M. Fractures of the odontoid process. Treatment with anterior screw fixation. *Spine* 1989;14:1065–1070.
67. Ryan MD, Taylor TK. Odontoid fractures. A rational approach to treatment. *J Bone Joint Surg* 1982;64:416–421.
68. Anderson PA, Budorick TE, Easton KB, et al. Failure of halo vest to prevent in vivo motion in patients with injured cervical spines. *Spine* 1991;16S:501–505.
69. Southwick WO. Management of fractures of the dens (odontoid process). *J Bone Joint Surg* 1980;62:482–486.
70. Jeanneret B, Magerl F. Primary posterior fusion C1/2 in odontoid fractures: indications, technique, and results of transarticular screw fixation. *J Spinal Disord* 1992;5:464–475.
71. Bohler J. Anterior stabilization for acute fractures and non-unions of the dens. *J Bone Joint Surg* 1982;64:18–27.
72. Geisler FH, Cheng C, Poka A, et al. Anterior screw fixation of posteriorly displaced type II odontoid fractures. *Neurosurgery* 1989;25:30–38.
73. Montesano PX, Anderson PA, Schlehr F, et al. Odontoid fractures treated by anterior odontoid screw fixation. *Spine* 1991;16:S33–S37.
74. Magerl F, Seeman PS. Stable posterior fusion of the atlas and axis by transarticular screw fixation. In: Weidner PA, ed. *Cervical spine*. New York: Springer-Verlag, 1987:322–327.
75. Harms J, Melcher RP. Posterior C1-C2 fusion with polyaxial screw and rod fixation. *Spine* 2001;26:2467–2471.
76. Brooks AL, Jenkins EB. Atlanto-axial arthrodesis by the wedge compression method. *J Bone Joint Surg* 1978;60:279–284.
77. Gallie WE. Fractures and dislocations of the cervical spine. *Am J Surg* 1939;46:494–499.
78. Heller JG, Alson MD, Schaffler MB, et al. Quantitative internal dens morphology. *Spine* 1992;17:861–866.
79. Jenkins JD, Coric D, Branch CL. A clinical comparison of one- and two-screw odontoid fixation. *J Neurosurg* 1998;89:366–370.
80. McBride AD, Mukherjee DP, Kruse RN, et al. Anterior screw fixation of type II odontoid fractures. A biomechanical study. *Spine* 1995;20:1855–1860.
81. Sasso R, Doherty BJ, Crawford MJ, et al. Biomechanics of odontoid fracture fixation. Comparison of the one- and two-screw technique. *Spine* 1993;18:1950–1953.
82. Polin RS, Szabo T, Bogaev CA, et al. Nonoperative management of types II and III odontoid fractures: the Philadelphia collar versus the halo vest. *Neurosurgery* 1996;38:450–457.
83. Spivak JM, Weiss MA, Cotler JM, et al. Cervical spine injuries in patients 65 and older. *Spine* 1994;19:2302–2306.
84. Andersson S, Rodrigues M, Olerud C. Odontoid fractures: high complication rate associated with anterior screw fixation in the elderly. *Eur Spine J* 2000;9:56–59.
85. Schneider RC, Livingston KE, Cave AJE, et al. Hangman's fracture of the cervical spine. *J Neurosurg* 1965;22:141–154.
86. Francis WR, Fielding JW, Hawkins RJ, et al. Traumatic spondylolisthesis of the axis. *J Bone Joint Surg (Br)* 1981;63:313–318.
87. Effendi B, Roy D, Cornish B, et al. Fractures of the ring of the axis. A classification based on the analysis of 131 cases. *J Bone Joint Surg (Br)* 1981;63:319–327.
88. Levine AM, Edwards CC. The management of traumatic spondylolisthesis of the axis. *J Bone Joint Surg Am* 1985;67:217–226.
89. Muller EJ, Wick M, Muhr G. Traumatic spondylolisthesis of the axis: treatment rationale based on the stability of the different fracture types. *Eur Spine J* 2000;9:123–128.
90. Starr JK, Eismont FJ. Atypical hangman's fractures. *Spine* 1993;18:1954–1957.
91. Grady MS, Howard MA, Jane JA, et al. Use of the Philadelphia collar as an alternative to the halo vest in patients with C-2, C-3 fractures. *Neurosurgery* 1986;18:151–156.
92. Greene KA, Dickman CA, Marciano FF, et al. Acute axis fractures. Analysis of management and outcome in 340 consecutive cases. *Spine* 1997;22:1843–1852.
93. Moon MS, Moon JL, Moon YW, et al. Traumatic spondylolisthesis of the axis: 42 cases. *Bull Hosp J Dis* 2001–2002;60(2):61–66.
94. Verheggen R, Jansen J. Hangman's fracture: arguments in favor of surgical therapy for type II and III according to Edwards and Levine. *Surg Neurol* 1998;49:253–261, discussion 261–262.
95. Arand M, Neller S, Kinzl L, et al. The traumatic spondylolisthesis of the axis. A biomechanical in vitro evaluation of an instability model and clinical relevant constructs for stabilization. *Clin Biomech* 2002;17:432–438.
96. Fujimura Y, Nishi Y, Kobayashi K. Classification and treatment of axis body fractures. *J Orthop Trauma* 1996;10:536–540.
97. Ferrera PC, Bartfield JM. Traumatic atlanto-occipital dislocation: a potentially survivable injury. *Am J Emerg Med* 1996;14:291–296.
98. Friedman D, Flanders A, Thomas C, et al. Vertebral artery injury after acute cervical spine trauma: rate of occurrence as detected by MR angiography and assessment of clinical consequences. *AJR Am J Roentgenol* 1995;164:443–447.

CHAPTER 34

Lower Cervical Spine Injury

Kamran Aflatoon and John J. Carbone

Spine fractures and spinal cord injury were first reported more than 5,000 years ago in the Edwin surgical papyrus (1). This injury was described as an ailment that should not be treated because of its grave prognosis. Until the first century A.D., therefore, such injuries, primarily the result of direct blows to the spine, were usually managed only with nonoperative, supportive care. The result was usually paralysis and eventual death because there was no way to stabilize the injured spine and prevent additional damage to the neural elements. However, in 600 A.D., Paul of Aegina reported the first spinal laminectomy; he found that removing spinal lamina splinters from the cord decompressed it, allowing healing (2).

By the mid-twentieth century, the perceived mechanism of injury began to change from direct blows and sword-induced trauma (producing bone splinters that penetrated the cord) to high-energy, indirect forces (e.g., high-energy motor vehicle crashes and diving accidents), resulting in ligamentous and bony injuries (3). This change in etiology resulted in a change in treatment focus: the philosophy of laminectomy for spinal fracture and cord injury evolved to a philosophy of stabilization. Despite recent advances in diagnostic and treatment techniques, such traumatic injuries to the spine and spinal cord are common causes of substantial disability and death.

The purpose of this chapter is to define the epidemiology, types, treatment, and outcome of subaxial spine injury.

BACKGROUND: INCIDENCE AND DIAGNOSIS

Although traumatic spinal injuries are common worldwide, the exact incidence is difficult to determine. In the United States, more than 50,000 spinal fractures occur per year; one-fifth (10,000) of those injuries involve neurologic compromise. Approximately 75% of all spinal fractures occur in the cervical spine (4).

The diagnosis of spinal injury is often delayed, and the treatment is not uniformly established. The delay in diagnosis may occur because of the lack of obvious deformity on physical or radiographic examination. One study reported that of 300 cervical spine injuries, 100 were missed initially; the delays in diagnosis ranged from 1 day to 1 year (5). Other studies have confirmed these findings (6,7). The most common causes for misdiagnosis are concomitant head injury or alcohol intoxication.

The pattern of cervical spine injury differs according to a patient's age primarily because of differences in bone quality, mechanism of injury, and presence of degenerative changes, resulting in altered biomechanics (8,9). Upper cervical spine injury is more common in the elderly than in younger patients (10).

ANATOMY AND BIOMECHANICS

Subaxial Anatomy

The vertebral bodies in the subaxial spine are oval and have an anterior inferior slope. The superior surface of the body is concave because of the projection of bony ridges (the uncinate process) from the superior lateral aspects. The facet joints are oriented at an angle, with the inferior facet of the vertebra above covering the superior facet of the vertebra below. All spinous

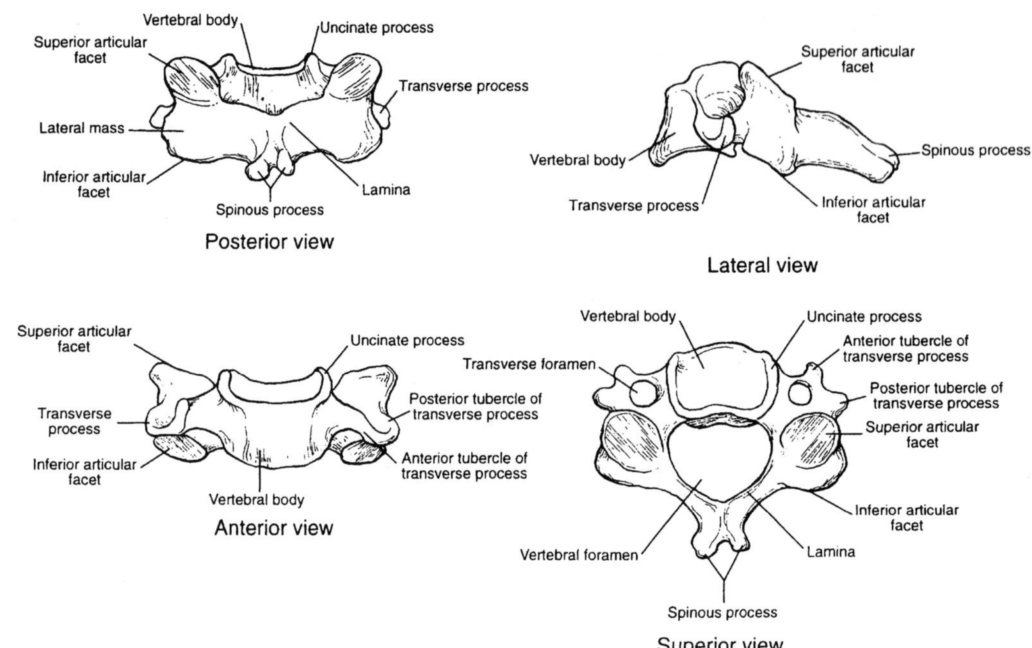

FIG. 1. The cervical vertebra in posterior, anterior, lateral, and superior views. (From An HS, Cotler JM, eds. *Spinal instrumentation*, 2nd ed. Philadelphia, Lippincott Williams & Wilkins, 1999:13, with permission.)

processes are directed posteriorly and inferiorly. The spinous process of C-7 (the vertebra prominens, the largest in the cervical spine) is not bifid. The last cervical vertebra, C-7, is a transitional vertebral body from the cervical spine to the thoracic spine. The lateral mass of C-7 is usually smaller than those of vertebrae in levels above (Fig. 1).

The vertebral artery is the first branch off the subclavian artery on either side. It travels through the foramen transversarium within the transverse processes of the cervical spine. At C-7, the artery passes through the foramen in only 10% of cadaveric specimens (11). The nerve roots pass just posterior to the vertebral artery (Fig. 2).

The anterior and posterior longitudinal ligaments are immediately opposed to the vertebral bodies anteriorly and posteriorly. The ligamentum nuchae starts from base of the skull and forms a broad ligament that acts as part of the posterior tension band. It becomes the supraspinous ligament distal to the C-7 spinous process. The ligamentum flavum travels between the adjacent laminas (Fig. 3).

The spinal cord begins as the continuation of the brainstem, extending from the foramen magnum and terminating at the upper lumbar spine (L1-2). There are eight cervical nerve roots exiting on each side of the cord. The first cervical nerve root exits above the ring of C-1. The eighth cervical nerve root exits between C-7 and T-1. Nerve roots exit directly lateral, passing over the pedicle, posterior to the joint of Luschka (or uncovertebral joint) and vertebral artery.

The cervical spine has several common anatomic anomalies. Failure of bony vertebral segmentation leading to large block vertebra (Klippel-Feil syndrome) is most frequently encountered between C3-4, C4-5, and C5-6. A hemivertebra and congenital absence of the posterior ring of C-1 may also be present. When one vertebral anomaly is identified, other defects, perhaps on other levels, may be present (12).

Stability

In 1983, Denis published his three-column theory of spinal stability for thoracolumbar injuries, which has proven useful in studying the cervical spine (13). According to this theory, each

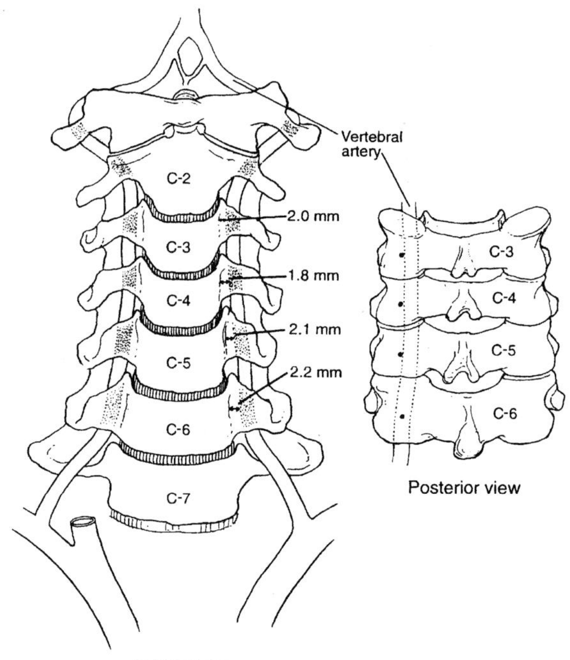

FIG. 2. The location of the transverse foramina on the anterior and posterior aspects of the cervical spine. (From An HS, Cotler JM, eds. *Spinal instrumentation*, 2nd ed. Philadelphia, Lippincott Williams & Wilkins, 1999:14, with permission.)

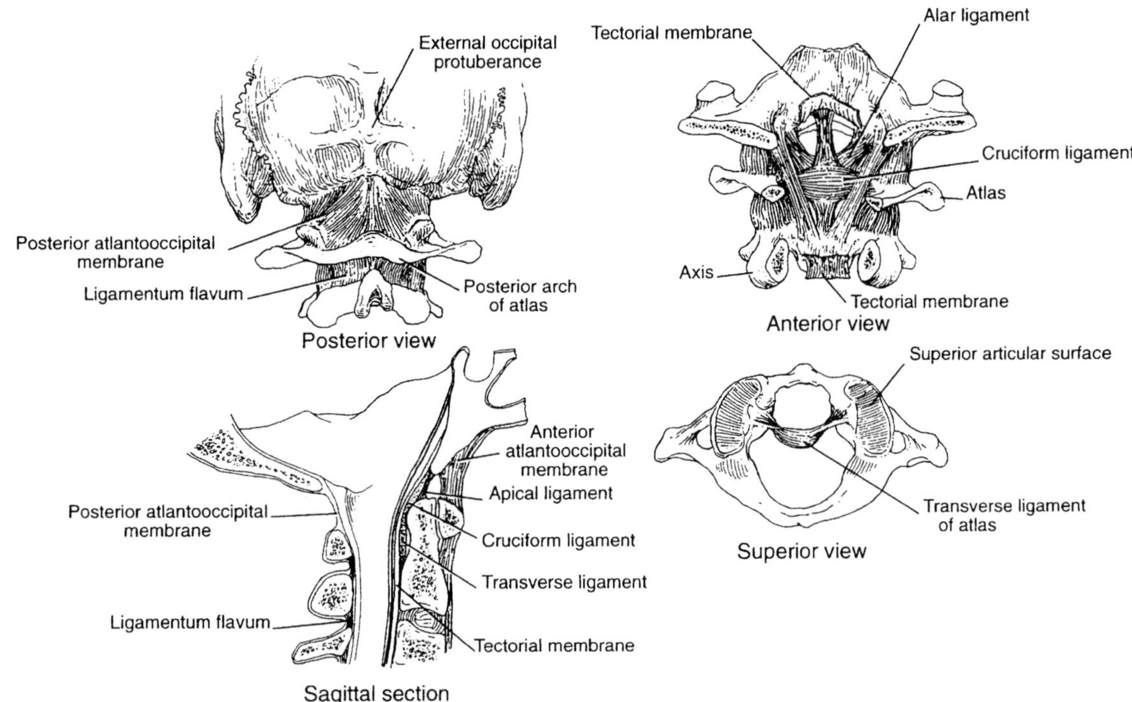

FIG. 3. The ligaments in the occipitocervical region in posterior, anterior, lateral, and superior views. (From An HS, Cotler JM, eds. *Spinal instrumentation*, 2nd ed. Philadelphia, Lippincott Williams & Wilkins, 1999:20, with permission.)

motion segment can be divided into anterior, middle, and posterior columns.

The middle column plays a critical role in providing stability for each motion segment. White and Panjabi showed that sectioning the posterior or anterior ligamentous structures alone did not render the spine unstable (14). Instability in flexion became evident only after the middle column (posterior longitudinal ligament, posterior annulus) was disrupted in conjunction with disruption of one of the other two columns. Similarly, instability in extension became evident after both anterior and middle columns were disrupted. Conceptually, instability is related to the compromise of any two columns.

EVALUATION OF THE INJURED PATIENT

At the Scene

Care of a patient with traumatic spinal injury starts at the scene of the accident. Rescue team members are taught to assume that every patient has a spinal injury. When injury is possible, the patient's neck is stabilized in a cervical collar, and the patient is transported on a rigid spine board or stretcher.

In the Emergency Room

Physical and Radiographic Assessment

Patients with possible spine injury (as determined by mechanism of injury or history of loss of consciousness, presence of closed head injury, etc.) should undergo systematic evaluation in the emergency department. A standard trauma protocol should be implemented, followed by radiographic screening (anteroposterior and lateral cervical spine, chest, and pelvis) and physical examination (15). When possible, the history and mechanism of injury should be obtained from the patient and from the rescue team members.

The spine is examined from the cervical to the sacral region. The anterior portion of the cervical collar is removed, and the neck is examined for tenderness or bruises. The posterior aspect of the neck is palpated for spinal tenderness. The patient may be asked for voluntary movement of his neck. If such movement causes pain, the collar is replaced and no additional manipulation or neck motion is allowed until imaging has documented the absence of injury. The patient is then log rolled for inspection of the rest of the spine. After complete assessment, including neurologic rectal evaluation, the patient is gently rolled back to the resting supine position. Pressure sore precautions should begin immediately in the patient with neurologic impairment.

Neurologic Examination

A thorough neurologic examination, including sensory, motor, and reflex evaluation, should be documented. The examiner should be familiar with sensory dermatomes of the upper and lower extremities. The sensory examination should include: pinprick, temperature, and light touch for spinothalamic tracts; and vibration and proprioception for assessment of the posterior column. An important part of this examination is the sensory and motor examinations of the perianal region, which is supplied by the lower sacral roots (S2-5). For patients with partial neurologic deficit, perianal sensation may be a prognostic indicator (16,17).

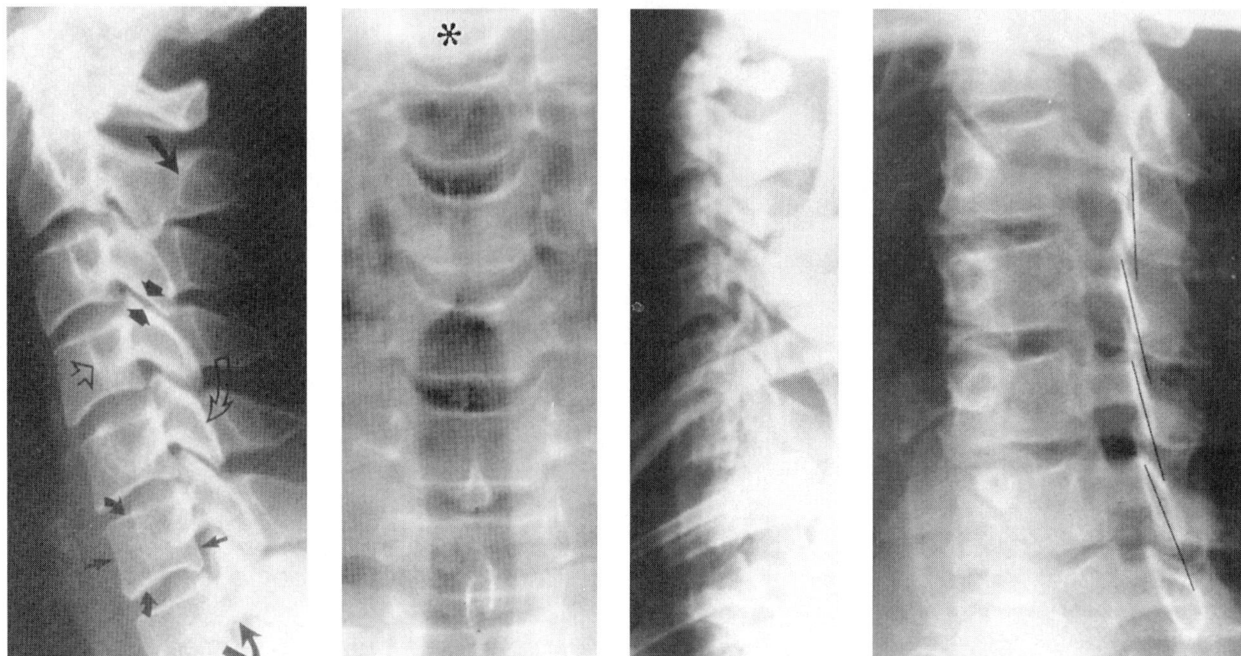

FIG. 4. A: Lateral view. Note anterior longitudinal, posterior longitudinal, and sublaminar lines. In the left column, from top to bottom, the open arrow indicates the vertebral body, the downward curved filled arrow indicates the end-plate, the small filled arrow shows the anterior longitudinal line, and the upward curved arrow shows the end-plate. In the right column, from top to bottom, the large filled arrow indicates the sublaminar line, the pair of filled arrows designates the facet joint, the curved open arrow shows the lateral mass, the small filled arrow indicates the posterior longitudinal line, and the large curved filled arrow indicates the pedicle. **B:** Anteroposterior view. Note the spacing of the uncovertebral joints and the alignment of the spinous process. Asterisk denotes the midline for alignment comparison. **C:** The swimmer's view allows observation of the cervicothoracic junction. **D:** Trauma oblique view highlights the foramen and facet joints.

A complete motor examination of the upper and lower extremities should be documented. Motor strength is evaluated and recorded according to a 0- to 5-point grading scale of the American Spinal Injury Association (18). Rectal examination, including sensory and resting tone and volitional contractility, is an integral part of motor examination.

Reflex examination completes the neurologic examination. The bulbocavernosus reflex may be helpful while evaluating patients for spinal shock. This reflex can be elicited by stimulating the glans penis or clitoris with the one hand, while examining for anal sphincter contraction with the other. A patient presenting with complete neurologic deficit (lack of motor, sensory, and reflex functions) may be suffering from spinal shock, which may be present during the first 24 to 48 hours after spinal injury. The neurologic status of a patient in spinal shock cannot be reliably determined. The return of the bulbocavernosus reflex signifies the resolution of spinal shock. In patients with conus level injuries, the reflex may never return.

Diagnostic Studies

Plain Radiographs

Radiographic series include anteroposterior (AP), open mouth, and lateral views. Lateral radiograph of the cervical spine should visualize the entire region from the occipitocervical to cervicothoracic junction. If the cervicothoracic area is not well visualized because of the patient's body habitus, a swimmer's view should be obtained. The swimmer's view is obtained by abducting one arm to 180 degrees and the other arm pulled down along the side with the x-ray beam directed at a 60-degree oblique angle (Fig. 4).

Radiographic imaging of the cervical spine may be limited, and detection of the injury is often subtle. Woodring and Lee (19) reported that 67% of cervical spine fractures and 45% of cervical spine subluxations and dislocations were not detected by routine cross-table lateral radiographs in the emergency department.

Plain radiographic findings that may provide clues for spinal instability include facet joint widening, tear-drop fracture (shear fracture of the anterior 20% of the vertebral body), angulation more than 11 degrees between adjacent segments, anterior or posterior translation more than 3.5 mm, spinous process widening on the lateral view, malalignment of the spinous processes on the AP view, rotation of the facets on the lateral view (bow tie sign), or tilting of the vertebrae on the AP view. There are several radiographic findings that indicate the need for magnetic resonance imaging (MRI) or computed tomography (CT) scans: precervical soft-tissue widening, minimal compression fracture of the vertebral body, nondisplaced fracture through the vertebra, or avulsion fractures at the insertion of spinal ligaments. Precervical soft-tissue widening may be a clue to occult spinal fracture that is not visualized radiographically. One retrospective study of patients presenting to a level I trauma center showed a 66% sensitivity when the soft tissue in front of C-3 measured more than 4 mm (20). There were no differences between soft-tissue expansion anterior to C-3 for upper versus lower cervical spine injuries (20).

Dynamic Radiographs

In some institutions, stress radiographs are obtained only when the patient continues to have neck pain after the spine has been found to be free of major injuries. Before obtaining the films, a delay of 7 to 14 days may be necessary to allow resolution of acute muscle spasm. Ligamentous injuries may be assessed using lateral flexion/extension radiographs. The radiographs should be closely scrutinized for slippage of one vertebra over the other (>3.5 mm), angulation of one body compared with the other (11 degrees), facet joint widening, and nonuniform interspinous widening.

Computed Tomography Scan

If a patient has substantial pain and the plain radiographs are negative, then a CT scan may be obtained to identify fractures not visualized on plain radiographs. Two-dimensional reconstruction images may also clearly highlight fractures that were not obvious on routine axial images. High rates of false-negative findings in the acute trauma setting have been reported [46% in one study (21)]; therefore, an experienced physician should evaluate these images.

Magnetic Resonance Imaging Scan

MRI may help identify injuries to the disc, ligaments, and spinal cord, as well as help exclude other fractures (22,23). It is the imaging study of choice for patients with ankylosing spondylitis.

Ligamentous abnormalities are evaluated on sagittal T2-weighted images. Focal hyperintensity in the region of the interspinous ligaments and splaying of the spinous processes may reflect injury to the posterior ligamentous structures. Disruption of the posterior longitudinal ligament is suggested when there is an abrupt discontinuity of the linear signal void directly behind the vertebral body (22).

Patients with facet dislocation and intact neurologic status may undergo MRI before reduction. If a large disc herniation is present, the process of reduction may decrease the available space for the cord and cause neurologic injury.

Types of Injuries

Several classifications have been proposed for determining the mechanism of injury to the spine. The commonly used classification by Allen and colleagues is based on the position of the neck at the time of the injury and is divided into six categories (24) (Table 1). Because injuries to the spine may take place in multiple planes, others suggest there is no single universal classification for cervical spine injuries (25).

Compression Fracture

Compression-flexion forces may cause an anterior wedge fracture. This injury is commonly seen in the lower cervical spine (C4-5 or C5-6). A subtle radiographic feature is a 3-mm difference in the anterior height of the vertebral body compared with the posterior height. The deformity is most commonly secondary to failure of the superior end-plate (stage 1). The degree of compression and deformity is a result of the magnitude of the injuring force and the strength of the bone. These injuries generally do not compromise the neural canal.

Compressive injuries to the spine are based on the specific force vectors producing the injury. When compression is combined with flexion, the typical compression fracture is produced,

TABLE 1. *Types and characteristics of injuries*

Type/ stages	Characteristics
Compression flexion (CF)	
CFS1	Intact posterior ligaments with blunting of the anterior/superior vertebral end-plate
CFS2	CFS1 plus beaking of the anterior/inferior vertebral body with decreased body height
CFS3	CFS2 plus beak fracture
CFS4	All above injuries plus <3-mm displacement at the fracture site
CFS5	CFS3 with displacement of the vertebral body into the canal. Complete ligamentous disruption
Vertical compression (VC)	
VCS1	Superior or inferior end-plate fracture with cupping of the central portion
VCS2	Fracture of both end-plates with minimal displacement
VCS3	VCS2 with fragmentation and displacement of the vertebral body
Distraction flexion (DF)	
DFS1	Facet subluxation with divergence of the spinous process
DFS2	Unilateral facet dislocation
DFS3	Bilateral facet dislocation
DFS4	Complete vertebral body displacement anterior to the level below
Compression extension (CE)	
CES1	Unilateral vertebral arch fracture
CES2	Bilateral lamina fracture at contiguous levels
CES3	Bilateral arch fracture without displacement of the body
CES4	Bilateral arch fracture with partial displacement of the body
CES5	Bilateral arch fracture with complete vertebral body displacement
Distraction extension (DE)	
DES1	Widened disc space or transverse fracture through the vertebral body
DES2	DES1 with posterior ligamentous disruption
Lateral flexion (LF)	
LFS1	Unilateral arch fracture with an asymmetric compression fracture of the body
LFS2	Ipsilateral arch fracture with displacement and contralateral ligamentous disruption

most commonly affecting C-4, C-5, and C-6. Five stages are identified as shown in Table 1; increasing stages above stage III are associated with an increased risk of instability. Stage I is a subtle injury and may sometimes only be identified by comparing the anterior to the posterior height of the vertebral body. A 3-mm reduction in the anterior height is suggestive of the injury that is commonly secondary to failure of the superior end-plate with blunting. Stage II has the characteristic anterior vertebral body wedging and beaking of the anterior/inferior vertebral body. Stage III fractures have all of the features of stage II, but a beak fracture is evident. Stage IV and stage V injuries are associated with translational deformities and represent three-column disruptions. In stage IV, there is a beak fracture with subluxation greater than 3 mm, whereas in stage V, the subluxation exceeds 5 mm, and there is ligamentous instability and the vertebral body is displaced into the canal.

Stage I and II as purely bony injuries can be treated effectively with a rigid cervical orthosis for a period of 8 to 12 weeks. Stage III and IV injuries can also be treated by bracing but require careful monitoring to assess any further displacement. If that occurs, fusion is recommended. Stage V fractures are highly unstable and are best treated initially in skeletal traction followed by surgical fusion.

Vertebral Compression Fractures

Vertebral compression fractures are caused by direct axial loading with the injury vector vertically oriented, as opposed to an element of flexion or extension. Three stages have been identified. Stage I affects only the superior or inferior end-plate of the affected vertebra; stage II indicates fractures of both the superior and inferior end-plates, whereas stage III is associated with bursting of the vertebral body in a centrifugal pattern. This injury mechanism is much more common in upper cervical spine fractures and accounts for only 15% of the injuries affecting the lower cervical spine (26). Stages I and II are stable and can be managed with cervical orthosis. Stage III is similar to a burst fracture and when associated with neurologic defects is best managed with vertebral corpectomy and arthrodesis.

Treatment of Compression Fracture

The first two stages of compression fractures are bony injuries rather than ligamentous and may be treated effectively with a rigid cervical orthosis for 8 to 12 weeks. The third stage of this injury, with disruption and displacement of the vertebral body, requires anterior corpectomy and arthrodesis. If the patient has posterior tenderness, ligament injury should be suspected as well.

Vertebral Body Burst Fracture

Vertebral body burst fractures may be a result of compression-flexion or vertical compression forces. The unstable cervical flexion tear-drop fracture (the "quadrangular" fracture) is characterized by anterior column failure in flexion and posterior column failure in tension. This fracture pattern consists of a coronal split through the ventral portion of the vertebral body, with dorsal displacement of the remaining vertebral body that leads to narrowing of the spinal canal. The posterior column failure through tension leads to disruption of posterior ligamentous structures and possible dislocation of the facet joints.

In a retrospective study, Koivikko and colleagues (27) compared outcomes in patients with burst injuries treated surgically versus those treated nonoperatively. They reported that patients in the operative group had at least one more Frankel grade of improvement than did patients in the nonoperative group, as well as statistically significant improvements in kyphotic deformity and spinal canal encroachment.

Fractures with cord compression and neurologic deficit should be managed with anterior corpectomy and fusion. The defect may be filled with a mesh cage, structural allograft, or autograft. Autograft has been shown to have high risk for nonunion compared with other types of structural grafts (27–29). Burst fractures without neurologic deficit may be managed either with anterior corpectomy and arthrodesis or posterior arthrodesis with lateral mass screws to the adjacent levels.

Distraction-Flexion Injuries

Distraction-flexion force may lead to facet dislocation in the lower cervical spine. This injury pattern is often seen as a result of motor vehicle accident or fall from a height. The lower cervical spine is the most common location (C5-6 or C6-7) (30). The spectrum of injury includes joint subluxation, perched facets, unilateral dislocation, and bilateral dislocation. A facet fracture and vertebral body fracture may also be present as part of these injuries.

Unilateral Facet Dislocation

On dislocation of the facet joint, the facet of the cephalad vertebra comes to rest anterior to the superior caudad vertebra and within the neuroforamen at that level. Associated facet fractures are reported to occur in 47 to 73% of patients (31–33). Radiculopathy is present in as many as 73%, whereas spinal cord injury is present in 12% (34).

Disc herniation is reported in as many as 46% of patients with facet subluxation and unilateral facet dislocation (35,36). Neurologic deterioration may occur after closed reduction when a herniated cervical disc is part of the injury (35,37). In a study of 68 patients with subluxation or dislocation of a cervical facet, six patients (9%) had marked protrusion of disc material into the spinal canal (37). All six patients suffered a neurologic injury after attempted reduction of the facet joint. Narrowed disc space, nonreduced dislocations, or increasing symptoms, especially during attempted reduction, may be valuable indicators of the presence of an extruded disc. One multicenter pilot study on the surgical treatment of acute spinal cord injury reported an 8.1% rate of neurologic deterioration after reduction; however, it is not clear if any of those cases were related to disc herniation (38). Shapiro and colleagues (34) showed immediate improvement of radicular symptoms after reduction and gradual improvement in those who sustained spinal cord injury secondary to cord compression caused by disc herniation.

After closed reduction, halo immobilization has been reported to have a 38 to 100% risk for failure (39–42). In general, unilateral facet injuries have substantial associated soft-tissue disruption, hence the high frequency of failure with halo management. Internal fixation is a better treatment alternative (34,43). For patients with large extruded disc herniation, anterior corpectomy or discectomy should be performed before reduction and arthrodesis of the affected motion segment. The reduction may be done through the anterior or posterior approach (4,34,44,45).

Bilateral Facet Dislocation

Among all cervical fractures, bilateral facet dislocation has the highest rate of neurologic compromise. Razack and colleagues reported an 87% risk for spinal cord injury and a 9% risk of radiculopathy at presentation (45). There are reports of neurologic worsening after closed reduction (37,46,47).

Patients with incomplete spinal cord injury or progressive neurologic deficit present a special challenge to the surgeon because recovery of neurologic function is time-dependent. In a retrospective study of 82 patients with facet dislocation who underwent immediate closed reduction before MRI imaging, Grant and colleagues found that 58% of their patients had spinal cord injury, 13% had cervical radiculopathy, 9% had transient deficit, and 22% were neurologically intact (36). Only one patient had neurologic deterioration 6 hours after closed reduction. The prevalence of disc herniation and disruption were 22% and 24%, respectively. Those authors did not recommend obtaining MRI images before reduction in patients with neurologic deficit.

These injuries should be treated with closed reduction. Closed reduction may be performed with the patient awake as follows: Longitudinal traction with Gardner-Wells or halo ring applied. Initially, 10 to 15 lb of traction are applied, and a lateral cervical spine radiograph is obtained. Weights are added in 10-lb increments with a 10- to 15-minute fatigue time between additions. Neurologic and radiographic examinations are performed after each increment. Direct manipulation of the neck should be avoided, except by those experienced in that technique. To facilitate the reduction and change the force vector, bolsters may be used under each or both shoulders. If the closed reduction maneuver fails, an operative reduction should be performed. After posterior exposure, an elevator may be placed between the facet joints. The dislocated vertebra is manipulated by its spinous process. The reduction maneuver is first rostral traction and then posterior and caudal traction of the spinous process, which permits bilateral reduction of the facet joints. If there is any difficulty in achieving reduction, the superior aspect of the inferior facet may be resected.

Fracture of Posterior Elements

Fracture of posterior elements as a mechanism for injury is variable and may result from lateral flexion or be a component of hyperextension injury. A floating lateral mass or articular process fracture is a result of ipsilateral pedicle and lamina fracture. When combined with ligamentous and disc injury, this fracture may be unstable, with forward or rotational subluxation of the vertebral body. Some patients may experience radicular symptoms secondary to compression of the exiting nerve root.

Plain radiographs are not very sensitive in detecting this type of injury (19,43). In a retrospective study of 24 patients with unilateral facet fracture, Halliday and colleagues found that only 6 patients had evidence of bony abnormality on the initial radiographs (43). They found CT scan to be most sensitive in detection of the fracture pattern and MRI to be the most sensitive for detection of soft-tissue injury.

In another retrospective study, Lifeso and colleagues reported that no patient healed who was treated nonoperatively (rigid cervical collar or halo), whereas Bucholz and colleagues reported a 17% failure rate (failure defined as subluxation of the vertebral body after removal of the vest) with the use of a halo vest for facet fractures (4,41). Lifeso et al. also showed that posterior cervical arthrodesis with lateral mass screws resulted in 45% inadequate outcomes with respect to progression (loss of correction) of kyphotic deformity or continued instability. In contrast, all patients who had anterior arthrodesis for this fracture pattern had satisfactory functional outcomes and complete fusion.

Hyperextension Injury

A hyperextension injury results from a distraction-extension (DE) force and is commonly associated with an anterior blow to the head and face secondary to a fall or a motor vehicle accident. This injury accounts for 8 to 22% of subaxial injuries (29,48,49). According to the classification of Allen et al., there are two stages of injury pattern (24). Distraction-extension stage (DES) 1, the mildest form of this injury, is a disruption of the anterior longitudinal ligament and the anterior portion of the disc. Radiographs may show a small avulsion fracture from the anterior-inferior aspect of the vertebral body, which is secondary to failure of the anterior longitudinal ligament at its insertion to the bone. MRI is useful in identifying the extent of the soft-tissue injury.

Continued DE force may lead to failure of the posterior column, causing a greater instability pattern referred to as *DES 2*. The vertebral body may dislocate posteriorly with compression of the spinal cord between the stable lamina below and the mobile posterior inferior edge of the vertebral body above (50). Patients with ankylosing spondylitis or diffuse idiopathic skeletal hyperostosis are predisposed to this injury because of reduced spinal mobility.

DES 1 with minimal disc disruption may be treated nonoperatively (rigid cervical collar). When there is complete disc disruption, anterior cervical arthrodesis may yield superior results (30). In a comparison of halo treatment versus anterior corpectomy and arthrodesis, Fisher and colleagues reported that 24 patients treated with a halo had a mean kyphotic deformity of 11.4 degrees; five of the 24 failed, and four of these ultimately required a corpectomy and arthrodesis (51). The kyphotic deformity in the corpectomy group was 3.5 degrees; no patient had construct failure (51).

DES 2 is an extensive injury that may require arthrodesis. Vaccaro and colleagues recommended approaching this injury posteriorly first to obtain the reduction, then performing anterior discectomy and arthrodesis (30). The authors warned against excessive anterior distraction: two patients suffered from neurologic deterioration intraoperatively because the spine was overdistracted by the graft.

Fractures in Patients with Ankylosing Spondylitis

Ankylosing spondylitis is a seronegative inflammatory disorder affecting the axial skeleton. Patients with this condition develop autofusion of the spine through the discovertebral joints, leading to decreased range of motion of the spine. Radio-

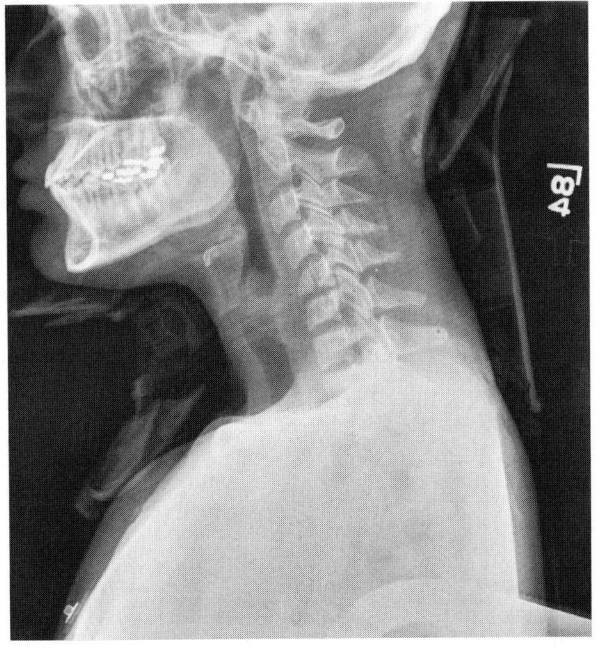

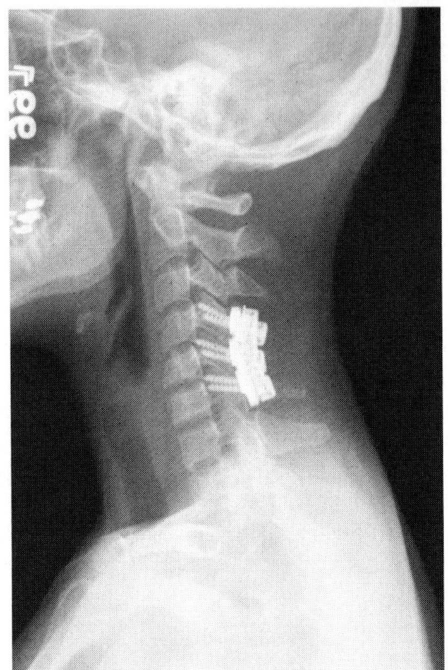

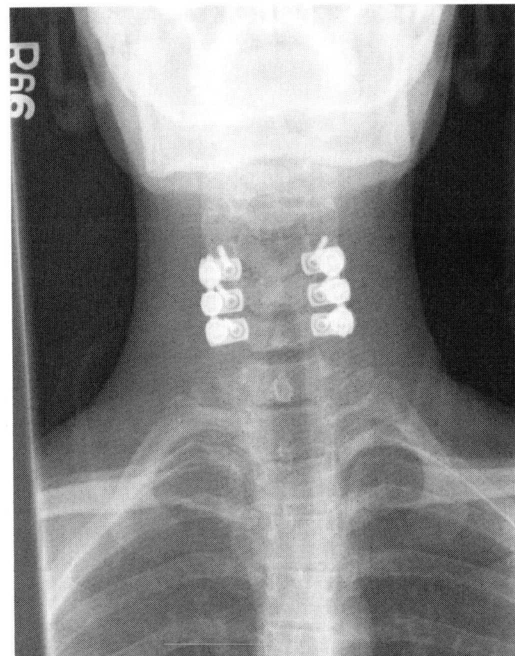

FIG. 5. C-5 burst fracture. **A:** Lateral preoperative view. **B:** Lateral postoperative view of the fracture stabilized with posterior instrumentation. **C:** Posterior fixation.

graphic examination shows an abundance of bone, but it is osteoporotic (52).

Patients with ankylosing spondylitis have a much higher (3.5 times) risk of spinal fractures than the normal population (53). Such patients also have a 11.4 times higher risk of spinal cord injury after sustaining a spine fracture (54,55). The most common cause of spinal fracture in this group is a low-energy fall. Neck pain in such patients should mandate additional study despite the history of minor trauma.

The fracture pattern is commonly transverse and may not be apparent on plain radiographs. An MRI best defines this injury. It is also important to obtain a sagittal screening MRI of the entire spine to exclude fractures at other levels.

TREATMENT OPTIONS

Operative Modalities and Indications

The first recorded operative treatment for spinal injury was a laminectomy in the seventh century. Today, improved operative techniques have led to major advances in spinal stabilization. The development of dedicated spinal cord injury centers and improved postoperative rehabilitation have led to significant improvement in functional outcome.

The treatment of cervical spine fractures and dislocations has several goals, including reduction of the deformity and stabilization, minimizing or decreasing neurologic injury, and early

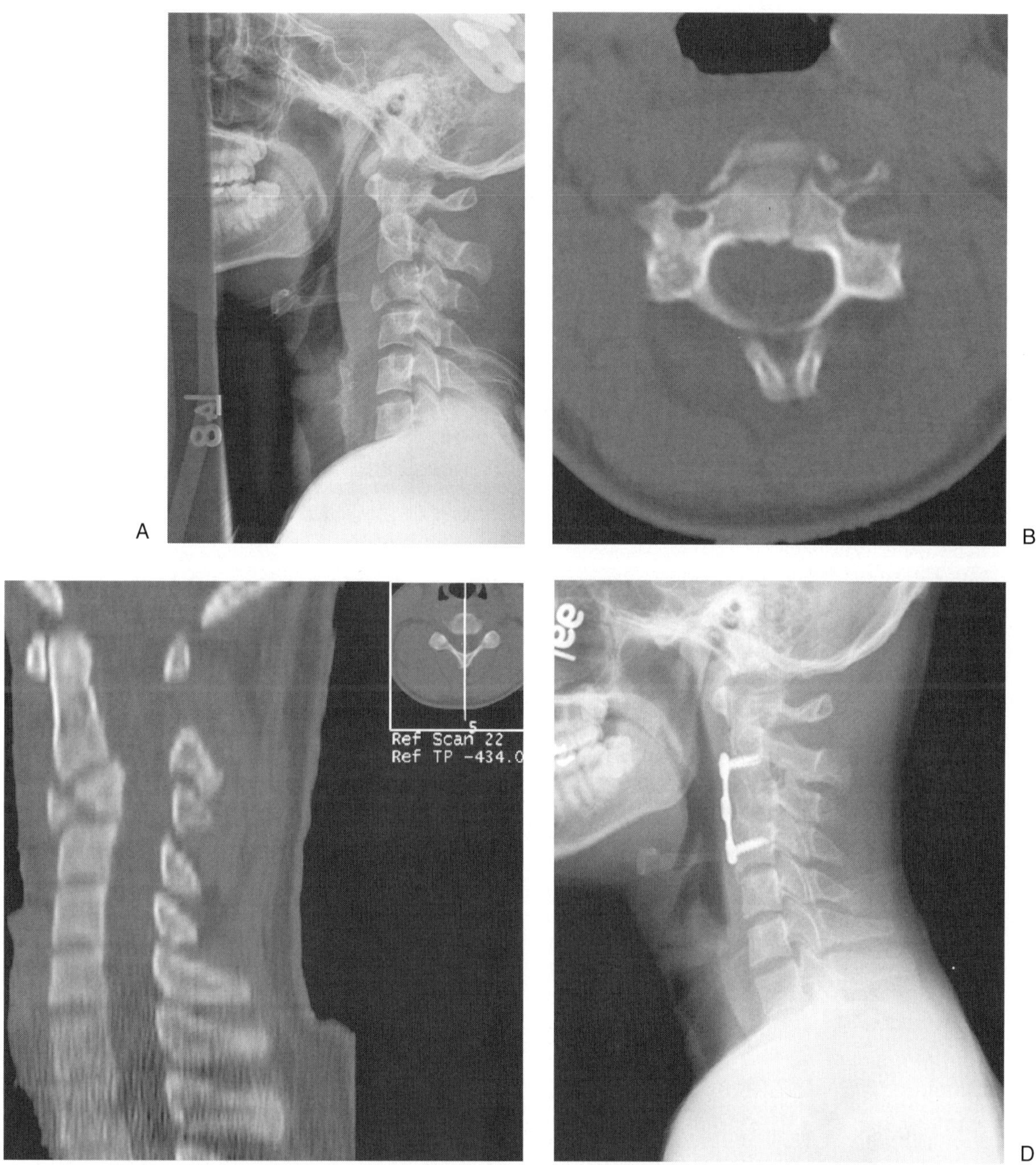

FIG. 6. C-3 burst fracture. **A:** Preoperative lateral view. **B:** Preoperative axial computed tomography (CT) scan. **C:** CT reconstruction. **D:** Healing after anterior corpectomy and plating.

rehabilitation. The choice of treatment modality is based on the anatomy of the fracture and the experience of the surgeon.

Posterior Segmental Fixation

Modern posterior segmental fixation provides stable flexion tension band with cantilever support, increased rotational stability, and buttressing in extension. The principal indications for its use include ligamentous or osseous instability of the vertebral elements. The instability may be due to failed prior surgery, trauma, or tumor.

Koh and colleagues evaluated the biomechanical strength of posterior lateral mass screw fixation and anterior arthrodesis in patients with distraction-flexion injury (56). They showed superior biomechanical advantages with posterior fixation for patients with distraction injuries or burst fractures.

The approach is through a midline incision at the levels of injury. If the midline exposure is kept within the ligamentum nuchae, blood loss can be minimal in this relatively avascular region.

During the exposure, subperiosteal dissection should extend to the lateral edge of each lateral mass, taking care to protect the joint capsule superior and inferior to the level of injury. The medial border is the groove formed by the junction of the lamina and the lateral mass. The pilot hole for the insertion of the screw should start lateral to this groove using techniques as described by Jeanneret et al. (Magerl's technique) and Roy-Camille et al. (57,58).

Roy-Camille and colleagues described the original technique for insertion of lateral mass screw (58). The pilot hole is drilled at the junction of the upper and middle third of the lateral mass in the midline and is directed 10 degrees laterally and perpendicular to the posterior cortex of the lateral mass in sagittal direction. The major disadvantage of this technique is that the screw length is relatively short. With the Magerl technique (as described by Jeanneret et al.), the pilot hole is drilled 2 mm medial to the center of the lateral mass (57). The screw is oriented 30 to 40 degrees cranially and 20 to 25 degrees laterally as verified with lateral fluoroscopic guidance. Penetration of the facet joint with the screw should be avoided. An described an alternative technique (59). Both of the latter two techniques offer a longer screw and purchase in the bone compared with the Roy-Camille technique (60).

After the starting point is identified, the path is drilled in unicortical or bicortical fashion. The screw length is identified using a depth gauge. The outer cortex is tapped using an appropriate tap. The proper length screw is then inserted in the same direction as the drill. Each step may be checked under fluoroscopy.

To prepare for the arthrodesis, the facet joints, spinous processes, and laminar are denuded of cartilage with a high-speed burr or curette. Appropriate-length rods or plates are contoured for each side and then inserted with appropriate surgical technique for the posterior cervical or lateral mass system selected. Although plates or rods may be used to connect the screws, the authors prefer segmental rods/screws for their ease of application (Fig. 5). An iliac crest bone graft is then placed over the lamina and denuded facets. The wound is closed over a suction drain.

Postoperatively, the patient's neck is immobilized using a rigid cervical orthosis for a period of time, based on the pathology and the quality of fixation. The patient may perform physical therapy exercises while in the cervical collar, which can be removed for hygienic purposes.

Anterior Fixation

Anterior plating may be used for anterior column support for patients with severe compression fracture or instability or with burst fractures. The plate functions as a tension band in extension and as a buttress plate in flexion. After corpectomy for decompression of the spinal canal, the area is filled with a strut graft or a cage, and a plate is used as a load-sharing mechanism. Anterior plating alone offers less rigid fixation for distraction-flexion injuries in which there is disruption of the posterior elements (56).

When cervical spine instability is associated with a minimal vertebral body compression, a standard anterior approach is used. Discectomy above or below the compressed vertebral body is followed by placement of grafts in the appropriate disc spaces. It is critical to fashion the graft in lordosis, correcting the deformity. An appropriately sized plate is used in the construct to obtain rigid stability.

Burst fracture with canal compromise is best treated with corpectomy for canal decompression (Fig. 6). The defect may be filled using a cage, structural allograft, or autograft (61). Of the several available plating systems, the authors prefer plates that can be locked to the screw. Such plates permit the use of unicortical screws and offer better biomechanical stability than non-locking plates (62,63). The disadvantage of a fixed-angle locking plate is that no axial compression is possible.

Wiring Techniques

Although recent advancements in posterior cervical fixation have decreased the use of wiring techniques, wiring techniques offer the advantages of ease of application and safety. In addition, they may be used to enhance other posterior fixation techniques.

A hole is made on each side of the spinous process at its base, and a towel clamp is used to connect the holes. A 1.2-mm wire is passed through the hole, brought around the spinous process of the lower level, and tightened. After decortication of the arthrodesis segment, bone graft is added and the wound is closed over a suction drain (64).

CONCLUSION

The use of spinal instrumentation in the treatment of subaxial cervical spine instability and deformity is a rapidly evolving area in spinal surgery. The expanded use of posterior fixed-angle segmental systems shows great promise of improved care for patients with bony and neurologic injury to the cervical spine.

REFERENCES

1. Garfin SR, Blair B, Eismont FJ, et al. Thoracic and upper lumbar spine injuries. In: Browner BD, Jupiter JB, Levine AM, Trafton PG, eds. *Skeletal trauma: fractures, dislocations, ligamentous injuries*, 2nd ed. Philadelphia: WB Saunders, 1998:947–1034.
2. Shannon E, MacMillan M. Fractures and dislocations of the cervical spine. In: Rockwood CA Jr, Green DP, Bucholz RW, Heckman JD, eds. *Rockwood and Green's fractures in adults*, 4th ed. Philadelphia: JB Lippincott Co, 1996:1473–1571.
3. Fife D, Kraus J. Anatomic location of spinal cord injury. Relationship to the cause of injury. *Spine* 1986;11(1):2–5.
4. Lifeso RM, Colucci MA. Anterior fusion for rotationally unstable cervical spine fractures. *Spine* 2000;25(16):2028–2034.
5. Bohlman HH. Acute fractures and dislocations of the cervical spine. An analysis of three hundred hospitalized patients and review of the literature. *J Bone Joint Surg Am* 1979;61A(8):1119–1142.
6. Schenarts PJ, Diaz J, Kaiser C, et al. Prospective comparison of admission computed tomographic scan and plain films of the upper cervical spine in trauma patients with altered mental status. *J Trauma* 2001;51(4):663–668.
7. Stabler A, Eck J, Penning R, et al. Cervical spine: postmortem assessment of accident injuries—comparison of radiographic, MR imaging, anatomic, and pathologic findings. *Radiology* 2001;221(2):340–346.
8. Hu R, Mustard CA, Burns C. Epidemiology of incident spinal fracture in a complete population. *Spine* 1996;21(4):492–499.
9. Hanson JA, Blackmore CC, Mann FA, et al. Cervical spine injury: a clinical decision rule to identify high-risk patients for helical CT screening. *AJR Am J Roentgenol* 2000;174(3):713–717.
10. Lomoschitz FM, Blackmore CC, Mirza SK, et al. Cervical spine injuries in patients 65 years old and older: epidemiologic analysis regarding the effects of age and injury mechanism on distribution, type, and stability of injuries. *AJR Am J Roentgenol* 2002;178(3):573–577.
11. Erbil KM, Sargon MF, Celik HH, et al. A study of variations of transverse foramens of cervical vertebras in human: accessory foramina in shape and number. *Morphologie* 2001;85(269):23–24.

12. Evans JA, Vitez M, Czeizel A. Congenital abnormalities associated with limb deficiency defects: a population study based on cases from the Hungarian Congenital Malformation Registry (1975–1984). *Am J Med Genet* 1994;49(1):52–66.
13. Denis F. The three-column spine and its significance in the classification of acute thoracolumbar spinal injuries. *Spine* 1983;8:817–831.
14. White AA III, Panjabi MM. Update on the evaluation of instability of the lower cervical spine. *AAOS: Instructional Course Lectures* 1987;36:513–520.
15. American College of Surgeons Committee on Trauma. *Advanced trauma life support program for doctors*, 6th ed. Chicago: American College of Surgeons, 1997.
16. Stauffer ES. Neurologic recovery following injuries to the cervical spinal cord and nerve roots. *Spine* 1984;9(5):532–534.
17. Stauffer ES. Spinal cord injury syndromes. *Semin Spine Surg* 1991;3(1):87–90.
18. American Spinal Injury Association. *International standards for neurological and functional classification of spinal cord injury, revised 1992*, Chicago: American Spinal Injury Association, 1992.
19. Woodring JH, Lee C. Limitations of cervical radiography in the evaluation of acute cervical trauma [see comments]. *J Trauma* 1993;34(1):32–39.
20. Herr CH, Ball PA, Sargent SK, Quinton HB. Sensitivity of prevertebral soft tissue measurement of C3 for detection of cervical spine fractures and dislocations. *Am J Emer Med* 1998;16(4):346–349.
21. Woodring JH, Lee C. The role and limitations of computed tomographic scanning in the evaluation of cervical trauma. *J Trauma* 1992;33(5):698–708.
22. el Khoury GY, Kathol MH, Daniel WW. Imaging of acute injuries of the cervical spine: value of plain radiography, CT, and MR imaging. *AJR Am J Roentgenol* 1995;164(1):43–50.
23. Katzberg RW, Benedetti PF, Drake CM, et al. Acute cervical spine injuries: prospective MR imaging assessment at a level 1 trauma center. *Radiology* 1999;213(1):203–212.
24. Allen BL Jr, Ferguson RL, Lehmann TR, et al. A mechanistic classification of closed, indirect fractures and dislocations of the lower cervical spine. *Spine* 1982;7(1):1–27.
25. Cusick JF, Yoganandan N, Pintar F, et al. Cervical spine injuries from high-velocity forces: a pathoanatomic and radiologic study. *J Spinal Disord* 1996;9(1):1–7.
26. Koivikko MP, Myllynen P, Karjalainen M, et al. Conservative and operative treatment in cervical burst fractures. *Arch Orthop Trauma Surg* 2000;120(7–8):448–451.
27. Fernyhough JC, White JI, LaRocca H. Fusion rates in multilevel cervical spondylosis comparing allograft fibula with autograft fibula in 126 patients. *Spine* 1991;16[10 Suppl]:S561–S564.
28. Zdeblick TA, Ducker TB. The use of freeze-dried allograft bone for anterior cervical fusions. *Spine* 1991;16(7):726–729.
29. Vaccaro AR, Cook CM, McCullen G, et al. Cervical trauma: rationale for selecting the appropriate fusion technique. *Orthop Clin North Am* 1998;29(4):745–754.
30. Vaccaro AR, Klein GR, Thaller JB, et al. Distraction extension injuries of the cervical spine. *J Spinal Disord* 2001;14(3):193–200.
31. Shapiro SA. Management of unilateral locked facet of the cervical spine. *Neurosurgery* 1993;33:832–837.
32. Benzel EC, Kesterson L. Posterior cervical interspinous compression wiring and fusion for mid to low cervical spinal injuries. *J Neurosurg* 1989;70(6):893–899.
33. Shanmuganathan K, Mirvis SE, Levine AM. Rotational injury of cervical facets: CT analysis of fracture patterns with implications for management and neurologic outcome. *AJR Am J Roentgenol* 1994;163:1165–1169.
34. Shapiro S, Snyder W, Kaufman K, et al. Outcome of 51 cases of unilateral locked cervical facets: interspinous braided cable for lateral mass plate fusion compared with interspinous wire and facet wiring with iliac crest. *J Neurosurg* 1999;91[1 Suppl]:19–24.
35. Rizzolo SJ, Piazza MR, Cotler JM, et al. Intervertebral disc injury complicating cervical spine trauma. *Spine* 1991;16:S187–S189.
36. Grant GA, Mirza SK, Chapman JR, et al. Risk of early closed reduction in cervical spine subluxation injuries. *J Neurosurg* 1999; 90[1 Suppl]:13–18.
37. Eismont FJ, Arena MJ, Green BA. Extrusion of an intervertebral disc associated with traumatic subluxation or dislocation of cervical facets. Case report. *J Bone Joint Surg Am* 1991;73A:1555–1560.
38. Weis JC, Cunningham BW, Kanayama M, et al. In vitro biomechanical comparison of multistrand cables with conventional cervical stabilization. *Spine* 1996;21(18):2108–2114.
39. Anderson PA, Budorick TE, Easton KB, et al. Failure of halo vest to prevent in vivo motion in patients with injured cervical spines. *Spine* 1991;16[10 Suppl]:S501–S505.
40. Beyer CA, Cabanela ME, Berquist TH. Unilateral facet dislocations and fracture-dislocations of the cervical spine. *J Bone Joint Surg Am* 1991;73B(6):977–981.
41. Bucholz RD, Cheung KC. Halo vest versus spinal fusion for cervical injury: evidence from an outcome study. *J Neurosurg* 1989;70 (6):884–892.
42. Sears W, Fazl M. Prediction of stability of cervical spine fracture managed in the halo vest and indications for surgical intervention. *J Neurosurg* 1990;72(3):426–432.
43. Halliday AL, Henderson BR, Hart BL, et al. The management of unilateral lateral mass/facet fractures of the subaxial cervical spine: the use of magnetic resonance imaging to predict instability. *Spine* 1997;22(22):2614–2621.
44. Abumi K, Shono Y, Kotani Y, et al. Indirect posterior reduction and fusion of the traumatic herniated disc by using a cervical pedicle screw system. *J Neurosurg* 2000;92[1 Suppl]:30–37.
45. Razack N, Green BA, Levi ADO. The management of traumatic cervical bilateral facet fracture-dislocations with unicortical anterior plates. *J Spinal Disord* 2000;13(5):374–381.
46. Ludwig SC, Vaccaro AR, Balderston RA, Cotler JM. Immediate quadriparesis after manipulation for bilateral cervical facet subluxation. A case report. *J Bone Joint Surg Am* 1997;79A(4):587–590.
47. Mahale YJ, Silver JR. Progressive paralysis after bilateral facet dislocation of the cervical spine. *J Bone Joint Surg Am* 1992;74B(2): 219–223.
48. de Oliveira JC. Anterior plate fixation of traumatic lesions of the lower cervical spine. *Spine* 1987;12(4):324–329.
49. Nazarian SM, Louis RP. Posterior internal fixation with screw plates in traumatic lesions of the cervical spine. *Spine* 1991;16:S64–S71.
50. Taylor AR. The mechanism of injury to the spinal cord in the neck without damage to the vertebral column. *J Bone Joint Surg Am* 1951;33B(4):543–547.
51. Fisher CG, Dvorak MFS, Leith J, et al. Comparison of outcomes for unstable lower cervical flexion teardrop fractures managed with halo thoracic vest versus anterior corpectomy and plating. *Spine* 2002;27(2):160–166.
52. Maillefert JF, Aho LS, El Maghraoui A, et al. Changes in bone density in patients with ankylosing spondylitis: a two-year follow-up study. *Osteoporos Int* 2001;12(7):605-609.
53. Hunter T, Dubo HI. Spinal fractures complicating ankylosing spondylitis. A long-term followup study. *Arthritis Rheum* 1983;26(6):751–759.
54. Fox MW, Onofrio BM, Kilgore JE. Neurological complications of ankylosing spondylitis. *J Neurosurg* 1993;78(6):871–878.
55. Weinstein PR, Karpman RR, Gall EP, et al. Spinal cord injury, spinal fracture, and spinal stenosis in ankylosing spondylitis. *J Neurosurg* 1982;57(5):609–616.
56. Koh YD, Lim TH, Won YJ, et al. A biomechanical comparison of modern anterior and posterior plate fixation of the cervical spine. *Spine* 2001;26(1):15–21.
57. Jeanneret B, Magerl F, Ward EH, et al. Posterior stabilization of the cervical spine with hook plates. *Spine* 1991;16:S56–S63.
58. Roy-Camille R, Saillant G, Mazel JC. Internal fixation of the unstable cervical spine by a posterior osteosynthesis with plates and screws. In: The Cervical Spine Research Society EC, ed. *The cervical spine*, 2nd ed. 1989:390–412.
59. An HS. Cervical spine trauma. *Spine* 1998;23(24):2713–2729.
60. Choueka J, Spivak JM, Kummer FJ, et al. Flexion failure of posterior cervical lateral mass screws. Influence of insertion technique and position. *Spine* 1996;21(4):462–468.
61. Das K, Couldwell WT, Sava G, et al. Use of cylindrical titanium mesh and locking plates in anterior cervical fusion. Technical note. *J Neurosurg* 2001;94[1 Suppl]:174–178.
62. Grubb MR, Currier BL, Shih JS, et al. Biomechanical evaluation of anterior cervical spine stabilization. *Spine* 1998;23(8):886–892.
63. Spivak JM, Chen D, Kummer FJ. The effect of locking fixation screws on the stability of anterior cervical plating. *Spine* 1999;24(4):334–338.
64. Ulrich C, Arand M, Nothwang J. Internal fixation on the lower cervical spine--biomechanics and clinical practice of procedures and implants. *Eur Spine J* 2001;10(2):88–100.

CHAPTER 35

Cervical Disc Disease

A. Axial-Mechanical Neck Pain and Cervical Degenerative Disease

Nicholas U. Ahn, Uri M. Ahn, Glenn M. Amundson, and Howard S. An

Axial or *mechanical neck pain* refers to neck pain that does not radiate into the upper extremities but is confined to the cervical area. Axial neck pain may take many forms; it may be unilateral or bilateral, cause headaches, or lead to stiffness in one or all directions of cervical motion. Although the vast majority of cases involve injury to the muscle or paraspinal soft tissues and resolve within 6 weeks of onset with conservative treatment alone, large population studies have demonstrated that chronic neck pain persists in 10 to 34% of adults in the general population (1–3). These refractory cases provide a great dilemma for the spine surgeon.

The patient with axial neck pain and cervical degenerative disc disease may be difficult to treat. The unique anatomy of the cervical spine with joint complexes both anteriorly and posteriorly have made isolating a pain generator difficult. In addition, the success of cervical fusion is unpredictable for the treatment of axial neck pain alone. As in all clinical syndromes, the correct diagnosis must be made before any treatment is initiated. The differential diagnosis for axial neck pain is broad, and the most common conditions that do not require surgery should always be ruled out first. The clinician must take great care to consider the psychosocial issues and examine the patient thoroughly for nonorganic signs. Attempting operative intervention in such cases may spell disaster for both the patient and the treating physician.

The cornerstone for caring for the patient with axial neck pain is patience. The only indications for immediate operative intervention are severe instability with risk of neurologic compromise, significant or worsening neurologic deficits, or an abscess causing sepsis or systemic symptoms. If the patient does not fall into one of these categories, reassurance must be given that the vast majority of cases improve with conservative treatment alone, and that surgery is reserved only for cases of severe, unrelenting pain unresponsive to treatment that has lasted many months.

ANATOMY AND PATHOPHYSIOLOGY

The cervical spine is comprised of the cervical vertebrae, ligamentous supporting structures, intervertebral joints, and the spi-

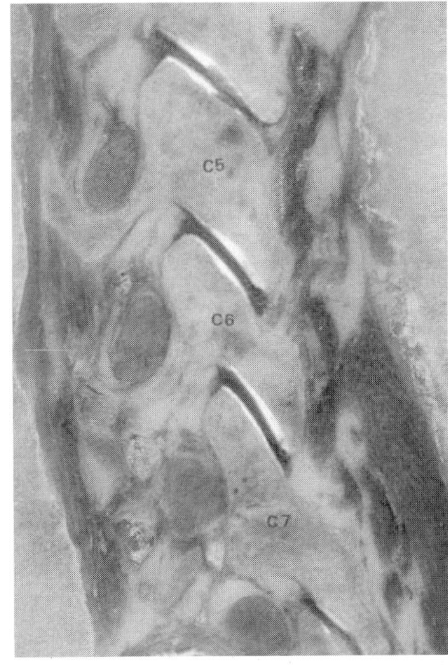

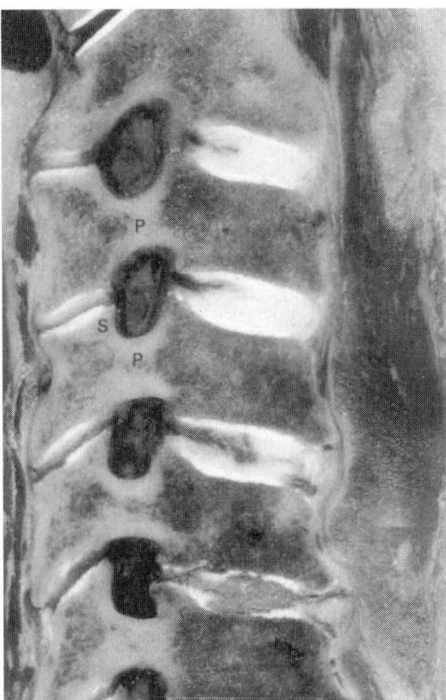

A,B

FIG. 1. A: Parasagittal freezing microtome section of the facet joint showing an angle approximately 45 degrees cephalad from the transverse plane in the middle region and a greater angle in the lower region **B:** A 45-degree oblique freezing microtome showing the intervertebral foramina that are bounded anteriorly by the vertebral bodies and intervertebral discs, posteriorly by the facets and superior articular process, and cephalad and caudad by the pedicles. Note that in both images, the facet, or zygapophyseal joints, appear as oblique slits. (From An HS, Simpson JM. *Surgery of the cervical spine*. London: Martin Dunitz Ltd, 1994, with permission.)

nal cord itself. Anteriorly, the spinal cord is protected by the vertebral bodies and discs; posteriorly, the laminae and ligamentum flavum form the roof of the spinal canal. Motion at the intervertebral level is conferred by the joints at each segment as well as by the intervertebral discs. The intervertebral discs, along with the uncovertebral joints anteriorly and the facet joints posteriorly, comprise what is thought of as a five-joint complex at each level.

At each intervertebral level from C-2 to C-7, there are two sets of paired joints. The facet or zygapophyseal joints are located posteriorly, and their oblique orientation confers stability in the anteroposterior plane (4) (Fig. 1). The uncovertebral joints, also called *joints of Luschka* or *neurocentral joints*, are false joints formed by the curved edges of the vertebral bodies at their lateral edges (5) (Fig. 2). The nerve roots exit their associated foramen just anterior to the facet joints and just lateral to the lateral edges of the uncovertebral joints (Fig. 3). As cervical spondylosis is associated with degenerative changes and osteophyte formation in the cervical joints, cervical radiculopathy is common in patients with degenerative cervical disease and axial neck pain (6–9).

The intervertebral discs lie anteriorly between the vertebral bodies and confer the majority of the mobility and structural integrity between each motion segment. The discs are composed of the annulus fibrosus and inner nucleus pulposus. The latter is rich in proteoglycans, which attract water and maintain the height and integrity of the disc (10) (Fig. 4).

It is thought that cervical spondylosis begins with disc degeneration that results from desiccation of the inner nucleus. Some have hypothesized that a tear in the outer annulus may lead to a nuclear leakage, but the disc dehydration may also occur without such a tear. As the disc dehydrates, the mechanical properties of the disc change as height and volume are lost and annular tension decreases. These events may lead to instability at the intervertebral level with increased motion under physiologic loads of the anterior uncovertebral and posterior facet joints. Increased motion and abnormal stresses cause these joints to degenerate and form osteophytes, which may cause central canal impingement or foraminal stenosis. The end-plates are now exposed to an increase in stresses, which results in osteophyte formation and sclerosis (11,12).

Posteriorly, the ligamentum nuchae attaches to the spinous processes at each level at the midline and confers additional stability between each of the intervertebral levels. The surrounding

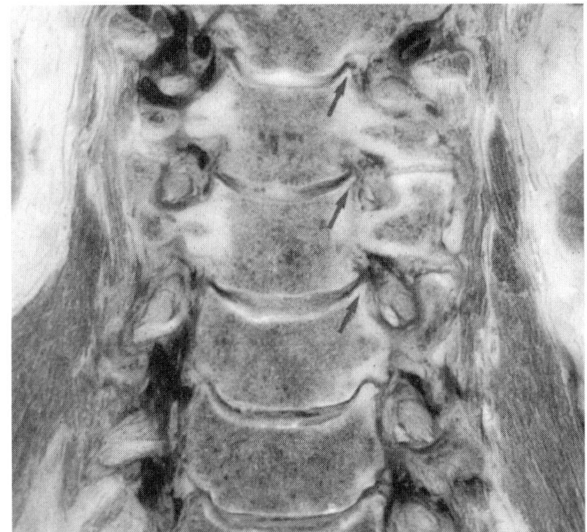

FIG. 2. Midcoronal freezing microtome of the cervical spine. Note the arrows that indicate the uncovertebral or neurocentral joints (joints of Luschka). These anterior joints are adjacent to the vertebral body and curve cephalad along the lateral borders. (From An HS, Simpson JM. *Surgery of the cervical spine*. London, Martin Dunitz Ltd, 1994, with permission.)

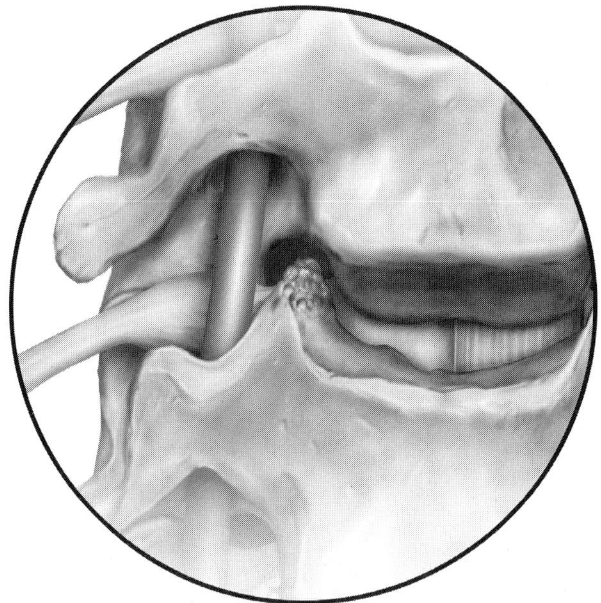

FIG. 3. Relationship between the uncovertebral joint and the exiting nerve root and vertebral artery. Note that the root and artery lie just lateral to the lateral wall of the joint. It is mandatory to understand this relationship when performing surgery in the cervical spine to minimize the chances of a vascular accident or neurologic injury. (From An HS, Simpson JM. *Surgery of the cervical spine.* London: Martin Dunitz Ltd, 1994, with permission.)

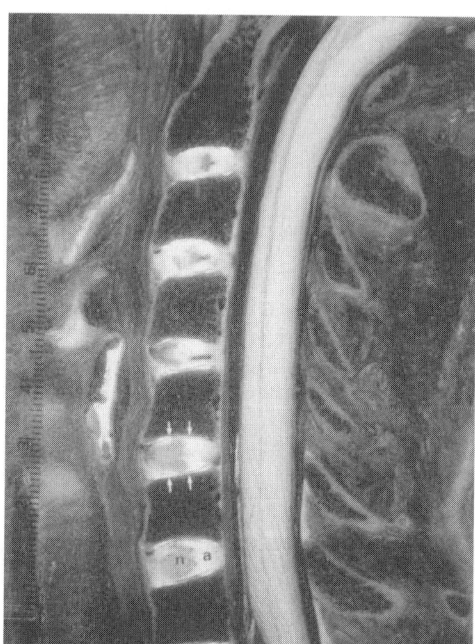

FIG. 4. A midsagittal freezing microtome of cervical spine showing the intervertebral disc consisting of the nucleus pulposus at the interior of the disc, the outer annulus fibrosus, and the cartilaginous end-plates (*arrows*) adjacent to the vertebral surfaces. (From An HS, Simpson JM. *Surgery of the cervical spine.* London: Martin Dunitz Ltd, 1994, with permission.)

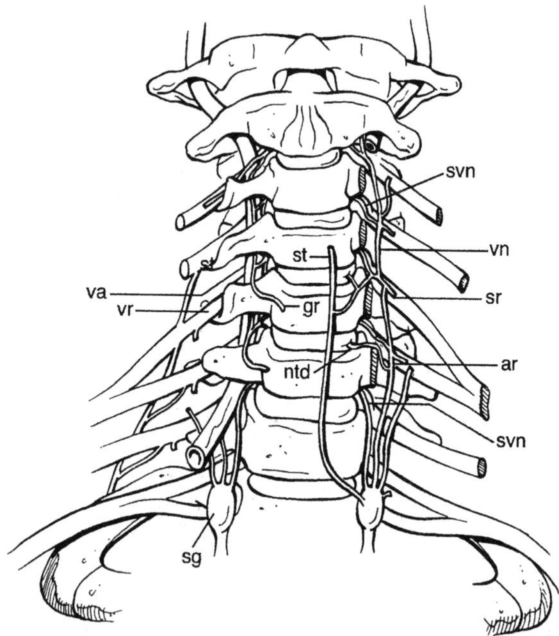

FIG. 5. Anterior view of the cervical spine. The right vertebral artery (va) is seen running through the foramina transversaria and in front of the C-3 to C-7 rami (vr), accompanied by the vertebral nerve (vn), which is formed by grey rami communicantes (gr) from the sympathetic trunk (st) and the stellate ganglion (sg). On the left, the costal parts of the transverse processes and the vertebral artery have been resected to reveal the vertebral nerve and the origins of the C-3 to C-7 sinuvertebral nerves (svn). Each nerve arises from a somatic root (sr) from a ventral ramus and an autonomic root (ar) from elements of the vertebral nerve. Also shown are nerves (ntd) to the C4-5 and C5-6 discs from the vertebral nerve. (From Bogduk N, Windsor M, Inglis A. The innervation of the cervical intervertebral discs. *Spine* 1988;13:2–8, with permission.)

posterior cervical musculature includes the trapezius superficially, as well as the deeper paraspinal cervical muscles (semispinalis, splenius, longissimus, and interspinalis muscles) (13).

What exactly causes axial pain is not clearly understood, although it is most likely multifactorial. The annulus is supplied by the sinuvertebral nerve, which is a branch of the ventral root and sympathetic plexus (14) (Fig. 5). An annular tear may directly stimulate the nerve, or disc dehydration with stiffening of the disc may predispose the annulus to injury. Either of these mechanisms may stimulate the sinuvertebral nerve and cause neck pain. Some investigators have suggested that pain patterns elicited with discographic stimulation indicate the significance of the disc as causing mechanical neck pain. The observation that injection of analgesics during discography can cause relief of pain in some subjects has also strengthened the notion the disc is a significant pain generator (15).

It is also thought the facet or zygapophyseal joints may mediate a significant component of mechanical neck pain. As the five-joint complex degenerates, the facets are predisposed to increased and, perhaps, abnormal motions (4,16). This may lead to altered stresses on the joint capsules, which are innervated by branches of the dorsal rami (17). Dwyer et al. injected contrast material into the cervical facet joints of five healthy volunteers and elicited typical mechanical neck pain that radiated into the posterior scapular and proximal shoulder regions (18). The fact that facet blocks and ablations of the dorsal primary rami cause at least temporary improvement of symptoms is further proof that the facets may mediate a significant portion of axial neck discomfort (19–21).

Finally, and perhaps most nebulous, is the effect of injury to the paraspinal musculature and ligamentous complexes on the production of mechanical neck pain. Ulig et al. studied biopsied neck muscles of 64 patients with mechanical neck pain and found increased amounts of type IIC fibers (22). McPartland et al. compared magnetic resonance image (MRI) findings in seven patients with and without a history of chronic neck pain and demonstrated atrophy and fatty infiltration in the suboccipital muscles in the patients with axial symptoms (23,24). Larsson (24) demonstrated changes in blood flow and innervation to the trapezius muscles in patients with chronic neck pain. In addition, postmortem studies of trauma victims with chronic mechanical neck pain have shown a high prevalence of ligamentous injuries (25). Whether these changes have anything to do with the chronic neck pain or whether these changes are a result rather than a cause of the axial pain is not known (26).

All of this information suggests that the discs, facet joints, ligaments, and muscles may be disrupted from acute traumatic events or insidious deterioration, which may subsequently result in axial neck pain. Most likely, mechanical neck pain is multifactorial. This may also explain why patients may have differing pain responses despite similar MRI findings of cervical disc degeneration (27).

HISTORY AND PHYSICAL EXAMINATION

Although the history and physical examination for the cervical spine patient has been described in an earlier chapter, a number of points bear reemphasis. Although the vast majority of patients with axial neck pain should undergo an initial trial of conservative treatment, exceptions do exist for more emergent radiographic evaluation and more aggressive intervention. Red flags include the presence of night or unrelenting pain, weight loss, fevers, chills, or night sweats, which are suggestive of a neoplastic or infectious process (28–30). Other red flags include significant head and neck trauma and the presence of a neurologic deficit (31).

Many patients with axial neck pain present with associated symptoms of radiculopathy or myelopathy because the same degenerative changes that appear to cause axial neck pain may also cause nerve root or cord impingement (6–9). Thus, a complete neurologic examination is of utmost importance in any patient complaining of axial neck pain. A motor and sensory examination as well as testing for normal and abnormal upper motor neuron reflexes is mandatory in all patients (3). In some instances, the axial neck pain may be so severe as to mask pain, weakness, or numbness in the extremities, and thus, simply asking the patient if he or she has had any peripheral deficits is not sufficient.

The full range of motion should be tested with special emphasis on flexion-extension, left and right rotation, and left-side and right-side bending. It is best to estimate motion based on degrees from midline. Active and passive motion should be examined separately, and any motion that reproduces pain should be noted. Axial compression should be performed to determine if this reproduces the pain. In addition, provocative maneuvers that apply tension on the nerve roots should be performed, such as Spurling's and Lhermitte's signs (3).

Many cases of C-4 radiculopathy may mask as axial neck pain because the dermatomes are located in the posterior scapular and proximal neck regions (32). Sensation should be tested in these distributions, and the patient should be questioned as to whether paresthesias are present in these areas. All patients should be tested for nonorganic signs. A pain response even to light touch performed in a random distribution is usually a good nonorganic sign. An examination that changes when the examiner retests specific elements should also be suspect. Cogwheeling or jerking motions when strength is tested actually requires more strength than holding a stable position, because it requires deceleration against resistance. Finally, the patient's demeanor and overall facial expression should correlate with the amount of pain the patient states is being experienced (33).

DIFFERENTIAL DIAGNOSIS OF AXIAL NECK PAIN

Cervical Strain

By far, the most common diagnosis of axial neck pain is cervical strain, thought to result from an injury to the soft-tissue structures of the neck, including muscles, tendons, and ligaments. When the injury results from an acceleration-deceleration–type trauma, it is often referred to as *whiplash.* It is unclear whether the changes in the paraspinal muscles and ligaments that occur in patients with cervical strain are a cause or a result of the chronic pain syndrome. Some authors have hypothesized that muscle or ligament injury leads to vessel tears and small bleeds within the muscle tissue, resulting in muscle irritation and spasm (34). Fibrosis may occur later, which could alter the muscle structure and lead to continuing spasm and pain. Others feel the primary injury affects discs or facets, and the soft-tissue alterations are secondary to pain. The etiology of cervical strain remains mostly speculative and is the subject of controversy, but its causation is most likely multifactorial and may include biochemical or biomechanical factors sometimes modulated by psychosocial and behavioral influences.

Typically, the physical examination reveals diffuse tenderness along the paraspinal cervical musculature with diminished range of motion in all directions. The neurologic examination should be normal, and the patient should not display any changes in gait or coordination. Focal areas, often referred to as *trigger points,* may be hypersensitive to palpation and may be associated with localized areas of muscle spasm (35). The presence of trigger points may also be associated with fibromyalgia, which is thought by many to be a common cause of cervical neck pain. When that diagnosis is made, trigger point injections often are recommended.

The vast majority of cervical strain injuries improve over a 6-week period of time with conservative measures alone. The Quebec Task Force noted that whiplash associated disorder is nearly always self limited and rarely results in permanent disability (36). However, it has been noted in some long-term follow-up studies that there is a 20 to 40% rate of persistent neck pain after whiplash-type cervical trauma (37–39). Persistent and progressive neck pain in patients without nonorganic signs suggests that cervical degenerative disease has resulted from the traumatic incident.

Cervical Degenerative Disc Disease

Patients with neck pain that has lasted longer than 12 weeks usually have cervical degenerative disease. This is thought to result from a cascade of changes starting with dehydration and incompetence of the disc, resulting in lost disc height and increased forces on the adjacent end-plates. Abnormal stresses result in end-plate sclerosis, osteophyte formation, and hypertrophy of the uncovertebral and facet joints (11,12). The decreased anterior disc height may also result in loss of cervical lordosis (10,40–42).

The actual pain generator in cervical degenerative disease is currently unknown. Although many investigators believe that the incompetent disc is the causative structure (10,16,42a), others believe facet joint degeneration may also contribute significantly (17–19). Cervical discography does not accurately predict if a cervical disc is a major source of pain, and outcomes from cervical fusion do not always correlate with preoperative discography findings (42a–45). In addition, cervical facet blocks have had mixed results in the patient with axial neck pain and cervical disc disease, and thus, it is not clear that the facets are the major pain generators in this degenerative process (46–48). Another hypothesis suggests that the overall loss of cervical lordosis from the disc degeneration may cause muscle spasm and subsequent axial neck pain (40–42). However, many successfully treated patients of cervical degenerative disc disease do not have complete restoration of cervical lordosis but have a good outcome (49). It is likely that the mechanical neck pain caused by cervical degenerative disease is multifactorial and that the discs, facets, and alignment all play a role.

Although the initial insult in disc degeneration is generally felt to be the result of increased mechanical stresses, others suggest that alterations in blood supply and disc nutrition are potential risk factors. The annulus receives more of a direct blood supply than does the nucleus, which is nourished via an ultrafiltrate of the plasma diffused through the vertebral end-plates (50). Nonetheless, the nucleus appears to be more sensitive to changes in nutrient concentration and thus more dependent on blood supply (although indirect) than the annulus tissue. Alterations in nutrient supply may result in cell deterioration in the nucleus followed by disc dehydration and degenerative disc disease (51).

The patient with cervical degenerative disc disease typically complains of axial neck pain that is worsened by flexion, which increases stress on the discs. Axial compression may also reproduce or exacerbate pain (3,6,52). Neurologic examination may also be abnormal because of the association of degenerative cervical disc disease with cervical radiculopathy or myelopathy (3,7,8). Often, these patients also have severe headaches that radiate into the occipital areas. These occipital headaches are thought to be secondary to severe spasm in the paraspinal musculature and are often relieved when the cervical disc disease is treated (4,42a).

C-4 Radiculopathy

The C-4 dermatomes distribution include the proximal trapezial areas and the posterior scapular areas, and, thus, root impingement at the C3-4 level may cause apparent axial neck pain (3). It is important to be able to distinguish between C-4 radiculopathy and true axial neck pain, which guides the appropriate operative treatment if surgery becomes necessary. Unilateral neck or posterior scapular pain suggests a C-4 radiculopathy because axial pain from degenerative disc disease is usually bilateral.

A full sensory examination should always be performed in the C-4 distributions (Fig. 6). The patient should always be asked about paresthesias in the C-4 distributions as well. However, the C-4 nerve root does not have a distinct motor unit, and strength and reflex testing is not possible (32).

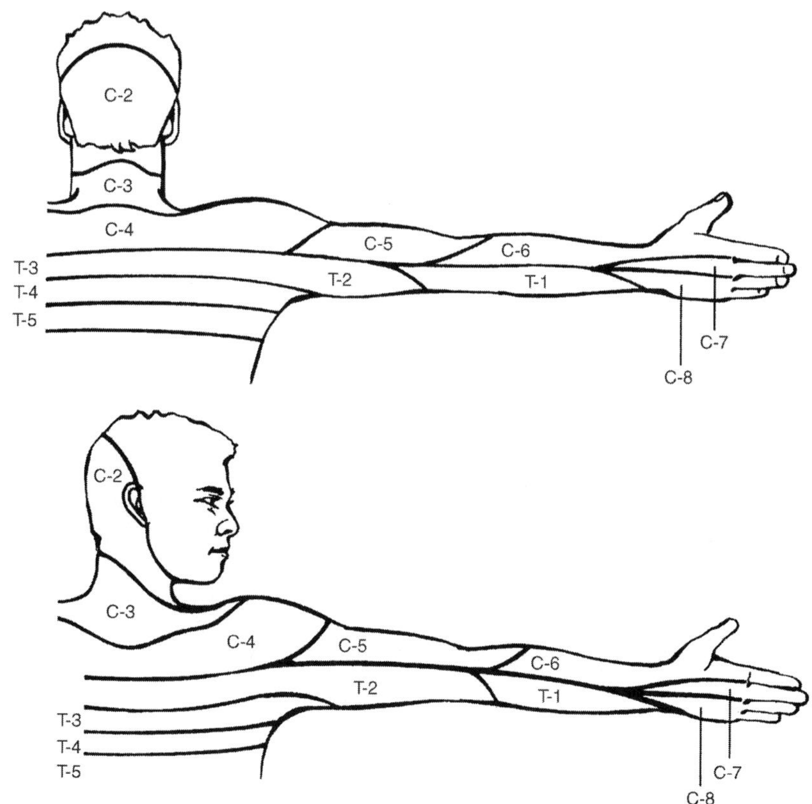

FIG. 6. The C-4 nerve root distribution according to Keegan (1947). (From Dvorak J. Epidemiology, physical examination and neurodiagnostics. *Spine* 1998;23:2663–2672, with permission.)

Pseudarthrosis

An increasingly common cause of axial neck pain is failed cervical surgery. Poor surgical technique or host factors (e.g., smoking, steroid medication, and noncompliance with postoperative immobilization) may predispose the patient to a postoperative nonunion. Many cases of fibrous unions are stable and thus asymptomatic and do not require refusion. Occasionally, enough motion is present at the nonunion site that axial neck pain is present (25,53,54).

Pseudarthrosis is most frequently seen after failed anterior cervical disc fusion (ACDF), presumably because ACDF is the most common cervical operation. With the advent of instrumentation and the widespread use of anterior cervical plates, the rate of nonunion has decreased; however, pseudarthroses still do occur, although less frequently (6,55). Graft collapse usually occurs, and it is not uncommon for the foramen to become narrowed with a resultant radiculopathy in conjunction with the neck pain (56). Other hallmarks of pseudarthrosis are broken instrumentation or progressive deformity (57).

MRI can be difficult to interpret if instrumentation is present. In these instances, computed tomography (CT) myelography gives the best bony definition, aids in determining the site and magnitude of the nonunion, and also clarifies sites of neural compression. In addition, plain films, including flexion and extension laterals, are invaluable in determining instability. If the immediate postoperative images are available, they also help the clinician to determine the amount of later graft collapse and increase in angular deformity (56,57).

Pathologic Processes in the Cervical Spine (Tumors, Trauma, and Infection)

Cervical tumors, trauma, and infection are covered in Chapters 10, 11, 33, and 34. These conditions are suspect when any red flags are elicited by history or on the physical examination (29).

Rheumatologic Disorders (Rheumatoid Arthritis, Ankylosing Spondylitis, Reiter's Syndrome, Psoriatic Arthritis)

Rheumatoid arthritis and seronegative spondyloarthropathies are discussed in Chapter 9. However, the clinician evaluating the patient with axial neck pain must keep a rheumatologic disorder in mind, especially if systemic or multiple other joint complaints are present (30). Specific evaluation includes blood testing for human leukocyte antigen B27 antibody or rheumatoid factor; however, these tests have a relatively high false negative rate. Thus, if the clinical suspicion is high enough, appropriate referral to a rheumatologist is necessary to rule out a seropositive or seronegative spondyloarthropathy.

Shoulder Pathology and Rotator Cuff Disease

The patient with shoulder pain often complains of associated neck pain or mistakes it to be coming from the cervical spine. When pain complaints about the shoulder or proximal deltoid are prominent, a complete shoulder examination should be performed. Rotator cuff pathology can be tested with Neer and Hawkins tests for impingement as well as with testing abductor strength from zero degrees. If the physical examination is equivocal, injection of local anesthetic into the subacromial space may aid in the diagnosis.

Acromial-clavicular joint arthritis usually presents with palpable osteophytes or tenderness localized over the region. Degenerative arthritis in the glenohumeral joint generally presents with decreased range of motion in all directions. Imaging studies, such as MRI, and injection of local anesthetic aid in the diagnosis of these conditions (58,59).

RADIOGRAPHIC EVALUATION

In the patient complaining mainly of pain with no neurologic deficit and who presents with no red flags (28,30,31), it is reasonable to wait 6 weeks before radiographs or other imaging studies are obtained and to start conservative treatment. If symptoms do not resolve after a 6- to 8-week interval, however, it is helpful to obtain radiologic studies (16).

Imaging studies should start with anteroposterior and neutral lateral view radiographs as well as flexion-extension views if there is any evidence of instability or listhesis. The overall lordotic contour should be evaluated. Loss of cervical lordosis may be a primary structural problem due to severe disc degeneration and loss of disc height, or it may be secondary to cervical muscle spasm from pain. Although the discs cannot be directly imaged on plain radiographs, degenerative levels can often be determined by loss of disc height, bone spurs, end-plate irregularities, and sclerosis (29,60).

Flexion and extension laterals are invaluable in determining stability, particularly in patients with trauma, tumor, or pseudarthrosis. If the patient has a degenerative spondylolisthesis, it is also useful to know how much motion is occurring with flexion and extension (28,31,60).

MRI is very useful in cervical spine discs when plain radiographs are normal. The sagittal T2-weighted images are usually useful in determining if any of the discs are dehydrated and diseased, as they will appear black. In addition, severely degenerative levels may demonstrate a vacuum disc sign, which indicates gas attracted from surrounding tissues that accumulates within clefts of the degenerated disc or in unstable facet joints. Annular tears, which may be a painful entity in and of itself or which may be a precursor to degenerative cervical disease, may also be identified. Finally, the presence of facet or uncovertebral joint arthropathy may be clarified with hypertrophy and osteophytic spur formation (29,60).

CT scans may give more information on the amount of bony destruction that has occurred in cases of tumor, infection, or trauma but in general are not as useful in the evaluation of the patient with axial neck pain. CT scan with 45-degree oblique reconstructions that best visualize the foramen is often helpful in cases of axial neck pain with a component of radicular pain (60,61). However, regular sagittal reconstructions oriented at 90 degrees rather than 45 degrees add little information as to the foraminal space available for the exiting nerve roots.

Imaging studies should not be delayed in the patient presenting with a neurologic deficit, particularly if the deficit is severe, if myelopathy is present, or if the patient has any changes in bowel or bladder. In such patients, conventional radiographs as well as MRI and 45-degree oblique CT scans should be obtained in a timely fashion, as it is generally accepted that optimum neurologic recovery occurs when decompression of neural structures is not delayed.

TREATMENT

Cervical Strain

The treatment for the patient with cervical strain is conservative. The vast majority of cases improve or resolve within a 6- to 8-week period of time, and thus, the treating physician's primary responsibility is to keep the patient comfortable until the symptoms resolve. Nonsteroidal antiinflammatory medications are often beneficial. Muscle relaxants may provide some temporary pain relief, but use for more than a week is discouraged because the long-term efficiency is not established, and these medications have a central sedating effect rather than a direct effect on the muscles (62). Soft cervical collars should generally be avoided except for the initial 2 to 3 days after an injury because they interfere with early mobilization (63,64).

It is of utmost importance that the patient's overall conditioning be maintained while recovering from a soft tissue injury. Patients should be encouraged to do as much as possible and reassured that the neck will not worsen and that they will not become paralyzed. Once the pain has started to abate, the patient should be encouraged to discontinue use of the cervical collar and resume an active lifestyle. Numerous studies support early mobilization and maintaining fitness as the most important factors for a good long-term outcome after cervical strain. McKinney studied 247 consecutive patients with acute neck sprain and found those patients who received advice for early mobilization improved more rapidly and had fewer persistent symptoms at 2-year follow-up than those who did not (65). Likewise, Mealy et al. found in 61 patients with whiplash injuries, those who underwent early mobilization had greater cervical motion and less pain (23). Cervical physiotherapy, which includes range of motion, strengthening, and endurance exercises, may be beneficial in the short term, as it helps to encourage motion initially after the injury or onset of pain (66–68).

Narcotic medications should be avoided if at all possible, as they may be habit-forming and often discourage the patient from remaining active. This may result in the patient becoming deconditioned, which often prolongs or impedes recovery (62).

The authors also discourage the use of steroid medications because the condition is usually self-limiting, as well as the fact that these medications may have potentially devastating side effects. Long-term improvement is similar with and without administration of steroids, although short-term improvement may be accelerated (69). Cervical epidural steroid injections have not been found to be effective in cervical strain (70) and are associated with significant risks (71–78). If the clinician does decide to administer steroids, even in the form of a methylprednisolone (Medrol) dose pack (prednisone taper), the patient must be informed of the potential risks including osteonecrosis and addisonian crisis (79). An exception to these concerns is the use of local steroid and anesthetic injections sometimes advocated in the treatment of trigger points, particularly in patients with the diagnosis of fibromyalgia.

Cervical Degenerative Disease

The patient with axial neck pain and cervical degenerative disc disease in the absence of radiculopathy or myelopathy should first be treated with an extensive regimen of conservative treatments. Surgery for axial neck pain and cervical degenerative disc disease has traditionally been less predictable than surgery for neural compression and should be avoided if at all possible.

The first line of treatment is similar to the treatment for cervical strain and includes nonsteroidal antiinflammatory drugs, early mobilization, and maintenance of fitness (62). Physical therapy, including stretching and strengthening exercises to help reduce muscle spasm, may provide significant relief, and a home program should be started (66,67,80). Early mobilization should be explicitly encouraged. Once again, narcotics should be avoided if at all possible, and muscle relaxants should be prescribed only in the short term. Soft cervical collars may provide some relief initially by limiting painful motion but should not be used for more than a few days because they prevent mobilization. Many clinicians believe a soft collar is appropriate for patients with cervical radiculopathy; however, there is no compelling evidence that these devices provide traction or speed recovery. Although oral steroids may allow a quicker return to work (69), the patient must be advised of the potential consequences and that the long-term outcomes in patients treated with or without a course of oral steroids are not different. The authors therefore do not routinely prescribe oral steroids for axial neck pain.

Epidural steroids for the treatment of cervical degenerative disease has been associated with poor results with little improvement in symptoms (70). In addition, recent studies have described potentially devastating complications occurring after cervical epidural steroid injections, including hematoma formation, inadvertent intrathecal or intravascular injection, cord damage, and development of complex regional pain syndrome (71–78). Botwin et al., in a study of 345 injections, found a complication rate of nearly 17% (81). Given the minimal benefit in these patients and the significant risks, it is our feeling that cervical epidural steroid injections have no place in the treatment of patients with mechanical neck pain.

Other anesthetic injection techniques that have been described for the treatment of neck pain include facet (zygapophyseal) blocks and radiofrequency neurotomy. Facet blocks involve the administration of a steroid and local anesthetic in the joint capsules at the suspected levels and are performed under fluoroscopic guidance. Although some authors have noted anecdotally that facet injections have shown some promise for cervical degenerative disease (82,83), all published trials have shown little long-term benefit (46–48). Hove and Gyldensted noted that in 11 patients, cervical facet blocks led to temporary improvement and served as a diagnostic guide for surgery but did not provide permanent pain relief (47). Barnsley et al. noted in a series of 41 patients that facet blocks offered little long-term pain relief (46). Radiofrequency neurotomy is a procedure that involves using radiofrequency heat to destroy the medial branch nerves that branch off the dorsal rami and innervate the zygapophyseal joints (84). Positive response rates nearing 60% have been reported with this procedure, but the effect may wear off within 9 to 12 months as the nerves regenerate from the dorsal rami (62,82,84). The procedure can be repeated, but second injections have been associated with poorer outcomes (84).

Surgical treatment for axial neck pain and cervical degenerative disc disease is generally discouraged because the success rates have traditionally been unpredictable. Williams et al. found, in their series of 15 patients undergoing ACDF, that 73% of patients with preoperative radicular symptoms had a good to excellent result; however, in those patients with mechanical neck pain alone, a good to excellent result was achieved in only 27% (85). Likewise, Rothman and Rashbaum did a 5-year follow-up of 88 patients with

TABLE 1. *Series studying the results of ACDF for mechanical neck pain*

Author	Number of patients	Reported outcome	Discography performed?
Andrews et al. (7)	23 with neck pain	57% good or excellent, 17% fair, 26% poor	No
Dohn (87)	34	62% good or excellent, 24% fair, 15% poor	No
Garvey et al. (52)	87	82% good or excellent, 16% fair, 2% poor	Yes
Palit et al. (88)	38	79% satisfactory, 21% not satisfactory	Yes
Riley et al. (8)	93	72% good or excellent, 18% fair, 10% poor	No
Robinson et al. (9)	56	73% good or excellent, 22% fair, 5% poor	No
Roth (15)	71	93% good or excellent, 1% fair, 6% poor	Yes
Siebenrock et al. (113)	29	73% good or excellent, 23% fair, 4% poor	Yes
Simmons et al. (89)	30 with neck pain; 51 with neck and arm pain	78% good or excellent, 18% fair, 7% poor	Yes
White et al. (86)	28	62% good or excellent, 23% fair, 23% poor	No
Whitecloud and Seago (114)	34	70% good or excellent, 12% fair, 18% poor	Yes
Williams et al. (85)	15	27% good or excellent, 33% fair, 40% poor	No

mechanical neck pain. There were no significant functional differences between those treated operatively and nonoperatively (15). Similar series by White et al. (86) and Dohn (87) showed good to excellent results in 62% of patients treated with ACDF for mechanical neck pain. All authors thought the inferior results after fusion for neck pain were because adequate identification of the painful level was difficult, particularly in patients with diffuse pain and multilevel disease.

However, newer studies have shown that if the appropriate indications have been met, surgery can be associated with high success rates. Palit et al. studied 38 patients who underwent one- to three-level ACDF for mechanical neck pain after provocative discography to determine pain generators (88). These authors demonstrated a 79% satisfaction rate and significant improvements in pain and functional scores postoperatively. Likewise, Garvey et al. studied the clinical outcome for 87 patients who underwent ACDF for the primary indication of neck pain with average follow-up greater than 4 years. Pain improvement was reported by 93% of the patients, and the average visual analog rating changed from 8.4 before surgery to 3.8 after surgery. The self-rated functional status improved approximately 50% on both the Oswestry and the modified Roland-Morris disability indexes (52). The authors concluded that, especially for single or two-level cervical disease, surgical management is associated with more reliable outcomes than had previously been reported. The studies published to date regarding success rates after anterior cervical fusion for mechanical neck pain are summarized in Table 1.

If surgical treatment for cervical degenerative disc disease and axial neck pain is performed, the goal is to limit the fusion to one or two levels. Numerous studies have demonstrated that patients with multilevel cervical fusions do not do as well as those who have fusion at a single level, and the success rates decline as the number of levels fused increases. These poor results may be due to the loss of motion, biomechanical changes, and increased stress on the remaining discs that occur with multilevel fusions, rather than a higher risk of pseudarthrosis. Robinson et al. studied 55 patients who had undergone ACDF for cervical spondylosis and reported good to excellent results occurred in 94% of those who had undergone a one-level fusion. In comparison, good to excellent results were found in 73% of patients who had undergone a two-level fusion and only 50% of patients who had undergone a three-level fusion (9). Simmons and Bhalla noted that the only three results after ACDF with the Keystone procedure occurred with fusions involving more than two levels (89). Likewise, Andrews et al. found good to excellent results in only 50% of patients who underwent ACDF involving three or more levels, as opposed to 63% in patients who had one- or two-level fusions (7).

Cervical discography is a topic of much debate regarding its use in determining pain generators in the cervical spine. Some studies have shown a good correlation between discographic findings and success rates after surgery (15,52,88–91), whereas others have demonstrated poor correlation with clinical outcomes (43–45,85,92). In addition, cervical discography may be associated with rare but serious complications such as disc infection or hematoma, which have occurred in 0.6 to 2.5% of patients (93,94). Although the relative risk is low, the potential for major neurologic dysfunction is greater because the injections are administered at cord level. Furthermore, the available evidence indicates little difference in outcomes between patients undergoing fusion for mechanical neck pain with and without preoperative discography (85,95). The authors believe that fusion should be considered for patients with one- or two-level degenerative disease that is clearly defined on MRI and with sparing of the remaining levels. Cervical discography should be reserved for patients with severe, unrelenting pain in whom MRI changes involve multiple levels as a means to limit the number of levels fused. Cervical discography may also be considered if MRI is not possible, such as in patients with pacemakers or metallic objects implanted in the eye. If discography is considered, the patient must be warned of the risks of discography before it is used. In addition, the patient must be advised that the use of cervical discograms is questionable and that even in the best of series, fusion based on discographic findings is associated with a failure rate of 20% or higher (52,88). The current conventional wisdom is that the true value of cervical discography most likely lies in determining when and where not to fuse rather than which level to treat (95,96). Table 1 summarizes the success rates of studies that have and have not used discography for identification of the target levels before ACDF for mechanical neck pain.

Operative Treatment

Operative treatment usually entails anterior cervical discectomy and fusion of the involved level(s). As the cervical disc is thought to be the major pain generator in cervical degenerative disease, this procedure eliminates the diseased disc and hopefully relieves axial neck pain. Anterior fusion also eliminates motion at the uncovertebral and facet joints, thereby neutralizing these joint complexes as potential sources of pain (Figs. 7–9).

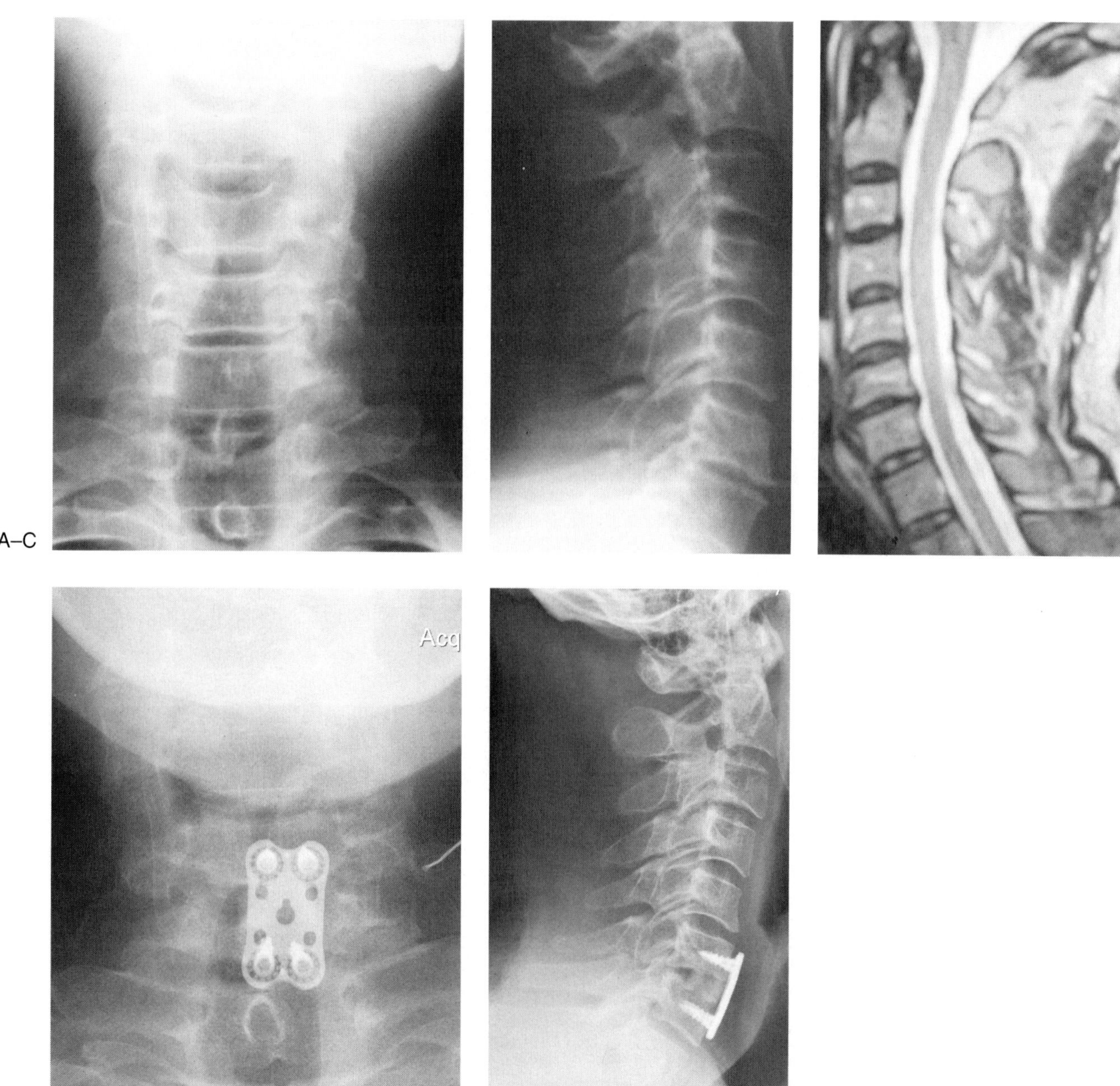

FIG. 7. C.A. is a 45-year-old man with severe neck pain that radiates into the posterior scapular areas. He had no arm pain, numbness, or weakness. His symptoms had lasted more than 1 year and persisted despite appropriate treatment with nonsteroidal antiinflammatory drugs and physical therapy. He did not opt to undergo steroid injections. His neurologic examination was normal. Anteroposterior and lateral radiographs demonstrate severe degenerative disc disease at one level, C6-7. The other levels were spared with good maintenance of disc height. **A,B:** The magnetic resonance image confirmed that the C6-7 level was black and desiccated with reactive changes in the adjacent vertebral end-plates and that the rest of the discs looked normal. **C:** Because only one level was clearly involved, discograms were not felt to be indicated. The patient underwent anterior cervical disc fusion at the C6-7 level. Postoperative anteroposterior and lateral radiographs are shown. **D,E:** The patient is now 5 months out, and his preoperative pain has completely resolved.

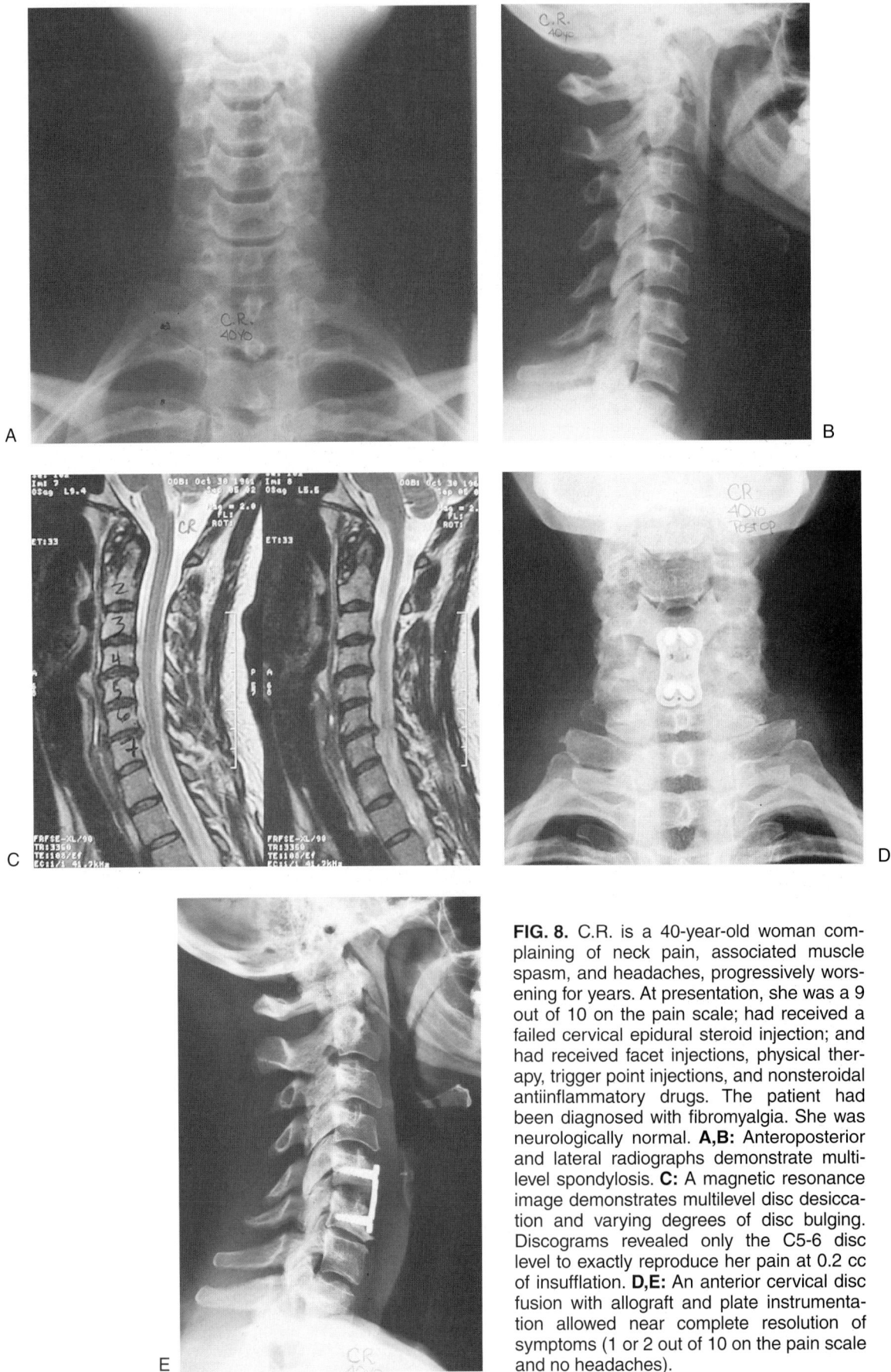

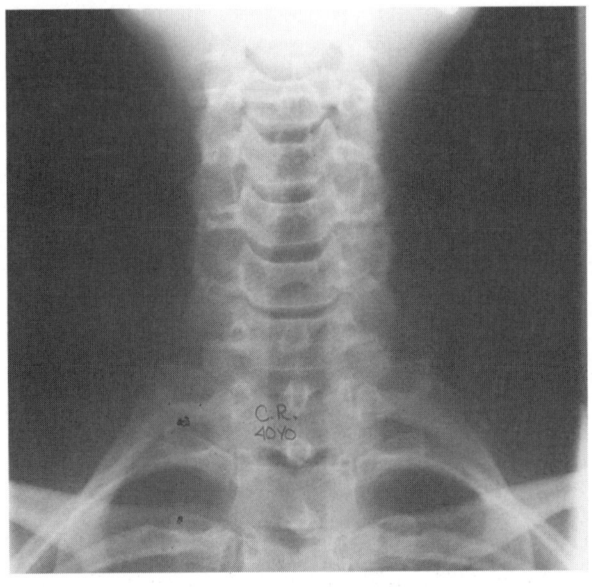

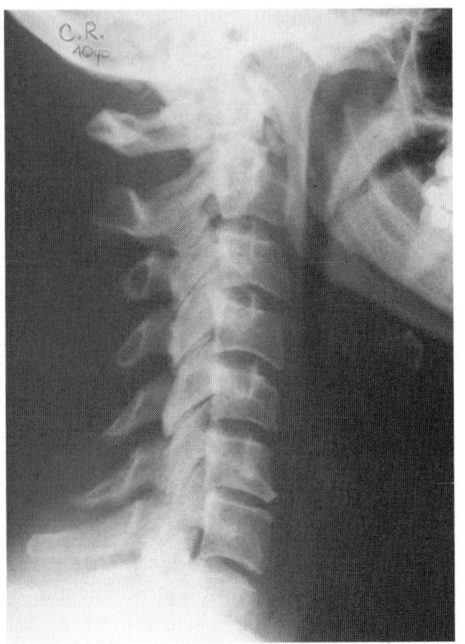

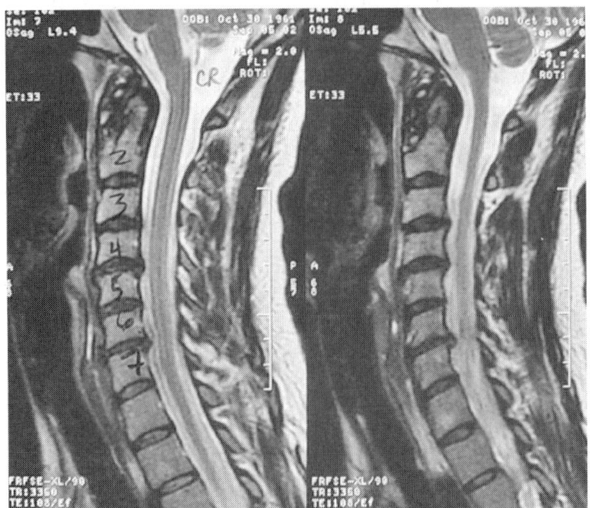

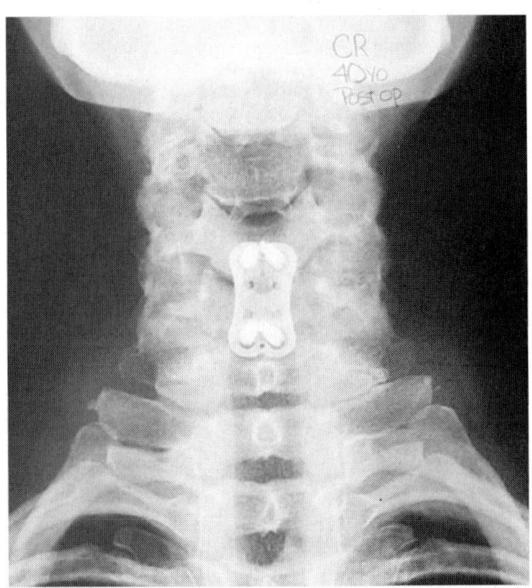

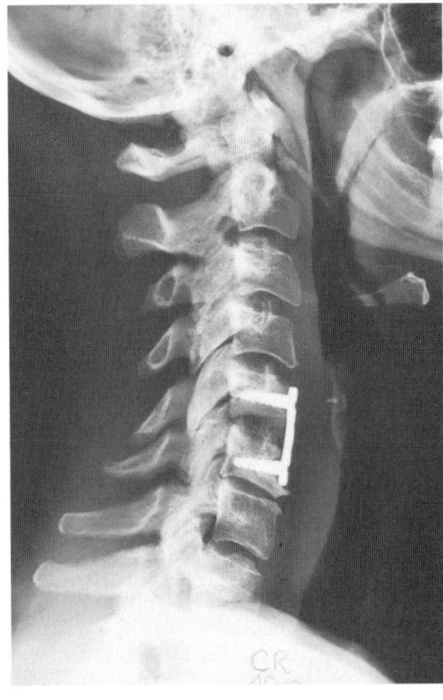

FIG. 8. C.R. is a 40-year-old woman complaining of neck pain, associated muscle spasm, and headaches, progressively worsening for years. At presentation, she was a 9 out of 10 on the pain scale; had received a failed cervical epidural steroid injection; and had received facet injections, physical therapy, trigger point injections, and nonsteroidal antiinflammatory drugs. The patient had been diagnosed with fibromyalgia. She was neurologically normal. **A,B:** Anteroposterior and lateral radiographs demonstrate multilevel spondylosis. **C:** A magnetic resonance image demonstrates multilevel disc desiccation and varying degrees of disc bulging. Discograms revealed only the C5-6 disc level to exactly reproduce her pain at 0.2 cc of insufflation. **D,E:** An anterior cervical disc fusion with allograft and plate instrumentation allowed near complete resolution of symptoms (1 or 2 out of 10 on the pain scale and no headaches).

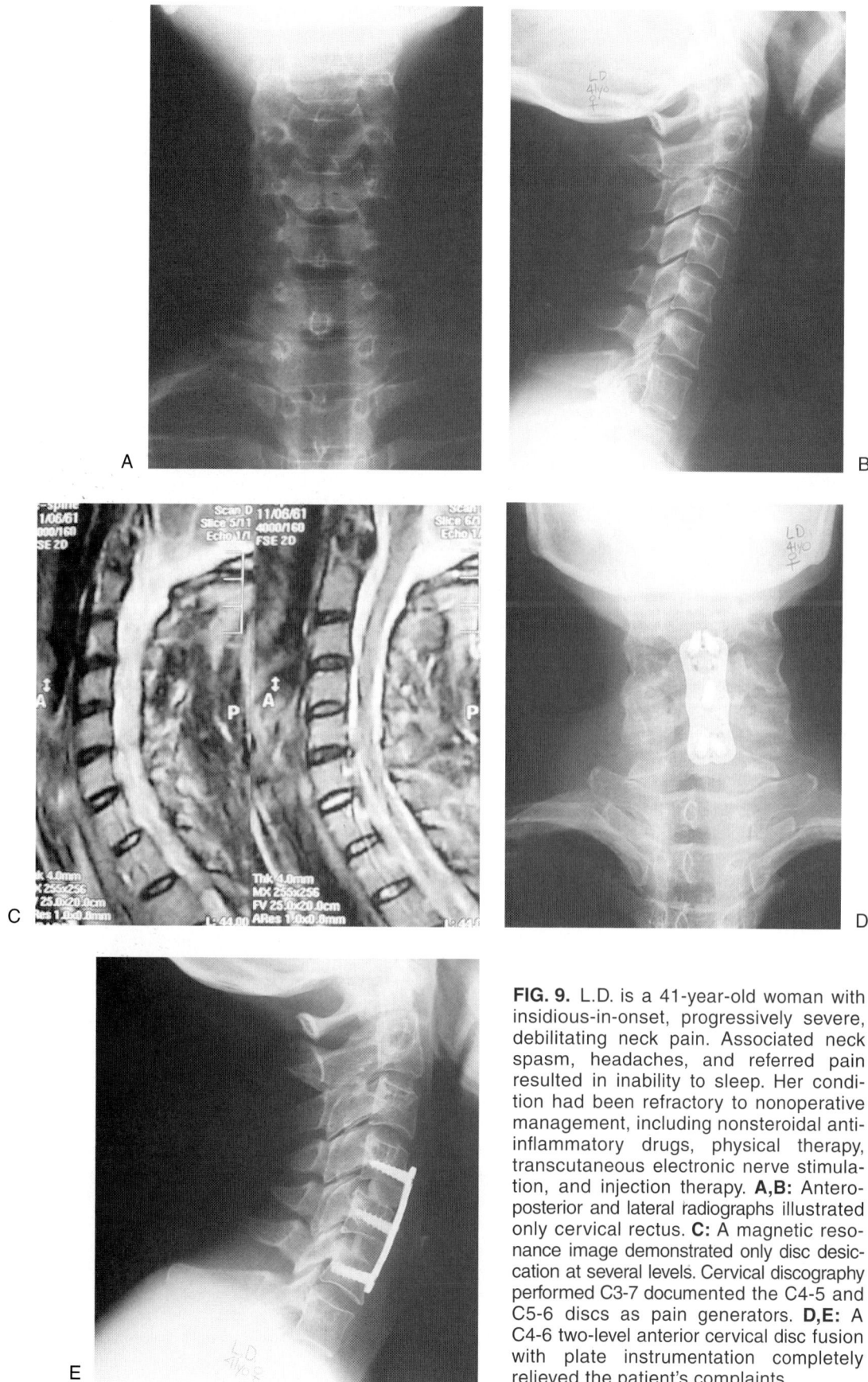

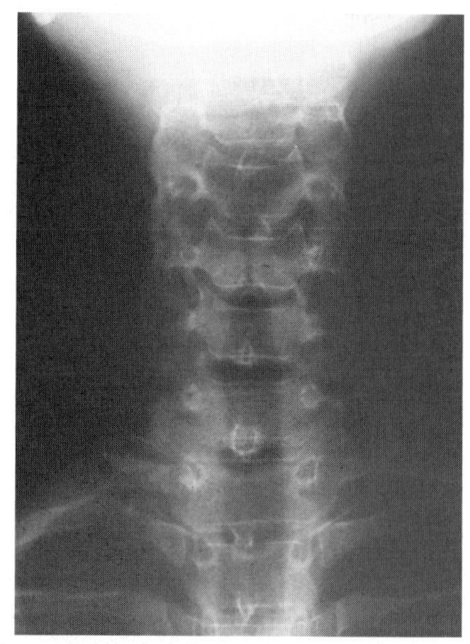

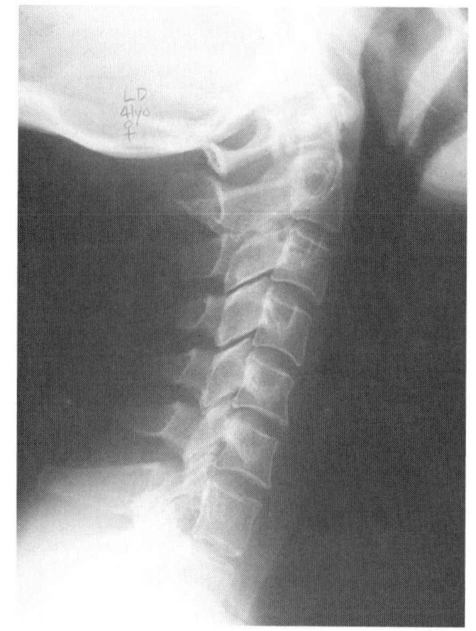

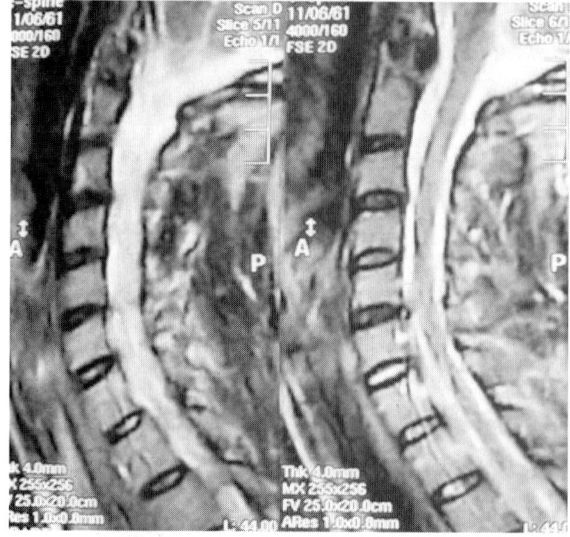

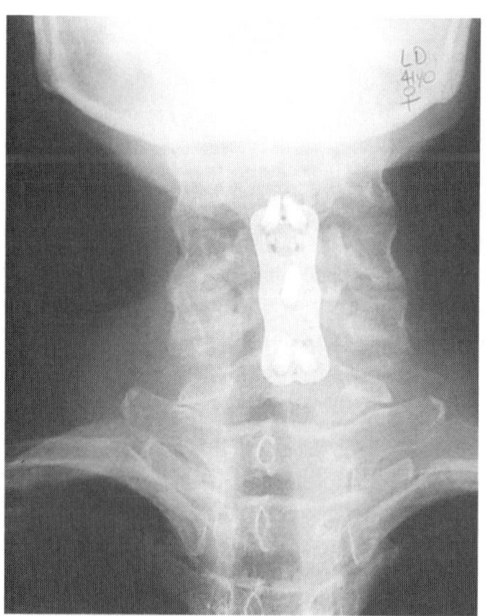

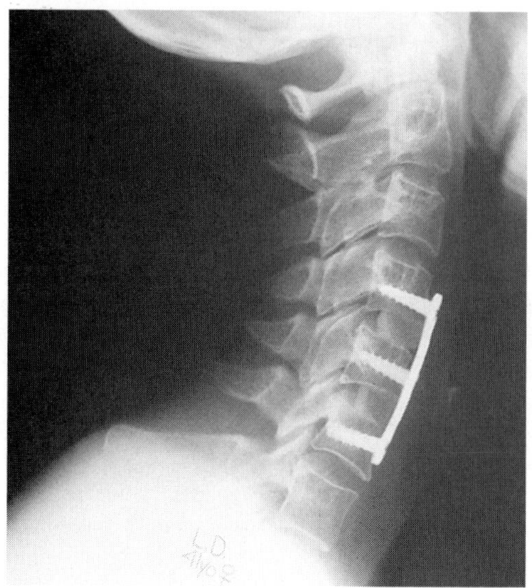

FIG. 9. L.D. is a 41-year-old woman with insidious-in-onset, progressively severe, debilitating neck pain. Associated neck spasm, headaches, and referred pain resulted in inability to sleep. Her condition had been refractory to nonoperative management, including nonsteroidal anti-inflammatory drugs, physical therapy, transcutaneous electronic nerve stimulation, and injection therapy. **A,B:** Anteroposterior and lateral radiographs illustrated only cervical rectus. **C:** A magnetic resonance image demonstrated only disc desiccation at several levels. Cervical discography performed C3-7 documented the C4-5 and C5-6 discs as pain generators. **D,E:** A C4-6 two-level anterior cervical disc fusion with plate instrumentation completely relieved the patient's complaints.

Posterior cervical fusion may offer an alternative treatment (55,97). Although the diseased discs are not actually removed, a successful posterior fusion may stabilize the painful levels and eliminate axial neck pain. Posterior fusions are usually reserved for patients who have had a failed anterior fusion or for the patient in whom a posterior decompression is advocated for relief of multilevel radiculopathy or myelopathy. Another relative indication for posterior surgery includes a short, wide neck where anterior exposure may be difficult.

The anterior approach is generally favored because the exposure is simple and straightforward, whereas the posterior approach to the cervical spine necessitates stripping muscle off the posterior elements and is associated with increased pain and blood loss. There are also more reported complications from placement of lateral mass screws than from anterior graft placement with or without plating. Interspinous wiring is associated with a fairly high rate of pseudarthrosis. Finally, with the anterior approach, the diseased discs are removed in their entirety, giving at least a theoretical advantage of completely eliminating the pain generators. Indeed, no current studies in the literature specifically address the efficacy of posterior fusions as a primary operative intervention for cervical degenerative disc disease and mechanical neck pain.

C-4 Radiculopathy

As with any patient with radiculopathy, conservative treatment is the appropriate initial treatment. Nonsteroidal antiinflammatory medications, muscle relaxants, and physical therapy with traction exercises and a home treatment program are all appropriate options (62). If these fail to provide improvement or relief of symptoms over a 6- to 12-week period of time, other treatment options, including surgical intervention, should be considered. Oral steroids and narcotics should be avoided if at all possible. Cervical epidural steroid injections may be of benefit (70,98,99), but as mentioned previously, these injections may be associated with significant complications (71–77).

If conservative treatment fails to adequately relieve symptoms, surgical intervention is warranted. Patients with C-4 radicular symptoms alone may be treated with ACDF or posterior foraminotomies (6,97,100). Because it is often difficult to differentiate whether or not the diseased disc is contributing to the overall clinical presentation, the authors prefer an ACDF; if the clinician is certain that pain is only from radiculopathy, posterior foraminotomies may be appropriate.

Jenis and An studied 12 consecutive patients with severe C-4 radiculopathy unresponsive to conservative treatment. The patients underwent either anterior cervical discectomy and fusion or posterior laminoforaminotomy at the C3-4 segment. The authors achieved a good to excellent clinical result in 92% of their patients, similar to the results found with ACDF or posterior foraminotomies for the treatment of cervical radiculopathy at other levels of the lower cervical spine (32). However, posterior foraminotomies are most appropriate for unilateral and multilevel disease. Performing bilateral foraminotomies is not recommended, because removal of more than 50% of the total facet at any level may result in destabilization (100,101). In addition, patients with loss of cervical lordosis are also poor candidates for foraminotomy, as the posterior decompression may lead to increased instability and a kyphotic deformity. In these cases, an anterior procedure or a posterior procedure with fusion should be considered.

If the pain is bilateral, if there is loss of cervical lordosis, or if there is question that some of the pain may be mechanical secondary to disc degeneration and not radicular in nature, ACDF should be performed. In most cases of one- or two-level disease, including the C3-4 level, ACDF is the treatment of choice.

Pseudarthrosis of the Cervical Spine

Pseudarthrosis is fairly common after anterior cervical fusion, particularly if instrumentation is not used and if multiple levels are fused (53,102). For that reason, anterior plate and screw instrumentation has become more popular. Instrumentation is particularly helpful if the patient is unwilling to tolerate or unlikely to be compliant with a hard collar postoperatively (6,55). Thus, even for single-level ACDF, the use of instrumentation has become increasingly common. Nonetheless, pseudarthrosis can still occur, particularly in cases of smokers, diabetics, those taking steroids, or where poor surgical technique was performed (6).

It must be emphasized that asymptomatic cervical pseudarthrosis does not necessarily require surgical repair. Many cervical fibrous unions are stable and are not associated with pain or disability. Phillips et al. studied 48 patients with radiographically documented cervical pseudarthroses and noted that 33% remained asymptomatic at a mean 5.1 years follow-up. An additional 12% initially had a symptom-free period of at least 2 years after the index ACDF before cervical symptoms redeveloped after a traumatic episode. However, 46% of the patients required reoperation for continued severe symptoms (54). In a similar study, Newman followed 23 patients with pseudarthrosis after ACDF and found that 16 (69%) ultimately required revision surgery (25). Thus, surgical management of cervical pseudarthrosis should be reserved for patients with significant pain and disability rather than radiographic abnormalities.

If surgery is required, using instrumentation improves the fusion rates and outcomes (66,103). Tribus et al. achieved an 81% fusion rate and a 75% improvement rate when iliac crest graft and anterior plate instrumentation were used (104).

There has been some disagreement, however, on whether anterior refusion with instrumentation or posterior instrumented fusion is superior for the treatment of anterior cervical pseudarthrosis. Phillips et al. treated 22 patients, 16 with an anterior and 6 with a posterior repair. All patients achieved a good or excellent result (54). Lowery et al. compared 20 patients who underwent an anterior refusion with a plate to 17 who underwent posterior cervical fusion with articular pillar plating. The authors found the fusion rate was significantly better in the posteriorly instrumented group (94% vs. 45%) than in the anterior group (102). Similarly, Brodsky compared 17 patients who underwent posterior pseudarthrosis repair with interspinous wiring with 17 patients who underwent anterior pseudarthrosis repair without instrumentation. The fusion rate was superior in the posterior group and good to excellent results were achieved in 88% of the posterior fusion group and only 59% of the anterior repair group (103).

Although posterior fusion appears to be superior for pseudarthrosis repair, there still is a contingent of surgeons who prefer the anterior procedure (Figs. 10–12). Their major argument is that posterior cervical instrumentation is associated with a fairly high complication rate (105,106). Heller et al. studied 78 patients whose

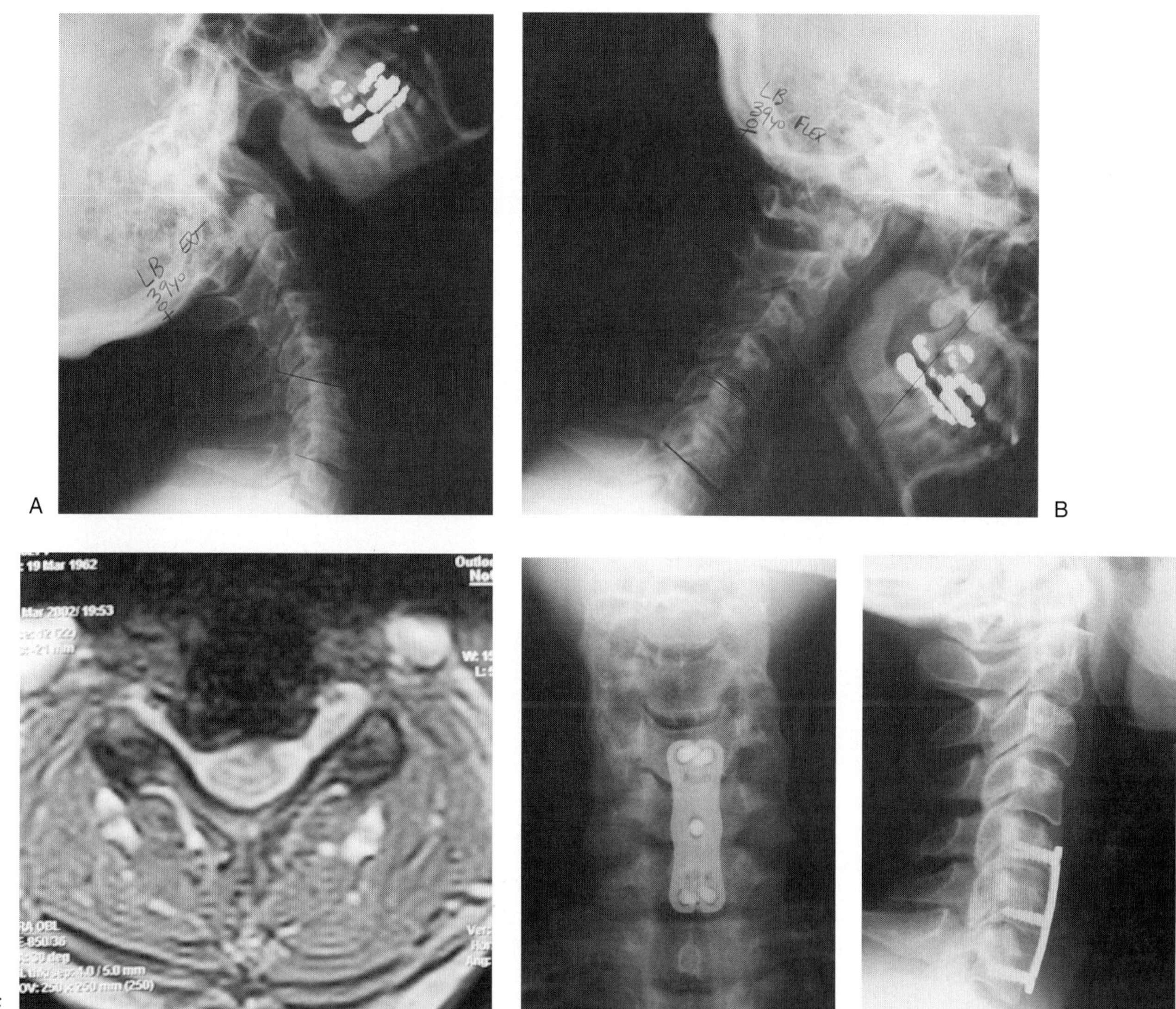

FIG. 10. L.B. is a 39-year-old woman smoker with several-year history of neck pain status post C5-6 anterior cervical disc fusion (ACDF). One year before evaluation, she developed left arm radicular pain. Associated numbness, tingling, and neck pain (8/10) were present. The patient had failed all nonoperative treatment. **A,B:** Flexion-extension lateral radiographs demonstrated motion and vacuum disc phenomenon at the C5-6 levels characteristic of pseudarthrosis. **C:** A magnetic resonance image documented a C6-7 herniated nucleus pulposus. **D,E:** The patient's pseudarthrosis was addressed by another ACDF at C5-6, and the C6-7 herniated disc was removed and treated with ACDF with C-5 to C-7 plate instrumentation.

treatment included posterior lateral mass plating, which involved the placement of 654 screws. Complications, although few, included nerve root injury, spinal cord injury, iatrogenic foraminal stenosis, broken instrumentation, infection, and pseudarthrosis (105). Interspinous wiring obviates the need for lateral mass screw placement, but the general consensus is that lateral mass screw instrumentation is superior and significantly stronger than posterior wiring techniques (107–112).

The potential risks of revising the scarred pseudarthrosis site anteriorly should not be ignored, even if the anterior cervical spine is approached from the contralateral side. These risks include dysphagia, damage to the anterior structures, recurrent laryngeal nerve injury, and anterior swelling that may compromise the airway (6). It is for these reasons (and because the overall success rates appear to be higher with posterior surgery) that the authors recommend posterior revision surgery for anterior cervical pseudarthrosis.

CONCLUSION

Axial neck pain can be the presentation of many different cervical spine disorders, and often, the cause can be nebulous and difficult to sort out. As in any disease process, it is of utmost importance for the clinician first to make the correct diagnosis. Because the differential diagnosis in the patient with axial neck pain is wide, a full history and physical examination, as well as appropriate imaging studies, are critical before implementing a treatment plan.

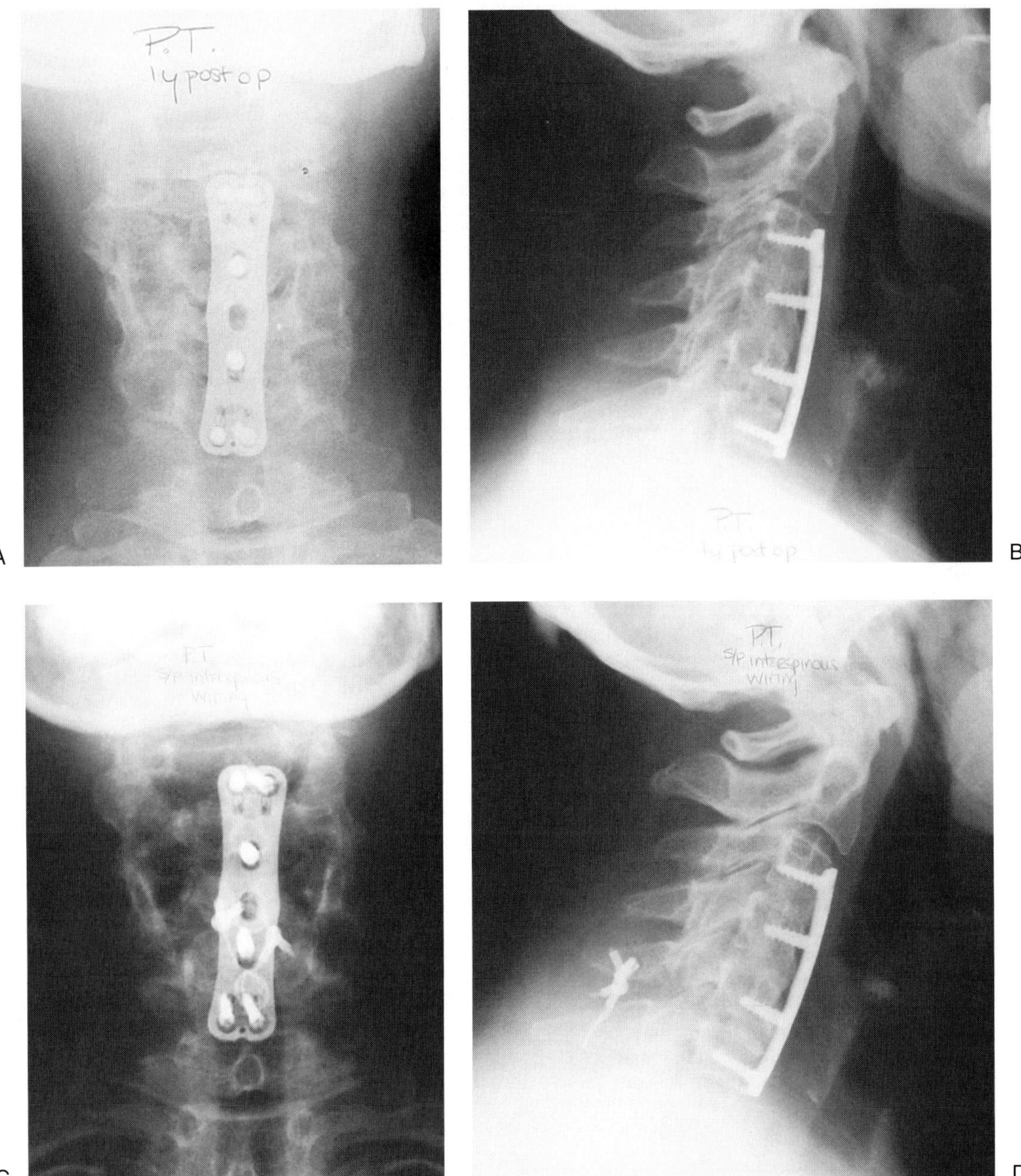

FIG. 11. P.T. is a 54-year-old woman with complaint of severe neck pain, secondary spasm, and headaches. The patient was referred 11 months after undergoing a three-level C-3 to C-6 anterior cervical disc fusion with plate instrumentation for herniated discs and spondylosis-related radiculopathy. She had no upper extremity symptoms. **A,B:** Anteroposterior and lateral radiographs revealed graft resorption and interface lucencies 1 year postoperatively. **C,D:** Anteroposterior and lateral radiographs obtained after posterior cervical wiring at C5-6 to address the pseudarthrosis confirmed at surgery. Consolidation is radiographically confirmed. Clinically, the patient is nearly asymptomatic and satisfied.

The most common cause of axial neck pain is cervical strain, which is a poorly defined soft tissue injury of the paraspinal ligaments and musculature. It is fortunate that the vast majority of patients with cervical strain resolve within 6 weeks, and the treatment is always nonoperative.

Cervical degenerative disc disease is the most common cause of neck pain that has not responded to conservative treatments. Unless associated with a neural compression, the treatment for axial neck pain is generally conservative. Nonoperative treatment is the rule, because fusion for axial neck pain alone has, in many series, been associated with less predictable results.

However, if a patient has severe, unrelenting neck pain that has lasted many months despite appropriate conservative care, operative intervention may be indicated. If imaging studies demonstrate one- or two-level disease with sparing of the remaining

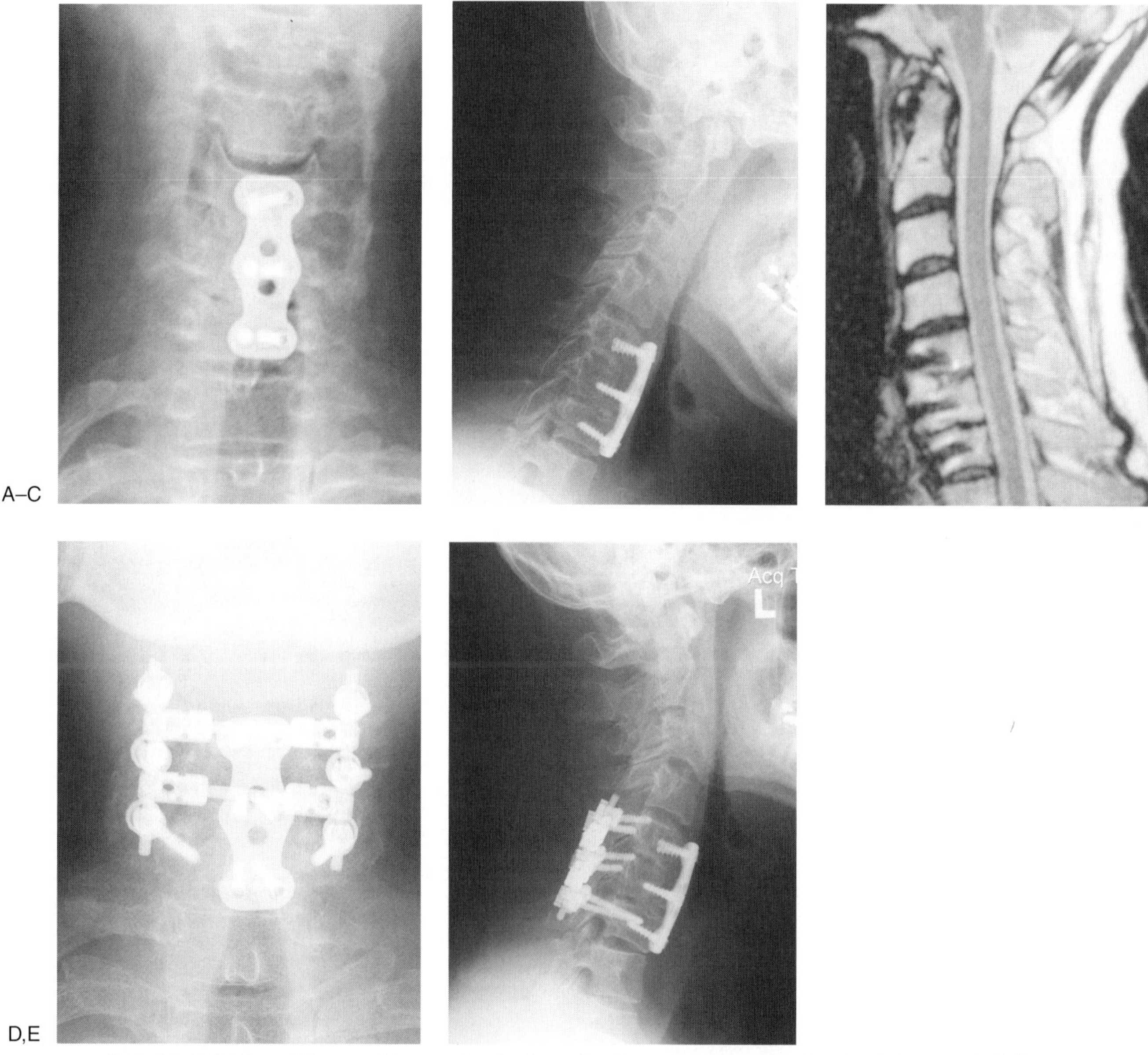

FIG. 12. B.M. is a 48-year-old man who had previously undergone a two-level anterior cervical disc fusion at C5-6 and C6-7 for mechanical neck pain and right upper extremity pain, numbness, and tingling. His symptoms improved initially after surgery, but he had recurrent and severe mechanical neck pain and occipital headaches 12 weeks after surgery. He worsened with time despite epidural steroid injections, facet blocks, and radiofrequency neurotomy. **A,B:** Anteroposterior and lateral radiographs taken 2 years after surgery revealed graft resorption and interface lucencies. The graft had clearly not consolidated at either level and had most likely collapsed significantly. **C:** Magnetic resonance imaging demonstrated no significant stenosis. The patient underwent posterior cervical fusion with lateral mass screw instrumentation. At C-7, pedicles were present and quite large, so it was possible to place pedicle screws at this level. **D,E:** Postoperative anteroposterior and lateral radiographs demonstrate appropriate placement of all screws and formation of fusion mass posterolaterally. Clinically, the patient is markedly improved, with minimal residual axial symptoms.

cervical discs, selective fusion has, in more recent studies, been found to be of benefit.

Other potential causes of axial neck pain include C-4 radiculopathy or cervical pseudarthrosis. C-4 radiculopathy should be suspected if the patient has paresthesias or numbness in this distribution or if the symptoms are unilateral. Often, it may be hard to distinguish C-4 radiculopathy from axial neck pain, and thus, ACDF is generally the treatment of choice. Cervical pseudarthrosis should be suspected in the patient with persistent symptoms despite previous ACDF. A thorough course of conservative treatment must always be prescribed for these conditions also, and surgery must be considered only if all nonoperative options have been exhausted.

REFERENCES

1. Bovim G, Schrader H, Sand T. Neck pain in the general population. *Spine* 1994;19:1307–1309.
2. Makela M, Heliovaara M, Sievers K, et al. Prevalence, determinants and consequences of chronic neck pain in Finland. *J Epidemiol* 1991;134:1356–1367.
3. Dvorak J. Epidemiology, physical examination and neurodiagnostics. *Spine* 1998;23:2663–2672.
4. Rappoport LH, O'Leary PF. Cervical disc disease. In: Bridwell KH, DeWald RL, eds. *The textbook of spinal surgery*. Philadelphia: Lippincott–Raven, 1997:1371–1396.
5. Riew KD, McCulloch JA, Delamarter RB, et al. Microsurgery for degenerative conditions of the cervical spine. *Instr Course Lect* 2003;52:497–508.
6. An HS. Anterior cervical spine procedures. In: An HS, Riley LH III, eds. *An atlas of surgery of the spine*. London: Martin Dunitz Ltd, 1998:2–13.
7. Andrews ET, Gentchos EJ, Beller ML. Results of anterior cervical spine fusions done at the Hospital of the University of Pennsylvania: a nine year follow up. *Clin Orthop Rel Res* 1971;81:15–20.
8. Riley LH, Robinson RA, Johnson KA, et al. The results of anterior interbody fusion of the cervical spine. *J Neurosurg* 1969;30:127–133.
9. Robinson RA, Walker E, Ferlic DC, et al. The results of anterior interbody fusion of the cervical spine. *J Bone Joint Surg Am* 1962; 44:1569–1587.
10. Smith MD. Cervical spondylosis. In: Bridwell KH, DeWald RL, eds. *The textbook of spinal surgery*. Philadelphia: Lippincott–Raven, 1997:1397–1420.
11. Lestini WF, Wiesel SW. The pathogenesis of cervical spondylosis. *Clin Orthop Rel Res* 1989;239:69–93.
12. Connell MD, Wiesel SW. Natural history and pathogenesis of cervical disc disease. *Orthop Clin North Am* 1992;23:369–380.
13. Winkelstein BA, McLendon RE, Barbir A, et al. An anatomical investigation of the human cervical facet capsule, quantifying muscle insertion area. *J Anat* 2001;198:455–461.
14. Bogduk N, Windsor M, Inglis A. The innervation of the cervical intervertebral discs. *Spine* 1988;13:2–8.
15. Roth DA. Cervical analgesic discography: a new test for the definitive diagnosis of the painful disc syndrome. *JAMA* 1976;235:1713–1714.
16. Emery SE. Cervical disc disease and cervical spondylosis. In: An HS, ed. *Principles and techniques of spine surgery*. Baltimore: Williams and Wilkins, 1998:401–412.
17. Bogduk N, Marsland A. The cervical zygapophysial joints as a source of neck pain. *Spine* 1988;13:610–617.
18. Dwyer A, Aprill C, Bogduk N. Cervical zygapophyseal joint pain patterns I: a study in normal volunteers. *Spine* 1990;15: 453–457.
19. Aprill C, Dwyer A, Bogduk N. Cervical zygapophyseal joint pain patterns II: a clinical evaluation. *Spine* 1990;15:458–461.
20. Barnsley L, Lord SM, Wallis BE, et al. False-positive rates of cervical zygapophysial joint blocks. *Clin J Pain* 1993;9:124–130.
21. Lord SM, Barnsley L, Bogduk N. The utility of comparative local anesthetic blocks versus placebo-controlled blocks for the diagnosis of cervical zygapophysial joint pain. *Clin J Pain* 1995;11:208–213.
22. Ulig Y, Weber BR, Grob D, et al. Fiber composition and fiber transformation in neck muscles of patients with dysfunction of the cervical spine. *J Orthop Res* 1995;13:240–249.
23. Mealy K, Brennan H, Frenelon GC. Early mobilization of acute whiplash injuries. *BMJ* 1986;292:656–657.
24. Larsson SE, Alund M, Cai H, et al. Chronic pain after soft tissue injury of the cervical spine: trapezius muscle blood flow and electromyography at static load and fatigue. *Pain* 1994;57:173–180.
25. Newman M. The outcome of pseudoarthrosis after cervical anterior fusion. *Spine* 1993;18:2380–2382.
26. Nadler S, Cooke P. Myofascial pain in whiplash injuries: diagnosis and treatment. *Spine State Art Rev* 1998;12:357–376.
27. Boden SD, McCowin PR, Davis DO, et al. Abnormal magnetic resonance scans of the cervical spine in asymptomatic subjects: a prospective investigation. *J Bone Joint Surg Am* 1990;72:1178–1184.
28. Abdu WA, Provencher M. Primary bone and metastatic tumors of the cervical spine. *Spine* 1998;23:2767–2776.
29. Kaiser JA, Holland BA. Imaging of the cervical spine. 1998; 23:2701–2712.
30. Reitner MF, Boden SD. Inflammatory disorders of the cervical spine. *Spine* 1998;23:2755–2756.
31. An HS. Cervical spine trauma. *Spine* 1998;23:2713–2729.
32. Jenis LG, An HS. Neck pain secondary to radiculopathy of the fourth cervical root: an analysis of 12 surgically treated patients. *J Spinal Disord* 2000;13:345–349.
33. Sobel JB, Sollenberger P, Robinson R, et al. Cervical nonorganic signs: a new clinical tool to assess abnormal illness behavior in neck pain patients: a pilot study. *Arch Phys Med Rehabil* 2000;81:170–175.
34. Taylor JR, Finch P. Acute injury of the neck: anatomical and pathological basis of pain. *Ann Acad Med Singapore* 1993;22:187–192.
35. Sola AE, Rodenberger ML, Getlys BB. Incidence of hypersensitive areas in posterior shoulder muscles. *Am J Phys Med Rehabil* 1955; 34:585–590.
36. Quebec Task Force on Spinal Disorders. Scientific approach to the assessment and management of activity-related spinal disorders: a monograph for clinicians. Report of the Quebec Task Force on Spinal Disorders. *Spine* 1987;12S:S1–S59.
37. MacNab I, McCulloch J. *Neck ache and shoulder pain*. Baltimore: Williams & Wilkins, 1994;54–78.
38. Hohl M. Soft tissue injuries of the neck in automobile accidents: factors influencing prognosis. *J Bone Joint Surg Am* 1974;56:1675–1682.
39. Gargan MF, Bannister GC. Long-term prognosis of soft tissue injuries of the neck. *J Bone Joint Surg Br* 1990;72:901–903.
40. Pellengahr C, Pfahler M, Kuhr M, et al. Influence of facet joint angles and asymmetric disc collapse on degenerative olisthesis of the cervical spine. *Orthopedics* 2000;23:697–701.
41. Helliwell PS, Evans PF, Wright V. The straight cervical spine: does it indicate muscle spasm? *J Bone Joint Surg Br* 1994;76:103–106.
42. Kristjansson E, Jonsson H Jr. Is the sagittal configuration of the cervical spine changed in women with chronic whiplash syndrome? A comparative computer-assisted radiographic assessment. *J Manipul Physiol Ther* 2002;25:550–555.

42a. Grob D. Surgery in the degenerative cervical spine. *Spine* 1998; 23:2674–2683.

43. Collins HR. An evaluation of cervical and lumbar discography. *Clin Orthop Rel Res* 1975;107:133–138.
44. Holt EP. Fallacy of cervical discography. *JAMA* 1964;188:799–801.
45. Holt EP. Further reflections on cervical discography. *JAMA* 1975;231:613–614.
46. Barnsley L, Lord SM, Wallis BJ, et al. Lack of effect of intraarticular corticosteroids for chronic pain in the cervical zygapophyseal joints. *N Engl J Med* 1994;330:1047–1050.
47. Hove B, Gyldensted C. Cervical analgesic facet joint arthrography. *Neuroradiology* 1990;32:456–459.
48. Kwan O, Friel J. Critical appraisal of facet joint injections for chronic whiplash. *Med Schi Monit* 2002;8:191–195.
49. Laing RJ, Ng I, Seeley HM, et al. Prospective study of clinical and radiological outcome after anterior cervical discectomy. *Br J Neurosurg* 2001;15:319–323.
50. Kauppila LI, Penttila A. Postmortem angiographic study of degenerative vascular changes in arteries supplying the cervicobrachial region. *Ann Rheum Dis* 1994;53:94–99.
51. Ahn NU, Imai Y, An HS, et al. Effect of nutrient concentration and OP-1 on intervertebral disc metabolism: an *in vitro* organ culture study. Presentation at the North American Spine Society Annual Meeting, Montreal, October 2002.
52. Garvery TA, Transfeldt EE, Malcolm JR, et al. Outcome of anterior cervical discectomy and fusion as perceived by patients treated for dominant axial-mechanical cervical spine pain. *Spine* 2002;27:1887–1894.
53. Lindsey RW, Newhouse KE, Leach J, et al. Nonunion following two-level anterior cervical discectomy and fusion. *Clin Orthop Rel Res* 1987;223:155–163.
54. Phillips FM, Carlson G, Emery SE, et al. Anterior cervical pseudoarthrosis: natural history and treatment. *Spine* 1997;22:1585–1589.
55. An HS. Internal fixation of the cervical spine: current indications and techniques. *J Am Acad Orthop Surg* 1995;3:194–206.

56. Hilibrand AS, Dina TS. The use of diagnostic imaging to assess spinal arthrodesis. *Orthop Clin North Am* 1998;29:591–601.
57. Cannada LK, Scherping SC, Yoo JU, et al. Pseudoarthrosis of the cervical spine: a comparison of radiographic diagnostic measures. *Spine* 2003;28:46–51.
58. Fongemie AE, Buss DD, Rolnick SJ. Management of shoulder impingement syndrome and rotator cuff tears. *Am Fam Phys* 1998;57:667–682.
59. Clarke HD, McCann PD. Acromioclavicular joint injuries. *Orthop Clin North Am* 2000;31:177–187.
60. Maus TP. Imaging of the spine and nerve roots. *Phys Med Rehabil Clin N Am* 2002;13:487–544.
61. Chevrot A, Drape JL, Godefroy D, et al. Imaging of the painful cervical spine. *J Radiol* 2003;84:181–239.
62. Dreyer SJ, Boden SD. Nonoperative treatment of neck and arm pain. *Spine* 1998;23:2746–2754.
63. Maimaris C, Barnes MR, Allen MJ. Whiplash injuries of the neck: a retrospective study. *Injury* 1988;19:393–396.
64. Squires B, Gargan MF, Bannister GC. Soft-tissue injuries of the cervical spine. *J Bone Joint Surg Br* 1996;78:955–957.
65. McKinney LA. Early mobilization and outcome in acute sprains of the neck. *BMJ* 1989;299:1006–1008.
66. Bronfort G, Evans R, Nelson B, et al. A randomized clinical trial of exercise and spinal manipulation for patients with chronic neck pain. *Spine* 2001;26:788–797.
67. McKinney LA, Dornan JO, Ryan M. The role of physiotherapy in the management of acute neck sprains following road traffic events. *Arch Emerg Med* 1989;6:27–33.
68. Stovner LJ. The nosologic status of the whiplash syndrome: a critical review based on a methodological approach. *Spine* 1996;21:2735–2746.
69. Pettersson K, Toolanen G. High-dose methylprednisolone prevents extensive sick leave after whiplash injury: a prospective, double blind study. *Spine* 1998;23:984–989.
70. Ferrante FM, Wilson SP, Iacobo C, et al. Clinical classification as a predictor of therapeutic outcome after cervical epidural steroid injection. *Spine* 1993;18:730–736.
71. Field J, Rathmell JP, Stephenson JH, et al. Neuropathic pain following cervical epidural steroid injection. *Anesthesiology* 2000;93:885–888.
72. Furman MB, Giovanniello MT, O'Brien EM. Incidence of intravascular penetration in transforaminal cervical epidural steroid injections. *Spine* 2003;28:21–25.
73. Hodges SD, Castleberg RL, Miller T, et al. Cervical epidural steroid injection with intrinsic spinal cord damage. Two case reports. *Spine* 1998;23:2137–2142.
74. Reitman CA, Watters W 3rd. Subdural hematoma after cervical epidural steroid injection. *Spine* 2002;27:E174–E176.
75. Siegfried RN. Development of complex regional pain syndrome after a cervical epidural steroid injection. *Anesthesiology* 1997;86:1394–1396.
76. Stoll A, Sanchez M. Epidural hematoma after epidural block: implications for its use in pain management. *Surg Neurol* 2002;57:235–240.
77. Waldman SD. Complications of cervical epidural nerve blocks with steroids: a prospective study of 790 consecutive blocks. *Reg Anesth* 1989;14:149–151.
78. Williams KN, Jackowski A, Evans PJ. Epidural haematoma requiring surgical decompression following repeated cervical epidural steroid injections for chronic pain. *Pain* 1990;42:197–199.
79. Mankin HJ. Nontraumatic necrosis of bone (osteonecrosis). *N Engl J Med* 1992;326:1473–1479.
80. Vendrig AA, van Akkerveeken F, McWhorter KR. Results of a multimodal treatment program for patients with chronic symptoms after a whiplash injury of the neck. *Spine* 2000;25:238–244.
81. Botwin KP, Castellanos R, Rao S, et al. Complications of fluoroscopically guided interlaminar cervical epidural injections. *Arch Phys Med Rehabil* 2003;84:627–633.
82. Schellhas KP. Facet nerve blockade and radiofrequency neurotomy. *Neuroimag Clin N Am* 2000;10:493–501.
83. Silbergleit R, Mehta BA, Sanders WP. Image-guided injection techniques with fluoroscopy and CT for spinal pain management. *Radiographics* 2001;21:927–942.
84. Lord SM, Barnsley L, Wallis BJ, et al. Percutaneous radio-frequency neurotomy for chronic cervical zygapophyseal joint pain. *N Eng J Med* 1996;335:1721–1726.
85. Williams JL, Allen MB, Harkess JW. Late results of cervical discectomy and interbody fusion: some factors influencing the results. *J Bone Joint Surg Am* 1968;50:277–286.
86. White AA III, Southwick WO, Deponte RJ, et al. Relief of pain by anterior cervical spine fusion for spondylosis: a report of sixty-five patients. *J Bone Joint Surg Am* 1973;55:252–534.
87. Dohn D. Anterior interbody fusion for treatment of cervical disc condition. *JAMA* 1966;197:897–900.
88. Palit M, Schofferman J, Goldwaite N, et al. Anterior discectomy and fusion for the management of neck pain. *Spine* 1999;24:2224–2228.
89. Simmons EH, Bhalla SK. Anterior cervical discectomy and fusion: a clinical and biomechanical study with eight-year follow up. *J Bone Joint Surg Br* 1969;51:225–237.
90. Colhoun EI, McCall W, Williams L, et al. Provocation discography as a guide to planning operations on the spine. *J Bone Joint Surg Br* 1988;70:267–271.
91. Kikuchi S, McNab I, Moreau P. Localisation of the level of symptomatic cervical disc degeneration. *J Bone Joint Surg Br* 1981;63:272–277.
92. Sneider SE, Winslow OP, Pryor TH Cervical discography: is it relevant? *JAMA* 1963;185:163–165.
93. Guyer RD, Ohnmeiss DD, Mason SL, et al. Complications of cervical discography: findings in a large series. *J Spinal Disord* 1997;10:95–101.
94. Zeidman SM, Thompson K, Ducker TB. Complications of cervical discography: analysis of 4400 diagnostic disc injections. *Neurosurgery* 1995;37:414–417.
95. Bogkuk N. Point of view. *Spine* 2002;27:1895.
96. Garfin SR. Editorial. Spine focus: cervical spine. *Spine* 1998;23:2661–2662.
97. An HS, Xu R. Posterior cervical spine procedures. In: An HS, Riley LR III, eds. *An atlas of surgery of the spine*. London: Martin Dunitz Ltd, 1998:13–54.
98. Cicala RS, Thoni K, Angel JJ. Long-term results of cervical epidural steroid injections. *Clin J Pain* 1989;5:143–145.
99. Mulligan KA, Rowlingson JC. Epidural steroids. *Curr Pain Headache Rep* 2001;5:495–502.
100. An HS, Ahn NU. Posterior decompressive procedures for the cervical spine. *Instr Course Lect* 2003;52:471–477.
101. Zdeblick TA, Zou D, Warden KE, et al. Cervical stability after foraminotomy. A biomechanical *in vitro* analysis. *J Bone Joint Surg Am* 1992;74:22–27.
102. Lowery GL, Swank ML, McDonough RF. Surgical revision for failed anterior cervical fusions: articular pillar plating or anterior revision? *Spine* 1995;20:2436–2441.
103. Brodsky AE, Khalil MA, Sassard WR, et al. Repair of symptomatic pseudoarthrosis of anterior cervical fusion: posterior versus anterior repair. *Spine* 1992;17:1137–1143.
104. Tribus CB, Corteen DP, Zdeblick TA. The efficacy of anterior cervical plating in the management of symptomatic pseudoarthrosis of the cervical spine. *Spine* 1999;24:860–864.
105. Heller JG, Silcox DH III, Sutterlin CE III. Complications of posterior cervical plating. *Spine* 1995;20:2442–2448.
106. Wellman BJ, Follett KA, Traynelis VC. Complications of posterior articular mass plate fixation of the subaxial cervical spine in 43 consecutive patients. *Spine* 1998;23:193–200.
107. Panjabi MM. Cervical spine models for biomechanical research. *Spine* 1998;23:2684–2700.
108. Papagelopoulos PJ, Currier BL, Neale PG, et al. Biomechanical evaluation of posterior screw fixation in cadaveric cervical spines. *Clin Orthop* 2003;411:13–24.
109. Shad A, Shariff SS, Teddy PJ, et al. Craniocervical fusion for rheumatoid arthritis: comparison of sublaminar wires and the lateral mass screw craniocervical fusion. *Br J Neurosurg* 2002;16: 483–486.
110. Lindsey RW, Miclau T. Posterior lateral mass plate fixation of the cervical spine. *J South Orthop Assoc* 2000;9:36–42.
111. Mihara H, Cheng BC, David SM, et al. Biomechanical comparison of posterior cervical fixation. *Spine* 2001;26:1662–1667.
112. Siambanes D, Miz GS. Treatment of symptomatic anterior cervical nonunion using the Rogers interspinous wiring technique. *Am J Orthop* 1998;27:792–796.
113. Siebenrock KA, Aebi M. The value of discography in disc related pain syndrome of the cervical spine for evaluation of indications for sponydlodesis. *Z Orthop Ihre Grenzgeb* 1993; 131:220–224.
114. Whitecloud TS III, Seago RA. Cervical discogenic syndrome: results of operative intervention in patients with positive discography. *Spine* 1987;12:131–316.

CHAPTER 35

Cervical Disc Disease

B. Cervical Radiculopathy

Louis G. Jenis, David H. Kim, and Howard S. An

Treatment of cervical radiculopathy is based on a clear understanding of its natural history and available therapeutic options for this disorder. This chapter reviews the pathophysiology of cervical spondylosis and nerve root compression and relates it to the development of clinical manifestations. It also discusses clinical evaluation and nonoperative and operative management of such problems.

CERVICAL ANATOMY AND PATHOANATOMY

Management of the symptomatic patient is based on an understanding of normal and pathologic cervical anatomy. The subaxial vertebral bodies increase in size from cephalad to caudad and are greater in the transverse than the anteroposterior dimension (1). The superior end-plate surface is concave, whereas the inferior surface is convex. Uncovertebral joints of Luschka or uncinate processes project from the superior posterior corner of each vertebral body and form a synovial-lined articulation with the corresponding vertebra (2). Short, small pedicles arise from the posterior vertebral body and extend posterolaterally to the lateral masses. The lateral masses are unique to the cervical spine and form superior and inferior articulations through synovial-lined facet joints. The laminae extend posteromedially from the lateral masses and form the spinous process, which in the cervical spine is ordinarily bifid.

A clinically important area of the cervical spine is the neuroforamen. The neuroforamina are confined zones for the exiting nerve roots bordered anteriorly by the lateral aspect of the intervertebral disc and uncovertebral joint, superiorly and inferiorly by the pedicles, and posteriorly by the articular masses, notably the superior articular facet. Pathologic conditions involving these structures can lead to stenosis of the foramen and nerve root compression.

The lordosis that is typically present in the cervical spine is the result of the shape and configuration of the intervertebral disc. The discs make up nearly 22% of the overall length of the cervical spine (1) and are thicker in height anteriorly, which promotes the lordosis. The intervertebral discs increase range of motion between the vertebral bodies and distribute forces over the length of the spine.

The change from normal anatomy to an aging spondylotic cervical spine is subtle and is part of the degenerative cascade. The initial biochemical alterations are suspected to occur within the intervertebral disc, leading to secondary mechanical changes in the surrounding facet joints and soft tissue structures. Diminished water content, along with changes in the ratio of proteoglycan to collagen and keratin sulfate to chondroitin sulfate, are early manifestations of degeneration (3). The nucleus pulposus is no longer able to generate the hydro-

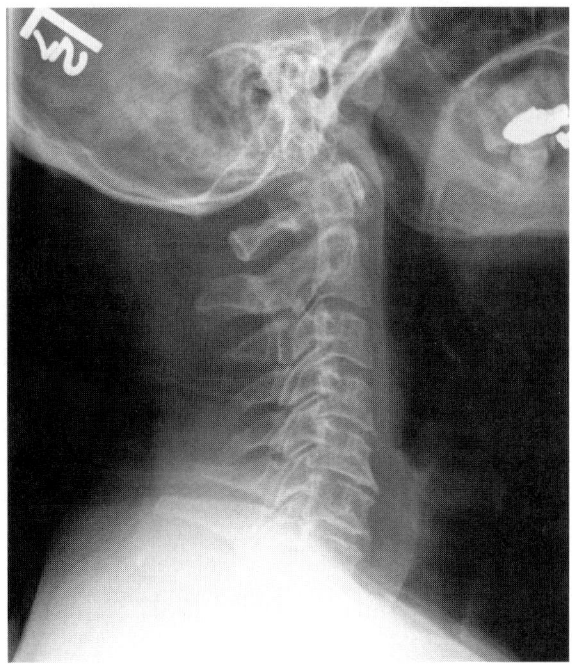

FIG. 1. Lateral radiograph depicting spondylosis and multiple-level disc height loss. Note loss of cervical lordosis.

static intradiscal force required to expand the annular fibers. This subjects the annular fibers to excessive compression and shear forces, causing weakening and tearing of their outer layers. Weakened external annular fibers may still be sufficiently strong to contain a nucleus bulging, or frank protrusion or rupture may intrude into the spinal canal. This is often referred to as a *soft disc herniation*.

Disc dehydration also results in loss of height. This is more prominent in the anterior disc space because the uncovertebral joints impact on the posterior vertebral bodies as collapse occurs, preventing further posterior disc height loss. The combined effect leads to the characteristic loss of cervical lordosis, observed in lateral plain radiographs (4) (   ).

Approximation of the vertebral bodies alters the biomechanical forces placed on the uncovertebral joints and articular facet joints. Osteophytic spurring, often referred to as *hard disc*, may develop, leading to encroachment on the neuroforamina. Similarly, reactive bone forms along the posterior vertebral bodies that is thought to be the result of increased compressive loads. A spondylotic transverse bar may subsequently form, combined with bulging of the posterior disc and stretching of the posterior longitudinal ligament (PLL). Further collapse of the anterior column height leads to buckling of the ligamentum flavum into the spinal canal, most notably during neck extension. This combination of events may lead to spondylosis-induced compromise of the anterior-posterior diameter of the canal.

There are several sites within the spinal canal where neurocompression may occur. Radiculopathy may occur from posterolateral soft disc herniation contained by the PLL or free material extruded into and sequestered within the canal. In addition, foraminal stenosis from the degenerative changes described previously may also lead to impingement on the exiting nerve root.

NATURAL HISTORY

The natural history of cervical radiculopathy has been studied. Progression from radiculopathy to myelopathy is unusual, and it appears that these are distinct entities (5). Lees and Turner reported on the long-term surveillance of patients with spondylosis and confirmed that 30% experienced intermittent radicular symptoms, whereas 25% had a persistent radiculopathy (6). In general, there is agreement that nonoperative treatment may alleviate symptoms of cervical spondylotic radiculopathy in the short term, but over a long period of time, symptoms frequently recur. Gore and colleagues retrospectively reviewed patients with cervical radiculopathy treated conservatively and noted 50% with persistent symptoms at 15-year follow-up (7). It appears that most patients with arm pain improve over time; however, recurrence of symptoms is common.

A common clinical dilemma is separating normal aging changes seen on plain radiographs from degenerative changes that produce symptoms. The natural history of cervical spine aging has been studied in a variety of population-based cohorts. Degenerative changes evaluated radiographically have included disc space narrowing and osteophytes. As a rule of thumb, the prevalence of significant radiographic changes parallels the decade of age. For example, in the 50-year cohort, approximately 50% demonstrate degenerative change independent of any history of cervical spine complaints. The severity of these changes also increases with age. These observations mean the clinician cannot immediately assume the radiographic changes observed are the cause of the patient's symptoms.

CLINICAL EVALUATION

Clinical evaluation of patients with cervical degenerative disorders requires interpretation of the patient's complaints, meticulous examination, and appropriate selection of diagnostic tests. A detailed history is the initial step. A complete description of the symptoms includes the onset, quality, and location of pain; inciting and alleviating factors; temporal nature; degree of impairment; and any associated symptoms. Axial neck pain may be discogenic or musculogenic in origin, or related to shoulder, occipitocervical, myofascial, or visceral pathology. To differentiate potential multiple sources of neck pain, it is necessary to establish whether the symptoms are mechanical (i.e., increased with activity and diminished with rest or positioning) or nonmechanical (i.e., no relief with positional changes or rest). Nonmechanical neck pain may be related to tumor or infection, and such processes should be carefully sought out. A history of deep-seated aching pain that occurs only at night and is absent or markedly diminished during the day is suggestive of neoplasm or infection. Mechanical neck pain is commonly discogenic in origin and exacerbated with neck extension and rotation toward the side that is more symptomatic. Patients may describe pain referred to the shoulder, upper-arm region, or interscapular area. Patients with upper cervical degeneration may also experience occipital or temporal pain, or retroocular headaches. Musculogenic pain, most frequently associated with acute or chronic muscle strain, is more often exacerbated with neck flexion and rotation leading to increased symptoms on the opposite side of head rotation.

Radiculopathy may present in a single or multiple nerve root distribution. Symptoms consist of variable degrees of sharp, boring, or lancinating radiating arm pain associated with various degrees of dysesthesias, paresthesias, and numbness along a dermatomal pat-

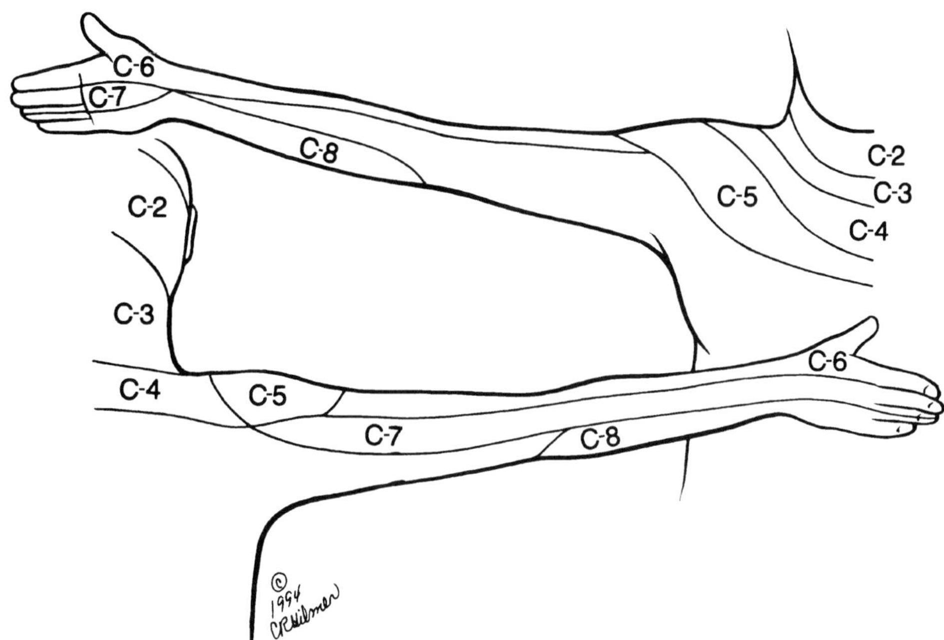

FIG. 2. An illustration of dermatomal patterns that corresponds to a distribution of cervical radicular symptoms consisting of variable degrees of sharp, boring, or lancinating radiating arm pain associated with various degrees of dysesthesias, paresthesias, and numbness of the involved nerve root or nerve roots.

tern of the involved nerve root (   ). The symptoms may be exacerbated or relieved by several tests. Typically, patients describe an increase in pain with the Valsalva maneuver. *Spurling's sign* is elicited by neck hyperextension and rotation toward the symptomatic side, resulting in reproduction of the arm pain (   ). This test proposes to diminish the available area in an already compromised neuroforamen, leading to further nerve root compression. A less reliable provocative sign is the axial compression test, in which compression on the vertex of the skull may diminish the height of the foramen and also reproduce symptoms. The *shoulder abduction sign* is a test that relieves symptoms of compression by lessening nerve root stretch with placement of the ipsilateral hand on top of the head (8) (   ). Patients may relate this as the only upper-extremity position that provides relief or comfort.

Upper cervical nerve root compression is less common than at lower levels, but it must be considered in the differential diagnosis of recalcitrant neck pain (9). Radiculopathy of the C-3 or C-4 roots manifests as neck pain radiating to the trapezial, shoulder, and anterolateral area of the chest. The symptoms are described as pain with variable degrees of paresthesias but without a specific motor deficit. The more classic presentations occur with compression of the lower cervical nerve roots.

A C-5 radiculopathy produces radiating pain down the lateral aspect of the shoulder and proximal arm with associated sensory changes and increased fatigue or weakness of shoulder abduction. The C-5 root solely innervates the deltoid, whereas the biceps have dual innervations from C-5 and C-6.

A C-6 radiculopathy produces neck pain radiating down the biceps and anterior arm to the radial aspect of the forearm and index finger and thumb. The biceps and wrist extensors may demonstrate weakness. The extensor carpi radialis longus and brevis are innervated by C-6, whereas the extensor carpi ulnaris is primarily C-7. Therefore, wrist extensor weakness may reflect compression of C-6 or C-7. The brachioradialis reflex is most directly affected with C-6 compression, with subtle changes noted in the biceps reflex owing to its dual innervations.

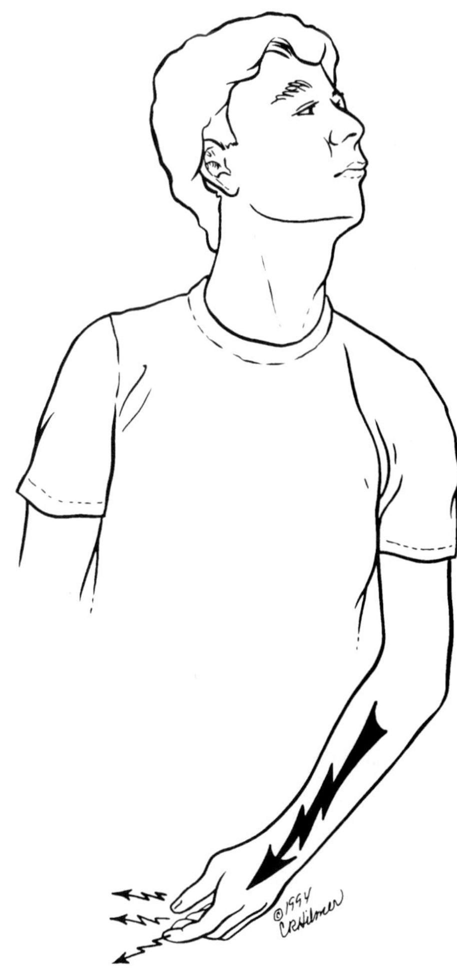

FIG. 3. A diagram of Spurling's sign, elicited by neck hyperextension and rotation toward the symptomatic side and resulting in reproduction of the arm pain.

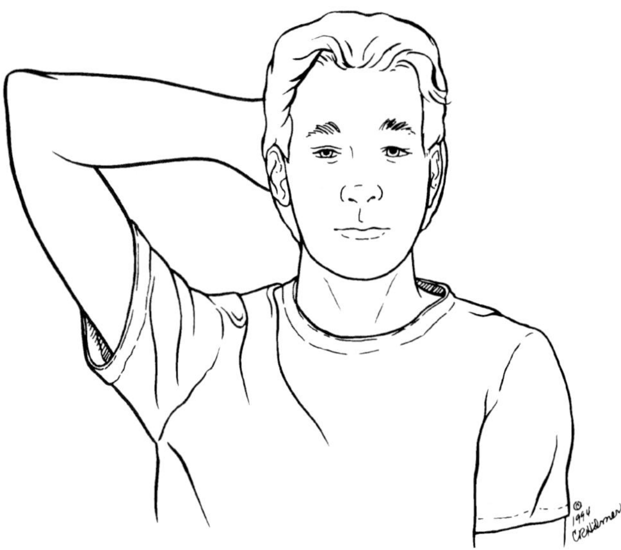

FIG. 4. A diagram of the shoulder abduction sign, which relieves symptoms of compression by lessening nerve root stretch with placement of the ipsilateral hand on top of the head.

Compressive pathology of the C-7 nerve root presents with pain along the posterior shoulder and arm, radiating to the posterolateral aspect of the forearm to the long finger. Inconsistent symptoms involving the index and ring digits as well as the first web space may also be detected. The triceps muscle is affected, resulting in a diminished reflex and elbow extensor weakness.

C-8 radiculopathy is characterized by pain referred to the ulnar aspect of the forearm, small finger, and ulnar half of the ring finger. The findings are primarily below the elbow, with most dysfunction noted as numbness along the ulnar digits and weakness in finger adduction and abduction and flexion. In chronic C-8 root compression, intrinsic muscle atrophy may be seen in the affected hand.

DIAGNOSTIC TESTING

Improved neuroradiologic imaging has led to a better understanding of the pathologic process of cervical radiculopathy and myelopathy. Several techniques are available for the evaluation of the symptomatic patient. Each modality has its own inherent strengths and weaknesses, and often combinations of examinations are required.

The initial radiographic evaluation includes anteroposterior, lateral, and oblique views, and, when instability is suspected, dynamic lateral images in flexion-extension may be obtained. Findings such as disc space narrowing, developmental canal stenosis, subluxations and malalignments, and vertebral osteophyte formation must be evaluated in light of the patient's symptoms. Abnormal findings on plain radiographs may not be the cause of the clinical picture, and may simply reflect age-related changes. Further correlative studies may be necessary before recommending specific treatment. Changes on plain radiographs may reassure the clinician and the patient that the clinical suspicion of typical degenerative disease is correct.

The anteroposterior view on water-soluble myelography demonstrates the exiting nerve roots to the level of the pedicle. A filling defect is a typical finding of nerve root compression. The lateral view may detect spinal cord compression caused by the disc or posterior vertebral osteophytes or hypertrophied ligamentum flavum, or both. Current practice favors myelographically enhanced computed tomography (CT), which improves visualization of osseous compressive structures especially in the neuroforamina (4). CT-myelography infers neural compression by deformity of the dural sac or nerve roots, however, and cannot directly determine the etiology of contrast blockade.

Magnetic resonance imaging (MRI) provides direct information about nerve root or spinal cord compression. The advantage of MRI in detecting direct compression is the intrinsic "contrast" available from the cerebrospinal fluid as seen on T2-weighted images ( ). This is the most sensitive modality for assessing

A

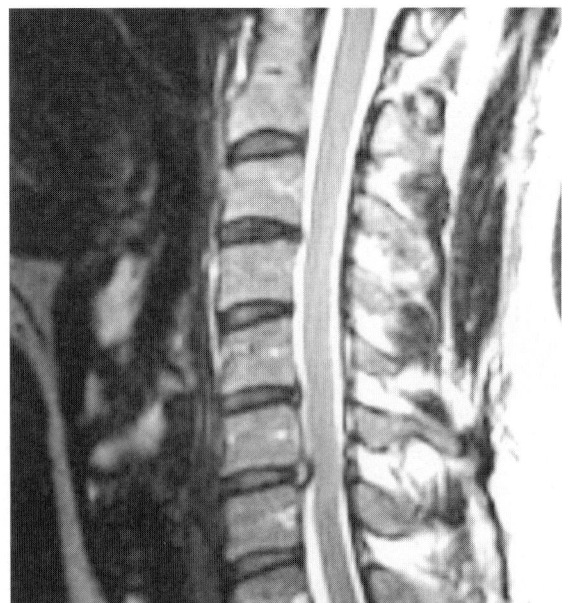

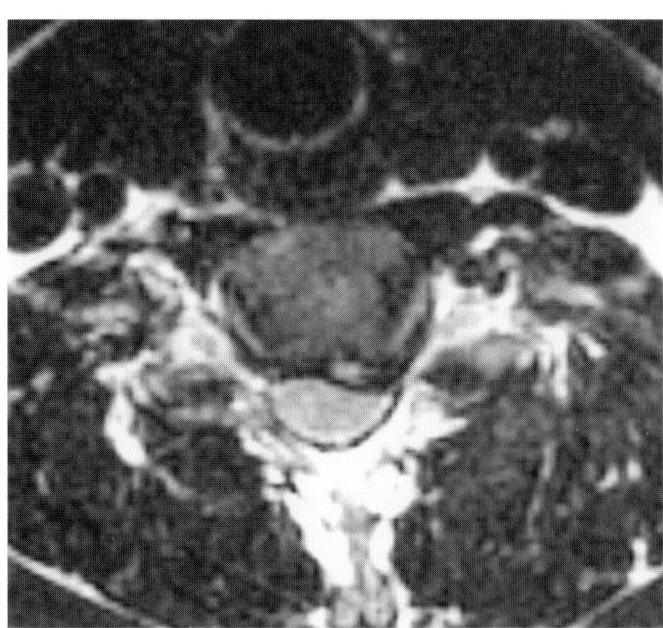

B

FIG. 5. Midsagittal **(A)** and axial **(B)** T2-weighted magnetic resonance images depicting left paracentral herniation extending into the neuroforamen.

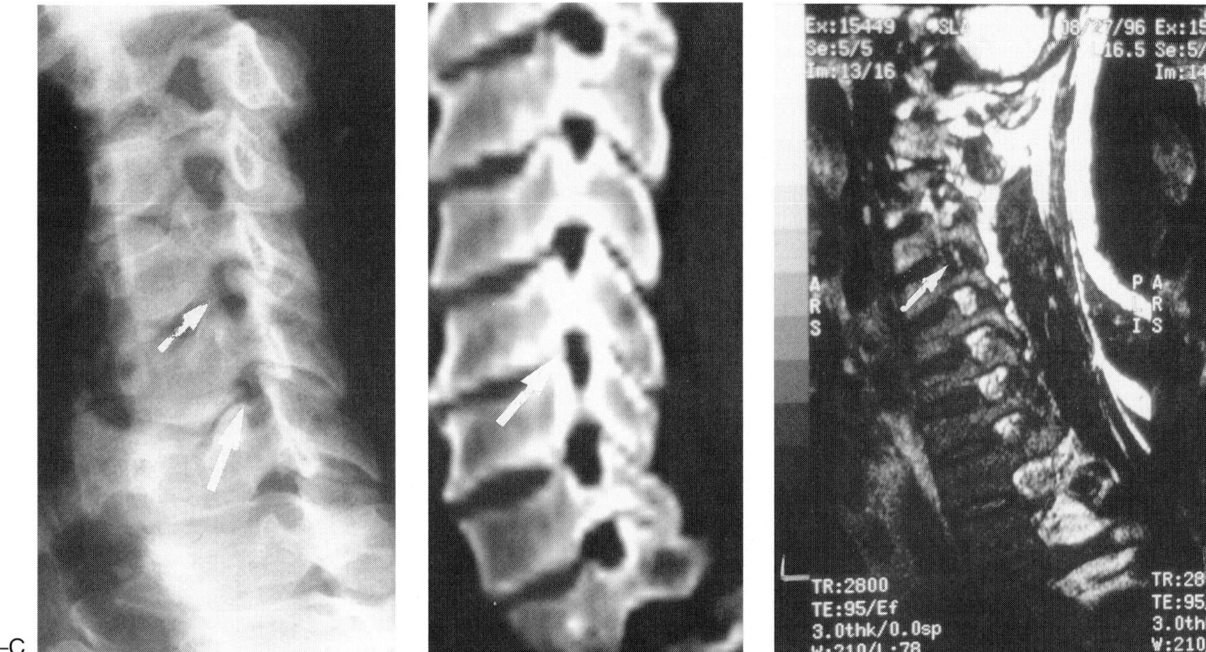

FIG. 6. Oblique radiograph **(A)**, 45-degree oblique sagittal reconstruction computed tomography image **(B)**, and direct 45-degree oblique magnetic resonance image showing foraminal stenosis **(C)** (*arrows*).

the morphology of the spinal cord and its relation to the spinal canal. MRI also shows intramedullary cord changes that may relate to disease prognosis. MRI is less sensitive in detecting foraminal stenosis, however, and does not demonstrate cortical margins as well as CT-myelography. Because the diagnosis of symptomatic foraminal stenosis may be elusive, special scans and procedures may be necessary, such as oblique radiographs, 45-degree oblique sagittal reconstruction CT images, direct oblique MRI, and foraminal nerve root block (10) ( ).

Electromyography/nerve conduction studies may be used to confirm suspected radiculopathy or may be used as an additional diagnostic method to further elucidate the cause of symptoms in a patient with atypical findings. These tests are most useful in differentiating root compression from a peripheral neuropathy. Bone scans, local trigger or facet injections, discography, and cerebrospinal fluid analysis have a limited diagnostic role in most patients.

NONOPERATIVE TREATMENT

In general, the natural history of cervical radiculopathy is considered to be favorable. The majority of patients experience resolution or acceptable improvement in symptoms without surgical intervention. A large number of published studies support the efficacy of a wide variety of nonoperative treatment modalities. Most studies suffer from serious methodologic flaws, however, such as lack of appropriate control groups, small numbers, and retrospective design. Heterogeneous patient populations and inconsistent use of validated functional outcome measures further limit interstudy comparisons. The absence of a so-called gold standard for diagnosis of cervical radiculopathy or even a professional consensus regarding diagnostic criteria is an additional impediment.

Most patients experiencing an acute episode of unilateral radiculopathy without a major motor deficit and no evidence of spinal cord compression can be well managed by nonoperative measures. In these patients, the most common treatments are activity modification, nonsteroidal antiinflammatory drugs, physical therapy, and steroid injections.

Activity Modification

The efficacy of bed rest has been well studied in acute low back pain. A brief period of bed rest may be appropriate for patients with an acute lumbar radiculopathy that is aggravated by work or moderate activity. Two days of bed rest appears just as effective as 7 days and is thought to be preferable given the risk of deconditioning and learned "sick behavior" with more extended periods of bed rest (11). If patients can tolerate continuation of their work and routine daily activity with only mild pain, this should be encouraged. In these patients, a soft collar can be used to reduce muscle spasm and pain. Collars should be worn for a few days only, followed by a period of weaning (12).

Medication

Analgesic medication may be prescribed to reduce pain and improve activity tolerance. First-line medication consists of acetaminophen or a nonsteroidal antiinflammatory drug. Treatment with nonsteroidal antiinflammatory drugs has the added theoretical benefit of addressing the inflammatory component of radiculopathy. Elderly patients should be warned of the risk of gastrointestinal bleeding and renal toxicity. Physicians should also be aware of the possibility of mental status deterioration, particularly in a patient with a history of dementia or prior episodes of confusion. If an acute episode of radiculopathic pain is particularly severe, narcotic medication may be appropriate. Concerns regarding the risk of respiratory depression and addiction have limited the use of narcotic analgesia. The vast majority of patients readily discontinue narcotics once an acute pain episode has resolved (13).

Significant paraspinal muscle spasm can usually be adequately treated with a soft cervical collar. A minority of patients may benefit from a brief trial of muscle relaxants, such as cyclobenzaprine or diazepam. These mediations may have a higher addiction profile than narcotics, however, and treatment should not be prolonged. In the subpopulation of patients with pain-induced depression, antidepressant medication, such as amitriptyline, may also reduce neuropathic pain (14).

The use of oral corticosteroid medications for treatment of acute radiculopathy is controversial. Theoretically, their efficacy is due to a potent antiinflammatory effect on irritated nerve roots. Patients often demonstrate rapid and dramatic reduction in acute pain levels. The toxicity of corticosteroids is limited when these drugs are used for short periods; however, behavioral changes, such as depression and peptic ulceration, can occur. Rarely, osteonecrosis has also been associated with short courses of oral steroid use.

Physical Therapy

Physical therapy is a component of many early treatment paradigms for cervical radiculopathy, but there have been no well-designed studies unequivocally demonstrating the superiority of any specific physical therapy modality compared to no treatment at all (15). In general, the most popular treatments include traction, superficial/deep heat or cold therapy, ultrasonography, and ergonomic instruction. These can be started within 3 to 5 days and are of variable benefit to individual patients (12). Often, selection of specific modalities is left to the discretion of the therapist based on available resources and their trial-and-error experience.

An active exercise program typically begins with isometric stabilizing exercises involving the major neck and shoulder girdle muscles. These exercises are performed to maintain muscle strength during the early acute period when more complete range of motion exercises may still cause pain. Low-impact or no-impact aerobic exercise, such as a treadmill or stationary bicycle, should also be initiated as early as possible to avoid deconditioning. Once pain is controlled, active and active-assisted range of motion exercises may promote regaining functional neck motion. Progressive resistance exercises can safely begin once a pain-free range of motion has been established. After successful completion of outpatient therapy, a home therapy program should be designed and rigorously maintained. Whether this reduces the risk of recurrence is unknown.

Injection Therapy

Corticosteroid cervical epidural or nerve root injections have been proposed as a nonoperative treatment alternative for cervical radiculopathy, but their use remains controversial (16,17). Reported success rates have ranged from 40 to 71%. Analysis of the available literature is complicated by difference in techniques, medications, and the patient populations studied, as well as flawed study designs (16–19). At least two prospective randomized studies of cervical epidural or nerve root corticosteroid injection have reported positive results in patients with cervical radiculopathy (19,20).

Complication rates associated with cervical epidural nerve root injection have been reported to occur in 3 to 35% of patients. Most are minor, such as nausea, bloating, vomiting, local pain, neck stiffness, and facial flushing (18,21,22). Dural puncture, infection, and upper-extremity weakness appear to be relatively uncommon (21,22).

There are no prospective randomized well-controlled studies demonstrating efficacy of trigger point or facet injections in treatment of patients with acute cervical radiculopathy, although in one study no significant difference was found between trigger-point injection and a dry-needle placebo (23).

Manipulation

Despite widespread concern regarding the potential hazards of cervical spine manipulation, the chiropractic literature contains several reports of high-velocity–low-amplitude manipulation for cervical disc herniation (24–28). Such manipulation has been associated with increased pain and neurologic injury, as well as catastrophic vascular complications (27,29). Given the lack of strong evidence supporting the efficacy of neck manipulation for treatment of cervical radiculopathy and numerous reports of serious complications, this form of treatment cannot be recommended (30,31).

OPERATIVE TREATMENT

The indications for operative intervention in cervical radiculopathy include failure of a 3-month trial of conservative methods of treatment to relieve persistent or recurrent radicular arm pain with or without neurologic deficit and a progressive neurologic deficit (32,33). Neuroradiographic findings must be consistent with the clinical signs and symptoms, and the duration and magnitude of symptoms must be sufficient to justify surgery.

The operative approaches used for radiculopathy include anterior decompression with discectomy with or without interbody fusion (ACDF/ACD), anterior corpectomy with fusion (ACF), posterior laminotomy with foraminotomy, and laminectomy or laminoplasty with or without fusion.

Surgical exposure of the anterior aspect of the cervical spine is a relatively safe procedure and takes advantage of normal anatomic fascial planes during the approach (34–36) (see Chapter 38). The superficial anatomic landmarks for incision include the hyoid bone overlying C-3, thyroid cartilage overlying the C4-5 interspace, and cricoid cartilage overlying the C-6 level. A transverse incision is used for exposure in most patients when one or two discs are to be exposed. When three or more levels are approached, a longitudinal incision along the anterior border of the sternocleidomastoid muscle is recommended.

Anterior Cervical Discectomy and Fusion

In ACDF, the intervertebral space is localized and incised with an annulotomy blade, and the disc contents and end-plate carti-

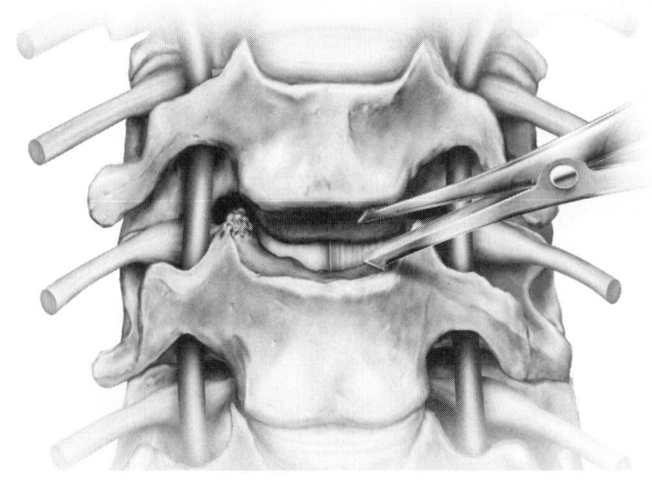
A

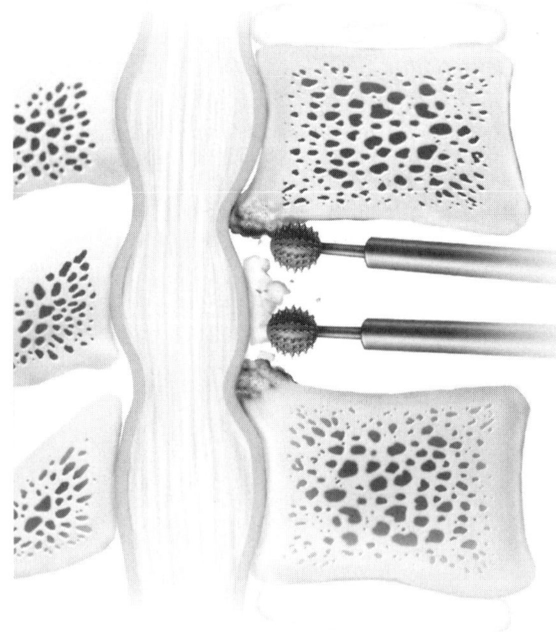
B

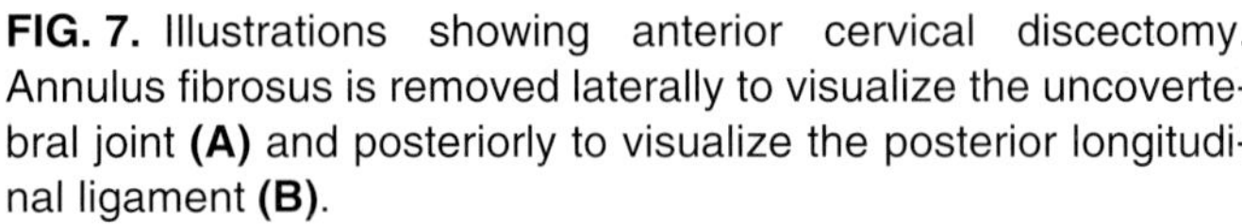
FIG. 7. Illustrations showing anterior cervical discectomy. Annulus fibrosus is removed laterally to visualize the uncovertebral joint **(A)** and posteriorly to visualize the posterior longitudinal ligament **(B)**.

lage are removed to the PLL ( ). The proper technique of discectomy involves removal of disc material in a posterior to anterior direction and lateral to medial away from the vertebral arteries. Preoperatively, it is important to evaluate imaging studies to determine the presence of a sequestered disc behind the PLL. Intraoperative palpation of the PLL may reveal a rent that also indicates a sequestered fragment. In the event that a rent is noted, or if an expected disc fragment is not identified, then the PLL is removed with Kerrison rongeurs or curettes and the fragment identified.

Removal of end-plate and uncovertebral osteophytes is controversial. The proposed benefits of fusion without spur resection are that disc space distraction reduces ligamentum flavum buckling and increases neuroforaminal area. Many believe fusion arrests spur progression and stability may allow for osteophyte resorption over time. This is not a consistent phenomenon, however, and the location and size of the offending spur must be carefully considered when performing decompression for spondylotic radiculopathy. Exposure of the uncinate processes is critical to safely remove osteophytes.

Several techniques of anterior cervical interbody fusion have been described that differ mainly in their graft configuration. The *Robinson interbody fusion technique* involves the placement of a tricortical iliac crest wedge graft into the disc space ( ). The graft height should be 2 mm greater than the preexisting disc height or have a minimum thickness of at least 5 mm to assure adequate compressive strength and to enlarge the neural foramina (37). Overdistraction of the disc space by greater than 4 mm of the preexisting height may result in overcompression, graft collapse, and pseudarthrosis.

After measuring the depth and width of the disc space, a tricortical graft is harvested from the anterior iliac crest. The graft is obtained with an oscillating bone saw, as the risk of bone weakening is greater when osteotomes are used (38). The graft is contoured to fit into the disc space and then inserted with the leading cortical edge anteriorly. The final graft position should be inset 2 mm within the vertebral bodies. The end-plate preparation is important. Too vigorous removal of the end-plate might increase the fusion rate, but the risk of subsidence is higher. Too little removal of the end-plate results in a higher rate of pseudarthrosis. The authors burr the end-plate to create flat surfaces, and then make a 3- to 4-mm central hole, which increases vascularity while preserving the strength of the end-plates (39) ( ). The graft may also be inserted in the reverse position, with the leading cortex directed posteriorly to maximize the posterior disc space height and gain foraminal distraction. Reports have shown that this is an acceptable alternative to the more traditional graft position (40).

Other configurations of bone grafts exist, each with its own proposed advantages. The *Cloward technique* uses a bicortical dowel-shaped graft (41). The technique requires the use of specialized instruments, including drills, guards, and a dowel cutter.

The *Simmons technique* for interbody fusion uses a "keystone"–shaped graft (42). After completion of the discectomy, bone is removed from the inferior aspect of the superior vertebral body and superior aspect of the inferior vertebral body with specialized osteotomes. The end of the vertebra is beveled to a 14- and 18-degree angle, as recommended by Simmons and Bhalla (42). A rectangular iliac crest graft is harvested and contoured to match the beveled surfaces of the vertebral bodies. The graft is impacted in the host bed, thus locking the graft in place.

The *Bailey and Badgley technique* involves developing an anterior trough in the vertebral bodies (43). The trough is 1/2 in. wide and 3/16 in. in depth along the full length of the vertebrae to be fused. The intervening disc and end-plate cartilage are removed to a depth of 3/16 in., and a unicortical iliac crest graft is impacted into place.

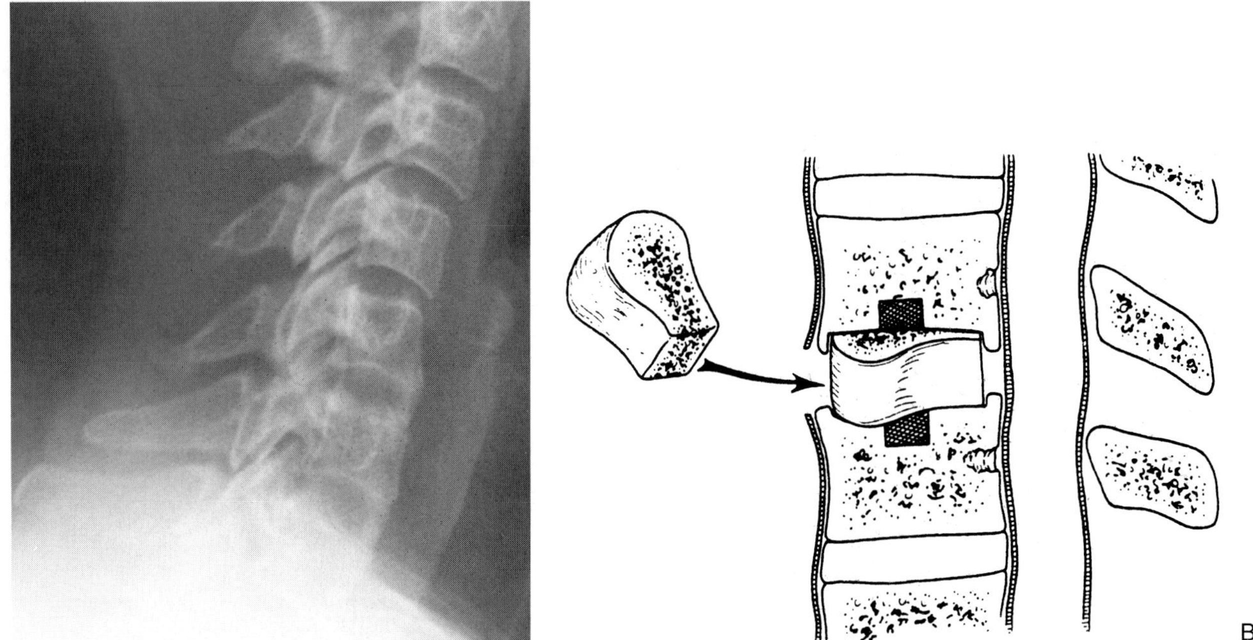

FIG. 8. A: Lateral radiograph of anterior C5-7 fusion using Robinson tricortical iliac crest autograft. Note incorporation into the vertebral end-plates and maintenance of cervical lordosis. **B:** Illustration of the end-plate preparation by making flat surfaces and creating central holes in the end-plates to preserve end-plate strength and vascularity.

Because autogenous iliac crest bone harvesting has an associated morbidity, the use of allograft bone has become a popular alternative. Nonunion rates and graft collapse are more common in ACDF, however. One study with freeze-dried tricortical iliac crest allograft produced clinical results similar to ACDF with autogenous bone graft (44). Fibular allograft has also been shown to provide results similar to autograft with acceptable single-level fusion rates and the absence of donor site pain (45). Other studies have found a higher radiographic nonunion rate with allograft and greater clinical improvement when autograft is used. Therefore, the results of using allograft bone are difficult to evaluate.

Anterior Cervical Corpectomy

ACF may be necessary in situations in which disc herniation is associated with a sequestered fragment that has migrated behind the vertebral body. Subtotal anterior corpectomy and fusion may also be performed when two-level radiculopathy is present. The theoretical advantage of ACF over two-level ACDF is based on the number of sites that must fuse.

Laminotomy and Laminectomy

Posterior decompression for cervical radiculopathy can be performed with laminotomy and foraminotomy, laminectomy, or laminoplasty. Careful patient positioning is required to minimize the risk of neurologic injury and to maximize exposure of the required level.

Laminoforaminotomy involves removal of portions of the inferior and superior laminae at the level of the specific nerve root compression, and partial facetectomy with a high-speed burr. To prevent iatrogenic instability, no more than 50% of the facet is removed (46). The lamina and thinned bone should be gently lifted off the nerve and spinal cord with small angled curettes. Before discectomy, the nerve root is retracted and the surrounding venous plexus is cauterized ( ). Remember that discectomy or removal of osteophytes is generally not necessary to obtain good clinical outcome. Decompression by laminoforaminotomy alone is enough to relieve radicular symptoms in the majority of patients.

Laminectomy is an option for treating multilevel spondylotic radiculopathy with anterior bony ankylosis when cervical lordosis has been preserved. Laminoplasty may be used in the treat-

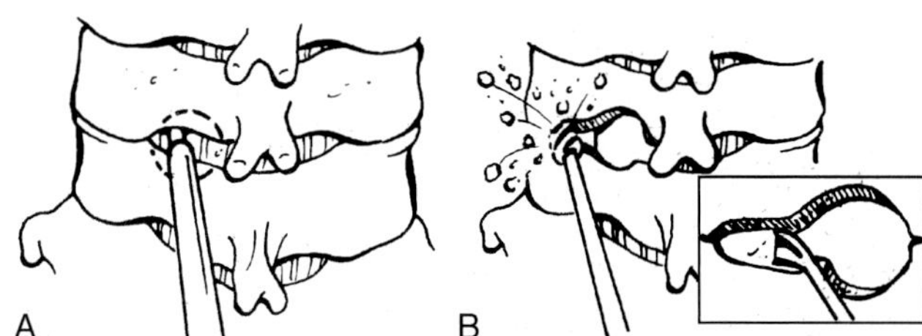

FIG. 9. Illustrations of laminoforaminotomy involving removal of portions of the inferior and superior laminae at the level of the specific nerve root compression, and partial facetectomy with a high-speed burr **(A)**. The lamina and thinned bone should be gently lifted off the nerve and spinal cord with small angled curettes **(B)**. If discectomy is chosen, the nerve root is retracted after the surrounding venous plexus is cauterized.

ment of multilevel spondylotic radiculopathy with predominantly unilateral symptoms. Several methods of laminoplasty exist and vary by location of the hinge and means of maintaining the open position (47).

Spinal Instrumentation

The role of instrumentation in the surgical management of cervical radiculopathy is less clear than it is for traumatic conditions. In degenerative disc disease, various studies suggest nonunion rates and graft dislodgment increase with the number of operated levels (32,48). The goals of instrumentation are to provide immediate stability, increase fusion rate, prevent loss of fixation of the bone graft, improve postoperative rehabilitation, and possibly avoid the requirements for an external orthosis (49).

Animal studies have not demonstrated an improved fusion rate in a three-level ACDF with plating (48). Avascularity beneath the plate has also been detected, although its significance is unclear. It is controversial whether anterior plating for single-level ACDF increases fusion rate (50) ( ). The potential benefits of instrumentation may not outweigh the risks

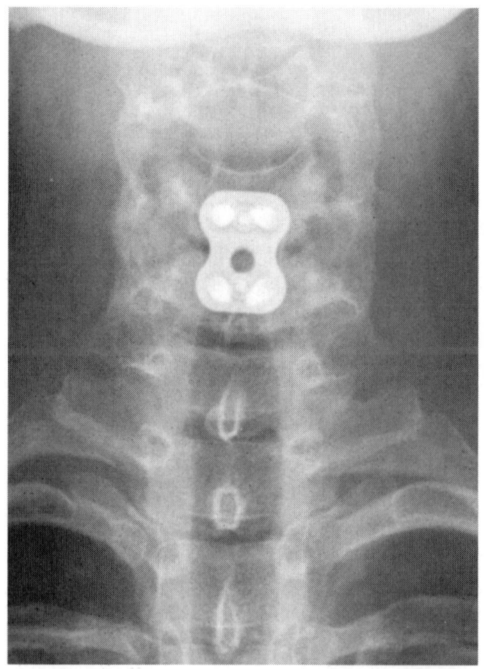

A

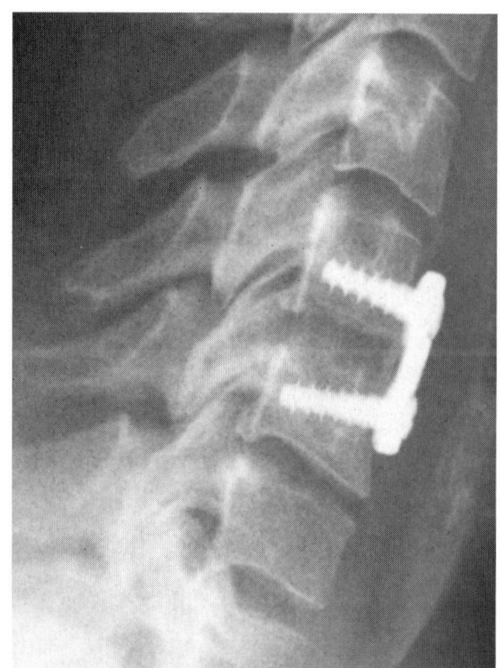

B

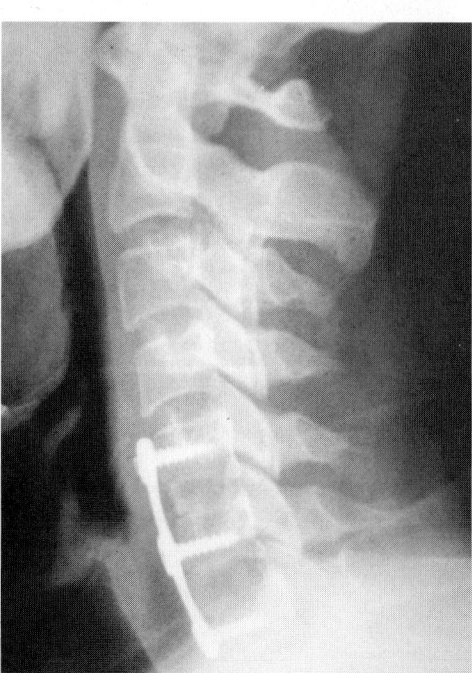

C

FIG. 10. Anteroposterior **(A)** and lateral **(B)** radiographs of interbody bone graft with an anterior plate (Atlantis Plate, Medtronics Sofamor-Danek, Memphis, TN). **C:** Lateral radiograph of interbody grafts and rigid segmental plating (Peak Polyaxial Plate, DePuy Acromed, Raynham, MA).

in these situations. Whether multiple-level ACDF fusion is improved by instrumentation remains to be determined, and presently no guidelines are available for its use. Two-level ACDF has a higher pseudarthrosis rate than single-level, and instrumentation is often used in certain clinical situations, such as a patient who is actively smoking ( ).

More recently, several cervical cage designs have been developed. The most common is the threaded titanium device (51). Potential advantages of the cervical cage include similar fusion rates as ACDF with minimal complications, while circumventing the need for autograft or allograft.

The role of posterior instrumentation in degenerative conditions is also controversial. Posterior decompressive laminectomy may require concomitant fusion in patients with preexisting instability based on preoperative imaging studies. Whether the additions of instrumentation such as lateral mass plating or facet joint wiring increase fusion rate while improving the postoperative course is unknown.

SURGICAL OUTCOMES

Postoperative results of surgical treatment of cervical radiculopathy vary depending on the type of approach used and severity of the disease (32,35,52–61). Limitations in drawing firm conclusions from previous reports stem from the lack of uniform patient population, inclusion of different disease processes in the same analysis (e.g., soft vs. hard disc), and inconsistency of outcome criterion. Overall, the surgical treatment of cervical radiculopathy yields satisfactory results in greater than 90% of patients. Although controversial, it appears that patients who attain a solid fusion do have better outcomes than those with a pseudarthrosis.

Complications

A variety of potential complications exist, some of which are the function of the operative approach, whereas others are generic. The anterior approach to the cervical radiculopathy involves dissection and retraction of numerous vital vascular, respiratory, and neural structures. An overall 0.2% frequency of neck site complications based on an extensive review of published series has been reported (62). The risk of vocal cord paralysis from recurrent laryngeal nerve injury ranges from 1 to 11% of all neurologic injuries (63). Possible etiologies include traumatic division, stretch injury, compression from postoperative swelling, and injury from thermal necrosis. The injury is manifested as a hoarse, weak voice with a risk of postoperative aspiration due to the inability to completely close the larynx. When symptoms persist for more than 6 weeks, referral to an otolaryngologist is recommended for evaluation and possible vocal cord injection. Sympathetic chain injury is uncommon and manifests as ipsilateral miosis, ptosis, and anhidrosis. Treatment options are limited.

Midline soft tissue injury to the trachea, esophagus, and pharynx are unusual. Dysphagia after anterior cervical surgery is common and is estimated to occur transiently in 8% of patients. When persistent symptoms develop, evaluation should include lateral radiograph to check bone graft position. Esophageal lacerations occur in 0.25 to 0.70% (64). When identified, immediate primary repair should be performed, the wound appropriately drained, and the patient started on broad-spectrum antibiotics.

Vascular injuries during the surgical approach or decompression are rare but can have devastating sequelae. The structures that may potentially be injured include the carotid sheath contents, superior and inferior thyroid arteries, and vertebral artery. Avoidance of overzealous retraction and the use of blunt-edged retractors reduces the risk of injuries to these vessels. Knowledge of the anatomy of the vertebral artery and its relationship to the lateral disc space and vertebral body, as well as maintaining midline orientation during decompression, serve to minimize the risk of injury estimated to occur in 0.3 to 0.5% (65).

Spinal cord injury is perhaps the most devastating complication and is reported to occur in 0.10 to 0.64% of patients treated for anterior spinal injury (66). A review of the literature suggests that the drill and dowel technique and the presence of myelopathy are the major risk factors for this neurologic injury. In addition, neck manipulation during intubation, cervical malalignment after decompression and grafting, and postoperative epidural hematoma must all be considered in the evaluation of the patient with postoperative neurologic deterioration. Management should include maintenance of normotensive blood pressure, administration of steroids, and imaging studies to assess for possible graft dislodgment (66). If compressive pathology is identified, then rapid reexploration and decompression is indicated.

Pseudarthrosis rates after anterior grafting procedures range from 0 to 26% (34,35,41,52,54,60,61). Estimates for fusion for single-level, two-level, and three-level ACDF are respectively 88 to 90%, 73 to 80%, and 70% (32,48). Although bony union may not occur, a stable fibrous union can develop and account for the lack of symptoms in some patients with pseudarthrosis. Several studies reported better clinical results when solid fusion is attained, how-

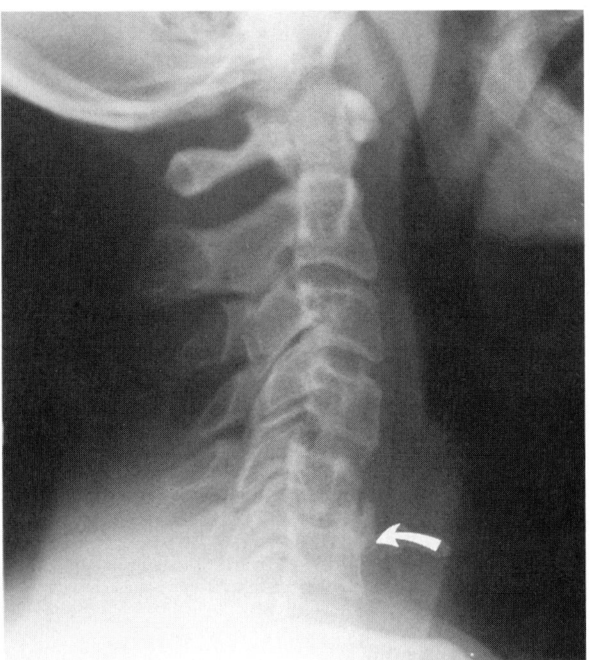

FIG. 11. Lateral radiograph of anterior C5-7 fusion and collapsed C6-7 interbody graft (*arrow*) with slight anterior graft migration.

ever (32,35,60). Graft collapse may precede pseudarthrosis, and this complication is higher in patients with osteoporosis, overdistraction of the disc space, and no plating ( ).

Bone graft site complications are not infrequent, with a near 20% reported prevalence (62). Injury to superficial nerves may result in numbness or pain with neuroma formation. Superior gluteal artery injury has also been reported in iliac crest bone harvest and iliac crest fracture.

Complications associated with the posterior approach to cervical radiculopathy may also occur. The risk of hematoma can be diminished with strict attention to dissection within the ligamentum nuchae and subperiosteally along the laminae. Reattachment of the paraspinal muscles, especially to the C-2 spinous process, may prevent loss of cervical lordosis after posterior decompression (67).

Neurologic injuries are rare during the posterior approach, although they are more common than with anterior surgery (66). Avoidance of placement of instruments into the spinal canal and thinning of the cortex with a high-speed burr followed by the use of curettes during decompression may diminish the risk of neurologic injury.

SUMMARY

Cervical radiculopathy is a common problem owing to various etiologies. Appropriate selection of imaging and other diagnostic tests is important for making the correct diagnosis and for cost-effectiveness. The treatment of patients with cervical disc disease is largely nonoperative. Only those patients who failed conservative treatment should undergo surgery for symptomatic relief of radicular arm pain or improvement of neurologic deficits.

REFERENCES

1. Lestini W, Weisel S. The pathogenesis of cervical spondylosis. *Clin Ortho Rel Res* 1989;239:69–93.
2. Hayashi K, Yabuki T. Origin of the uncus and of Luschka's joint in the cervical spine. *J Bone Joint Surg* 1985;67A:788.
3. Simpson J, An H. Degenerative disc disease of the cervical spine. In: An H, ed. *Surgery of the cervical spine*. Baltimore: Williams & Wilkins, 1994:181.
4. McNab I. Symptoms in cervical disc degeneration. In: Sherk H, ed. *The cervical spine*, 2nd ed. Cervical Spine Research Society. Philadelphia: Lippincott, 1989:599-606.
5. Dillin W, Booth R, Cuckler J, et al. Cervical radiculopathy—a review. *Spine* 1988;11:988–991.
6. Lees F, Turner J. Natural history and prognosis of cervical spondylosis. *BMJ* 1963;2:1607–1610.
7. Gore D, Sepic S, Gardner G. A long-term follow-up of 205 patients. *Spine* 1987;12:1–5.
8. Davidson R, Dunn E, Metzmaker J. The shoulder abduction test in the diagnosis of radicular pain in cervical extradural compressive monoradiculopathies. *Spine* 1981;6:441–446.
9. Jenis L, An H. Neck pain secondary to radiculopathy of the fourth cervical root: an analysis of 12 surgically treated patients. *J Spinal Disord* 2000;13:345–349.
10. Humphreys SC, An HS, Lim TH, et al. Oblique MRI as a useful adjunct in evaluation of cervical foraminal impingement *J Spin Dis* 1998;11:295–299.
11. Deyo R, Diehl A, Rosenthal M. How many days of bed rest for acute low back pain? *N Engl J Med* 1986;315:1064.
12. Kurz LT. Nonoperative treatment of degenerative disorders of the cervical spine. In: The Cervical Spine Research Society Editorial Committee, ed. *The cervical spine*. Philadelphia: Lippincott–Raven, 1998.
13. Kaplan FS, et al. The cluster phenomenon in patients who have multiple vertebral compression fractures. *Clin Orthop Rel Res* 1993;297:161–167.
14. Ward N. Tricyclic antidepressants for chronic low back pain: mechanisms of action and predictors of response. *Spine* 1980;11:661.
15. Wainner RS, Gill H. Diagnosis and nonoperative management of cervical radiculopathy. *J Orthop Sports Phys Ther* 2000;30:728–744.
16. Purkis IE. Cervical epidural steroids. *Pain Clin* 1986;1:3–7.
17. Rowlingson JC, Kirschenbaum LP. Epidural analgesic techniques in the management of cervical pain. *Anesth Analg* 1986;65:938–942.
18. Shulman M. Treatment of neck pain with cervical epidural steroid injection. *Reg Anesth* 1986;11:92.
19. Castagnara L, et al. Long-term results of cervical epidural steroid injection with and without morphine in chronic cervical radicular pain. *Pain* 1994;58:239–243.
20. Fukusaki M, et al. The role of nerve blocks to deal with pain associated with cervical radiculopathy. *Pain Clin* 1995;8:219–225.
21. Waldman SD. Complications of cervical epidural nerve blocks with steroids: a prospective study of 790 consecutive blocks. *Reg Anesth* 1989;14:149–151.
22. Cicala RS, Westbrook L, Angel JJ. Side effects and complications of cervical epidural steroid injections. *J Pain Symptom Manage* 1989;4:64–66.
23. Gunn C, et al. Dry needling of muscle motor points for chronic low back pain: a randomized clinical trial with long-term follow-up. *Spine* 1980;5:279.
24. BenEliyahu DJ. Magnetic resonance imaging and clinical follow-up: study of 27 patients receiving chiropractic care for cervical and lumbar disc herniations. *J Manipulative Physiol Ther* 1996;19:597–606.
25. Brouillette DL, Gurske DT. Chiropractic treatment of cervical radiculopathy caused by a herniated cervical disc. *J Manipulative Physiol Ther* 1994;17:119–123.
26. Eriksen K. Management of cervical disc herniation with upper cervical chiropractic care. *J Manipulative Physiol Ther* 1998;21:51–56.
27. Hubka MJ, et al. Rotary manipulation for cervical radiculopathy: observations on the importance of the direction of the thrust. *J Manipulative Physiol Ther* 1997;20:622–627.
28. Polkinghorn BS. Treatment of cervical disc protrusions via instrumental chiropractic adjustment. *J Manipulative Physiol Ther* 1998; 21:114–121.
29. Hurwitz EL, et al. Manipulation and mobilization of the cervical spine: a systematic review of the literature. *Spine* 1996;21:1746–1760.
30. LaBan M, Taylor R. Manipulation: an objective analysis of the literature. *Orthop Clin North Am* 1992;23:451.
31. Livingston M. Spinal manipulation causing injury: a three-year study. *Clin Orthop* 1971;81:82.
32. Bohlman H, Emery S, Goodfellow D, et al. Robinson anterior cervical discectomy and arthrodesis for cervical radiculopathy. *J Bone Joint Surg* 1993;75A:1298–1307.
33. Fischgrund J, Herkowitz H. Anterior surgical procedures for cervical spondylotic radiculopathy and myelopathy. In: An H, ed. *Surgery of the cervical spine*. Baltimore: Williams & Wilkins, 1994:195.
34. Riley L, Robinson R, Johnson K. The results of anterior interbody fusion of the cervical spine. *J Neurosurg* 1969;30:127.
35. Robinson R, Walke A, Ferlic E, et al. The results of anterior interbody fusion of the cervical spine. *J Bone Joint Surg* 1962;44A:1569–1587.
36. Robinson R, Riley L. Techniques of exposure and fusion of the cervical spine. *Clin Ortho Rel Res* 1975;109:78–84.
37. An H, Evanich C, Nowicki B, et al. Ideal thickness of Smith-Robinson anterior cervical fusion. *Spine* 1993;18:2043–2047.
38. Jones A, Dougherty P, Sharkey N, et al. Iliac crest bone graft: osteotome versus saw. *Spine* 1993;18:2048–2053.
39. Lim TH, Kwon H, Jeon CH, et al. The effect of end-plate conditions and bone mineral density on the compressive strength of the graft-end-plate interface in anterior cervical spine fusion. *Spine* 2001; 26:951–956.
40. Jenis L, An H, Simpson J. A prospective study of the standard and reverse Robinson cervical grafting techniques: radiographic and clinical analyses. *J Spinal Dis* 2000;13:369–373.
41. Cloward R. The anterior approach for removal of ruptured cervical discs. *J Neurosurg* 1958;15:602.

42. Simmons E, Bhalla S. Anterior cervical discectomy and fusion. *J Bone Joint Surg* 1969;51B:255–337.
43. Bailey R, Badgley C. Stabilization of the cervical spine by anterior fusion. *J Bone Joint Surg* 1960;42A:565–594.
44. Zdeblick T, Ducker T. The use of freeze-dried allograft bone for anterior cervical fusions. *Spine* 1991;16:726–729.
45. Young W, Rosenwasser R. An early comparative analysis of the use of fibular allograft versus autograft iliac crest graft for interbody fusion after anterior cervical discectomy. *Spine* 1993;18:1123–1124.
46. Zdeblick T, Zou D, Warden K, et al. Cervical stability after foraminotomy: a biomechanical in-vitro analysis. *J Bone Joint Surg* 1992;74A: 22–27.
47. Hirabayashi K, Watanabe K, Wakano K, et al. Expansive open-door laminoplasty for cervical spinal stenotic myelopathy. *Spine* 1983;8: 693–699.
48. Zdeblick T, Cooke M, Wilson D, et al. Anterior cervical discectomy, fusion, and plating—a comparative animal study. *Spine* 1993;18:1974–1983.
49. Herkowitz H. Internal fixation for degenerative cervical spine disorders. In: Weisel S, ed. *Seminars in spine surgery—cervical disc disease*. Philadelphia: WB Saunders, 1995:57–60.
50. Connolly P, Esses S, Kostuik J. Anterior cervical fusion outcome. Analysis of patients fused with and without anterior cervical plates. *J Spinal Dis* 1996;9:202–206.
51. Hacker R, Cauthen J, Gilbert T, et al. A prospective randomized multicenter clinical evaluation of an anterior cervical fusion cage. *Spine* 2000;25:2646–2655.
52. Connolly E, Seymore R, Adams J. Clinical evaluation of anterior cervical fusion for degenerative cervical disc. *J Neurosurg* 1965;23:431–437.
53. Krupp W, Schatke H, Muke R. Clinical results of the foraminotomy as described by Frykholm for the treatment of lateral cervical disc herniation. *Acta Neurochir* 1990;107:22–29.
54. DePalma A, Rothman R, Lewinneck R. Anterior interbody fusion for severe cervical disc degeneration. *Surg Gynecol Obstet* 1972;134:755–758.
55. Herkowitz H, Kurz L, Overholt D. Surgical management of cervical soft disc herniation: a comparison between the anterior and posterior approach. *Spine* 1990;15:1026.
56. Gore D, Sepic S. Anterior cervical fusion for degenerated or protruded discs. *Spine* 1984;9:667.
57. Aronson N. The management of soft cervical disc protrusions using the Smith-Robinson approach. *Clin Neurosurg* 1973;20: 253–258.
58. Bosacco D, Berman A, Levenberg R, et al. Surgical results in anterior cervical discectomy and fusion using a countersunk interlocking autogenous iliac crest bone graft. *Orthopedics* 1992;15:923–925.
59. Brigham C, Tsahakis P. Anterior cervical foraminotomy and fusion: surgical technique and results. *Spine* 1995;20:766–770.
60. White W, Southwick W, Deponte R. Relief of pain by anterior cervical spine fusion for spondylosis. *J Bone Joint Surg* 1973;55A:525–534.
61. Williams J, Allen M, Harkess J. Late results of cervical discectomy and interbody fusion: some factors influencing results. *J Bone Joint Surg* 1986;50A:277–286.
62. Whitecloud T. Complications of anterior cervical fusion. In: *American Academy of Orthopaedic Surgeons, Instructional course lectures*, vol. 30, 1978.
63. Heeneman H. Vocal cord paralysis following approaches to the anterior cervical spine. *Laryngoscope* 1973;83:17–21.
64. Kelley M, Rizzo K, Spigel J, et al. Delayed esophageal perforation: a complication of anterior spine surgery. *Ann Otol Rhinol Laryngol* 1991;100:201–205.
65. Smith M, Emery S, Dudley A, et al. Vertebral artery injury during anterior decompression of the cervical spine—a retrospective review of ten patients. *J Bone Joint Surg* 1993;75B:410–415.
66. Flynn T. Neurologic complications of anterior cervical interbody fusion. *Spine* 1982;7:536–539.
67. Nolan J, Sherk H. Biomechanical evaluation of the extensor musculature of the cervical spine. *Spine* 1988;13:9–11.

CHAPTER 35

Cervical Disc Disease

C. Cervical Spondylotic Myelopathy

P. Justin Tortolani and S. Tim Yoon

In the strictest definition, *cervical spondylotic myelopathy* (CSM) is spinal cord dysfunction accompanying typical age-related degeneration of the cervical spine. Upper-motor neuron findings, such as hyperreflexia and gait disturbance, are typical manifestations of this disease process, the final common pathway of which is compression of the spinal cord. Debate remains regarding whether the primary etiology is direct pressure-induced injury or ischemia as a result of spinal cord blood supply compression.

Although CSM is reported to be the most common cause of spinal cord dysfunction in individuals older than 55 years of age (1,2), the exact prevalence is unknown. This lack of epidemiologic data stems not only from the paucity of prospective studies on this entity, but also from the difficulty clinicians have in making a timely and accurate diagnosis. The clinical signs and symptoms of CSM are often obscure or difficult to illicit; may be overshadowed by other concurrent conditions, such as a radiculopathy; or may masquerade as other diseases, such as amyotrophic lateral sclerosis or multiple sclerosis (3). Furthermore, the natural history appears highly variable and is not predictable.

This chapter aims to resolve the conflicts in the pathophysiology as well as the natural history of CSM through evidence based in the current literature, with the ultimate goal of elucidating the most modern, yet clinically tested methods of evaluation and treatment.

PATHOPHYSIOLOGY

Similar to the lumbar and thoracic spine, the cervical spine undergoes a slowly progressive yet stereotypical process of degeneration in all individuals as they age. This process involves biomechanical and biochemical changes affecting the intervertebral disc, facet joints, uncovertebral joints, and ligamentum flavum. Most investigators agree the cascade of cervical spine degeneration begins with loss of integrity of the intervertebral disc (2,4,5), which then leads to reduced load-bearing capability, disc bulging, and loss of disc height. Abnormal motions and forces may then lead to osteophyte formation and inflammation of the uncovertebral and facet joints. The ligamentum flavum thickens as it loses tension and folds into the spinal canal as the intervertebral disc loses height. These events ultimately lead to a circumferential narrowing of the spinal canal and compromise of the spinal cord.

Despite the ubiquitous presence of cervical spondylosis in the aging spine, most patients do not develop myelopathy, as a certain amount of narrowing is tolerated before cervical cord impingement. Based on plain radiographic evaluations of healthy volunteers (6–8), the normal sagittal diameter of the spinal canal from C-3 to C-7 is 17 to 18 mm, whereas the diameter of the cervical spinal cord itself measures approximately 10 mm (4,9). This leaves a "buffer zone" of approximately 6 to 7 mm in the anteroposterior dimension before significant cord compression is a risk. It is important to note that a sagittal canal diameter of less than 12 mm has been shown to be a risk factor for myelopathy in patients with cervical spondylosis (10). Patients with congenital narrowing of the cervical canal or ossification of the posterior longitudinal ligament (OPLL) tolerate far less spondylotic narrowing before cord compression occurs. In a study of myelopathic subjects evaluated postmortem, Ogino and colleagues demonstrated that the degree of cervical cord destruction correlated well with the anteroposterior (AP) compression ratio (sagittal cord diameter/transverse cord diameter × 100), and they also demonstrated the importance of congenitally narrowed canal and multilevel spondylosis in the pathogenesis of cervical myelopathy (11). In fact, some authors have suggested that almost all patients with CSM have some degree of antecedent congenital stenosis (5,7).

In addition to the AP compression ratio, Okada and colleagues developed a complimentary measurement termed the *canal-occupying ratio* (transverse area of the cord/transverse area of the spinal canal × 100) (12). Using magnetic resonance imaging (MRI), they demonstrated that patients with CSM had significantly higher canal-occupying ratios than healthy age-matched adults, and that the severity of cord compression significantly correlated with neurologic symptoms.

Although the critical AP sagittal diameter, the compression ratio, and the canal-occupying ratio are important considerations when evaluating patients, CSM is not a necessarily a static phenomenon (13,14). In fact, cervical spine alignment and dynamic factors contribute to the pathogenesis of CSM. A neutral neck position usually provides the most space available for the cord. Biomechanical (15) and cadaveric studies have shown that neck flexion results in tension forces on the spinal cord and concomitant ventral spinal cord compression against vertebral osteophytes and disc material (16,17). Conversely, in extension, the cervical cord shortens and its cross-sectional area increases (16). At the same time, the ligamentum flavum folds inward to further reduce the area available for the cord (18). A pincer effect in neck extension has been described in which the cord is compressed between the hard disc anteriorly and ligamentum posteriorly (15). Neck extension may pose the greatest risk of cord injury, therefore, because the space available is narrowed simultaneously with expansion of the cervical cord. "Dynamic" MRI in flexion, neutral, and extension may more accurately detail cord impingement as a function of position (13,14), but it has not been available for widespread clinical use.

Cervical cord damage has been hypothesized to be manifest on MRI as increased signal intensity on T2-weighted images. Numerous investigators have sought to determine the prognostic significance of such findings in CSM. In a retrospective review of CSM patients undergoing decompressive surgery, however, Morio and colleagues have shown the postoperative outcome was the same regardless of the presence or absence of spinal cord signal changes evident on preoperative MRI (19). Similarly, in a group of 109 patients with CSM or OPLL, the presence of high-intensity signal on preoperative MRI did not correlate with the degree of myelopathy or postoperative functional outcome (20). In contrast, Singh and colleagues' retrospective analysis suggested that high-intensity signal on preoperative MRI correlated with improved surgical outcome in patients with CSM (21). Their results were confounded by the fact that the patients with high-intensity signal MRI also had the worst preoperative ambulatory status, and that this poor preoperative ambulation demonstrated the greatest postsurgical improvement. Finally, Wada and colleagues have shown that patients with multisegmental regions of high-intensity signal changes demonstrate poorer postoperative outcomes, but a solitary region of high intensity had no predictive value (22). Note that the transverse area of the spinal cord at the most compressed level was the strongest predictor of postoperative recovery: the smaller the transverse area, the less likelihood of neurologic recovery. Of the patients with poor surgical outcome (i.e., less than average improvement), nearly 80% had a minimal transverse area of the spinal cord of less than 40 mm (10,22). Taken together, these data suggest that MRI findings do not accurately predict the severity of myelopathy or recovery after surgical decompression but are useful in identifying the exact location and degree of compression.

Although spinal cord compression is the final denominator, it is not yet clear how extrinsic compression is translated into neuronal injury. It may be due to pressure-induced apoptosis of the spinal cord neurons, spinal cord ischemia and infarction, or a combination of multiple different factors. Several animal studies suggest that interruption of blood flow combined with extrinsic compression of the spinal cord accounts for the histopathologic changes seen in patients with CSM (11,23–26). More recent data suggest prolonged ischemia may induce programmed cell death or apoptosis, a phenomenon distinguished from necrosis by the lack of inflammation (27). Oxygen free radical formation in response to compression may be a second pathway toward neuron injury (28). A clearer understanding of these cellular mechanisms may enable us to intervene at the molecular level, or at least more accurately predict the natural history and postoperative recovery of patients with CSM.

NATURAL HISTORY

Rational decisions about the treatment of CSM are possible only with a clear understanding of its natural history and the limitations of those data. The current trend is to surgically decompress the spinal cord in patients demonstrating moderate to severe myelopathy to halt progression of the disease. However, consensus regarding the natural history of CSM remains elusive despite numerous published reports. After Brain's initial characterization of CSM as a clinical entity (29,30), Clark and Robinson (31) published the first natural history study. Of the 120 patients they followed, none had reversal of their symptoms or remission to a normal neurologic status. Clark and Robinson demonstrated that motor symptoms progressed slowly over time. Acute exacerbations were more common than a steady, unrelenting neurologic decline. Lees and Turner reviewed 44 patients with documented symptoms and signs of CSM. Twenty-two of the 44 had a minimum surveillance of 3 years, while an additional 22 patients were followed for a minimum of 10 years. They concluded CSM follows a prolonged clinical course, with lengthy periods of relatively stable symptoms (32). In similar fashion, Nurick retrospectively assessed 37 patients. Although patients may deteriorate early on, their clinical presentation follows a static clinical course for many years (33). In this study, patients were classified according to six grades of disability (Table 1) based on the degree of difficulty encountered in walking at the time of admission (34). Lees and Turner as well as Nurick considered CSM a benign disorder in which old age was the only risk factor for future neurologic decline, and they concluded that no significant difference in outcome could be found in patients treated with laminectomy versus nonoperative care. In contrast, Symon and Lavender argued that CSM is not a "benign" condition, and in their review, 67% of patients demonstrated a relentless progression of neurologic deterioration without stable clinical plateau periods (35).

More recent studies confirm that a significant percent of patients with CSM progress in neurologic function. Sadasiv-

TABLE 1. *Nurick grades of disability*

Grade	Description
0	Signs or symptoms of root involvement but without evidence of spinal cord disease.
1	Signs of spinal cord disease but no difficulty in walking.
2	Slight difficulty in walking that does not prevent full-time employment.
3	Difficulty in walking that prevents full-time employment or the ability to do all housework, but that is not so severe as to require someone else's help to walk.
4	Able to walk only with someone else's help or with the aid of a frame.
5	Chairbound or bedridden.

From Nurick S. The pathogenesis of the spinal cord disorder associated with cervical spondylosis. *Brain* 1972;95:87–100, with permission.

ian's retrospective evaluation of 22 patients classified according to the Nurick grades suggests progressive deterioration in CSM is the rule with no stabilization of symptoms, as Lees and Turner reported. In addition, they demonstrated a mean delay from onset of symptoms to diagnosis of 6.3 years and a decline in two Nurick grades in the majority of patients (36). Matsunaga and colleagues reviewed 37 patients with myelopathy due to compression from OPLL (37). They found that 40% of patients had clear neurologic deterioration over a mean 10.3-year follow-up period. These more recent works are subject to the same criticisms as the older studies, however. They are all retrospective, and therefore, subject to observation bias and lacking standardized outcome measurements.

Prospective studies on the effectiveness of surgery in altering the natural history of CSM are few and inconclusive, highlighting the difficulty in performing controlled studies in these patients. In a metaanalysis study by Fouyas and colleagues, no significant differences between conservative care and surgery were discernible 2 years after treatment. However, Fouyas and colleagues did not limit the inclusion criteria to myelopathy, and therefore, the results are confounded by patients with predominantly radicular symptoms (38). Kadanka and colleagues performed a randomized prospective study of surgical versus nonsurgical treatment of patients with mild and moderate degrees of myelopathy from cervical spondylosis and found no discernible difference between the two groups at 3-year follow-up (39). In contrast, Sampath and colleagues reported a prospective, multicenter, nonrandomized trial that demonstrated the superiority of surgical versus nonsurgical treatment of patients with CSM. Despite the fact that surgically treated patients had worse neurologic and functional status before treatment, surgically treated patients had better outcomes (40). A plethora of noncontrolled reports document substantial improvement after surgery. However, good controlled studies that document long-term benefit of surgical decompression are still needed.

In 1976, in an attempt to objectively classify the functional status of patients with cervical myelopathy, the Japanese Orthopaedic Association published a scoring system that provides a comprehensive assessment of upper- and lower-extremity function as well as sensory and bladder disturbance (Table 2) (41). This system goes well beyond the Nurick classification, which

TABLE 2. *Japanese Orthopaedic Association classification of myelopathy*

Upper-extremity function
0 = impossible to eat with chopsticks or spoon
1 = possible to eat with spoon, but not with chopsticks
2 = possible to eat with chopsticks, but inadequate
3 = possible to eat with chopsticks, but awkward
4 = normal
Lower-extremity function
0 = impossible to walk
1 = need cane or aid on flat ground
2 = need cane or aid only on stairs
3 = possible to walk without cane or aid, but slow
4 = normal
Sensory
Upper extremity
0 = apparent sensory loss
1 = minimal sensory loss
2 = normal
Lower extremity
Same as upper extremity
Trunk
Same as upper extremity
Bladder function
0 = complete retention
1 = severe disturbance (inadequate evacuation, straining, or dribbling of urine)
2 = mild disturbance (urinary frequency, urinary hesitancy)
3 = normal

Maximum score = 17 points.

From Hirabayashi K, Miyakawa J, Satomi K, et al. Operative results and postoperative progression of ossification among patients with ossification of cervical posterior longitudinal ligament. *Spine* 1981;6:354–364, with permission.

focuses primarily on gait dysfunction. Importantly, the Japanese Orthopaedic Association scoring system has been validated as an accurate assessment of the severity of myelopathy (42). Other validated outcome measures, such as the Short Form 36 and Oswestry Scores, should allow future investigators to more accurately determine the role of surgery in the treatment of CSM as measured by overall function.

SYMPTOMS AND PHYSICAL FINDINGS

The diagnosis of CSM early in its course can be very difficult, as the clinical symptoms may be subtle. Also, there are a number of specific neurologic tests that strongly suggest CSM but typically are not performed as part of the routine examination. Furthermore, isolated myelopathy is relatively rare in patients with cervical spondylosis. Typically, the presentations include nerve root impingement and radiculopathy (7). Classically, patients present with difficulty performing fine upper-extremity functions, such as buttoning clothes and using a zipper, or loss of penmanship. In addition, they may complain of stumbling and easy fatigue with walking. Confirmation of clinical suspicion is made by a complete motor, sensory, and reflex examination on every patient, with special attention to confirmatory tests, as discussed below.

Certain key symptom complexes should be evaluated. *Myelopathy hand* (43) describes wasting of the intrinsic muscles with associated spasticity. To test for this, the patients are asked to hold their fingers extended and adducted. If the ulnar two digits drift into abduction and flexion, they have a positive finger escape sign. Cervical myelopathy is also suggested when a patient is unable to make and release a fist more than 20 times in 10 seconds (grip release sign). This loss of coordination, in a task that is easy for healthy subjects, requires upper-motor neuron function. Loss of vibratory sensation due to damage to the posterior columns may be the earliest sign of myelopathy. This can be detected by tuning fork examination of the great toes or by testing perception of toe or ankle position.

Injury to upper-motor neurons in the cervical cord is manifested by hyperreflexia below the level of compression. For example, hyperreflexia noted in the brachioradialis and triceps, but normal or diminished biceps reflexes, implies compression at the C-5 level. Other pathologic reflexes, such as Hoffman's sign and inverted radial reflex, should also be tested (44). Hoffman's sign is considered present when sudden extension of the distal interphalangeal joint of the middle finger causes reflexive flexion of the thumb or index finger. An inverted radial reflex occurs when tapping the distal brachioradialis tendon induces reflexive flexion of the one or more of the fingers and a diminishment of the normal wrist extension. These pathologic reflexes, which result from a loss of the inhibitory function of upper-motor neurons, are the clinical findings associated with the term *spasticity*, so often used to describe patients with myelopathy.

In the lower extremities, reflexive extension and abduction of the toes after gentle, sharp stimulation of the lateral aspect of the sole of the foot, the Babinski response, as well as more than two beats of clonus after rapid Achilles stretch, also suggest upper-motor neuron pathology. It is important to note that the presence of spasticity is not specific for myelopathy; however, its presence helps corroborate the diagnosis of CSM and warrants further investigation.

Gait disturbance may be extremely subtle and is often the first physical symptom of CSM (45). Patients may not notice changes in their walking pattern because they occur gradually over time and are only slowly progressive. One of the earliest gait disturbances is increased sensation of imbalance or coordination walking around corners. Other patients may complain of unsteadiness on uneven terrain or inability to walk distances as they once could. Physical examination consistent with myelopathy gait is broad-based and hesitant, with difficulty performing heel-toe walking in a straight line. Loss of motor coordination is further demonstrated by difficulty maintaining balance with toe walking and heel walking. Finally, a positive Romberg test is demonstrated by a loss of balance while standing with the eyes closed and the arms elevated in front of the body. Taken together, these findings help pinpoint the presence and extent of myelopathy.

Symptoms of loss of control (incontinence) or retention in the urinary or gastrointestinal system may herald the diagnosis of CSM. Bladder and bowel dysfunction may ultimately affect 20 to 50% of patients with CSM (41,45,46). This is rare in early myelopathy, however. Changes in the pattern of bowel and bladder function are key components of the history.

CERVICAL CORD SYNDROMES

Several syndromes of incomplete spinal cord injury have been described in patients with CSM (47,48). The most prevalent is the *central cord syndrome*, which is characterized by motor and sensory deficits more pronounced in the upper extremities than the lower extremities. The typical patient is elderly, with preexisting cervical spondylosis, who has sustained a hyperextension neck injury during a fall from standing height. This hyperextension causes an acute compression of an already narrowed spinal canal. These patients can have profound neurologic deficits despite a paucity of radiographic findings. As the name implies, the motor system syndrome involves compression of purely motor tracts and affects corticospinal tract and anterior horn cells. These patients should be differentiated from those with multiple sclerosis and amyotrophic lateral sclerosis. The Brown-Séquard syndrome can be conceptualized as a hemitransection of the cord, although it is never as clear cut as would occur with a knife wound to the cord. Patients manifest ipsilateral sensory loss of proprioception, and vibration, ipsilateral motor loss, and contralateral loss of pain and temperature sensation. The brachialgia cord syndrome (47) occurs when compression in the caudal cervical cord leads to radiculopathy in the upper extremities and spasticity in the lower extremities.

IMAGING STUDIES

Anteroposterior and lateral plain radiographs can provide a wealth of information and should be ordered before MRI when evaluating patients with CSM (Fig. 1). The anteroposterior view may demonstrate uncovertebral joint space narrowing or scoliosis. The lateral view delineates disc space narrowing, presence of end-plate osteophytes, as well as alterations in sagittal plane alignment, such as loss of lordosis or spondylolisthesis (or both). Radiographs should be taken in the upright position and are critical to document the extent of subluxation or degree of kyphosis. These postures may reduce from a subluxed location when the patient's neck is in the supine position. Evidence of congenital cervical stenosis and OPLL can also be evaluated on these views. A Torg ratio (49) (vertebral body diameter/space available for the cord) of less than 0.8 or overlap of the spinolaminar line with the posterior edge of the facets suggests congenital stenosis. OPLL may be evident as a solid line of bone immediately posterior to the vertebral bodies. Flexion-extension radiographs help to determine whether increased motion is occurring at levels with spondylosis or spondylolisthesis.

MRI should be ordered on patients with myelopathy who present with severe and unremitting neck pain, and/or progressive neurologic deficits. The sagittal T2-weighted images provide excellent visualization of the spinal cord, which appears gray (intermediate signal intensity) in contrast to the cerebrospinal fluid, which appears white (high signal intensity) (Fig. 2). The cervical level and location (anterior versus posterior) of compression, as well as the space available for the cord, can be measured directly from these sagittal images. Pathologic changes within the cord appear as regions of high signal inten-

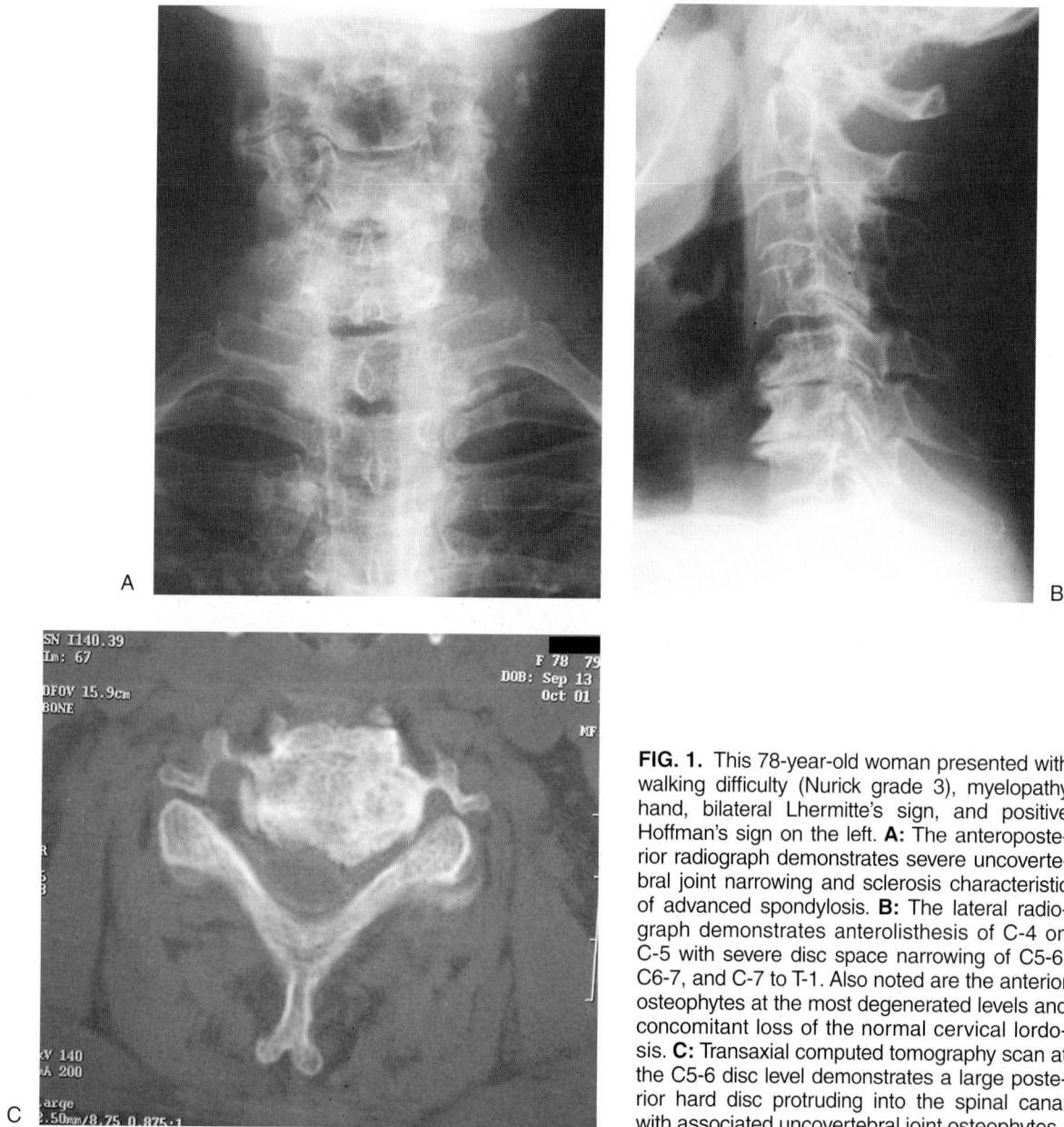

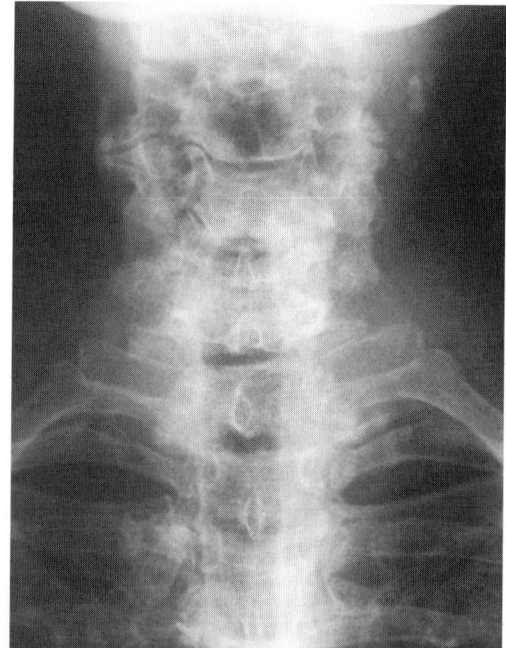

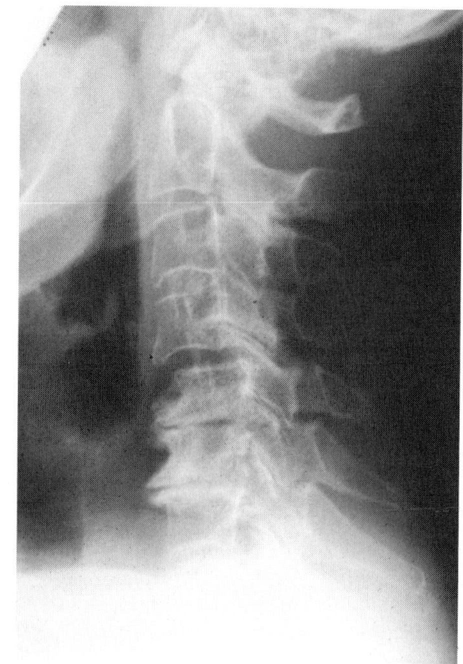

FIG. 1. This 78-year-old woman presented with walking difficulty (Nurick grade 3), myelopathy hand, bilateral Lhermitte's sign, and positive Hoffman's sign on the left. **A:** The anteroposterior radiograph demonstrates severe uncovertebral joint narrowing and sclerosis characteristic of advanced spondylosis. **B:** The lateral radiograph demonstrates anterolisthesis of C-4 on C-5 with severe disc space narrowing of C5-6, C6-7, and C-7 to T-1. Also noted are the anterior osteophytes at the most degenerated levels and concomitant loss of the normal cervical lordosis. **C:** Transaxial computed tomography scan at the C5-6 disc level demonstrates a large posterior hard disc protruding into the spinal canal with associated uncovertebral joint osteophytes.

sity on T2-weighted images. Although the presence of these cord changes does not correlate with preoperative function or postoperative outcomes (19–22,44), their presence may suggest compression of longer duration. Axial MRI allows circumferential evaluation of structures surrounding the cervical cord. Foraminal narrowing is best seen in 45-degree oblique views designed to achieve true cross-sectional views of the foramina (50). The relative contributions of the disc, facet joints, and ligamentum flavum to cervical cord compression should be evaluated in preparation for decompressive surgery. The degree of flattening of the cord, the anteroposterior compression ratio (50), and canal-occupying ratio (50) can only be accurately determined on the axial images.

Computed tomographic myelography is most powerful in its application as a surgical road map. It gives precise assessment of the most stenotic levels, as well as unparalleled detail of the osseous anatomy, which can be particularly helpful if instrumentation is being considered as a component of surgical treatment. Some authors believe that computed tomographic myelography demonstrates facet joint hypertrophy, foraminal stenosis, and the distribution and extent of OPLL more accurately than MRI.

NONOPERATIVE TREATMENT

Nonoperative treatment is indicated in patients with mild myelopathy (i.e., mild hyperreflexia without functional impairments), or in whom medical comorbidities make the risk of surgery too great (51). Asymptomatic patients with evidence of cervical cord compression on MRI are also candidates for nonoperative management. For these patients, immobilization and isometric exercises may reduce the neural irritation and provide some relief from

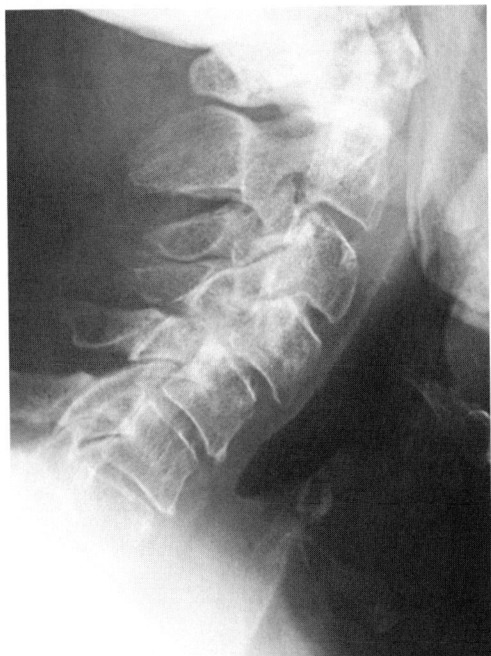

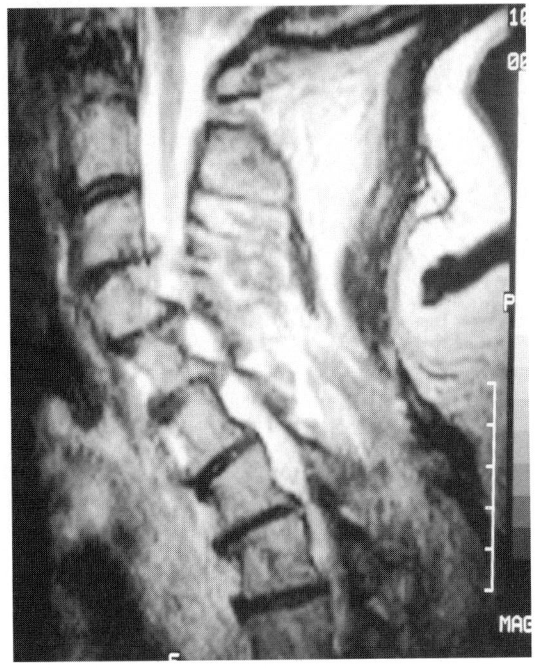

A B

FIG. 2. This 61-year-old man presented to the authors' clinic with severe gait disturbance (Nurick grade 4) and severe intrinsic muscle wasting in the hands. Inverted radial reflexes and Hoffman's sign were elicited in bilateral upper extremities. **A:** The lateral radiograph demonstrates spondylolisthesis of C-4 on C-5 and C-5 on C-6 with preservation of lordosis in the upper cervical region. **B:** T2-weighted sagittal magnetic resonance imaging demonstrates multiple areas of spinal cord compression from degenerative discs anteriorly and from ligamentum flavum buckling posteriorly at C3-4, C4-5, C5-6, and C6-7.

myelopathic symptoms (52). Nonsteroidal antiinflammatory medications may provide symptomatic relief early in the disease course as well. Epidural steroids and cervical traction do not reduce the symptoms of myelopathy, in contrast to the dramatic relief seen in some patients with radiculopathy (see Chapter 35B).

OPERATIVE TREATMENT

The natural history of CSM seems to be one of persistent deterioration over time, so certain relative surgical indications are justified. Factors to consider are the severity and rate of neurologic deterioration, the amount of pain, and the magnitude of cord compression seen on imaging studies. Patients with moderate to severe symptoms, including disruption of gait; changes in bowel, bladder, and sexual function; and significant hand dysfunction, should be offered surgery, especially if their symptoms significantly impact their quality of life or employment potential. It is also appropriate to suggest urgent surgery for individuals whose neurologic decline is rapidly progressive. Patients with intractable arm pain due to coexisting radiculopathy despite nonoperative treatment are also candidates for operative intervention. Because the severity of cord compression has been shown to predict a negative postoperative prognosis (53), patients with milder symptoms should be considered for surgery if marked canal stenosis is evident on their imaging studies. The goal of surgery in each of these situations is to halt the neurologic progression of the disease and to reduce pain. Although improvement in neurologic function is possible, it may not occur (53–56). The choice of surgical technique and approach is based on the location of the compression, the number of involved levels, the presence of instability, and the overall sagittal plane alignment.

Anterior Surgery

Bohlman and others have championed the use of anterior decompression and fusion for CSM (15,54,55,57–65). Anterior options include single or multiple anterior discectomies and fusion, partial corpectomy, or subtotal corpectomy at one or more levels followed by arthrodesis with autogenous or allogeneic bone grafts with or without the use of instrumentation. As cervical spondylosis most typically involves compression of the cord by anterior structures, the anterior approach allows for direct decompression of these pathologic elements. Other advantages of the anterior approach are that it allows for better restoration of sagittal plane alignment in patients with loss of cervical lordosis or frank kyphosis. Sagittal plane deformity correction is more difficult to achieve posteriorly. Patients with evidence of cord compression solely at the disc levels are candidates for anterior cervical discectomy and fusion (ACDF) with structural bone graft or cages at each level. Most surgeons do not perform an ACDF at greater than three disc levels due to the risk of pseudarthrosis (54).

When osteophyte formation, disc herniation, or OPLL extends above or below the disc space, partial or subtotal corpectomy is indicated. A single-level corpectomy may also be considered as a substitute for a two-level ACDF to reduce the number of healing surfaces from four to two, with the concomitant theoretical advantage of reducing the risk of pseudarthrosis. Partial corpectomy involves removal of a portion of the top or bottom of the vertebral body, whereas subtotal corpectomy involves removal of the entire proximal-to-distal extent of the vertebral body with the exception of the lateral walls, which are left intact to protect the vertebral arteries and stabilize the graft. The corpectomy defects, be they one, two, or three levels, can then be reconstructed and arthrodesed with a combination of structural bone graft, metal cages, and cancellous bone. Despite numerous bone graft substitutes and extenders, tricortical iliac crest autograft remains the gold standard in terms of providing the fastest and most consistent arthrodesis. Donor site morbidity, including pain, fracture of the ilium, and lateral femoral cutaneous nerve palsy, is the main disadvantage to its use. Bone morphogenetic proteins and other growth factors, although not currently U.S. Food and Drug Administration–approved for use in the cervical spine, are emerging technologies that may obviate the need for autograft harvest in the future.

Anterior plate and screw constructs may provide enhanced stability and maintenance of deformity correction. For multilevel ACDF procedures, plate fixation has been shown to increase the probability of fusion compared to no plates and may eliminate the need for rigid collar immobilization postoperatively (66–68). The use of plates for single-level ACDF, however, is controversial. Improved fusion rates and outcomes have not been demonstrated convincingly (69).

The use of anterior cervical plates in patients undergoing multilevel corpectomy is also controversial. Vaccaro and colleagues have shown a high rate of screw loosening and plate dislodgement in two- and three-level corpectomy (70–72). To prevent the complications of a long plate, an "anti–kick-out" plate has been described (Fig. 3). Here, a small plate is secured to the vertebral body at the caudal end of a long fusion, with the cephalad portion of the plate providing a buttress against anterior displacement of the graft. These plates are also not without complications (73). In summary, plate fixation is not indicated in all anterior cervical procedures and its associated complications and cost require critical evaluation.

Complications of anterior cervical surgery are multiple. Dysphagia has been reported to affect as many as 50% of patients after anterior cervical surgery. This may be related to retraction on the esophagus, swelling, hematoma, or on occasion, a prominent plate. Most dysphagia is mild and self-limited, however. Dysphonia can arise from injury to the recurrent laryngeal nerve. Its frequency has been reported at approximately 3% of all anterior cervical cases. Because the anatomy of the right recurrent laryngeal nerve is relatively more varied than the left, many surgeons prefer to perform the surgical approach on the left side of the neck. However, no convincing clinical correlation has been demonstrated between the side of approach and recurrent laryngeal nerve injury. There are some surgeons who feel that recurrent laryngeal nerve injury is related to the endotracheal tube.

Pseudarthrosis after anterior surgery can result in neck pain, recurrent radicular or myelopathic symptoms owing to osteophyte reformation, or deformity owing to graft subsidence. With ACDF, the risk of pseudarthrosis increases with each additional level of surgery. Whereas fusion rates with single-level ACDF are very high using modern techniques, two-level ACDF can result in up to a 20% pseudarthrosis rate, and the rate increases to up to 50% with three-level ACDF. Therefore, corpectomy is often preferred in multilevel anterior cervical fusion (54). Cervical fusion rates are also diminished by the use of nonsteroidal antiinflammatory drugs and nicotine products, and these should be stopped before surgery and during healing, if possible.

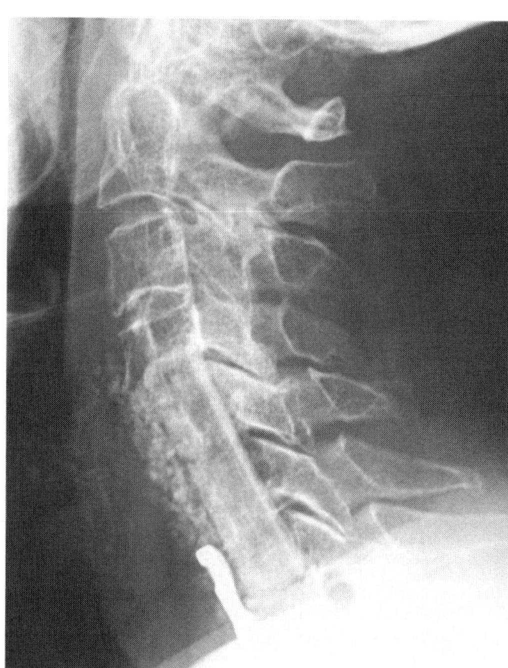

FIG. 3. This lateral radiograph was taken after anterior corpectomy of C5-7 and fusion with a fibular allograft. Local autograft was packed adjacent to the fibula and an anti–kick-out buttress plate, which can be seen at the C-7 to T-1 level. Note the maintenance of sagittal plane alignment.

Graft subsidence, graft dislodgement, or plate loosening can occur. This is more problematic with multilevel corpectomy (i.e., three or more levels). Careful preparation of the graft bed and strut graft is important in preventing these complications. Anterior cervical plates that span multilevel corpectomies have a high rate of failure due to the lack of segmental fixation. Some surgeons have preferred to perform corpectomy with an adjacent ACDF to allow for an extra point of fixation with the plate while reducing the number of fusion surfaces as compared to multilevel ACDFs. Although the idea is attractive, the effectiveness of this strategy has yet to be rigorously demonstrated.

Posterior Surgery

Posterior surgery is indicated in patients with dorsal spinal cord compression, such as buckling of the ligamentum flavum. Other indications include diffuse canal stenosis, multilevel spondylosis, OPLL, or, rarely, synovial cysts (Fig. 4). Compared to long anterior exposures, posterior decompressions are technically less demanding and do not place key anterior structures, such as the esophagus, trachea, and recurrent laryngeal nerve, at risk. Note that to treat anterior pathology with a posterior decompression, the spinal cord must shift dorsally in the thecal sac. If the patient's spine is kyphotic in the sagittal plane, the spinal cord is less likely to move posteriorly after the decompression. For

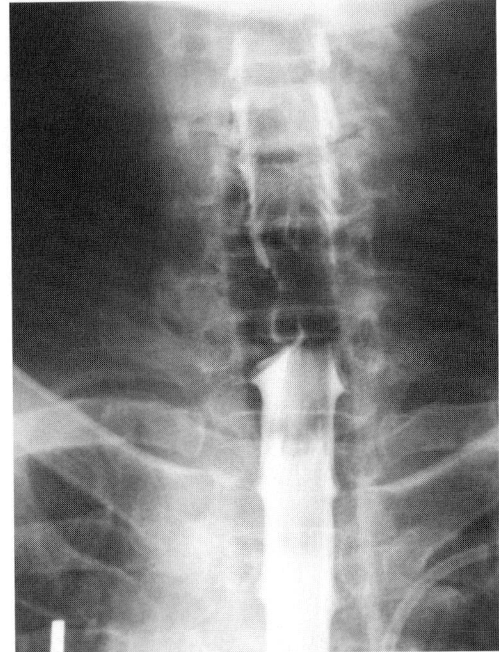

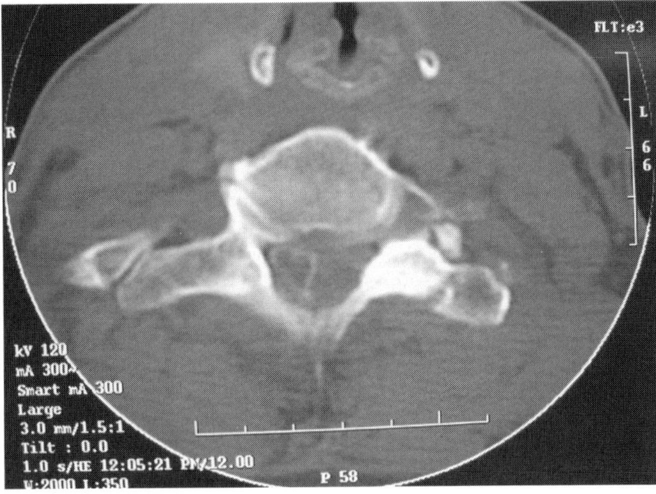

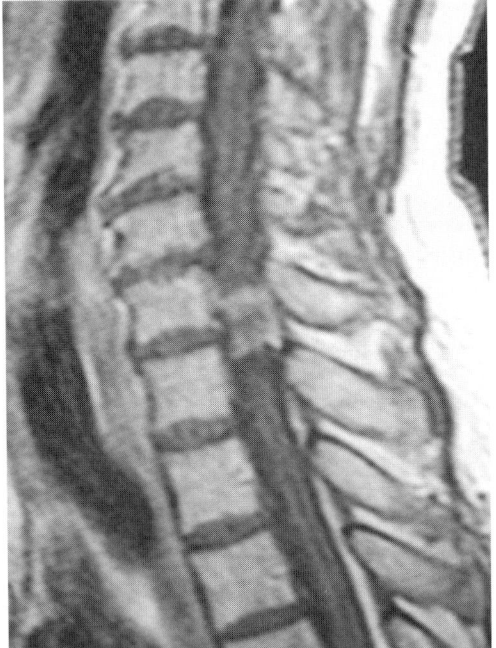

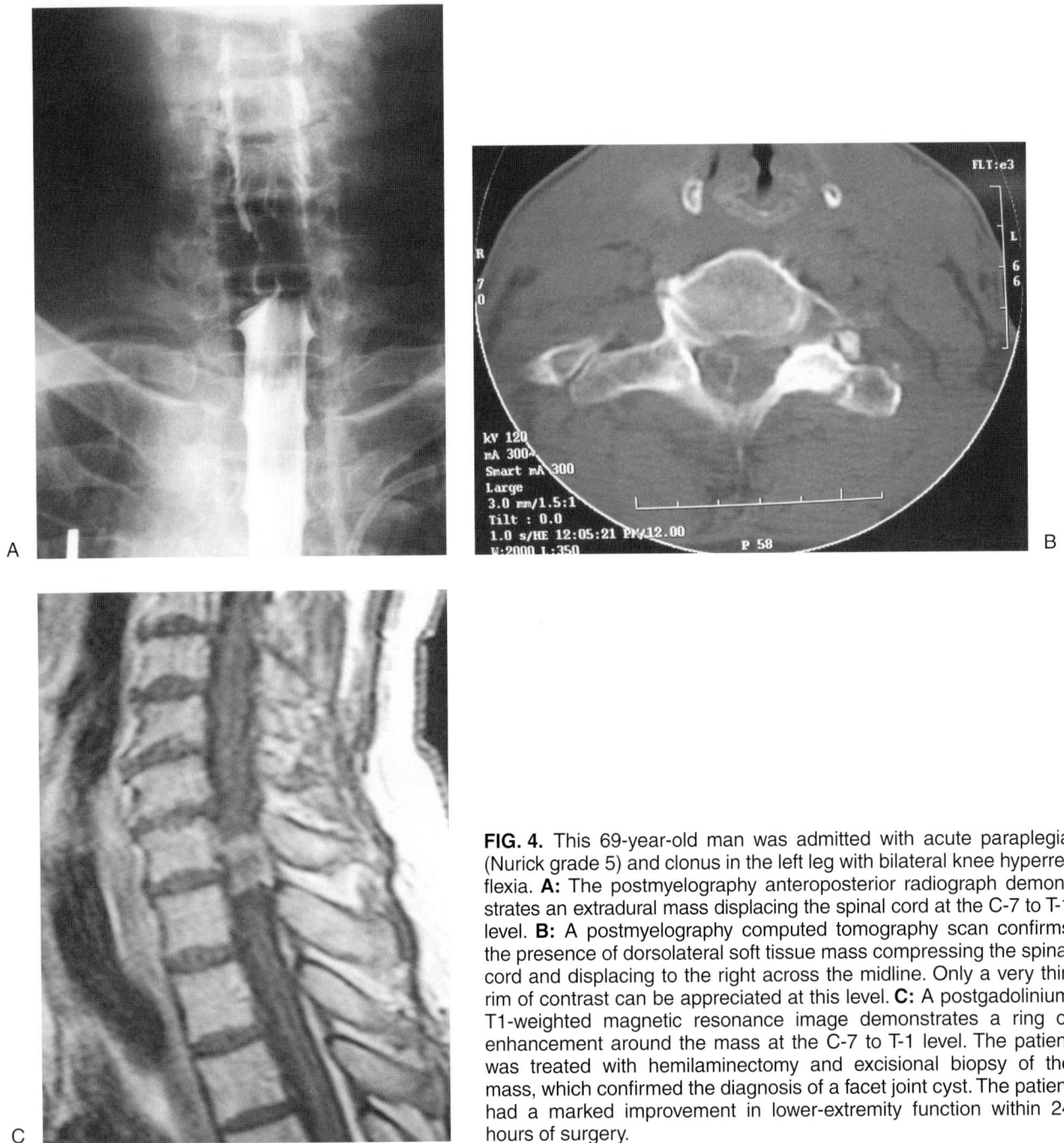

FIG. 4. This 69-year-old man was admitted with acute paraplegia (Nurick grade 5) and clonus in the left leg with bilateral knee hyperreflexia. **A:** The postmyelography anteroposterior radiograph demonstrates an extradural mass displacing the spinal cord at the C-7 to T-1 level. **B:** A postmyelography computed tomography scan confirms the presence of dorsolateral soft tissue mass compressing the spinal cord and displacing to the right across the midline. Only a very thin rim of contrast can be appreciated at this level. **C:** A postgadolinium T1-weighted magnetic resonance image demonstrates a ring of enhancement around the mass at the C-7 to T-1 level. The patient was treated with hemilaminectomy and excisional biopsy of the mass, which confirmed the diagnosis of a facet joint cyst. The patient had a marked improvement in lower-extremity function within 24 hours of surgery.

this reason, one relative contraindication to posterior surgery is preoperative kyphosis in the sagittal plane.

The posterior surgical options include laminectomy with or without fusion or laminoplasty. The relative merits of each of these methods remain controversial. Single- or multilevel laminectomy was originally the only procedure available for the treatment of CSM (46,74). The main disadvantages of laminectomy alone are development of postoperative kyphosis, increase in instability, increased progression of OPLL, and neurologic deterioration (75–78). Although historically significant, laminectomy alone currently has very narrow indications, and it should probably be offered only to patients with single-level posterior compressive lesions and normal sagittal plane alignment.

Adding a fusion to the laminectomy theoretically eliminates the disadvantages associated with laminectomy alone (79). In a long-term follow-up of patients treated with laminectomy and fusion, Kumar and colleagues have shown that instability, progression of spinal deformity, and late clinical deterioration are not clinically significant. Originally, posterior fusions after laminectomy involved wiring of autogenous bone graft to the facet joints or spinous processes. Lateral mass screw fixation with plates or rods and autogenous bone graft has been developed, which makes the posterior instrumentation more effective biomechanically. In fact, for multilevel corpectomy, posterior fixation is superior to anterior fixation in the improvement of mechanical stiffness and pain. Three popular techniques of lateral mass screw insertion have been described: the Magerl technique, the Roy-Camille technique, and the An technique. In the Magerl technique, the entry point (starting hole) for drilling is 1 mm medial and inferior to the center of the lateral mass. Drilling is angled 25 degrees laterally and 45 degrees superiorly (80). The Roy-Camille technique uses the center of the lateral mass for the drill entry point. Drilling is angled 10 degrees laterally and perpendicular (0 degrees) to the coronal plane of the lateral mass (81). An entry point 1 mm medial to the center of the lateral mass is used in the An technique. The trajectory for drilling is 25 to 30 degrees laterally and 15 degrees superiorly (82). Surgeon preference typically dictates the chosen technique. Unicortical lateral mass screws are nearly as good as bicortical screws from a biomechanical perspective, and they may minimize the most common risks, such as injury of facet joint and cervical root injury. The risk of injury of the vertebral artery is extremely low. At C-7, the lateral mass is typically smaller than the other subaxial levels, resulting in a poorer substrate for screw fixation. In situations in which a biomechanically strong fixation is desired at C-7 (e.g., end of a long cervical fusion), C-7 pedicle screws can be placed.

Laminoplasty

Since the late 1980s, the laminoplasty technique has become more popular. The technique was originally developed to reduce postoperative instability while maintaining spinal motion (83–85). Various techniques have been described, each with the common goal of expanding the area of the spinal canal while simultaneously preserving the posterior elements, which serve as anchors for muscle reattachment. The "open door" technique and its variations involve opening the posterior arch on one side with a contralateral hinge (83) (Fig. 5). The "french door" technique involves opening the lamina in the midline with bilateral hinges (85,86).

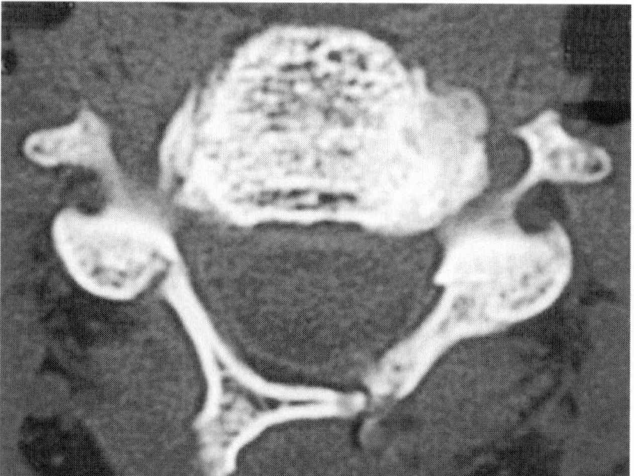

FIG. 5. Axial computed tomography scan image demonstrates the long-term anatomic result after open-door expansive laminoplasty. The hinge is well healed, and the graft that holds the laminoplasty open is incorporated into the lateral mass.

One theoretical advantage of muscular reattachment is the maintenance of cervical stability and alignment. Based on the work of Yonenobu et al. (87) and Inoue et al. (88), cervical alignment is maintained in approximately 90% of laminoplasty patients at 8-year follow-up. Although laminoplasty techniques result in a loss of approximately 30 to 50% of cervical mobility (56,83,84,87,89), this compares favorably to techniques involving multilevel arthrodesis in which the goal of surgery is the elimination of all motion. Despite the theoretical advantages of laminoplasty, long-term follow-up studies comparing laminoplasty with laminectomy reveal no significant differences with respect to segmental instability and recovery rates (90,91). In a matched cohort analysis of laminoplasty and laminectomy with lateral mass plate fusion, Heller and colleagues demonstrated improved results with significantly fewer complications with laminoplasty (92). In an effort to combine the best of all worlds, laminoplasty with limited lateral mass plate fusion at one or two high risk levels can also be offered as a surgical alternative.

The complication rate of cervical laminoplasty is relatively low. However, a monoradicular palsy typically involving the C-5 root has been noted in up to 5% of patients within the first postoperative day. It is usually painless and often resolves significantly. The etiology is unclear, although some surgeons have suggested it is related to the shift in the cord, which stretches the fifth cervical root. Persistent neck pain has been reported in up to 50% of patients. This has been hypothesized to be related to the length of retraction, cervical facet joint injury, and soft tissue scarring. However, this problem is usually not severe.

In summary, posterior surgery can be very effective in certain situations. It does have a higher rate of wound complications and infection than anterior cervical surgery, however. Usually, posterior surgery is more painful for the patient and recovery is longer than the short-segment anterior surgery.

Anterior-Posterior Surgery

Combined anterior and posterior approaches may be required in patients with postlaminectomy kyphosis. Patients with a combination of severe sagittal plane kyphosis and multilevel stenosis may require combined procedures as well. Posterior multilevel decompression and fusion combined with anterior corpectomy and strut grafting as a staged procedure may be required in these challenging circumstances. The anterior procedure is aimed at restoring sagittal plane alignment and spinal cord decompression. Typically, this entails a corpectomy with a long strut graft over two to three levels. The goal of the posterior procedure is enhanced stability to minimize anterior graft complications and enhance the chances of arthrodesis. Lateral mass screws with plates or rod fixation and bone graft help compensate for the absent posterior arch and any facet joint disruption. A circumferential approach may also be indicated in patients with osteoporosis. In the severely osteoporotic patient, an ACDF risks end-plate fractures, and supplemental posterior fixation may minimize the chances of this complication.

SUMMARY

Myelopathy is a potentially devastating sequelae of age-related cervical spondylosis. Despite recent advances in the understanding of neuron function and cell death, the precise pathophysiology and natural history of CSM remain elusive. It is the responsibility of the physician to make an accurate and timely diagnosis based initially on certain signs and symptoms, such as walking difficulty, loss of fine motor control of the hands, and hyperreflexia, and subsequently confirm the diagnosis with appropriate imaging modalities, including plain radiographs and MRI.

Traditional approaches to therapy have focused on surgical decompression of the spinal cord for patients with moderate or severe disease of at least 6 months' duration with an unsatisfactory impact on their quality of life. Prospective, controlled studies are needed and may challenge this dogma, however. Anterior surgery has the advantages of direct decompression of the offending structures and sagittal plane deformity correction. Posterior options include laminoplasty or laminectomy with or without fusion. These techniques afford the benefit of safe, multilevel, cervical decompression; however, sagittal plane lordosis is a prerequisite and the decision regarding technique (laminoplasty vs. laminectomy) remains controversial. Anterior-posterior surgery is reserved for patients with complex kyphotic sagittal plane deformities and for those with severe osteoporosis.

REFERENCES

1. Crandall PH, Gregoriuis FK. Long-term follow-up of surgical treatment of cervical spondylitic myelopathy. *Spine* 1977;2:139–146.
2. Orr RD, Zdeblick TA. Cervical spondylotic myelopathy. Approaches to surgical treatment. *Clin Orthop* 1999;359:58–66.
3. Burgerman R, Rigamonti D, Randle JM, et al. The association of cervical spondylosis and multiple sclerosis. *Surg Neurol* 1992;38:265–270.
4. Bohlman HH, Emery SE. The pathophysiology of cervical spondylosis and myelopathy. *Spine* 1988;13:843–846.
5. Lestini WF, Wiesel SW. The pathogenesis of cervical spondylosis. *Clin Orthop* 1989;239:69–93.
6. Burrows EH. The sagittal diameter of the spinal canal in cervical spondylosis. *Clin Radiol* 1963;14:77–86.
7. Murone I. The importance of the sagittal diameters of the cervical spinal canal in relation to spondylosis and myelopathy. *J Bone Joint Surg Br* 1974;56:30–36.
8. Wolf BS, Khiinani M, Malis LI. The sagittal diameter of the bony cervical spinal canal and its significance in cervical spondylosis. *J Mt Sinai Hosp* 1956;23:283–292.
9. Payne EE. The cervical spine and anatomico-pathological study of 70 specimens (using a special technique) with particular reference to the problem of cervical spondylosis. *Brain* 1957;80:571–597.
10. Arnold JG Jr. The clinical manifestations of spondylochondrosis (spondylosis) of the cervical spine. *Ann Surg* 1955;141:872–889.
11. Ogino H, Tada K, Okada K, et al. Canal diameter, anteroposterior compression ratio, and spondylotic myelopathy of the cervical spine. *Spine* 1983;8:1–15.
12. Okada Y, Ikata T, Katoh S, et al. Morphologic analysis of the cervical spinal cord, dural tube, and spinal canal by magnetic resonance imaging in normal adults and patients with cervical spondylotic myelopathy. *Spine* 1994;19:2331–2335.
13. Epstein NE, Hyman RA, Epstein JA, et al. "Dynamic" MRI scanning of the cervical spine. *Spine* 1988;13:937–938.
14. Muhle C, Metzner J, Weinert D, et al. Classification system based on kinematic MR imaging in cervical spondylitic myelopathy. *AJNR Am J Neuroradiol* 1998;19:1763–1771.
15. White AA III, Panjabi MM. Biomechanical considerations in the surgical management of cervical spondylotic myelopathy. *Spine* 1988;13:856–860.
16. Breig A, Turnbull I, Hassler O. Effects of mechanical stresses on the spinal cord in cervical spondylosis. A study on fresh cadaver material. *J Neurosurg* 1966;25:45–56.
17. Panjabi M, White A III. Biomechanics of nonacute cervical spinal cord trauma. *Spine* 1988;13:838–842.
18. Parke WW. Correlative anatomy of cervical spondylotic myelopathy. *Spine* 1988;13:831–837.
19. Morio Y, Yamamoto K, Kuranobu K, et al. Does increased signal intensity of the spinal cord on MR images due to cervical myelopathy predict prognosis? *Arch Orthop Trauma Surg* 1994;113:254–259.
20. Yone K, Sakou T, Yanase M, et al. Preoperative and postoperative magnetic resonance image evaluations of the spinal cord in cervical myelopathy. *Spine* 1992;17:S388–S392.
21. Singh A, Crockard HA, Platts A, et al. Clinical and radiological correlates of severity and surgery-related outcome in cervical spondylosis. *J Neurosurg* 2001;94:189–198.
22. Wada E, Yonenobu K, Suzuki S, et al. Can intramedullary signal change on magnetic resonance imaging predict surgical outcome in cervical spondylotic myelopathy? *Spine* 1999;24:455–461.
23. Doppman JL. The mechanism of ischemia in anteroposterior compression of the spinal cord. *Invest Radiol* 1975;10:543–551.
24. Gledhill RF, Harrison BM, McDonald WI. Demyelination and remyelination after acute spinal cord compression. *Exp Neurol* 1973;38:472–487.
25. Gooding MR, Wilson CB, Hoff JT. Experimental cervical myelopathy. Effects of ischemia and compression of the canine cervical spinal cord. *J Neurosurg* 1975;43:9–17.
26. Shimomura Y, Hukuda S, Mizuno S. Experimental study of ischemic damage to the cervical spinal cord. *J Neurosurg* 1968;28:565–581.
27. Kato H, Kanellopoulos GK, Matsuo S, et al. Neuronal apoptosis and necrosis following spinal cord ischemia in the rat. *Exp Neurol* 1997;148:464–474.
28. Braughler JM, Hall ED. Involvement of lipid peroxidation in CNS injury. *J Neurotrauma* 1992;9[Suppl 1]:S1–S7.
29. Brain WR. Discussion on rupture of the intervertebral disc in the cervical spine [Part I: CSM as a clinical entity]. *Proc R Soc Med* 1952;41:509–511.
30. Brain WR, Northfield D, Wilkinson M. The neurological manifestations of cervical spondylosis. *Brain* 1952;75:187–225.
31. Clarke E, Robinson PK. Cervical myelopathy: a complication of cervical spondylosis. With a surgical note by L.S. Walsh and Ian Mackenzie. [first natural history study of CSM as a clinical entity]. *Brain* 1956;79:483–510.
32. Lees F, Turner JW. Natural history and prognosis of cervical spondylosis. *Br Med J* 1963;2:1607–1610.
33. Nurick S. The natural history and the results of surgical treatment of the spinal cord disorder associated with cervical spondylosis. *Brain* 1972;95:101–108.
34. Nurick S. The pathogenesis of the spinal cord disorder associated with cervical spondylosis. *Brain* 1972;95:87–100.
35. Symon L, Lavender P. The surgical treatment of cervical spondylotic myelopathy. *Neurology* 1967;17:117–127.
36. Sadasivan KK, Reddy RP, Albright JA. The natural history of cervical spondylotic myelopathy. *Yale J Biol Med* 1993;66:235–242.
37. Matsunaga S, Sakou T, Taketomi E, et al. The natural course of myelopathy caused by ossification of the posterior longitudinal ligament in the cervical spine. *Clin Orthop* 1994;305:168–177.
38. Fouyas IP, Statham PF, Sandercock PA. Cochrane review on the role of surgery in cervical spondylotic radiculomyelopathy. *Spine* 2002;27:736–747.
39. Kadanka Z, Mares M, Bednanik J, et al. Approaches to spondylotic cervical myelopathy: conservative versus surgical results in a 3-year follow-up study. *Spine* 2002;27:2205–2210.
40. Sampath P, Bendebba M, Davis JD, et al. Outcome of patients treated for cervical myelopathy. A prospective, multicenter study with independent clinical review. *Spine* 2000;25:670–676.
41. Hukuda S, Mochizuki T, Ogata M, et al. Operations for cervical spondylotic myelopathy. A comparison of the results of anterior and posterior procedures. *J Bone Joint Surg Br* 1985;67:609–615.
42. Yonenobu K, Abumi K, Nagata K, et al. Interobserver and intraobserver reliability of the Japanese Orthopaedic Association scoring system for evaluation of cervical compression myelopathy. *Spine* 2001;26:1890–1894.
43. Ono K, Ebara S, Fuji T, et al. Myelopathy hand. New clinical signs of cervical cord damage. *J Bone Joint Surg Br* 1987;69:215–219.
44. Shimizu T, Shimada H, Shirakura K. Scapulohumeral reflex (Shimizu). Its clinical significance and testing maneuver. *Spine* 1993;18:2182–2190.

45. Lunsford LD, Bissonette DJ, Zorub DS. Anterior surgery for cervical disc disease. Part 2: Treatment of cervical spondylotic myelopathy in 32 cases. *J Neurosurg* 1980;53:12–19.
46. Epstein N, Epstein JA, Carras R. Cervical spondylostenosis and related disorders in patients over 63: current management and diagnostic techniques. *Orthopedic Transactions* 1987;11:15–16.
47. Crandall PH, Batzdorf U. Cervical spondylotic myelopathy. *J Neurosurg* 1966;25:57–66.
48. Ferguson RJ, Caplan LR. Cervical spondylitic myelopathy. *Neurol Clin* 1985;3:373–382.
49. Torg JS, Pavlov H, Genuario SE, et al. Neurapraxia of the cervical spinal cord with transient quadriplegia. *J Bone Joint Surg Am* 1986;68:1354–1370.
50. Humphreys SC, An HS, Eck JC, et al. Oblique MRI as a useful adjunct in evaluation of cervical foraminal impingement. *J Spinal Disord* 1998;11:295–299.
51. Matsumoto M, Chiba K, Ishikawa M, et al. Relationships between outcomes of conservative treatment and magnetic resonance imaging findings in patients with mild cervical myelopathy caused by soft disc herniations. *Spine* 2001;26:1592–1598.
52. Murphy MJ, Lieponis JV. Nonoperative treatment of cervical spine pain. In: Sherk HH, Cervical Spine Research Society, eds. *The cervical spine*. Philadelphia: JB Lippincott Co, 1989:670–677.
53. Fujiwara K, Yonenobu K, Ebara S, et al. The prognosis of surgery for cervical compression myelopathy. An analysis of the factors involved. *J Bone Joint Surg Br* 1989;71:393–398.
54. Emery SE, Bohlman HH, Bolesta MJ, et al. Anterior cervical decompression and arthrodesis for the treatment of cervical spondylotic myelopathy. Two- to seventeen-year follow-up. *J Bone Joint Surg Am* 1998;80:941–951.
55. Onari K, Akiyama N, Kondo S, et al. Long-term follow-up results of anterior interbody fusion applied for cervical myelopathy due to ossification of the posterior longitudinal ligament. *Spine* 2001;26:488–493.
56. Seichi A, Takeshita K, Ohishi I, et al. Long-term results of double-door laminoplasty for cervical stenotic myelopathy. *Spine* 2001;26:479–487.
57. Bernard TN Jr, Whitecloud TS III. Cervical spondylotic myelopathy and myeloradiculopathy. Anterior decompression and stabilization with autogenous fibula strut graft. *Clin Orthop* 1987;221:149–160.
58. Boni M, Cherubino P, Denaro V, et al. Multiple subtotal somatectomy. Technique and evaluation of a series of 39 cases. *Spine* 1984;9:358–362.
59. Connolly ES, Seymour RJ, Adams JE. Clinical evaluation of anterior cervical fusion for degenerative cervical disc disease. *J Neurosurg* 1965;23:431–437.
60. Emery SE, Bolesta MJ, Banks MA, et al. Robinson anterior cervical fusion comparison of the standard and modified techniques. *Spine* 1994;19:660–663.
61. Hanai K, Fujiyoshi F, Kamei K. Subtotal vertebrectomy and spinal fusion for cervical spondylotic myelopathy. *Spine* 1986;11:310–315.
62. Hirabayashi K, Bohlman HH. Multilevel cervical spondylosis. Laminoplasty versus anterior decompression. *Spine* 1995;20:1732–1734.
63. Simmons EH, Bhalla SK. Anterior cervical discectomy and fusion. A clinical and biomechanical study with eight-year follow-up. *J Bone Joint Surg Br* 1969;51:225–237.
64. Smith GW, Robinson RA. The treatment of certain cervical-spine disorders by anterior removal of the intervertebral disc and intervertebral disc and interbody fusion. *J Bone Joint Surg* 1958;40-A:607–624.
65. White AA III, Southwick WO, Deponte RJ, et al. Relief of pain by anterior cervical-spine fusion for spondylosis. A report of sixty-five patients. *J Bone Joint Surg Am* 1973;55:525–534.
66. Connolly PJ, Esses SI, Kostuik JP. Anterior cervical fusion: outcome analysis of patients fused with and without anterior cervical plates. *J Spinal Disord* 1996;9:202–206.
67. Wang JC, McDonough PW, Endow KK, et al. Increased fusion rates with cervical plating for two-level anterior cervical discectomy and fusion. *Spine* 2000;25:41–45.
68. Wang JC, McDonough PW, Kanim LE, et al. Increased fusion rates with cervical plating for three-level anterior cervical discectomy and fusion. *Spine* 2001;26:643–646.
69. Wang JC, McDonough PW, Endow K, et al. The effect of cervical plating on single-level anterior cervical discectomy and fusion. *J Spinal Disord* 1999;12:467–471.
70. Vaccaro AR, Falatyn SP, Scuderi GJ, et al. Early failure of long segment anterior cervical plate fixation. *J Spinal Disord* 1998;11:410–415.
71. Vaccaro AR, Kreidl KO, Pan W, et al. Usefulness of MRI in isolated upper cervical spine fractures in adults. *J Spinal Disord* 1998;11:289–293.
72. Vaccaro AR, Urban WC, Aiken RD. Delayed cortical blindness and recurrent quadriplegia after cervical trauma. *J Spinal Disord* 1998;11:535–539.
73. Riew KD, Sethi NS, Devney J, et al. Complications of buttress plate stabilization of cervical corpectomy. *Spine* 1999;24:2404–2410.
74. Epstein JA, Janin Y, Carras R, et al. A comparative study of the treatment of cervical spondylotic myeloradiculopathy. Experience with 50 cases treated by means of extensive laminectomy, foraminotomy, and excision of osteophytes during the past 10 years. *Acta Neurochir (Wien)* 1982;61:89–104.
75. Albert TJ, Vacarro A. Postlaminectomy kyphosis. *Spine* 1998;23:2738–2745.
76. Herkowitz HN. Cervical laminaplasty: its role in the treatment of cervical radiculopathy. *J Spinal Disord* 1988;1:179–188.
77. LaRocca H, Macnab I. The laminectomy membrane. Studies in its evolution, characteristics, effects and prophylaxis in dogs. *J Bone Joint Surg Br* 1974;56B:545–550.
78. Yonenobu K, Fuji T, Ono K, et al. Choice of surgical treatment for multisegmental cervical spondylotic myelopathy. *Spine* 1985;10:710–716.
79. Kumar VG, Rea GL, Mervis LJ, et al. Cervical spondylotic myelopathy: functional and radiographic long-term outcome after laminectomy and posterior fusion. *Neurosurgery* 1999;44:771–777.
80. Jeanneret B, Magerl F, Ward EH, et al. Posterior stabilization of the cervical spine with hook plates. *Spine* 1991;16:S56–S63.
81. Heller JG, Carlson GD, Abitbol JJ, et al. Anatomic comparison of the Roy-Camille and Magerl techniques for screw placement in the lower cervical spine. *Spine* 1991;16:S552–S557.
82. An HS, Gordin R, Renner K. Anatomic considerations for plate-screw fixation of the cervical spine. *Spine* 1991;16:S548–S551.
83. Hirabayashi K, Satomi K. Operative procedure and results of expansive open-door laminoplasty. *Spine* 1988;13:870–876.
84. Hirabayashi K, Toyama Y, Chiba K. Expansive laminoplasty for myelopathy in ossification of the longitudinal ligament. *Clin Orthop* 1999;359:35–48.
85. Tomita K, Nomura S, Umeda S, et al. Cervical laminoplasty to enlarge the spinal canal in multilevel ossification of the posterior longitudinal ligament with myelopathy. *Arch Orthop Trauma Surg* 1988;107:148–153.
86. Tomita K, Kawahara N, Toribatake Y, et al. Expansive midline T-saw laminoplasty (modified spinous process-splitting) for the management of cervical myelopathy. *Spine* 1998;23:32–37.
87. Inoue H, Ohmori K, Ishida Y, et al. Long-term follow-up review of suspension laminotomy for cervical compression myelopathy. *J Neurosurg* 1996;85:817–823.
88. Yonenobu K, Hosono N, Iwasaki M, et al. Laminoplasty versus subtotal corpectomy. A comparative study of results in multisegmental cervical spondylotic myelopathy. *Spine* 1992;17:1281–1284.
89. Hirabayashi K, Miyakawa J, Satomi K, et al. Operative results and postoperative progression of ossification among patients with ossification of cervical posterior longitudinal ligament. *Spine* 1981;6:354–364.
90. Hukuda S, Ogata M, Mochizuki T, et al. Laminectomy versus laminoplasty for cervical myelopathy: brief report. *J Bone Joint Surg Br* 1988;70:325–326.
91. Nakano N, Nakano T, Nakano K. Comparison of the results of laminectomy and open-door laminoplasty for cervical spondylotic myeloradiculopathy and ossification of the posterior longitudinal ligament. *Spine* 1988;13:792–794.
92. Heller JG, Edwards CC, Murakami H, et al. Laminoplasty versus laminectomy and fusion for multilevel cervical myelopathy: an independent matched cohort analysis. *Spine* 2001;26:1330–1336.

CHAPTER 36

Evaluation and Management of Cervical Instability and Kyphosis

Jonathan N. Grauer, John M. Beiner, and Todd J. Albert

The cervical spine provides stability and protection to the neural elements while maintaining a high degree of flexibility. This is achieved by a precise interaction of the bony, ligamentous, and muscular elements. Perturbations to the normal anatomy can lead to imbalances that, if left uncorrected, may progress to significant deformities. Such deformities can have adverse biomechanical, clinical, and neurologic sequelae.

Many of the pathologic conditions that result in deformities have been introduced in earlier chapters. These are outlined in Table 1. This chapter reviews the normal anatomy and biomechanics, as well as the management, of rare deformities.

ANATOMY AND ALIGNMENT OF THE NORMAL CERVICAL SPINE

The cervical spine is composed of anterior and posterior elements. The anterior column is made up of the vertebral bodies, discs, and anterior longitudinal ligament. The posterior column is made up of the posterior longitudinal ligament, facets, lamina, and the interspinous ligaments. The normal weight-bearing axis of the head passes through the C-1 and T-1 vertebral bodies in the sagittal plane, falling behind the C-2 to C-7 vertebral bodies. This lordotic posture of the cervical spine compensates for thoracic kyphosis and allows the head to be positioned over the trunk with level gaze and maximum flexibility (Fig. 1).

Many models have been used to describe and study the function of the cervical spine. These include *in vivo*, *in vitro*, physical, and computer models. These can be used together to characterize the precise behavior of this complex anatomic region (1).

The average cervical lordosis in asymptomatic patients is approximately 15 to 35 degrees (2,3). In this posture, Pal and colleagues found 36% of the compressive loads to pass through the anterior column, whereas 64% of the loads passed through the posterior column (32%/side) (4). With shared weight bearing, competence of both columns of the cervical spine is crucial for normal load distribution.

The height of the anterior column is clearly important in maintaining normal sagittal alignment. The cervical discs are slightly trapezoidal, with a greater height anteriorly than posteriorly and an average height of approximately 5 mm (3). The cervical vertebrae are biconcave with similar anterior and pos-

TABLE 1. *Causes of cervical deformity*

Congenital and developmental cervical deformities
Neoplastic cervical deformities
Neurologic abnormalities
Metabolic and degenerative cervical deformities
Inflammatory-induced cervical deformities
Infection-induced cervical deformities
Iatrogenically induced cervical deformities
Traumatically induced deformities

terior heights of approximately 10 to 15 mm (3,5). Loss of disc height due to degenerative arthritis or collapse of a vertebral body secondary to a fracture can shorten the anterior column, leading to a kyphotic deformity.

Many investigators have studied the importance of the posterior elements to cervical stability. Cusick and colleagues found unilateral facetectomy decreased the flexion-compression strength of a motion segment by 32%, whereas bilateral facetectomies decreased the strength by 53% (6). Facetectomies also were associated with anterior displacement of the instantaneous axis of rotation in the sagittal plane, leading to increased compressive loads on anterior column structures. Using a finite element analysis of the cervical spine, Kumaresan et al. confirmed this increased anterior cervical loading after graded facetectomies (7).

How much of the facets are required to maintain normal kinematics has also been studied by several investigators. Resection of 25 to 50% of the facet has been shown to significantly increase cervical motion in several cadaveric studies (8,9). Kumaresan et al. again confirmed these findings using finite element analyses (7). Raynor et al. studied the effects of a 50% and 70% facetectomy on the ultimate strength of the cervical motion segment (10). Fifty percent facetectomies, which allowed exposure of only 3 to 5 mm of the nerve roots, did not result in facet failure. Conversely, 70% facetectomies, which allowed exposure of 8 to 10 mm of the nerve roots, did result in facet fracture when shear loads were applied.

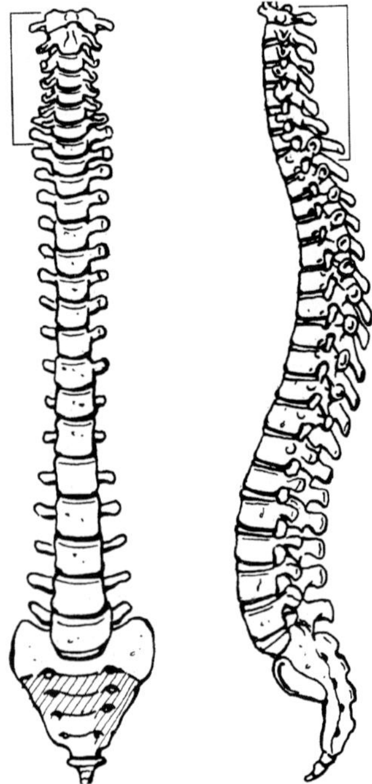

FIG. 1. In a normally aligned spine, the cervical spine is straight in the coronal plane and lordotic in the sagittal plane.

The facet capsules also directly contribute to cervical stability. Zdeblick et al. studied cadaveric specimens in which a laminectomy was performed, followed by graded facet capsule resections and retention of the facet joint (11). Increased torsion was noted after 50% of the facet capsule was resected, and increased flexion was noted after 75% of the facet capsule was resected.

The complex ligamentous structures act as further static stabilizers of the cervical spine. Increased intervertebral motion has been noted after laminectomies without any violation of the facets or facet capsules by most investigators (12–14), but not all (9). This increased motion is presumably due to the disruption of posterior interspinous ligaments. This presumption is supported by finite element analyses of Saito et al., which found that kyphosis or lordosis of the cervical spine develops after disruption of the posterior ligaments depending on the location of the gravitational center of the head (15).

Biomechanical ligament sectioning studies by Panjabi and White have further linked the loss of ligamentous restraints to the loss of cervical stability (16,17). These investigations noted that the cervical ligaments acted as a unit; the risk of instability gradually increased as more ligaments were sacrificed. They observed that there was the potential for catastrophic instability when 3.5 mm of horizontal displacement or 11 degrees of rotational displacement were present. As expected, anterior ligaments were important in resisting extension, and posterior ligaments were important in resisting flexion.

The muscles act as essential dynamic stabilizers to the cervical spine. The neck is subjected to approximately 1,200 N with activities involving maximal isometric muscle contractions (18). Nevertheless, *in vitro* experiments have shown that the osteoligamentous cervical spine is not able to carry even the compressive load of the head without the balancing effect of muscle forces. At approximately 10 N (one-fourth of the mass of the head), the cervical column buckles (19). The stability of the cervical spine is regained in the laboratory as muscle forces are replicated (20,21). In particular, semispinalis cervicis and capitus are responsible for extension of the cervical spine and head (22). For this reason, Nolan et al. emphasized the importance of preserving the attachment of the muscles to the C-2 arch whenever possible (22).

PATHOGENESIS OF CERVICAL DEFORMITIES

Deformities may develop when there is disruption of the anterior or posterior elements of the spine as a result of congenital deformities, tumor, trauma, surgery, osteoporosis, or inflammatory or degenerative processes. The extent of the resultant deformities is a function of the nature and extent of the underlying mechanical imbalances. The most common deformity seen in the cervical spine is kyphosis. The most commonly reported symptoms include neck pain, muscle fatigue, loss of forward gaze, radiculopathy, and myelopathy.

Regardless of the initial pathomechanics, cervical kyphosis initiates a vicious cycle of pathologic forces that can result in the development of a progressive deformity. As the head shifts forward, the weight-bearing axis translates anteriorly, and this causes the anterior column to be loaded with increased compression while the posterior column is placed under increased tension (23). Posterior ligamentous structures and facet capsules become attenuated. Posterior extensor muscles are placed at a mechanical disadvantage and become less effective at holding the head upright (22).

Cervical laminectomy provides a classic example in which imbalances can lead to kyphotic deformities. This operation involves removal of the spinous processes, inter- and supraspinous ligaments, laminae, and ligamentum flavum, and possibly compromise of the facet joints. Furthermore, there is stripping of the extensor muscles (22,24). Even if not detached, these muscles may be denervated or may become fibrotic secondary to aggressive surgical retraction (25). With the loss of posterior stability and continued normal flexion forces, kyphosis can result.

Neck pain and gaze difficulty can cause significant disability for patients with kyphosis. The forward position of the head necessitates constant contraction of the neck extensor muscles to balance the weight of the head against gravity. This leads to muscle fatigue, and occipital and neck pain often worsen as the day progresses. Gaze difficulty is encountered in patients with severe, fixed cervical kyphotic deformities, especially in patients with ankylosing spondylitis (AS). To look forward, patients must compensate with hyperextension at another level, such as the occipital-cervical junction. If compensatory hyperextension is not possible, forward gaze may be limited.

As kyphosis develops, the spinal cord is pulled against the apex of the kyphotic deformity, resulting in irritation or dysfunction of the cord or nerve roots. A finite amount of spinal cord lengthening can occur without a significant rise in internal tensile stresses, such as occurs with normal cervical flexion. However, in pathologic kyphosis, the posterior cord becomes stretched beyond its elastic limit. The anterior spinal cord concomitantly becomes compressed as it is pulled against the posterior vertebral osteophytes and protuberant intervertebral discs (26,27). These stresses result in complex changes within the spinal cord. Cord flattening and internal stresses may lead to compromise of cord microvasculature and neuronal ischemia, as well as increased susceptibility to injury from trauma. Variations in cord stresses and ischemia are partly responsible for the wide spectrum of neurologic manifestations observed in patients with cervical kyphotic deformities (28).

In summary, cervical imbalance can lead to the triad of progressive deformity, attenuation of soft-tissue restraints, and neurologic compromise. One of the primary goals for the management of cervical deformity must be to relieve neurologic compression. This can be achieved indirectly by correction of a deformity or directly by removal of the elements compressing the cord or nerve roots. The other primary goal for the management of cervical deformity is to restore the head to a forward directed, upright posture without the need for excessive muscle compensation and fatigue. This can be achieved externally with the aid of braces or internally with deformity correction and arthrodesis. A discussion of the individual causes of deformity is included in the following sections.

CONGENITAL AND DEVELOPMENTAL CERVICAL DEFORMITIES

Congenital abnormalities of the cervical spine are detailed in Chapter 33. These can lead to cervical deformity secondary to abnormal formation or development of the spine or supporting structures.

Congenital Abnormalities

Congenital deformities of the upper cervical spine include os odontoideum, atlantoaxial rotatory subluxation, and torticollis. Os odontoideum most likely represents an unrecognized fracture at the base of the odontoid but nonetheless is usually considered in the category of congenital deformity. The presence of os odontoideum may lead to instability, but fixed deformity is uncommon. Treatment can be conservative, but surgical intervention is indicated if instability, neurologic symptoms, or signal change in the spinal cord on T2-weighted magnetic resonance imaging (MRI) are present.

Atlantoaxial rotatory instability usually follows retropharyngeal inflammation or minor trauma. Conservative treatment with traction and immobilization is usually sufficient, with posterior fusion reserved for recalcitrant cases (29). *Torticollis* is a combined rotatory and head-tilting deformity. The etiology of this deformity may be atlantoaxial rotary subluxation or a variety of other conditions, including intrauterine trauma to the sternocleidomastoid muscle. Again, treatment is generally conservative. It is important to rule out underlying disorders. Treatment is aimed at increasing neck range of motion, relieving neck pain, and occasionally correcting cosmetic deformity (30).

Cervical instability and deformities are frequent in patients with skeletal dysplasias, affecting up to 48% (31). However, the natural history for children with the different syndromes varies. For example, marked cervical kyphosis frequently resolves spontaneously in children with diastrophic dysplasia (32). Conversely, early posterior stabilization has been recommended for kyphotic deformities in children with Larsen's syndrome (33), because of the likelihood of progression. In general, the cervical spines of all children with skeletal dysplasias must be screened and monitored for signs or symptoms of instability or deformity. Treatment of any finding is tailored to the individual condition and patient.

Klippel-Feil deformities result from congenital fusions of the cervical vertebrae. Although it is reported that less than one-half of these patients have the classic triad of short neck, low posterior hair line, and limitation of neck motion, 60 to 70% of the patients do have significant scoliosis (34,35). As noted in Chapter 17, close observation of these curves is recommended, with bracing or surgery if progression occurs. Associated issues, such as renal and cardiac abnormalities, must also be evaluated.

Developmental Abnormalities

A later developmental cause of cervical deformity is associated with idiopathic scoliosis. This topic is detailed in Chapter 16, but the cervical aspects of this are reviewed here. In particular, the proximal component of King type II and V curves can be balanced by compensatory curves at the cervical-thoracic junction.

Considerable research has been invested in determining the appropriate proximal extent of fusion for thoracic scoliosis. Criteria for including the proximal thoracic curve in adolescent idiopathic cases have traditionally been based on Harrington rod instrumentation for a King V double thoracic curve pattern (36). These indications included an elevated left shoulder or first rib, relative stiffness of the upper curve, and a positive T-1 tilt. Later authors noted proximal kyphosis after posterior spinal fusion (37). Further work by Lenke et al. established specific radiographic criteria for including the proximal curve in the instrumented fusion of idiopathic scoliosis treated with Cotrel-Dubousset instrumentation (38). In general, there seems to be a consensus that nonstructural proximal curves will correct spontaneously. In contrast to the dangers of fusing too short in the lumbar spine, fusing too long or achieving too much correction in the proximal thoracic spine can cause problems. Too much correction of a type II right thoracic curve can result in left shoulder elevation, coronal imbalance, and an apparent increase in the cervical component of the curve (39–41). Lenke et al. stress the importance of clinical as opposed to radiographic balance as the main goal in fusion in these patients; deliberate undercorrection of the curve can affect a better clinical balance (38).

Furthermore, changes in the sagittal alignment of the thoracic spine of patients with idiopathic scoliosis may hold implications for the cervical spine (42). Idiopathic scoliosis is a lordoscoliosis with relative hypokyphosis of the thoracic spine. A subjective observation of flattening or kyphosis of the cervical spine has been made in some patients fused for scoliosis who have relative thoracic lordosis (43,44). In the only study correlating the degree of deformity of the cervical spine with that of the thoracic spine in idiopathic scoliosis, Hilibrand et al. demonstrated that there is a positive relationship between the magnitude of preoperative thoracic lordosis and cervical kyphosis (45). The authors were not able to determine if cervical kyphosis is a compensatory mechanism to keep gaze level or an intrinsic part of the disease. Furthermore, all surgery for fusion of the scoliosis increased the cervical kyphosis, perhaps as a consequence of the amount of muscle and soft tissue stripping needed for the surgical exposure.

NEOPLASTIC CERVICAL DEFORMITIES

Spinal neoplasms are covered in Chapter 11. The topic is briefly revisited here in regard to cervical neoplasms and their resultant deformities.

Primary Spinal Tumors

Only 17% of primary spinal tumors are cervical (46). The most common malignant tumors in this region are chordoma and plasmacytoma (47,48). These have a predilection for the anterior spinal elements. Resultant deformities are dependent on the patterns of bony destruction, but kyphosis due to destruction of the vertebral bodies is most common. Wide resection of these lesions would be ideal, but treatment is often limited to intralesional excision secondary to anatomic constraints (48). Reconstruction generally involves anterior structural grafts with supplemental posterior stabilization. Adjuvant therapy is based on the specific tumor type and the extent of resection.

Benign lesions have a predilection for the posterior spinal elements of younger patients and are more common than primary malignant lesions in the cervical spine (49). The most common tumors in this category are osteoid osteoma and osteoblastoma (47,50). These lesions are generally treated by excisional biopsy or marginal excision. Osteoid osteoma is the classic example of a lesion that leads to painful scoliosis. Ozaki et al. presented a series of patients with spinal osteoid osteomas (51). Twenty-five percent of these were in the cervical spine, and all cervical lesions presented with scoliosis. This cervical scoliosis improved with excision of two of the three cervical lesions.

Metastatic Spinal Tumors

Eight percent to 20% of metastatic spinal lesions are cervical (52). These lesions typically begin in the anterior spinal elements. Vertebral body destruction leads to the potential for kyphotic collapse in the subaxial cervical spine. In the upper cervical spine, destruction of the lateral articular masses and transverse ligament are more common and predispose to rotary instability (52).

Radiation with or without chemotherapy is often appropriate treatment for metastatic spinal disease if there is no instability. However, as discussed in Chapter 12, surgical stabilization is necessary in patients with instability, deformity, progressive neurologic deficit or collapse, intractable pain, or failure of less invasive treatment modalities.

Asdourian et al. described the pathogenesis of vertebral body collapse and outlined a treatment algorithm for a group of patients with metastatic breast cancer (53). Their work described a progression from stability to axial instability to translational instability. They recommend decompression and anterior stabilization for single-level cases of axial instability, posterior stabilization for multilevel axial instability, and combined anterior and posterior approaches for translational instability. For focal metastatic lesions of C-1 and C-2, Nakamura et al. reported good results from posterior fusions to the occiput for metastatic lesions of C-1 and C-2 (54).

NEUROGENIC CERVICAL DEFORMITIES

A host of neurologic disorders, such as syringomyelia, syphilitic tabes dorsalis, and diabetes, can lead to deformities known as Charcot's arthropathy. Similar to neuropathic deformities elsewhere in the body, these spinal deformities are a consequence of the insensate nature of the vertebral elements.

Charcot's arthropathy after a spinal injury involves bony hypertrophy subadjacent to a cord lesion or can occur just below a previous fusion level (55,56). Abnormal movement between the vertebrae leads to destruction of the cartilage, fracture of the subchondral bone, and ultimately to collapse of the vertebrae (57). This can lead to instability, kyphosis, and loss of vertebral body height (Fig. 2). Common presenting symptoms included back pain, loss of a preexistent spasticity, change in bladder function, and audible noises with motion (56).

In general, this constellation of symptoms is seen most often after a previous traumatic spinal cord injury. Vaccaro and Silber pointed out the various characteristics of this rare problem (57). It can be seen after operative or nonoperative treatment of the spinal cord injury and can present quite late (55,58). It often occurs at a relatively high-stress area in the spine, such as at the transitional cervicothoracic or thoracolumbar zones, or just caudal to a previously fused segment.

Of the other neurologic diseases associated with Charcot's arthropathy, syringomyelia is the most common. The classic clin-

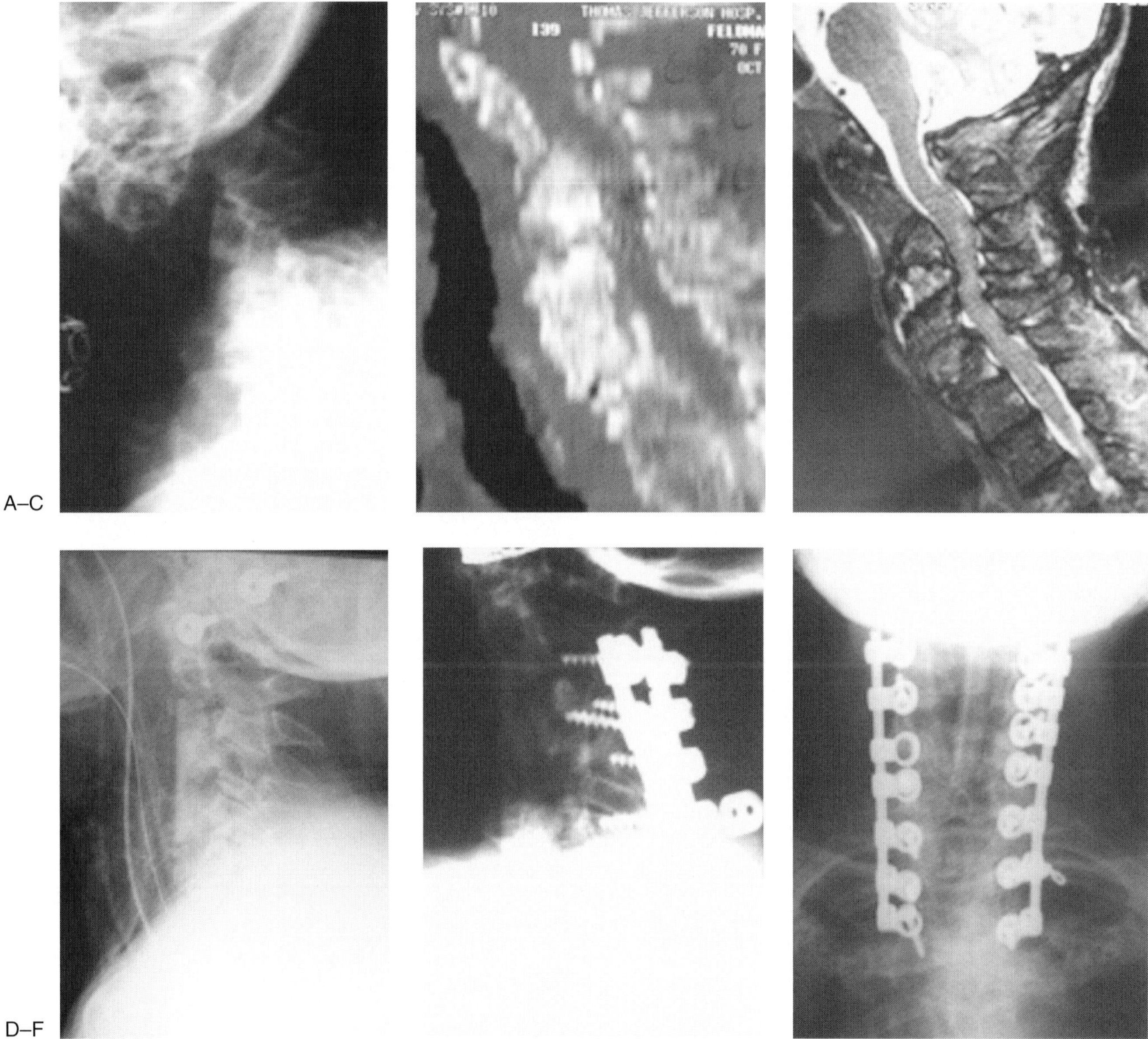

FIG. 2. Seventy-year-old woman with history of Parkinson's disease presented with Charcot's arthropathy. Lateral radiograph **(A)** and computed tomography reconstruction **(B)** revealed kyphotic deformity with destruction of C3-5 vertebral bodies. **C:** Magnetic resonance imaging demonstrated significant cord compression. Anterior deformity correction with C2-7 strut grafting **(D)** was followed by posterior instrumented fusion **(E,F)**.

ical features of this disorder can be described as segmental dissociative loss of sensory function in the upper extremities, which most commonly consists of the loss of distal sensation to pain and temperature and the preservation of proprioceptive sensation and light touch (59). Pain in the cervical-occipital area, weakness in the upper extremities, and lower extremity spasticity are common. The etiology of syrinxes is not fully known; they can occur after trauma, as a congenital abnormality in association with Chiari I malformations of the brainstem, or secondary to neoplastic disease. In patients with scoliosis, factors that provoke an MRI evaluation of the cervical spinal cord for possible syringomyelia are abnormally high curves, rapid curve progression, or bony anomalies of the upper cervical or occipital region. The presence of cervical spondylosis may exacerbate the clinical findings of syringomyelia, but a definitive correlation has not been found (60).

Charcot's arthropathy is much less common in the cervical than in the thoracolumbar region. In fact, limited reports are identified in the literature (61). Once initiated, rapid progression may occur. Therefore, frequent follow-up of these patients is necessary. If found early, the underlying neurologic disorder should be corrected if possible. For example, many forms of syrinxes can be shunted. Once the Charcot's arthropathy has developed, stabilization of the deformity should be performed as early as possible to preserve bone stock and prevent pain and instability.

METABOLIC AND DEGENERATIVE CERVICAL DEFORMITIES

Metabolic and degenerative processes can have a significant impact on the spine. The aspects relevant to the cervical spine and the potential for deformity are reviewed.

Cervical Disc Disease

Cervical disc disease is detailed in Chapter 37. This process begins with disc space narrowing and is followed by hypertrophic degenerative changes of the uncovertebral and facet joints. Loss of anterior column height leads to tensile forces in the posterior column and ultimately laxity of the posterior soft tissue structures. Spondylolisthesis or excess mobility in the sagittal plane may accompany this process and further contribute to neural compression and irritation. Ultimately, the combination of degenerative narrowing of the spinal canal, kyphotic deformity, and sagittal plane instability can lead to spinal cord dysfunction and long tract findings (62). The magnitude of kyphosis seen in degenerative conditions is generally less severe than seen in postlaminectomy kyphosis.

In patients with straight or lordotic cervical spines, anterior and posterior surgery can successfully provide decompression of the spinal cord. Ebersold et al. reported on 84 patients after decompression for spondylotic myelopathy (63). Thirty-three patients were treated by anterior decompression and fusion, whereas 51 patients underwent posterior decompression only. Although no differences in outcome were found between the two surgical approaches, patients with a longer duration of symptomatic myelopathy all had statistically significant worse outcome after surgery.

However, in patients with a fixed kyphotic deformity, posterior decompression alone is contraindicated. Therefore, anterior decompression alone or anterior surgery combined with a posterior decompression is required to provide satisfactory outcomes. In treating patients with senile cervical kyphosis due to degenerative disease, it is important for the surgeon to use different surgical techniques to address the specific pathology that is encountered.

In general, the treatment of cervical spondylotic myelopathy associated with kyphosis is dependent on the number of levels

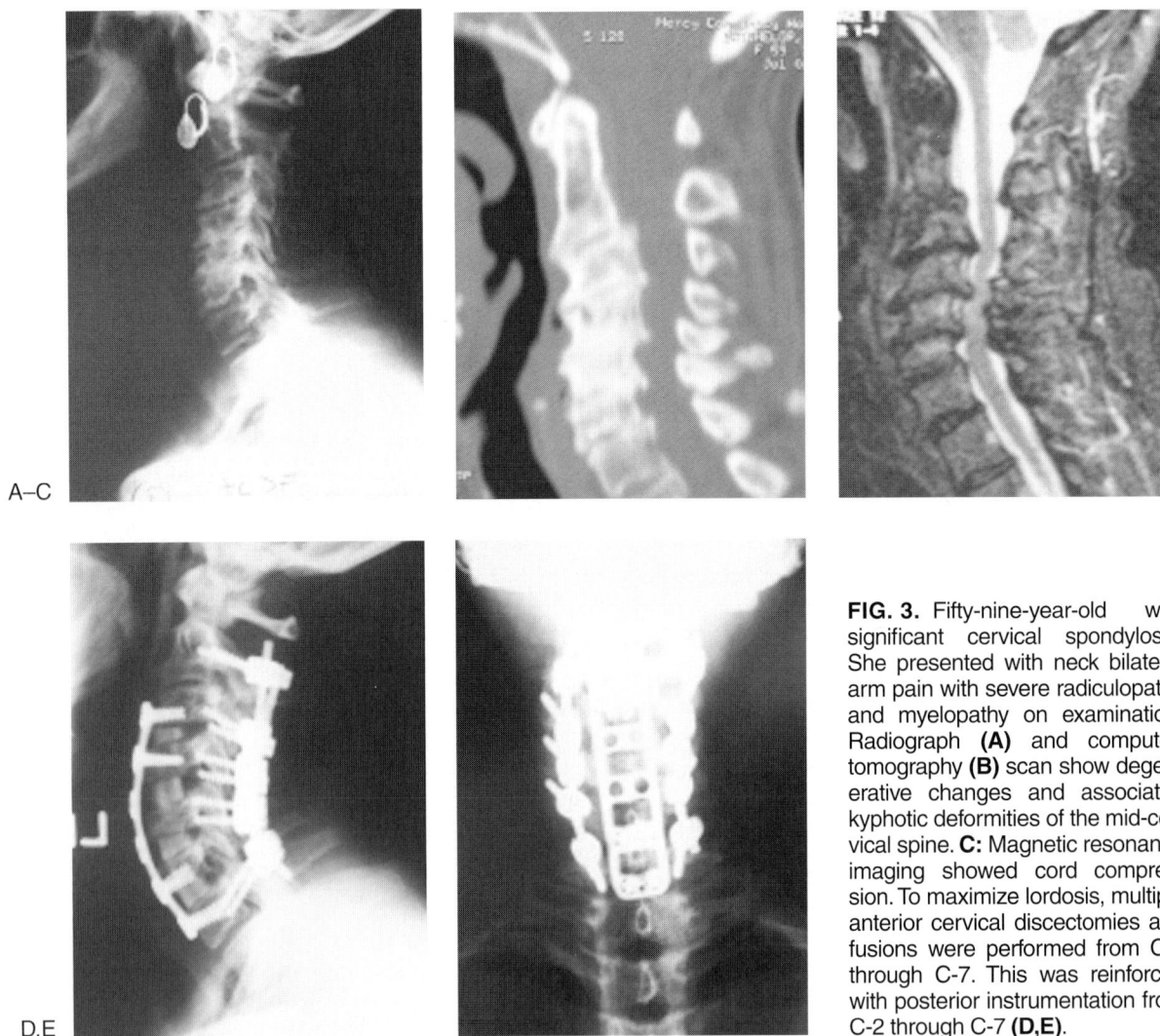

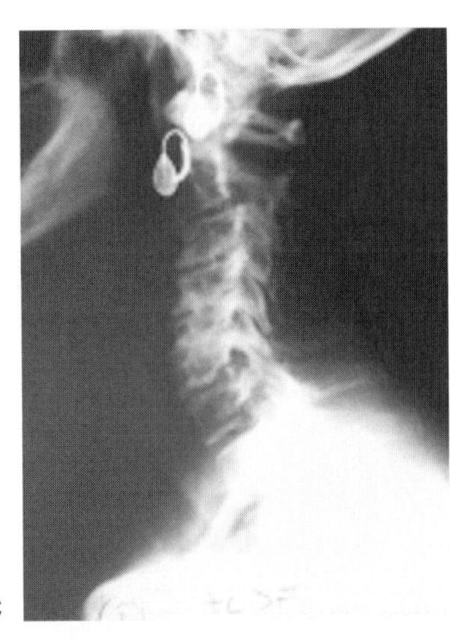
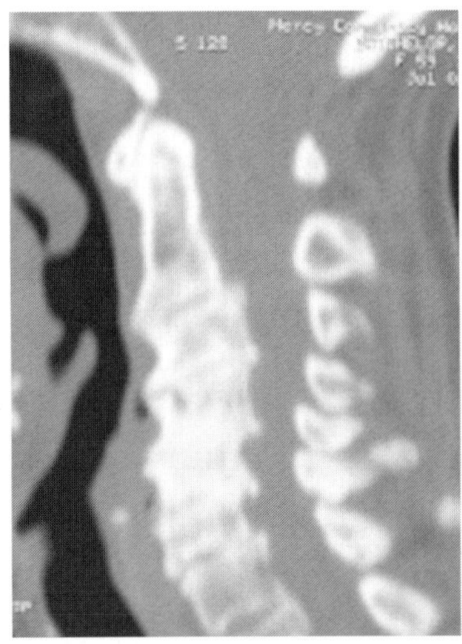
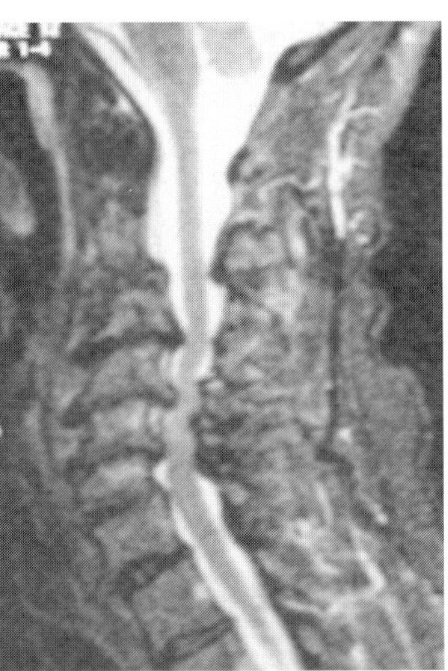

A–C

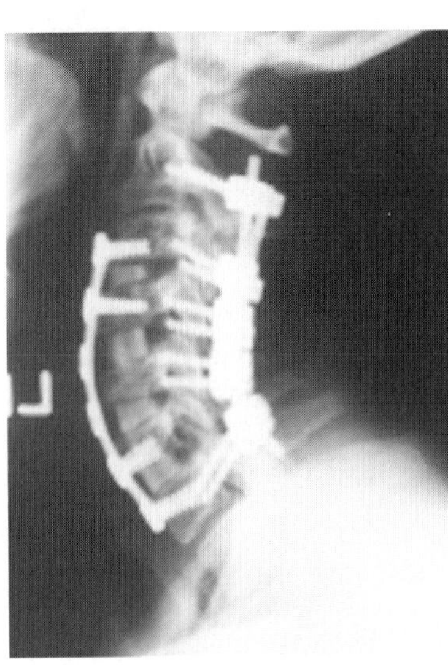

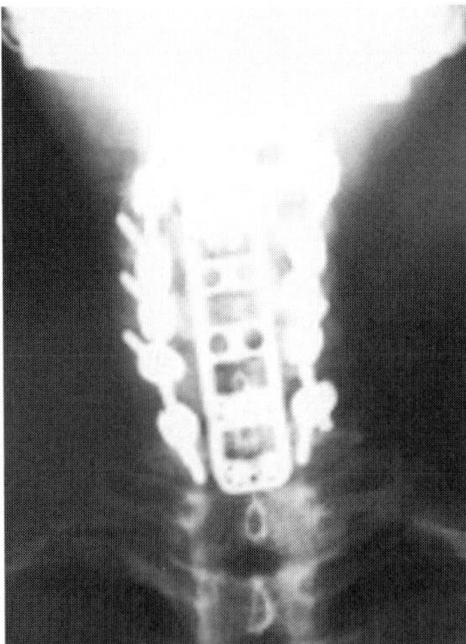

D,E

FIG. 3. Fifty-nine-year-old with significant cervical spondylosis. She presented with neck bilateral arm pain with severe radiculopathy and myelopathy on examination. Radiograph **(A)** and computed tomography **(B)** scan show degenerative changes and associated kyphotic deformities of the mid-cervical spine. **C:** Magnetic resonance imaging showed cord compression. To maximize lordosis, multiple anterior cervical discectomies and fusions were performed from C-3 through C-7. This was reinforced with posterior instrumentation from C-2 through C-7 **(D,E)**.

requiring decompression, the degree and flexibility of the kyphotic deformity, and the anatomic causation of the neural compression (disc or vertebral body). Because the spinal cord is nearly always compressed anteriorly, the authors most often use an anterior approach to achieve decompression of the neural elements. Anterior discectomies with fusion can be used to decompress pathology limited to the disc space at one or two levels. More extensive pathology requires removal of the vertebral bodies or a combination of vertebrectomy and discectomy. Structural grafting is used to lengthen the anterior column and correct the kyphotic deformity and, if possible, leaving the posterior longitudinal ligament intact to act as a hinge. Anterior plating or junctional plating is used to provide construct stability. When three or more vertebral bodies are removed or when a large deformity is corrected supplemental posterior instrumentation and fusion are performed under the same anesthetic. The most powerful strategy for kyphosis correction is intersegmental correction using wedged-shaped lordosing interbody grafts at each level if corpectomies are not necessary for decompression. If three or more interbody grafts are required, use of posterior fixation should be considered (Fig. 3).

Osteoporosis

As discussed in Chapter 8, the National Institutes of Health Consensus Conference defined *primary osteoporosis* as an age-related disorder characterized by decreased bone mass and increased susceptibility to fractures in the absence of other recognizable causes of bone loss (64). Resultant problems are widespread in the spine: Seventy-five percent of women with scoliosis older than the age of 65 years have at least one osteopenic wedge fracture (65).

The disease is characterized by trabeculae of decreased size and number, cortical thinning, and weakening of the internal structure of the vertebral bodies. The diagnosis of osteoporotic fractures of the spine can be difficult. The technique of Genant requires a 25% change in vertebral density in one dimension or a 40% change in total cross section (66). Once osteopenia is suspected, bone densitometry can be used to quantify its extent.

The prevalence of vertebral compression fractures increases during menopause. The normal centrifugal shift of long bone increases the diameter, which protects against torque and bending stress. These changes are not found in the vertebral bodies, which lose their axial load-bearing capacity. Nevertheless,

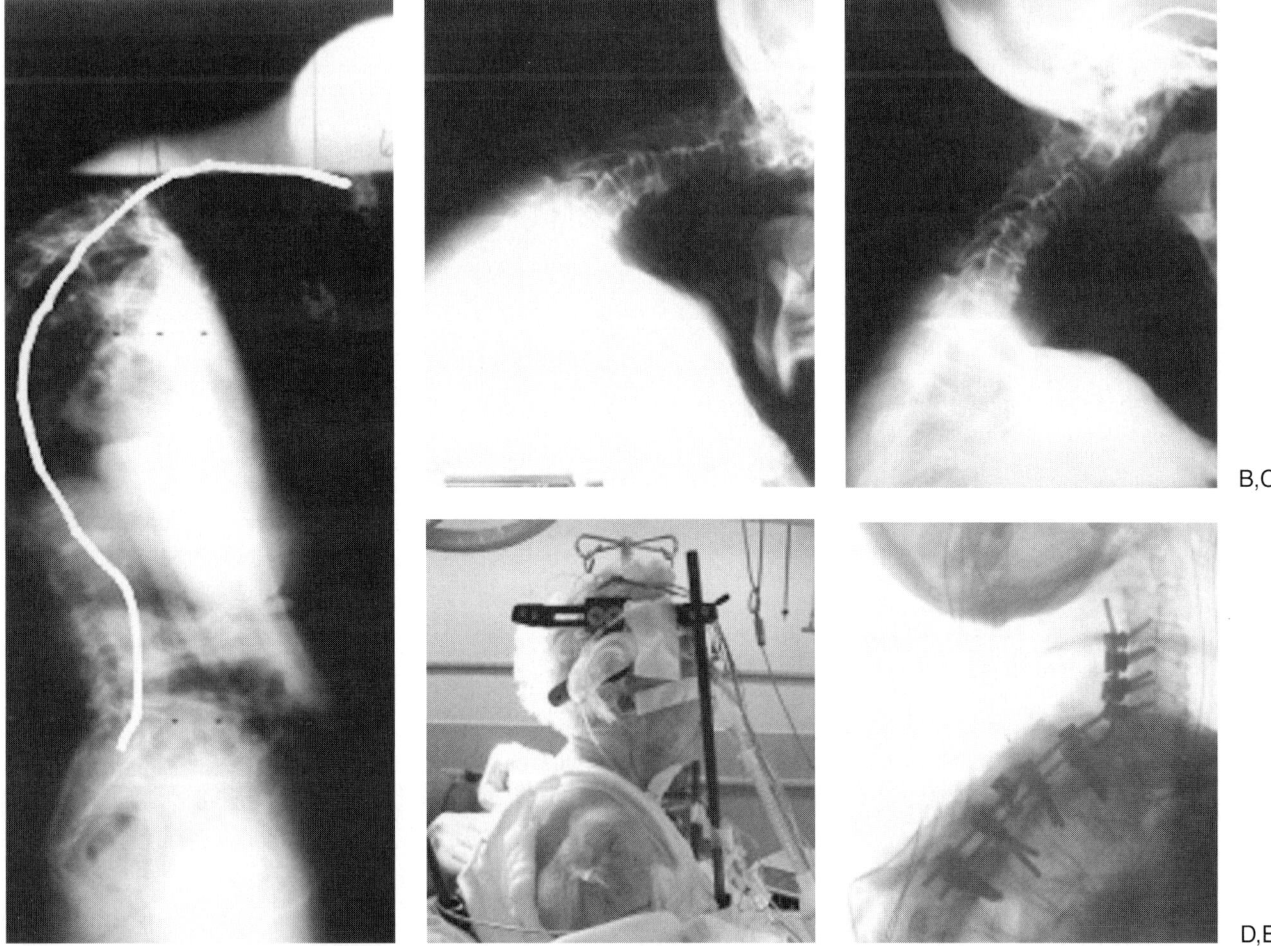

FIG. 4. Seventy-nine-year-old with senile kyphosis. This progressive deformity was associated with significant discomfort and lack of ability to achieve forward gaze, which interfered with activities of daily living. Preoperative standing **(A)**, flexion **(B)**, and extension **(C)** radiographs are shown. Postoperative clinical **(D)** and lateral radiographs **(E)** are shown after anterior discectomy/release, posterior C-7 Smith-Petersen osteotomy, and posterior instrumented fusion.

unlike the thoracic spine, the cervical spine is not a common place for osteoporotic compression fractures. This is probably due to a combination of two factors: relatively less overall axial loading in the cervical spine compared to the more caudal spine and the further load sparing of the anterior cervical vertebral bodies due to the lordotic curvature in this region of the spine. However, compression fractures and progression of kyphotic deformities may occur (Fig. 4) when a kyphotic deformity is present or develops in the cervical spine or if osteoporosis sufficiently weakens the vertebrae. The authors are unaware of any published patient series that gives information to specifically evaluate and treat osteoporotic compression fractures.

Paget's Disease

Paget's disease is a chronic disturbance of the adult skeleton resulting in softening, enlargement, and bowing of bones due to disorganization of osseous architecture. Although it is often present in the skull and thoracolumbar spine, the disease rarely affects the cervical spine. Schmorl's classic study was one of the first to report this disease in the cervical spine (67). He observed that when adjacent vertebrae are affected, Paget's disease may lead to ossification of the intervertebral disc and subsequent osseous fusion.

Other authors stress the importance of considering this disease in the differential diagnosis of patients with abnormal radiographic findings, particularly suspected tumors. Paget's disease almost always involves the entire vertebral body as well as the neural arch, and it should be present in other bones of the axial and appendicular skeleton. Absence of these findings suggests metastatic disease or other neoplastic conditions.

Relatively few cases of cervical Paget's disease have been reported in the literature since Schmorl's study. Feldman and Seaman conducted a review of all cases in the literature (68). They describe the characteristic coarse trabeculation and bony overgrowth of the vertebral bodies but mention that these findings may be obscured by degenerative changes. They note that the most striking feature of the disease in the cervical spine is the associated high rate of neurologic compromise (28%). The bony overgrowth narrows the spinal canal and intervertebral foramen, which is postulated to compromise the blood supply to the neural elements. In addition, the weakened bone predisposes to fracture or subluxation, which may worsen the neurologic state.

With multilevel involvement, significant kyphotic deformities may develop. Particularly when combined with degenerative changes, operative intervention may be required. There are no studies to date evaluating the best approach to this difficult problem.

INFLAMMATORY-INDUCED CERVICAL DEFORMITIES

The systemic and physiologic aspects of the inflammatory conditions of the spine, such as rheumatoid arthritis and AS, were presented in Chapter 9. These can also lead to cervical deformities.

Rheumatoid Arthritis

Rheumatoid arthritis is a chronic systemic autoimmune disease characterized by erosive synovitis that infiltrates and destroys multiple joints in the body. The cervical spine is the focus of involvement in the axial skeleton. The prevalence of spinal involvement in rheumatoid arthritis has been correlated to the severity of the peripheral manifestations (69). In the spine, three common patterns of deformity occur: (a) atlantoaxial instability (AAI) or subluxation, (b) cranial settling, and (c) subaxial subluxation. The reason the upper cervical spine is affected most commonly is because the occiput C-1 and the C1-2 articulations are purely synovial, whereas in the subaxial spine, only the facet articulations are synovial.

AAI, reported to occur in up to 49% of rheumatoids (70), can be fixed or reducible. The direction of instability is most commonly anterior but can be lateral or posterior. Erosion of the C1-2 articulations, combined with a lack of bony restraint of motion due to their axial orientation, can cause compression of the brainstem and superior spinal cord between the anterior pannus and the posterior ring of C-1. Cranial settling, also called superior migration of the odontoid or basilar invagination, is caused by erosion of these same joints, combined with those of the occiput C-1 articulation. The result is loss of height and intrusion of the odontoid into the foramen magnum. This can lead to static or dynamic compression of the brainstem (71). Subaxial subluxation is less common and can mimic osteoarthritic degeneration at multiple levels, with resultant kyphosis or instability (Fig. 5) (72).

Clinical manifestations most commonly include neck pain, occipital headaches, and stiffness. Other symptoms can be related to the onset of myelopathy: weakness, loss of endurance, gait disturbance, loss of dexterity, and radicular symptoms (73). Vertebrobasilar insufficiency may also occur related to AAI. Because of the multitude of diseases that can produce these findings, imaging has become the mainstay of evaluation for these patients.

Studies on the natural history of rheumatoid arthritis in the cervical spine are difficult to interpret. Overall, the course is one of progressive disease, but it is difficult to predict with certainty which patients will have progression of their deformity or will experience neurologic sequelae (73). Several investigators have shown that upper cervical lesions typically progress from AAI to cranial settling (74,75), but which of these will go on to neurologic sequelae is unclear. The presence of AAI has been correlated with a high mortality rate (76). In addition, once myelopathy develops, progression of disease and death are common without treatment. However, newer pharmacologic treatments have made an impact on the disease. Early combination therapy with disease-modifying antirheumatic drugs is significantly effective in preventing the onset of cervical spine subluxation but may not affect the instability once present (77). Surgical treatment algorithms are discussed in Chapter 10.

Ankylosing Spondylitis

The epidemiology, pathogenesis, and extraskeletal manifestations of AS are discussed in Chapter 10. Similar to patients with rheumatoid arthritis, those with AS can exhibit a wide range of symptoms and deformities. The diseases are, however, quite different in their clinical features and treatment. In this section, the particular aspects of the disease as they pertain to the cervical spine are discussed, with emphasis on the management of cervical deformities.

The characteristic deformities of AS are loss of lumbar lordosis and thoracic hyperkyphosis. There can also be involvement

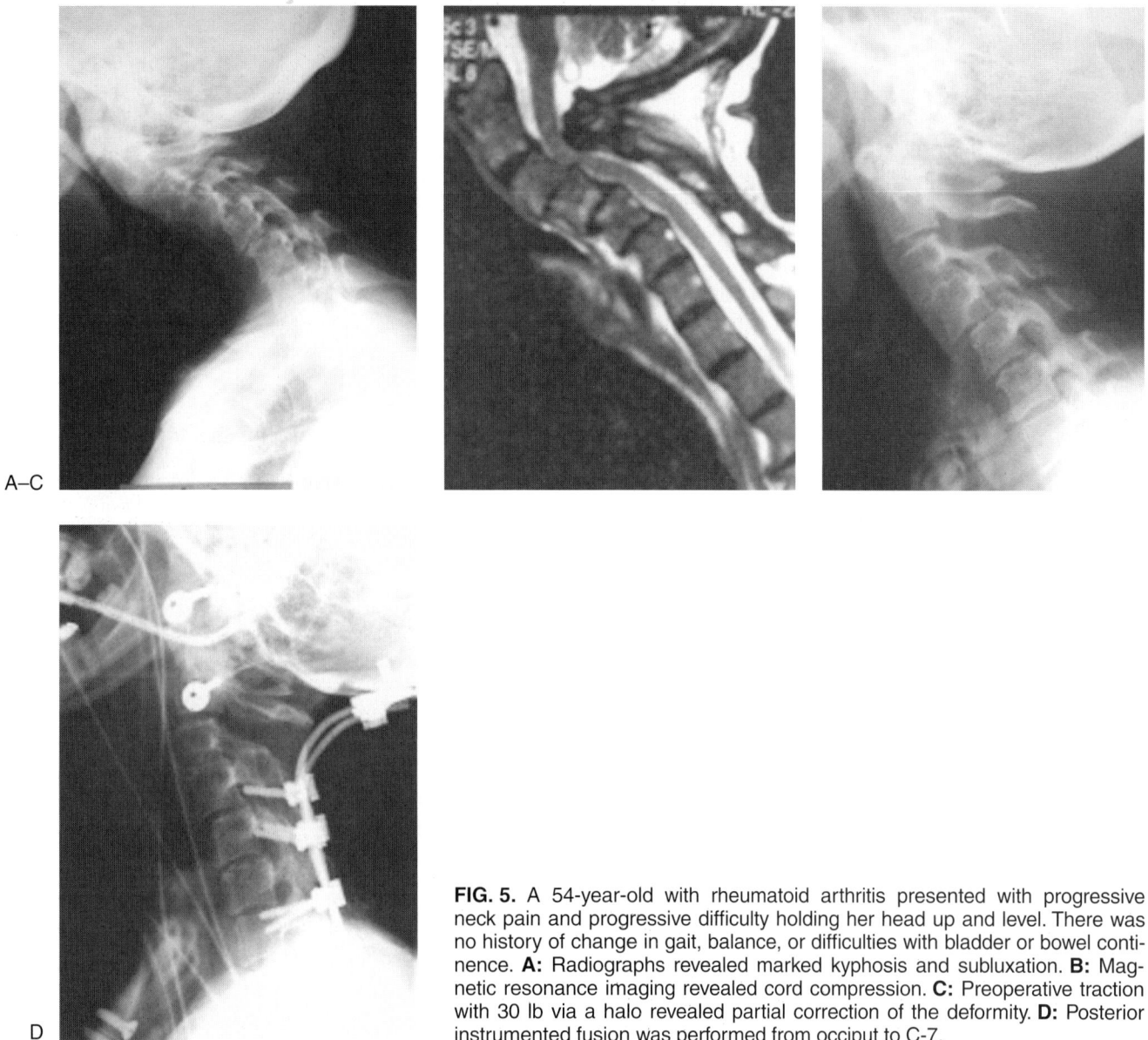

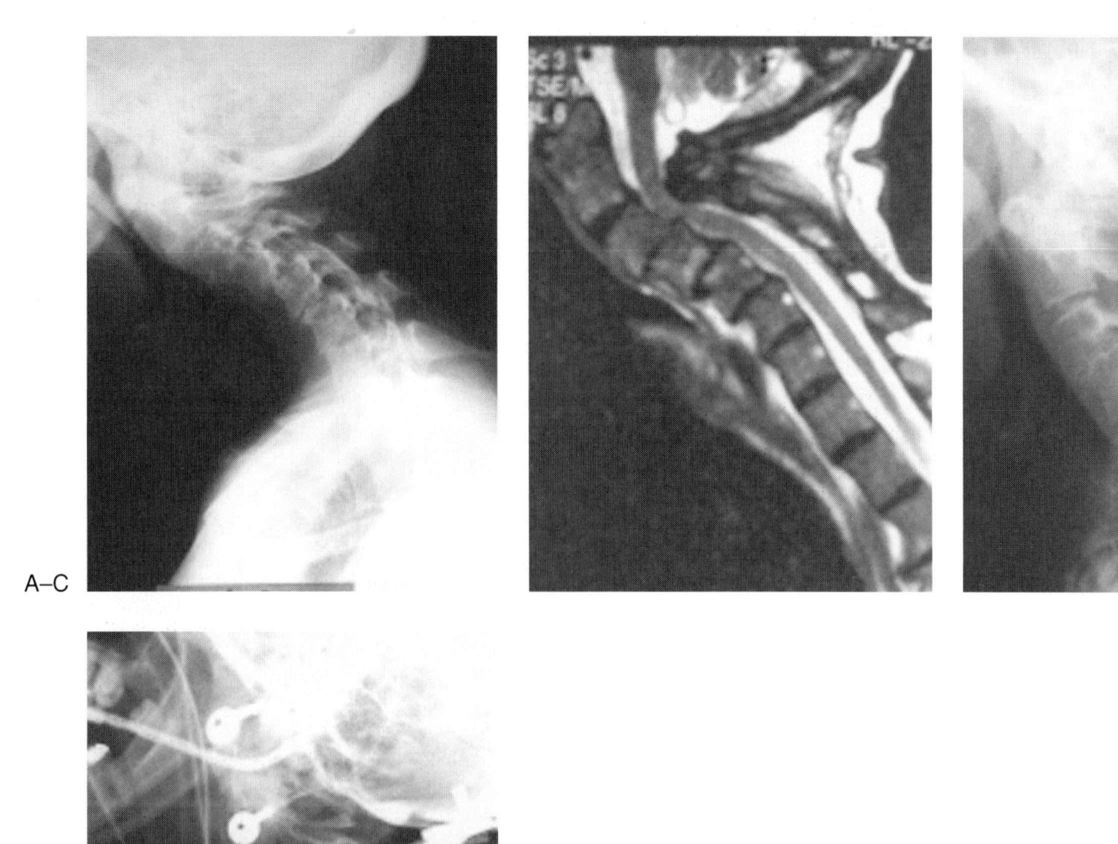

FIG. 5. A 54-year-old with rheumatoid arthritis presented with progressive neck pain and progressive difficulty holding her head up and level. There was no history of change in gait, balance, or difficulties with bladder or bowel continence. **A:** Radiographs revealed marked kyphosis and subluxation. **B:** Magnetic resonance imaging revealed cord compression. **C:** Preoperative traction with 30 lb via a halo revealed partial correction of the deformity. **D:** Posterior instrumented fusion was performed from occiput to C-7.

of the cervical region that can range from loss of flexibility in extension to fixed gross deformity. In the extreme form, "chin on chest" deformity can result, with the face pointing towards the floor. This can cause disabling restriction of the field of vision, interference with skin care and hygiene of the neck area, difficulty opening the mouth, and severe swallowing disorders.

As the cervical spine becomes a single column of bone, movement at the occiput C-1 or C1-2 articulations can increase as a compensatory mechanism. These patients can demonstrate instability and spinal cord compression, with signs of myelopathy. Attention to this possibility should be directed toward all patients with AS undergoing general anesthesia. As mobility is lost and movement is concentrated to the craniocervical or cervicothoracic junctions, the risk of fracture rises.

The indications and techniques for correction of cervical kyphosis in this patient population are not as clear as those for the lower spine. The chin-brow to vertical angle is a useful measurement to determine the amount of deformity present, track progression of deformity, and determine the amount of correction needed when planning surgery. Simmons described a measurement technique using the angle of the face with respect to the vertical as an estimate of the amount of correction needed to return the gaze to a functional position (10 degrees downward) (78).

The technique of cervical osteotomy originated with Urist (79), but it was Simmons who first reported the more modern technique of an osteotomy at C-7 to T-1 in 42 patients (80). The author stressed that the correction not be overzealous. Under local anesthetic in the sitting position, he relied on patient cooperation and used very gentle maneuvers to fracture the anterior spine after posterior decompression. Using this technique, he reported no major complications. Modern techniques with more advanced intraoperative monitoring have allowed prone positioning and the safer use of general anesthesia. The Stagnara wake-up test is still used commonly. Using the Simmons technique but with general anesthesia in the prone position, McMaster reported a series of 15 patients corrected a mean of 54 degrees (81). He reported quadriparesis in one patient at 1 week postoperatively, with symptoms of nerve root compression in two additional patients, both of which partially or fully resolved. Other methods of performing the osteotomy have been developed, but the Simmons method continues to be popular (82). Internal fixation has added to the stability of the spine but has not replaced the use of halo body jackets or vests.

The ankylosed spine is unusually susceptible to fracture, particularly at the cervicothoracic junction. This is due to the combination of vertebral body osteoporosis and intervertebral disc ossification, with resultant stress concentration. Fractures usually occur through the bodies and not through the disc spaces. The most common mechanism in AS or diffuse idiopathic skeletal hyperostosis patients is an extension distraction mechanism. The majority of these fractures occurs in the cervical spine and can result in severe neurologic injury. In a report of 15 patients with AS sustaining fractures by Graham et al., 12 were cervical, 11 had neurologic compromise, and 9 had major cord injury (83).

These fractures can be missed on initial evaluation because they are difficult to detect, and the shoulders can obscure the anatomy at the lower cervical levels. A delay in diagnosis has been reported in multiple studies. Such delay often leads to neurologic compromise due to instability or epidural hematoma formation (84–87). The history of pain with or without deformity progression in the neck is highly suggestive of fracture. Until proven otherwise, these symptoms should be treated as a fracture. Due to poor results with surgical stabilization with fractures in this patient population, nonoperative immobilization is recommended by many (83,86) but not all authors (84).

Rowed reviewed 21 patients with AS and cervical fractures, reporting that 76% had spinal cord injury at presentation (86). Neurologic deterioration occurred in 19% of patients. Patients treated with urgent decompression and stabilization for worsening deficits did not improve; the results for nonoperatively managed patients were variable. These authors stress the value of nonoperative management. In contrast, Fox et al., based on a retrospective review of 23 patients with cervical fractures in AS, recommend decompressive surgery for all patients with progressive neurologic deficits. They believe the early mobilization of patients was facilitated by internal fixation combined with postoperative halo vest immobilization (84).

Overall, cervical fractures in patients with AS are fraught with complications, both related to the initial injury as well as the associated medical problems inherent to the disease, regardless of treatment method. Because these fractures usually heal with conservative treatment, operative intervention must be proven to offer a significant benefit to outweigh the risks of the surgery. Newer, improved fixation techniques may allow more stable fixation and decompression, allowing faster mobilization of these patients with a decrease in the associated medical morbidity. More rigorous studies are required to assess this promising but as yet unproven possibility.

INFECTION-INDUCED CERVICAL DEFORMITIES

Spinal infections are covered in Chapter 10. Their potential to cause cervical deformity and the subsequent management is reviewed.

Pyogenic Infection

Approximately 3 to 14% of spinal infections are cervical (88,89). This incidence is increased in certain populations, such as diabetics, drug abusers, and those with human immunodeficiency virus (90). The source of pyogenic infections can be postsurgical, traumatic, or hematogenous.

The most common complaint in patients with cervical infections is neck pain. Other complaints include fever, chills, night sweats, malaise, radiculopathy, myelopathy, and dysphagia. The primary diagnostic tools used in the diagnosis of cervical infections are laboratory and diagnostic imaging studies (88). Once the diagnosis is strongly suspected, it can be confirmed with biopsy done at the time of surgical irrigation and débridement if an abscess is present. Acute management involves prolonged courses of intravenous antibiotics.

Deformity is associated with infections when they become chronic. The infectious process, which initially leads to disc collapse, can advance to involve destruction of the vertebral bodies and secondary kyphosis. At this stage, débridement of the infected tissue must be accompanied by decompression of neural elements, correction of deformity, and stabilization with autograft and often instrumentation (Fig. 6) (88). Antibiotic therapy then follows. The authors generally do not recommend the use of instrumentation or allograft anteriorly in the cervical spine in the face of an active (or even chronic) pyogenic infection.

Tuberculosis Infection

Spinal tuberculosis presents differently from pyogenic infection. Large paraspinal abscesses are more common, and the disc is more resistant. However, in the modern era of antituberculous antibiotics, abscesses of all kinds are less frequent. The cervical spine is less commonly involved than the thoracic or lumbar.

Tuberculosis typically occurs in three major types of involvement: peridiscal, central, and anterior, in decreasing order of prevalence (91). In the central form, the disease begins within the middle of the vertebral body and remains isolated to one vertebra. Central lesions tend to lead to vertebral collapse and, therefore, are most likely to produce spinal deformity in the cervical spine (91). Anterior abscesses can form in the retropharyngeal space and cause deformity as well.

Operative débridement plays a primary role in the cervical spine. Neurologic compromise is common, and the prognosis for patients treated operatively is clearly better than those with nonoperative management (92,93). When surgical treatment is necessary, radical débridement and anterior strut graft fusion in association with antituberculous therapy is recommended (Hong Kong operation) (94,95). The decompression should expose the dura when significant neurologic compression is evident. Kyphotic deformity is corrected by insertion of a strut graft; autograft or allograft bone healing is reliable in adults and children (96–98). Considerations for supplemental posterior fusion are identical to those in other disease processes creating instability. However, posterior fusion should not be used in lieu of anterior surgery. Rezai et al. concluded that anterior débridement and bone grafting with supplemental posterior instrumented fusion minimized neurologic deterioration and spinal deformity, allowed early mobilization, and resulted in excellent neurologic outcome (99).

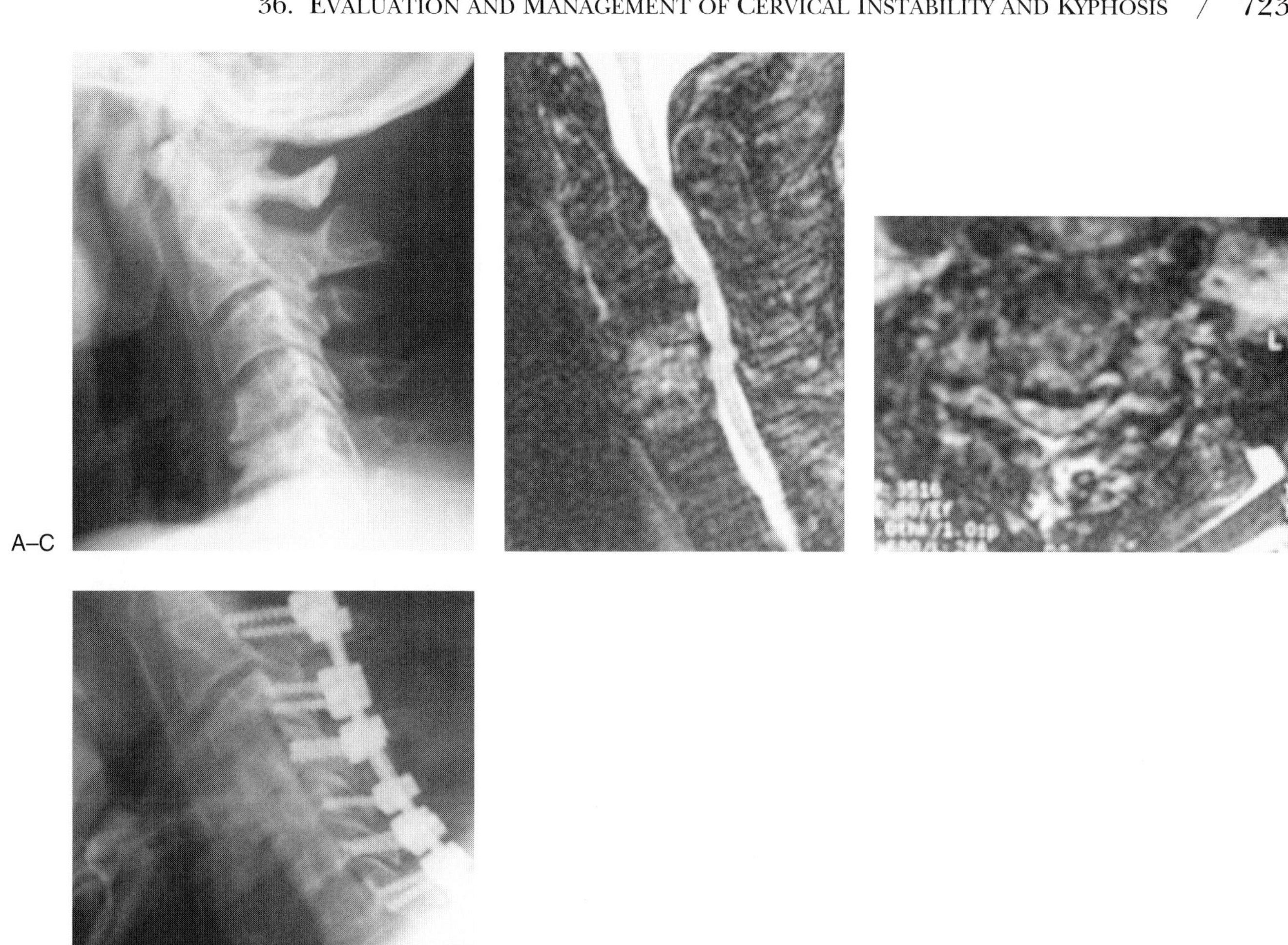

A–C

D

FIG. 6. Sixty-seven-year-old man with a kyphotic deformity secondary to chronic osteomyelitis. This patient had continued pain despite antibiotics. Collapse **(A)** and abnormal signal **(B)** were seen in vertebral bodies of C4-6 **(B)** with no epidural abscess **(C)**. **D:** He underwent anterior C4-6 corpectomies, autogenous fibula strut grafting, and posterior instrumented fusion.

IATROGENICALLY INDUCED CERVICAL DEFORMITIES

Iatrogenic instability after cervical laminectomy often follows a characteristic clinical course (100). In the early postoperative period, there is often good resolution of radicular or myelopathic symptoms due to the decompression of the neural elements. As kyphosis begins to develop, the patient will often complain of axial neck pain associated with easy fatigability of neck musculature. As the kyphotic deformity worsens, there may be a recurrence of the prior neurologic symptoms, or the development of new neurologic complaints. The true frequency of postlaminectomy kyphosis is difficult to ascertain from the literature due to the heterogeneous nature of the patients who have undergone laminectomy, but it does appear to be the most common cause of cervical kyphosis.

In general, postlaminectomy kyphosis in the subaxial cervical spine is seen much more frequently in growing children than adults, with a reported frequency of 37 to 100% (14,101,102). Laminectomies in this juvenile population are most frequently performed for the treatment of Arnold-Chiari malformations, syringomyelia, and tumors. Yasuoka and colleagues reported the development of kyphosis without preexisting deformity or violation of the facet joints and speculated that the development of kyphosis in children occurs secondary to the effects of growth when there are disrupted stabilizing structures (103). In contrast, 0 to 9% of juvenile patients developed kyphosis after laminectomy in the upper cervical spine (102,104).

Adults have a much lower frequency of kyphosis after cervical laminectomy. A change in cervical curvature is reported in 21 to 47% of patients (24,105–108), but not all are clinically significant. Zdeblick and Bohlman speculated that this decreased risk of postoperative kyphosis in adults, as compared to children, might be due to the presence of narrowed discs, osteophytes, and hypertrophied facets in the degenerative spine (62).

Kato et al. studied patients after multilevel cervical laminectomy for ossification of the posterior longitudinal ligament (107). A postoperative change in cervical alignment (with the cervical spine variably becoming straight, S-shaped, or kyphotic) was seen in 47% of the patients. None of the patients had neurologic worsening attributed to the presence of the deformity. Mikawa et al. reviewed a series of patients after multilevel cervical laminectomy for a variety of pathologies (108). In their adult population, 33% demonstrated a change in cervical alignment, and a kyphotic deformity was observed in 11%. Those who developed kyphosis did not exhibit neurologic worsening and thus did not require treatment.

INSTABILITY

Risk factors for the development of instability have been evaluated by many studies. Factors that consistently appear to predispose to postoperative deformity include the following: younger age (102,105,109), lack of preoperative lordosis (24,106,109), and disruption of the facet joints (109). Some have noted laminectomy of C-2 to be a risk factor (105,109), whereas others have not (102,108). Some have specifically noted that more levels of laminectomy are correlated with risk of kyphosis (109), whereas others have not (101,102,104,105). Similarly, some have noted preoperative range of motion to be a risk factor (105), whereas others have not (109). Gender does not appear to be a risk factor (101,102,105,109). Kasumi et al. were able to directly correlate the number of risk factors for kyphosis with the need for later stabilization procedures (109).

Prophylactic fusion should be considered at the time of the initial surgery for those who are at significant risk for developing kyphosis, because prevention of a deformity is much easier than its treatment. Facet fusion and lateral mass fixation can be performed in conjunction with laminectomy to provide stability and prevent the development of a progressive deformity (108–110). Kumar et al. found excellent long-term neurologic improvement in 25 patients undergoing laminectomy, fusion, and lateral mass fixation for spondylotic myelopathy (111).

The other technique designed to prevent postlaminectomy instability is cervical laminoplasty. Although several forms of laminoplasty have been described, the common goal of these procedures is to expand the size of the cervical spinal canal while maintaining the integrity of the posterior vertebral arch. Nowinski and colleagues compared laminoplasty to multilevel laminectomy in a cadaver model and found laminoplasty maintained motion characteristics similar to the intact spine (8). Matsunaga et al. reported a significantly lower frequency of cervical kyphotic deformity with laminoplasty compared to laminectomy (112). Herkowitz compared laminoplasty, laminectomy, and anterior decompression and found a higher rate of good and excellent outcomes in the laminoplasty group (86%) compared to those who had only the laminectomy (66%) (113).

A laminectomy patient who does go on to develop postoperative kyphosis may return to using a cervical collar or may begin to manually support his chin. Return of neurologic symptoms may be noted, or new symptoms may be noted. Once progression of a deformity is noted, especially if accompanied by neurologic deterioration or intractable neck pain, fusion is clearly advisable (101,109,114). This can be a surgical challenge.

The goals of correcting postlaminectomy kyphosis include decompression of the neural elements, reestablishment of the normal sagittal vertical axis, and stabilization of the spine. Preoperatively, the flexibility of a curve should be assessed by flexion and extension radiographs. If flexibility is limited, partial correction can be attempted in the conscious patient with traction before surgical fusion.

In myelopathic patients with a significant kyphotic deformity, correction of the spine deformity may place the spinal cord at significant risk. Therefore, spinal cord monitoring is imperative. Some patients will not tolerate complete correction of the deformity, and in these cases, decompression of the neural elements should take precedence over deformity correction. If myelomalacia and severe compression are present, there can be a significant risk of catastrophic deterioration with induction of anesthesia and mild to moderate hypotension. Therefore, mean arterial pressure should be carefully observed and kept at or above the patient's waking levels.

As with kyphosis correction in general, deformity correction can be achieved operatively by lengthening the anterior column, shortening the posterior column, or both (100). Specific to the postlaminectomy patient is the fact that the posterior portion of the vertebral ring and the normal posterior tension band of the cervical spine are disrupted. This must be considered in any treatment algorithm. As a consequence, the posterior longitudinal ligament becomes even more important as a hinge for the correction and should be preserved.

Corpectomy at the level of prior laminectomy was suggested for postlaminectomy instability as early as 1960 by Bailey and Badgley (115). However, this technique dissociates the left and right halves of the involved segments and can lead to significant forces on an anterior strut grafts. Riew et al. hypothesized that these abnormal forces are the cause of an unacceptably high complication rate for noninstrumented corpectomy and strut graft constructs (116). In their series of 18 patients who were treated with one- to four-level corpectomies, nine patients had graft-related complications despite postoperative immobilization. These complications included graft extrusion, graft collapse, and pseudarthrosis. Based on their review, this group changed their earlier recommendation for not instrumenting postlaminectory kyphosis correction (62) to recommending circumferential arthrodesis and instrumentation in the setting of multilevel postlaminectomy kyphosis (116). These new studies have led us to perform multiple discectomies, intersegmental graft correction, and anterior or anterior/posterior instrumentation if the cord compression is due to the deformity and not pathology behind the vertebral bodies (Fig. 7).

Herman and Sonntag reported on 20 patients who had postlaminectomy kyphosis treated with anterior decompression and strut grafting over an average of 3.8 levels accompanied by anterior cervical plate stabilization (117). One-half of the patients also received supplemental halo fixation. The preoperative kyphosis was an average of 38 degrees and was corrected to an average of 16 degrees; most patients experienced neurologic improvement. They concluded that this procedure is a viable option for patients treated for symptomatic postlaminectomy kyphosis.

Other authors have advocated circumferential surgery for patients with postlaminectomy kyphosis. Advocates of this approach emphasize the biomechanical superiority of rigid posterior instrumentation in reconstructing the deficient posterior tension band (100). In a biomechanical study, Foley et al. showed that anterior and posterior instrumentation could significantly decrease the loading of anterior strut grafts in multiple level strut graft constructs (118). Vanichkachorn et al. reported no failures among 11 patients with cervical myelopathy and a postlaminectomy kyphosis treated with long corpectomy constructs, a junctional plate, and posterior instrumentation (119).

The presently recommended approach to postlaminectomy kyphosis in a patient without a fused spine begins with an anterior decompression of the kyphotic segment, often including a multi-

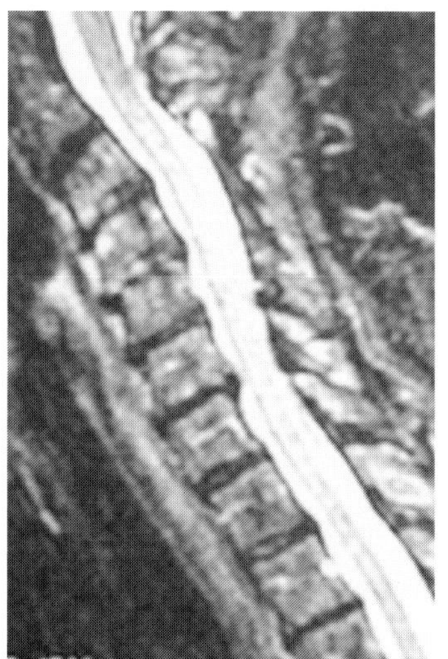
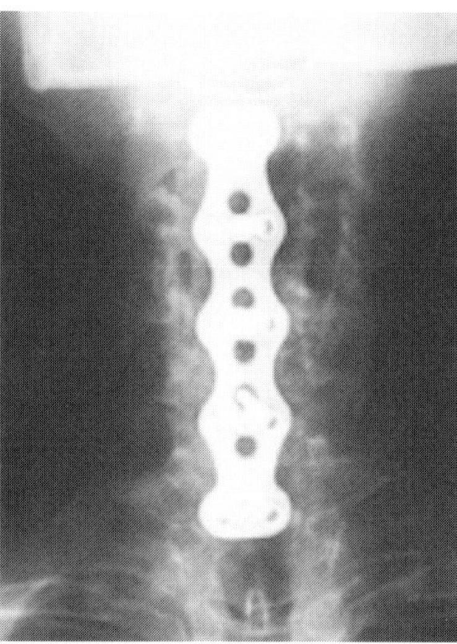
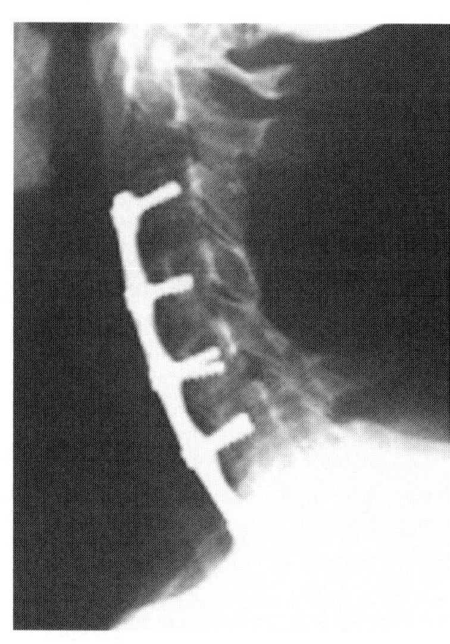

A–C

FIG. 7. Seventy-year-old woman with postlaminectomy kyphosis. She had temporary improvement after her initial operation but then developed neck pain and myeloradiculopathy. Sagittal magnetic resonance image is shown **(A)**. She underwent segmental correction from C3-7, with multiple anterior cervical discectomies and autogenous iliac crest fusion to regain maximal lordosis **(B,C)**.

level corpectomy. A structural strut graft is used to reconstruct the compressive strength of the anterior column and regain anterior height while allowing kyphosis correction about the axis of the posterior longitudinal ligaments. Depending on the length of the anterior construct, a cervical plate or a buttress plate is often applied to prevent graft extrusion, which can occur during positioning for the posterior procedure. Under the same anesthesia, a posterior facet fusion is performed using rigid segmental lateral mass instrumentation. When decompression of the entire body is not required for decompression, segmental correction can be obtained by interbody grafting in conjunction with anterior plating. In situations in which a significant deformity is corrected, the authors believe posterior instrumentation and facet fusion significantly decrease the rate of construct failure. The authors additionally recommend C-7 or T-1 pedicle screws at the terminal end of the construct to enhance construct stability and decrease pullout (100). It is reasonable to consider supplemental halo fixation postoperatively for patients with circumferential instability and very large kyphosis corrections or poor bone quality.

TRAUMATICALLY INDUCED CERVICAL DEFORMITIES

Traumatic injuries of the cervical spine can lead to the development of a cervical deformity. As with the other classes of deformity discussed above, this can be due to tension failure of posterior column structures or compression failure of the anterior column structures. These deformities can be seen acutely after an injury, later after inadequate or lack of treatment, or after chronic insidious microtrauma.

Acute Traumatic Injuries

The mechanism of injury is critical to understand when analyzing the direction and degree of instability of a given injury. This issue is addressed by classification systems as detailed by Allen et al., who describe the anatomic structures likely to be disrupted in a given injury (120). For example, the injury mechanisms most prone to the development of kyphosis include flexion-distraction and flexion-compression due to the disruption of the posterior stabilizing structures. The acute management of such injuries is discussed in Chapters 33 and 34 and is not revisited here.

Delayed Sequelae of Traumatic Injuries

Most cervical injuries are recognized early and definitively managed at that time. However, if the initial treatment of cervical injuries is inadequate or less obvious injuries are missed, delayed deformities may be seen (57). It is, thus, imperative to visualize the entire cervical spine and cervicothoracic junction on initial screening radiographs.

For those injuries that are not acutely surgically stabilized, kyphosis may progress due to inability or inadequacy of external immobilization. Even in seemingly innocuous injuries, it is important to be vigilant to the possibility of a developing deformity. This subacute instability has been described by Herkowitz and Rothman in patients who initially appeared to have a stable cervical spine but were subsequently noted to develop instability and a cervical deformity secondary to an occult ligamentous injury (121). To avoid missing these injuries, the authors recommended maintaining immobilization until muscle spasm has subsided, followed by good quality flexion-extension lateral radiographs taken to rule out instability (121). In addition, patients with continued neck symptoms should be followed at regular intervals for up to1 year to avoid missing late instability.

Many high-grade injuries cannot be adequately stabilized nonoperatively. For example, high-grade distractive and compressive flexion injury patterns tend to be highly unstable and may displace even in a halo-vest orthosis (122,123). This is generally due to the loss of the posterior stabilizing structures. High-grade distraction-extension injuries also tend to demonstrate a high frequency of progressive instability when treated nonoperatively (124). The vertical compression injury pattern often demonstrates segmental kyphosis due to loss of the structural integrity of the anterior vertebral body in association with retropulsion of bone into the spinal canal.

If traumatic instabilities or deformities present with progression of deformity, symptoms, or neurologic exam, surgical correction and stabilization must be considered. In this setting, the length of time since the injury is an important variable. Recent injuries often remain mobile, allowing significant correction with the use of preoperative cervical traction.

Injuries older than 4 to 6 weeks are more challenging to treat and may require surgical release to obtain correction (Fig. 8). The location of neural compression, the magnitude of deformity, and the neurologic status of the patient must all be considered when designing a treatment plan. Old traumatic deformities generally are not flexible and, therefore, require a release of the ankylosed segments before attempting any correction. It is also crucial to adequately decompress the spinal cord before attempting a deformity correction. Therefore, the operation may begin with a release of the deformity on one side of the spine, followed by a decompression and release of the deformity on the opposite side of the spine. This allows the deformity to be corrected, followed by appropriate grafting, fusion, and circumferential instrumentation. For example, some patients may require a "back, front, back" approach. Good spinal cord monitoring is advisable in neurologically intact patients or those with incomplete neurologic injuries undergoing significant deformity corrections. Postoperative immobilization is generally required to supplement the overall surgical construct and minimize the chance of failure.

For those injuries that are surgically corrected, deformity may persist or recur if not adequately managed. For example, in a series of trauma patients undergoing anterior, posterior, or combined cervical fusions, Jenkins et al. found that 20% of the patients ended up with kyphosis greater than or equal to 20 degrees (125). They could not identify a significant difference in the frequency of kyphosis and surgical approach used, but the number of patients was small. Nonetheless, a persistent or recurrent deformity was correlated with worse clinical outcomes. Other groups have similarly described kyphosis remaining in 21 to 27% of patients with anterior fusions (126,127). Progression

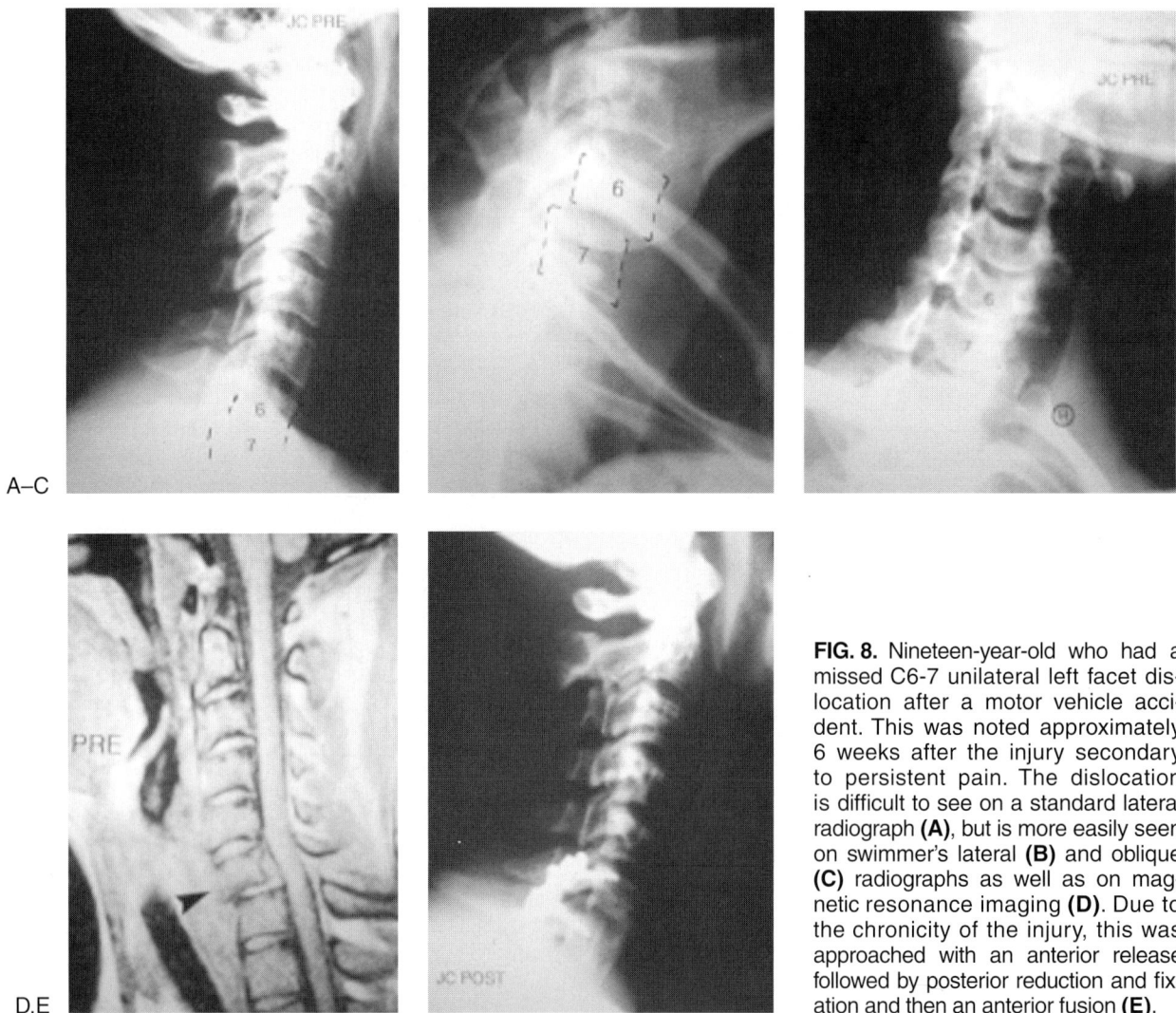

A–C

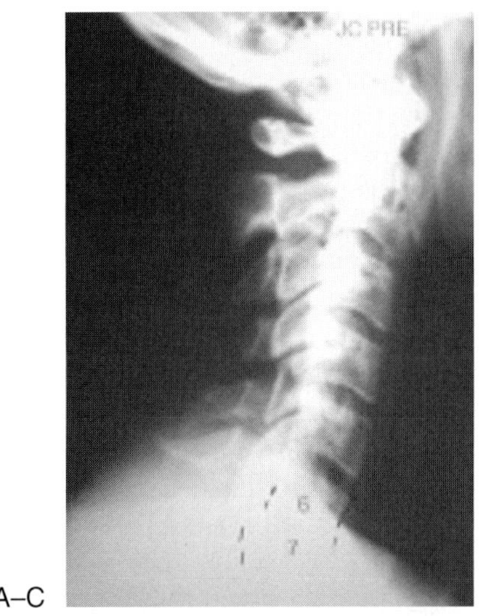

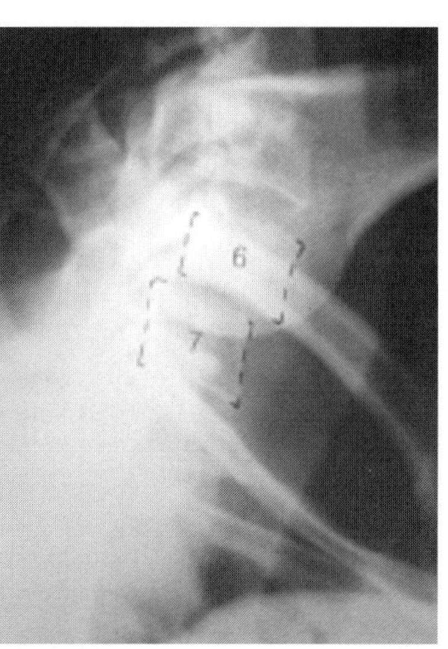

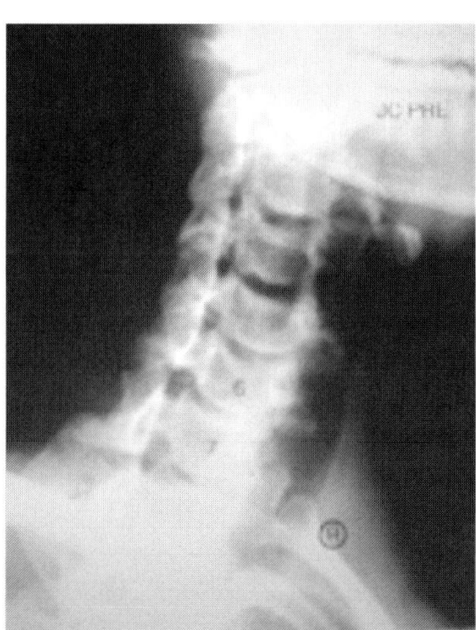

D,E

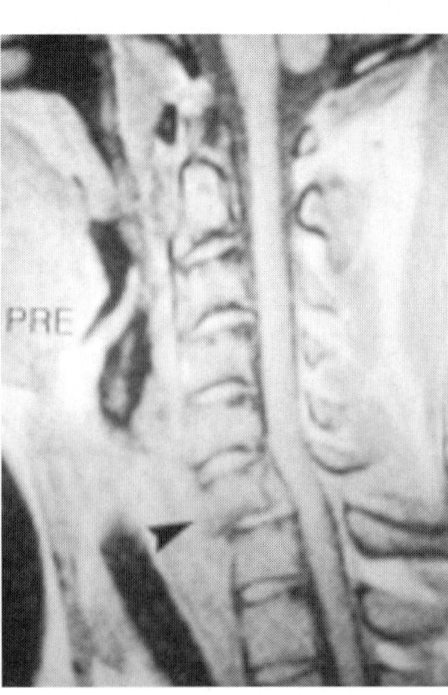

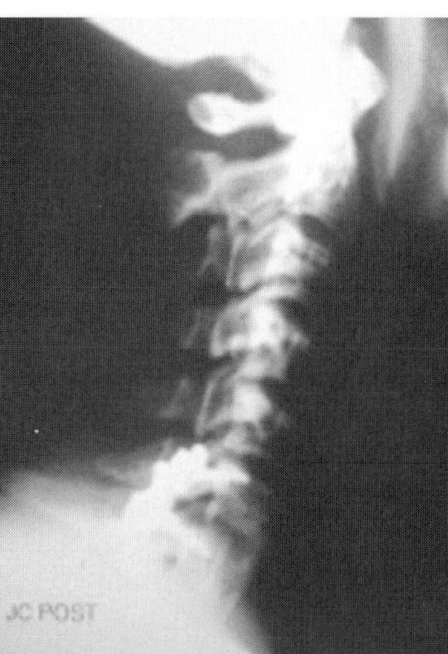

FIG. 8. Nineteen-year-old who had a missed C6-7 unilateral left facet dislocation after a motor vehicle accident. This was noted approximately 6 weeks after the injury secondary to persistent pain. The dislocation is difficult to see on a standard lateral radiograph **(A)**, but is more easily seen on swimmer's lateral **(B)** and oblique **(C)** radiographs as well as on magnetic resonance imaging **(D)**. Due to the chronicity of the injury, this was approached with an anterior release followed by posterior reduction and fixation and then an anterior fusion **(E)**.

of kyphosis was related to the settling of the strut grafts and was noted up to 16 months postoperatively (126). These data argue for aggressive use of instrumentation in these patients.

In addition to deformity at the site of fusion, others have described instability and deformity adjacent to fusion constructs. This may be due to stress concentration at the adjacent levels or to unrecognized trauma at the time of the initial injury. Whitehill and Schmidt reported a series of patients with posterior interspinous wiring, 23% of whom developed flexible kyphosis adjacent to fused regions averaging 16 degrees (128).

In summary, vigilance should be applied to cervical injuries, so that progressive deformity can be detected early. Acute management of a cervical injury should be based on the good understanding of the disrupted anatomy. Delayed management of such injuries should be based on an understanding of why initial management failed, the current nature of the deformity, and reconstructive options (57).

Repetitive Microtrauma Injuries

There are many reports of occupational hazards resulting in acute cervical trauma. These injuries are discussed in Chapters 3A and 3B. Posttraumatic instability may progress to deformity if not appropriately addressed. However, there are additional reports of repetitive cervical microtrauma in the workplace causing cervical deformity.

Kelkar et al. reported on several cases of extreme kyphosis in railway porters (129). These patients had severe, asymptomatic deformities with a history of normal preemployment cervical films (no congenital abnormalities), no history of infection, and no evidence of rheumatoid arthritis. They concluded that the repetitive trauma of heavy lifting experienced by these patients resulted in chronic physical strains, disc degeneration, and a secondary premature degenerative kyphosis.

Others have found mining in tunnels to correlate with marked cervical extension secondary to the need to maintain forward gaze in a stooped position (130). Additionally, miners working on the seam face are subjected to vibrations that exacerbate degenerative processes (131). Similarly, people who perform load-carrying on their heads have an accelerated course of degeneration (132). The best initial management of these conditions is to stop the activity leading to the microtrauma.

CONCLUSION

Cervical deformities, regardless of their cause, result in a pathologic shift in the normal balance of the head. The clinical result is often severe axial neck pain and progressive neurologic compromise. Treatment strategies are based on decompressing the neural elements and restoring normal cervical biomechanics by correction of the deformity. To achieve success, a thorough understanding of anterior and posterior cervical decompression, instrumentation, and fusion techniques is required.

REFERENCES

1. Panjabi MM. Cervical spine models for biomechanical research. *Spine* 1998;23:2684–2700.
2. Gore DR, Sepic SB, Gardner GM. Roentgenographic findings of the cervical spine in asymptomatic people. *Spine* 1986;11:521–524.
3. Kandziora F, Pflugmacher R, Scholz M, et al. Comparison between sheep and human cervical spines: an anatomic, radiographic, bone mineral density, and biomechanical study. *Spine* 2001;26:1028–1037.
4. Pal GP, Sherk HH. The vertical stability of the cervical spine. *Spine* 1988;13:447–449.
5. Panjabi MM, Duranceau J, Goel V, et al. Cervical human vertebrae. Quantitative three-dimensional anatomy of the middle and lower regions. *Spine* 1991;16:861–869.
6. Cusick JF, Yoganandan N, Pintar F, et al. Biomechanics of cervical spine facetectomy and fixation techniques. *Spine* 1988;13:808–812.
7. Kumaresan S, Yoganandan N, Pintar FA, et al. Finite element modeling of cervical laminectomy with graded facetectomy. *J Spinal Disord* 1997;10:40–46.
8. Nowinski GP, Visarius H, Nolte LP, et al. A biomechanical comparison of cervical laminoplasty and cervical laminectomy with progressive facetectomy. *Spine* 1993;14:1995–2004.
9. Zdeblick TA, Zou D, Warden KE, et al. Cervical stability after foraminotomy: a biomechanical in vitro analysis. *J Bone Joint Surg* 1992;74A:22–27.
10. Raynor RB, Pugh J, Shapiro I. Cervical facetectomy and its effect on spine strength. *J Neurosurg* 1985;63:278–282.
11. Zdeblick TA, Abitol JJ, Kunz DN, et al. Cervical stability after sequential capsule resection. *Spine* 1993;18:2005–2008.
12. Cusick JF, Pintar FA, Yoganandan N. Biomechanical alterations induced by multilevel cervical laminectomy. *Spine* 1995;20:2392–2399.
13. Goel VK, Clark CR, Harris KG, et al. Kinematics of the cervical spine: effects of multiple total laminectomy and facet wiring. *J Orthop Research* 1988;6:611–619.
14. Lonstein JE. Post-laminectomy kyphosis. *Clin Orthop Rel Research* 1977;128:93–100.
15. Saito T, Yamamuro T, Shikata J, et al. Analysis and prevention of spinal column deformity following cervical laminectomy. I. Pathogenetic analysis of postlaminectomy deformities. *Spine* 1991;16:494–502.
16. Panjabi MM, White AA, Keller D, et al. Stability of the cervical spine under tension. *J Biomechanics* 1978;11:189–197.
17. White AA, Johnson RM, Panjabi MM, et al. Biomechanical analysis of clinical stability in the cervical spine. *Clin Orthop Rel Research* 1975;109:85–96.
18. Moroney SP, Schultz AB, Miller JAA. Analysis and measurement of neck loads. *J Orthop Res* 1988;6:713–720.
19. Panjabi MM, Cholewicki J, Nubu K, et al. Critical load of the human cervical spine: an *in vitro* experimental study. *Clin Biomech* 1988;13:11–17.
20. Panjabi MM, Miura T, Cripton PA, et al. Development of a system for *in vitro* neck muscle force replication in whole cervical spine experiments. *Spine* 2001;26:2214–2219.
21. Patwardhan AG, Havey RM, Ghanayem AJ, et al. Load-carrying capacity of the human cervical spine in compression is increased under a follower load. *Spine* 2000;25:1548–1554.
22. Nolan JP, Sherk HH. Biomechanical evaluation of the extensor musculature of the cervical spine. *Spine* 1988;13:9–11.
23. White AA, Panjabi MM, Thomas CL. The clinical biomechanics of kyphotic deformity. *Clin Orthop* 1977;128:8–17.
24. Ishda Y, Suzuki K, Ohmori K, et al. Critical analysis of extensive cervical laminectomy. *Neurosurgery* 1989;24:215–222.
25. Epstein JA. The surgical management of cervical spinal stenosis, spondylosis and myeloradiculopathy by means of the posterior approach. *Spine* 1988;13:864–869.
26. Breig A, El-Nadi F. Biomechanics of the cervical spinal cord. Relief of contact pressure on and over stretching of the spinal cord. *Acta Radiol Diag* 1966;4:602–624.
27. Reid JD. Effects of flexion-extension movements of the head and spine upon the spinal cord and nerve roots. *J Neurol Neurosurg Psych* 1960;23:214–221.
28. Panjabi M, White A. Biomechanics of nonacute cervical spinal cord trauma. *Spine* 1988;13:838–842.
29. Fielding JW, Francis WR, Hawkins RJ, et al. Atlantoaxial rotatory deformity. *Semin Spine Surg* 1991;3:33–38.
30. Wolfort FG, Kanter MA, Miller LB. Torticollis. *Plastic Reconstr Surg* 1989;84:682–692.

31. Skeletal Dysplasia Group. Special report: instability of the upper cervical spine. *Arch Dis Child* 1989;64:283–288.
32. Remes V, Marttinen E, Poussa M, et al. Cervical kyphosis in diastrophic dysplasia. *Spine* 1999;24:1990–1995.
33. Johnston CE, Birch JG, Daniels JL. Cervical kyphosis in patients who have Larsen syndrome. *J Bone Joint Surg* 1996;78A:538–545.
34. Hensinger RN, Lang JE, MacEwen GD. Klippel-Feil syndrome: a constellation of associated anomalies. *J Bone Joint Surg* 1974;56A:1246–1253.
35. Thomsen MN, Schneider U, Weber M, et al. Scoliosis and congenital anomalies associated with Klippel-Feil syndrome types I-III. *Spine* 1997;22:396–401.
36. King HA, Moe JH, Bradford DS, et al. The selection of fusion levels in thoracic idiopathic scoliosis. *J Bone Joint Surg* 1983;65A:1302–1313.
37. Lee GA, Betz RR, Clements DH, et al. Proximal kyphosis after posterior spinal fusion in patients with idiopathic scoliosis. *Spine* 1999;24:795–799.
38. Lenke LG, Bridwell KH, O'Brien MF, et al. Recognition and treatment of the proximal thoracic curve in adolescent idiopathic scoliosis treated with Cotrel-Dobousset instrumentation. *Spine* 1994;19: 1589–1597.
39. Winter RB. The idiopathic double thoracic curve pattern: its recognition and surgical management. *Spine* 1989;14:1287–1292.
40. Winter RB, Denis F. The King V curve pattern: its analysis and surgical treatment. *Orthop Clin North Am* 1994;25:353–362.
41. Arlet V, Marchesi D, Papin P, et al. Decompensation following scoliosis surgery: treatment by decreasing the correction of the main thoracic curve or "letting the spine go." *Eur Spine J* 2000;156–160.
42. Cochran T, Irstam L, Nachemson A. Long-term anatomic and functional changes in patients with adolescent idiopathic scoliosis treated by Harrington rod fusion. *Spine* 1990;15:644–649.
43. Rechtman AM, Border AGB, Gershon-Cohen J. The lordotic curve of the cervical spine. *Clin Orthop* 1961;20:208–216.
44. Winter RB, Lovell WW, Moe JH. Excessive thoracic lordosis and loss of pulmonary function in patients with idiopathic scoliosis. *J Bone Joint Surg* 1975;57A:972–976.
45. Hilibrand AS, Rannenbaum DA, Graziano GP, et al. The sagittal alignment of the cervical spine in adolescent idiopathic scoliosis. *J Ped Orthop* 1995;15:627–632.
46. Boriani S, Biagini R, DeIure F, et al. Focus on the spine: primary bone tumors of the spine: a survey of the evaluation and treatment at the istututo ortopedico Rizzoli. *Orthopaedics* 1995;18:993–1000.
47. Abdu WA, Provencher M. Primary bone and metastatic tumors of the cervical spine. *Spine* 1998;23:2767–2777.
48. Bohlman HH, Sachs BL, Carter JR, et al. Primary neoplasms of the cervical spine. Diagnosis and treatment of twenty-three patients. *J Bone Joint Surg* 1986;68A:483–493.
49. Weinstein JN, McLain RJ. Primary tumors of the spine. *Spine* 1987;12:843–851.
50. Levine AM, Boriani S, Donati D, et al. Benign tumors of the cervical spine. *Spine* 1992;17:S399–S406.
51. Ozaki T, Liljenqvist U, Hillmann, et al. Osteoid osteoma and osteoblastoma of the spine: experience with 22 patients. *Clin Ortho Rel Research* 2002;397:394–402.
52. Jennis LG, Dunn EJ, An HS. Metastatic disease of the cervical spine. *Clin Orthop* 1999;359:89–103.
53. Asdourian P, Mardjetko S, Raushning W, et al. An evaluation of spinal deformity in metastatic breast cancer. *J Spinal Disord* 1990;3:119–134.
54. Nakamura M, Toyama Y, Suzuki N, et al. Metastases to the upper cervical spine. *J Spinal Disord* 1996;9:195–201.
55. McBride GG, Greenberg D. Treatment of Charcot spinal arthropathy following traumatic paraplegia. *J Spinal Disord* 1991;2:212–220.
56. Standaert C, Cardenas DD, Anderson P. Charcot spine as a late complication of traumatic spinal cord injury. *Arch Phys Med Rehabil* 1997;2:221–225.
57. Vaccaro AR, Silber JS. Post-traumatic spinal deformity. *Spine* 2001;26:S111–S118.
58. Brown CW, Jones B, Donaldson DH, et al. Neuropathic (Charcot) arthropathy of the spine after traumatic spinal paraplegia. *Spine* 1992;6:S103–S108.
59. Madsen PW, Green BA, Bowen BC. Syringomyelia. In: *The spine*, 4th ed. Rothman & Simeone, 1999.
60. Yu YL, Moseley IF. Syringomyelia and cervical spondylosis: a clinicoradiological investigation. *Neuroradiology* 1987;29:143–151.
61. Cutting PJE. A case of Charcot's disease of the cervical spine. *Br Med J* 1949;1:311–313.
62. Zdeblick TA, Bohlman HH. Cervical kyphosis and myelopathy: treatment by anterior corpectomy and strut-grafting. *J Bone Joint Sur* 1989;71A:170–182.
63. Ebersold MJ, Pare MC, Quast LM. Surgical treatment for cervical spondylitic myelopathy. *J Neurosurg* 1995;82:745–751.
64. National Institutes of Health Consensus Development Conference: statement on osteoporosis. *JAMA* 1984;252:799.
65. Healey JG, Lane JM. Structural scoliosis in osteoporotic women. *Clin Orthop* 1985;1985:216–223.
66. Storm T, Thamsborg G, Steiniche T, et al. Effects of intermittent cyclical etidronate therapy on bone mass and fracture rate in women with postmenopausal osteoporosis. *N Engl J Med* 1990;322:1265–1271.
67. Schmorl G. Über ostitis deformans paget. *Virchows Arch Path Anat* 1932;283:694–751.
68. Feldman F, Seaman WB. The neurologic complications of Paget's disease in the cervical spine. *AJR Am J Roentgenol* 1969;105:375–382.
69. Oda T, Fujiwara K, Yonenobu K, et al. Natural course of cervical spine lesions in rheumatoid arthritis. *Spine* 1995;20:1128–1135.
70. Morizono Y, Sakou T, Kawaida H. Upper cervical involvement in rheumatoid arthritis. *Spine* 1987;12:721–725.
71. Reijnierse M, Bloem JL, Dijkmans BA, et al. The cervical spine in rheumatoid arthritis: Relationship between neurologic signs and morphology of MR imaging and radiographs. *Skeletal Radiol* 1996; 25:113–118.
72. Gurley JP, Bell GR. The surgical management of patients with rheumatoid cervical spine disease. *Rheum Dis Clin North Am* 1997;23: 317–332.
73. Reiter MF, Boden SD. Inflammatory disorders of the cervical spine. *Spine* 1998;23:2755–2766.
74. Casey A, Crockard H, Geddes J, et al. Vertical translocation: the enigma of the disappearing atlandodens interval in patients with myelopathy and rheumatoid arthritis. Part I: Clinical radiological and neuropathological features. *J Neurosurg* 1997;87:856–862.
75. Casey A, Crockard H, Stevens J. Vertical translocation, Part II: Outcomes after surgical treatment of rheumatoid cervical myelopathy. *J Neurosurg* 1997;87:863–869.
76. Riise T, Jacobsen BK, Gran JT. High mortality in patients with rheumatoid arthritis and atlantoaxial subluxation. *J Rheum* 2001;28:2425–2429.
77. Neva MH, Kauppi MJ, Kautiainen H, et al. Combination drug therapy retards the development of rheumatoid atlantoaxial subluxations. *Arthr Rheum* 2000;43:2397–2401.
78. Simmons EH. Kyphotic deformity of the spine in ankylosing spondylitis. *Clin Orthop* 1977;128:65–77.
79. Urist MR. Osteotomy of the cervical spine: report of a case of ankylosing rheumatoid spondylitis. *J Bone Joint Surg* 1958;40A:833–843.
80. Simmons EH. The surgical correction of flexion deformity of the cervical spine in ankylosing spondylitis. *Clin Orthop* 1972;86:132–143.
81. McMaster MJ. Osteotomy of the cervical spine in ankylosing spondylitis. *J Bone Joint Surg* 1997;79B:197–203.
82. Bouchard JA, Feibel RJ. Gradual multiplanar cervical osteotomy to correct kyphotic ankylosing spondylitic deformities. *Can J Surg* 2002; 45:215–218.
83. Graham B, Van Peteghem PK. Fractures of the spine in ankylosing spondylitis. Diagnosis, treatment, and complications. *Spine* 1989; 14:803–807.
84. Fox MW, Onofrio BM, Kilgore JE. Neurologic complications of ankylosing spondylitis. *J Neurosurg* 1993;78:871–878.
85. Hunter T, Dubo HI. Spinal fractures complicating ankylosing spondylitis: a long-term follow-up study. *Arthritis Rheum* 1983;26: 751–759.
86. Rowed DW. Management of cervical spinal cord injury in ankylosing spondylitis: the intervertebral disc as a cause of cord compression. *J Neurosurg* 1992;77:241–246.
87. Farmer J, Vaccaro A, Algert TJ, et al. Neurologic deterioration after cervical spinal cord injury. *J Spinal Disord* 1998;11:192–196.

88. Ghanayem AJ, Zdeblick TA. Cervical spine infections. *Ortho Clinics North Am* 1996;27:53–67.
89. Griffiths HED, Jones DM. Pyogenic infections of the spine: a review of twenty-eight cases. *J Bone Joint Surg* 1971;53B:383–391.
90. Hanley EN, Phillips EO. Profile of patients who get spine infections and the type of infections that have a predilection for the spine. *Semin Spine Surg* 1990;2:257–264.
91. Forsythe M, Rothman RH. New concepts in the diagnosis and treatment of infections of the cervical spine. *Orthop Clin North Am* 1978;9:1039–1051.
92. Fang D, Leong JC, Fang HS. Tuberculosis of the upper cervical spine. *J Bone Joint Surg* 1983;65B:47–50.
93. Martin NS. Pott's paraplegia: a report of 120 cases. *J Bone Joint Surg* 1971;53B:596–608.
94. Fang SY, Ong GB. Direct anterior approach to the upper cervical spine. *J Bone Joint Surg* 1962;44A:1588–1593.
95. Hodgson AR, Stock FE. Anterior spinal fusion. A preliminary communication on the radical treatment of Pott's disease and Pott's paraplegia. *Clin Orthop Rel Res* 1994;300:16–23.
96. Kemp HB, Jackson JW, Jeremiah JD, et al. Anterior fusion of the spine for infective lesions in adults. *J Bone Joint Surg* 1973;55B: 715–34.
97. Govender S. The outcome of allografts and anterior instrumentation in spinal tuberculosis. *Clin Orthop* 2002;398:60–66.
98. Sing J, DeWald CJ, Hammerberg KW, et al. Long structural allografts in the treatment of anterior spinal column defects. *Clin Orthop* 2002;394:121–129.
99. Rezai AR, Lee M, Cooper PR, et al. Modern management of spinal tuberculosis. *Neurosurgery* 1995;36:87–97.
100. Albert TJ, Vacarro A. Postlaminectomy kyphosis. *Spine* 1998;23: 2738–2745.
101. Bell DF, Walker JL, O'Conner G, et al. Spinal deformity after multiple-level cervical laminectomy in children. *Spine* 1994;19:406–411.
102. Yasuoka S, Peterson HA, MacCarty CS. Incidence of spinal deformity after multilevel laminectomy in children and adults. *J Neurosurg* 1982;57:441–445.
103. Yasuoka S, Peterson HA, Laws ES, et al. Pathogenesis and prophylaxis of postlaminectomy deformity of the spine after multiple level laminectomy: difference between children and adults. *Neurosurgery* 1981;9:145–152.
104. McLaughlin MR, Wahlig JB, Pollack IF. Incidence of postlaminectomy kyphosis after Chiari decompression. *Spine* 1997;22:613–617.
105. Guigui P, Benoist M, Deburge A. Spinal deformity and instability after multilevel cervical laminectomy for spondylotic myelopathy. *Spine* 1998;23:440–447.
106. Kaptain GJ, Simmons NE, Replogle RE, et al. Incidence and outcome of kyphotic deformity following laminectomy for cervical spondylotic myelopathy. *J Neurosurg* 2000;93:S199–S204.
107. Kato Y, Iwasaki M, Fuji T, et al. Long-term follow-up results of laminectomy for cervical myelopathy caused by ossification of the posterior longitudinal ligament. *J Neurosurg* 1998;89:217–223.
108. Mikawa Y, Shikata J, Yamamuro T. Spinal deformity and instability after multilevel cervical laminectomy. *Spine* 1987;12:6–11.
109. Katsumi Y, Honma T, Nakamura T. Analysis of cervical instability resulting from laminectomies for removal of spinal cord tumor. *Spine* 1989;14:1171–1176.
110. Cattell HS, Clark GL. Cervical kyphosis and instability following multiple laminectomies in children. *J Bone Joint Surg* 1967;49A:713–720.
111. Kumar VGR, Rea GL, Mervis LJ, et al. Cervical spondylotic myelopathy: functional and radiographic long-term outcome after laminectomy and posterior fusion. *Neurosurgery* 1999;44:771–778.
112. Matsunaga S, Sakou T, Nakanisi K. Analysis of the cervical spine alignment following laminoplasty and laminectomy. *Spinal Cord* 1999;37:20–24.
113. Herkowitz HN. A comparison of anterior cervical fusion, cervical laminectomy, and cervical laminaplasty for the surgical management of multiple level spondylotic radiculopathy. *Spine* 1988;13: 774–780.
114. Sim FH, Svien HJ, Bickell WH. Swan-neck deformity following extensive cervical laminectomy. *J Bone Joint Surg* 1974;56A:564–580.
115. Bailey RW, Bagdley CE. Stabilization of the cervical spine by anterior fusion. *J Bone Joint Surg* 1960;42A:565–594.
116. Riew KD, Hilibrand AS, Palumbo MA, et al. Anterior cervical corpectomy in patients previously managed with a laminectomy: short-term complications. *J Bone Joint Surg* 1999;81A:950–957.
117. Herman J, Sonntag V. Cervical corpectomy and plate fixation for postlaminectomy kyphosis. *J Neurosurg* 1994;80:963–970.
118. Foley KT, DiAngelo DJ, Rampersaud YR, et al. The *in vitro* effects of instrumentation on multilevel cervical strut-graft mechanics. *Spine* 1999;24:2366–2376.
119. Vanichkachorn JS, Vaccaro AR, Silveri CP, et al. Anterior junctional plate in the cervical spine. *Spine* 1998;23:2462–2467.
120. Allen BL, Ferguson RL, Lehmann TR, et al. A mechanistic classification of closed, indirect fractures and dislocations of the lower cervical spine. *Spine* 1982;7:1–27.
121. Herkowitz HN, Rothman RH. Subacute instability of the cervical spine. *Spine* 1984;9:348–357.
122. Sears W, Fazl M. Prediction of stability of cervical spine fracture managed in the halo vest and indications for surgical intervention. *J Neurosurg* 1990;72:426–432.
123. Glaser JA, Whitehill R, Stamp WG, et al. Complications associated with the halo-vest: a review of 245 cases. *J Neurosurg* 1986;65: 762–768.
124. Lifeso RM, Colucci MA. Anterior fusion for rotationally unstable cervical spine fractures. *Spine* 2000;25:2028–2034.
125. Jenkins LA, Capen DA, Zigler JE, et al. Cervical spine fusions for trauma. A long-term radiographic and clinical evaluation. *Orthop Rev* 1994;S13–S19.
126. Capen DA, et al. Surgical stabilization of the cervical spine: a comparative analysis of anterior and posterior spine fusions. *Clin Orthop* 1985;196:229–237.
127. Foley MJ, et al. Radiologic evaluation of surgical cervical spine fusion. *Amer J Roentgenol* 1982;138:79–89.
128. Whitehill R, Schmidt R. The posterior interspinous fusion in the treatment of quadriplegia. *Spine* 1983;8:733–740.
129. Kelkar P, O'Callaghan B, Lovblad KO. Asymptomatic grotesque deformities of the cervical spine: an occupational hazard in railway porters. *Spine* 1998;23:737–740.
130. Friedrich M, Kranzl A, Kirtley C, et al. Spinal posture during stooped walking under vertical space constraints. *Spine* 2000;25: 1118–1125.
131. Kolesov VG. Cervical osteochondrosis in miners [Russian]. *Gigiena Truda I Professionalnye Zabolevaniia* 1992;6:19–22.
132. Jagar HJ, Gordon-Harris L, Mehring UM, et al. Degenerative change in the cervical spine and load-carrying on the head. *Skeletal Radiol* 1997;26:475–481.

CHAPTER 37

Disorders at the Cervicothoracic Junction

Raj D. Rao and Jeffrey S. Fischgrund

The cervicothoracic spine is a region of transitional morphology and function between the mobile and lordotic cervical spine and the stiff and kyphotic thoracic spine. The anatomy of the vertebrae in this region is quite different from a typical cervical or thoracic vertebra. Routine radiographs do not allow good visualization of the cervicothoracic spine, making it more difficult to diagnose disorders of the region. These factors, coupled with the difficult surgical access to the region, increase the risk of misdiagnosis and, sometimes, the avoidance of appropriate surgery.

Historically, surgeons have tended to treat lesions involving the cervicothoracic spine with a halo orthosis, primarily because of the challenge of surgical reconstruction. The sternum, clavicle, rib cage, scapula, and great vessels in the superior mediastinum are intimidating obstacles to an anterior approach to the region. Posterior instrumentation of the cervicothoracic vertebral bodies involves risk because of the narrow spinal canal, narrow pedicles, and proximity of spinal cord, nerve roots, and vertebral artery. Injury or other unstable lesions affecting this region often increase the local kyphosis, making access even more difficult.

We define the *cervicothoracic region* as the region from the superior aspect of the C-7 vertebral body to the disc space between T-4 and T-5. This chapter reviews the relevant mediastinal and spinal anatomy of the region. We evaluate the pertinent biomechanics, radiographic techniques, and surgical approaches available. Finally, we review some common disorders that affect the cervicothoracic region.

ANATOMY

Mediastinal Anatomy

The superior mediastinum is the midline cleft between the two sides of the chest cage, extending from the thoracic inlet to an imaginary horizontal plane between the angle of the sternum and the T4-5 intervertebral disc (Fig. 1). The inlet to the mediastinum is bounded by the superior aspect of the manubrium sterni, the inner border of the first rib, and the body of the first thoracic vertebra posteriorly (Fig. 2). The anterior-posterior diameter of the

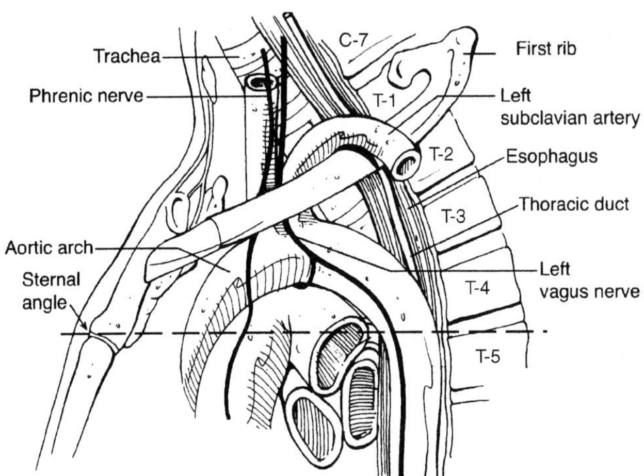

FIG. 1. Sagittal section showing margins and key contents of superior mediastinum, from the thoracic inlet to an imaginary line drawn from the sternal angle to the T4-5 intervertebral disc.

inlet is 6 cm in the midsagittal plane, and the widest transverse diameter is 11 cm. The scalenus anterior muscle attaches to a tubercle on the inner border of the first rib at the junction of the anterior and middle thirds. The subclavian vein crosses the superior aspect of the rib anterior to the tubercle, whereas the subclavian artery and brachial plexus cross posterior to the tubercle.

Within the mediastinum, the encapsulated fatty lymphoid mass of the thymus lies immediately posterior to the sternum in loose areolar tissue (Fig. 3). The thymus involutes rapidly after puberty and is small in most adults. The physiologic role of the thymus gland in adults is unclear, and surgical resection is generally felt to be inconsequential. The loose areolar tissue provides a natural plane for dissection in the retrosternal region. The left brachiocephalic vein, formed by the confluence of the left jugular and subclavian veins, descends obliquely behind the thymus posterior to the upper portion of the manubrium to unite with the right brachiocephalic vein and form the superior vena cava at the first right intercostal space. The superior vena cava descends behind the right margin of the manubrium to the third right intercostal space, where it empties into the right atrium.

The brachiocephalic veins are closely related to the vagus and phrenic nerves, with both nerves on either side lying posterior to the respective brachiocephalic vein. Both nerves enter the superior mediastinum posterior to the first rib. They are anterior to the arterial trunks, with the left vagus and phrenic nerves lying anterior to the aortic arch and the right-sided nerves anterior to the subclavian artery. The vagus nerves then descend posterior to the root of the lung, whereas the phrenic nerves course anterior to the root of the lung. The recurrent laryngeal nerve on the left branches from the left vagus nerve and passes below the arch of the aorta before ascending into the neck between the trachea and esophagus. The right recurrent laryngeal nerve arises from the right vagus nerve as it descends anterior to the right subclavian artery. It then arches beneath this artery to ascend back into the neck, reaching the groove between the trachea and esophagus at a variable location.

Three large vessels arise from the superior aspect of the aortic arch—the brachiocephalic trunk, the left common carotid, and the left subclavian arteries. The left brachiocephalic vein is anterior to all three of these vessels (Fig. 4). The brachiocephalic

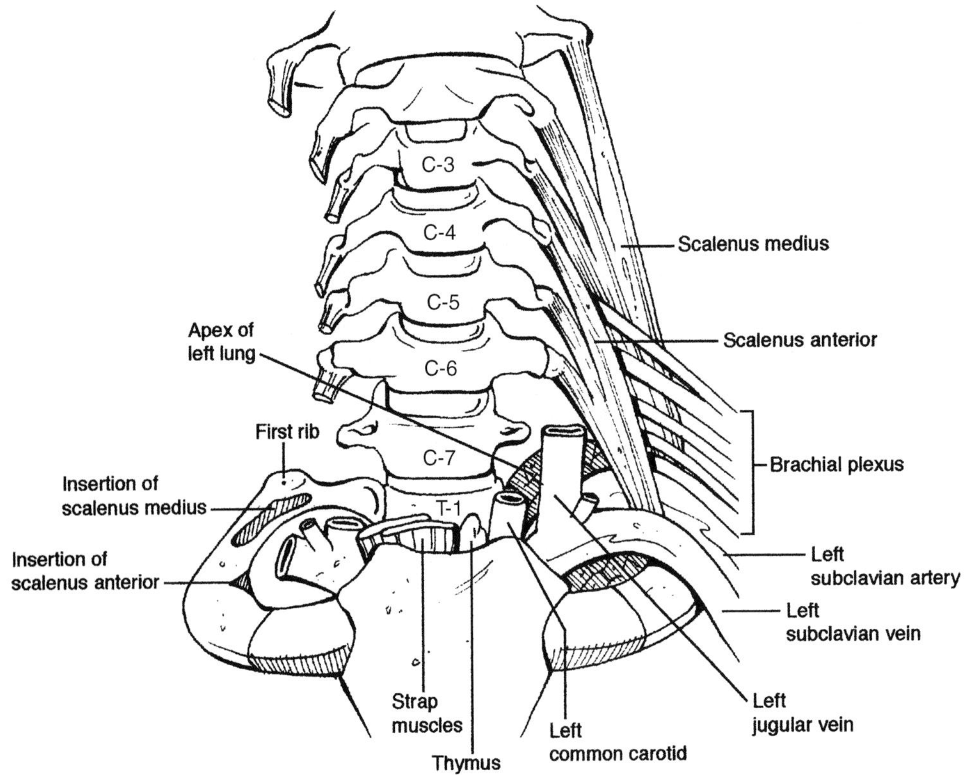

FIG. 2. Bony margins of thoracic inlet, showing relationship of the first rib and manubrium with exiting vessels, apex of the lung, and muscle attachments.

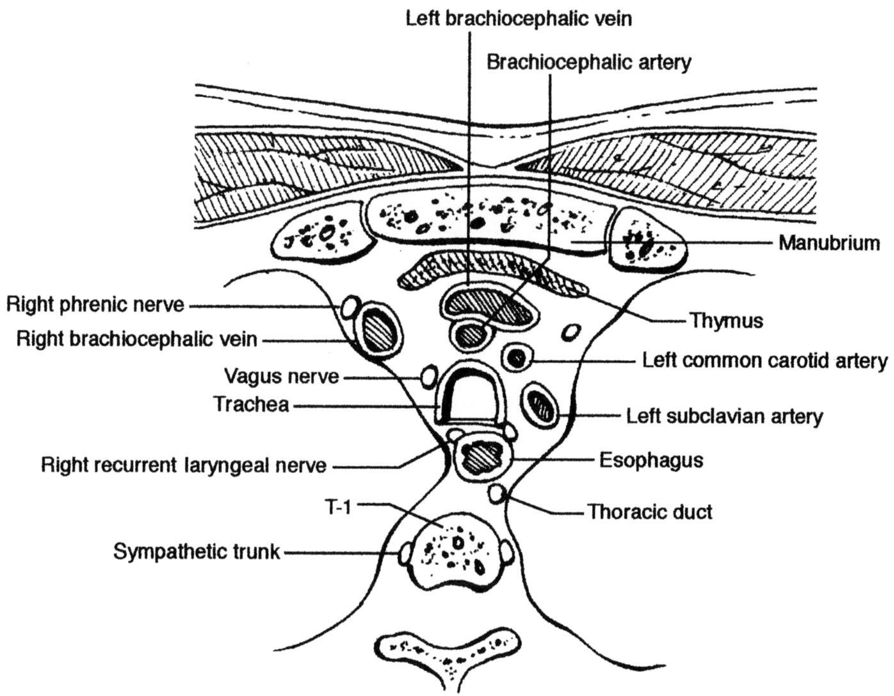

FIG. 3. This transverse section at the level of T-1 clearly shows the anterior-posterior relationship of the contents of superior mediastinum.

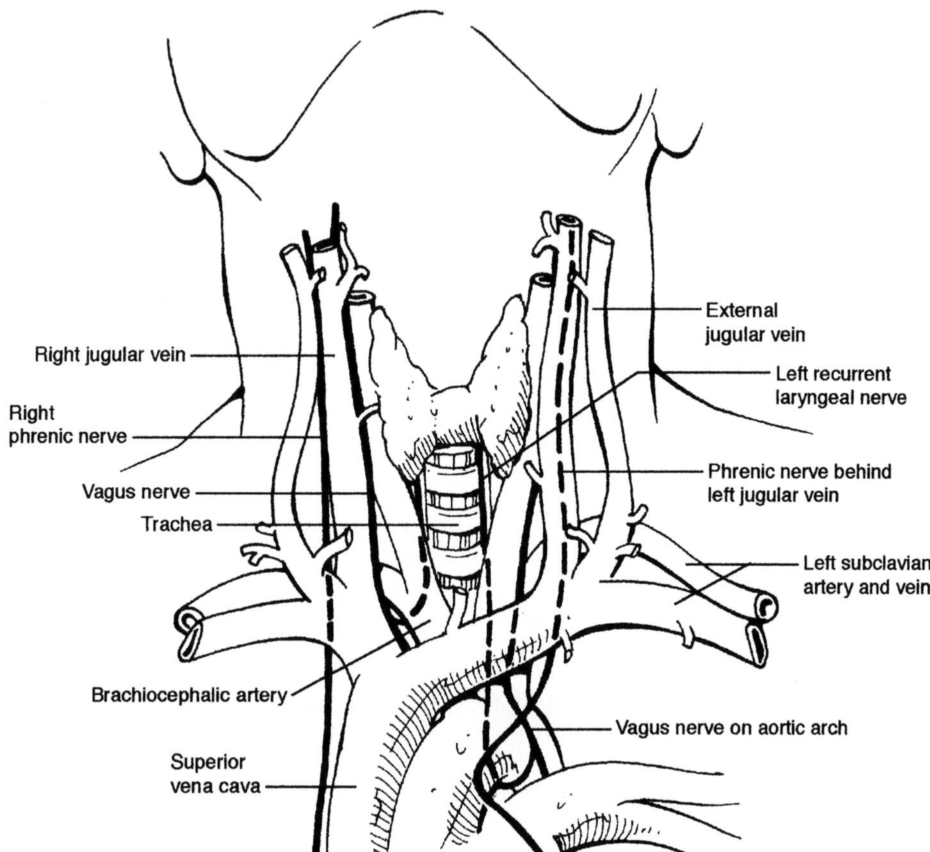

FIG. 4. Great vessels in superior mediastinum and their relationship with the vagus and phrenic nerves.

trunk ascends to the posterior aspect of the right sternoclavicular joint, where it splits into the right common carotid and subclavian arteries. The left common carotid artery climbs to the posterior aspect of the left sternoclavicular joint, where it passes into the carotid sheath along with the internal jugular vein and vagus nerve. The left subclavian artery arches superiorly and posteriorly behind the first costal cartilage to enter the axilla on its way to the left upper extremity.

The suprapleural membrane is a dense fascial layer attached to the first rib peripherally and medially to the investing fascia around the structures passing from the mediastinum into the neck. The apex of the lung, with its pleural layers, and the suprapleural membrane project superiorly into the root of the neck up to 1 in. above the clavicle.

The larynx continues as the trachea from below the cricoid cartilage to the T4-5 disc, where it divides into the two main bronchi. The esophagus is posterior to the trachea from C-7 to T-4, lying in a trough created by the U-shaped tracheal cartilaginous rings. The thoracic duct lies directly posterior to the esophagus in the superior mediastinum and anterior to the vertebral bodies. It crosses to the left, where it empties into the junction between the left internal jugular and subclavian veins behind the left first rib.

Spinal Anatomy

The cervicothoracic junction is a transitional region, with C-7 morphology resembling T-1 and T-2. When compared to the midcervical vertebrae, C-7 has a larger vertebral body, nonbifid and prominent spinous process, larger transverse process, and a small or absent foramen transversarium. The lateral mass of C-7 thins out in the anterior posterior direction, but the pedicle is larger. In 3.5% of the population, the vertebral artery enters the foramen transversarium at C-7 instead of C-6 (1). The thoracic vertebral bodies are also larger and broader than the midcervical vertebrae and have long spinous and transverse processes. The first thoracic vertebra is distinguished from the other upper thoracic vertebrae by having on either side of its body a complete facet for articulation with the first rib head and a second hemifacet for articulation with a portion of the second rib.

Stanescu and colleagues, in a study of the vertebral morphology of the cervicothoracic region, found that pedicle height increased steadily from C-5 (6.7 mm) to T-5 (10.4 mm) (2). Pedicle width increased from C-5 (5.2 mm) to T-1 (7.8 mm) and then decreased to 4.4 mm at the T-5 level. Medial angulation of the pedicle steadily decreased from C-5 (49.8 degrees) to T-4 (15.1 degrees). Lateral mass thickness, as measured from the posterior face to the posterior margin of the neuroforamen, decreased from C-5 (11 mm) to C-6 (10.5 mm). The lateral mass of C-7 was significantly thinner at 8.7 mm. Dimensions of the lower cervical vertebral bodies stayed relatively constant, with the upper end-plate increasing in sagittal diameter from C-5 (14.8 mm) to T-1 (15.6 mm). The upper thoracic levels increased significantly in size, reaching 19.9 mm at the T-5 level.

An and colleagues did an anatomic study of the pedicle dimensions in this region (3). The medial to lateral pedicle outer diameters average 6.9 mm at C-7, 8.5 mm at T-1, and 7.5 mm at T-2. The superior to inferior outer diameters at these levels are 6.4 mm, 8.8 mm, and 10.7 mm, respectively. Medial angulation of the pedicles was 34, 32, and 26 degrees at C-7, T-1, and T-2, respectively. The thoracic pedicles gradually get narrower, and the transverse and sagittal diameters are smallest at the T-5 or T-6 level (4).

The spinal canal is at its narrowest in the upper thoracic spine. At C-7, the canal is oval from side to side and measures 24 mm by 15 mm. The shape of the canal gradually becomes circular and reaches an average 16 mm by 16 mm in the midthoracic spine. The posterior extradural space is almost absent at the C-7 to T-1 level, with the dura almost in direct contact with the ligamentum flavum (5). Approximately two-thirds of the spinal canal through the cervicothoracic region is occupied by the spinal cord. A region of bulbous thickening of the spinal cord between C-3 and C-6 corresponds to where the nerves innervating the upper extremities attach to the cord. The nerve roots occupy approximately two-thirds of the intervertebral foramina in the lower cervical spine but one-fifth of the foramen in the upper thoracic spine. This may explain why radicular symptoms are less common in the upper thoracic spine. The blood supply to the spinal cord is through the anterior spinal artery and two posterior spinal arteries, all three of which originate at the base of the brain. These vessels are the main blood supply for the upper cervical spinal cord, but they taper as they descend. The lower cervical and upper thoracic spinal cord are supplied primarily by radicular branches that arise from the vertebral, deep cervical, ascending cervical, and highest intercostal arteries.

BIOMECHANICS SPECIFIC TO THE REGION

The cervical spine serves primarily to position the sense organs in our head in different directions. There is accordingly little inherent osseous stability to the lower cervical spine, and the intervertebral ligaments are the main determinants of cervical stability. The anterior and posterior longitudinal ligaments, with the intervening discs, the supraspinous and interspinous ligaments, the ligamentum flavum, and the facet joint capsule provide stability to the lower cervical spine. In contrast, the thoracic spine is designed primarily to (a) provide the rigidity necessary for erect posture, (b) protect the spinal cord and other vital organs in the thoracic cavity, and (c) facilitate the mechanical activities of respiration.

Biomechanical terminology used in other areas of the spine may not apply to the cervicothoracic because of the presence of costovertebral junctions. The basic spinal unit in the spine typically consists of two vertebral bodies with intervening ligaments and disc. In the thoracic spine, this basic unit would include the rib articulations with the vertebral bodies, rib cage, and sternum. The three-column theory of spinal stability proposed by Denis may not be valid in thoracic spine fractures (6). Berg has suggested that the sternum-rib complex be considered a fourth column (7).

The region from C-6 to T-3 bears the brunt of the transitional responsibility between the cervical and thoracic spine. The impedance of the rib cage and clavicles exacerbates this transition. There are several ways in which the ribs add to thoracic spine stiffness: (a) The ribs are attached to the vertebral bodies and transverse processes via the strong costovertebral ligaments and costotransverse ligaments, respectively; (b) the thoracic vertebral bodies are attached to the adjacent vertebrae via the rib articulations; and (c) the very presence of the rib cage increases the mechanical dimensions of the spine in the transverse plane. This, in turn, increases the moment of inertia, resulting in increased resistance to bending and rotation. This increased resistance to deformation is greatest in extension, followed by lateral bending and flexion (8). Pal and Routal investigated the role of the neural arch in weight transmission in the cervical and upper thoracic spine (9). They felt that compressive forces in the spine abruptly shifted from the posterior columns to the anterior column at the cervicothoracic region. In contrast, data from Boyle et al. demonstrated that the biomechanical transition between the cervical and thoracic spine was gradual (10). Their data also indicated there was no significant craniocaudal increase in the end-plate surface area below T-1.

As a transitional zone, the upper thoracic spine resembles the cervical spine, whereas the lower thoracic spine resembles the lumbar spine. The upper thoracic vertebrae are smaller, and the kinematics and kinetics are slightly different from those in the middle and much different from the lower thoracic spine. The pattern of motion in the upper thoracic vertebrae is relatively similar to that of the cervical vertebrae, with the arc formed by the instantaneous center of motion in flexion and extension being moderately acute. Coupled motions in the upper thoracic spine are similar to those in the cervical spine, with lateral bending accompanied by axial rotation of the spinous process toward the convexity of the curve. This pattern of coupling is less consistently seen in the middle and lower thoracic spine (11).

Most segmental motion in the subaxial cervical spine typically occurs at the C5-6 segment. Median segmental motion in this region is 20 degrees of flexion or extension, 8 degrees of lateral bending, and 7 degrees of axial rotation. There is an abrupt change in segmental motion at the C-7 to T-1 level, with flexion and extension, lateral bending, and axial rotation all showing a sharp decrease that continues into the upper thoracic spine (11) (Table 1). The median range of segmental flexion and extension in the upper thoracic spine is 4 degrees, lateral bending 6 degrees, and axial rotation 8 degrees.

Some authors have studied the biomechanics of instrumentation through the cervicothoracic region. Posterior hook or pedicle screw constructs at the cervicothoracic junction appear to have greater stiffness than anterior plating systems (12). When three-column instability of the cervicothoracic junction is present, Kreshak et al. recommend anterior plate fixation to supplement posterior stabilization (13). Sublaminar wires are likely to pull through weak bone, and the use of other posterior implants would be recommended in an osteoporotic spine (14). Butler et al. reported that the pedicles of T-2 (and, by inference, T-1) were stronger than those at lower levels (14). This increased strength was related to the increased width of these pedicles. They recommend that instrumentation constructs include these levels if possible.

TABLE 1. *Representative angles of ranges of motion from C-5 to T-7*

Level	Combined flexion-extension (degrees)	One-side lateral bending (degrees)	One-side axial rotation (degrees)
C5-6	20	8	7
C6-7	17	7	6
C-7 to T-1	9	4	2
T1-2	4	5	9
T2-3	4	6	8
T3-4	4	5	8
T4-5	4	6	8
T5-6	4	6	8
T6-7	5	6	7

Adapted from White AA III, Panjabi MM. *Clinical biomechanics of the spine*, 2nd ed. Philadelphia: JB Lippincott Co, 1990.

CLINICAL EXAMINATION OF THE CERVICOTHORACIC JUNCTION

Examination of the cervicothoracic spine includes the following: (a) gross assessment of skin, posture, and range of motion of the spinal column and (b) clinical detection of nerve root or spinal cord involvement in the C-7 to T-4 region. The patient's spine should be adequately exposed to allow a thorough examination.

Adult patients often present with chronic pain in the posterior lower neck or interscapular region. In a significant number, this axial pain is likely the result of muscular or ligamentous factors related to posture, poor ergonomics, stress, and chronic muscle fatigue. Pain in the posterior cervicothoracic spine can also develop secondarily as a result of postural adaptations to a primary source of pain in the shoulder. Tumors and infection in the region can present with severe local pain. Patients with ankylosing spondylitis who sustain a fracture through their cervicothoracic spine present with an abrupt increase in their kyphotic alignment and may subjectively feel that they are unable to hold their head up. The chin-brow angle, formed by the intersection of a vertical line and the line between the chin and brow, is an indicator of the patient's overall balance and measure of clinical deformity.

Neurologic sequelae due to cervicothoracic lesions are common and were reported in 80% of patients in one series (15). The predilection to neurologic deficits is likely a result of the smaller canal size, with less free space available for the cord; smaller vertebral bodies, resulting in earlier extension of tumors or infections into the foraminal regions; and, possibly, the tenuous vascularity of the spinal cord in this region.

C-8 radiculopathy is uncommon but can occur with nerve root impingement at the C-7 to T-1 level. The patient presents with pain and paresthesias going down the medial arm and forearm into the medial hand and ulnar digits. Numbness usually involves the dorsal and volar aspects of the ulnar two digits and hand and may extend up the medial forearm. The long finger flexors are weak, and difficulty using the hand for routine daily activities is reported. Differentiating C-8 radiculopathy from ulnar nerve weakness is important: flexor digitorum profundus function in the index and middle fingers and flexor pollicis longus function in the thumb can be affected in C-8 radiculopathy but not by ulnar nerve entrapment (16). With the exception of the adductor pollicis, the short thenar muscles are spared in ulnar nerve involvement but involved in C-8 to T-1 radiculopathy. Anterior interosseus nerve entrapment may masquerade as C-8 radiculopathy but lacks the sensory changes and thenar muscle involvement. Motor involvement of T-1 results in weakness in finger abduction, but motor involvement of the remaining upper thoracic roots below T-1 cannot be demonstrated clinically.

Identifying a level of involvement through sensory evaluation is difficult in the cervicothoracic region. Involvement of the T-1 root may cause paresthesia or numbness over the medial arm, whereas T-2 affects the medial arm and axillary regions. Sensory involvement of T-3 cannot be verified because the supraclavicular nerves cross into the area. Sensory involvement of T-4 may lead to sensory disturbances just below the nipple line.

Horner's syndrome, or oculosympathetic paralysis, manifests clinically as unilateral ptosis, miosis, and anhidrosis of the face. It can result from interruption of the sympathetic pathway at any point from the brain to the end organs, but it usually results from tumors of the upper lobe of the lung affecting the stellate ganglion. Lateral herniation of upper thoracic discs or other pathology of the cervicothoracic vertebrae that spreads to involve the sympathetic chain can also result in a Horner's syndrome (17).

Myelopathy results in long tract signs below the site of spinal cord involvement. The upper extremities will be spared when the pathology is below T-1. The legs are weaker, and the gait has elements of both ataxia and spasticity from involvement of the posterior and lateral columns, respectively. Hyperreflexia below the level of pathology and an extensor Babinski sign are pathognomonic. Superficial abdominal and cremasteric reflexes are lost.

RADIOGRAPHIC IMAGING

Routine lateral radiographs of the cervical spine fail to visualize the cervicothoracic junction in 26% of cases (18). The difficulty with imaging is particularly pronounced in obese or muscular patients. When the lateral view of the cervical spine does not allow adequate evaluation of the C-7 to T-1 junction, additional imaging must be obtained.

A swimmer's view is intended to visualize the cervicothoracic junction when the shoulders obscure this area on the lateral radiograph. The patient lays in the lateral position, with one upper extremity extended cranially and abducted 180 degrees and the other extremity extended posteriorly. This complex patient positioning is contraindicated if an unstable injury is suspected. When such an injury is clinically suspect, the best option is computed tomography (CT) with sagittal reconstructions. Bilateral supine oblique radiographs to evaluate injury at the cervicothoracic junction have been proposed as a cost-effective alternative to CT (18). When possible, traction views with the shoulders pulled down may help to visualize the cervicothoracic junction.

The soft tissues may provide another indication of underlying pathology. Mediastinal widening seen on a chest radiograph is usually interpreted as aortic injury but may be seen in fractures of the upper thoracic spine. The tracheal shadow is visibile typically down to the T4-5 disc space, and the prevertebral soft-tissue shadow measures 6 to 10 mm (19). An increase in this prevertebral shadow may suggest hematoma from fracture or abscess from infection.

Flexion and extension radiographs are not advised when there has been acute trauma. Varying levels of alertness may preclude completely controlled motion of the neck, and the accompanying muscle spasm may prevent translation between vertebral bodies. Anterior-posterior radiographs must be carefully assessed and will occasionally reveal trauma, erosions, or absence of the spinous processes or pedicles (Fig. 5).

Magnetic resonance imaging (MRI) provides excellent imaging capability for the cervicothoracic junction. Ligament, disc, and neural tissue can be defined clearly, and bone pathology can be recognized. In patients with trauma, the biggest drawback is the length of time it takes for the study. Magnetic field interference with life-support systems prevents the use of MRI in these patients.

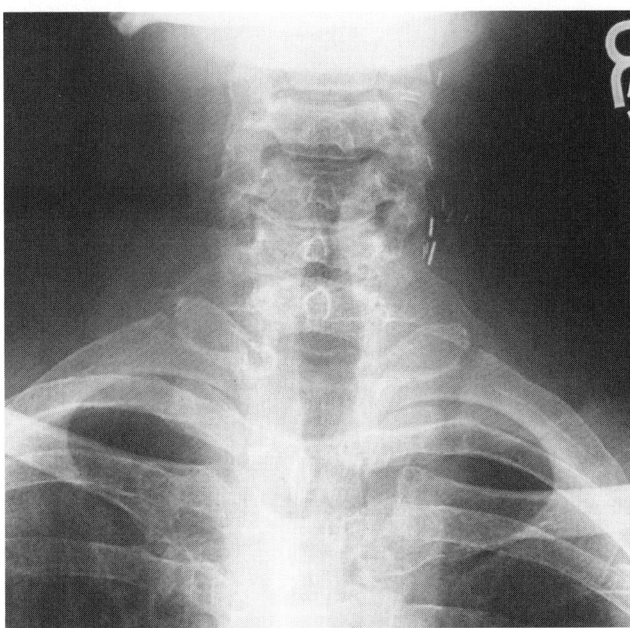

FIG. 5. Bony landmarks must be carefully evaluated at all levels on the anterior-posterior radiographs. In this patient with metastatic tumor involving the posterior elements of T-1, the spinous process cannot be visualized—the only clue in an apparently negative radiographic examination.

Sagittal MRI images may help to determine the surgical approach in the treatment of cervicothoracic disorders. In cases in which the pathology is noted on MRI to be above the sternal notch, a low anterior sternocleidomastoid approach may suffice. If the pathology is below the sternal notch, consideration needs to be given to anterior mediastinal or posterior approaches.

SURGICAL APPROACHES

The level and intravertebral location of the pathology, body habitus, general health of the patient, and the individual surgeon's preference dictate the choice of approach in disorders of the cervicothoracic spine. A variety of approaches to the cervicothoracic junction are reviewed.

Low Anterior Neck Approach

Distal extension of the anterior-medial cervical approach, commonly referred to as the *Smith-Robinson approach*, is useful in approaching the cervicothoracic junction anteriorly. The approach is inadequate in muscular individuals with large shoulders, but in slender individuals with long necks, the anterior aspect of T-2 may occasionally be accessed. Sagittal MRI scanning allows a determination as to whether this suprasternal approach will suffice. A line drawn tangential to the superior aspect of the sternum and extending posteriorly to the spinal column will usually indicate the lowest level that may be accessed.

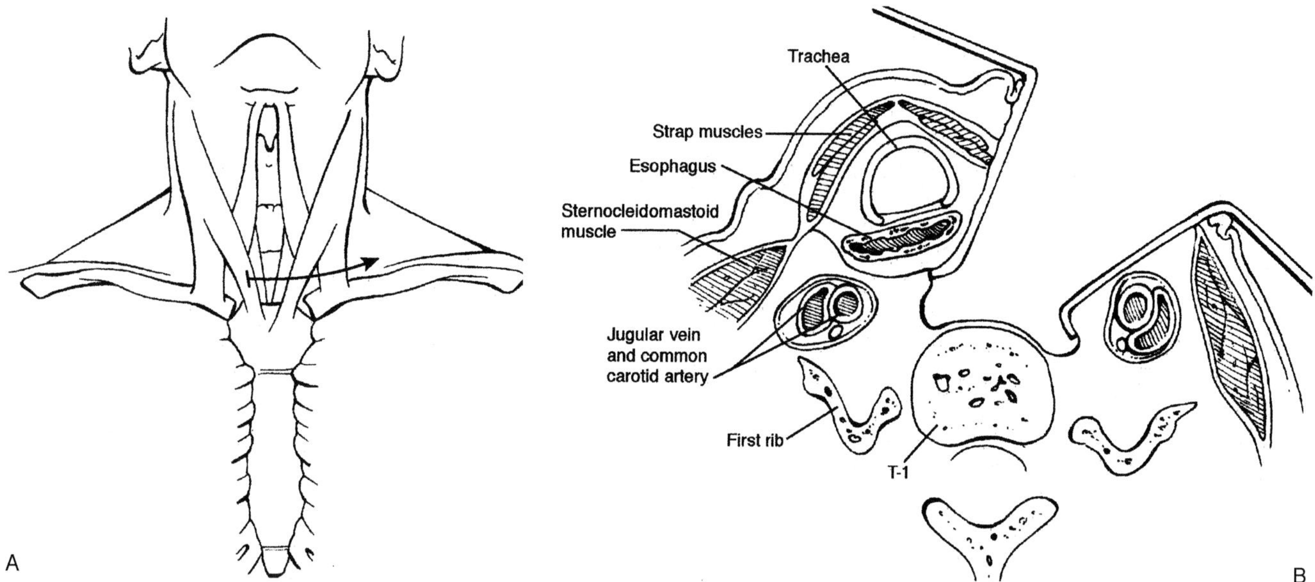

FIG. 6. A: Optional transverse skin incision for low cervical approach to cervicothoracic junction. **B:** Transverse section showing plane of dissection in low cervical approach, medial to carotid sheath and sternocleidomastoid muscle and lateral to trachea, esophagus, and strap muscles.

The standard skin incision anterior to the sternocleidomastoid is extended distally to the suprasternal notch (Fig. 6A). The platysma is divided, and the medial fibers of the sternocleidomastoid, sternohyoid, and sternothyroid muscles attaching to the upper sternum and medial clavicle are divided. The loose areolar tissue of the superior mediastinum is bluntly dissected, and the interval between the tracheoesophageal structures medially and the carotid sheath laterally is used to approach the anterior aspect of the cervicothoracic spine (Fig. 6B). A deep retractor provides exposure and protects the superior mediastinal structures. A left-sided approach is commonly used because the course of the recurrent laryngeal nerve is less variable on this side.

Fielding reported exposure down to T-4 using this approach (20). He advocated a right-sided approach to avoid the thoracic duct and to obtain better control of the innominate artery and vein. Retraction of the innominate vessels inferiorly and the trachea and esophagus medially provided exposure down to the level of T-4. Although visualization at the more distal levels may be obtained using this approach, the ability to decompress or reconstruct the spine is limited, and it is recommended that the surgeon be prepared to extend to a sternotomy if necessary. Potential complications of the approach include postoperative hematoma formation, dysphagia, vocal cord paralysis, and Horner's syndrome.

Upper Thoracotomy

A third-rib thoracotomy can be used to access the cervicothoracic junction. The approach is relatively safe, but it does not allow direct anterior access to the spinal column. The shorter ribs and converging rib cage limit the working area. Thoracotomy above the third rib is impractical, as the shorter first and second ribs restrict the scope of the incision, and the scapula impedes the incision posteriorly. Kirkaldy-Willis favored this approach for the evacuation and débridement of cervicothoracic tuberculosis (21).

The approach is generally carried out in conjunction with a thoracic surgeon. The patient is placed in a lateral decubitus position, with the left side up. A J-shaped incision parallel and medial to the medial border of the scapula is made through skin and fascia. The trapezius and latissimus dorsi muscles and the deeper rhomboid muscles are identified and incised in the line of the incision. The scapula is retracted laterally. The third rib is identified, and the periosteum over it is incised. The intercostal muscles and periosteum are then detached from the rib, and the rib is divided posteriorly at the lateral border of the transverse process and anteriorly at the junction with the costal cartilage. The lung cavity is entered by incising the deeper layer of rib periosteum and parietal pleura. The lung is medially displaced to identify the arch of the aorta. The parietal pleura overlying the vertebral bodies medially is then incised longitudinally to expose the upper two thoracic vertebral bodies. Careful dissection proximally through the dome of the pleura exposes the seventh cervical vertebra.

Cervical Approach Combined with Sternotomy

In 1957, Cauchoix and Binet described an anterior approach to the cervicothoracic region that included a median sternotomy (22). They felt the approach was useful in approaching compressive lesions directly anterior to the spinal cord. The skin incision is along the anterior border of the sternocleidomastoid, extending distally over the midline of the sternum to the xiphoid process (Fig. 7A). The cervical spine is exposed in standard fashion, medial to the carotid sheath and lateral to the trachea, esophagus, and strap muscles. After the cervical spine has been exposed, the sternum is divided longitudinally in the midline and held apart

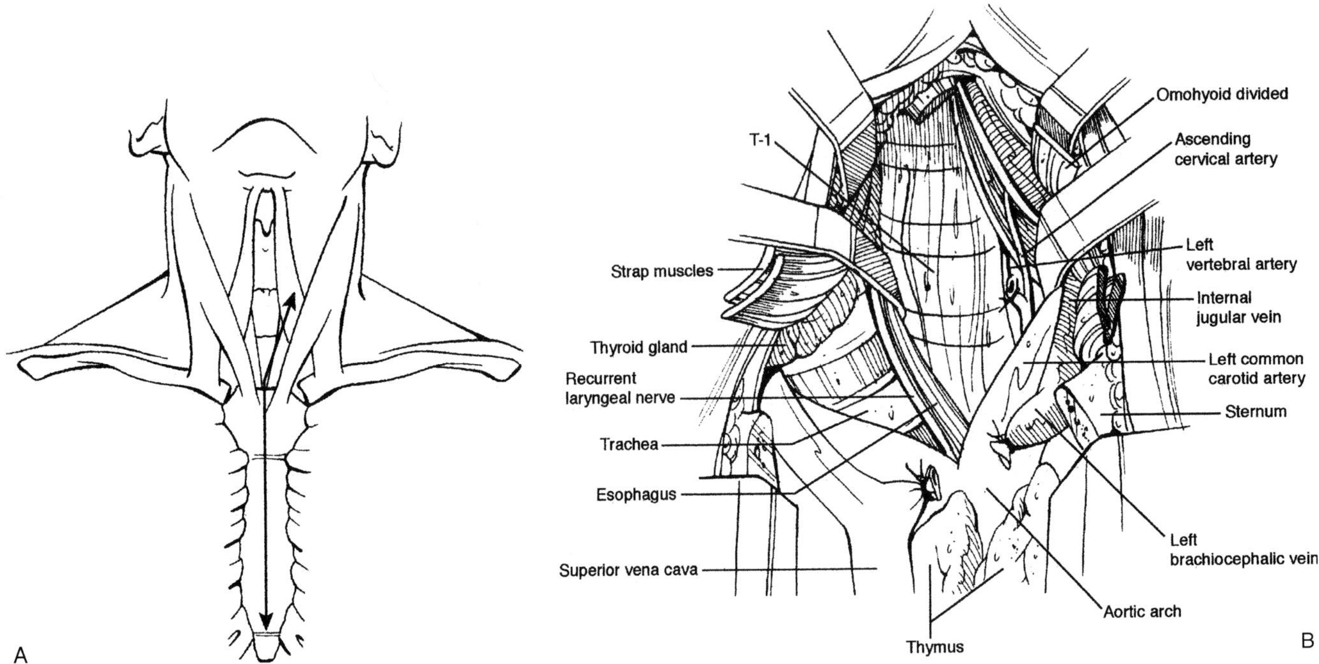

FIG. 7. A: Skin incision for cervical approach combined with complete sternotomy. **B:** Deep exposure after sternotomy, with retractors holding apart the divided sternum and left brachiocephalic vein ligated.

with self-retaining retractors. The cervical and thoracic areas are joined together by dividing the sternothyroid and sternohyoid attachments to the proximal sternum. The left brachiocephalic vein is divided between ligatures, and the upper border of the aortic arch is exposed (Fig. 7B). The trachea and esophagus are retracted to the right, and the upper thoracic vertebral bodies are exposed in the interval between the brachiocephalic artery and left carotid artery.

In 1960, Hodgson and colleagues reported a 40% operative mortality with this approach in a series of ten patients (23). Thoracic surgeons now perform sternotomy routinely, and the complications are similar to other approaches. Complications specific to the approach include persistent pain at the sternotomy site in as many as one-third of patients and venous congestion in the left upper extremity from ligation of the left brachiocephalic vein carried out to visualize below the third thoracic body.

Radek et al. state that a complete sternotomy is the best option to gain access to lesions of the upper thoracic spine (24). They believe that the modifications that rely on a manubriotomy or clavicle osteotomy provide more limited access and may cause upper-extremity dysfunction.

Combined Cervical and Upper Sternal Approaches

Several modifications to a complete sternotomy have been proposed that divide the manubrium or upper sternum alone. The aim of these modifications is to reduce the morbidity of sternotomy. In addition, not much can be done through the lower half of the sternotomy, because the heart and great vessels impair access.

Sundaresan et al. proposed a partial resection of the manubrium and clavicle. A T-shaped incision is made, with the horizontal limb 1 cm above the clavicles, extending beyond the lateral margin of the sternocleidomastoid muscle on either side (25) (Fig. 8A). The vertical limb extends down in the midline to the midbody of the sternum. The platysma is divided in the line of the skin incision. The sternocleidomastoid and strap muscles on the side of the approach are detached at their insertions on the clavicle and proximal sternum and reflected upward. The medial clavicle and manubrium are stripped subperiosteally. The medial one-third of the clavicle is divided with a Gigli saw, and the clavicle is resected after curetting and detaching its attachment at the sternoclavicular joint. A rectangular block of the manubrium is then resected, leaving a peripheral rim of bone. The underlying subclavian vein is dissected free. The plane develops between the carotid sheath laterally and the trachea and esophagus medially to expose the spinal column. The resected clavicle and sternum can serve as autologous structural grafts if needed. The authors report no complications specific to the approach. The recurrent laryngeal nerve is less variable in its course on the left side, and approaching via the left clavicle may better protect the nerve. Kurz and Herkowitz proposed a similar approach for lesions from C-3 to T-4 (26). The approach differs in that the transverse part of the skin incision is made only on the side of the approach, and the manubrium is left intact (Fig. 8B). The authors felt that osteotomy of the manubrium did not add to the exposure, and removal of the medial clavicle alone was adequate. Sar et al. felt that resection of the medial clavicle could lead to eventual shoulder dysfunction and recommended replantation of the osteotomized segment of manubrium and clavicle (27). They recommend the manubrium and clavicle be fixed to the sternum and lateral clavicle with Kirschner wires at the completion of the case.

Several authors propose a unilateral (L-shaped) or bilateral (inverted T-shaped) manubriotomy as a way of avoiding the potential shoulder morbidity associated with disruption of the sternoclavicular joint (28–31). The anterior medial cervical approach is extended over the manubrium and upper sternum. A

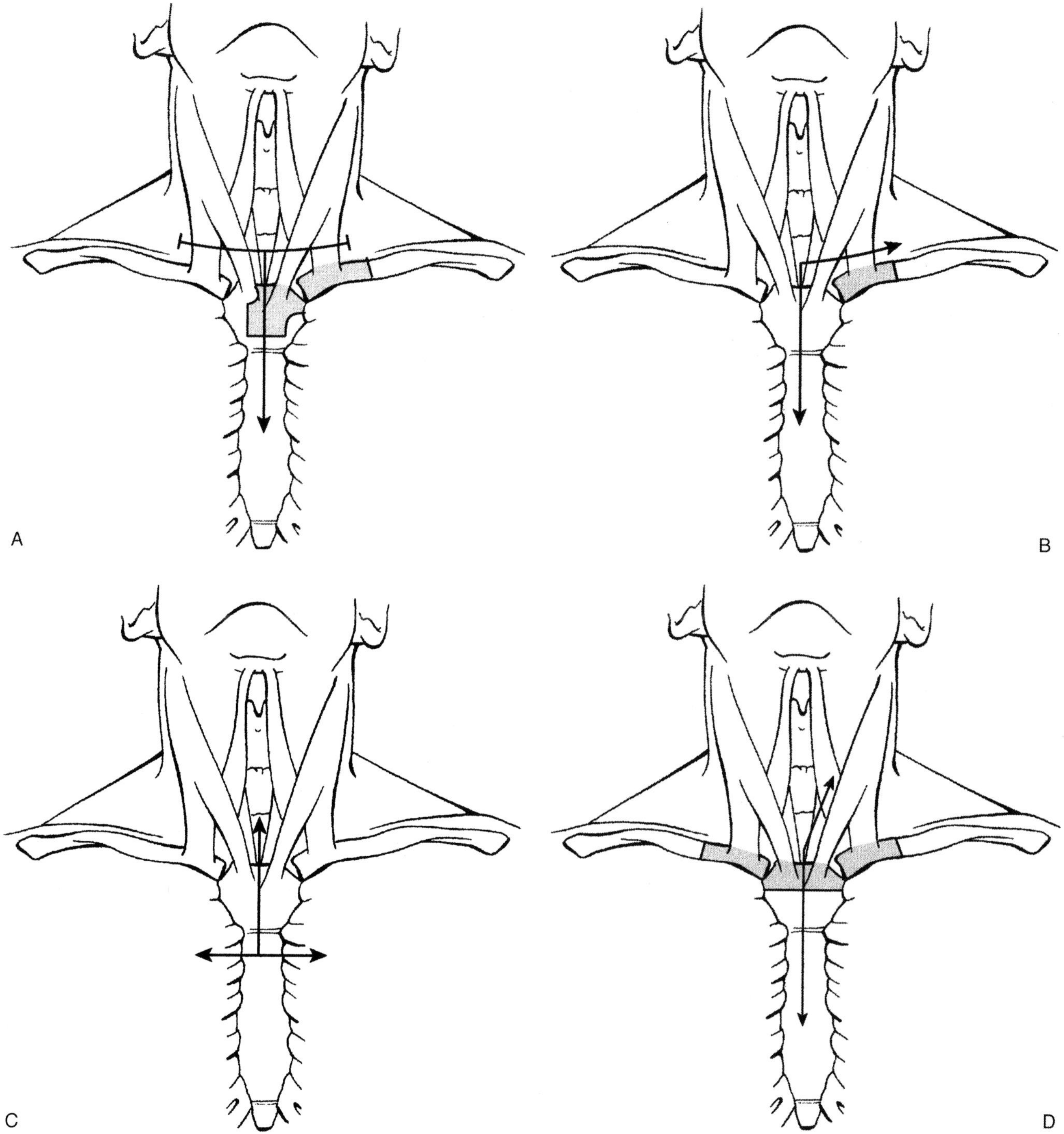

FIG. 8. Skin incision and bone resection of different partial sternotomy techniques. **A:** Sundaresan technique with resection of medial clavicle and rectangular block of manubrium. **B:** Herkowitz and Kurz technique with resection of medial clavicle alone. **C:** L- or inverted T-shaped upper sternal osteotomy. **D:** Lesoin technique with transverse osteotomy of upper manubrium and bilateral medial clavicles and upward reflection of this bone block with the muscles still attached.

midline osteotomy is made through the manubrium and upper sternum. The transverse limb of the osteotomy exits at the second intercostal space and can be unilateral or bilateral (Fig. 8C). With the unilateral manubriotomy, 4 cm of exposure is obtained, as compared to 8 cm with a bilateral manubriotomy. A retractor holds apart the vertical cuts of the manubrium to provide access to the superior mediastinum. The authors report access down to the T4-5 level through this approach.

Lesoin et al. felt that detachment of the sternocleidomastoid muscle from the clavicle could weaken thoracic movements during respiration (32). They recommend dividing a block of bone (including the medial clavicle) bilaterally and the intervening manubrium, leaving the sternoclavicular muscles attached (Fig. 8D). This block of bone with its attached muscles is then reflected upward. Deep dissection is carried out, as with the other approaches in the region. At the end of the procedure, wire sutures are used to reattach the clavicles. A similar modification was proposed by Birch et al., in which the medial half of one clavicle, upper outer corner of the manubrium, and an intact sternoclavicular joint are reflected proximally in a block, along with the attached sternocleidomastoid muscle (33).

Common problems with all of these combined approaches include superficial wound infections over the sternum and persistent pain at the sternotomy site. Healing of the sternal or clavicular osteotomy in most cases proceeds uneventfully, but occasionally, it may result in nonunion, necessitating further surgery. Disruption of shoulder mechanics is a concern when the clavicle is excised or the sternoclavicular joint disrupted. Recurrent laryngeal nerve palsy is possible and is more likely with right-sided approaches.

Separate Cervical and Thoracic Approaches

Micheli and Hood described a combination of cervical and thoracic approaches to this region (34). They used the approach in six patients with ages ranging from 13 to 22 years, all of whom had severe cervicothoracic kyphoscoliosis.

The patient is positioned in the lateral decubitus position, with the convexity of the scoliosis up and the upper extremity draped free and included in the sterile field. The neck incision is above and parallel to the clavicle. The lower cervical vertebral bodies are accessed posterior to the carotid sheath. A second incision is then made in the axillary region overlying the third rib. Mobilizing the scapula and dividing the chest wall muscles directly overlaying it exposes the third rib. The rib is detached anteriorly at its attachment to the sternum and posteriorly at its attachment to the transverse process. The thoracic vertebral bodies are approached through this thoracotomy.

The authors reported no major complications with this technique. The approach is particularly suited to deformity in the region, whereas a midline anterior approach in the thoracic region may not allow access to the apex of the lateral curve. Anterior release of deformity and grafting of the disc spaces can be easily carried out through this approach. The approach is extensile, and additional ribs may be excised to access the middle and lower thoracic spine. Disadvantages of this approach are that it does not allow for direct anterior exposure of the nonscoliotic thoracic spine and that most spine surgeons are unfamiliar with the cervical approach posterior to the carotid sheath.

Posterior Approaches

A posterior approach is used for direct resection of posterior pathology or when posterior stabilization is contemplated. The patient is positioned prone, with care taken to tuck arms and pad all bony prominences in the upper and lower extremities. The head is preferentially held with a Mayfield clamp. Using image intensification, the head holder is aligned to obtain anatomic alignment at the cervicothoracic spine before being clamped down to the table. The approach is carried out through a midline posterior skin incision. The fascia is incised and the paraspinal muscles retracted laterally. The posterior vertebral elements are exposed and laminotomy or laminectomy is performed as planned. Hook, screw, or wire fixation of the cervical and thoracic vertebrae can be obtained, and posterior bone graft fusion can be carried out.

A costotransversectomy is an extrapleural posterolateral approach used for drainage of tubercular abscesses or anterolateral decompression of the upper thoracic vertebrae. The approach is useful in individuals who cannot tolerate a more extensive thoracotomy or who require limited anterior column work in addition to posterior surgery. The skin incision is either midline or curved laterally, extending three levels above and below the level of the pathology. The chest wall muscles are incised and retracted laterally, whereas the paraspinal muscles are retracted medially. The transverse process and 2 to 3 in. of underlying rib are resected. This allows direct access to the anterolateral aspect of the vertebral bodies and disc. Limited resection and decompression and fusion may be carried out through this approach. Anterior visualization is limited, control of bleeding may be difficult, and it is difficult to insert large structural bone graft in the anterior column. Using a 30- or 70-degree angled endoscope within the cavity may help provide better light and magnification anterior to the spinal cord (35).

Minimally Invasive Approaches

Rubino and associates developed a pig model for an endoscopic approach to the anterior cervical and upper thoracic spine (36). They were able to perform discectomies from C-1 to T-3 with good visualization and no complications. A partially endoscopic approach to the cervicothoracic spine has also been described, with the aim of minimizing the morbidity of the sternal osteotomy (37). The lower cervical spine is approached through a Smith-Robinson incision. Finger dissection is then performed posterior to the manubrium. Endoscopes are then inserted above the manubrium and through the second rib space. Visualization through these endoscopes allowed the authors to perform vertebral body resection of T-1 and T-2 and subsequent reconstruction. The endoscopes allowed good visualization while obviating the need for a sternotomy.

Minimally invasive video-assisted techniques are currently being used to provide access to the thoracic spine without the morbidity of an open thoracotomy and have been reported to provide access from T-2 to T-12 (38). There is a steep learning curve associated with the video-assisted technique. Cervicothoracic sympathectomy is routinely being carried out through a thoracoscopic approach (39). Disc removal, anterior release, fusion, and instrumentation are being increasingly carried out with these techniques. Longer follow-up is needed to ensure that fusion and morbidity rates are comparable with the open technique. Huang et al. reported on eight patients who underwent video-assisted thoracoscopic spinal surgery with "extended channels" to treat infections and metastatic lesions between T-1 and T-4 (40). Hertlein et al. used thoracoscopic techniques for unstable fractures of the upper thoracic spine (41). The fracture was initially stabilized with a posterior pedicle screw construct. Minimally invasive thoracoscopic technique was used a few days later to perform anterior discectomy and bone grafting.

Transpedicular approaches to the cervicothoracic spine are often percutaneously carried out for needle biopsy of the vertebral bodies. A similar approach can be used for placement of pedicle screws in the region. The procedure is carried out with fluoroscopic or CT assistance. A thorough knowledge of the anatomy of the pedicles and adjacent vascular and nerve structures is essential. Surface landmarks for the pedicles are discussed in the next section.

RECONSTRUCTION OF THE CERVICOTHORACIC SPINE

Reconstruction of the cervicothoracic junction is indicated for potential or existing instability that follows injury, disease, or surgical resection. Several alternatives are available to restore mechanical integrity of the anterior column after partial or total corpectomy. In most cases, autologous structural bone graft can be obtained from nondiseased autologous iliac crest or fibula. When the clavicle has been osteotomized as part of the approach, this provides a good source for graft. Allograft fibula or mesh cages packed with autograft or other commercially available and approved bone extenders are satisfactory alternatives for anterior column support. Postoperatively, the halo vest is still widely used to provide immobilization and is an excellent option. The trend is to use internal fixation when the potential for instability at the cervicothoracic junction exists and also to avoid the later development of a kyphosis.

When instrumentation is contemplated, the surgeon must clearly recognize the advantages and potential risks of the different implants and must have a thorough understanding of the local anatomy. Whether anterior or posterior instrumentation or a combination of both is selected depends on the location of the pathology and the operative approach. Anatomic constraints play a role in surgical decision at the cervicothoracic junction: Difficulty with anterior plating of C-7 or T-1 through a low cervical approach may favor halo vest application; small pedicles may preclude pedicle screw fixation; and sublaminar wiring may increase the risk of paraplegia with a congenitally small canal and is less effective in patients with osteoporosis. This section reviews the different instrumentation options available for stabilization of the cervicothoracic spine.

Posterior Reconstruction

Posterior reconstruction techniques use wires, hooks, and screws, connected by rods or plates and are biomechanically superior to anterior plates (12). Because of the transitioning anatomy and variations in anatomy imposed by previous surgery, a hybrid construct using multiple types of implants is usually necessary. At any given level, the implant chosen provides secure fixation to that level while minimizing risk of neurologic or vascular injury. Careful preoperative assessment of the radiographic studies helps determine which particular implant is most appropriate at each level.

When the spinous processes are intact, interspinous wiring techniques provide a safe and easy option for posterior fusion and stabilization. Using the triple-wire technique with compression of bone graft against the laminae is superior to wiring alone (42). There are considerable deforming forces acting at the cervicothoracic region, and if a wiring technique is used, the patient should be immobilized postoperatively in a halo vest or other cervicothoracic orthosis until the fusion has consolidated. The most common complication from posterior wiring is loss of fixation and recurrence of deformity. Other complications include cord injury, dural tears, and extension of fusion beyond the desired levels.

Laminar hooks may be used in the lower cervical spine and upper thoracic spine but have significant disadvantages. The hooks are inherently small to accommodate for the narrow spinal canal and have the potential for dislodgement due to weak bone or excessive forces. When the hook is not rigidly seated on the bone, dislodgement may occur as a result of extension and torsion. Also, the hook encroaches into the spinal canal, risking the possibility of cord injury, especially in individuals with a stenotic canal. Transverse process hooks are a good alternative for the upper thoracic spine when bone quality is not compromised.

When the spinous process and lamina are fractured or resected by laminectomy, the anchors available for posterior fixation are primarily the lateral masses and pedicles. Lateral mass screw fixation is frequently used from C-3 to C-6, and it may be combined with hooks or pedicle screws inserted in the upper thoracic spine. The lateral mass at C-7 is thin and typically does not allow for placement of a screw. If it is large enough, the screw needs to be angled more cephalad than elsewhere in the cervical spine to avoid injury to the inferior facet and C-8 nerve root. Anderson et al. reported using the lateral mass screw technique at C-7, T-1, and T-2 with good results (43). However, the thoracic vertebrae do not have a well-defined lateral mass, and other fixation options are necessary. Chapman et al. reviewed their experience in 23 patients, using lateral mass fixation in the cervical spine combined with pedicle screw fixation in the upper thoracic spine (44). They had no neurovascular or pulmonary complications and concluded that this hybrid technique was a satisfactory method of treatment of cervicothoracic instability.

Pedicle screw fixation of C-7 through T-4 is a good option in some cases of posterior instability, but it is technically challenging for several reasons: (a) The pedicles are narrow and often more tall than wide; (b) the internal architecture of the pedicle is not predictable based on external diameter; (c) intraoperative imaging of the pedicle can be difficult because of kyphotic alignment of the spinal column and the interposition of the shoulders; (d) the spinal canal is narrow, and violation of the medial pedicle can result in cord injury; (e) vertebral arteries may occasionally be anomalous and enter the foramen transversarium of C-7 or have a tortuous path and, thus, are at risk when the lateral cortical is violated; and (f) starting points for the screws are not well defined and can be obscured by local pathology or degenerative changes.

The preoperative CT scan is particularly useful in evaluating pedicle dimensions and inclination. The CT scan is also used to better orient where the starting point for the screw should be and to rule out an anomalous vertebral artery. Abumi et al. reported on 180 patients who underwent reconstructive surgery using cervical pedicle screws (45). The prevalence of neurovascular complications from the use of these screws was equivalent to that with lateral mass screws. They found that 1.7% of patients developed root or vertebral artery injury. No patients sustained spinal cord injury.

The entry point for cervicothoracic pedicle screws is located using surface landmarks. These landmarks may be distorted by local degenerative changes or injury and must be meticulously reviewed on the preoperative CT scan. An et al. recommended that the entry point for the C-7 and T-1 pedicle screws be at the intersection of a horizontal line through the middle of the trans-

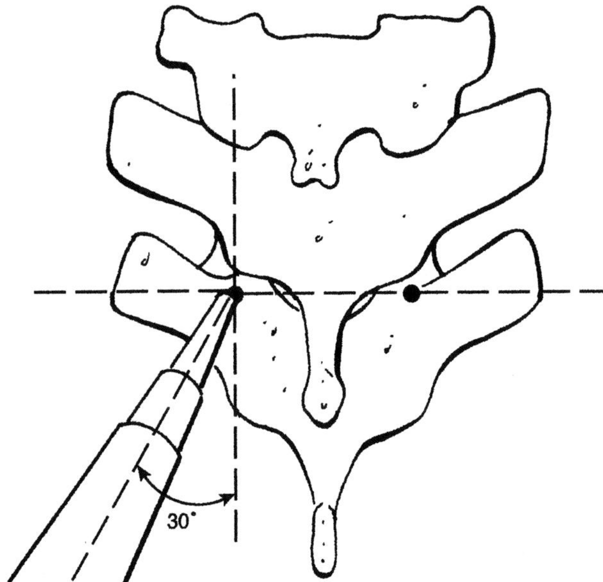

FIG. 9. Pedicle insertion into upper thoracic levels. The entry point is at the intersection of a transverse line drawn 1 to 2 mm inferior to the caudal edge of the facet joint and 2 to 3 mm medial to the outer edge of the lateral mass. The screw is angled 25 to 30 degrees medially, and sagittal angulation is determined with the help of intraoperative fluoroscopy.

verse process and a vertical line through the middle of the facet joint (46). There is concern that this entry point may result in medial cortical penetration, and we prefer going 1 to 2 mm inferior to the caudal edge of the facet joint and 2 to 3 mm medial to the outer edge of the lateral mass (Fig. 9). The pedicle cavity is directly exposed with a burr and then probed with a small Kirschner wire or curette. Sagittal orientation is determined by intraoperative fluoroscopy. The medial angulation of the screw is usually 25 to 30 degrees. Direct palpation of the pedicle with a right-angled nerve hook through a small laminoforaminotomy may help with insertion of the pedicle screw. Computer-assisted navigation systems may assist with insertion of pedicle screws in the cervicothoracic region, but they cannot substitute for a poor grasp of the anatomy. Pedicle screw instrumentation should not be attempted when the outer diameter of the pedicle measures less that 4.5 mm.

Anterior Instrumentation

Anterior cervical locking plates and anterior lateral thoracic plates are frequently used for reconstruction of the lower cervical and upper thoracic spine. These implants function as buttress or tension band plates when used in conjunction with anterior column structural support. The choice of plate is determined by the pathology and approach selected. A low cervical or upper sternotomy approach is conducive to the anterior cervical plate, whereas a thoracotomy allows placement of the anterior lateral thoracic plate. However, the upper thoracic vertebral bodies are frequently too small to allow placement of the anterior lateral thoracic plate. In this situation, a single screw inserted from left to right across the vertebral body may be placed at the proximal and distal ends of the fusion construct and connected with a rod.

CERVICOTHORACIC INJURY

There is little information on the incidence of injury at the cervicothoracic junction. Nichols et al. found that 9% of cervical injuries involved the C-7 to T-1 articulation (47). The majority of cervical injuries occur at the lower three levels, with approximately 23% of injuries occurring at C-6 and 16% each at C-5 and C-7 (48). The actual number may be even higher, with a large number of injuries at the C-7 to T-1 junction being missed initially (49,50). Reasons for undiagnosed injury include the following: (a) Radiographs do not include the C-7 to T-1 level, or the injury is obscured by overlying tissues; (b) there is an overlooked injury in a patient with multiple trauma, head injury, or other altered state of consciousness; and (c) there is a low index of suspicion by the examining physician. To rule out injury, all cervical spine radiographs must visualize the C-7 to T-1 interspace clearly. If these images show no fracture, but injury is believed to be present, CT or MRI scans must be obtained, depending on whether primarily bone or soft tissue injury is suspected. If a vertebral fracture is identified at the cervicothoracic region, associated injuries at other spinal levels must be sought. Multiple-level noncontiguous fractures appear to occur at a disproportionately greater frequency when the primary vertebral fracture is at the cervicothoracic or upper thoracic region (51,52).

The C-7 to T-1 segment is subject to the same injuries as the lower cervical spine. Treatment for injury at C-7 or the C-7 to T-1 articulation is similar to injury in the lower cervical spine. In most cases, this involves early realignment of the spinal column, decompression in cases of residual neurologic compromise, and stabilization to prevent further injury and to allow rehabilitation (Fig. 10). Evans has addressed treatment of dislocations or fracture dislocations at the cervicothoracic junction (49). He reports that these injuries usually require open reduction. He suggests that the neurologic status is largely independent of treatment and recommends open reduction only if the cord lesion is incomplete and less than 24 hours old, and the reduction can be done quickly and safely. The authors recommend a more vigorous treatment of cervicothoracic facet dislocations, with initial closed traction using skull traction. Up to 140 lb. may be necessary for closed reduction (53). If closed realignment of the spinal column cannot be achieved rapidly, open reduction is advocated. This approach offers a better chance of cord recovery in incomplete neurologic injuries and allows additional root recovery.

Injuries involving T1-4 are less common, possibly as a result of the increased stability of the region from the ribs and associated rib cage. Injury at the upper thoracic spine must be suspected in all cases in which the upper ribs or sternum are fractured and in cases with severe lung injury. Most of these injuries are relatively stable, do not need operative stabilization, and can be managed with orthotic support. Capen et al. reported on 49 patients with fractures between T-1 and T-8 who underwent nonsurgical management at Rancho Los Amigos Medical Center between 1966 and 1989 (54). All patients were treated with orthoses. One patient had neurologic worsening. Brace-related skin necrosis occurred in eight patients. They found that rib fractures did not affect stability of the fracture. They concluded that brace management was successful for treating fractures between T-1 and T-8,

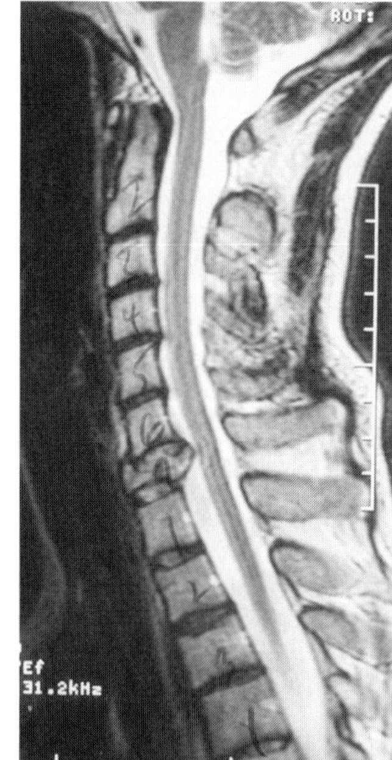

A

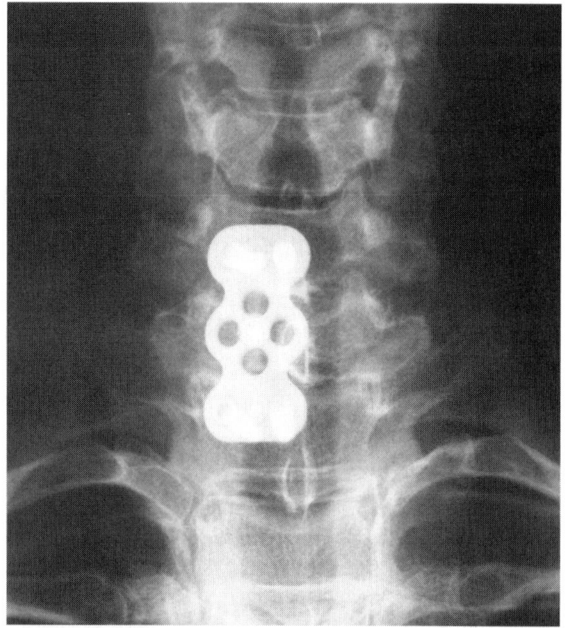

B

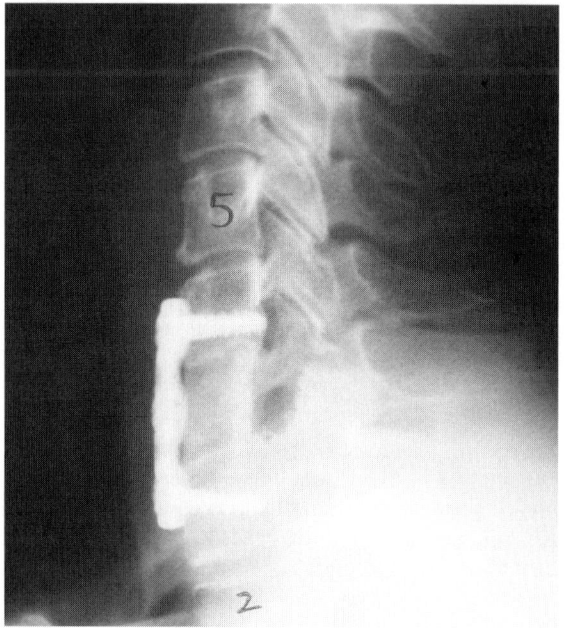

C

FIG. 10. A–C: Preoperative magnetic resonance imaging scan and postoperative radiographs of a 45-year-old nurse with C-7 burst fracture and partial cord injury. The patient underwent a C-7 corpectomy through a low cervical approach, with strut grafting using allograft bone, and anterior plating from C-6 to T-1. She recovered complete cord function and resumed her regular job.

especially in patients in whom early surgery was not possible. The exception to brace treatment would be the patient with complete dislocation of the spinal column, which requires open reduction, internal fixation, and arthrodesis (55).

The upper thoracic spinal canal is narrow and has diminished blood supply. Both of these factors predispose to neurologic injury when the fractures occur. If residual compression of the anterior spinal cord is evident on MRI or CT scans, anterior decompression is recommended. Bohlman reported neurologic improvement after anterior transthoracic decompression in eight patients with incomplete cord injury, up to 16 months after trauma (55). He also concluded that laminectomy was contraindicated in patients with incomplete lesions of the upper thoracic spinal cord.

Fractures of one or more of the spinous processes in the lower cervical and upper thoracic spine are referred to as *clay shoveler's fracture*. The injury was initially felt to be a result of forces transmitted to the spinous processes via the ligamentum nuchae and supraspinous ligaments. Currently, the injury is felt to be more likely from pull of the trapezius, rhomboid, and posterior serratus muscles, which originate at these spinous processes. The injury may be preceded by symptoms in the region for a while before the actual fracture occurs. This initial period of pain may be indicative of fatigue of the muscles attached to these spinous processes. The injury can be satisfactorily treated by analgesics, a short period of rest, and immobilization in a soft cervical brace.

Orthoses

A variety of orthoses are used in the management of cervicothoracic injury. Motion allowed by cervicothoracic and even cervical orthoses diminishes significantly at the C-7 to T-1 level, a result of the diminished mobility of the T-1 vertebral body (56). A halo is necessary to immobilize extension-type injuries below C-5, but other cervicothoracic braces may be adequate to immobilize flexion-type injuries from C-5 to T-1. The intact rib cage provides adequate stability to satisfactorily immobilize most minor injuries to the upper thoracic spine.

DEGENERATIVE CONDITIONS OF THE CERVICOTHORACIC SPINE

Degenerative changes within the cervicothoracic discs may contribute to axial neck or interscapular pain. Nerve fibers and nerve endings found in the peripheral portions of the peripheral disc offer a possible mechanism by which these degenerative discs directly produce pain (57,58). The cervicothoracic facet joints do not have the classic referred pain patterns seen elsewhere in the cervical spine. Fukui et al. injected the facet joints of the cervicothoracic and thoracic spine to determine if reproducible pain patterns were present (59). Pain in the suprascapular area and the superior angle of the scapula was referred from the facet joints of C-7 to T-1 and T1-2. Pain in the midscapula region was referred from C-7 to T-1, T1-2, and T2-3. They established that axial upper back pain could originate from changes at the facet joints, but these referred pain patterns showed significant overlap and could not be clinically distinguished.

Radicular pain from the C-7 to T-1 disc is not common. Murphey et al. found the frequency of cervical radiculopathy to be 26% at C-6, 61% at C-7, and 8% at C-8 (60). Henderson et al. did a retrospective review of patients who underwent surgery for cervical radiculopathy (61). Among the 456 patients who had a radicular component to their symptoms, only 21 (4.6%) presented with pain or paresthesia in a C-8 distribution. Of 846 patients who underwent surgery for cervical disc pathology, the C-7 to T-1 disc was involved in ten patients (1.2%). The relative lower frequency of symptomatic C-8 radiculopathy may be partly explained by the fact that the C-8 nerve root has little contact with the C-7 to T-1 disc in the intervertebral foramen (62). The C-7 to T-1 foramen is also larger than the other cervical foramina (63). It is not clear whether the relatively stiffer T-1 vertebral body provides any protection against degenerative changes at C-7 to T-1 disc.

Symptomatic thoracic disc herniations are also uncommon, with less than 1% of all disc herniations occurring in the thoracic spine. Only 7% of thoracic disc herniations occur at the upper four thoracic disc levels, with most occurring below T-8 (64). Most patients who have upper thoracic disc herniations are middle-aged and present with interscapular pain. Radicular pain in a C-8 distribution may result from T1-2 disc herniation, or patients may have vague paresthesias around their medial arms and anterior chest (65). Patients can present with a spastic paraparesis with bladder disturbances or Horner's syndrome (17,66).

MRI scans are excellent for diagnosis of disc pathology in the cervicothoracic spine, but they must be interpreted with caution because of the high incidence of asymptomatic radiographic disc pathology in the cervical and thoracic disc spaces. Wood et al. found a 73% prevalence of disc-related pathology on thoracic MRI scans of asymptomatic individuals, including disc bulging, annular tears, herniation, Scheuermann end-plate changes, and cord deformation (67). These changes are seen at every level in the thoracic spine but are more common in the middle lower thoracic spine. Most of these disc herniations remain asymptomatic and tend to get smaller in size (68).

In most cases, axial and radicular pain arising from disc pathology in the cervicothoracic spine resolves with a regimen of antiinflammatory agents, analgesics, and modification of activities. A brief supervised regimen of physical therapy to include instruction in ergonomics, stretching, and isometric exercises is useful. When nonoperative measures are unsuccessful, and the pain is intractable, anterior discectomy and fusion are preferred for C-7 to T-1 disc pathology. Posterior cervical foraminotomy is not recommended for disc pathology at C-7 to T-1. Adequate decompression of the C-8 root requires greater than 50% resection of the facet joint, because of the longer and more lateral direction of the root below the C-7 pedicle (62).

Surgery for upper thoracic spine disc herniations is best carried out via an anterior approach when feasible. A low anterior cervical approach may be possible in asthenic individuals. The lowest disc to be easily accessed through this approach is at or above the top of the sternum on the MRI scan in these individuals. When the sternum is high riding, anterior exposure is obtained through a manubriotomy or thoracotomy. The disc and cartilaginous endplate are removed, osteophytes resected if necessary, and fusion carried out with a block of autogenous bone. Other surgical approaches for removal of refractory symptomatic thoracic disc herniations have included laminectomy with facetectomy and costotransversectomy. Video-assisted thoracoscopic surgery has been recently reported as a safe and efficacious alternative for thoracic disc herniations from T1-2 to T-12 to L-1 (69).

Progression of the degenerative cascade at the disc and facet joints eventually narrows the spinal canal and can result in myelopathy. This is seen frequently in the middle cervical spine and occasionally in the lower thoracic spine but rarely in the cervicothoracic region. Chana and Afshar reported one case of paraparesis from T1-2 degenerative changes (70). The patient responded well to a decompressive cervicothoracic laminectomy. Patients with degenerative cervicothoracic spondylotic myelopathy who have no subjective symptoms and only very mild upper motor neuron findings on examination may be closely observed. If the patient presents with a greater degree of myelopathy, or symptoms or clinical examination suggest progression of myelopathy, surgical decompression is recommended. The choice of anterior versus posterior decompression is generally based on the location of the pathology, number of levels involved, ease of access, and subsequent reconstruction options. Decompression is accompanied by bone grafting and, in most cases, with stabilization using screws, hooks, rods, or plates. If instrumentation is not feasible, the spine is immobilized in a cervicothoracic orthosis for 8 weeks or until signs of early fusion are present.

Synovial cysts occasionally arise adjacent to the cervicothoracic facet joints in older patients. Patients present with radicular pain or may be myelopathic from a large cyst. Hemorrhage within the cyst may result in an acute exacerbation of back pain or radiculopathy. These cysts are more common at the C-7 to T-1 level than at any other level in the cervical spine and are suggestive of greater facet joint stresses at the C-7 to T-1 level (71). Histologically, these cysts resemble degenerative synovial cysts

(72). Resection of the cyst with laminectomy or hemilaminectomy results in positive relief of symptoms.

Ossification of the posterior longitudinal ligament is common from C-4 to C-6 but may occasionally involve C-7. Ossification of the posterior longitudinal ligament and the ligamentum flavum is also seen in the thoracic spine but more frequently involves the middle lower thoracic spine. Neurologic manifestations from ossification of the spinal ligaments in the cervicothoracic region are rare. Diffuse idiopathic skeletal hyperostosis is another disorder of the spine characterized by large flowing osteophytes along contiguous vertebrae. The disorder is most commonly seen in the thoracic spine, but again, it has a predilection for the middle lower thoracic spine. Large osteophytes may result in gradual paraparesis or occasionally in acute weakness from trivial trauma.

INFECTIONS AT THE CERVICOTHORACIC JUNCTION

Thirteen percent of spinal tuberculosis involves the cervicothoracic region (73). This relatively high prevalence may be explained by the spread of the organism from the nearby upper lobe of the lung. The diagnosis of infection may be delayed because of difficulty with radiographic visualization of the cervicothoracic region. Widening of the superior mediastinum from a soft-tissue abscess may be evident on chest radiographs. Infection typically occurs initially in the vertebral bodies, and CT or MRI scans show involvement of one or more vertebral bodies with relative sparing of the discs. Granulation tissue and pus from the infection may result in anterior subligamentous or epidural abscesses and cord or root injury. A computer-guided needle aspiration of abscess fluid or vertebral body biopsy is necessary for microbiological and histologic confirmation of the diagnosis.

Patients present with pain, local deformity, or mass effects from the abscess on the trachea or esophagus. The cervicothoracic region is at higher risk for developing neurologic deficits from tuberculosis (74). Patients develop a C-8 radiculopathy (or, frequently, spastic paraparesis) when C-7 to T-1 is involved. The neurologic deficits most commonly result from the mechanical pressure of the disc, abscess, or kyphosis on the anterior spinal cord. The infected granulation tissue can occlude the blood vessels supplying the cord and result in myelopathy secondary to vascular insufficiency. Destruction of the anterior vertebral bodies results in a sharp local kyphosis, which may lead to delayed paraparesis from anterior pressure on the spinal cord. Arachnoiditis and intradural tuberculomas also result in neurologic sequelae. The predisposition to neurologic manifestations is higher in the cervicothoracic spine as a result of the smaller spinal canal, tenuous blood supply to the cord, and kyphotic upper thoracic spine.

Early tuberculosis of the cervicothoracic spine with minimal bone destruction is managed by a medical drug regimen combined with orthotic support. Patients with significant bone destruction and kyphosis are best managed by anterior débridement and arthrodesis. Nonoperative management results in progressive kyphosis, which can lead to delayed paraplegia even after the disease has been treated. The abscess can usually be approached through a low anterior cervical incision with detachment of the strap muscles distally if necessary. Patients with the disease are typically emaciated, and this, along with the tuberculous kyphosis, often allows access to T-3 or even T-4 through this approach. The abscess is drained, débridement and corpectomy are carried out as necessary to decompress the spinal cord, and reconstruction is performed with autogenous structural bone graft. The spine must be immobilized in a halo orthosis until signs of incorporation of the graft are visible. A costotransversectomy approach is useful for drainage of a large thoracic abscess in a patient who cannot tolerate a more extensive operation or in whom an anterior approach is technically difficult. Limited bone grafting is possible through this approach.

Both posterior (75) and anterior (76) instrumentation have been reported after radical débridement and grafting of the tuberculous spine. The instrumentation provides immediate stability and is felt to promote early fusion. There are no long-term studies on the role of instrumentation in tuberculosis of the cervicothoracic spine. When significant deformity exists from destruction of the vertebral bodies anteriorly, posterior stabilization may allow more secure correction of deformity and prevention of neurologic deficit. Treatment of the deformity with closed reduction in traction or in an orthosis is another option. Prolonged immobilization is necessary with this technique, and the long-term kyphosis is less predictable.

Pyogenic vertebral infections do not have a specific predilection for the cervicothoracic spine (77). In general, these infections result in osteomyelitis, discitis, or epidural abscess. The symptoms vary depending on the organism's virulence and host resistance. Most patients present with fever of unexplained origin, with or without local pain. Epidural abscesses or granulation tissue can result in marked radicular pain or myelopathy. Cervicothoracic involvement is more likely to be associated with paralysis than involvement of the lower thoracic or lumbar spine (78). MRI scan is the diagnostic modality of choice when infection is suspected.

Treatment of pyogenic vertebral osteomyelitis consists of intravenous antibiotics for 6 weeks followed by oral antibiotics until the disease is resolved. Patients are immobilized in a cervicothoracic orthosis to help with pain and prevent the development of deformity. Surgery is indicated (a) to relieve cord compression from epidural abscess, granulation tissue, or sequestered bone or disc fragments; (b) to drain large abscesses; (c) to obtain bacteriologic diagnosis; (d) for débridement of cases refractory to antibiotic management; and (e) to treat deformity or instability.

Infections managed with antibiotics and immobilization usually heal within 1 year, with spontaneous interbody fusion occurring in a significant number of patients. The tendency to spontaneous fusion after infection is most pronounced in the cervical and upper thoracic spine (79). In children, progressive kyphosis can result even after healing of cervicothoracic infections from a combination of cessation of growth at the involved levels, growth retardation in the anterior vertebral bodies above and below, and continued growth of the posterior vertebral elements (80).

TUMORS AT THE CERVICOTHORACIC REGION

Osseous Tumors

There are no specific bone tumors that have a proclivity for the cervicothoracic region. The frequency of bone tumors in the cervicothoracic spine was reviewed from records maintained at the Rizzoli Institute in Bologna, Italy. A total of 20,003 bone lesions, including benign, malignant, systemic, metastatic, and

TABLE 2. *Frequency of bone tumors at the cervicothoracic region (from C-7 to T-4) over a 102-year period at the Rizzoli Institute in Bologna, Italy*

Metastasis from carcinoma	68
Myeloma-plasmacytoma	13
Osteoblastoma	10
Osteoid osteoma	9
Giant-cell tumor	9
Non-Hodgkin's lymphoma	5
Hodgkin's lymphoma	1
Classic osteosarcoma	5
Radiation-induced osteosarcoma	2
Chondrosarcoma	3
Angioma	4
Fibrous dysplasia	1
Aneurysmal bone cyst	4
Osteochondroma	2
Histiocytosis X	4
Sarcoma (not otherwise specified)	4
Ewing's family	4
Hemangioendothelioma (low-grade angiosarcoma)	3

From Piero Picci, M.D., *personal communication*, September 2002.

pseudotumoral lesions, were diagnosed in a 102-year period from September 1900 to August 2002. Of these, 2,345 (11%) were in the spinal column from C-1 to the coccyx. There were 151 bone lesions in the region from C-7 to T-4 (6.4% of spine lesions) (Table 2) (personal communication from Piero Picci, M.D., September 2002). Metastatic tumors are most commonly from the lung, breast, myeloma, and thyroid in this region.

Patients typically present with pain directly over the involved region of the spine and interscapular area, with radiating pain in the shoulders, arms, or torso. Persistent nonmechanical radicular pain suggests underlying tumor. Some patients may present with symptoms and findings of cord compression with gait changes, bladder involvement, and hyperreflexia. Horner's syndrome may result from an expansile tumor involving the stellate ganglion. Pain generally precedes neurologic manifestations.

Bony lesions are not easily identified on radiographs of the cervicothoracic spine. The anterior posterior view may show an absent spinous process or distortion of the rounded pedicle outline. Widening of the interpedicular space may be present with intraspinal tumors. Eroded, lytic, or blastic lesions must be further studied. Any upper thoracic spine fracture in older patients must be viewed with suspicion. Isolated osteoporotic fractures are uncommon in this region. A more likely cause of upper thoracic fracture is metastatic disease (81). If malignancy is suspected and radiographs are negative, a further workup must be considered. MRI scans with and without gadolinium provide excellent visualization of the spine and spinal cord and are the investigation of choice in suspected cervicothoracic tumors.

The management of spinal tumors at the cervicothoracic region is similar to that of spinal tumors elsewhere. After establishing a tissue diagnosis and oncologic staging studies, treatment options consist of observation, adjuvant therapy (radiation and chemotherapy), surgical debulking or resection, and palliative procedures (e.g., vertebroplasty) designed to help with tumor pain. Combined anterior posterior approaches may be necessary for vertebrectomy, and aggressive posterior resection necessitates posterior stabilization (Fig. 11). If methylmethacrylate reconstruction is used anteriorly, this should be supplemented with posterior instrumentation. Problems specific to the cervicothoracic region are the following: difficulty with approach to anterior tumors at T-3 and T-4, challenges of reconstruction posteriorly, and exaggerated kyphosis from wide or multilevel laminectomy posteriorly and from anterior collapse of tumor-involved vertebral bodies.

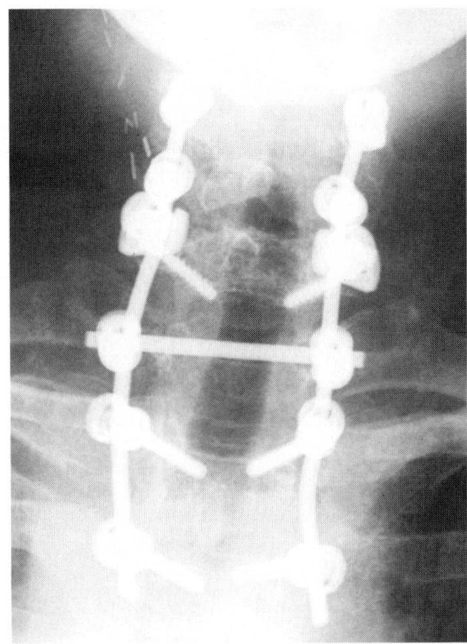
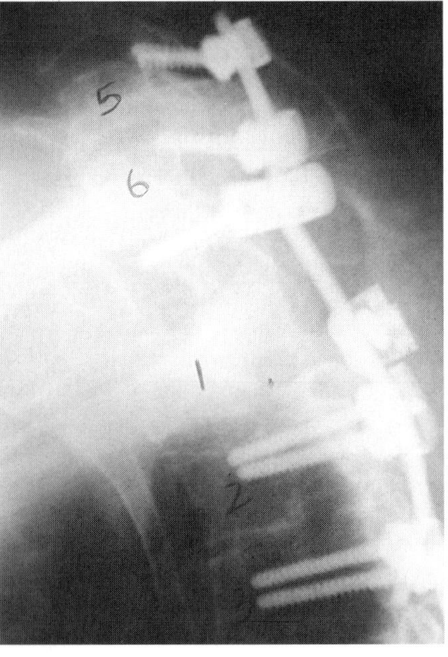

A,B

FIG. 11. A,B: Postoperative anterior posterior and lateral radiographs of a 70-year-old woman who underwent resection of a metastatic T-1 spinous process lesion with cord compromise. Reconstruction was carried out with a combination of lateral mass screws at C-5 and C-6 with pedicle screws at C-7, T-2, and T-3.

Neurogenic Tumors

In comparison to bony neoplasms, spinal cord tumors are common in the cervical and thoracic spine. There are three broad groups of these tumors: (a) extradural (55%), most of which are metastatic lesions; (b) intradural-extramedullary (40%), most commonly meningiomas or nerve sheath tumors; and (c) intramedullary (5%), arising within the substance of the spinal cord, and most commonly astrocytoma or ependymoma (82). Intramedullary glioblastomas are fast-growing astrocytomas that have a predilection for the cervicothoracic spinal cord. They tend to occur in younger individuals and become clinically evident early. Surgical resection of the tumor through a laminectomy is recommended, and a concomitant fusion may be necessary to prevent postlaminectomy kyphosis. Malignant tumors are given postoperative radiation. The prognosis depends on multiple factors (e.g., age at diagnosis, histology, and extent of resection) but is, in general, poor.

Pancoast's Tumors

Pancoast's tumors (or superior sulcus tumors) are bronchogenic carcinomas arising from the apex of the lung. They frequently invade the superior mediastinum, sympathetic chain, cervicothoracic spinal column, adjacent ribs, and chest wall. They result in a characteristic syndrome of pain around the shoulder and down the arm, Horner's syndrome, and C-8, T-1, or T-2 neurologic deficits. Radiographs show a shadow at the apex of the lung, with rib or vertebral infiltration. The degree of spinal involvement varies from none to minor involvement of the costovertebral junction to major involvement of the vertebral body. Spread of the tumor to the vertebral body is associated with poor prognosis (83), and in tumors that involve the vertebral body, survival is worse when the tumor has invaded the spinal canal (84). The value of surgery in these tumors is debated, and traditional management has involved radiotherapy or chemotherapy, with equivocal results. With advances in surgical technique and reconstruction options at the cervicothoracic spine, several authors have carried out aggressive resections of these tumors (85–87). The operation generally involves partial or complete resection of the vertebral body, upper lung, and chest wall, as necessary, through a thoracotomy, followed by a posterior approach with resection of the posterior elements of the involved vertebral levels. Reconstruction of the spinal column is carried out with methylmethacrylate or cages anteriorly, followed by posterior instrumentation using pedicle or lateral mass screws, hooks, rods, and spinous process wires. Surgical resection when combined with an aggressive multidisciplinary approach is associated with significant morbidity, but it appears to improve survival rates while preserving neurologic function and offering improved pain control (88).

DEVELOPMENTAL CONDITIONS

Klippel-Feil Syndrome

Patients with Klippel-Feil syndrome frequently present with anomalies at the cervicothoracic region. The classic clinical triad associated with the syndrome is a short neck, low posterior hairline, and limited motion of the neck. Webbing of the neck, torticollis, and facial asymmetry are present in many individuals. Renal and cardiovascular abnormalities and deafness are linked to the disorder. Radiographs typically show fusion of two or more cervical vertebrae, but in many patients, the congenital anomalies extend to the upper thoracic spine. Thomsen et al. reported that 40% of patients with Klippel-Feil syndrome had involvement of the upper thoracic spine (89). The group with involvement of the upper thoracic spine also had a higher propensity to develop a cervicothoracic scoliotic deformity. Most patients with Klippel-Feil syndrome remain asymptomatic throughout life. Some patients require stabilization for marked instability, deformity, or neurologic problems.

Vertebral Segmentation Abnormalities

Congenital vertebral segmentation anomalies at the cervicothoracic region are unusual but potentially disfiguring conditions. Head tilting, uneven shoulder heights, upper thoracic rotation, and torticollis occur relatively early. There is little normal spinal column above the area of segmentation defects to allow an effective compensatory curve. An unsegmented bar with contralateral hemivertebra is associated with a high likelihood of progressive deformity. These patients should be closely monitored for progressive deformity and, in most cases, will require a posterior spinal fusion (90). Early fusion in childhood prevents the development of rigid painful curves in the adult. Adolescent idiopathic cervicothoracic scoliosis is a rare, typically left-sided curve, running from C-5 to T-5. The curve is asymptomatic but causes cosmetic disfigurement in the shoulder levels. Treatment is usually not indicated.

Congenital Spondylolisthesis

Congenital spondylolisthesis occurs rarely in the cervicothoracic region, primarily as a result of dysplastic posterior vertebral elements. The neural arch may be absent, the laminae may be elongated, and the facet joints may be incompetent. Severe local kyphosis results, with compensatory cervical hyperlordosis. Patients with significant slip and neurologic deficit usually require combined anterior and posterior fusion (91).

Sprengel's Deformity

Sprengel's deformity, or congenital high scapula, results in a shoulder and scapula that are higher on one side. When the condition is bilateral, both shoulders are displaced upwards, and the neck appears shortened. A fibrous or bony band may be palpated, going from the upper angle of the scapula toward the neck. Outside of the cosmetic deformity, most cases are minimally symptomatic and do not require treatment. The deformity frequently accompanies Klippel-Feil syndrome (92). Rarely, in cases with significant restriction of shoulder abduction or marked deformity, the scapula can be released and retethered.

ANKYLOSING SPONDYLITIS

Patients with advanced ankylosing spondylitis frequently sustain fractures through the cervicothoracic region. These fractures can occur with relatively minor trauma and are associated with a higher frequency of spinal cord injury and a higher frequency of nonunion because of the greater biomechanical forces acting at the fracture site. In addition to the usual difficulty with radiographic imaging of the cervicothoracic junction, visualization of fractures is particularly difficult in these patients because of the diffuse osteoporosis and the fact that the fractures often occur through the ossified disc and ligament structures.

Individuals who sustain these fractures can present with a subjective sense of change in position of the head, with varying degrees of pain. If radiographs do not show a fracture, but the index of suspicion is high, CT scans with multiplanar reconstruction through the region are recommended. Neurologic deficits can occur in these patients as a result of the initial cord injury, delayed cord injury from unrecognized fractures, an epidural hematoma, or from traction on the poorly vascularized upper thoracic cord (93). If neurologic deficit is present, an MRI is obtained to differentiate these possibilities and as a guide to therapy.

In most cases, uncomplicated cervical or cervicothoracic fractures in ankylosing spondylitis are best treated with a halo vest. These patients have difficulty with anesthesia. The cervical spine deformity and rigidity necessitate fiberoptic intubation. The thoracic kyphosis and ossification of the costovertebral articulations result in reduced pulmonary function and make ventilation difficult. Surgery is complicated by poor bone quality, ossified ligamentous structures, and bleeding from bone surfaces. Patients who develop an epidural hematoma require rapid surgical evacuation through a laminectomy and subsequent immobilization in a halo vest. Patients with cord compression from residual bone or soft tissue require decompression, realignment, and stabilization.

The other presentation of patients with long-standing ankylosing spondylitis is a severe kyphosis at the cervicothoracic junction. They are unable to see the ground straight ahead, and in some cases, the proximity of the chin to the chest may interfere with eating. When the disability is severe, the only treatment available is an extension osteotomy of the spine, which is carried out at the cervicothoracic junction. The vertebral arteries are not tethered in the foramen transversarium at this level, and they are, therefore, less liable to kink when the neck is extended. The bulbous enlargement of the lower cervical spinal cord has ended at this level, and there is a slight increase in canal space. The procedure is done under local or general anesthetic. Spinal cord monitoring is carried out during the procedure. A complete laminectomy is carried out at C-7, with partial laminectomy of C-6 and T-1. The underlying nerve roots of C-8 are decompressed beyond the foraminal zones by removing the facet joints and lateral masses as needed. Extension is achieved by moving the head back while directly observing the spinal cord and roots for compression. Bone obtained during the decompression is used as graft for achieving fusion. The extended position is immediately stabilized with a halo or internal fixation.

Inflammatory arthritides besides ankylosing spondylitis can affect the cervicothoracic spine. In a review of 100 patients with severe rheumatoid arthritis who underwent occipitocervical fusion, arthritis of the upper thoracic spine with subluxation was reported in four patients (94). MRI examination in three of these patients revealed changes similar to those seen in the rheumatoid cervical spine, with subluxation of the vertebrae, encroachment on the anterior subarachnoid space, and compression of the spinal cord. Correction of severe cervical and cervicothoracic flexion deformity in rheumatoid disease was reported in four cases (95). The authors used progressive distraction while in a halo-dependent traction to correct the deformity and restore extension. An instrumented posterior spinal fusion was then carried out, and the corrected position held with a halo orthosis for 3 to 4 months.

POSTLAMINECTOMY KYPHOSIS

Laminectomy is a frequently performed operation in adults, and in most cases, it does not result in significant spinal deformity. In children and younger individuals, laminectomy is occasionally performed for the diagnosis and treatment of spinal tumors. In this subgroup, deformity frequently occurs after surgery. The most common deformity after laminectomy is kyphosis, and this is most likely to develop after surgery at the cervicothoracic region.

Multiple factors play a role in the development of postlaminectomy kyphosis (11). Gravity exerts a natural flexion-bending moment on the upright spine, which is most pronounced in the cervicothoracic and upper thoracic spine. With laminectomy, the tether provided by the supraspinous and interspinous ligaments and ligamentum flavum is lost. The facet joint capsules of the lower cervical and upper thoracic spine are thin and loose and do not play a significant role in resistance against flexion loads. After a laminectomy, the posterior erector spinae muscles reattach to scar tissue that is more anteriorly located, reducing the movement arm and decreasing the efficiency of the muscles. Development of kyphosis shifts the spinal sagittal balance further forward, predisposing to further deformity. Notwithstanding these biomechanical considerations, adult patients who undergo laminectomy without facet resection in most cases do not develop deformity.

The likelihood of deformity is linked to the number of levels involved and the width of the laminectomy. Resection of the facet joints is an important determinant as to the likelihood of developing deformity. Wide resection of the facet joints at any level will likely result in a sharp angular kyphosis at the level, whereas central laminectomy carried out over multiple levels may result in a gradual rounding of the spine. Asymmetric resection of the facet joints in children can result in a concomitant scoliosis. The incidence of postlaminectomy kyphosis varies, with one study reporting a 100% frequency of spinal deformity in young patients who underwent a multilevel cervical or cervicothoracic laminectomy (96). The chances of developing deformity are higher in younger patients with greater facet resection and in more cephalad laminectomies. Postoperative radiation can affect growth at the vertebral end-plates and exacerbate the deformity.

Patients present with increasing curvature at the site of their previous surgery or with what appears to be poor upper trunk posture noted by the parents or physician. With kyphosis, the paraspinal muscles of the neck and upper back have to work harder to maintain posture and a forward-looking gaze. This results in chronic muscle fatigue and pain. Increased loads on the facet joints after laminectomy can cause pain in some of these patients. Severe kyphosis may cause a myelopathy as a result of the mechanical deformation of the cord, as well as from vascular compromise of the anterior spinal arteries. The deformity is almost invariably progressive, and progression is most rapid during the adolescent growth spurt.

Patients who require laminectomy in the cervicothoracic region must be recognized to be at risk for development of kyphotic deformity after surgery. This risk is greater when multiple levels are included in the decompression, when facet resection is necessary, and in younger patients. There are no guidelines as to whether the spine should be fused at the time of the initial laminectomy, but an individual decision needs to be made based on the age of the patient, extent of decompression, preexisting instability, and the degree of physiologic kyphosis. Yasuoka recommended that all children undergoing multilevel laminectomy in the cervical or thoracic region should be monitored for developing deformity for 6 years after surgery (97). When the decision is made to observe the patient, radiographs must be carefully reviewed at frequent intervals. At the first sign of deformity, a cervicothoracic orthosis is applied. If the deformity progresses in the brace, surgical fusion should be carried out.

The decision as to whether to fuse the spine anteriorly, posteriorly, or with combined approaches is individualized. Posterior fusion is technically easier through the cervicothoracic region, but it is difficult to achieve when extensive bone resection has been carried out. A posterior fusion is subject to distractive forces and is at a disadvantage biomechanically. The use of instrumentation helps to counteract these forces. Posterior fusion with rigid instrumentation may in some patients result in spontaneous anterior interbody fusion, especially in the upper thoracic spine. Successful posterior fusion may also lead to partial correction of deformity by continued anterior growth of the vertebral bodies. Anterior fusion may be required in cases of severe deformity or extensive posterior resection, but it is accompanied by the risks of an additional mediastinal or upper thoracic approach.

CONCLUSION

The cervicothoracic region of the spine from C-7 to T4-5 is at the same time challenging and fascinating for spine surgeons. An improved understanding of the variety of conditions that can affect this part of the spine, coupled with the systematic use of investigations, allows better diagnosis and earlier treatment. Historically, unstable disorders of this region have been treated with a halo vest. With advances in surgical techniques and improved survival rates from severe injury or tumors, reconstruction of the unstable cervicothoracic spine is being performed with greater frequency by the spine surgeon today.

REFERENCES

1. Rene L. *Surgery of the spine: surgical anatomy and operative approaches*. New York: Springer-Verlag, 1983:120.
2. Stanescu, et al. Morphometric evaluation of the cervico-thoracic junction. *Spine* 1994;19:2082–2088.
3. An HS, Gordin R, Renner K. Anatomic considerations for plate-screw fixation of the cervical spine. *Spine* 1991;16(10S):S548–S551.
4. Scoles PV, Linton AE, Latimer B, et al. Vertebral body and posterior element morphology: the normal spine in middle life. *Spine* 1988;13 (10):1082–1088.
5. Hirabayashi Y, Saitoh K, Fukuda H, et al. Magnetic resonance imaging of the extradural space of the thoracic spine. *Br J Anesth* 1997;79(5):563–566.
6. Denis F. The three-column spine and its significance in the classification of acute thoracolumbar spinal injuries. *Spine* 1983;8(8):817–831.
7. Berg EE. The sternal-rib complex. A possible fourth column in thoracic spine fractures. *Spine* 1993;18(13):1916–1919.
8. Andriacchi T, Schultz A, Belytschko T, et al. A model for studies of mechanical interactions between the human spine and rib cage. *J Biomech* 1974;7:497–507.
9. Pal GP, Routal RV. A study of weight transmission through the cervical and upper thoracic regions of the vertebral column in man. *J Anat* 1986;148:245–261.
10. Boyle JJW, Singer KP, Milne N. Morphological survey of the cervicothoracic junctional region. *Spine* 1996;21(5):544–548.
11. White AA III, Panjabi MM. *Clinical biomechanics of the spine*, 2nd ed. Philadelphia: JB Lippincott Co, 1990.
12. Bueff HU, Lotz JC, Colliou OK, et al. Instrumentation of the cervicothoracic junction after destabilization. *Spine* 1995;20(16):1789–1792.
13. Kreshak J, Lindsey D, Kim D, et al. Posterior fixation at the cervicothoracic junction: a biomechanical analysis. Seattle: North American Spine Society, 16th annual meeting, November 3, 2001.
14. Butler TE, Asher MA, Jayaraman G, et al. The strength and stiffness of thoracic implant anchors in osteoporotic spines. *Spine* 1994; 19(17):1956–1962.
15. An HS, Vaccaro A, Cotler JM, et al. Spinal disorders at the cervicothoracic junction. *Spine* 1994;19:2557–2564.
16. Rao R. Pathophysiology, natural history and clinical features of neck pain, cervical radiculopathy and myelopathy. *J Bone Joint Surg Am* 2002;84A(10):1872–1881.
17. Lloyd TV, Johnson JC, Paul DJ, et al. Horner's syndrome secondary to herniated disc at T1-T2. *AJR Am J Roentgenol* 1980;134:184–185.
18. Kaneriya PP, Schweitzer ME, Spettell C, et al. The cost-effectiveness of oblique radiography in the exclusion of C7-T1 injury in trauma patients. *AJR Am J Roentgenol* 1998;171:959–962.
19. Jain AK, Kumar S, Tuli SM. Tuberculosis of spine (C1 to D4). *Spinal Cord* 1999;37:362–369.
20. Fielding JW, Stillwell WT. Anterior cervical approach to the upper thoracic spine: a case report. *Spine* 1976;1(3):158–161.
21. Kirkaldy-Willis WH, Allen PBR, Willox GL. Surgical approaches to the anterior elements of the spine: indications and techniques. *Canadian J Surg* 1966;9:294–308.
22. Cauchoix J, Binet JP. Anterior surgical approaches to the spine. *Ann R Coll Surg Engl* 1957;21:237–243.
23. Hodgson AR, Stock FE, Fang HSY, et al. Anterior spinal fusion. The operative approach and pathologic findings in 412 patients with Pott's disease of the spine. *Br J Surg* 1960;48:172–178.
24. Radek A, Maciejczak A, Kowalewski J, et al. Trans-sternal approach to the cervicothoracic junction. *Neurol Neurochir Pol* 1999;33(5): 1201–1213.
25. Sundaresan N, Shah J, Foley KM, et al. An anterior surgical approach to the upper thoracic vertebrae. *J Neurosurg* 1984;61:686–690.
26. Kurz LT, Pursel SE, Herkowitz HN. Modified anterior approach to the cervicothoracic junction. *Spine* 1991;16(10S):S542–S547.
27. Sar C, Hamzaoglu A, Talu U, et al. An anterior approach to the cervicothoracic junction of the spine (modified osteotomy of manubrium sterni and clavicle). *J Spinal Disord* 1999;12(2):102–106.
28. Luk KD, Cheung KM, Leong JC. Anterior approach to the cervicothoracic junction by unilateral or bilateral manubriotomy: a report of five cases. *J Bone Joint Surg* 2002;84A(6):1013–1017.
29. Darling GE, McBroom R, Perrin R. Modified anterior approach to the cervicothoracic junction. *Spine* 1995;20(13):1519–1521.
30. McDonald P, Letts M, Sutherland G, et al. Aneurysmal bone cyst of the upper thoracic spine. An operative approach through a manubrial sternotomy. *Clin Orthop* 1992;279:127–132.
31. LoCicero J. The combined cervical and partial sternotomy approach for thymectomy. *Chest Surg Clin North Am* 1996;6:85–93.
32. Lesoin F, Thomas CE III, Autricque A, et al. A transsternal biclavicular approach to the upper anterior thoracic spine. *Surg Neurol* 1986;26:253–256.
33. Birch R, Bonney G, Marshall RW. A surgical approach to the cervicothoracic spine. *J Bone Joint Surg* 1990;72B:904–907.
34. Micheli LJ, Hood RW. Anterior exposure of the cervicothoracic spine using a combined cervical and thoracic approach. *J Bone Joint Surg* 1983;65A(7):992–997.
35. McLain RF. Endoscopically assisted decompression for metastatic thoracic neoplasms. *Spine* 1998;23(10):1130–1135.
36. Rubino F, Deutsch H, Pamoukian V, et al. Minimally invasive spine surgery: an animal model for endoscopic approach to the anterior cervical and upper thoracic spine. *J Laparoendosc Adv Surg Tech A* 2000;10(6):309–313.
37. LeHuec JC, Lesprit E, Guibaud JP, et al. Minimally invasive endoscopic approach to the cervicothoracic junction for vertebral metastases: report of two cases. *Eur Spine J* 2001;10(5):421–426.
38. Ikard RW, McCord DH. Thoracoscopic exposure of intervertebral discs. *Ann Thoracic Surg* 1996;61(4):1267–1268.
39. Johnson JP, Obasi C, Hahn MS, et al. Endoscopic thoracic sympathectomy. *J Neurosurg* 1999;91:90–97.
40. Huang TJ, Hsu RW, Liu HP, et al. Video-assisted thoracoscopic surgery to the upper thoracic spine. *Surg Endosc* 1999;13(2):123–126.
41. Hertlein H, Hartl WH, Dienemann H, et al. Thoracoscopic repair of thoracic spine trauma. *Eur Spine J* 1995;4(5):302–307.

42. Bohlman HH. Acute fractures and dislocations of the cervical spine: an analysis of 300 hospitalized patients and review of the literature. *J Bone Joint Surg* 1979;61A:1119–1142.
43. Anderson PA, Henley MB, Grady MS, et al. Posterior cervical arthrodesis with AO reconstruction plates and bone graft. *Spine* 1991;16(3S):S72–S79.
44. Chapman JR, Anderson PA, Pepin C, et al. Posterior instrumentation of the unstable cervicothoracic spine. *J Neurosurg* 1996;84(4):552–558.
45. Abumi K, Shono Y, Ito M, et al. Complications of pedicle screw fixation in reconstructive surgery of the cervical spine. *Spine* 2000;25(8): 962–969.
46. An HS, Coppes MA. Posterior cervical fixation for fracture and degenerative disc disease. *Clin Orthop* 1997;335:101–111.
47. Nichols CG, Young DH, Schiller WR. Evaluation of cervicothoracic junction injury. *Ann Emerg Med* 1987;16:640–642.
48. Miller MD, Gehweiler JA, Martinez S, et al. Significant new observations on cervical spine trauma. *AJR Am J Roentgenol* 1978;130:659–663.
49. Evans DK. Dislocations at the cervicothoracic junction. *J Bone Joint Surg* 1983;65B:124–127.
50. Gisbert VL, Hollerman JJ, Ney AL, et al. Incidence and diagnosis of C7-T1 fractures and subluxations in multiple trauma patients: evaluation of the advanced trauma life support guidelines. *Surgery* 1989;106(4):702–708.
51. Rogers LF, Thayer C, Weinberg PE, et al. Acute injuries of the upper thoracic spine with paraplegia. *AJR Am J Roentgenol* 1980;134(1):67–73.
52. Calenoff L, Chessare JW, Rogers LF, et al. Multiple level spinal injuries: importance of early recognition. *AJR Am J Roentgenol* 1978;130 (4):665–669.
53. Cotler J, Herbison GJ, Nasuti JF, et al. Closed reduction of traumatic cervical spine dislocation using traction weights up to 140 pounds. *Spine* 1993;13:386–390.
54. Capen DA, Gordon ML, Zigler JE, et al. Nonoperative management of upper thoracic spine fractures. *Orthop Rev* 1994;23(10):818–821.
55. Bohlman HH, Freehafer A, Dejak J. The results of treatment of acute injuries of the upper thoracic spine with paralysis. *J Bone Joint Surg* 1985;67A(3):360–369.
56. Johnson RM, Hart DL, Simmons EF, et al. Cervical orthosis. A study comparing their effectiveness in restricting cervical motion in normal subjects. *J Bone Joint Surg* 1977;59A(3):332–339.
57. Ferlic DC. The nerve supply of the cervical intervertebral discs in man. *Bull Johns Hopkins Hosp* 1963;113:347–351.
58. Bogduk N, Windsor M, Inglis A. The innervation of the cervical intervertebral discs. *Spine* 1988;13:2–8.
59. Fukui S, Ohseto K, Shiotani M. Patterns of pain induced by distending the thoracic zygapophyseal joints. *Regional Anesth* 1997;22(4):332–336.
60. Murphey F, Simmons JC, Brunson B. Ruptured cervical discs, 1939 to 1972. *Clin Neurosurg* 1973;20:9–17.
61. Henderson CM, Hennessy RG, Shuey HM, et al. Posterior-lateral foraminotomy as an exclusive operative technique for cervical radiculopathy: a review of 846 consecutively operated cases. *Neurosurgery* 1983;13(5):504–512.
62. Tanaka N, Fujimoto Y, An HS, et al. The anatomic relationship among the nerve roots, intervertebral foramina, and intervertebral discs of the cervical spine. *Spine* 2000;25(3):286–291.
63. Ebraheim NA, An HS, Xu R, et al. The quantitative anatomy of the cervical nerve root groove and the intervertebral foramen. *Spine* 1996;21:1619–623.
64. Arce CA, Dohrmann GJ. Thoracic disc herniation: improved diagnosis with computed tomographic scanning and a review of the literature. *Surg Neurol* 1985;23:356–361.
65. Rossitti S, Stephensen H, Elkholm S, et al. The anterior approach to high thoracic (T1-T2) disc herniation. *Br J Neurosurg* 1993;7(2):189–192.
66. Arseni C, Nash F. Thoracic intervertebral disc protrusion: a clinical study. *J Neurosurg* 1960;17:418–430.
67. Wood KB, Garvey TA, Gundry C, et al. Thoracic MRI evaluation of asymptomatic individuals. *J Bone Joint Surg Am* 1995;77:1634–1638.
68. Wood KB, Blair JM, Aepple DM, et al. The natural history of asymptomatic thoracic disc herniations. *Spine* 1997;22:525–529.
69. Anand N, Regan JJ. Video-assisted thoracoscopic surgery for thoracic disc disease. *Spine* 2002;27:871–879.
70. Chana JS, Afshar F. Thoracic spondylosis presenting with spastic paraparesis. *Postgrad Med J* 1996;72(846):243–244.
71. Krauss WE, Atkinson JL, Miller GM. Juxtafacet cysts of the cervical spine. *Neurosurgery* 1998;43(6):1363–1368.
72. Lunardi P, Acqui M, Ricci G, et al. Cervical synovial cysts: case report and review of the literature. *Eur Spine J* 1999;8(3):232–237.
73. Tuli SM. *Tuberculosis of the spine*. New Delhi: Amerind Publishing Co., 1975.
74. Shunmugam G, Parbhoo AH, Suresh Kumar KP. Tuberculosis of the cervicodorsal junction. *J Pediatr Orth* 2001;21:285–287.
75. Moon MS, Woo YK, Lee KS, et al. Posterior instrumentation and anterior interbody fusion for tuberculous kyphosis of dorsal and lumbar spine. *Spine* 1995;20:1910–1916.
76. Yilmaz C, Selek HY, Gurkan I, et al. Anterior instrumentation for the treatment of spinal tuberculosis. *J Bone Joint Surg* 1999;81A(9):1261–1267.
77. Malawski SK, Lukawski S. Pyogenic infections of the spine. *Clin Orthop* 1991;272:58–66.
78. Eismont FJ, Bohlman HH, Soni PL, et al. Pyogenic and fungal vertebral osteomyelitis with paralysis. *J Bone Joint Surg* 1983;65A:19–29.
79. Collert S. Osteomyelitis of the spine. *Acta Orthop Scand* 1977;48(3): 283–290.
80. Fountain SS, Hsu LC, Yau AC, et al. Progressive kyphosis following solid anterior spine fusion in children with tuberculosis of the spine. A long-term study. *J Bone Joint Surg* 1975;57A(8):1104–1107.
81. Biyani A, Ebraheim NA, Lu J. Thoracic spine fractures in patients older than 50 years. *Clin Orthop* 1996;328:190–193.
82. Zeidman SM, Ellenbogen RG, Ducker TB. Intradural tumors. In: The Cervical Spine Research Society Editorial Committee, ed. *The cervical spine*, 3rd ed. Philadelphia: Lippincott–Raven, 1998.
83. Ginsberg RJ, Martini N, Zaman M, et al. Influence of surgical resection and brachytherapy in the management of superior sulcus tumor. *Ann Thorac Surg* 1994;57:1440–1445.
84. Martinod E, D'Audiffret A, Thomas P, et al. Management of superior sulcus tumors: experience with 139 cases treated by surgical resection. *Ann Thorac Surg* 2002;73:1534–1540.
85. Grunenwald D, Mazel C, Girard P, et al. Total vertebrectomy for en bloc resection of lung cancer invading the spine. *Ann Thorac Surg* 1996;61:723–726.
86. DeMeester TR, Albertucci M, Dawson PJ, et al. Management of tumor adherent to the vertebral column. *J Thorac Cardiovasc Surg* 1989;97:373–378.
87. York JE, Walsh GL, Lang FF, et al. Combined chest wall resection with vertebrectomy and spinal reconstruction for the treatment of Pancoast tumors. *J Neurosurg* 1999;91:74–80.
88. Gandhi S, Walsh GL, Komaki R, et al. A multidisciplinary surgical approach to superior sulcus tumors with vertebral invasion. *Ann Thorac Surg* 1999;68:1778–1785.
89. Thomsen MN, Schneider U, Weber M, et al. Scoliosis and congenital anomalies associated with Klippel-Feil syndrome types I-III. *Spine* 1997;22(4):396–401.
90. Smith MD. Congenital scoliosis of the cervical or cervicothoracic spine. *Orthop Clin North Am* 1994;25(2):301–310.
91. Tokgozoglu AM, Alpaslan AM. Congenital spondylolisthesis in the upper spinal column. *Spine* 1994;19(1):99–102.
92. Hensinger RN, Lang JE, MacEwen GD. Klippel-Feil syndrome. A constellation of associated anomalies. *J Bone Joint Surg* 1974;56A:1246–1253.
93. Foo D, Bignami A, Rossier AB. Two spinal cord lesions in a patient with ankylosing spondylitis and cervical spine injury. *Neurology* 1983;33(2):245–249.
94. Redlund-Johnell I, Larsson EM. Subluxation of the upper thoracic spine in rheumatoid arthritis. *Skel Radiol* 1993;22(2):105–108.
95. Graziano GP, Hensinger R, Patel CK. The use of traction methods to correct severe cervical deformity in rheumatoid arthritis patients. A report of five cases. *Spine* 2001;26(9):1076–1081.
96. Yasuoka S, et al. Incidence of spinal column deformity after multilevel laminectomy in children and adults. *J Neurosurg* 1982;57:441–445.
97. Yasuoka S, Peterson HA, Laws ER, et al. Pathogenesis and prophylaxis of postlaminectomy deformity of the spine after multiple level laminectomy: difference between children and adults. *Neurosurgery* 1981;9:145–152.

Operative Techniques

Editor: Howard S. An

CHAPTER 38

Surgical Approaches to the Craniocervical Junction and the Upper Cervical Spine

Bong-Soo Kim, Faheem Sandhu, Daniel Refai, and Richard G. Fessler

The *craniocervical junction* is defined as the region of the occipital bone surrounding the foramen magnum, the atlas, and the axis. Approaches to this region are impeded by the complex anatomy at the skull base, which renders surgery technically difficult and poses significant risk of complications. As a result of these challenges, surgeons have often approached the craniocervical junction via the "easier" posterior approach. New developments in skull-base operative techniques and improved instruments have made anterior, lateral, posterior, and combined approaches to the craniocervical junction safer and easier to perform (1). Approach selection aims to maximize operative exposure while minimizing morbidity and is dependent on several factors: (a) lesion location, (b) suspected pathology (i.e., osseous or traumatic pathology differs from that of neoplastic lesions, which may require gross total resection), (c) lesion size, (d) maintenance of stability, and (e) cosmetic results (2,3).

Anterior approaches to the craniocervical junction and upper cervical spine include transoral, transfacial, and anterolateral retropharyngeal approaches (Fig. 1) (1,4,5). The transoral or transfacial approach is best indicated for ventral, extradural lesions. Both approaches are performed through a transmucosal route; therefore, the risks of infection, meningitis, and cerebrospinal fluid (CSF) leak when treating intradural pathology are significant. In contrast, the anterolateral retropharyngeal approach is an extramucosal approach and is better suited for midline intradural lesions (5–7). Lateral approaches to the craniocervical junction include the retrosigmoid, transpetrosal, and infratemporal approaches. These approaches are superior to anterior approaches for intradural lesions because they avoid direct contamination with nasopharyngeal organisms (1,8,9). Posterior approaches consist of the midline suboccipital and transcondylar approaches. These two approaches can widely expose the foramen magnum and are well suited for dorsal and lateral intradural or extradural lesions (1,10).

This chapter describes the commonly used approaches to the craniocervical junction and upper cervical spine, with particular focus on the indications and technical nuances of each. The choice of a single or combined technique is made in accordance with the risks and benefits that each approach provides.

ANTERIOR APPROACH

Transoral Approach

The transoral approach, performed through an open mouth, provides access to the lower clivus, craniocervical junction, and upper cervical vertebrae. This approach is ideally suited for removal of ventral extradural midline lesions. It can be used for ventral intradural lesions; however, its use is limited for intradural pathology because of serious procedural related complications, such as meningitis and CSF leak (3,11).

In most circumstances, the surgeon can expose the lower one-third of the clivus to the third cervical vertebra in the rostral-caudal direction and 2 cm laterally to either side of the midline by retracting the tongue and the soft palate (Fig. 2A). Various modifications of the transoral approach have been introduced to extend the exposure superiorly and inferiorly, including transmaxillary, transpalatal, and transmandibular approaches (Fig. 2B) (1,4,6,12). Although these extended transoral approaches provide wider exposures for extensive lesions, they should be performed in properly selected patients because of morbidities associated with the procedures, such as dysphagia, dysphonia, and nasal regurgitation of fluids (3).

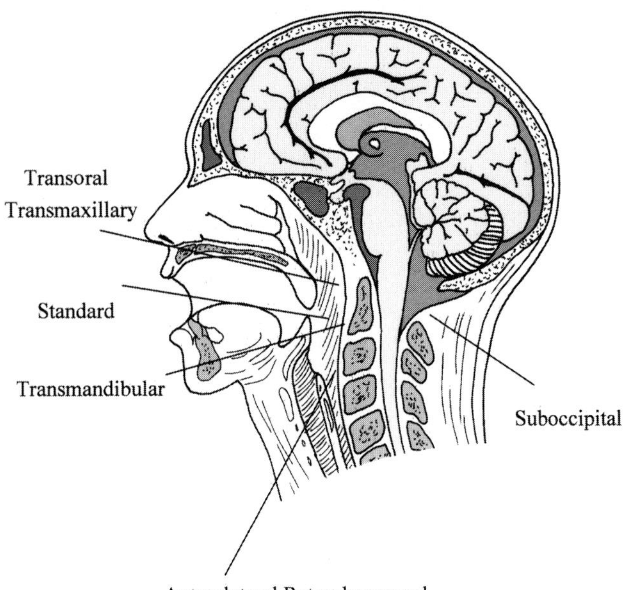

FIG. 1. Various approaches to the craniocervical junction and upper cervical spine.

Indications

Indications for the transoral approach include extradural tumor, translocation of the odontoid process in rheumatoid arthritis, basilar impression, congenital atlantoaxial subluxation, fracture-dislocation at the craniocervical junction, vertebrobasilar aneurysm, and anterior compression of the neural structures. Although some authors have successfully used the transoral approach for intradural lesions, it is not generally recommended for intradural lesions because of the risk of complications related to dural opening, such as CSF leak and meningitis (4). In addition, the transoral procedure is contraindicated in patients with an ectatic vertebral or basilar artery that transgresses the operative field, or if an active infectious process is present in the nasopharyngeal cavity (6).

Preoperative Assessment

Preoperative evaluation of the oral cavity is extremely important before performing the transoral procedure. An interdental length of 2.5 cm is the minimum distance required for adequate exposure using the transoral route; therefore, in any patient with less than 2.5 cm of interdental space, splitting the mandible and glossectomy usually provides the additional room necessary for performing surgery (Fig. 2B). A culture of the nasal and oropharyngeal cavities is obtained preoperatively to identify unusual organisms and guides perioperative antibiotic selection. Alternatively, triple-antibiotic therapy can be used routinely.

Operative Technique

The patient is positioned supine on the operative table with the head slightly extended and fixated rigidly with a head holder. Rigid fixation of the head is not used by some surgeons, however, to avoid potential injury during the procedure that may result from distal segment movement away from a fixed cranio-

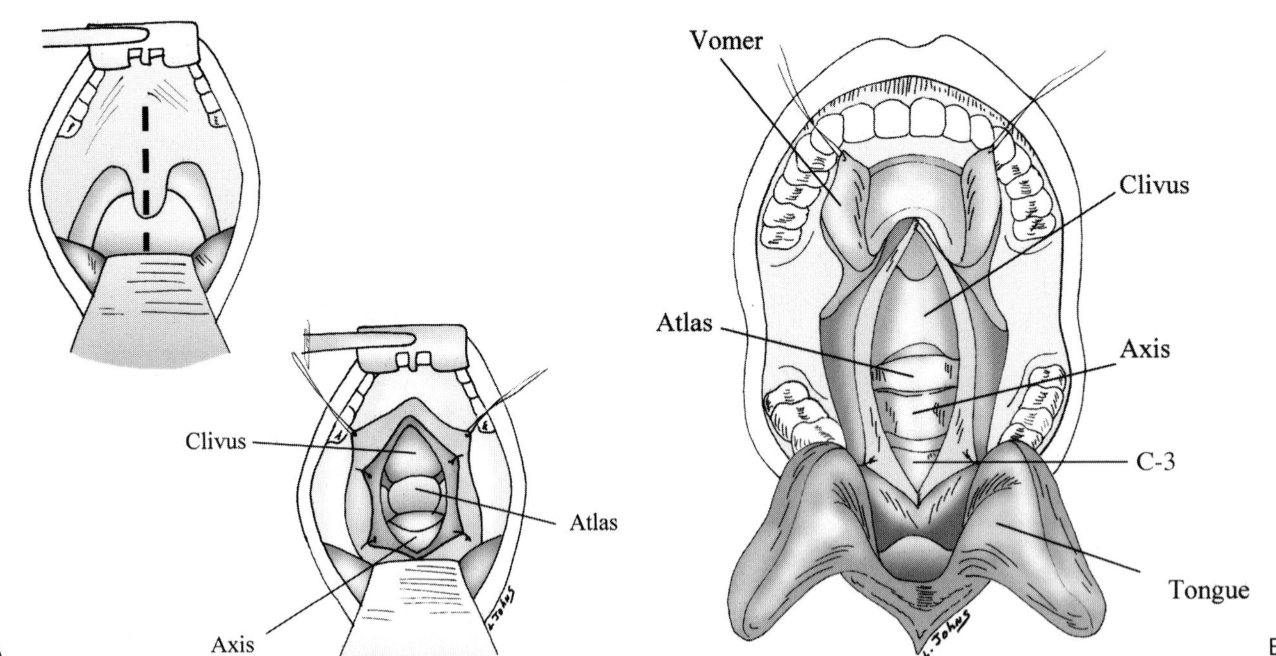

FIG. 2. A: The transoral approach, which provides exposure from the clivus to C-2. The incision (*dotted line*) can include the soft palate to expose more of the clivus or, more typically, be limited to posterior pharyngeal wall. **B:** By performing a glossectomy and mandibular osteotomy, exposure can be extended to C-3.

cervical junction (3,6). If the patient has preoperative spinal instability, a halo brace can be used and awake, fiberoptic oral intubation is indicated. Tracheostomy is generally reserved for patients with severe respiratory disturbance or lower cranial nerve deficits that require prolonged postoperative ventilatory support. Various self-retaining retractor systems, such as the modified Dingman, can be used to facilitate the exposure and secure the endotracheal tube. The oropharyngeal cavity is sterilized with 10% povidone iodine solution and hydrogen peroxide after placement of retractors and a throat pack. The tubercle of C-1 is identified for orientation to the midline by its surface landmark or with aid of intraoperative radiography. A linear midline incision, centered on the C-1 tubercle, is created in the median raphe of the posterior pharyngeal wall and is then carried down to bony structures with the monopolar diathermy. This single-layer tissue flap is elevated from the anterior surfaces of the clivus, the C-1 arch, and the C-2 vertebral body subperiosteally and retracted laterally to provide a wide exposure. To expose the base of the odontoid process, the anterior arch of C-1 may be removed partially or totally using a high-speed drill and a Kerrison rongeur. The soft tissue ventral to the odontoid is removed with a rongeur. After the odontoid process is transected at the level of its base, the dens is pulled caudally and ventrally to decompress the medulla and cervical spinal cord before the ligaments are detached. The apical and alar ligaments are dissected and detached meticulously from the dens using angled curettes. Then the odontoid process is freed and removed completely. The tectorial membrane and transverse portion of the cruciate ligament may be removed to decompress the dura if they are thickened. The ligaments can adhere tightly with attenuated dura, however, and extreme caution is needed to avoid a dural tear. If the surgeon sees good pulsations of dura after removal of the odontoid and adequate decompression has been achieved, no further ligamentous resection is necessary.

If the dura is opened, primary closure of dura with a fascial graft and fat pad should be attempted. Fibrin glue can also be used to reinforce dural closure. A lumbar drain and intravenous antibiotics are maintained for 7 to 10 days after the procedure to prevent CSF leak and fistula formation. The posterior pharyngeal wall is closed in a single layer with running or interrupted suture after hemostasis is obtained.

Postoperative Care

The patient remains intubated for 1 to 3 days after surgery while tongue swelling subsides. Topical steroids may help reduce soft-tissue swelling of the oral cavity. Nutritional support is important during the immediate postoperative period and starts with feeding through a nasogastric tube. The diet can be advanced to clear liquids at the end of postoperative week 1 and then to a soft diet the following week.

Postoperative spinal stability should be evaluated carefully because the odontoidectomy may create instability at the craniocervical junction. Menezes considers all patients with rheumatoid arthritis that undergo transoral odontoidectomy as unstable (6). If the craniocervical junction is unstable, patients must be immobilized with a cervical orthosis and an occipitocervical fusion needs to be performed. Some surgeons advocate performing the odontoidectomy and posterior fusion on the same day (4,13). Tuite et al. have demonstrated successful fusion in pediatric patients who underwent perioperative posterior fusion after transoral decompression (14).

Anterolateral (Transcervical) Retropharyngeal Approach

Indications

The transcervical or anterolateral retropharyngeal approach is an extrapharyngeal approach and directed through the fascial plane of the neck to the craniocervical junction and the upper cervical vertebrae. By way of the anterolateral retropharyngeal approach, the lower clivus, anterior foramen magnum, anterior C-1 arch, odontoid, vertebral bodies of C-2 and C-3 and corresponding intervertebral disc, and superior epiphysis of C-4, can be exposed without significantly increasing the risks of CSF leak and infection (Fig. 3) (5,15). Therefore, the anterolateral retropharyngeal approach is an effective alternative to the transoral approach in selected cases.

Operative Technique

The patient is placed in the supine position. The head is resting on a sponge doughnut or horseshoe headrest, rotated 30 degrees to the contralateral side with the neck extended. The side of approach depends on the surgeon's preference when the pathology is midline. If a unilateral lower cranial nerve deficit exists, the approach should be performed from the same side of impairment. The incision is dependent on the required extent of the craniocervical exposure. A transverse incision is made 2 cm below the lower edge of the mandible from the angle of the mandible to the base of the mental protuberance across the midline. The key to adequate exposure is wide dissection of each plane of the cervical fascia, beginning with the dissection of the subcutaneous flap. Dissection is then made in the subplatysmal plane after transection of the platysma. The facial artery and vein are dissected along their courses. Dissection of the facial artery leads to the carotid sheath, the lateral limit of the exposure. After retraction of the submandibular gland superiorly, the dissection is carried down deep to expose the digastric muscle. The posterior belly of the digastric muscle is followed to its tendon at the hyoid bone and is transected to allow for digastric muscle retraction towards the mandible. The hypoglossal nerve is gently dissected along its course and mobilized superiorly. At this point, the retropharyngeal space can be accessed by blunt dissection. The medial edges of the longus coli muscles are dissected and elevated from the C-2 and C-3 vertebral body. The tubercle of C-1 is identified and aids to identify midline orientation. The anterior decompression is performed similar to the transoral procedure. Once decompression is completed, fusion, if necessary, may be carried out with a bone graft between the caudal clivus and the upper cervical vertebral body.

Postoperative Care

Patients should remain intubated for 3 to 5 days until soft-tissue swelling in the oropharynx and retropharyngeal space diminish (15). Mechanical ventilation is then weaned. Nutritional support

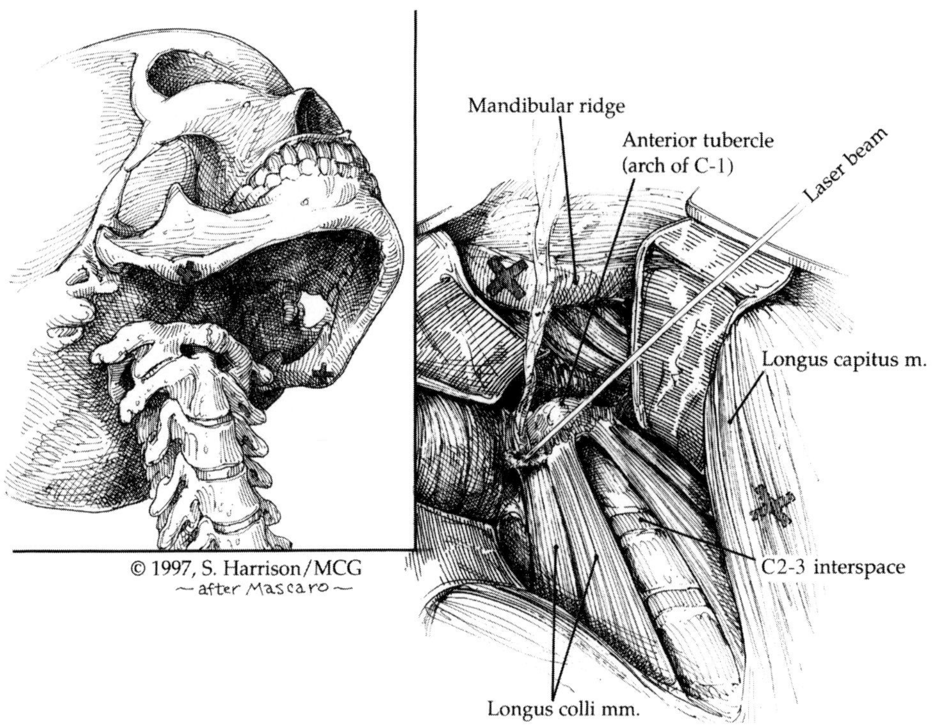

FIG. 3. The position of the skull relative to the spine *(inset)* and the operative exposure provided by the anterolateral retropharyngeal approach is depicted. The angles of the mandible are marked with an X. (From Vender JR, Harrison SJ, McDonnell DE. Fusion and instrumentation at C1-3 via the high anterior cervical approach. *J Neurosurg Spine* 2000;92:26, with permission.)

is important during the immediate postoperative period and starts with feeding through a nasogastric or nasojejunal tube. The diet can be advanced to clear liquids as the patient begins to tolerate oral feeding. Postoperative spinal stability has been demonstrated successfully in small studies with instrumentation or arthrodesis (15,16).

LATERAL APPROACH

Petrosal Approach

Indications

The transpetrosal approach is designed to reach the middle one-third of the clivus. This approach, with a combined transcondylar technique, can provide a wide exposure of anterior and lateral aspects of the brain stem, clivus, and anterolateral foramen magnum while minimizing retraction of neural structures. The combined approach is best suited for extensive intra- and/or extradural pathology that involves the upper clivus and the jugular foramen (10,17,18).

Operative Technique

The patient is placed in the supine position with the head turned or in the modified park-bench position. A reverse question-mark incision begins at the zygoma at 1 cm anterior to the tragus, circles above the ear, and descends just behind the mastoid process. If combined with a transcondylar approach, the incision is made more medial to midline and down to C-3 or C-4. The skin flap is elevated and reflected anteriorly and inferiorly. Four burr holes are made, with two on each side of the transverse sinus, and a temporal suboccipital craniotomy is performed with special care of the sinus. The mastoid cortex overlying the atrium is drilled out. Once the atrium is identified, the drilling is carried out posteriorly. Care should be taken to avoid injury to the sigmoid sinus and the facial nerve inferiorly during the mastoidectomy. After identification of the semicircular canals, the facial canal is skeletonized at the inferior edge of the lateral semicircular canal and the stylomastoid foramen. The sigmoid sinus is also skeletonized down to the jugular bulb. The dura is incised along the anterior margin of the sigmoid sinus, and then the incision extends over the temporal lobe in the anterior portion of the craniotomy. Citelli's sinodural angle, in which the superior petrosal sinus enters the sigmoid sinus, is then exposed. The superior petrosal sinus is clipped or coagulated and divided, which allows the dural incision to be continued on the tentorium. Special care should be taken to preserve the vein of Labbe to prevent a postoperative venous infarction. Another dural incision in the posterior fossa allows access from the supratentorial and infratentorial direction.

The petrosal approach is usually chosen for petroclival lesions involving the middle one-third of the clivus, but it yields limited access to the craniocervical junction near the jugular tubercle and the jugular bulb. However, combining it with approaches such as the transcondylar technique allows access from the upper clivus to the upper cervical region (18,19).

Postoperative Care

The postoperative course of patients undergoing lateral approaches to the craniovertebral junction is less complicated than in the anterior approach. The risk of CSF leak or infection is low. Despite bone resection, spinal stability is not an issue if the joints are not disturbed (20).

Transcondylar Approach

Indications

The transcondylar approach is suitable for intradural pathology located anterior or lateral to the brain stem and the upper spinal cord, where transoral access is difficult because of the occipital condyle, jugular bulb, vertebral artery, and upper spinal cord (6,9). Various transcondylar approaches have been described in the literature, including the extreme lateral transcondylar and transjugular approach, the dorsolateral transcondylar approach, the lateral suboccipital approach, and the far-lateral suboccipital approach (10,21–23). Each approach differs slightly; nevertheless, all of them provide excellent access to the lower one-third of the clivus, the pontomedullary junction, the anterolateral foramen magnum, the craniocervical junction, and the upper cervical spine (Fig. 4). The transcondylar approach requires removal of the lateral rim of the foramen of magnum and the dorsal aspect of occipital condyle. This approach can be combined with exposures such as the subtemporal, infratemporal, petrous, and cervical approaches for extended exposure (10,17,18).

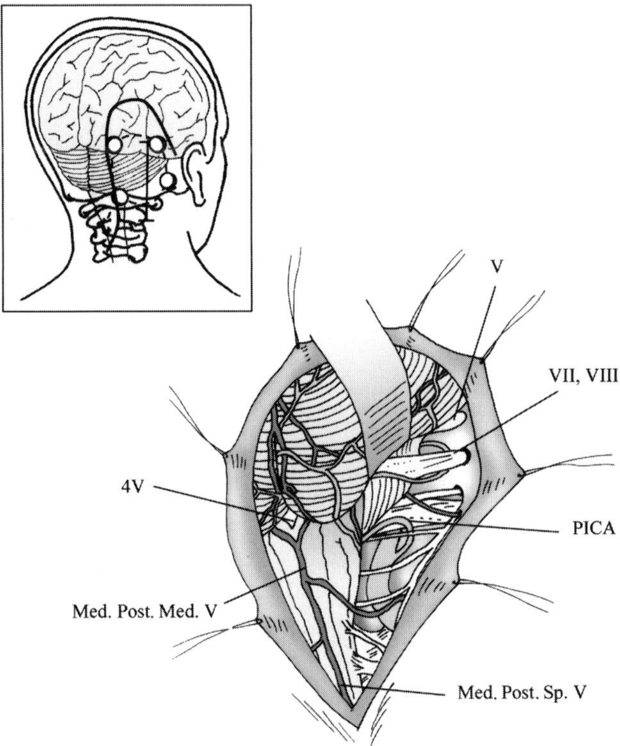

FIG. 4. A schematic depicting the hockey-stick skin incision (*inset*) and exposure for the transcondylar approach to the craniocervical junction. Exposure of the anterolateral brainstem, cranial nerves, and cerebropontine angle is possible after unilateral suboccipital craniectomy and removal of the posterior rim of the foramen magnum. The posterior inferior cerebellar artery (*PICA*) can be seen coming off the vertebral artery. The trigeminal (*V*) nerve is seen just under the cerebellar hemisphere; the facial (*VII*) and vestibulocochlear (*VIII*) nerves are centered in the operative field just superior to the PICA artery. Important venous structures include median posterior medullary vein (*Med. Post. Med. V*) and the median posterior spinal vein (*Med. Post. Sp. V*). The fourth ventricle (*4V*) is located in the midline between the cerebellar tonsils.

Operative Technique

The patient is placed in the lateral decubitus or modified park-bench position with the head in a Mayfield head holder. An inverted hockey-stick or inverted U-shaped fashion incision begins at the tip of the mastoid process and extends superiorly to the superior nuchal line and then continues medially to the inion and downward to the spinous processes of the upper or middle cervical spine. A myocutaneous flap is elevated along the subperiosteal plane and reflected laterally. A cuff of muscle and fascia is left attached to the superior nuchal line to enable a watertight closure at the end of the procedure, which aids in preventing CSF leak postoperatively.

The vertebral artery is dissected subperiosteally from the superior lamina of C-1, and then the dissection continues laterally to the foramen transversarium of the C-1 lateral mass. The dissection is carried along the course of the vertebral artery medially to the entry point of the vertebral artery into the dura. Bleeding from the paravertebral venous plexus is controlled by gentle tamponade. Vigorous coagulation of the venous plexus around the vertebral artery should be avoided because of the risk of vertebral artery occlusion. To limit venous bleeding for inadequate drainage, proper patient positioning without excessive neck rotation and flexion should be performed. The retrosigmoid suboccipital craniotomy and C-1 laminectomy are performed using a high-speed drill and a Kerrison rongeur. The foramen transversarium of C-1 can be opened to mobilize the vertebral artery. The posterior one- to two-thirds, depending on the need of exposure, of the occipital condyle and C-1 lateral mass is removed using a high-speed drill. The hypoglossal nerve is located just superior to the anterior third of the occipital condyle. Care should be taken to avoid injury of this structure during removal of the posterior two-thirds of the occipital condyle. If necessary, the mastoid process can be removed up to the vertical segment of the facial nerve and the entire occipitoatlantal facet joint drilled out. The curvilinear dural opening extends from the sigmoid sinus and is carried down medial to the vertebral artery. Section of the dentate ligament facilitates access to the inferior clivus, anterolateral medulla, and the cervicomedullary junction.

Postoperative Care

The risk of postoperative instability associated with the extent of the occipital condyle removal is debatable. Some investigations report that two-thirds of the occipital condyle can be removed without postoperative instability of the craniocervical junction, whereas greater resection may necessitate fusion (24). Based on results of biomechanical testing after unilateral occipital condyle resection, Visteh and colleagues found significant hypermobility in the occiput–C-1 joint with removal of 50% of the condyle; they recommend fusion after resection of 50% or more of the occipital condyle (25). If stabilization is necessary, occipitocervical fusion is performed as a part of the primary procedure (24,26).

POSTERIOR APPROACH

Suboccipital Approach

Indications

The posterior approach has been the long-standing procedure for access to the craniocervical junction and the upper cervical spine. The suboccipital approach is still the procedure of choice for most intradural pathology located posterior or lateral to the cervicomedullary junction and upper spinal cord (1,3). The suboccipital approach provides direct access to the midline and paramedian structures in the posterior fossa and can be easily modified to extend the incision from the transverse sinus down to the cervical spine (Fig. 5).

Operative Technique

The patient is placed in the prone or sitting position. The sitting position provides a good surgical view, but it carries the risk of venous air embolism and consequent hemodynamic instability. Special care is required to prevent air embolism, including the use of end-tidal carbon dioxide monitoring, precordial Doppler recording, and central venous access in the right atrium. Because of the potential for catastrophic air embolism, most surgeons prefer to perform the suboccipital approach in the prone position.

A midline incision is made from the inion to C-3 or C-4, depending on the extent of exposure required. The muscle dissection is carried out through the avascular midline plane. The muscle attachments of C-2 are left intact unless C-2 laminectomy is required for adequate exposure. The suboccipital craniotomy or craniectomy is performed using a high-speed drill and rongeurs. The C-1 arch is dissected subperiosteally as far laterally as needed. As the dissection proceeds laterally, brisk venous bleeding from paravertebral venous structures is often encountered. This bleeding is easily controlled with the bipolar diathermy and Gelfoam. The dura is usually opened in a Y-shaped fashion based on the transverse sinus to avoid the midline occipital sinus. Care is taken to adequately control bleeding from the marginal sinus, which is located at the level of foramen magnum (27).

Postoperative Care

The posterior approach may require spinal cord retraction to visualize the pathology, and thus, special care must be taken to avoid injury to the neural elements. Spinal stability is not as challenging as in lateral or transoral approaches because posterior fusion can be easily accomplished if necessary.

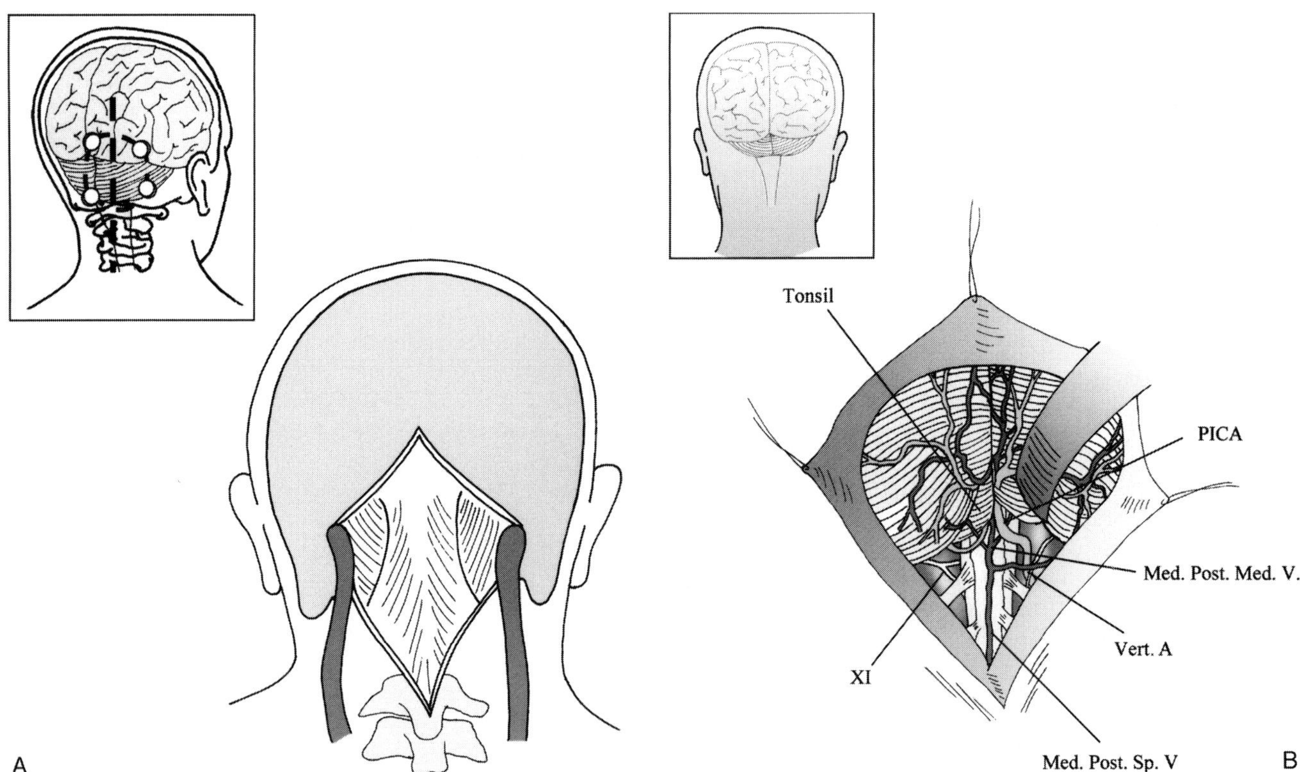

FIG. 5. A: A schematic of the midline skin incision and craniotomy (*inset*) and the incision of the musculature surgical exposure after the suboccipital approach to the craniocervical junction. **B:** After suboccipital craniotomy and C-1 laminectomy, the operative exposure is shown. Dorsal and dorsolateral access (after division of the dentate ligament) to the medulla, upper cervical spinal cord, and fourth ventricle is provided by this approach. PICA, posterior inferior cerebellar artery; Med. Post. Med. V., median posterior medullary vein; Med. Post. Sp. V., median posterior spinal vein; Vert. A, vertebral artery; XI, accessory nerve.

CONCLUSION

Advances in surgical techniques and instrumentation provide the surgeon with many options for approaching the craniovertebral junction. The choice of approach is made with several factors in mind, including the location of the lesion, the size of the lesion, the pathology, the desired exposure, and the postoperative stability of the spine. These factors are measured with the technical challenges and perioperative risks to finalize the approach selection. Finally, prompt recognition and management of postoperative complications is essential for optimal patient outcome.

REFERENCES

1. Long DM. Surgical approaches to tumors of the skull base: an overview. In Wilkins RH, Rengachary SS, eds. *Neurosurgery*, 3rd ed. New York: McGraw-Hill, 1996:1573–1583.
2. Menezes AH, VanGilder JC, Graf CJ, et al. Craniocervical abnormalities, a comprehensive surgical approach. *J Neurosurg* 1980;53:444–455.
3. Menezes AH, Traynelis VC. Tumors of the craniovertebral junction. In: Youmans JR, ed. *Neurological surgery*, 6th ed. Philadelphia: WB Saunders, 1996:3041–3072.
4. James D, Crockard HA. Surgical access to the base of the skull and upper cervical spine by extended maxillotomy. *Neurosurgery* 1991;29.
5. McDonnell DE, Harrison SJ. Anteriolateral cervical approach to the craniovertebral junction. In: Wilkins RH, Rengachary SS, eds. *Neurosurgery,* 3rd ed. New York: McGraw-Hill, 1996:1641–1653.
6. Menezes AH, Van Gilder JC. Transoral-transpharyngeal approach to the anterior craniocervical junction: ten year experience with 72 patients. *J Neurosurg* 1988;69:895–903.
7. Spetzler RF, Selman WR, Nash CL. Transoral microsurgical odontoid resection and spinal cord monitoring. *Spine* 1979;4:506–510.
8. Al-Mefty O, Fox J, Smith R. Petrosal approach to petroclival meningiomas. *Neurosurgery* 1988;22:510–516.
9. Haddad GF, Al-Mefty O. Approaches to petroclival tumors. In: Wilkins RH, Rengachary SS, eds. *Neurosurgery*, 3rd ed. New York: McGraw-Hill, 1996:1695–1706.
10. Sen C, Sekhar LN. An extreme lateral approach to intradural lesions of the cervical spine and foramen magnum. *J Neurosurg* 1990;27:197–204.
11. Hadley MN, Spetzler RF, Sonntag VK. The transoral approach to the superior cervical spine: a review of 53 cases of extradural cervicomedullary compression. *J Neurosurg* 1989;71:16–23.
12. Arbit E, Patterson RH Jr. Combined transoral and median labiomandibular glossotomy approach to the upper cervical spine. *Neurosurgery* 1981;8:672–674.
13. Dickman CA, Locantro J, Fessler RG. The influence of transoral odontoid resection on stability of the craniovertebral junction. *J Neurosurg* 1992;77:525–530.
14. Tuite GF, Veres R, Crockard HA, et al. Pediatric transoral surgery: indications, complications, and long-term outcome. *J Neurosurg* 1996;84:573–583.
15. Vender JR, Harrison SJ, McDonnell DE. Fusion and instrumentation at C1-3 via the high anterior cervical approach. *J Neurosurg* 2000;92:24–29.
16. Behari S, Banerji D, Trivedi P, et al. Anterior retropharyngeal approach to the cervical spine. *Neurol India* 2001;49:342–349.
17. Sen CN, Sekhar LN. The subtemporal and preauricular infratemporal approach to intradural structures ventral to the brain stem. *J Neurosurg* 1990;73:354.
18. Spetzler RF, Daspot CP, Pappas CTE. The combined supra- and infratentorial lesions of the petrous and clival regions: experience with 46 cases. *J Neurosurg* 1992;76:588–599.
19. Baldwin HZ, Miller CG, Van Loveren HR. The far lateral/combined supra- and infratentorial approach. A human cadaveric prosection model for routes of access to the petroclival region and ventral brain stem. *J Neurosurg* 1994;81:60–68.
20. Shucart W, Borden J. Lateral approaches to the cervical spine. In: Menezes AH, Sonntag VK, eds. *Principles of spinal surgery*. New York: McGraw-Hill, 1996:1325–1332.
21. Babu RP, Sekhar LN. Extreme lateral transcondylar approach: technical improvements and lessons learned. *J Neurosurg* 1994;81:49–59.
22. Bertalanffy H, Seeger W. The dorsolateral, transcondylar approach to the lower clivus and anterior portion of the craniocervical junction. *Neurosurgery* 1991;29:815–821.
23. Heros RC. Lateral suboccipital approach for vertebral and vertebrobasilar artery lesions. *J Neurosurg* 1986;64:559–562.
24. Bejjani G, Sekhar LN, Riedel C. Occipitocervical fusion following the extreme lateral transcondylar approach. *Surg Neurol* 2000;54: 109–116.
25. Vishteh AG, Crawford NR, Melton MS, et al. Stability of the craniovertebral junction after unilateral occipital condyle resection: a biomechanical study. *J Neurosurg* 1999;90:91–98.
26. Al-Mefty O, Borba LA, Aoki N, et al. The transcondylar approach to extradural nonneoplastic lesions of the craniovertebral junction. *J Neurosurg* 1996;84:1–6.
27. Rhoton AL. The far-lateral approach and its transcondylar, supracondylar, and paracondylar extensions. *Neurosurgery* 2000;47:S195–S209.

CHAPTER 39

Surgical Approaches to the Subaxial Cervical Spine

Timothy R. Kuklo, Ronald A. Lehman, Jr., Brett A. Taylor, and K. Daniel Riew

Indications for cervical spine surgery include compression of the spinal cord or nerve roots, trauma, instability, and degenerative conditions (1–8). Various surgical approaches for these conditions have been described (2,8–10).

Historically, the posterior approach was used for decompression and fusion in the cervical spine. The development of the anterior approach to the cervical spine by Bailey and Badgley (3), Smith and Robinson (2), and Cloward (4) defined this technique for various cervical pathologies (11). The Smith-Robinson approach was originally described for the treatment of degenerative conditions of the cervical spine by stabilization of the involved segment with the use of a cortical cancellous horseshoe-shaped graft inserted into the prepared disc space (2). These authors did not describe decompression of neurologic structures at the time of the anterior disc excisions, but most subsequent investigators recommended that procedure if indicated by neurologic signs and symptoms.

The Cloward technique makes use of a drill to open the disc space posteriorly to the level of the posterior longitudinal ligament, which allows for better visualization of the neural canal and its contents. Both of these procedures have yielded good results, but they do not permit good exposure over multiple segments. As a result, some surgeons have adapted these techniques to include partial corpectomy.

This chapter reviews the standard anterior and posterior approaches to the subaxial cervical spine (Fig. 1). In addition to surgical landmarks and key neurovascular structures, the common indications and complications are also reviewed.

ANTERIOR APPROACH TO THE CERVICAL SPINE

One of the most commonly used approaches for exposure of the anterior cervical spine is the Smith-Robinson approach (2). It is generally considered for exposure of the subaxial cervical spine from C-3 to T-1, but extension to the upper cervical spine has also been described by McAfee and Bohlman (12). The approach provides access to vertebral bodies and discs in the subaxial spine, and it can be performed on the left or right side, although right-handed surgeons may prefer a right-sided approach. The authors' preference is for a left-sided approach for index procedures, because of the variable course of the right recurrent laryngeal nerve, which can cross the surgical field around C5-6 (13). This nerve branches from the vagus nerve inferiorly near the level of the aortic arch and runs alongside the trachea after looping around the right subclavian artery (Fig. 2). In the subaxial spine, it crosses from lateral to medial to reach the midline trachea (14). On the left-sided approach, the thoracic duct may be encountered at the cervical thoracic region (Fig. 3) (15).

The approach requires proper identification of the medial border of the sternocleidomastoid muscle and the interval between the carotid sheath laterally and the trachea and esophagus medially. Care must be taken to identify the superior laryngeal, glossopharyngeal, and hypoglossal nerves. The superior laryngeal nerve usually crosses into the operative field at C3-4 (16,17). It travels with the superior thyroid artery and vein, which arise from the carotid sheath, and passes through the pretracheal fascia near the midline. Injury to the superior laryngeal nerve may result in dysphasia, voice

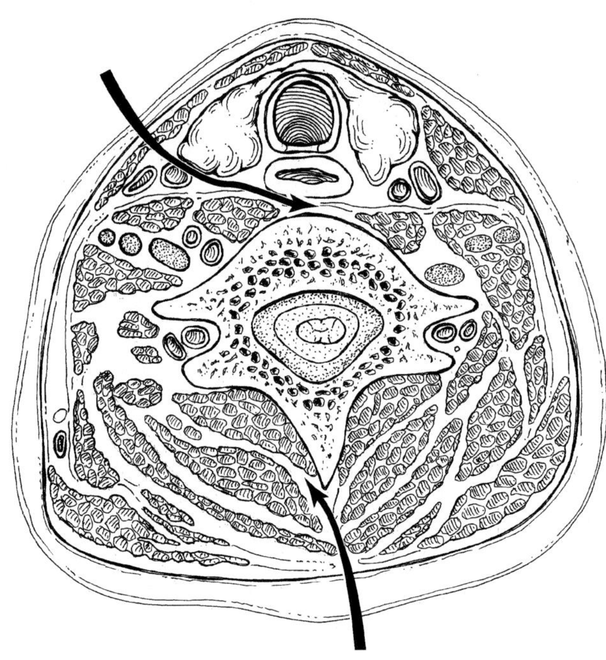

FIG. 1. Anterior and posterior approaches to the subaxial cervical spine.

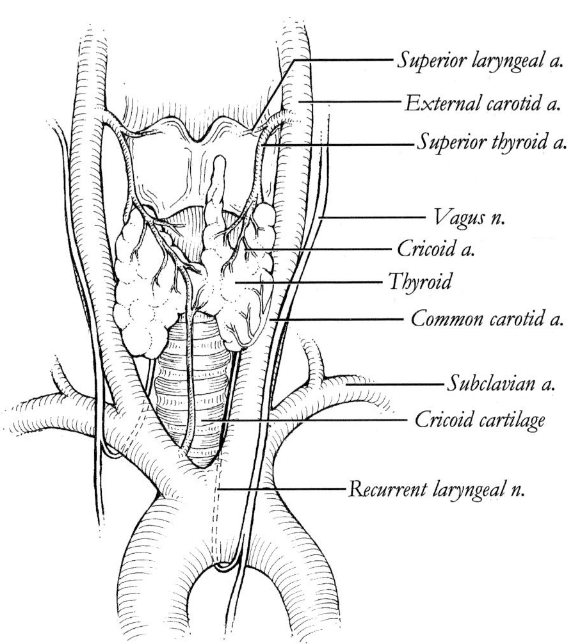

FIG. 2. The right recurrent laryngeal nerve crosses the surgical field variably around C5-6. a, artery; n, nerve.

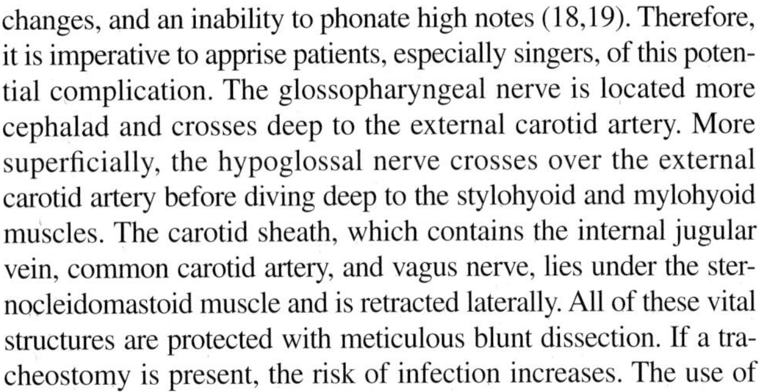
changes, and an inability to phonate high notes (18,19). Therefore, it is imperative to apprise patients, especially singers, of this potential complication. The glossopharyngeal nerve is located more cephalad and crosses deep to the external carotid artery. More superficially, the hypoglossal nerve crosses over the external carotid artery before diving deep to the stylohyoid and mylohyoid muscles. The carotid sheath, which contains the internal jugular vein, common carotid artery, and vagus nerve, lies under the sternocleidomastoid muscle and is retracted laterally. All of these vital structures are protected with meticulous blunt dissection. If a tracheostomy is present, the risk of infection increases. The use of intraoperative electrodiagnostic techniques to avoid injury to the facial nerve have been described; however, the authors have not found this practice necessary (20).

Positioning and Dissection

The patient is placed supine on the operating room table with the head and neck rotated slightly away from the intended operative side, or straight midline. The endotracheal tube is taped opposite from the operative field. A soft roll or folded towel is placed

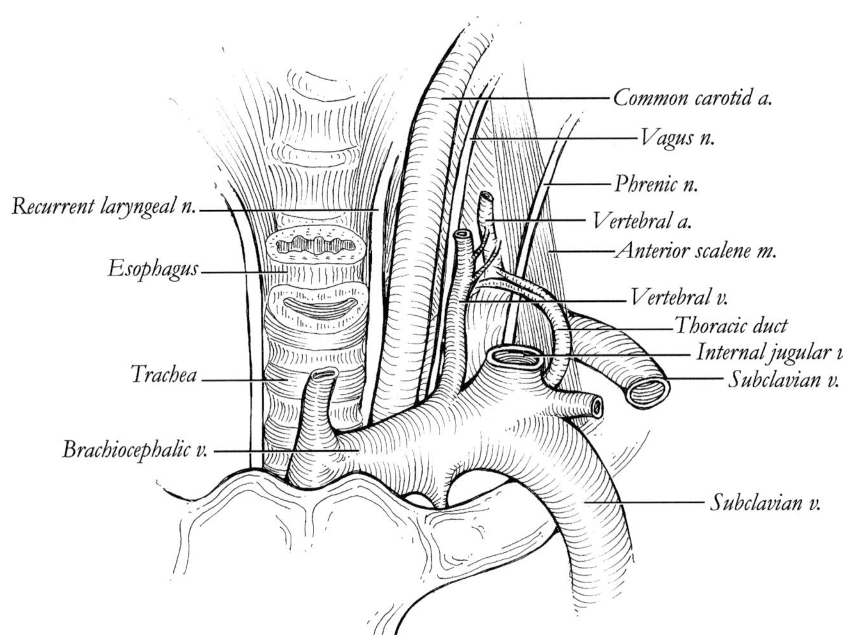

FIG. 3. The thoracic duct may be encountered during the lower left-sided approach. a, artery; n, nerve; v, vein.

under the scapulae to provide slight extension of the cervical spine. The table may be placed in slight reverse Trendelenburg position to reduce venous bleeding during the procedure.

The application of a distractive force may be appropriate, especially when performing an interbody fusion. Traction is generally applied with the use of Gardner-Wells tongs with applied weights of 10 to 15 lb. Gardner-Wells tongs may be beneficial because they can be used to provide continuous traction and stability to the spine, especially after a multilevel corpectomy or trauma. Also, Gardner-Wells tongs can be used to distract the discectomy or corpectomy space just before graft insertion. The authors routinely use Gardner-Wells tongs for a multilevel anterior cervical discectomy and fusion or for a corpectomy, but do not use the tongs for single-level fusions. Alternatively, head-halter traction may be applied, thus obviating the need for skeletal traction. Before the Gardner-Wells tongs are placed, the authors typically use 3-in. tape to secure the shoulders to the Jackson table. This provides countertraction for symmetric distraction of the cervical spine and may help with radiographic visualization of the subaxial cervical spine. Care must be taken to avoid excessive traction to the brachial plexus with this method.

After the area is prepared and draped and prophylactic antibiotics are administered, a 3-cm transverse incision is made in line with the skin creases at the selected level of the pathology. This results in a more cosmetically pleasing scar postoperatively. A left-side incision is preferred to decrease the incidence of recurrent laryngeal nerve injury. The authors also recommend use of the transverse incision for multilevel cases, but the incision must be longer to provide greater cephalad-caudad access. Some authorities, however, prefer a more vertical or oblique incision along the medial border of the sternocleidomastoid muscle when more than two levels are to be addressed.

Once the skin is incised, the superficial fascia anterior to the platysma is gently elevated off the muscle. It is important to appreciate the vascularity of the skin and platysma muscle. For this reason, some surgeons advocate injection with diluted epinephrine before incising the skin. The platysma muscle is then divided longitudinally in line with its fibers or transversely. The authors' practice is to divide the platysma horizontally. Next, the interval between the strap muscles and the anterior border of the sternocleidomastoid muscle is identified, and the fascia lying anterior to the muscle is bluntly dissected. This can be done with gentle finger dissection or with the use of a surgical instrumentation. Dissection in a cephalad and caudal direction at each level significantly enhances visualization when using a transverse skin incision. In addition, adequate mobilization helps prevent excessive pressure from retraction, which may decrease the risk of postoperative dysphagia and laryngeal edema (18,19).

Small vessels may traverse the operative field in this interval and should be ligated or cauterized. After incision of this deep cervical fascia, the pretracheal fascia is identified and dissected medial to the carotid sheath. Palpation of the carotid artery aids in the identification of the carotid sheath and its contents. This structure should remain lateral during the approach. Dissection just lateral to the thyroid gland, between the alar and visceral fascia, leads directly to the anterior aspect of the vertebral bodies posterior to the esophagus. If the approach is errant within or lateral to the sternocleidomastoid muscle, hemostasis may be difficult. Hand-held retractors are use to protect vital structures. The superior and inferior thyroid arteries, which connect the

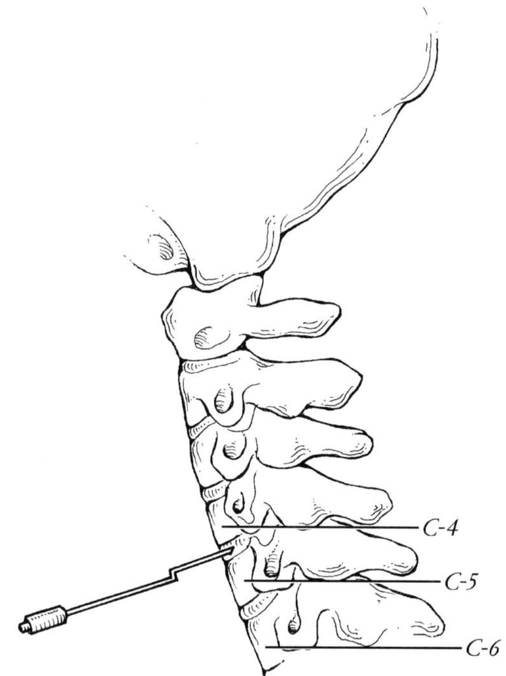

FIG. 4. A prebent 18-gauge spinal needle is placed into the disc space as a radiographic marker.

carotid sheath with the midline structures, may limit the superior extent of the dissection. They can be ligated to enhance exposure if necessary, as the thyroid gland has rich collateral vascularization.

The cervical vertebrae can be visualized with the longus colli muscles and the prevertebral fascia covering them. Additionally, the anterior longitudinal ligament can be seen in the midline as a gleaming white structure. The sympathetic chain lies on the longus colli, just lateral to the vertebral bodies. It is important to discern between the alar fascia, which invests the carotid sheath (superficial to the prevertebral fascia), and the visceral fascia, which envelops the esophagus and the recurrent laryngeal nerve. The plane between the alar and visceral fascia should be developed to widen the exposure. A Kitner can be used to tease off the fascia from the vertebral bodies, but it is important to stay in the midline. A prebent 18-gauge spinal needle (14-mm depth) is then placed into the disc space and the proper level is confirmed fluoroscopically (Fig. 4). With the use of electrocautery or Cobb elevators, the longus colli is split longitudinally over the midline of the vertebral bodies, and the medial edge of the muscle is subperiosteally dissected laterally from themidline (Fig. 5). This allows for exposure of the anterior surface of the vertebral bodies. Remember, the sympathetic nerve lies over the longus colli muscle and should not be disturbed, as injury may result in Horner's syndrome (6,21,22). The disc spaces, or "hills," can be differentiated from the vertebral bodies, or "valleys." Long retractors are placed deep to the longus colli muscles on the lateral edge of the vertebral body (Fig. 6). This places the retractors anterior to the transverse processes and provides for better visualization while protecting the recurrent laryngeal nerve, trachea, and esophagus. The authors routinely use the Caspar pins and distractor for added disc exposure and distraction.

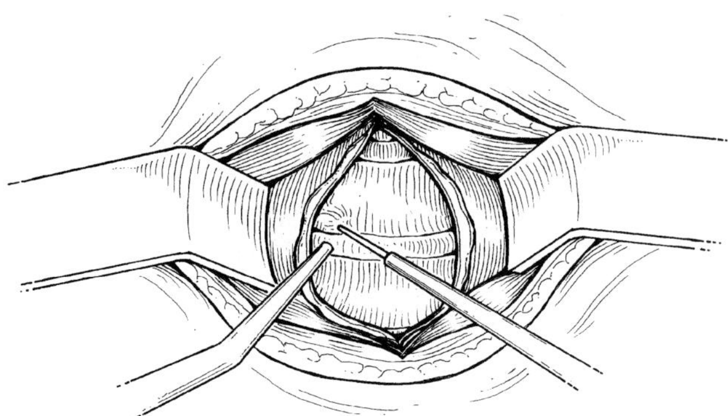

FIG. 5. The longus colli is subperiosteally dissected lateral from midline.

Transverse Incisions

As noted earlier, a transverse incision allows for a more cosmetically pleasing scar. This incision may be extended to allow for a three-, four-, or five-level corpectomy (1,2,15). Common palpable landmarks are used to localize the incision. Generally, the lower border of the mandible is at C2-3 and the hyoid bone is located at the C-3 vertebrae. The thyroid cartilage is at the C4-5 level, whereas the cricoid cartilage is anterior to C-6. The carotid tubercle (Chassaignac's tubercle) can be palpated adjacent to the carotid pulse on the anterior part of the transverse process of C-6 (Fig. 7). These landmarks are especially important for transverse incisions. A single lateral fluoroscopic image can be used to confirm the intended level of the skin incision, as well as confirm that the intended level can in fact be visualized, as it can be particularly difficult to visualize C6-7 in short-necked individuals. A technique the authors have found useful is to use a radiopaque marker, such as a self-adhesive electrocardiograph sticker or hemostat, and place it at the level of the intended skin incision. The incision is placed along the inferior one-third of the planned surgical levels because it is easier to mobilize the skin in a cephalad direction.

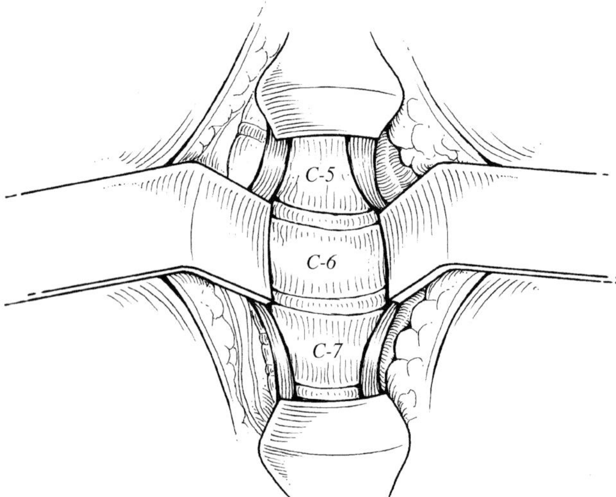

FIG. 6. Retractors are placed deep to longus colli muscle on lateral edge of vertebral body.

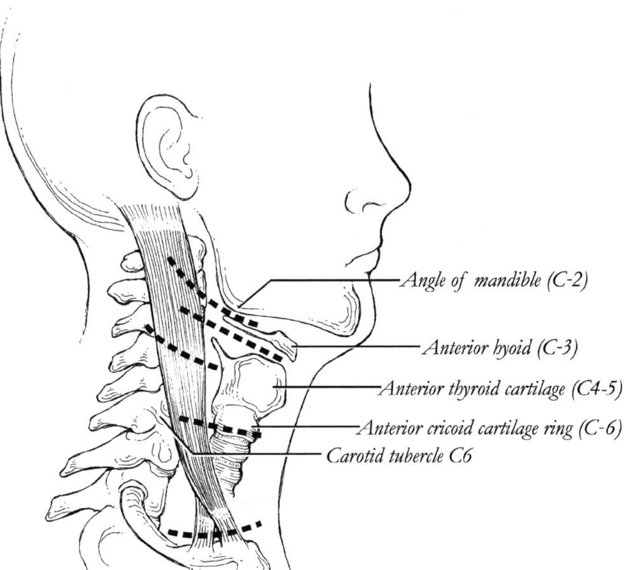

FIG. 7. Palpable landmarks used to localize the incision include the lower border of the mandible, hyoid bone, thyroid cartilage, cricoid cartilage, and Chassaignac's tubercle.

The omohyoid muscle is often encountered with extensive caudal dissection. It can be retracted out of the operative field or transected with electrocautery if it is well developed or hinders the surgical approach. If the omohyoid is transected, it is generally not primarily repaired during closure. The superior and inferior thyroid vessels may also be ligated. As previously mentioned, the superior laryngeal nerve courses with the superior thyroidal vessels and needs to be identified and protected. With a left-sided approach, the course of the recurrent laryngeal nerve is more consistent and, thus, more easily avoided. Decompression can be performed with or without microscopic visualization.

Difficulties with an Anterior Approach

One of the main difficulties that surgeons encounter with the use of the anterior approach is that the amount of root decompression is easily overestimated (23). The lateral limits of the decompression must be beyond direct visualization to equal that obtained posteriorly. Furthermore, some nerve roots leave the dural tube a significant distance above the interspace; thus, a soft disc fragment may migrate out of the interspace and behind the body to compress the root (23). As a result, this fragment may be missed using the anterior approach unless the root anatomy is carefully evaluated.

Complications

One of the most frequent complications involves injury to the recurrent laryngeal nerve (13,20). Injury to the nerve may result in unilateral vocal cord paralysis (20,22,24). The nerve can be protected by using long-blade retractors and ensuring that they are placed well under the medial edges of the longus colli muscles. Some authors advocate a left-sided approach because the course of the nerve is more predictable. However, there is also a higher learning curve for right-handed surgeons (16). Ebraheim et al. showed that the recurrent laryngeal nerve on the right side is highly vulnerable to injury if ligature of the inferior thyroid vessels is not performed as laterally as possible or if retraction of the midline structures along with the recurrent laryngeal nerve is not performed intermittently (13).

Hoarseness may also be secondary to irritation of the trachea, injury to the larynx, or during endotracheal intubation (5,21,24,25). The external laryngeal nerve, which crosses the neck adjacent to the superior thyroid artery and innervates the cricothyroid muscle, may also produce hoarseness. Another potential pitfall involves injury to a sympathetic nerve and stellate ganglion. These may be protected by subperiosteal dissection from the midline and avoiding extension of the dissection laterally to the transverse processes. Injury or irritation can result in Horner's syndrome (i.e., miosis, ptosis, and anhydrosis) (22).

Several vessels are also encountered during the dissection. The carotid sheath and its contents lie just posterior to the border of the sternocleidomastoid muscle. Avoid placing self-retaining retractors in the area of the carotid sheath. The use of blunt dissection of hand-held retractors may aid in the exposure. The vertebral artery is at particular risk during uncovertebral joint decompression or corpectomy (26). It should not be routinely visualized, although it is thought to be only approximately 4 to 5 mm anterior and lateral to the uncovertebral joint where it lies in the anterolateral transverse process. In the case of injury, tamponading the artery with Gelfoam appears to be the prudent approach because repair is difficult. Most injuries to the vertebral arteries are the result of the use of an air drill (26).

The inferior thyroid artery may also cross into the operative field during dissection to the subaxial cervical spine (16). If incidentally ligated, it may retract posterior to the carotid sheath and may be difficult to find. The thoracic duct may also be encountered on the left side during the approach to the subaxial cervical spine just lateral to the esophagus within the prevertebral fascia. It loops around the subclavian artery at the level of the first thoracic vertebrae. For this reason, some surgeons prefer to perform a right-sided approach if the ultimate site of surgery is at the cervicothoracic junction.

Potentially, one the most catastrophic complications involves injury to the esophagus or trachea (27). Injury may result in dysphasia with esophageal leak and resultant mediastinitis. This risk may be reduced by the anesthesiologist inserting a small, soft nasogastric tube to allow for proper visualization of the esophagus during the procedure. If the esophagus is accidentally perforated, it should be repaired primarily in several layers and irrigated, usually with the aid of a general or thoracic surgeon. Injury to the esophagus, or postoperative hematoma, may result in local compression of the trachea or "thirst hunger." This usually occurs on the first night after surgery, and the authors therefore recommend inserting a drain to bulb suction and admitting the patient overnight to an intensive care unit for observation with the head of the bed elevated to 60 degrees. This position permits postoperative bleeding that is not collected in the bulb suction to drain into the mediastinum. Should this potentially devastating complication occur, intubation should be avoided on the surgical ward and the patient should be taken back to the operative suite, where the wound can be decompressed in a controlled environment.

Injury to the trachea has been reported to occur in 0.25% of the cases, with nearly one-third of these occurring at the time of surgery (27). Late perforations, however, have been reported with the use of plates and screws. Particular care should be used with a cortical burr, keeping the burr within the confines of the disc space while turning it on and off during the procedure.

The most feared complication involves injury to the spinal cord and a resultant permanent or partial spinal cord deficit (11,28,29). Reasons for injury to the cord include vascular insult or cord syndrome secondary to cervical stenosis, mechanical insult, graft position, or extrusion. Graft extrusion can be minimized by placing the graft at least 2 mm beyond the edge of the vertebra. Anterior graft extrusion is minimized by use of an anterior cervical plate. Postoperative immobilization in a cervical collar can also minimize flexion and extension, which may lead to graft extrusion.

There is also an associated morbidity from the bone graft donor site if autologous graft is used. For iliac crest grafts, the most common donor site complications include infection, bleeding, injury to the lateral femoral cutaneous nerve, bowel perforation, iliac crest fracture, and unremitting pain (6,7,9,30,31). Careful attention to the anatomic landmarks, meticulous dissection, and watertight closure help prevent many of these complications.

ANTERIOR CERVICOTHORACIC APPROACHES

General Approach

Pathology located at the cervicothoracic junction presents certain challenges to the surgeon. The sternum and clavicle inhibit direct access, which is particularly difficult in individuals with short, stout necks. There are also significant mechanical forces present at the cervicothoracic junction, which tend to lead to kyphosis and collapse. Resultant kyphosis further decreases surgical access by standard anterior approaches. In general, specific anterior approaches to the upper thoracic spine and cervicothoracic junction are used for these special circumstances (32–36).

As with the other anterior approaches, a towel is used between the scapulae to hyperextend the neck and Gardner-Wells tongs are used for traction. For a left-sided approach, a transverse incision is placed approximately 2 cm proximal to the clavicle; however, some surgeons prefer a longitudinal incision. The incision is from lateral to the insertion of the sternocleidomastoid muscle to the midline, where it turns inferiorly and extends to the manubriosternal junction. The dissection is carried through the platysma muscle transversely, and the sternocleidomastoid muscle is subperiosteally dissected from the sternum and retracted proximally and laterally. The middle one-third of the clavicle is also dissected subperiosteally after the strap muscles are disconnected posterior to the clavicle. The clavicle is transected with a saw at the medial one-third and disarticulated from the manubrium. Blunt dissection is used to develop the plane between the carotid sheath laterally and the trachea and esophagus medially. During the development of this plane, the recurrent laryngeal nerve may be seen between the trachea and esophagus on the left-sided approach. The inferior thyroid vein may need to be ligated to improve access and visualization.

The prevertebral fascia is then visualized, and hand-held retractors are placed deep to enlarge the interval. Once the vertebral bodies are adequately identified, a spinal needle is placed into a disc space and intraoperative radiography is used to confirm the vertebral level. After completion of the procedure, a deep drain is placed and the strap muscles and medial clavicle are reapproximated. The sternocleidomastoid is sutured to the periosteum on the clavicle and the platysma is repaired.

Alternative Approaches

Other described techniques include median sternotomies, medial clavicle resection, partial sternal osteotomies, and combinations of these approaches (32,34–36). The median sternotomy approach was described by Cauchoix and Binet, and it includes a proximal extension of the Smith-Robinson approach (15). Although this approach gives excellent exposure to the T3-4 level, there is significant morbidity associated with this technique. As a result, there have been a number of less radical approaches described for exposure of the cervicothoracic junction (30,33).

Sundaresan proposed performing osteotomies of the medial portion of the left clavicle and the upper portion of the sternum (9,35,37). With this approach, it is important to identify and retract the brachiocephalic vein medially or laterally, while the midline structures are retracted to the right. Other authors have advocated a medial clavicle resection without a sternal osteotomy. This provides for an adequate exposure but is somewhat limited to a right-sided approach to the cervicothoracic junction, as caudal extension is difficult. In addition, the medial clavicle resection may have a detrimental effect on shoulder mechanics.

Darling advocated avoiding a proximal clavicle resection by making an L-shaped sternal cut (10,34). The advantage of this approach is that it allows for wide centralization of the upper thoracic vertebra without the associated morbidity of a sternotomy or a medial clavicle resection.

Considerations

The anterior cervicothoracic approach allows for extensive bony resection, spinal cord decompression, correction of deformity, spinal reconstruction, and stabilization (36). When increased exposure is needed, a medial one-third osteotomy is performed. Care must be taken when performing the osteotomy, as failure to remain subperiosteal during the dissection may result in vascular compromise. It may also be prudent to mobilize the great vessels to aid in the dissection, and particular attention should be given to identifying the thoracic duct during the left-sided approach. Accidental violation of the thoracic duct may lead to a chylothorax and the need for placement of a chest tube. Furthermore, the course of the recurrent laryngeal nerve, as previously discussed, must be taken into consideration.

POSTERIOR APPROACH TO THE CERVICAL SPINE

Specific pathology should be considered before choosing the anterior or posterior approach to the cervical spine. One drawback of the posterior approach is that one-fourth to one-half of the facet joint must be removed to unroof the neural foramen and provide access for surgical decompression (23). Anterior osteophytes in the region of the uncovertebral joint are also difficult to resect from a posterior approach unless they are very large (23).

Standard indications for the posterior approach include cervical myelopathy with spinal cord compression at three or more levels without associated kyphosis, unilateral radiculopathy at one or more levels, spinal cord compression secondary to degenerative subluxation, and spinal cord compression secondary to congenital spinal stenosis or acquired stenosis from posterior compression (10,37,38). In a patient without a previous laminectomy, exposure of the posterior cervical spine is relatively straightforward (8,16,39). However, if surgery is acutely performed after trauma, care must be taken not to depress or manipulate the fracture fragments, especially if there is a concomitant laminar fracture or instability. In this instance, electrocautery and sharp scalpel dissection may be safer than using a periosteal elevator. Dissection along the midline between the paraspinal muscles further minimizes bleeding and iatrogenic muscle trauma. In the subaxial cervical spine, dissection should be performed to the lateral margin of the lateral masses. Further dissection laterally only promotes increased bleeding.

Surgical Approach and Positioning

The midline approach to the posterior cervical spine is the most commonly used approach because it allows for safe and expedient access to the posterior cervical spine for the following indications: posterior cervical spine fusion, treatment of facet joint dislocations, treatment of tumors, excision of herniated discs, and nerve root exploration (17,40,41).

The patient is placed prone on an open table, with the neck flexed slightly to facilitate opening of the interspinous spaces. The head is usually secured in a Mayfield headrest or Gardner-Wells tongs. Alternatively, the patient may be seated upright with the use of a special brace; however, this method of positioning has been associated with air emboli and is not routinely used. The operating room table is tilted in reverse Trendelenburg position to ensure that the cervical spine is held roughly parallel to the floor. This allows for compression or collapse of the epidural vessels, thereby decreasing the risk of air emboli (Figs. 8–11).

Surgical landmarks include the C-2, C-7, and T-1 spinous processes, which are easily palpable as the most prominent

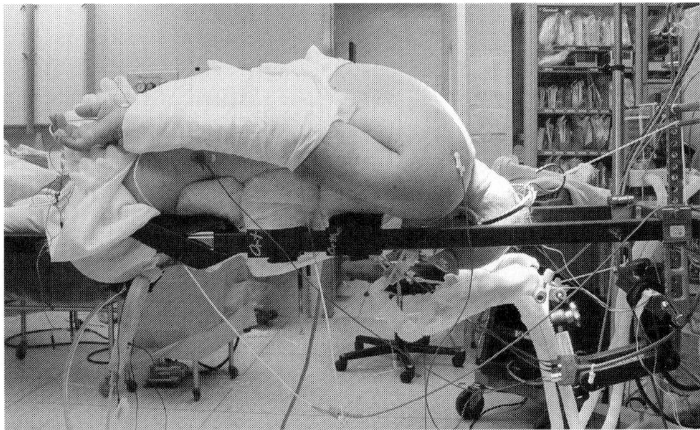

FIG. 8. This patient has ankylosing spondylitis and severe cervical kyphosis. He has been placed on a Jackson frame with his head suspended using Gardner-Wells tongs. This keeps the face and eyes completely free but allows for the repositioning of the neck intraoperatively without having to adjust the Mayfield headrest. The head is suspended with 15 to 20 lb of Gardner-Wells tong traction.

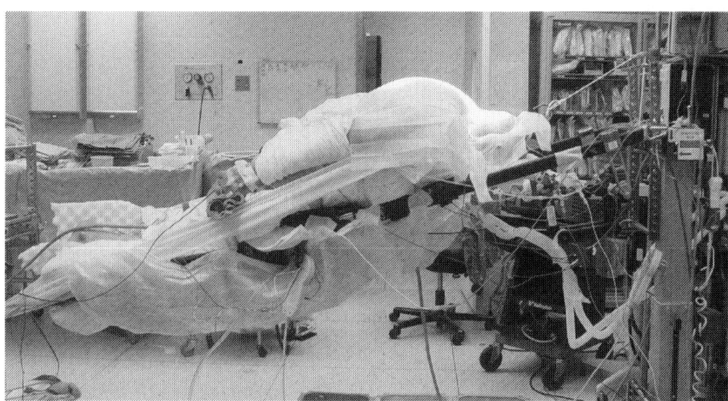

FIG. 9. The patient is placed in a reverse Trendelenburg position. A body-warming blanket is taped to the undersurface of the table such that the hot air rises and keeps the patient warm. The shoulders are gently taped down, and the arms are tucked. Using three bolsters on either side decompresses the abdomen, which reduces intraoperative bleeding.

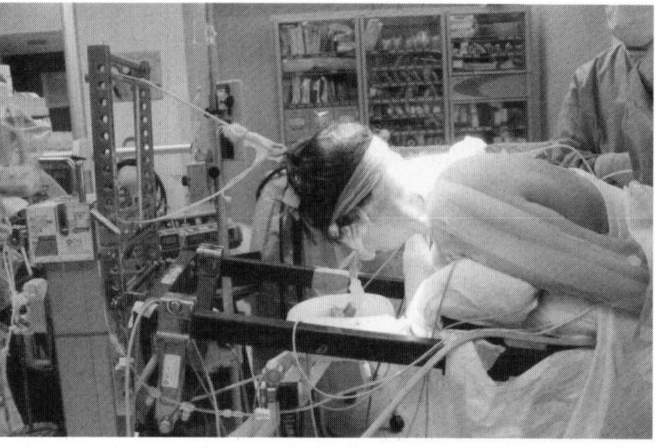

FIG. 11. After the foraminotomy, the weight is switched to the top rope. This restores the neck to a normal lordotic position, in which the fusion should be performed.

spinous processes. Although the C-7 spinous process is generally thicker, it is often difficult to differentiate C-7 from T-1; therefore, placement of a spinal needle in the one of the spinous processes with radiographic confirmation determines the proper level. Also, C-7 is thicker, is not bifid, and has a tubercle at its end.

A straight-midline incision is centered over the spinous processes. The skin over the posterior cervical spine is much thicker than that of the anterior aspect of the neck and is generally very vascular. The internervous plane is between the left and right paracervical muscles, which run in three layers and are segmentally innervated by the left and right posterior rami of the cervical nerves. The superficial layer consists of the trapezius muscle, whereas the splenius capitis comprises the intermediate layer. The deep layer consists of three parts—the semispinalis capitis superficially, the semispinalis cervicis in the middle, and the multifidus muscles, short and long rotator muscles deep.

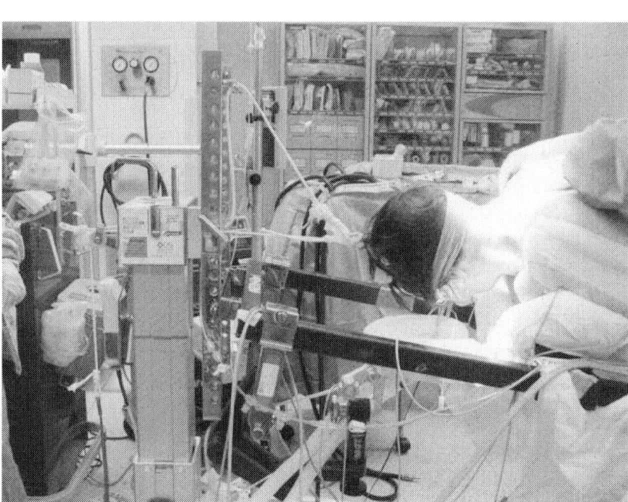

FIG. 10. When the patient requires a posterior cervical foraminotomy as well as a fusion, the authors use two ropes to suspend the head and neck. In this figure, the head is being suspended from the lower of the two ropes. This places the neck into a more flexed position, opening up the facet joints so it is easier to perform a foraminotomy procedure.

The paraspinal muscles should be dissected subperiosteally with electrocautery or a Cobb elevator to minimize bleeding. Bilateral exposure is performed for posterior cervical fusions and cord decompression, whereas unilateral exposure is generally reserved for foraminotomies and herniated disc excisions. The dissection can be carried as far laterally as needed to visualize the lamina, facet joints, and the transverse processes, but dissection beyond the lateral masses only increases unnecessary bleeding. The segmental arteries may need to be cauterized, as they run between the transverse processes in proximity to the facets.

The ligamentum flavum can be identified between the lamina of adjacent vertebrae. It takes origin from the leading edge of the lower lamina and inserts proximally into the ridges on the anterior surface of the superior vertebra. Each ligamentum flavum extends laterally from the midline to the joint capsule. Of note, the spinal cord is directly anterior to the ligamentum flavum, so care must be taken while removing this structure. When necessary, sharp dissection is used to remove it from the leading edge of the lamina of the inferior vertebra while a Woodson #3 or Penfield #1 may be used to protect the cord during sharp dissection. In addition, a laminectomy may be performed to expose the epidural fat and dura. Laterally, the dura may be gently retracted a few millimeters to expose the posterior portion of the vertebral body and disc space for disc excision. In this area, the epidural veins may bleed profusely and can be difficult to control between the anterior aspect of the cord and the posterior part of the vertebral body.

It is also important to appreciate that the laminae of the cervical vertebrae are angled from medial to lateral at approximately 45 degrees. The joint capsules lie lateral to the laminae and completely encompass the cervical facet joints. Unless a fusion is planned, care should be taken to avoid the joint capsules.

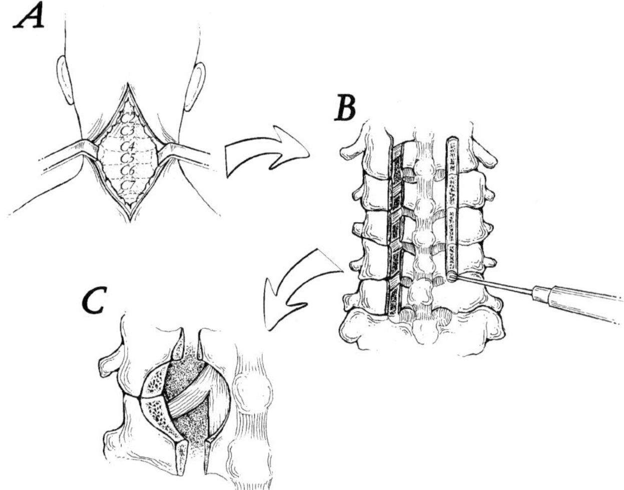

FIG. 12. A: Posterior spine exposed subperiosteally. **B:** The laminoplasty can be performed by creating two bone gutters with a burr, medial to the facets. **C:** Foraminotomies can be performed with laminoplasty to decompress the nerve root.

Posterior Nerve Root Decompression and Foraminotomy

As noted earlier, precise localization is performed with placement of a spinal needle and a lateral fluoroscopic image. A posterior midline incision, approximately 3 to 4 cm long, is made between the two spinous processes at the desired level, and the dissection is carried down to the laminae. Retractors are placed, and the operating microscope (authors' preferred method) or loupe magnification is used to enhance visualization. A small circular defect is made at the lateral intersection of adjacent lamina with a high-speed air drill or Kerrison rongeur. The bone is then thinned near the level of the nerve root. The working area for drilling proceeds interpedicularly, thus forming the rectangular portion of the "keyhole." Once the lamina has been thinned, the extension of this hole is completed with the use of a curette or Kerrison rongeur. This prevents thermal or mechanical damage to the neurovascular structures in the area. The area of decompression is explored with a Woodson elevator or nerve hook as the instrument is passed between the tissues surrounding the nerve root and foramen. If resistance or "tightness" is noted, the foraminotomy should be enlarged. Failure to adequately decompress the nerve root is the most common postoperative complaint (Fig. 12).

Complications

Several structures are at risk during the posterior approach to the cervical spine. These include the spinal cord, which can be injured as a result of compression during resection of the posterior elements or undue retraction (10). This can be obviated by obtaining additional exposure with a larger laminectomy. The nerve roots should also be gently retracted to prevent postoperative tethering due to adhesions.

Although somewhat less morbid if injured, the vasculature of around the spinal cord can be somewhat problematic. The venous plexus in the cervical canal has a very thin wall and may bleed profusely. The use of bipolar cautery is helpful in this region to control venous bleeding. The segmental blood supply is also plentiful to the paracervical muscles and can result in significant bleeding. These vessels should be aggressively ligated to stop bleeding. Occasionally a nutrient vessel from the spinous process may bleed, and this can be controlled with cautery or bone wax.

REFERENCES

1. Robinson RA, Smith GW. Anterolateral cervical disc removal and interbody fusion for cervical disc syndrome. *Bull Johns Hopkins Hosp* 1955;96:223–224.
2. Smith GW, Robinson RA. The treatment of certain cervical-spine disorders by anterior removal of the intervertebral disc and interbody fusion. *J Bone Joint Surg* 1958;40A(3):607–623.
3. Bailey R, Badgley C. Stabilization of the cervical spine by anterior fusion. *J Bone Joint Surg* 1960;42A:565.
4. Cloward R. The anterior approach for removal of ruptured cervical disks. *J Neurosurg* 1958;15:602.
5. Herkowitz HN. Anterior cervical surgery in cervical spondylosis. Presented at the American Academy of Orthopaedic Surgeons annual meeting, Washington, DC, 1992.
6. Riley L. Anterior cervical spine surgery. *Instr Course Lect* 1978;27: 154–158.
7. Rothman RH, Simeone FA. Cervical disc disease. In: Rothman RH, Simeone FA, eds. *The spine*, 2nd ed. Philadelphia: WB Saunders, 1982:440–449, vol. 1.
8. Mayfield FH. Cervical spondylosis: a comparison of the anterior and posterior approaches. *Clin Neurosurg* 1965;13:181–188.
9. Simmons EH, Bhalla SK. Anterior cervical discectomy and fusion (keystone technique). *J Bone Joint Surg Br* 1969;51:225–237.
10. Herkowitz HN. A comparison of anterior cervical fusion, cervical laminectomy, and cervical laminoplasty for the surgical management of multiple level spondylotic radiculopathy. *Spine* 1988;13: 774–780.
11. Whitecloud TS. Anterior surgery for cervical spondylotic myelopathy: Smith-Robinson, Cloward and vertebrectomy. *Spine* 1988;13 (17):861–863.
12. McAfee PC, et al. The anterior retropharyngeal approach to the upper cervical spine. *J Bone Joint Surg* 1987;(69A):1371–1383.
13. Ebraheim NA, Lu J, Skie M, et al. Vulnerability of the recurrent laryngeal nerve in the anterior approach to the lower cervical spine. *Spine* 1997;22(22):2664–2667.
14. Southwick WO, Robinson RA. Surgical approaches to the vertebral bodies in the cervical and lumbar regions. *J Bone Joint Surg Am* 1957;39:631–644.
15. Cauchoix J, Binet J. Anterior surgical approaches to the spine. *Ann R Coll Surg Engl* 1957;27:237–243.
16. Yaeger VL, Cooper MH. Surgical anatomy of the cervical spine surrounding structures. In: Young PH, ed. *Microsurgery of the cervical spine*. New York: Raven Press, 1991:1–17.
17. Reference deleted.
18. Bulger RF, Rejowski JE, Beatty RA. Vocal cord paralysis associated with anterior cervical fusion: consideration for prevention and treatment. *J Neurosurg* 1985;62:657–661.
19. Welch LW, Welsh JJ, Chinnici JC. Dysphagia due to cervical spine surgery. *Ann Otol Rhinol Laryngol* 1987;96:112–115.
20. Weisberg NK, Spengler DM, Netterville JL. Stretch induced nerve injury as a cause of paralysis secondary to the anterior cervical approach. *Otolaryngol Head Neck Surg* 1997;116(3):316–317.
21. Whitecloud TS. Complications of anterior cervical fusion. *Instr Course Lect* 1978;27:223–227.
22. Tew JM, Mayfield FH. Complications of surgery of the anterior cervical spine. *Clin Neurosurg* 1976;23:424–434.
23. Raynor RB. Anterior or posterior approach to the cervical spine: an anatomical and radiographic evaluation and comparison. *Neurosurgery* 1983;12(1):7–13.

24. Brodsky A. Management of radiculopathy secondary to acute cervical disk degeneration and spondylosis by the posterior approach. In: Cervical Spine Research Society, ed. *The cervical spine*. Philadelphia: Lippincott , 1983:395–402.
25. Herkowitz HN. The surgical management of cervical spondylotic radiculopathy and myelopathy. *Clin Orthop* 1994;239:94–108.
26. Smith MD, Emery SE, Dudley A, et al. Vertebral artery injury during anterior decompression of the cervical spine. A retrospective review of ten patients. *J Bone Joint Surg Br* 1993;75:410–415.
27. Newhouse K, Lindsey R, Clark C, et al. Esophageal perforation following anterior cervical spine surgery. *Spine* 1989;14:1051–1056.
28. Bohlman H. Cervical spondylosis with moderate to severe myelopathy. *Spine* 1977;2:151–162.
29. Kraus FR, Stauffer ES. Spinal cord injury as a complication of elective anterior cervical fusion. *Clin Orthop* 1975;112:1310.
30. Kurz LT, Pursel SE, Herkowitz HN. Modified anterior approach to the cervicothoracic junction. *Spine* 1991;5:542–549.
31. DePalma A, Rothman RH, Lewinnek G, et al. Anterior interbody fusion for severe cervical disk degeneration. *Surg Gynecol Obstet* 1972;134:777.
32. An HS, et al. Spinal disorders at the cervicothoracic junction. *Spine* 1994;19(22):2557–2564.
33. Charles R. Anterior approach to the upper thoracic vertebrae. *J Bone Joint Surg* 1989;71:81–84.
34. Darling GE, McBroom R, Perrin R. Modified anterior approach to the cervicothoracic junction. *Spine* 1995;20(13):1519–1521.
35. Sundaresan N, et al. An anterior surgical approach to the upper thoracic vertebrae. *J Neurosurg* 1984;61:686–690.
36. Kurz LT, Pursel SE, Herkowitz HN. Modified anterior approach to the cervicothoracic junction. *Spine* 1991;16(10):S542–S547.
37. Hase HT, Watanabe, Hirasawa Y. Bilateral open laminoplasty using ceramic laminas for cervical myelopathy. *Spine* 1991;16:1269–1276.
38. Hirabayashi K, Watanabe, Wakano K. Expansive open-door laminoplasty for cervical spinal stenotic myelopathy. *Spine* 1983;8:693–699.
39. Epstein JA. The surgical management of cervical canal stenosis, spondylosis, and myeloradiculopathy by means of the posterior approach. *Spine* 1988;13:864–869.
40. Rogers WA. Treatment of fracture dislocations of the cervical spine. *J Bone Joint Surg* 1942;24:245.
41. Holdsworth FW. Fractures, dislocations and fracture dislocations of the spine. *J Bone Joint Surg Br* 1963;45:6.

CHAPTER 40

Internal Fixation of the Cervical Spine

A. Occiput and Upper Cervical Spine*

Jonathan J. Baskin, Paul J. Apostolides, Curtis A. Dickman, and Volker K. H. Sonntag

The craniovertebral junction (CVJ) is comprised of the occipital bone, the first two cervical vertebrae (atlantoaxial complex), and their soft-tissue articulations. Traumatic disruption of these osseous elements, their tethering ligaments, or both can cause immediate instability of this most rostral region of the axial skeleton. Alternatively, these bony and soft-tissue structures can be compromised over a more prolonged and insidious course. Patients with degenerative, inflammatory, infectious, developmental, or neoplastic processes involving the CVJ typically have progressive clinical symptoms related to worsening mechanical incompetence and compression of the upper cervical spinal cord and lower brainstem. The surgical management of patients with instability of the CVJ must, therefore, achieve neural decompression and structural stabilization. Technical considerations related to the latter topic are the primary concern of this chapter.

Most contemporary spine surgeons use stabilization techniques that rely on titanium-based materials (magnetic resonance imaging–compatible) to establish immediate rigid internal fixation of the occipitocervical junction and the C1-2 complex. These techniques have significantly increased the frequency of arthrodesis compared to earlier methods that used only onlay autologous bone to promote fusion in this particularly mobile region of the spine. The use of internal rigid fixation limits the need for routine postoperative external bracing with a halo orthosis. Consequently, convalescence is more comfortable and patients can resume productive activities more rapidly after surgery.

Hardware fatigue and its eventual failure are time-dependent certainties when a solid arthrodesis is absent. Therefore, regardless of the particular instrumentation used, meticulous attention to the biologic and mechanical principles that influence the fusion response is crucial to attain a successful clinical outcome. This chapter focuses on the authors' preferred method of performing posterior atlantoaxial arthrodesis using a combination of transarticular facet fixation and interspinous wiring and also their preferred method of occipitocervical fusion using a contoured, threaded Steinmann pin or titanium grooved rod that is anchored with suboccipital and sublaminar wires. Alternative methods of stabilizing the occipitocervical junction with screw plates are also discussed.

INDICATIONS

Atlantoaxial fusion is indicated for patients with C1-2 instability. Occipitocervical fusion is indicated for patients with occipitocervical instability, including those with rheumatoid settling, primary basilar invagination, occipitoatlantal dislocation, or primary or metastatic neoplastic disease that involves the CVJ. Occipitocervical fusion can also be used as a "salvage" procedure for a failed C1-2 arthrodesis or for complex atlantoaxial fractures in which interspinous wiring or transarticular screw fixation is unfeasible or contraindicated.

*Adapted from Baskin JJ, Apostolides PJ, Dickman CA. Posterior atlantoaxial and occipitocervical fixation and fusion techniques. In: Tornetta P III, O'Brien M, Sandhu H, eds. *Techniques in fracture surgery*. St. Louis: Mosby, 2000, with permission.

OPERATIVE TECHNIQUE

Preoperative Preparation and Positioning

Typically, patients with occipitocervical or atlantoaxial instability arrive in the operating room wearing an external cervical orthosis, such as a hard collar or halo vest. Preoperatively, the patient's hair is shaved in the occipitocervical midline from the inion to over the spinous process of C-5. Intravascular access is secured, and a prophylactic dose of antibiotic (i.e., cefuroxime, 1.5 g, or cefazolin, 2.0 g) is administered. The patient is intubated, often using an awake fiberoptic technique to minimize the risk of neurologic injury from an inadvertent occipitocervical or atlantoaxial dislocation. Paralytic medications are not used with the anesthetic agents to avoid exacerbating instability of the CVJ. Clinical evidence of spinal cord or nerve root irritation can then also be monitored during the procedure.

Intraoperatively, somatosensory, motor, and brainstem auditory evoked potentials are assessed. Baseline waveforms are often recorded before the patient is rotated into the prone position. If patients have severe preoperative myelopathy or instability, or if the evoked potentials change significantly during surgery, methylprednisolone may be administered in accordance with the North American Spinal Cord Injury Study (NASCIS III) guidelines. Postoperatively, the steroid is discontinued if the patient's neurologic examination is stable.

If the patient is wearing a cervical collar, the Mayfield headholder (Codman, Inc., Raynham, MA) is applied before prone positioning. If the patient is wearing a halo brace, the Mayfield adaptor is connected to the halo ring to fixate the patient to the operating table (Fig. 1). A lateral cervical radiograph is obtained after the patient is positioned to assess the atlantoaxial or craniovertebral alignment. Intraoperative fluoroscopy is used if closed manipulation of the vertebral column is required before the procedure begins or for performing open reduction before instrumentation is placed. For atlantoaxial arthrodesis, transarticular screws are inserted under direct, continuous fluoroscopic guidance.

Autologous bone is the substrate of choice to promote posterior cervical arthrodesis, and an allograft bone is an unreliable secondary choice. The donor site must be prepared in a sterile fashion at the start of the procedure, and it must be accessible after draping. Interspinous wiring of the C1-2 complex relies on a bicortical strut graft fashioned from a tricortical graft obtained from the posterior iliac crest. The authors have seldom found a surgical drain to be necessary at this site if meticulous attention is directed toward hemostasis. Iliac crest bone (cortical and cancellous grafts) is preferred for occipitocervical fusion. Autologous rib provides an excellent alternative to the iliac crest for onlay corticocancellous bone. With its use, fusion rates have been comparable to those associated with iliac crest grafts, and morbidity at the donor site is minimal (1).

Skin Incision and Soft-Tissue Dissection

The surgical exposures necessary for performing posterior atlantoaxial and occipitocervical fusions are similar. The rostral aspect

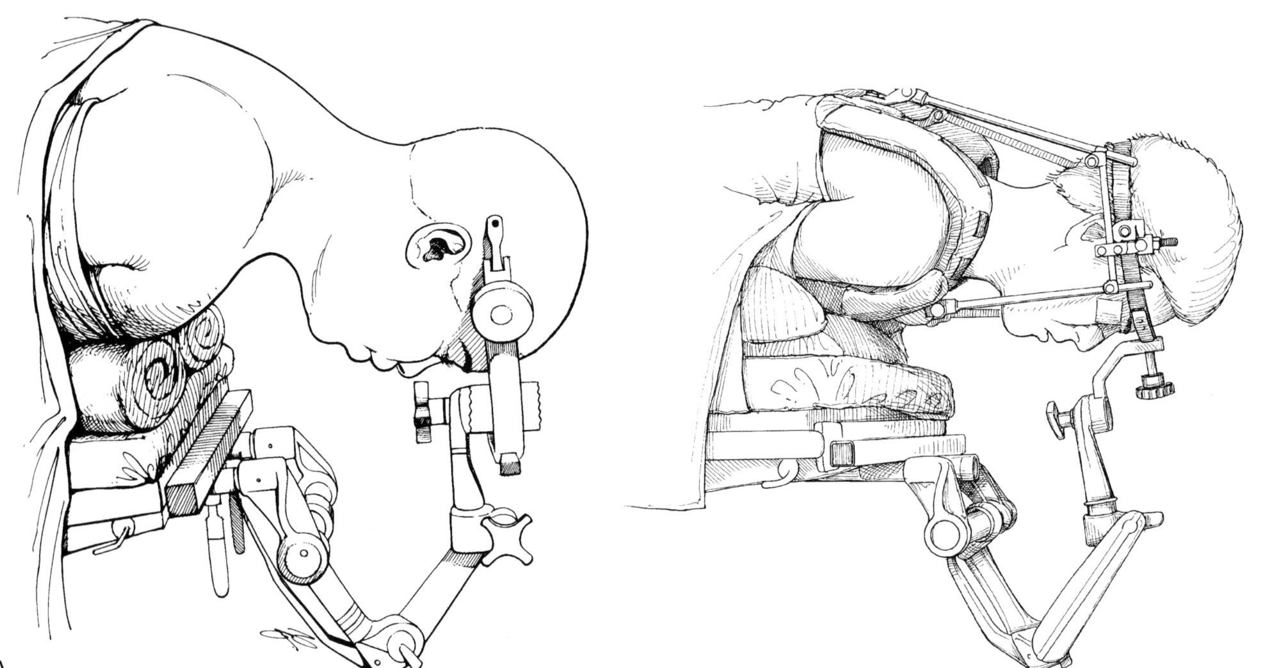

FIG. 1. A: Patients are placed in the prone position and secured to the surgical table using the Mayfield headholder (Codman, Inc., Raynham, MA). Patients with craniovertebral instability are positioned while wearing a hard cervical collar to minimize the risk of a harmful loss of reduction. **B:** The Mayfield halo adaptor is used to stabilize patients wearing a halo brace. The posterior aspect of the halo vest can be removed to allow access to the iliac crest for autologous bone graft material. The posterior bars of the halo apparatus can be removed from the surgical field. Alternately, they function well as hand rests for surgeons during the procedure. (From Barrow Neurological Institute, with permission.)

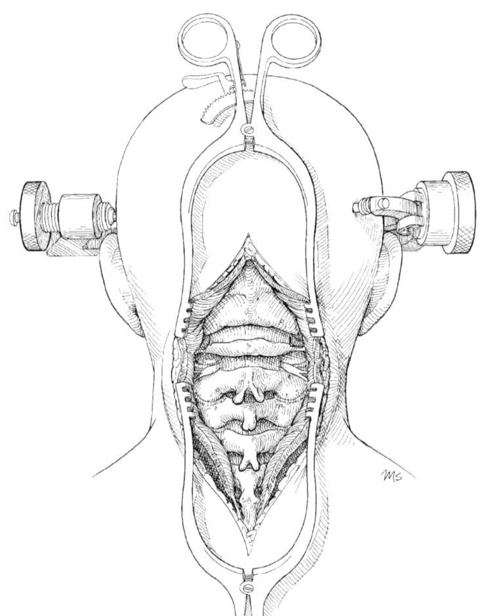

FIG. 2. The posterior midline surgical exposure for both occipitocervical and atlantoaxial fusion techniques. For occipitocervical fusion, slightly more of the occipital bone needs to be exposed to allow placement of burr holes for suboccipital wire passage. (From Barrow Neurological Institute, with permission.)

of exposure is the external occipital protuberance. The minimum extent of caudal dissection includes the complete exposure of the dorsal elements of the first three cervical vertebrae. Further caudal dissection may be necessary if additional fixation points are warranted to maximize the stability of the construct. Soft-tissue dissection is limited to the levels of craniovertebral instability to avoid inadvertent fusion or potential destabilization of normal motion segments.

After a standard sterile preparation, the inscribed midline incision is infiltrated with 0.5% lidocaine with epinephrine for hemostasis. The skin and subcutaneous tissues are incised down to the dorsal cervical fascia, and this plane is mobilized laterally to facilitate closure. The avascular midline plane between the cervical paraspinal muscles is dissected using monopolar cauterization to expose the underlying occipital squama and the spinous processes of the cervical vertebrae.

Sharp dissection and cauterization are used to elevate this muscle laterally in a subperiosteal plane along the occipital bone and cervical laminae. Adequate soft-tissue retraction and bony exposure provide unimpeded visualization of the foramen magnum and the upper three cervical laminae bilaterally as far as the lateral aspect of their respective facet joints (Fig. 2). For occipitocervical fusion procedures, the occipital bone is exposed slightly more to allow the Steinmann pin to be seated and the appropriate burr holes to be placed for suboccipital wire passage. During the course of dissecting and retracting soft tissues, meticulous care should be exerted to avoid dislocation of unstable vertebral segments.

Atlantoaxial Fixation and Fusion

At the authors' institution, the treatment of choice for atlantoaxial instability entails a combination of interspinous wiring (2) and transarticular facet screw placement (3). The immediate rigid three-point internal fixation provided by this construct eliminates the need for a routine postoperative halo orthosis.

Not all patients with C1-2 instability are candidates for both techniques, however. Interspinous wiring requires the presence of intact posterior elements at C-1 and C-2. These structures can be compromised as a consequence of trauma, degenerative processes, or the laminectomy performed for neural decompression. If interspinous wiring is impossible, the C1-2 complex can be stabilized by the isolated placement of transarticular screws or by performing an occipitocervical fusion that extends to the adjacent vertebrae. Finally, anteriorly placed C1-2 transarticular screws are available as a "salvage" procedure to secure atlantoaxial stability when circumstances prevent placement of posterior fixation devices (4).

Prospective analysis has demonstrated that almost 20% of patients harbor regional anatomy that contraindicates transarticular screw placement on at least one side (5), usually owing to a unilateral anomaly. Of 94 patients in this same study, the anatomy of three (3.2%) was unsuitable bilaterally for transarticular screw placement. Thus, when C1-2 transarticular screws are contemplated, the workup should include fine-cut computed tomographic scans in the plane of the transarticular screw with sagittal reconstructions. These studies permit the width of the pars interarticularis and the proximity of the vertebral artery to the proposed screw course to be assessed. Other contraindications to unilateral placement of a transarticular screw include fractures of the C-1 lateral mass or C-2 pars interarticularis. The inability to realign C-1 on C-2 before surgery also precludes transarticular screw placement and is associated with a high risk for vertebral artery injury.

In addition to the risks for neurovascular injury, screw malpositioning is also associated with a high risk for screw fracture. If interspinous wiring and transarticular screw placement are deemed feasible, the latter procedure is performed first. A single transarticular screw in conjunction with interspinous atlantoaxial wiring confers sufficient stability to obtain excellent fusion outcomes after immobilization in a hard collar (6).

As noted, fluoroscopy is used to direct patient positioning to achieve an appropriate atlantoaxial reduction and to estimate the proper trajectories for drill and screw passage. Cervical flexion is usually required to facilitate transarticular screw placement. However, the degree of flexion needed to insert the screw from within the operative wound is sometimes impossible to achieve due to the associated risk of dislocating the atlantoaxial junction. Rather than extending the skin incision and muscle dissection caudally, the screws are delivered percutaneously along the necessary trajectory through the pars interarticularis of C-2 and the lateral mass of C-1 (Fig. 3). Before the patient is draped, the locations of the stab incisions for percutaneous placement are estimated using fluoroscopy and must be included within the sterile field.

The key anatomic landmarks for transarticular screw placement include the posterior elements and facet joints between C1-2 and C2-3. The C1-2 facet is directly visualized by using a Penfield dissector to gently retract the C-2 nerve root and its associated venous plexus rostrally. The medial border of the pars interarticularis of C-2 is also visualized directly to ensure that screw placement does not violate its medial border and encroach on the vertebral canal. In preparation for subsequent interspinous wiring, soft tissues between the posterior elements of C-1 and C-2 are removed using curettes and rongeurs before any instrumentation is placed.

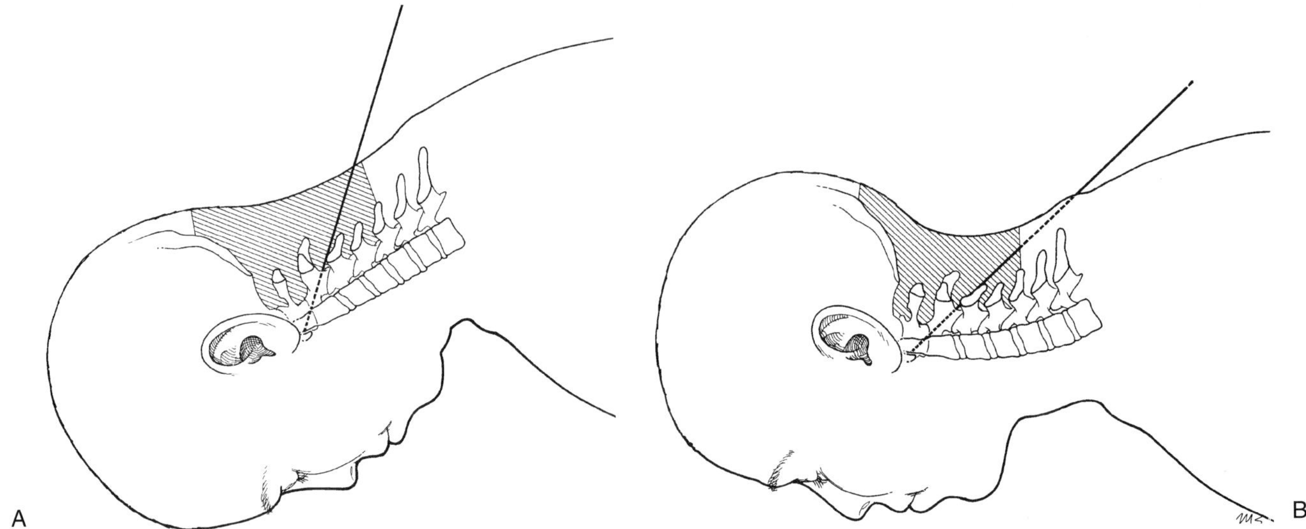

FIG. 3. Some element of cervical flexion is necessary to achieve the proper trajectory for transarticular screw placement. The shaded area illustrates the typical extent of soft-tissue dissection (inion to the C-5 spinous process). **A:** In some circumstances, adequate flexion can be performed safely so that the transarticular screw can be inserted from within the surgical site. **B:** The more common percutaneous technique used to compensate when a lesser degree of cervical flexion is possible. (From Barrow Neurological Institute, with permission.)

Transarticular Screw Placement

The authors prefer a cannulated screw technique for C1-2 fixation using the Universal Cannulated Screw System (Sofamor-Danek, Memphis, TN). A long, thin Kirschner (K)-wire is used to drill the initial path across the C1-2 facet. The wire fixates the adjacent unstable segments and guides screw placement. Because its diameter is narrow, the K-wire can be repositioned to optimize screw location without sacrificing potential screw purchase.

The atlas and axis must be realigned before the transarticular screw is placed. If the atlas has been dislocated anteriorly, open manipulation can be performed by applying tension to a sublaminar wire at the C-1 level (which can later be used for interspinous wiring). An Allis clamp applied to the C-2 spinous process can further facilitate open reduction of C-1 on C-2.

The screw entry point is 2 to 3 mm above the caudal edge of the C-2 inferior facet and 2 to 3 mm lateral to the medial border of the C2-3 facet (Fig. 4). A high-speed drill is used to penetrate the cortical bone at the entry point to help seat and direct the K-wire.

The screw trajectory is estimated with fluoroscopy by holding a long instrument adjacent to the patient's neck and thorax. If screw insertion cannot proceed directly through the incision and percutaneous delivery is necessary, a tunneling instrument (i.e., a tissue sheath and stylet) is passed carefully through the paraspinal soft tissues and positioned adjacent to the C2-3 facet. The C-2 pars interarticularis and C1-2 facet joint should be visualized directly to achieve the proper mediolateral screw trajectory during K-wire and screw insertion.

The stylet is removed from the tissue sheath and the K-wire drill guide is inserted. A 50-cm long, 1.2-mm diameter, end-threaded K-wire is attached to a reversible pneumatic drill and passed through the drill guide to the screw entry point. The medial surface of the C-2 pars interarticularis is defined with a No. 4 Penfield dissector (Fig. 5). The C-2 nerve root and venous plexus are retracted upward to provide direct visualization of the C-2 pars and the posterior aspect of the C1-2 facet joint. The K-wire is aimed between 0 and 10 degrees medial to the point of screw entry through the central axis of the pars interarticularis (Fig. 6). Lateral fluoroscopic monitoring is used to adjust the trajectory of the K-wire so that its tip is aimed at the middle of the C-1 tubercle (Fig. 7). The anterior C-1 tubercle is a crucial landmark for directing transarticular screw placement. Other investigators have reported an association between screw malposition

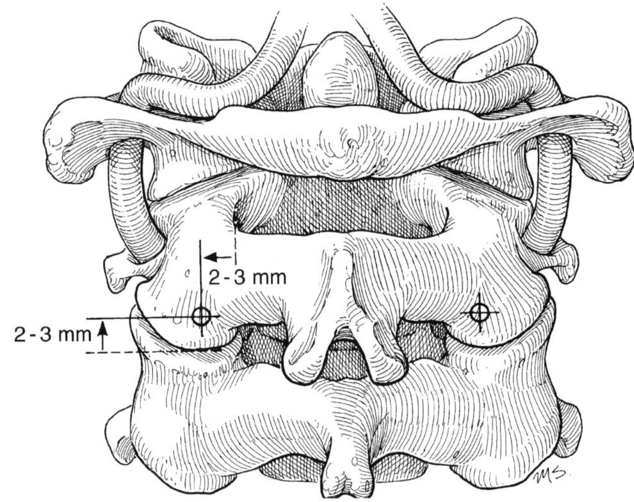

FIG. 4. The entry point for transarticular screw placement is depicted. The anatomy of individual patients may require this entry point to be modified to avoid intercepting the vertebral artery. (From Barrow Neurological Institute, with permission.)

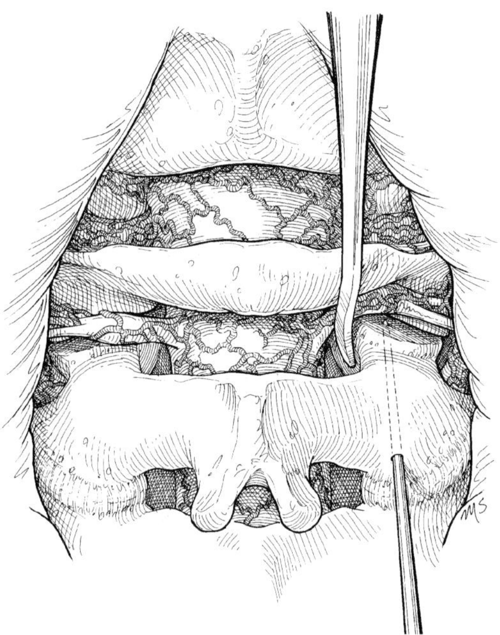

FIG. 5. Before the transarticular screws are placed, the most medial aspect of the C-2 pars interarticularis is visualized. The C1-2 facet joint is also visualized by rostral displacement of the C-2 nerve root and its accompanying venous plexus. A Kirschner wire has been placed through the entry point (see Fig. 4) and is about to cross the C1-2 facet joint. (From Barrow Neurological Institute, with permission.)

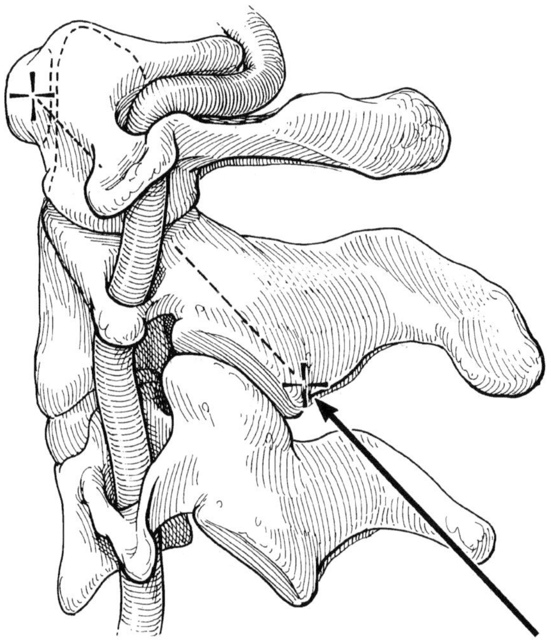

FIG. 7. The trajectory for C1-2 transarticular screw placement. A key landmark for deriving the trajectory is the anterior tubercle of the atlas. Failure to visualize this structure before the screw is placed under fluoroscopic guidance has been correlated with a substantially increased risk of positioning the screw suboptimally. (From Barrow Neurological Institute, with permission.)

and an absent C-1 tubercle (7). Thus, the authors attempt to preserve at least a portion of this structure during a transoral odontoidectomy in the event that transarticular screw fixation is necessary later.

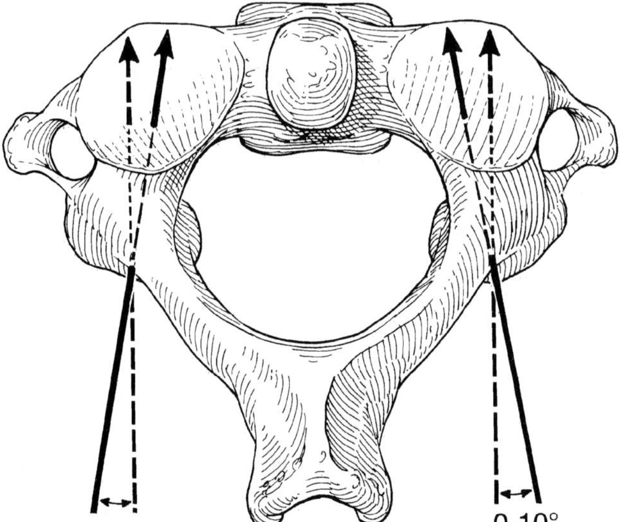

FIG. 6. The transarticular screw is placed along the longitudinal axis of the pars interarticularis. Slight medial angulation may be necessary to avoid the vertebral artery. Overcompensation can cause the screw to encroach on the vertebral canal. (From Barrow Neurological Institute, with permission.)

Once the proper screw trajectory has been determined, the K-wire is drilled through the C-2 pars interarticularis, across the posterior edge of the C1-2 facet joint, and into the lateral mass of C-1 under fluoroscopic guidance. To avoid creating excessive torque on the K-wire that could cause it to bend or break, the position of the drill guide and sheath should not be altered after the K-wire begins to engage the bone. If its trajectory is suboptimal, the K-wire should be removed completely by reversing the drill direction and reinserted along a new tract through a new entry point on the bone surface. Screws placed too ventrally can penetrate C-1 anteriorly and enter the pharynx. Screws placed too rostrally can cross the occipitoatlantal joint and injure the hypoglossal nerve or produce a painful occipitocervical joint. Screws placed too laterally can injure the vertebral arteries, and screws placed too medially can injure the spinal cord.

After the K-wire is positioned satisfactorily in the bone, a second K-wire of identical length is inserted into the tissue sheath until it contacts the bone surface. The difference between the ends of the K-wires is then measured with a ruler to determine the appropriate screw length. A fully threaded screw or an end-threaded screw can be used for fixation. In general, the widest diameter (3.5 vs. 4.0 mm), self-tapping cannulated screw that the patient's anatomy will accommodate should be used to fixate the C1-2 complex. If the patient's bone is soft, the self-tapping, self-drilling screw can be inserted directly over the K-wire. If the bone is normal, it often needs to be tapped before the screw is inserted. If the bone is hard, a pilot hole is made with a cannulated 2.0- or 2.5-mm drill and then tapped. The screw is placed over the K-wire and inserted into the bone using a hollow screwdriver (Fig. 8). The surgeon must carefully avoid

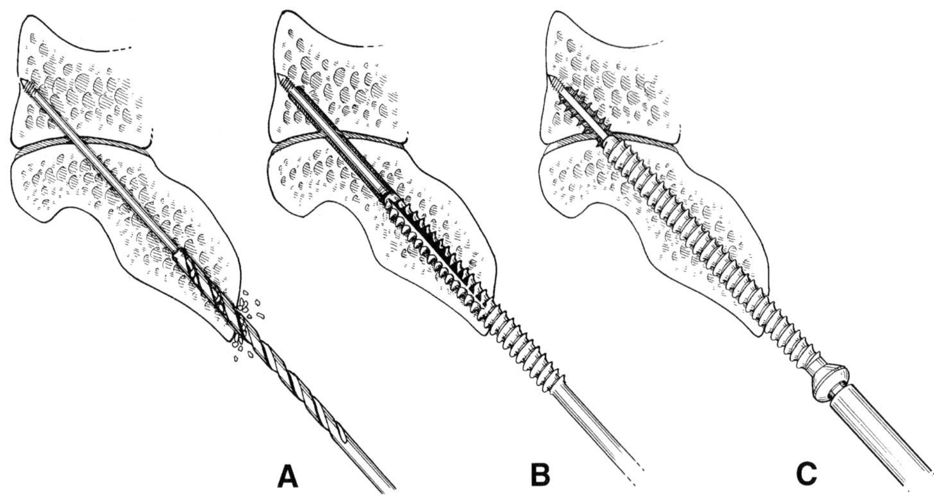

FIG. 8. A: After the Kirschner wire has crossed the C1-2 joint and has obtained adequate purchase of the C-1 lateral mass, a pilot hole is drilled with a cannulated drill bit. **B:** After the screw course has been tapped, the cannulated screw is placed **(C)**. (From Barrow Neurological Institute, with permission.)

advancing the K-wire while preparing the pilot holes or inserting the screws. The end of the K-wire should protrude beyond the end of the tap and screwdriver handles and be anchored by the surgical assistant with a needle holder. As the screw engages the bone, the positions of the K-wire and screw are monitored fluoroscopically. When the screw crosses the joint space into the lateral mass of C-1, the surgeon typically feels a characteristic stiffness as the atlas and axis lock together.

Once the screw has crossed the atlantoaxial articular surface and is satisfactorily seated within the distal bone, the K-wire is removed using the pneumatic drill. The screw head should be recessed slightly into the bone to prevent the screw from levering against the C2-3 joint space. An overtightened screw can shear through its thread track and destroy its purchase in the bone. The final position of the screw is verified with fluoroscopy in the anteroposterior and lateral planes. The contralateral screw is inserted in an identical manner. Suspicion of a vertebral artery injury during the initial screw insertion precludes placement of a contralateral screw. Of note, the successful application of frameless stereotactic navigational technology to spinal surgery currently enables transarticular screw insertion with enhanced accuracy and without the need for intraoperative fluoroscopy.

Interspinous Wiring

A variety of posterior atlantoaxial wiring techniques have been described, and each has its advocates (8). The authors believe that the advantage of the interspinous wiring method, as described by Sonntag (2,8), resides in its combination of excellent biomechanical characteristics for resisting rotational and translational forces and the safety of requiring sublaminar wire passage at only a single level (C-1). A partial invagination of the posterior C-1 ring into the foramen magnum can impede passage of the sublaminar wire. In that instance, rather than shave down (and weaken) the rostral aspect of the dorsal C-1 arch, the foramen magnum is enlarged to provide adequate room for safe sublaminar passage. The adjacent edges of the posterior caudal C-1 arch and rostral C-2 spinous process and lamina are decorticated with a high-speed drill or Kerrison rongeur. The inferior surface of the C-2 laminae is notched bilaterally to seat the wires at the spinolaminar junction (Fig. 9).

A tricortical bone graft (approximately 4 cm long × 3 cm high) is obtained from the posterior iliac crest. A bicortical, curved strut graft is created by removing the rounded cortical margin with a Leksell rongeur. The strut graft is sized to fit between the posterior arches of C-1 and C-2 under compression and to recreate the normal height of the C1-2 complex. The inferior margin of the bone graft is notched at its midpoint so that it straddles the C-2 spinous process. After the graft has been contoured adequately, it is removed from the field until the sublaminar wire is positioned.

A braided sublaminar cable, positioned under direct visualization of the epidural space, is used for interspinous wiring. The cable is passed beneath the posterior C-1 arch in the midline where the

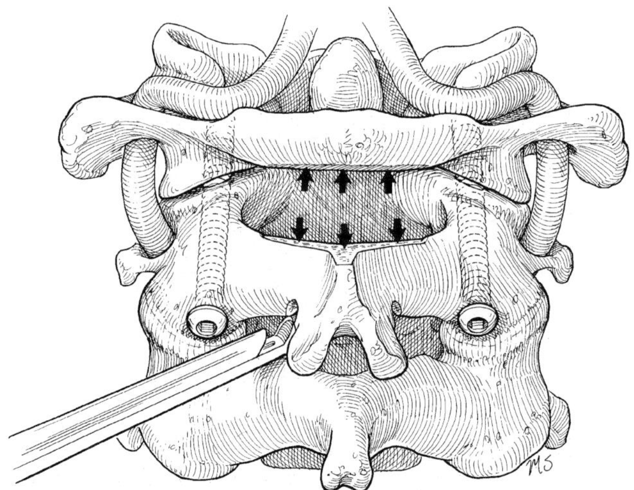

FIG. 9. Interspinous fusion is performed after the transarticular screws have been placed. The adjacent surfaces of the C1-2 posterior elements are decorticated to enhance the likelihood of integrating the autologous strut graft. A Kerrison rongeur is used to notch the spinolaminar junction bilaterally at the caudal aspect of the C-2 level to allow seating of the braided interspinous wires. (From Barrow Neurological Institute, with permission.)

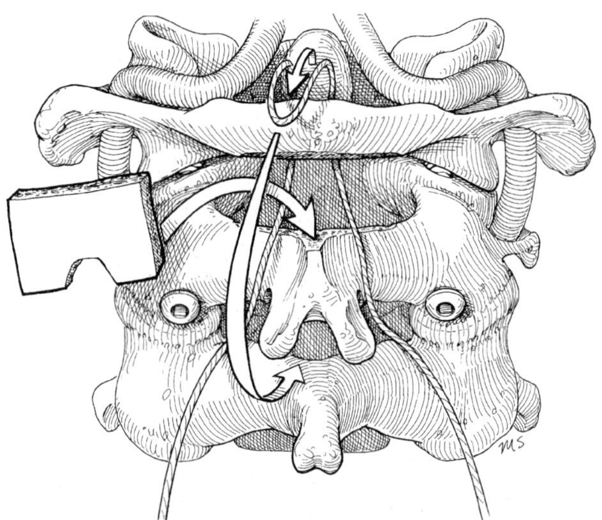

FIG. 10. A sublaminar wire is looped ventral to the posterior ring of C-1. It is passed in a caudal-to-rostral fashion with care exerted to avoid compressing the underlying dura. The autologous strut graft is then positioned between the lamina of C-1 and C-2, and the sublaminar loop is "doubled back" over the C-2 spinous process (Sonntag fusion). (From Barrow Neurological Institute, with permission.)

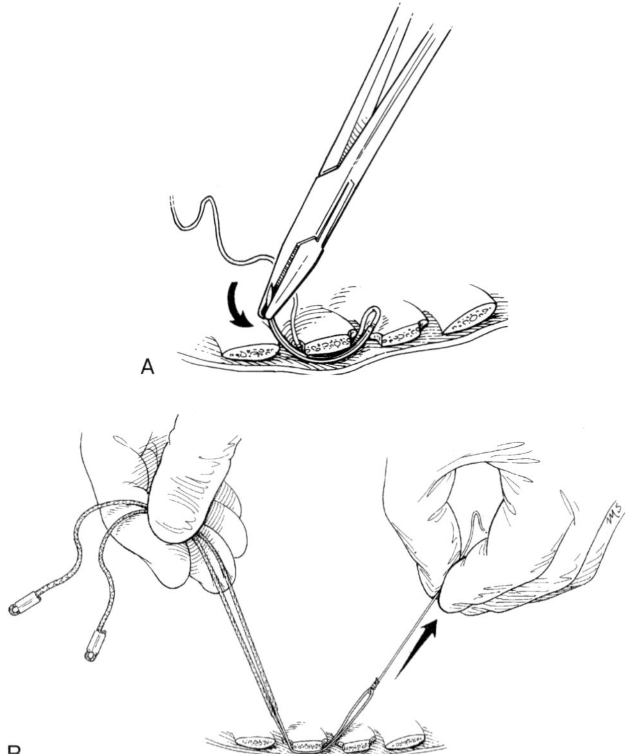

FIG. 11. Sublaminar wire passage. **A:** The blunt end of a needle is passed retrograde along the sublaminar course. The suture is pulled through, and the needle is removed. **B:** The suture is tied to the cable loop, and both are simultaneously "fed and pulled" to avoid developing slack in the wire that could compress the spinal cord. (From Barrow Neurological Institute, with permission.)

epidural space is widest (Fig. 10). Sublaminar wire passage is facilitated by passing the blunt end of a large needle attached to a 2-0 Vicryl suture under the posterior C-1 arch, tying it to the cable loop, and passing both under the C-1 arch with a simultaneous feeding-pulling technique (Fig. 11). Complications associated with sublaminar wire passage are related to allowing the wire to bow ventrally and compress the spinal cord. Every effort is therefore expended to ensure that the wire hugs the undersurface of the lamina during passage and maintains a low profile.

The graft is repositioned between the atlas and axis. The loop of cable is passed over the posterior C-1 ring, over the dorsal surface of the graft, and secured in the notches beneath the C-2 spinous process. The free ends of the cable are positioned anteriorly to the graft and are also seated beneath the notched C-2 spinous process. The cable is tightened and crimped with the bone graft secured between the surrounding cables and posterior elements of C-1 and C-2. At the time of cable tightening, careful observation is required to ensure that the wire does not cut through the laminae of C-1 or C-2. The surfaces of the dorsal atlantoaxial complex and bone graft are decorticated with a high-speed air drill (Fig. 12). Continuous irrigation is employed to minimize the risk of thermal injury to the fusion bed that could cause bone resorption or otherwise impede arthrodesis. Morcellized, cancellous bone graft from the iliac crest is compressed against the fusion surfaces. Curettes, osteotomes, or drills can also be used to remove the articular surfaces of the C1-2 facets, which can then be packed with autologous cancellous bone to further promote arthrodesis.

Occipitocervical Fixation and Fusion

Occipitocervical fusion is performed to treat occipitoatlantal instability or atlantoaxial instability that is not amenable to or has failed previous efforts at arthrodesis. Several metal implants are available for fixation of the occipitocervical junction. These include threaded/grooved titanium or steel rods, smooth steel templates, a titanium frame, and a variety of screw plates (Fig. 13). At the

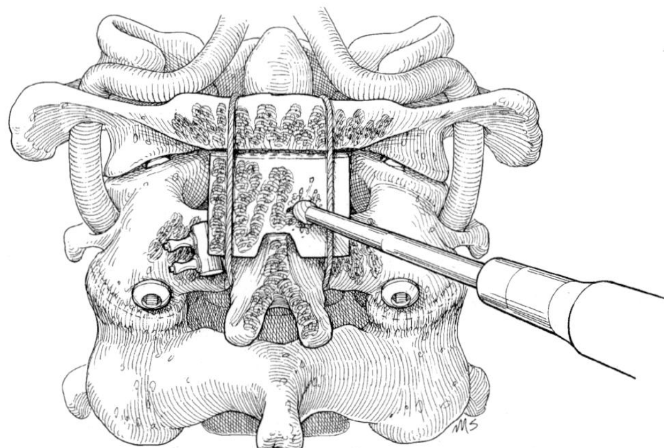

FIG. 12. After the interspinous wire has been tightened and crimped, the dorsal elements of C1-2 and the autologous graft are decorticated to maximize the surface area of exposed cancellous bone. (From Barrow Neurological Institute, with permission.)

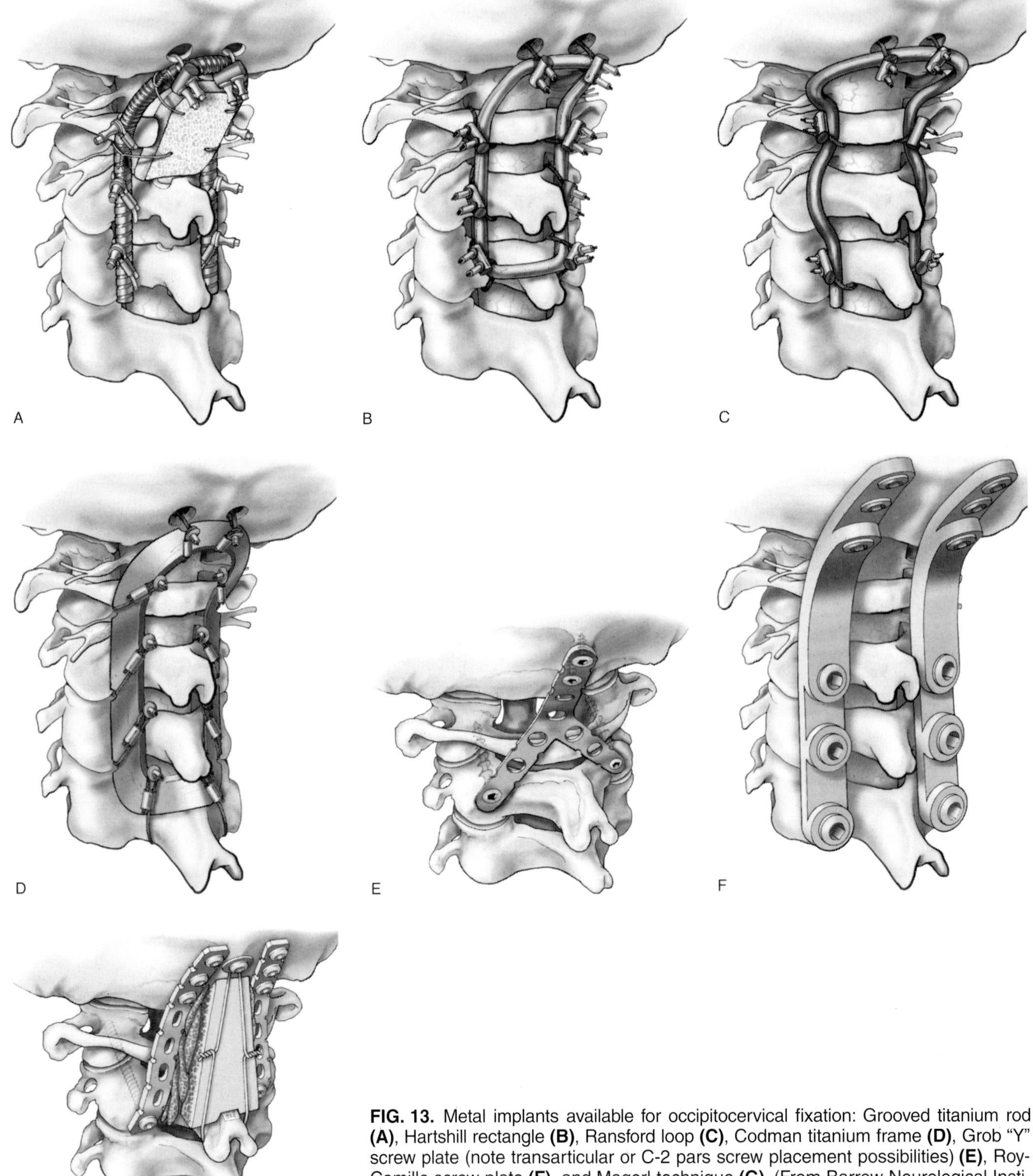

FIG. 13. Metal implants available for occipitocervical fixation: Grooved titanium rod **(A)**, Hartshill rectangle **(B)**, Ransford loop **(C)**, Codman titanium frame **(D)**, Grob "Y" screw plate (note transarticular or C-2 pars screw placement possibilities) **(E)**, Roy-Camille screw plate **(F)**, and Magerl technique **(G)**. (From Barrow Neurological Institute, with permission.)

authors' institution, a fully-threaded, $^5/_{32}$-in. diameter, grooved titanium rod is preferred to anchor the occipitocervical fusion mass (9). The grooved rod helps resist compaction or "telescoping" of the fusion construct, which can lead to vertical migration of the dens into the foramen magnum. Regardless of the surgeon's preference for implant, however, the cables or screws used to secure the device should be made of the same metal to avoid accelerated corrosion, early fatigue, and instrument failure.

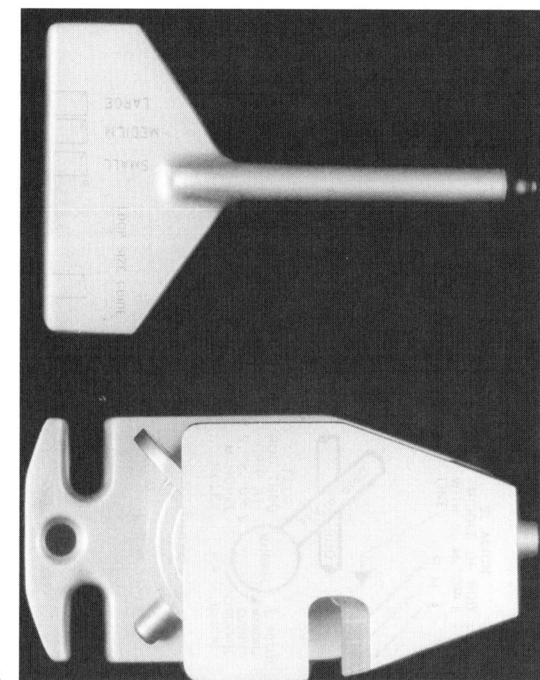

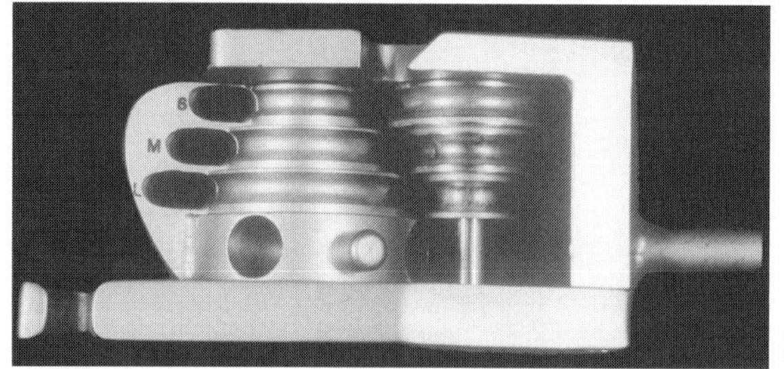

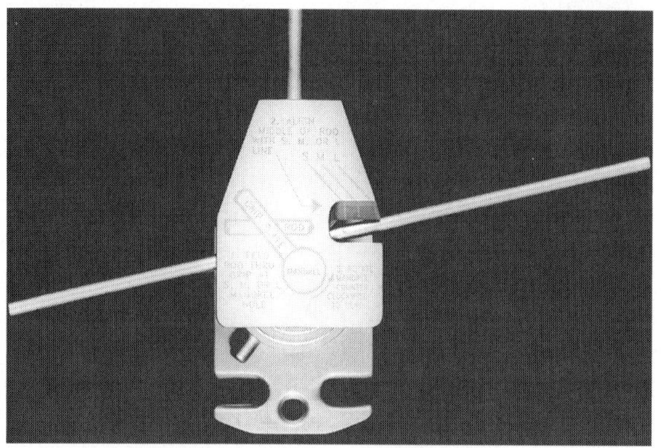

FIG. 14. A: The BendMeister Rod Bender has two components, including a Rod Bender handle (*top*) and the Rod Bender proper (*bottom*). **B:** Lateral view of the Rod Bender bending mandrel with the options for small (S), medium (M), and large (L) radii of curvature. **C:** Lateral surface of the rod bender with instructions for creating a primary curve in a pin. (From Apostolides PJ, Karahalios DG, Sonntag VKH. Use of the BendMeister Rod Bender for occipitocervical fusion. Technical note. *Neurosurgery* 1998;43:389–391, with permission.)

The authors rely on a unique rod bender (BendMeister, Sofamor-Danek, Memphis, TN) that permits easily reproducible contouring of the pins with smooth primary and secondary curves (10). In contrast, other methods of rod shaping (e.g., table vises, bending irons, French benders) can produce sharp angles and notch rods, thereby creating stress risers and diminishing the biomechanical strength of the metal. Smooth curves distribute forces more uniformly on the rod and help to optimize its strength and to increase its resistance to breaking. Use of the rod bender further simplifies the performance of occipitocervical fusion procedures, because only one size titanium rod or Steinmann pin is needed in the operating room at the time of custom sizing (Fig. 14A–C). In contrast, reliance on precontoured loops or rectangles requires the availability of multiple implant sizes and shapes (degrees of curvature) for any one patient.

In devising an occipitocervical fusion construct, achieving adequate rigidity must be balanced against minimizing the number of cervical motion segments sacrificed for that purpose ("as long as necessary, but as short as possible"). The number of levels that should be incorporated in a particular occipitocervical fusion is influenced by the degree of preoperative instability. For patients with occipitocervical instability, intact posterior laminar elements, and no anterior compressive pathology or basilar invagination, the authors perform the fusion procedure through the axial level (occiput C1-2). Patients who require an anterior decompressive transoral odontoidectomy usually require a subsequent occipitocervical fusion. These patients often require additional points of fixation to stabilize their fusion construct sufficiently, as do patients with evidence of basilar invagination. The authors usually immobilize these patients with a fusion mass that extends to C-3 or C-4. For patients with incompetent posterior elements, as a result of traumatic injury or a requirement for posterior decompression of the vertebral canal, the authors typically extend the occipitocervical fusion at least two levels below the unstable segment. If the lamina of a particular level is incompetent, facet wires can be used to anchor the titanium rod. Comparatively, sublaminar wires have greater strength to resist pulling out and provide more rigid immobilization than facet wires. Thus, they are the preferred fixation method. Occipitocervical screw plates provide an option for fixation that does not require sublaminar wire passage. They are especially useful if cervical laminae are incompetent or absent (Fig. 13F,G).

All soft tissues in the region of the proposed fusion site should be removed, including the occipitoatlantal membrane between the foramen magnum and C-1 and the interspinous ligaments and ligamentum flavum between C1-2 and C2-3. The posterior rim of the foramen magnum can be enlarged with a high-speed air drill to facilitate suboccipital epidural wire passage for anchoring the titanium rod to the skull base. Three burr holes are placed within the occipital bone approximately 1 cm away from the margin of the enlarged foramen magnum and off the midline. The burr holes are waxed, and the dura is dissected away from the inner table of the skull toward the foramen magnum. If the foramen magnum is relatively inaccessible because the patient's anatomy is anomalous or cervical flexion is limited, three sets of burr holes can be placed around the periphery of the foramen magnum, between which the suboccipital wires are passed. The laminae to be wired are often notched as medially as possible to facilitate wire passage (Fig. 15).

Suboccipital wires are passed between the occipital burr holes and foramen magnum in whichever direction appears to be easiest.

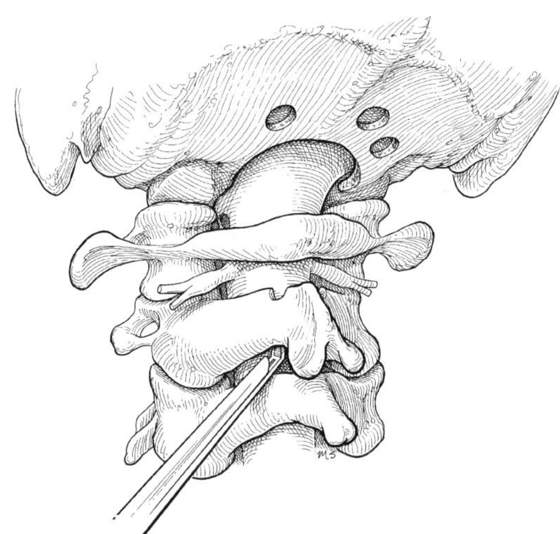

FIG. 15. Preparation for occipitocervical fusion. Suboccipital burr holes are placed for wire passage out through the foramen magnum. The most medial aspect of the lamina to receive a sublaminar wire is notched to facilitate wire passage. (From Barrow Neurological Institute, with permission.)

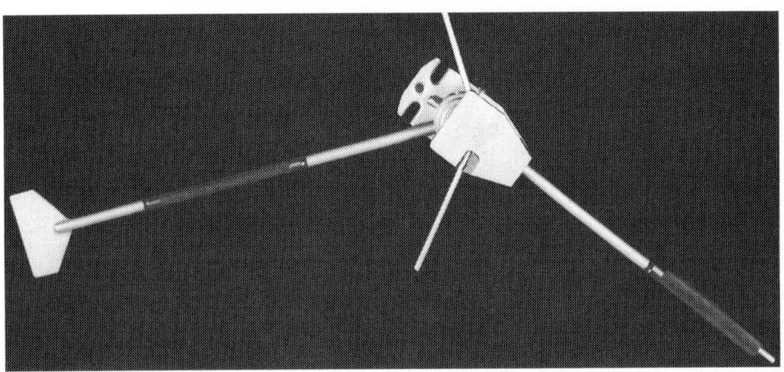

FIG. 16. Insertion of the handle into the Rod Bender with counterclockwise rotation and creation of a primary curve. (From Apostolides PJ, Karahalios DG, Sonntag VKH. Use of the BendMeister Rod Bender for occipitocervical fusion. Technical note. *Neurosurgery* 1998;43:389–391, with permission.)

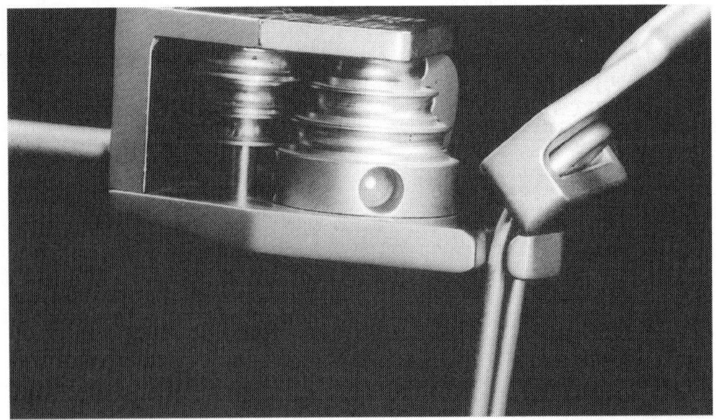

FIG. 17. At its end, the Rod Bender has a bending hole that holds the rod after its primary curve has been created. The secondary curve is formed using the paddle end of the Rod Bender handle. (From Apostolides PJ, Karahalios DG, Sonntag VKH. Use of the BendMeister Rod Bender for occipitocervical fusion. Technical note. *Neurosurgery* 1998; 43:389–391, with permission.)

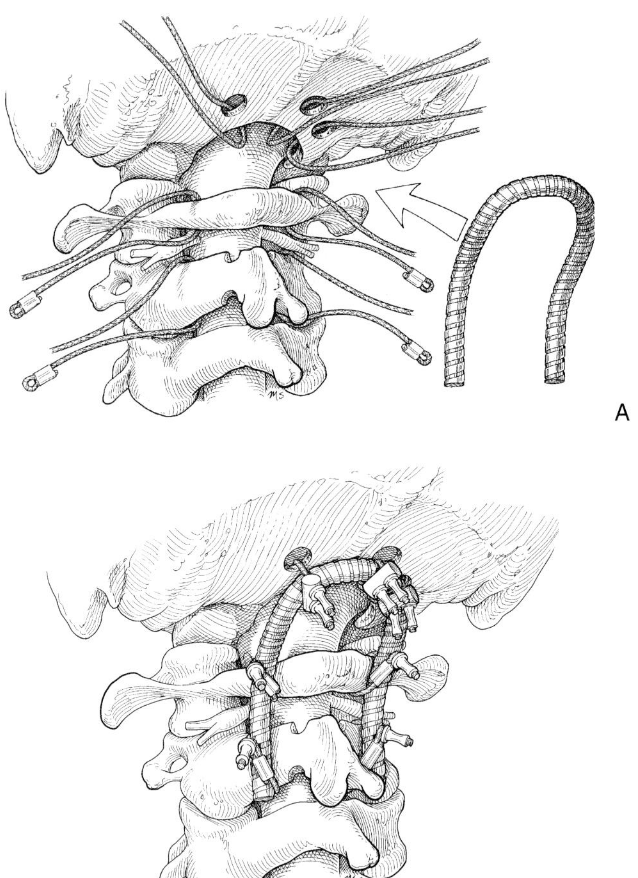

FIG. 18. A: Sublaminar and suboccipital wires have been positioned, and the contoured, grooved pin is seated flush against the osseous craniovertebral surfaces. The sublaminar wires were passed medially within the vertebral canal and then carefully mobilized laterally for fixation. Three suboccipital burr holes have been placed with the epidural wires brought through the foramen magnum. **B:** Final construct of Steinmann pin with suboccipital and sublaminar wires. (From Barrow Neurological Institute, with permission.)

The tip of the wire is bent into a blunt loop to help avoid violation of the dura. Using the technique described for interspinous wiring of the atlantoaxial complex, sublaminar wires are passed as medially as possible to minimize the risks of neurologic injury or cerebrospinal fluid leaks. Sublaminar wires are positioned at the most lateral aspects of the laminae when the construct is in final position.

A wide diameter (5/32-in.), threaded stainless steel Steinmann pin or titanium grooved rod is contoured to the anatomy of the patient's CVJ. The pin must be shaped precisely to maximize the area of metal-bone interface, which creates the most stable fixation construct. A sterile, malleable, endotracheal tube stylet is used to model the shape of the CVJ and to serve as a template for contouring the pin.

A primary U-shaped curve (Fig. 16) and smooth secondary curves (Fig. 17) are made with the BendMeister Rod Bender. When placed into the wound, the pin should lie flush against the occiput and laminae. Gaps between the pin and bone surfaces suboptimally fixate the unstable segments and can allow exces-

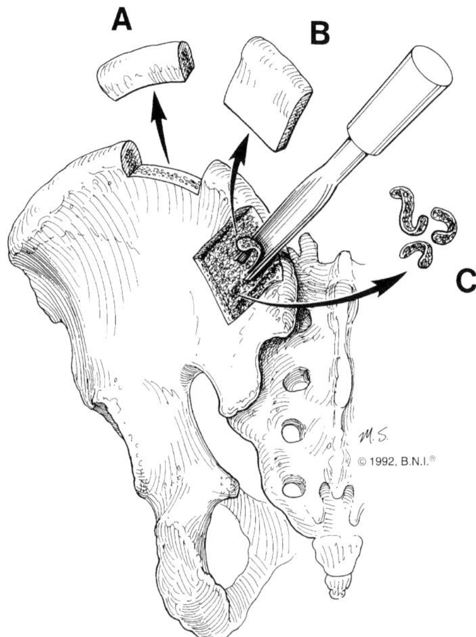

FIG. 19. Autologous iliac crest bone. Bone harvest is usually contained within 6 to 8 cm lateral to the sacroiliac joint to avoid injury to the cluneal nerves. The sacroiliac joint itself is left intact to avoid causing pelvic pain or instability. A tricortical bone graft (*A*) is harvested for the infraspinous C1-2 fusion and wiring procedure. The tricortical bone segment is modified to a bicortical strut graft and is sized to fit the interspinous space between C1-2 using a Leksell rongeur. Osteotomes can be used to cut a window in the posterior iliac crest to yield a unicortical plate (*B*) and cancellous bone (*C*) for occipitocervical fusion. (From Barrow Neurological Institute, with permission.)

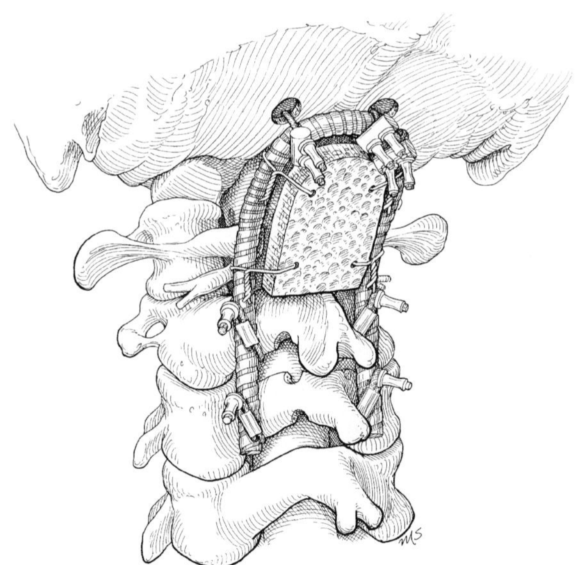

FIG. 20. In the case of a C-1 laminectomy, a unicortical graft can be sutured or wired to the Steinmann pin to function as a template for osseous integration and to preserve the decompression of the craniovertebral junction. (From Barrow Neurological Institute, with permission.)

sive motion that can lead to instrument failure and nonunion. The ends of the pin are cut so that they do not extend beyond the lowest segment to be fused. Failure to do so risks causing leverage on the hardware that can destabilize the fixation construct or unintentionally incorporate an additional motion segment within the fusion mass.

The pin is wired against the occiput and cervical laminae or facets (Fig. 18A,B). The occiput, facet joints, and posterior arches of the cervical levels to be fused are decorticated with curettes and a high-speed air drill to maximize the surface area for bone incorporation. Generous amounts of autologous, cancellous, iliac crest bone grafts are compressed against the levels to be fused (Fig. 19). If a suboccipital craniectomy or cervical laminectomy is required to decompress the neural elements, a unicortical plate of iliac crest bone can be sutured or wired to the central portion of the rod to act as a template for the fusion and to preserve the neural decompression (Fig. 20). A routine multilayered wound closure is performed.

ORTHOSES AND POSTOPERATIVE FOLLOW-UP

After atlantoaxial and occipitocervical fusion procedures, patients are usually maintained in a hard cervical collar. Patients are evaluated at 2- to 4-week intervals to assess their clinical progress and the healing of their fusion. After 10 to 12 weeks, dynamic radiographs with cervical flexion and extension are obtained to assess the stability of the construct. Patients with C1-2 instability who cannot have transarticular screws placed routinely have their interspinous wiring supplemented with a halo brace. Poor bone quality (e.g., rheumatoid arthritis), significant ligamentous instability (e.g., occipitoatlantal dislocation), and other individual patient characteristics that negatively impact the anticipated success of bone healing, such as malnutrition, cigarette smoking, metabolic disorders, exogenous steroid use, or a history of previously unsuccessful fusion attempts, are potential indications for halo bracing after rigid internal fixation to optimize the chances for fusion.

COMPLICATIONS

The potential risks associated with atlantoaxial or craniovertebral stabilization techniques include infection; bleeding requiring transfusion with the associated possibilities of transfusion reactions or infection (hepatitis or human immunodeficiency virus); medical complications (myocardial infarction, pneumonia, urinary tract infection, or deep venous thrombosis); high cervical myelopathy due to craniovertebral manipulation or sublaminar wire passage with its associated requirements for tracheostomy and placement of a feeding tube; lower cranial nerve injury; stroke related to injury of the vertebral artery; intracranial hemorrhage related to suboccipital wire passage; dural tear with a cerebrospinal fluid leak; suboccipital numbness; hardware failure with breakage of the screws, wires, or pin; and failure to obtain bony arthrodesis. Risks of surgery also include those related to donor site morbidity, such as infection, hematoma, cosmetic deformity, and prolonged pain or numbness.

The predominant concern regarding these procedures is to avoid a vertebral artery or spinal cord injury. A recent survey of 101 neurosurgeons who had placed transarticular screws in 1,318 patients (2,492 screws placed) reported the risk for vertebral artery injury at 2.2% per screw. Only two patients with a known or suspected vertebral artery injury manifested neurologic deficits. Only one patient, who sustained bilateral vertebral artery injuries, died (11). The well-recognized risk of myelopathy related to cervical sublaminar wire placement (12) can be minimized by carefully passing wires in a "push-pull" method as described and by exposing the dura widely so it can be visualized for distortion during wire passage.

CONCLUSION

Combining transarticular screw placement and interspinous wiring represents an excellent technique for rigidly fixating C1-2. Occipitocervical fixation with titanium or steel implants and sub-occipital and sublaminar wires confers immediate rigid internal fixation in patients with occipitocervical instability. The procedures are technically demanding. Absolute familiarity with the regional anatomy is mandatory for surgeons planning to perform these procedures. The great variability in CVJ anatomy among patients, particularly at C1-2, requires patients to undergo a thorough radiographic workup to insure accurate preoperative planning. The outcomes of arthrodesis with these techniques are excellent, and morbidity rates are low in experienced hands. Regardless of the internal fixation technique used, careful preoperative planning and adherence to time-proven surgical principles are fundamental to achieving successful arthrodesis.

REFERENCES

1. Sawin PD, Traynelis VC, Menezes AH. A comparative analysis of fusion rates and donor-site morbidity for autogeneic rib and iliac crest bone grafts in posterior cervical fusions. *J Neurosurg* 1998; 88:255–265.
2. Dickman CA, Sonntag VKH, Papadopoulos SM, et al. The interspinous method of posterior atlantoaxial arthrodesis. *J Neurosurg* 1991;74:190–198.
3. Marcotte P, Dickman CA, Sonntag VKH, et al. Posterior atlantoaxial facet screw fixation. *J Neurosurg* 1993;79:234–237.
4. Apostolides PJ, Karahalios DG, Sonntag VKH. Use of the Bend-Meister rod bender for occipitocervical fusion. *Neurosurgery* 1998;43:389–391.
5. Apostolides PJ, Dickman CA, Sonntag VKH. Anterior atlantoaxial facet screw fixation. In: Dickman CA, Sonntag VKH, Spetzler RF, eds. *Surgery of the craniovertebral junction.* New York: Thieme Medical Publishers, 1998:735–738.
6. Wright NM, Lauryssen C. Vertebral artery injury in C1-2 transarticular screw fixation: results of a survey of the AANS/CNS Section on Disorders of the Spine and Peripheral Nerves. American Association of Neurological Surgeons/Congress of Neurological Surgeons. *J Neurosurg* 1998;88:634–640.
7. Paramore CG, Dickman CA, Sonntag VKH. The anatomical suitability of the C1-2 complex for transarticular screw fixation. *J Neurosurg* 1996;85:221–224.
8. Geremia GK, Kim KS, Cerullo L, et al. Complications of sublaminar wiring. *Surg Neurol* 1985;23:629–635.
9. Song GS, Theodore N, Dickman CA, et al. Unilateral posterior atlantoaxial transarticular screw fixation. *J Neurosurg* 1997;87:851–855.
10. Madawi AA, Casey AT, Solanki GA, et al. Radiological and anatomical evaluation of the atlantoaxial transarticular screw fixation technique. *J Neurosurg* 1997;86:961–968.
11. Sonntag VKH, Dickman CA. Posterior atlantoaxial wiring techniques. In: Dickman CA, Sonntag VKH, Spetzler RF, eds. *Surgery of the craniovertebral junction.* New York: Thieme Medical Publishers, 1998:783–794.
12. Apostolides PJ, Dickman CA, Golfinos JG, et al. Threaded Steinmann pin fusion of the craniovertebral junction. *Spine* 1996;21: 1630–1637.

CHAPTER 40

Internal Fixation of the Cervical Spine

B. Anterior Lower Cervical Spine Instrumentation

Ashok Biyani and Howard S. An

The role of anterior spinal instrumentation for the treatment of disorders of the lower cervical spine has evolved significantly over the past several decades. The anterior approach to the lower cervical spine was initially reported by Abbott in 1952 (1). Smith and Robinson first described anterior cervical discectomy and fusion (ACDF) with autologous bone graft to achieve fusion and to maintain foraminal height as a treatment for radiculopathies (2). Their technique had an extremely high fusion rate and good clinical results for one level involvement, but multilevel discectomy with fusion was marred by significant nonunion rate and poorer outcomes. Morbidity associated with harvesting of iliac crest graft, need for postoperative immobilization after fusion without adjunct internal fixation, and higher pseudarthrosis rate associated with multilevel fusion and smoking are some of the factors that have led to an ever-increasing use of instrumentation in surgery of the subaxial cervical spine. Bohler introduced anterior plating in 1964 to create a more rigid construct and obviate the drawbacks of uninstrumented fusion (3). A variety of plates have since been developed to improve the biomechanical properties. Titanium implants have also become popular due to their compatibility with magnetic resonance imaging. Several dynamic plates and titanium cage systems are currently available.

This chapter reviews the general indications for anterior cervical spinal fusion patients with degenerative diseases and the multiple factors that indicate a benefit for supplemental anterior plating. It also reviews the authors' specific indications for these degenerative conditions, as well as the indications in trauma, neoplastic diseases, and revision surgery. Specific plate constructs are analyzed with respect to their clinical characteristics and biomechanical properties. Newer techniques of titanium cages also are presented. Finally, the technical considerations in the surgical use of these devices are detailed. The authors' overall perspective supports the view that internal fixation is effective in properly selected patients and has distinctive benefits in specific conditions.

INDICATIONS

The most common indication for anterior cervical surgery remains degenerative disc disease. In a multicenter study of 4,589 patients, Zeidman et al. observed that anterior cervical procedures were twice as common as posterior ones, and degenerative disc disease was the most common indication for surgical intervention (4). Trauma is the second most common indication and accounts for 17% of all cervical spine surgeries. In another study, 97% of all cervical spine fusions were for degenerative conditions, and 3% were performed for trauma (5). Other less common indications of anterior cervical instrumentation include reconstruction tumor surgery and revision surgery for pseudarthrosis or postlaminectomy kyphosis.

Degenerative Disc Disease

Most patients presenting with symptoms of axial neck pain with or without radiculopathy can be managed with conservative treatment, which usually includes nonsteroidal antiinflammatory agents, activity modification, and physical therapy. A soft collar may be used for a short duration to decrease the dynamic compression of an irritated nerve root and reduce pain from fatigue or spasm in the paraspinal muscles. Brief tapered course of oral cortisone may alleviate symptoms of radiculopathy. Cervical epidural steroid injections may also be used in patients with radiculopathy.

Operative Indications

The indications for operative intervention in patients with a cervical radiculopathy include failure of an adequate trial of nonoperative treatment to relieve persistent or recurrent radicular arm pain with or without neurologic deficit, or progressive neurologic deficit. Patients should have undergone several weeks of nonoperative measures without adequate pain relief or with worsening symptoms before being considered surgical candidates, providing the appropriate pathology is documented by neuroradiologic imaging studies. Patients presenting with progressive neurologic deficit require early intervention, particularly when profound motor weakness is present.

The surgical indications for the treatment of cervical myelopathy are not well defined. The natural history of myelopathy is that of slow and often stepwise deterioration. Patients with mild, nonprogressive, long-standing myelopathy that causes minimal symptoms and is unassociated with gait disturbance or pathologic reflexes may be observed closely. However, operative treatment may be necessary in patients with mild myelopathy when it adversely affects routine activities of daily living. Early operative intervention is recommended in patients with more rapid progressive myelopathy, or moderate to severe myelopathy, which is stable and of less than 1-year duration. Decompression of the affected neural elements is generally recommended to halt worsening of the neurologic status and to allow spinal cord recovery. The patients with mild to moderate myelopathy generally have a greater recovery of function, although some patients with severe myelopathy may also recover to a significant degree.

The indications for surgery in patients with axial neck pain secondary to spondylosis, canal stenosis, or discogenic neck pain are controversial. Patients with significant axial neck pain and moderate to severe canal stenosis may benefit from operative intervention. Whitecloud et al. reported 70% good to excellent results from anterior interbody fusion for patients with concordant neck pain provoked by discography (6). Palit et al. reported a 79% patient satisfaction rate and improved Oswestry scores at long-term follow-up of a group of patients with predominantly neck pain (7). Whether fusion for discogenic neck pain based on provocative testing favorably alters the natural history of the disorder remains unclear, however, and conservative management remains the treatment of choice.

Before embarking on operative treatment, several factors require careful consideration. The type, duration, and severity of symptoms and progression of neurologic deficit are foremost in determining whether surgical intervention is warranted. The underlying pathologic process dictates the extent and nature of decompression and number of levels to be fused. Other key questions include the following:

- What is the best surgical approach: anterior, posterior, or combined?
- What type of bone graft should be used?
- What technique is appropriate for fusion and reconstruction?
- Is instrumentation appropriate, and if so, what type?

A history of smoking and other comorbidities are important considerations in determining whether instrumentation should be added.

Anterior versus Posterior Approach

Once the decision has been made that surgical intervention is necessary, the next logical step in surgical planning is to determine if an anterior, posterior, or a circumferential approach is indicated. An anterior approach is typically preferred for posterolateral or central disc herniations with significant neck and arm pain, and in patients with spondylotic changes and radiculopathy. The disc and osteophytes can easily and safely be removed from an anterior approach, providing direct decompression of the neural elements. Further indirect decompression of the foramen is then achieved by slightly distracting the spondylotic segment.

Patients with cervical myelopathy often have cord compression from large osteophytes or ossification of the posterior longitudinal ligament, which frequently extends posterior to the vertebral body. Partial or complete corpectomy provides adequate decompression of the canal from an anterior approach in this situation. Preoperative sagittal alignment of the cervical spine and whether preoperative loss of cervical lordosis can be restored by extension also aid in determining whether an anterior or posterior approach is necessary. The presence of a cervical kyphosis mandates an anterior approach to achieve decompression and to restore cervical lordosis. A posterior approach is preferred for the treatment of congenital canal stenosis, ossification of posterior longitudinal ligament, and cervical spondylotic myelopathy at more than three levels when cervical lordosis is maintained.

General Considerations in the Choice of Instrumentation

Anterior plating alone affords biomechanically poor fixation in patients requiring multilevel corpectomy and strut grafting (Fig. 1). Concomitant or staged posterior segmental fixation with lateral mass plating is usually recommended in patients undergoing multilevel corpectomy and strut grafting or cage reconstruction. Complex postsurgical or other deformities of the cervical spine are also best stabilized with anterior and posterior fixation. A combined approach may sometimes be necessary in patients who cannot tolerate prolonged postoperative immobilization in a brace or a halo. Finally, circumferential surgical stabilization may also be beneficial in some patients when fixation is deemed to be inadequate due to poor bone quality or when suboptimal fixation is obtained due to technical difficulties encountered during surgery. A combined anterior and posterior approach appears to significantly decrease the incidence of graft related complications. For example, Epstein did not encounter any vertebral fractures and graft extrusions in 22 patients undergoing plated circumferential cervical surgery (8).

Type of Anterior Decompression and Fusion

Anterior decompression can be achieved with discectomy, corpectomy, or a combination of both. When osteophytes and

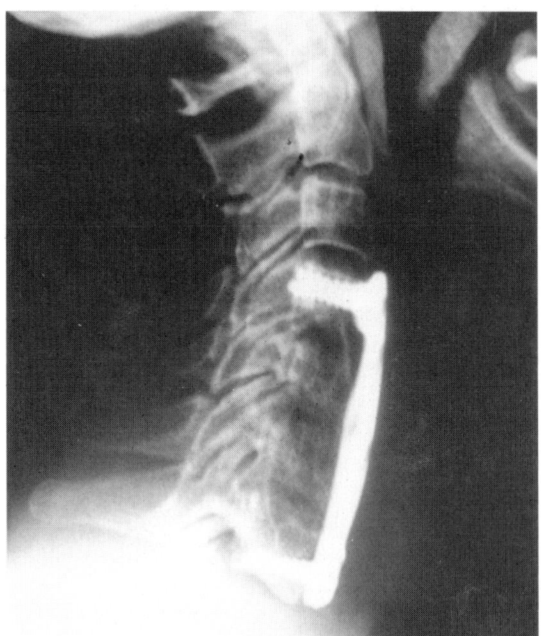

FIG. 1. Lateral radiograph showing nonsegmental plate screw fixation (Orion Cervical Plate, Sofamor-Danek, Memphis, TN) from C-4 to C-7 after corpectomy and strut grafting.

canal stenosis are present at multiple adjacent levels, determination of the extent of decompression and the selection of discectomy versus corpectomy is made. If the herniated disc or the osteophytes extend beyond the level of the disc space and cause spinal cord compression, corpectomy is usually recommended. If multilevel fusion is performed, the number of surfaces that must fuse is greatly increased, which causes a significant increase in the pseudarthrosis rate. Single- or multilevel subtotal corpectomy and strut graft fusion (ACF) are usually recommended for spondylotic myelopathy and myeloradiculopathy. A hemicorpectomy or corpectomy may be necessary when a sequestered disc fragment has migrated behind the vertebral body, or when stenosis is present at the level of the disc and vertebral body. A hybrid approach comprising corpectomy at the most severely involved segments and ACDF at less involved levels is also frequently chosen (Fig. 2). The corpectomy–discectomy approach decreases the length of the graft required and allows segmental fixation at one or more additional levels, thereby decreasing the risk of graft extrusion. Hemicorpectomy and discectomy may also be performed when appropriate, which again facilitates stronger segmental screw fixation and better restoration of lordosis.

Although numerous studies have been published in neurosurgical literature that support anterior discectomy without fusion (9–11), most orthopedic surgeons prefer a discectomy–fusion approach to maintain the cervical alignment and reduce the reoperation rate. The reported nonunion rate varies from 10 to 12% for single-level fusion and ranges from 20 to 27% for two-level fusion in degenerative disorders of the cervical spine (12–14). It is generally agreed that there is no difference in the fusion rate or clinical outcome with and without adjunct internal fixation in a single-level discectomy and fusion (12,13,15–19). Zdeblick et al. did not find any significant difference in histologic or

A–C

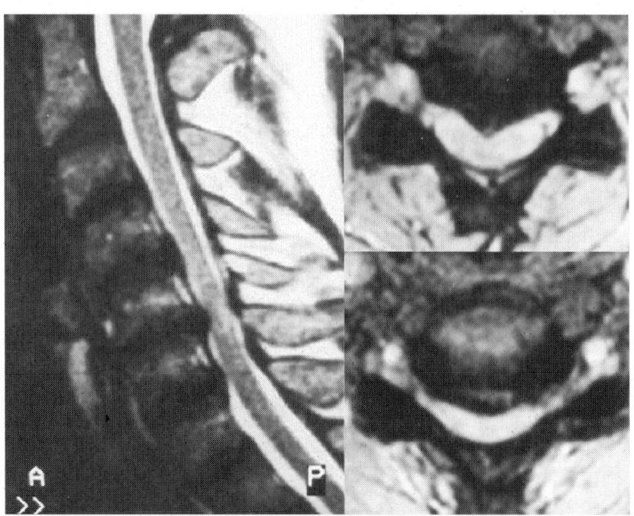

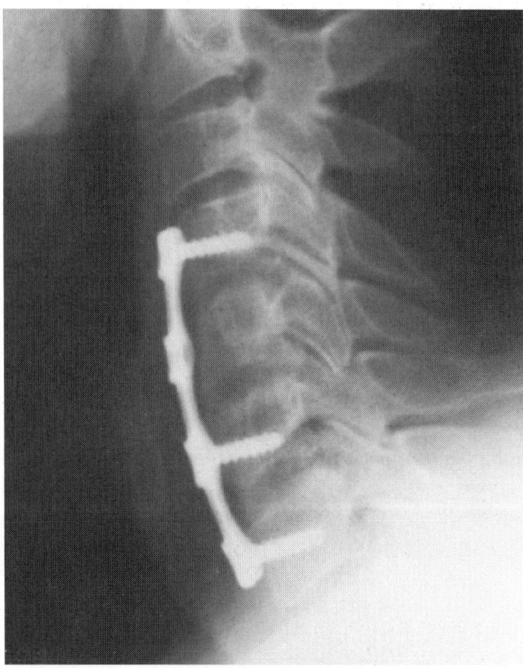

D

FIG. 2. Cervical spondylotic myelopathy due to herniated discs and stenosis. A: Sagittal magnetic resonance imaging (MRI) shows that stenosis is greatest at C5-6, followed by C4-5, and least at C6-7. B: Axial MRI at C4-5 shows moderate stenosis. C: Axial MRI at C5-6 shows severe stenosis. D: Lateral radiograph shows corpectomy and strut grafting at C-5 and discectomy and interbody grafting at C6-7 with "semi-segmental" rigid plate system (PEAK Polyaxial Plate, DePuy-AcroMed Inc., Raynham, MA). A, anterior; P, posterior.

radiologic fusion rate when internal fixation was added in a goat model (13). In fact, diminution of end-plate vascularity was noted in the plated animals, suggesting a decreased healing potential. Stress shielding caused by locked cervical plates and device-related osteopenia are also potential concerns (20).

Anterior Instrumentation: General Considerations

Allograft is increasingly being used for one-level discectomy and fusion and for strut grafting after corpectomy to avoid morbidity associated with harvesting of iliac crest graft. Internal fixation is recommended when allograft is used to improve the fusion rate. Plating also obviates the need for postoperative immobilization. Occurrence of a kyphotic deformity owing to collapse or settling of grafted bone into the vertebral end-plates is a common concern after anterior discectomy and fusion. Anterior cervical plate stabilization may preserve cervical lordosis better than an uninstrumented one-level fusion (15,21). Internal fixation also reduces the amount of disc space collapse and kyphotic deformity in the presence of a pseudarthrosis. Wang et al. reported 1.2 degrees of kyphotic deformity of the fused segment with plating compared with 1.9 degrees for patients without plating (22). Troyanovich et al. reported an overall reduction of 4.2 degrees in cervical lordosis between C-2 and C-7 and the segmental contribution to lordosis at the surgical site decreased by 2.5 degrees in the uninstrumented group (23). In comparison, overall cervical lordosis was preserved and the segmental lordosis at the surgical site increased by 5.67 degrees in the plated group. Zoega et al. performed radiodensitometric analysis in 27 patients who underwent one-level fusion with and without plating, and reported no difference in the fusion rate or outcome between the two groups; however, significant reduction in postoperative kyphotic deformation was noted with plating (18).

Number of Levels Fused

Previous studies have demonstrated that fusion rates decrease with increasing number of surgical levels included in the fusion. Two-level discectomy and fusion is associated with a higher rate of pseudarthrosis, and supplemental internal fixation is generally recommended to improve the fusion rate (24). Kaiser et al. reported 96% and 91% fusion rates, respectively, for one- and two-level ACDF with cortical allograft with anterior fixation, compared with 90% and 72% for one- and two-level ACDF without anterior fixation (17). Epstein reported pseudarthrosis with radiographic evidence of motion in 1% after one-level ACDF and in 10% after two-level ACDF without plating (25). She considered the addition of plate fixation for two-level ACDF a safe procedure with no significant increase in complication rates.

Connolly et al. reported a 70% fusion rate in the uninstrumented 2-level fusion group as compared to a 100% fusion rate in the instrumented group (16). They also encountered significantly lower graft complication rate in multilevel discectomy and fusion with anterior cervical plate fixation. In a retrospective review of 356 patients who underwent one- and two-level discectomy and fusion with and without plating, Caspar et al. reported a significantly lower reoperation rate of 2% for the instrumented group compared with a 10.4% reoperation rate for the uninstrumented group (26). The role of instrumentation in two-level discectomy and fusion is not universally agreed on, however, and some investigators have reported no difference in fusion rate with plating for two-level discectomy and fusion (19,27).

A single corpectomy and strut grafting have also been proposed as alternatives to performing a two-level adjacent discectomy and fusion because it decreases the number of fusion surfaces. However, addition of cervical plates to two-level discectomy and fusion appears to provide results similar to those attained with single-level corpectomy and fusion (28). Therefore, the authors usually perform two-level discectomy, and fusion is usually performed with supplemental internal fixation, unless stenosis is noted behind the vertebral body, in which case a one-level corpectomy may be more appropriate.

The rate of pseudarthrosis for three- or four-level discectomy and fusion is extremely high (25). The reported risk of nonunion with three-level discectomy and fusion varies from 30 to 63% (14). Wang et al. treated 59 patients with a three-level ACDF (29). Forty patients had cervical plates, whereas 19 had fusion without plating. The pseudarthrosis rates were 18% for the instrumented group and 37% for the noninstrumented group. Despite improved stability with anterior cervical plate fixation, a three- or more level discectomy and fusion procedure is still associated with a high nonunion rate (30). However, the risk of pseudarthrosis has, in general, been significantly reduced with the use of modern plating systems.

Anterior Cervical Corpectomy

Anterior cervical corpectomy is usually indicated in patients who require decompression at multiple levels, and when stenosis is present directly behind the vertebral body. The number of surfaces that must fuse is reduced with corpectomy and strut grafting, thereby decreasing the risk of pseudarthrosis. Hilibrand et al. reported a 93% fusion rate with corpectomy and uninstrumented strut grafting compared with 66% rate of arthrodesis with multilevel interbody grafting (31). More complications occurred among patients who had a postlaminectomy kyphosis.

Corpectomy provides safe and effective decompression in patients with cervical spondylotic myelopathy. It also improves the results in terms of myelopathy scores, compared with historical control subjects receiving no treatment or laminectomy (32). Corpectomy is usually recommended in myelopathic patients with loss or reversal of cervical lordosis, because a laminectomy is likely to worsen the kyphotic deformity. In contrast, an anterior decompression and fusion facilitates restoration of the cervical lordosis. Direct anterior decompression of ossification of the posterior longitudinal ligament is also possible with corpectomy, although the risk of dural laceration with this approach should be recognized.

A few studies have reported good results with corpectomy, uninstrumented fusion, and external brace wear or immobilization in a halo vest. Epstein did not find any difference in reoperation rates for graft extrusion and symptomatic pseudarthrosis after one-level anterior corpectomy and fusion with and without plate fixation (33). Saunders et al. performed a retrospective analysis of 31 cases of cervical spondylotic myelopathy treated with four-level subaxial cervical corpectomy without internal fixation (34). External orthoses (i.e., halo vest or a Philadelphia-type collar) were worn for 6 months after surgery. Three patients

(10%) had acute graft complications, and the overall morbidity rate was 25.8%.

Although the role of instrumentation in one-level corpectomy is debatable, there is growing consensus that most corpectomy and reconstruction cases should be stabilized with internal fixation. Mayr et al. reported their results on 261 patients with cervical stenosis who were treated with cervical corpectomy, allograft fibular strut placement, and instrumentation (35). A one-level corpectomy was performed in 133 patients, a two-level corpectomy in 96, and a three- or more level corpectomy in the remaining 32 patients. Successful fusion was observed in 226 patients (86.6%), and a stable, asymptomatic pseudarthrosis was present in 33 (12.6%) patients. Symptomatic improvement was achieved in 99.2% of patients. Eleraky et al. reported their experience with cervical corpectomy in 185 patients (36). Ninety-nine patients presented with myelopathy, 48 with myeloradiculopathy, 24 with radicular pain, and 14 with axial neck pain. One-level corpectomy was performed in 87 patients, two-level corpectomy in 70, and a three-level corpectomy in 28 patients. Iliac crest autograft was used in 141 patients and allograft fibular strut in 44. Adjunct anterior plate fixation was also performed in all but six patients. The reported fusion rate with this technique was 98.8%, and 86.5% of the patients demonstrated neurologic improvement.

Complications of Corpectomy

Reconstruction of the spine after multilevel corpectomy represents a significant challenge; nonunion and graft dislodgment are relatively common (Fig. 3). Vaccaro et al. reported a 50% rate of early postoperative graft or hardware dislodgment after three-level corpectomy and fusion, compared with 9% dislodgment rate for two-level corpectomy and fusion (37). Anterior cervical plating and bone grafting alone after a three-level cervical corpectomy appear to afford inadequate stability in the early postoperative period, regardless of external immobilization. Long-segment anterior cervical plates may reduce the incidence of graft displacement and migration, but they are still associated with a substantial risk for early failure of the construct.

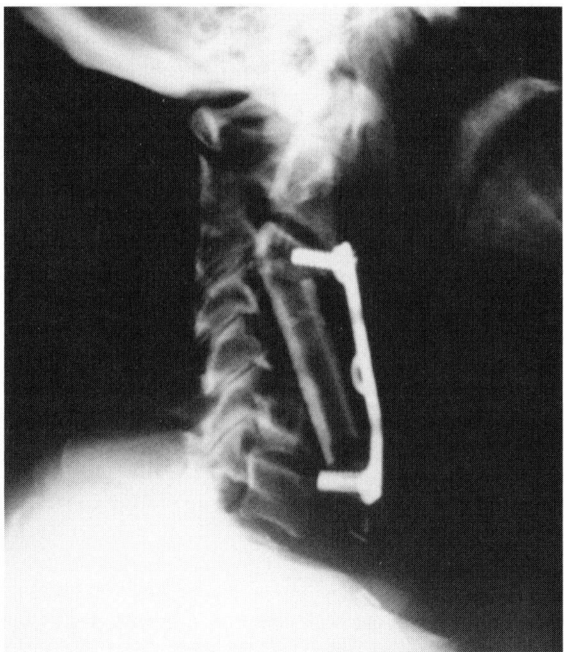

FIG. 3. Lateral radiograph showing strut grafting dislodgement and failure of the nonsegmental plate-screw construct.

The stresses applied to the construct usually tend to dislodge the graft at its lower end. An anterior plate spanning all fusion segments or a junctional "kick plate" at the inferior end of the construct have been recommended to provide a buttress effect and prevent acute graft dislodgment. Failures of a kick plate and graft dislodgment can cause catastrophic airway compromise, however, and are a major concern with this type of construct. Riew et al. have highlighted the significant complication rate associated with cervical corpectomy and short buttress plate fixation at the inferior end of the construct (38). Vanichkachorn et al. suggested posterior segmental fixation and fusion should be performed in addition to an anterior junctional plate to minimize graft and hardware migration in multilevel corpectomy cases (39).

Other modes of multilevel decompression and reconstruction are also being pursued to diminish the risk of graft subsidence, collapse, or extrusion. Posterior decompression and fixation may be a viable alternative in patients with preserved lordosis. Yonenobu et al. found no difference in Japanese Orthopaedic Association scores and recovery rate between laminoplasty and corpectomy, but the complication rate was 29% in the corpectomy group compared with 7% in the laminoplasty group (40). A combination of corpectomy, hemicorpectomy, and discectomy depending on the degree of stenosis present at a given level may facilitate improved segmental fixation.

Dynamic plates that allow controlled collapse have also recently become available. Epstein recently advocated dynamic (ABC, Aesculap, Center Valley, PA) plates, and suggested that they may be superior than constrained and semiconstrained plates (41). However, there is little evidence in the literature currently to recommend their widespread use. Furthermore, dynamic systems provide less stability of the construct, and postoperative construct failure and pseudarthrosis are potential problems. Other approaches that appear more promising include reconstruction of multilevel corpectomy with a fibular strut graft or a titanium cage, which is supplemented with posterior instrumentation. Schultz et al. reported a 100% fusion rate in patients who underwent one- to four-level anterior cervical corpectomy, allograft fibular strut, and lateral mass plating with iliac autograft (42). The authors' preference for a three-level corpectomy is allograft fibular strut or titanium cage reconstruction anteriorly followed by lateral mass plating for segmental posterior fixation (Fig. 4).

Type of Bone Graft

Several authors have reported favorable results with the use of allograft for discectomy–fusion. This approach avoids the need for harvesting iliac crest graft, shortens the duration of surgery and postoperative recovery, and decreases the donor site morbidity. Although one-level discectomy–fusion can be successfully performed with autograft without supplemental internal fixation, plating is recommended with the use of allograft to promote healing. Several investigators have previously reported autograft is superior to allograft in achieving cervical interbody fusion (43,44). A higher risk of graft collapse and pseudarthrosis has also been observed

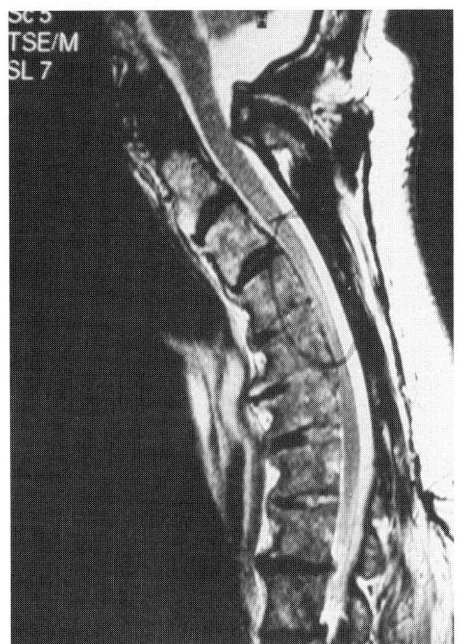

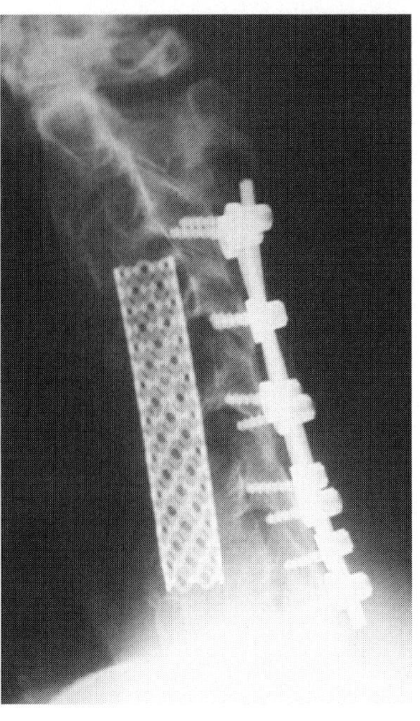

A,B

FIG. 4. Postlaminectomy kyphosis with myelopathy. **A:** Sagittal magnetic resonance imaging showing kyphosis with spinal cord stretched over the kyphotic vertebrae and cord edema with high signal intensity. **B:** Lateral radiograph shows multilevel corpectomy and strut grafting with Harm's cage (DePuy Acromed, Raynham, MA) filled with allograft and local autograft and posterior lateral mass screw rod fixation (Summit System, DePuy Acromed, Raynham, MA).

with the use of allograft (45,46). The risk of graft collapse and pseudarthrosis in one series involving two-level discectomy and fusion was 37% with allograft and 23.5% with autograft (45). However, the evolving consensus is that there is no difference in the fusion rate for one- or two-level surgery with the use of allograft or autograft when concomitant internal fixation is performed, but the allograft takes longer to incorporate. Use of allograft is associated with significantly fewer graft-related complications, and time until return to work is shorter than with autograft. (47,48). When technically properly performed, allograft in combination with rigid anterior plating gives equally good results as autografts.

There are a number of other graft alternatives. Thalgott et al. reported complete incorporation of coralline hydroxyapatite when used as a bone graft substitute in 26 patients who underwent anterior discectomy and instrumented fusion. (49). Shapiro and Bindal described the use of machined femoral ring allografts filled with allogeneic demineralized bone matrix for instrumented cervical interbody fusion (50). These bone grafting techniques are not popular, however, and currently there is a lack of long-term data that would support their widespread application.

A tricortical piece of iliac crest structural graft is typically used for one-level corpectomy, and a fibular allograft or autograft strut is frequently used for multilevel corpectomy. These techniques still are most commonly used. More recently, titanium cages filled with local autograft obtained from resected vertebral bodies have been used to restore structural integrity of the anterior column.

Common causes of bone graft–related complications include poor sizing, end-plate fracture, postoperative trauma, and inadequate immobilization (51). Clearly, meticulous grafting technique is paramount and as important as the type of graft chosen and internal or external immobilization in ensuring a successful outcome.

Smoking

Smoking has been shown to interfere with bone revascularization and metabolism, and to adversely affect bone healing in general. Several studies have also demonstrated a significant negative impact of smoking on healing and clinical recovery after cervical fusion (52–54). The reported rate of pseudarthrosis after ACDF varies from 27.9 to 47.1% in smokers; this is significantly higher than the rates reported for nonsmokers. For that reason, supplemental internal fixation is frequently recommended in smokers to negate the side effects of nicotine. When allografts are used, rigid internal fixation appears to improve the fusion rates for smokers and nonsmokers (55).

Bose reported a 97% fusion rate in a retrospective study of 106 patients treated with anterior cervical plating (56). The mean number of levels fused was 2.74, and majority of the patients received autograft. He found no difference between smokers, who constituted 45.5% of the study group, and nonsmokers, and concluded that anterior cervical plating markedly improved the fusion rate in smokers. Hilibrand et al. reported a 93% fusion rate in smokers and nonsmokers after corpectomy and strut-grafting, but smokers had a 50% rate of solid arthrodesis at all levels after multilevel interbody grafting compared with 75.8% fusion rate at all levels in nonsmokers (57). These authors, therefore, recommended subtotal corpectomy and autogenous strut grafting when multilevel anterior cervical decompression and fusion is necessary in smokers who are unable or unwilling to stop smoking before surgical treatment.

Authors' Indications for Anterior Plating for Degenerative Cervical Disorders

For the majority of single-level cases, anterior discectomy and Smith-Robinson type of fusion using the autologous iliac crest bone without plating is recommended. A high fusion rate is expected provided that the surgical techniques of thorough discectomy, meticulous end-plate preparation, appropriate amount of distraction of the disc space, and precise placement of the tricortical graft with 2 mm posterior to the anterior vertebral margin (58) (Fig. 5). These patients are advised to wear a hard

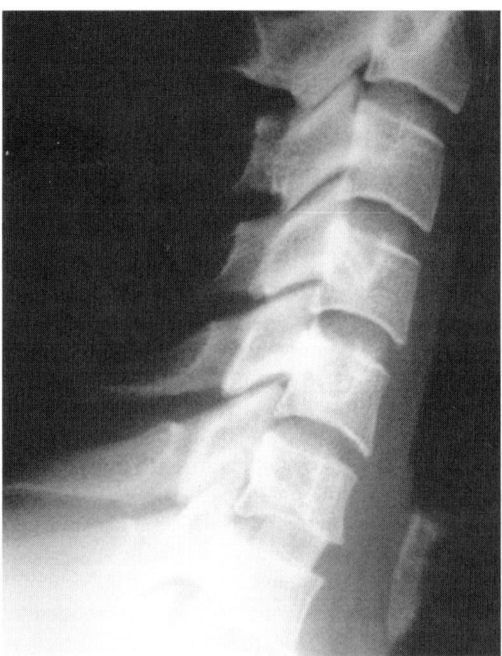

FIG. 5. Lateral radiograph showing the Smith-Robinson interbody graft at C6-7. The graft is countersunk approximately 2 mm.

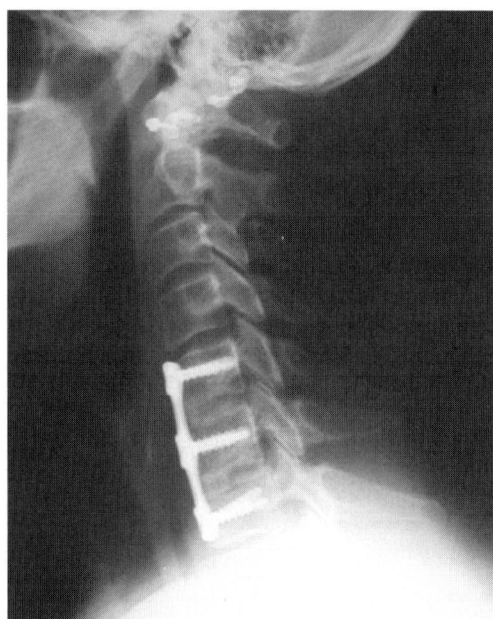

FIG. 7. Lateral radiograph shows interbody fusion and segmental screw plate fixation from C5-7 (Peak Polyaxial Plate System, DePuy Acromed Inc., Raynham, MA).

cervical brace for 6 weeks postoperatively. If the patient is unwilling to wear the brace or wishes to avoid autologous iliac crest grafting, anterior plating with allograft is recommended as a viable option (Fig. 6). For multilevel fusion, anterior plating is recommended with allograft or autograft, as the authors have found no difference in fusion rates between allograft and autograft using the rigid plating systems (55) (Fig. 7). The majority of these patients elects to have allograft to avoid autologous iliac crest grafting. For myelopathic patients undergoing multilevel decompression, a combination of discectomy and corpectomy is desirable whenever possible (Fig. 8). This "semi-segmental" construct gives better biomechanical stability over

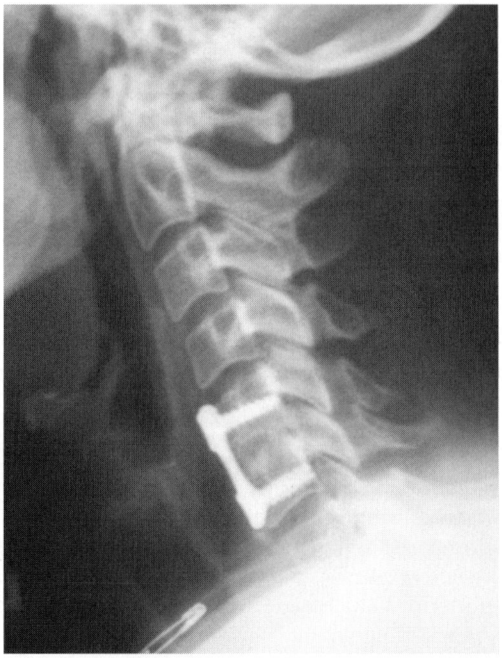

FIG. 6. Lateral radiograph showing a rigid plate-screw system (Peak Polyaxial Plate System, DePuy Acromed Inc., Raynham, MA) after allograft interbody fusion.

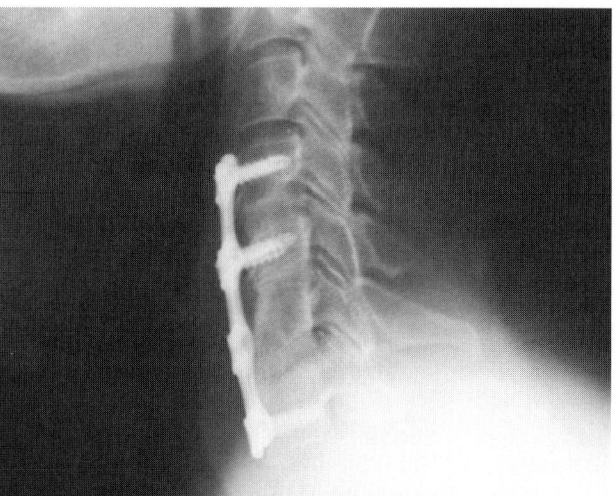

FIG. 8. Lateral radiograph showing discectomy and interbody fusion at C4-5 and corpectomy and strut grafting at C5-7 with "semi-segmental" rigid plate screw fixation (Peak Polyaxial Plate System, DePuy Acromed Inc., Raynham, MA).

that of long strut grafting with plating construct with screws only at the ends of the construct. If multilevel corpectomy must be performed, then a long strut grafting is performed using allograft iliac crest, fibula, or cage filled with allograft bone. The corpectomy bone is always saved and added as autogenous local bone grafts to enhance construct healing and incorporation of the allograft. In these long constructs, anterior plating is usually not performed, but posterior lateral mass fixation is added to provide the maximum stability.

Indications for Plating in Specific Pathologic Conditions

Trauma

The selection of an appropriate surgical approach in the management of unstable cervical spine injuries is dependent on the biomechanical deficiencies of the bony and ligamentous structures, age of the patient, experience of the surgeon, and medical comorbidities. Ideally, the approach should be the least invasive, provide the greatest benefit to risk ratio, and provide adequate stabilization to avoid cumbersome external immobilization and allow early rehabilitation. Anterior surgery is relatively atraumatic compared with a posterior approach that requires stripping of paraspinal muscles. An anterior approach avoids the risks of prone positioning in a traumatized cervical spine. Finally, the anterior approach allows direct anterior decompression at the site of the injury (59).

Uninstrumented anterior interbody fusion is associated with a high risk for later progressive instability and angular deformity in patients with posterior ligamentous instability (60). Late kyphotic deformity may occur in as many as 50% patients after cervical trauma (61,62). An anterior cervical plate in addition to bone graft provides immediate biomechanical stability to the injured area and produces nearly 70% reduction in motion in all loading modes (63). The addition of instrumentation to anterior decompression minimizes graft-related complications, reduces the number of levels fused, improves fusion rate, avoids the need for halo vest or rigid external immobilization, and significantly shortens the rehabilitation period (5). Anterior cervical plate instrumentation is also useful in the maintenance of cervical alignment and prevention of late deformity, and it potentially avoids the need for a secondary posterior cervical procedure.

Anterior interbody grafting and plating acts as an anterior tension band and provides excellent stability in distraction-extension injuries. However, anterior plate fixation is biomechanically inferior in comparison with posterior lateral mass plating for the treatment of flexion-distraction injuries or unstable cervical injuries. An anterior approach has, therefore, been recommended for anterior column injuries, and a posterior approach has been recommended for a predominantly posterior column cervical injury.

Koh et al. performed a biomechanical study to assess the stability provided by anterior, posterior, or combined cervical fixation in flexion-distraction injury and burst fracture models in fresh human cadavers (64). They observed that anterior plating alone failed to stabilize the cervical spine, particularly in the flexion-distraction injury model with failed posterior ligaments. Anterior plating fixation provided much greater fixation in the corpectomy model than in the flexion-distraction injury model, emphasizing the important role of the posterior ligaments in stability of the cervical spine. Koh et al. also noted that posterior plating with an interbody graft provides effective stabilization of the unstable cervical segments in all loading modes, and adjunct anterior fixation might not improve the stability significantly as compared with posterior grafting with lateral mass screws and interbody grafting (60). Richman et al. advocated the use of anterior grafting combined with posterior lateral mass plating to achieve maximum stability in patients with unstable cervical spine injury patterns involving anterior disruption (65). Spivak et al. noted that anterior or posterior plating alone may not provide sufficient stabilization in the absence of any additional external immobilization in patients with unstable cervical spine who have significant bilateral loss of posterior bony contact, and they suggested circumferential stabilization may be necessary in such patients (66).

Despite biomechanical data suggesting greater efficacy of posterior plate fixation for unstable injuries involving posterior column and stronger construct achieved with lateral mass plating, clinical results of anterior interbody fusion and plate fixation have been quite satisfactory. Anterior plating with load-sharing interbody graft provides sufficient stability; several clinical studies have shown additional posterior fixation is not routinely needed. If the anterior fixation is deemed inadequate, considerations should be given to secondary posterior fixation or to prolonged immobilization with a more rigid type of orthosis.

Aebi et al. treated 22 patients with burst fractures and 64 patients with flexion-distraction injuries with anterior instrumented fusion with a plate (59). They concluded that the operative technique of bone grafting and plating for cervical spine trauma was relatively straightforward, safe, and effective for anterior and predominantly posterior lesions. Caspar et al. observed solid fusion after 1 year in 60 patients with cervical trauma, and they concluded that the technique of anterior bone grafting and plating was reliable for anterior and posterior lesions of the cervical spine (67). Goffin et al. presented follow-up results 5 to 9 years after anterior cervical fusion and anterior plating for fractures or fracture dislocations of the cervical spine in 25 patients (68). Adequate bony fusion was obtained in all patients within 1 year after surgery. Similar results have been reported by others describing anterior plate fixation as a useful technique in the majority of patients with cervical trauma (69–75).

Specific compression-flexion cervical injuries that may be amenable to anterior decompression and plate stabilization include burst fractures and flexion teardrop fractures. Burst fracture without associated neurologic deficit may be treated in a halo vest or a rigid cervical orthosis. However, an anterior plate stabilization may be necessary if posttraumatic kyphosis develops, and instability is noted on subsequent flexion extension radiographs. In patients who present with burst fracture and associated neurologic deficit, steroids should be administered and traction should be applied. If cervical alignment does not improve with traction, then corpectomy, tricortical iliac crest graft and plate fixation are indicated (73,74).

The patients with traumatic disc herniation should be managed with anterior decompression of the spinal cord followed by anterior interbody fusion and stabilization (73). When an associated posterior ligamentous instability is present, additional posterior instrumentation is recommended. Direct anterior decompression in the form of corpectomy is recommended for patients with partial or complete neurologic injury. Bohlman and Anderson (76) demonstrated neurologic improvement in 71% of patients with incomplete quadriplegia, and 61% of patients were able to regain ambulation after anterior decompression and stabilization. An improvement in function of one or two nerve root levels distal to the injury was observed in 60% of patients with complete quadriplegia.

Common combined anterior and posterior column injuries include burst fracture with posterior ligamentous injury, flexion teardrop fracture, and fracture-dislocations. In neurologically intact patients presenting with burst fracture with significant loss of vertebral body height, an anterior approach is beneficial, but a posterior approach may be more appropriate when there is minimal body compromise. In patients with spinal cord injury secondary to an unstable burst fracture, anterior decompression and stabilization is indicated. Anterior cervical plating is also superior to halo vest in restoring and maintaining sagittal alignment of unstable cervical flexion teardrop fractures (77). When patients present with fracture-dislocation and complete quadriplegia, a posterior approach is often recommended after successful closed reduction, because there is usually no canal compromise left once the dislocation is reduced, and the severely damaged cord at the time of the injury is unlikely to improve with anterior decompression (78). Anterior plate fixation may be inadequate in patients with bilateral fracture dislocation or in patients with osteoporosis. These patients are best stabilized with lateral mass plating (79).

Patients with cervical trauma may occasionally have associated airway compromise that may require tracheostomy. Northrup et al. retrospectively reviewed 11 patients who had a tracheostomy before anterior cervical spine surgery for cervical trauma (80). Anterior instrumentation was used in more than one-half of the patients. They concluded that tracheostomy did not significantly increase the risk of infection in subsequent anterior cervical surgery in patients with cervical cord damage resulting from nonpenetrating trauma. A tracheostomy does not appear to be a contraindication to plate stabilization.

Tumors

The reported prevalence of metastasis in the cervical spine varies from 8.1 to 20.0% of all lesions involving the vertebral column (81–84). A multidisciplinary approach is necessary for treatment of cervical spine metastasis, and several factors that have a direct bearing on the patient's management must be carefully considered. These include age, general health, and overall life expectancy; location, type, and radiosensitivity of the tumor; degree of spinal instability, and neurologic compromise. The risks of surgery must be balanced against the benefits of improving the patient's quality of life and must be addressed on an individualized basis. Those patients with less than 8 to 12 weeks of remaining life expectancy are probably more appropriate candidates for palliative nonoperative measures. The mean survival time after diagnosis of cervical spine metastases of all tumor types is reported to be 14.7 months (83). The life expectancy for patients with lung and breast carcinomas with bony metastases are 7 to 9 months, and 30 months, respectively (85).

The treatment goals of cervical spinal metastases are to provide adequate pain control, improve the quality of remaining life, and prevent or improve neural deficit. Various nonoperative treatment methods are available, including radiotherapy, hormonal and chemotherapy, and high-dose steroid therapy. Radiation therapy is most appropriate in patients with significant neck pain secondary to epidural metastasis when there is no evidence of associated spinal instability, neurologic compromise, or history of radiation. Radiation therapy is also commonly used in patients with spinal cord compression and neurologic deficit. The ability to ambulate, rapidity of development of neurologic compromise, and duration of symptoms are some of the factors that have prognostic significance (86). Cord compression from soft-tissue metastases responds better to radiation therapy than canal compromise due to bony fragments (86,87).

Chemohormonal-sensitive tumors may also be treated with chemotherapy or hormonal therapy. Several chemotherapeutic agents are currently used to combat sensitive tumor types, including breast, thyroid, and small-cell lung carcinomas. Steroids are frequently administered preoperatively to diminish localized intramedullary spinal cord edema in patients with acute neurologic compromise due to spinal cord compression (88).

If surgery is considered, it is debatable whether to apply radiation or chemotherapy in the preoperative or postoperative period. Patients who present with significant deformity, progression of neurologic deficit, radio- or chemoresistant tumors, spinal instability, or previous maximum-dose radiation treatments are candidates for initial surgical management followed by appropriate radiation or chemotherapy to prevent tumor regrowth. The effect of perioperative radiation on the healing and incorporation of bone graft is a point of concern. Previous studies have suggested that preoperative radiation most likely does not affect strut graft incorporation (89,90); however, new information indicates immediate postoperative radiation has significant detrimental effects on the biomechanical and histologic properties of the bone grafts. Postoperative radiation is, therefore, generally delayed for 3 to 6 weeks. Similar recommendations exist for chemotherapeutic agents during the perioperative period (91).

The goals of operative intervention are to decompress the spinal cord, to prevent worsening of or (optimally) improve neurologic status, and to achieve or maintain stability with rigid fixation. Accordingly, the surgical indications for the treatment of cervical metastatic disease include spinal instability or progressive deformity from bone destruction or pathologic fracture, progressive neurologic deficit associated with significant spinal cord compression that is unresponsive to nonoperative treatment, and intractable neck pain recalcitrant to conservative means of therapy (92).

Anterior column involvement is nearly universal in metastatic disease of the lower cervical spine, and it is more likely to cause neurologic compression based on a relatively smaller canal size and greater volume of cancellous bone in the subaxial vertebral bodies (93). In an attempt to quantify mechanical instability of the spine, Kostuik et al. divided the vertebral body into six zones (94). They considered the spine to be unstable when the tumor involved three or more zones. DeWald et al. emphasized careful consideration of immunologic status of the patient, and they also considered the spine to be unstable if more than 50% of the vertebral body was destroyed or when both pedicles were involved (95).

Cervical corpectomy for metastatic disease is frequently associated with excessive bleeding, which may be controlled with thrombin-soaked gelatin sponges or bone wax. Massive intraoperative hemorrhage has been noted in metastatic thyroid and renal-cell carcinoma, and consideration should be given to preoperative embolization of these tumors (96). Surgical intervention should be carried out within 24 hours after angiography and embolization to avoid revascularization from collateral circulation (97,98).

After corpectomy, stabilization of the cervical spine is achieved with autograft or allograft struts from the iliac crest or of fibular origin depending upon the length of the construct needed. Allografts are generally preferred because the operative time and perioperative morbidity associated with harvesting of iliac crest graft are significantly diminished in this subset of patients, who have a limited life expectancy. Corpectomy and structural graft without instrumentation necessitates halo vest application, which may add to morbidity and delay postoperative mobilization. A titanium cage packed with morcellized bone graft is an attractive alternative to strut graft. Rigid internal fixation with anterior plates should also be carefully considered to improve the postoperative quality of life of the patient, with less reliance on cumbersome external immobilization (92).

The use of supplemental anterior plate fixation in metastatic cervical spine disease is not well established. Hall and Webb reported on five patients with neoplastic involvement of the cervical spine treated with decompression and vertebral body replacement with a strut graft or polymethylmethacrylate (PMMA) followed by AO plating (99). Caspar et al. conducted a retrospective study of 30 patients who were treated with cervical vertebral spinal neoplasms after they had undergone anterior decompression and plate stabilization with an autograft or polymethylmethacrylate as the anterior load-bearing support structure (100). Most patients received postoperative radiotherapy or chemotherapy, or both. The mean Kaplan-Meier survivorship estimate was 35.8 months. All but one patient achieved long-term or lifelong mechanical stability in the cervical spine.

Valid serious concerns do exist with anterior cervical plate stabilization, however, including adequacy of fixation in adjacent vertebral bodies for screw purchase and subsequent loss of fixation from postoperative irradiation of the surgical field that may compromise the fixation and spinal stability. When plates are used, the screws at the upper and lower ends of the construct should be placed in tumor-free vertebrae to minimize the risk of postoperative loss of fixation (92).

The use of PMMA combined with instrumentation has also been recommended as a means of achieving stability (101,102). Because PMMA provides immediate short-term stability only, its use should be judiciously considered only for those individuals with a relatively poor life expectancy. Sundaresan et al. and Clark et al. reported on the use of Steinmann pins inserted into the vertebral bodies incorporated into PMMA as a means of vertebral body replacement (103,104). Others have reported modifications of such techniques combined with PMMA in anterior spinal fixation, including Kirschner (K)-wires driven into the vertebral bodies or with use of rods (85,105,106).

The decision to perform a combined anterior and posterior approach to the cervical spine in tumor patients depends on the type, degree, and location of spinal cord compression. In instances in which a "napkin-ring" type of circumferential encroachment on the spinal canal is noted, consideration should be given to a combined decompressive and stabilization procedure. Other factors that must be taken into consideration include the patient's overall medical condition, his or her ability to withstand a same-day or staged procedure, life expectancy, and the tumor being treated. Patients with a long life expectancy from a relatively slow-growing tumor may be treated anteriorly with decompression and strut grafting without PMMA augmentation, then followed by an additional posterior stabilization procedure to avoid rigid external immobilization. The anterior approach and decompression along with realignment and stabilization is the initial procedure. This can then be followed by posterior stabilization with or without decompression, including laminectomy (92). Posterior decompression alone for circumferential compression has not been shown to be any more effective than radiation therapy alone and should not be considered as a sole means of treatment (107).

Repair of Pseudarthrosis and Postlaminectomy Kyphosis

A successful fusion is characterized by absence of lucency around the graft, evidence of bridging bone between the endplate and the graft, and the absence of movement on dynamic imaging scans. Several factors require careful consideration when fusion fails to occur. Surgical intervention for pseudarthrosis should be reserved only for patients with significant symptoms. A repeat anterior procedure can entail dissection in a scarred previously operated area, resection of a nonunion site, and regrafting. However, an approach from the intact contralateral side of the cervical spine is feasible in most cases. The presence of failed hardware also dictates the need for an anterior approach. Coric et al. successfully treated 19 patients with symptomatic pseudarthrosis after failed anterior cervical fusions with revision anterior cervical fusion using iliac crest allografts (108). Tribus et al. reported 81% fusion rate and 75% improvement in symptoms in 16 consecutive patients with symptomatic pseudarthrosis of the cervical spine, who were treated with anterior resection of the pseudarthrosis, autogenous iliac crest bone grafting, and stabilization with an anterior cervical plate (109).

However, posterior segmental fixation with lateral mass plating may be more appropriate for treatment of symptomatic anterior cervical pseudarthrosis in patients with well-fixed anterior instrumentation. Posterior fusion and articular pillar plating, whether alone or as a part of a circumferential procedure, has been demonstrated to provide the added fixation required to successfully repair failed anterior cervical fusion (110).

Surgical treatment of postlaminectomy kyphosis is technically very demanding and is associated with a significant complication rate. Riew et al. treated 18 patients with one- to four-level anterior cervical corpectomy and uninstrumented arthrodesis for postlaminectomy kyphosis (111). Eleven of these patients (60%) developed various complications, including pseudarthrosis and kyphosis. Graft extrusion is also common despite halo immobilization or anterior plating. Cervical corpectomy and anterior plate fixation (112) or corpectomy and reconstruction with a cage filled with local autograft or a strut graft and anterior plate are generally recommended for anterior decompression, restoration of sagittal alignment, and reconstruction of anterior column. Adjunct posterior lateral mass plating is almost universally recommended to improve the stability of the construct. In the long strut–grafting construct, the posterior lateral mass segmental construct offers the main stability, and the anterior plate does not significantly contribute to the biomechanical stability. If there is residual kyphosis after corpectomy and strut grafting, anterior plating is not recommended at all. Anterior plating over the kyphotic contour of the anterior cervical spine is not effective in stabilizing the construct and invites plate loosening and other complications associated with plate failure.

ANTERIOR CERVICAL INSTRUMENTATION

The goals of internal fixation in the cervical spine are stabilization, reduction and maintenance of alignment, early rehabilitation, and improvement in the fusion rate. The plate acts as a load-sharing device and eliminates the need for postoperative immobilization in a halo or an orthosis. Plate fixation improves fusion rate and decreases time to fusion after two- or more level discectomy. The use of a plate also helps to prevent late deterioration in the cervical spinal alignment obtained intraoperatively. Preservation of physiologic lordosis may minimize the long-term adverse effects of mechanical malalignment on adjacent disc segments (21), and it may prevent delayed neurologic deterioration. Plating in one- and two-level cervical degenerative disease also yields a lower reoperation rate (114).

Several plate systems and cages are currently available (Fig. 9). An appropriate device should be chosen based on the pathoanatomy of the lesion, biomechanics of the implant, and the surgeon's familiarity with the device. Some of the desirable features of an ideal plate design include the ease of use, unicortical fixation, flexibility for multidirectional screw placement, controlled compression capability without adversely affecting stiffness of the construct, and use of titanium implants for magnetic resonance imaging compatibility.

Some of the earliest plate systems, such as AO Orozco plate (Synthes, Paoli, PA) and Caspar trapezoidal plate (Aesculap, San Francisco, CA), were made of stainless steel and were secured with unlocked bicortical screws. Bicortical screws have been shown to be biomechanically superior to unicortical screws in one study (115), but Maiman et al. did not find any improvement in the pullout strength of Caspar screws with posterior cortical penetration in an isolated vertebral body model (116).

Even though the earlier results of anterior cervical plating were encouraging with the use of bicortical screws, several issues were raised, including the potential danger of spinal cord damage with posterior cortical penetration (117), occasional loosening of the screws, and construct failures. These concerns have led to the development of unicortical locking screw plate systems. The advent of constrained systems has eliminated the need for bicortical fixation and reduced the use of fluoroscopy.

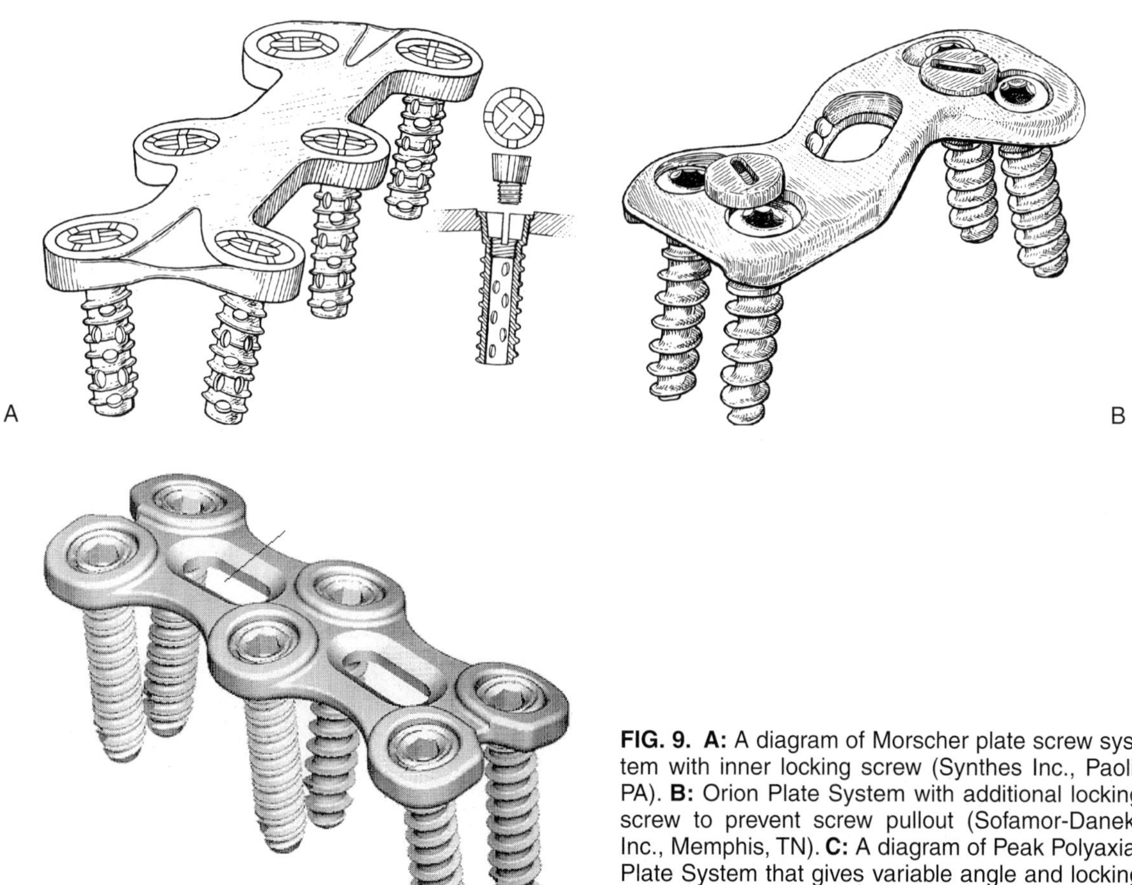

FIG. 9. A: A diagram of Morscher plate screw system with inner locking screw (Synthes Inc., Paoli, PA). **B:** Orion Plate System with additional locking screw to prevent screw pullout (Sofamor-Danek, Inc., Memphis, TN). **C:** A diagram of Peak Polyaxial Plate System that gives variable angle and locking mechanisms by a bushing that rotates and expands with final screw tightening (DePuy Acromed Inc., Raynham, MA).

Newer plate systems, such Morscher Cervical Spine Locking Plate (Synthes, Paoli, PA), the Orion Anterior Cervical Plate (Sofamor-Danek, Memphis, TN), and the Peak Polyaxial Anterior Cervical Plate (DePuy-Acromed, Raynham, MA), are made of titanium and are designed for unicortical screw fixation. Most current plate designs use 3.5- to 4.0-mm screws and allow variable placement of the screws through the holes of the plate to facilitate proper insertion of the screws within the vertebral bodies. Larger diameter "bail out" or rescue screws are also available with most systems.

Spivak et al. have shown that locking unicortical screws prevent screw backout and significantly increase the rigidity of the screw-plate interface initially and after cyclic loading (118). Some locking plates, such as the Orion plate, require insertion of blocking screws to prevent screw backout. Other plate systems use expansion-head screws, which have an expansible shoulder and the proximal portion of the screw is hollowed out. Initially, the expansion head screw is placed through the plate and into the vertebral body, and then locked to the plate with use of the smaller expansion screw. The locking mechanism is widening of the shoulder of the expansion head screw by the smaller expansion screw. Finally, some implant designs incorporate a locking plate feature without the need for an additional screw. The peak polyaxial anterior cervical plate has a rotational locking bushing in the plate hole that allows 25 degrees of freedom of motion in any direction, thus facilitating placement of unicortical screws in the desired trajectory while achieving a rigid locking interface between the plate and the screw. Some systems have locking rings, which are engaged as the screws are tightened and cause the screws to lock to the plate. More recently, a cam mechanism has been incorporated in some designs (Slim Lock, DePuy AcroMed, Raynham, MA), which is turned by 90 degrees to lock the plate after insertion of the screws.

Monocortical screw fixation is quicker, easier, and safer, and is currently favored for most anterior cervical fusion and plating procedures. Bicortical screw fixation may be beneficial in certain circumstances, such as multilevel stabilization, patients with poor bone quality due to osteoporosis or rheumatoid disease, unstable spine owing to trauma and tumor, and correction of kyphotic deformities (119).

The recommended length of unicortical screws varies from 12 to 16 mm. In a cadaveric study, Ebraheim et al. noted the mean depth of the superior end-plate increased consistently from C-3 to C-7, whereas that of inferior end-plate generally increased from C-2 to C-6, then decreased at C-7 (120). The mean sagittal and parasagittal middle vertebral body depths were both 14 mm. Xu et al. recommended convergent placement of screws 16 mm in length or less to avoid inadvertent penetration of posterior cortex (121). Although tapping of the screw hole does not significantly alter the pullout strength of the screw, some plate designs do not require pretapping.

Biomechanical Considerations of Anterior Cervical Plate Fixation

Several biomechanical factors, such as applied screw torque, screw pullout force, and plate geometry and strength, have been extensively evaluated. In a single-level procedure, an anterior cervical plate serves as a load-sharing device rather than a load-shielding device, which facilitates graft consolidation (122). However, the capability of an anterior cervical plate to stabilize the spine after multilevel corpectomy is significantly diminished with fatigue loading on biomechanical testing (123). Excessive screw-vertebra motion caused by fatigue also has been observed to occur at the lower end of the multilevel corpectomy model, which may explain why the caudal end of long anterior cervical plate constructs fails in clinical cases (124).

In a biomechanical study, DiAngelo et al. noted the application of an anterior plate significantly increased the global stiffness and decreased local motion at the instrumented levels (125). In a corpectomy model, flexion loaded the strut graft, whereas extension produced unloading of the graft in a corpectomy model. Anterior multilevel cervical plating effectively increases the stiffness and decreases the local cervical motion after corpectomy. Anterior cervical plating also reverses the graft loads, while unloading the graft occurs in flexion. Excessive loading of the graft in extension may promote pistoning and failure of multilevel constructs, however. In another study of corpectomy-strut graft–anterior plate model, the graft force decreased in flexion and increased in extension. Higher graft force increased, whereas fatigue decreased the stability of a three-level construct (126).

Load sharing is affected by the precision of the corpectomy and reconstruction, and postoperative events, such as graft resorption, end-plate fracture, and telescoping of the graft within the vertebral body (20). As the distance between superior end-plate of the cephalad vertebra and inferior end-plate of the caudal vertebra decreases, the stresses generated at the lower end of the construct increase significantly. Lowery and McDonough retrospectively compared 70 nonconstrained and 39 constrained plates, and they reported significantly fewer complications with constrained systems (127). Because of the increase rate of hardware failure in the unconstrained plate group, Lowery et al. recommended the use of constrained plate systems (127).

More recently, dynamization of cervical plates has been recommended to compensate for subsidence or resorption of the strut graft. Several plate designs, such DePuy AcroMed DOC system, Aesculap ABC plate, and Premiere plate (Medtronic Sofamor Danek, Memphis, TN), are available. Several biomechanical studies have reported the purported superiority of these translational plates over constrained designs. Brodke et al. compared two dynamic plate designs (DePuy AcroMed DOC and Aesculap ABC systems) and two constrained designs (Synthes CSLP and Medtronic Sofamor Danek Orion plates) in a corpectomy model (20). They concluded the locked constrained plates provide excellent load-sharing fixation in the absence of graft resorption or subsidence, but the dynamic plates provide superior load sharing with 10% graft subsidence. They also pointed out that the effect of dynamization on stiffness is dependent on plate design. Plates such as the DOC plate that act as a pure load-sharing device are less stiff than the ABC plate. DiAngelo et al. performed a biomechanical comparison of constrained Orion plate (Medtronic Sofamor Danek) with a semiconstrained translational Premiere plate (Medtronic Sofamor Danek) in a multilevel corpectomy and strut-grafting model (128). Both plated designs decreased the load motion and increased stiffness of the instrumented levels. They observed significant loading of the graft in extension with constrained plates, which may promote graft pistoning and eventual construct failure. Such loading of the graft in extension was not observed with the use of a translational plate. Despite these promising preliminary data, biomechanical superiority and clinical efficacy of the dynamic plates have not yet been fully established. Whether dynamization achieved at the expense of stiffness is able to provide a rigid enough construct that accommodates graft subsidence and improves fusion rate remains unresolved.

The biomechanical properties of circumferential and posterior instrumentation have also been evaluated by several authors. Kirkpatrick et al. performed a biomechanical study of various reconstruction techniques used after multilevel cervical corpectomy (129). The range of motion after reconstruction compared with a control group was decreased 24% after strut grafting, 43% after application of an anterior plate, and 62% after application of posterior plates. Posterior plate fixation was the least flexible followed by the anterior plate technique, and bone graft alone was the most flexible construct. The load to initial failure tended to be higher in posterior than in anterior plated specimens; screw pullout was the predominant mode of failure. In another study, Foley et al. demonstrated that although multilevel cervical instrumentation increases the stiffness following corpectomy, anterior or posterior plating alone excessively loads the graft with small degrees of motion, which may promote pistoning and failure of multilevel constructs (130).

The biomechanical characteristics of anterior cervical plate fixation are somewhat different in cervical trauma than those observed in degenerative spine, because posterior ligamentous structures are frequently torn in the former condition. An anterior cervical plate serves as a tension band during extension and as a buttress plate during flexion of the cervical spine (131). Sutterlin et al. observed significantly lower stiffness in Caspar anterior plate constructs compared with posterior cervical instrumentation in a distractive flexion bovine model (132). An anterior plate with bicortical screws restored the flexural stability to only one-half that of an intact specimen, with the lowest degree of stiffness in the axial flexural loading mode. In contrast, stability was restored to intact baseline with posterior instrumentation. Similar biomechanical findings have been observed in cadaveric human models (133). Anterior plate fixation provides poor rotational or flexural stability when posterior ligaments are compromised (134), and posterior segmental stabilization may be necessary in patients with circumferential bony or ligamentous injury (131). Posterior plating combined with an interbody graft also effectively stabilizes unstable cervical segments in all loading modes (60).

Titanium Mesh Cages

After their introduction for use in the lumbar spine, the application of titanium cages has recently been extended to the cervical spine for reconstruction after corpectomy and discectomy. The cages rely on the principle of ligamentotaxis to increase the spine stiffness and are best suited when the end-plates are preserved in a nonosteoporotic spine (135). They provide immediate strong noncollapsing anterior column load-bearing support and obviate the need for a structural bone graft. Donor site morbidity is minimized, and fusion rates are at least as good as those reported with allograft fibula (136,137). The pullout strength of cages has also been reported to be better than bone graft alone (135). When inserted without an adjunct anterior plate, the recessed cage does not leave any profile, thereby avoiding any risks related to the plate–esophageal interface (135).

Titanium cages have certain disadvantages. The cages are six to eight times more expensive than allograft (137), and they may also complicate the radiographic evaluation of fusion. The presence of bridging trabeculae and absence of motion between the spinous processes on flexion-extension radiographs may be the best indicators of fusion. Two degrees or less of motion with flexion and extension on lateral radiographs is considered to be indicative of solid fusion. A silhouette sign, which denotes the presence of bridging bone ventral and/or dorsal to the cage in lateral radiographs, usually represents successful fusion (135). Because the cages provide greater load bearing than bone graft, potentially higher stress shielding is also a concern. An extruded cage may lacerate the esophagus and potentially cause airway and neurovascular compromise. Finally, revision surgery may be difficult in the presence of an interbody cage, and titanium debris may also be generated in failed cases.

Although long-term data are not yet available for the results of cage reconstruction after corpectomy or discectomy and fusion, several authors have presented their early results. Riew and Rhee reported on 54 patients who underwent corpectomy-discectomy or hemicorpectomy-discectomy followed by titanium cage placement (136). There were no complications other than pseudarthrosis requiring revision in two patients (4%). They suggested the fusion rate with titanium cage appeared to be intermediary to that achieved with autograft and allograft. Das et al. reported a 100% fusion rate with titanium cage and anterior plating after corpectomy and discectomy. Majd et al. treated 34 patients with channel corpectomy followed by placement of a titanium cage packed with autogenous bone graft from the vertebral bodies to reconstruct the anterior column (137). Adjunct anterior cervical plating was performed in those patients requiring decompression of two or more levels. Radiographic evidence of fusion was attained in 97% of the patients 6 months after surgery. Hacker et al. performed one- or two-level discectomy and fusion with an iliac crest autograft or an interbody cage filled with local autograft in 54 patients for the treatment of radiculopathy with or without mild myelopathy (135). A 90% fusion rate was observed in both groups, with 97% good to excellent clinical results in the cage group and 88% in the iliac crest bone graft group.

Despite promising early results of the cages as stand-alone interbody fusion devices, their biomechanical characteristics have not been fully investigated. Early clinical data also need to be validated by further studies that evaluate the long-term results. Different cage designs are also available, and conflicting reports raise further questions. Kandziora et al. conducted an *in vitro* biomechanical study of cervical spine interbody fusion in a sheep model with different designs of cages (138). They concluded the cylindrical cages were able to control extension and bending more effectively than cages with a screw design. Greene et al. did not find any significant difference between threaded cervical cages and structural bone grafting for immediate *in vitro* stability after anterior cervical discectomy (139). The effects of cyclic loading, multilevel interbody cage placement, and presence of osteoporosis on the stability of a cage construct have also not been fully evaluated.

In a finite element model analysis, the authors' group has recently shown the stability achieved with a cage construct is slightly lower than that obtained with an interbody graft for one-level fusion, but substantially lower stability is achieved with the use of cages in a multilevel fusion construct (140). The stresses on intermediate vertebra in two-level fusion constructs with cages are significantly higher under all moment loads. Osteoporosis also exhibited pronounced effects at the caudal end of a multilevel construct with interbody cages. Kettler et al. also observed that simulated repeated neck movements increased the flexibility and subsidence of the implants into the adjacent vertebrae (141). Shimamoto et al. have also recommended that cervical interbody cages should be supplemented with additional internal fixation to prevent excessive motion in flexion-extension (142). Based on a prospective study, ElSaghir and Bohm concluded that lateral mass plating was superior and more stable than anterior plating after corpectomy and titanium cage reconstruction (143). Although pseudarthrosis was not encountered in either group, 23.3% patients had screw breakage after anterior plating, while there was no hardware failure with posterior plating.

SURGICAL TECHNIQUE

Proper preoperative planning, including consideration for intubation, positioning, and stabilization during the operative period, is imperative. Similar general principles apply to anterior subaxial cervical spine stabilization for degenerative disc disease, trauma, and tumor. The Stryker frame may be beneficial in patients with cervical trauma and in myelopathic patients when a circumferential fusion is planned. Awake fiberoptic intubation may be necessary in patients with myelopathy and fracture-dislocations, and excessive extension should be avoided during induction and positioning, particularly in patients with myelopathic symptoms. Insertion of an esophageal tube is frequently helpful in identifying and protecting the esophagus during surgery.

Positioning

Positioning and surgical exposure of the anterior aspect of the cervical spine are performed in a manner similar to that for anterior discectomy and fusion without plating. The patient is positioned in the supine position with the neck slightly extended to improve the access to the anterior aspect of the neck and to provide physiologic lordosis. A rolled towel may be placed under the scapulae to improve cervical alignment. If the preoperative pathology does not allow the neck to be safely extended, as in patients with myelopathy or trauma, the neck should be extended after appropriate decompression before application of the plate. Skeletal traction is applied via Gardner-Wells tongs to secure the patient's head and control the cervical spine in most situations, including fractures and dislocations, degenerative disorders, and tumors. Reverse Trendelenburg position is recommended to reduce venous bleeding. Prophylactic antibiotics are routinely given, and intravenous corticosteroids may be administered when necessary.

The surgical approach to the cervical spine and the details of anterior decompression and fusion are covered in Chapters 35 and 39.

Internal Fixation

The most important technical details in anterior cervical plating include a stable structural graft, maximum surface contact between the vertebral body and the plate, selection of appropriate length plate, and proper position of the screws. The process of instrumentation is started with selection of an appropriately sized cervical plate, which extends between the midportions of the superior and inferior vertebrae to be included in the fusion. Any anterior osteophytes should be removed with a high-speed burr or rongeur, and the plate should also be contoured appropriately to maximize bony contact with the plate and enhance stability of the construct. The plate is aligned mediolaterally and in a cephalad caudad direction, and fluoroscopic images may be obtained at this time to confirm length and orientation of the plate. With the plate stabilized in the desired location, holes are drilled to the appropriate depth using a drill guide with a stop allowing no more than 16 to 18 mm of penetration. The screw holes should be drilled parallel to the end-plates of the vertebral body and directed slightly toward the midline. The holes are tapped, and screws are initially placed loosely into the vertebral body before final tightening. Lateral radiograph or fluoroscopic image is obtained to assure correct placement and alignment of the plate and screws. Once satisfied with the implant position, the screws are firmly tightened, and any existing locking mechanism is activated to prevent screw migration.

Postoperative Care

Once the procedure is completed, Hemovac drains are placed, and the wound closed in a routine fashion. Postoperatively, consideration must be given to the patient's respiratory status. Patients undergoing prolonged and multilevel operative procedures are at significant risk of developing respiratory compromise due to pharyngeal edema, and careful consideration must be given to delayed extubation after 24 to 48 hours. Most patients are extubated immediately, however, with soft collar for comfort postoperatively. If the bone is osteoporotic and screw fixation is questionable, more rigid orthosis is recommended. External stabilization with rigid orthosis or halo should be considered when appropriate. The patients should be immobilized in a neutral position to avoid extension motion that could place excessive loads on the weaker posterior portion of the graft.

COMPLICATIONS

The complications attendant to anterior cervical procedures have also been detailed in Chapters 35 and 39. Here the authors consider those complications specific to anterior instrumentation. The surgeon should bear in mind potential complications specifically related to the instrumentation, which may occur in approximately 5 to 8% of patients (67,112). Paramore et al. recently reported hardware failure in 22% patients and concluded that plate length closely correlates with instrumentation-related problems (144). Such complications are likely to occur less frequently with better implant designs, improving surgeon experience, and meticulous operative technique. A drill guide is routinely used to prevent inadvertent posterior penetration, and insertion of excessively long screws should be avoided. Misplacement of the screw into the supra-adjacent or infra-adjacent disc space is a relatively common complication of anterior cervical plating. Selection of plate of an appropriate length that extends from the midportion of the vertebral bodies above and below the decompressed segment is critical. Orientation of the adjacent disc space and direction of the screws should be kept in mind, because intradiscal screw placement may compromise the stability of the construct and also lead to early degeneration of the violated disc space. Radiographs or fluoroscopic images should routinely be obtained intraoperatively after insertion of the screws, and screws that are malpositioned should be redirected in an appropriate trajectory. Visualization of the lower cervical spine in the lateral plane may be difficult, and the disc spaces may remain obscure despite obtaining radiographs with shoulders pulled. Nevertheless, every attempt should be made to ensure that screws are properly placed.

Besides the risk of intraoperative injury to the esophagus as discussed previously, esophageal erosion may also occur postoperatively. Gaundinez et al. reported 28 patients who had developed esophageal perforation after anterior cervical plating (145). Delayed oral extrusion of a screw (146) or elimination via rectal route have been also reported (147). The key to avoiding such a complication is to remove anterior osteophytes and contour the plate appropriately to allow placement of the plate flush with the anterior surface of the vertebral bodies without any hardware prominence. A construct should also be inherently stable to minimize the risk of subsequent graft or hardware migration. The patients with perforated esophagus present with crepitus, and radiographs reveal air and soft-tissue swelling. The diagnosis can be confirmed by contrast-swallow examination or magnetic resonance imaging. The treatment includes nutritional support, parenteral antibiotics, irrigation and débridement, and emergent surgical repair of the esophagus.

Hardware loosening may also occur as a result of insufficient bony purchase in patients with osteoporosis, multiple attempts at insertion leading to inadequate purchase, and improper postoperative immobilization of the patient. Graft dislodgment and plate failure are common complications of multilevel cervical corpectomy. A broken implant should arouse the suspicion of nonunion. The development of pseudarthrosis may or may not be related to the patient's symptoms, and routine removal of the failed hardware is not indicated. The risk of injury to tracheoesophageal structures by prominent hardware appears to be minimal at long-term follow-up. Minor asymptomatic loosening of the screws may simply be observed. After careful evaluation, if reoperation is deemed necessary for pseudarthrosis repair or kyphosis correction, the hardware may be revised. If the hardware is well fixed, and the patient's symptoms warrant repeat surgery for pseudarthrosis, posterior fusion with plating is usually recommended.

The risk of infection after anterior cervical spine surgery is quite low, unless there has been inadvertent perforation of the esophagus during surgery. Although there are no published studies that compare the risk of infection after instrumented and unistrumented anterior cervical fusion, internal fixation does not appear to increase the rate of infection.

Finally, multilevel corpectomy procedures require prolonged operative time and excessive retraction, which may lead to respiratory compromise and airway obstruction (148,149). Sagi et al. reported airway complication in 6.1% of 311 patients, six (1.9%) of whom required reintubation due to pharyngeal edema (149). History of myelopathy, spinal cord injury, pulmonary problems, smoking, anesthetic risk factors, and the absence of a drain did not correlate with an airway complication in that study. Overnight intubation and removal of the endotracheal tube after fiberoptic confirmation of reduction in swelling are recommended in patients undergoing prolonged multilevel surgery.

ADJACENT SEGMENT DEGENERATION

Arthrodesis of spinal motion segments leads to increased stresses at the unfused adjacent segments. Adjacent degeneration appears to be more common after anterior cervical fusion than posterior fusion. Capen et al. reported the presence of degenerative changes in 64% of patients after anterior fusion and in 2% patients who underwent posterior fusion at a 4-year follow-up (150). The reported prevalence of radiographic adjacent segment degeneration after anterior cervical arthrodesis varies from 25 to 89% (151). These radiographic changes may represent a natural progression of degenerative disease or increased stresses at the adjacent level after arthrodesis. Gore and Sepic reported a 50% frequency of radiographic changes consistent with progressive spondylosis, and 14% of patients experienced new level radicular symptoms (152). Bohlman et al. reported new onset radiculopathy in 9% patients after Smith-Robinson technique of ACDF without plating (12). Hilibrand et al. observed that symptomatic adjacent segment degeneration occurs at a relatively constant rate of 2.9% per year during the first 10 years after the operation (151). Whether instrumentation alters the incidence of adjacent segment degeneration in the cervical spine is unclear. Zaveri and Ford have recently suggested that the risk for adjacent segment degeneration after instrumented and uninstrumented anterior cervical spine fusion is similar (51).

Unlike in the lumbar spine, the risk of adjacent segment arthritis does not increase with multilevel arthrodesis in the cervical spine. This finding is attributable to the fact that most multilevel cervical fusion procedures are performed at the C5-6 and C6-7 levels, which are most mobile and most at risk of developing degenerative changes. In contrast, many patients undergoing one-level fusion have some degree of preexisting degeneration or may subsequently develop degenerative changes at the unfused segment. Therefore, careful preoperative evaluation of neuroradiologic imaging studies is imperative, and all degenerated segments producing symptoms should be included in the arthrodesis.

The reported reoperation rate for adjacent segment degeneration is 7 to 9% (153,154). Achieving fusion is more difficult when anterior cervical arthrodesis is performed adjacent to a prior fusion. Hilibrand et al. performed a retrospective review of 38 patients who underwent surgical treatment for adjacent segment degeneration of the cervical spine; they reported a 63% fusion rate with discectomy and interbody grafting and a 100% fusion rate with corpectomy and strut grafting (155).

Goffin et al. reported radiologically detectable evidence of late degenerative changes of the cervical spine at the disc levels adjacent to the fusion area in 60% of patients after internal fixation for cervical trauma (68). Fusion involving lower cervical spine or more than one disc level, Frankel class A to C neurologic deficit on admission, and hyperflexion injuries were some of the risk factors that were associated with a higher incidence of cervical adjacent segment degeneration.

COST EFFECTIVENESS AND OUTCOME ANALYSIS

The number of cervical fusion procedures performed in the United States continues to rise. The rate of cervical fusion has increased from 38,000 in 1985 to 110,000 in 1996, and cervical fusion now accounts for 48% of all spinal fusions performed (5). The number patients treated with instrumented cervical fusion is also growing with increasing availability of a wide variety of cervical implants. The enormous costs of health care and constrained resources are placing greater scrutiny on the cost effectiveness of surgical procedures. An increasing emphasis is also being placed on the outcome analysis.

In general, the literature supports the notion that a solid fusion appears to have a better outcome than those with a pseudarthrosis. Cauthen et al. performed an outcome analysis of noninstrumented anterior cervical discectomy and interbody fusion using the Cloward technique in 348 patients (156). They concluded better outcomes are associated with solid fusion, fewer fused levels, nonsmoking patients, higher education levels, and absence of secondary economic gain. Patients with greater neurologic deficits tend to experience less postoperative improvement in symptoms than patients with more acute and less severe neurologic findings.

McLaughlin et al. analyzed the cost effectiveness of rigid internal fixation for two-level ACDF (157). Thirty-nine patients were treated with allograft fusion and plating, and 25 were treated with uninstrumented allograft fusion. They observed that a two-level ACDF with anterior plating for radiculopathy is safe and effective, and it requires shorter convalescence period than conventional ACDF. The patients also have shorter duration of disability and are able to return to unrestricted work earlier. They concluded that increased cost of treatment for rigid internal fixation is more than offset by the benefits of earlier mobilization. In another study, Castro et al. compared the costs of ACDF using titanium cage, local autologous bone graft, and anterior plate instrumentation with ACDF using iliac crest bone graft and plate fixation (158). The three variables considered were cage cost, cost of the operating time, and hospitalization cost. The estimated costs for the two surgical procedures were not significantly different. Thus, the time saved by not harvesting an iliac crest bone graft was comparable to the cost of the cage. Harvesting ICBG also increased the morbidity rate by 22% in their study.

Anterior cervical instrumentation may also be highly cost effective in the surgical management of patients with cervical trauma. Rigid early fixation of cervical fracture with maintenance of alignment appears to significantly reduce the duration of acute hospital care, facilitate early rehabilitation and mobilization, minimize secondary kyphotic deformity, and decrease the need for additional posterior stabilization acutely or at a later date (131).

As the availability of modern implants has become more widespread, the number of instrumented fusion performed has tremendously increased. The indications and operative techniques will continue to be redefined over the next several years. More studies that focus on cost and outcome analysis of various cervical spine surgical procedures are necessary to clearly establish the indications and potential benefits of instrumentation.

SUMMARY

The surgical management of disorders of the cervical spine continues to evolve. The surgical treatment is individualized based on the patient's symptoms, location of pathology, number of levels involved, sagittal alignment, and surgeon's preference. Adequate decompression and fusion are necessary in relieving the patients' symptoms. Meticulous preparation of fusion bed and proper bone grafting technique are pivotal in achieving sound fusion.

The indications for the use of specific cervical spine implants have not been well established, and more clinical studies are needed to better elucidate the indications for modern spinal implants. The most critical factor for successful outcome of anterior cervical spinal instrumentation is proper patient selection. In discectomy cases, anterior cervical plating appears to be most useful in three-level discectomy and fusion. Segmental screw-plate fixation improves the biomechanical stability and fusion rate, and prevents graft settling and loss of sagittal alignment. The use of anterior plating for two-level discectomy and fusion is somewhat controversial, but many surgeons routinely recommend internal fixation, particularly in smokers. Anterior cervical plating for one-level discectomy and fusion is not justified in terms of enhancing fusion rates and improving clinical outcome, but plating is frequently performed to avoid complications of autograft harvesting and to minimize postoperative brace wear. Internal fixation is almost universally agreed on after one- or two-level corpectomy, but the controversy surrounds the type and extent of internal fixation, plate versus cage fixation, and anterior versus lateral mass plating. Reconstruction after three-level corpectomy continues to present a significant challenge to spine surgeons. A hybrid approach that combines corpectomy at more severely involved segments and a discectomy at less severely involved segments seems to offer the best approach in terms of enhancing rigidity of the construct and minimizing strut-graft related complications.

Anterior plate fixation also plays an important role in cervical spine stabilization in patients with cervical spine injury or tumors. Anterior decompression and fusion with plate fixation provides immediate stability to the affected area, reduces the risk of graft extrusion, avoids the need for extended postoperative external immobilization, and significantly shortens the rehabilitation period.

REFERENCES

1. Bailey RW, Badgley CE. Stabilization of the cervical spine by anterior fusion. *J Bone Joint Surg* 1960;42A:565–624.
2. Robinson RA, Smith GW. Anterolateral cervical disc removing and interbody fusion for cervical disc syndrome. *Bull Johns Hopkins Hosp* 1955;96:223–234.
3. Bohler J. Sofort—und Frubehandlung traumatischer Querschmnitt lahmungen. *Zeitschr Orthopad Grengebiete* 1967;103:512–528.
4. Zeidman SM, Ducker TB, Raycroft J. Trends and complications in cervical spine surgery: 1989–1993. *J Spinal Disord* 1997;10(6):523–526.
5. Abraham DJ, Herkowitz HN. Indications and trends in use in cervical spinal fusions. *Orthop Clin North Am* 1998;29(4):731–744.
6. Whitecloud T, Seago R. Cervical discogenic syndrome: results of operative intervention in patients with positive discography. *Spine* 1987;2:313–316.
7. Palit M, Schofferman J, Goldthwaite N, et al. Anterior discectomy and fusion for the management of neck pain. *Spine* 1999;24:2224–2228.
8. Epstein NE. The value of anterior cervical plating in preventing vertebral fracture and graft extrusion after multilevel anterior cervical corpectomy with posterior wiring and fusion: indications, results, and complications. *J Spinal Disord* 2000;13(1):9–15.
9. Gaetani P, Tancioni F, Spanu G, et al. Anterior cervical discectomy: an analysis on clinical long-term results in 153 cases. *J Neurosurg Sci* 1995;39(4):211–218.
10. Savolainen S, Rinne J, Hernesniemi J. A prospective randomized study of anterior single-level cervical disc operations with long-term follow-up: surgical fusion is unnecessary. *Neurosurgery* 1998;43(1):51–55.

11. Dowd GC, Wirth FP. Anterior cervical discectomy: is fusion necessary? *J Neurosurg* 1999;90[1 Suppl]:8–12.
12. Bohlman H, Emery S, Goodfellow D, et al. Robinson anterior cervical discectomy and arthrodesis for cervical radiculopathy. *J Bone Joint Surg* 1993;75A:1298–1307.
13. Zdeblick TA, Cooke ME, Wilson D, et al. Anterior cervical discectomy, fusion, and plating. A comparative animal study. *Spine* 1993;18(14): 1974–1983.
14. Parsons IM, Kang JD. Mechanism of failure after anterior cervical disc surgery. *Curr Opin Orthoped* 1998;9:2–11.
15. Wang JC, McDonough PW, Endow K, et al. The effect of cervical plating on single-level anterior cervical discectomy and fusion. *J Spinal Disord* 1999;12(6):467–471.
16. Connolly PJ, Esses SI, Kostuik JP. Anterior cervical fusion: outcome analysis of patients fused with and without anterior cervical plates. *J Spinal Disord* 1996;9(3):202–206.
17. Kaiser MG, Haid RW Jr, Subach BR, et al. Anterior cervical plating enhances arthrodesis after discectomy and fusion with cortical allograft. *Neurosurgery* 2002;50(2):229–236, discussion, 236–238.
18. Zoega B, Karrholm J, Lind B. One-level cervical spine fusion. A randomized study, with or without plate fixation, using radiostereometry in 27 patients. *Acta Orthop Scand* 1998;69(4):363–368.
19. Grob D, Peyer JV, Dvorak J. The use of plate fixation in anterior surgery of the degenerative cervical spine: a comparative prospective clinical study. *Eur Spine J* 2001;10(5):408–413.
20. Brodke DS, Gollogly S, Alexander Mohr R, et al. Dynamic cervical plates: biomechanical evaluation of load sharing and stiffness. *Spine* 2001;26(12):1324–1329.
21. Katsuura A, Hukuda S, Imanaka T, et al. Anterior cervical plate used in degenerative disease can maintain cervical lordosis. *J Spinal Disord* 1996;9(6):470–476.
22. Wang JC, McDonough PW, Endow KK, et al. Increased fusion rates with cervical plating for two-level anterior cervical discectomy and fusion. *Spine* 2000;25(1):41–45.
23. Troyanovich SJ, Stroink AR, Kattner KA, et al. Does anterior plating maintain cervical lordosis versus conventional fusion techniques? A retrospective analysis of patients receiving single-level fusions. *J Spinal Disord Tech* 2002;15(1):69–74.
24. Kostuik JP, Connolly PJ. Esses SI, et al. Anterior cervical plate fixation with the titanium hollow screw plate system. *Spine* 1993;18:1273–1278.
25. Epstein NE. Anterior cervical diskectomy and fusion without plate instrumentation in 178 patients. *J Spinal Disord* 2000;13(1):1–8.
26. Caspar W, Geisler FH, Pitzen T, et al. Anterior cervical plate stabilization in one- and two-level degenerative disease: overtreatment or benefit? *J Spinal Disord* 1998;11(1):1–11.
27. Zoega B, Karrholm J, Lind B. Plate fixation adds stability to two-level anterior fusion in the cervical spine: a randomized study using radiostereometry. *Eur Spine J* 1998;7(4):302–307.
28. Wang JC, McDonough PW, Endow KK, et al. A comparison of fusion rates between single-level cervical corpectomy and two-level discectomy and fusion. *J Spinal Disord* 2001;14(3):222–225.
29. Wang JC, McDonough PW, Kanim LE, et al. Increased fusion rates with cervical plating for three-level anterior cervical discectomy and fusion. *Spine* 2001;26(6):643–646.
30. Bolesta MJ, Rechtine GR 2nd, Chrin AM. Three- and four-level anterior cervical discectomy and fusion with plate fixation: a prospective study. *Spine* 2000;25(16):2040–2044.
31. Hilibrand AS, Fye MA, Emery SE, et al. Increased rate of arthrodesis with strut grafting after multilevel anterior cervical decompression. *Spine* 2002;27(2):146–151.
32. Fessler RG, Steck JC, Giovanini MA. Anterior cervical corpectomy for cervical spondylotic myelopathy. *Neurosurgery* 1998;43(2):257–265.
33. Epstein NE. Reoperation rates for acute graft extrusion and pseudarthrosis after one-level anterior corpectomy and fusion with and without plate instrumentation: etiology and corrective management. *Surg Neurol* 2001;56(2):73–80.
34. Saunders RL, Pikus HJ, Ball P. Four-level cervical corpectomy. *Spine* 1998;23(22):2455–2461.
35. Mayr MT, Subach BR, Comey CH, et al. Cervical spinal stenosis: outcome after anterior corpectomy, allograft reconstruction, and instrumentation. *J Neurosurg* 2002;96[1 Suppl]:10–16.
36. Eleraky MA, Llanos C, Sonntag VK. Cervical corpectomy: report of 185 cases and review of the literature. *J Neurosurg* 1999;90[1 Suppl]: 35–41.
37. Vaccaro AR, Falatyn SP, Scuderi GJ, et al. Early failure of long segment anterior cervical plate fixation. *J Spinal Disord* 1998;11(5):410–415.
38. Riew KD, Sethi NS, Devney J, et al. Complications of buttress plate stabilization of cervical corpectomy. *Spine* 1999;24(22):2404–2410.
39. Vanichkachorn JS, Vaccaro AR, Silveri CP, et al. Anterior junctional plate in the cervical spine. *Spine* 1998;23(22):2462–2467.
40. Yonenobu K, Hosono N, Iwasaki M, et al. Laminaplasty versus subtotal corpectomy. A comparative study of results in multisegment cervical spondylotic myelopathy. *Spine* 1992;17:1281–1284.
41. Epstein N. Anterior approaches to cervical spondylosis and ossification of the posterior longitudinal ligament: review of operative technique and assessment of 65 multilevel circumferential procedures. *Surg Neurol* 2001;55(6):313–324.
42. Schultz KD Jr, McLaughlin MR, Haid RW Jr, et al. Single-stage anterior-posterior decompression and stabilization for complex cervical spine disorders. *J Neurosurg* 2000;93[2 Suppl]:214–221.
43. Bishop RC, Moore KA, Hadley MN. Anterior cervical interbody fusion using autogeneic and allogenic bone graft substrate: a prospective comparative analysis. *J Neurosurg* 1996;85:206–210.
44. Heiple KG, Goldberg VM, Powell AE. Biology of cancellous bone grafts. *Orthop Clin North Am* 1987;18:179–185.
45. An HS, Simpson JM, Glover JM, et al. Comparison between allograft plus demineralized bone matrix versus autograft in anterior cervical fusion. A prospective multicenter study. *Spine* 1995;20:2211–2216.
46. Floyd T, Ohnmeiss D. A meta-analysis of autograft versus allograft in anterior cervical fusion. *Eur Spine J* 2000;9(5):398–403.
47. Shapiro S. Banked fibula and the locking anterior cervical plate in anterior cervical fusions following cervical discectomy. *J Neurosurg* 1996;84(2):161–165.
48. Shapiro S, Connolly P, Donnaldson J, et al. Cadaveric fibula, locking plate, and allogeneic bone matrix for anterior cervical fusions after cervical discectomy for radiculopathy or myelopathy. *J Neurosurg* 2001;95[1 Suppl]:43–50.
49. Thalgott JS, Fritts K, Giuffre JM, et al. Anterior interbody fusion of the cervical spine with coralline hydroxyapatite. *Spine* 1999;24(13):1295–1299.
50. Shapiro S, Bindal R. Femoral ring allograft for anterior cervical interbody fusion: technical note. *Neurosurgery* 2000;47(6):1457–1459.
51. Zaveri GR, Ford M. Cervical spondylosis: the role of anterior instrumentation after decompression and fusion. *J Spinal Disord* 2001;14(1):10–16.
52. Brown CW, Orme TJ, Richardson HD. The rate of pseudarthrosis (surgical nonunion) in patients who are smokers and patients who are non-smokers. *Spine* 1986;11:942.
53. Boden SD, Sumner DR. Biologic factors affecting spinal fusion and bone regeneration. *Spine* 1995;20:1025.
54. Hadley MN, Reddy SV. Smoking and human vertebral column: a review of the impact of cigarette use on vertebral bone metabolism and spinal fusion. *Neurosurgery* 1997;41:116–124.
55. Samartzis D, Matthews DK, Yoon ST, et al. Comparison of allograft to autograft in multi-level plated anterior cervical fusion. World Spine II, Chicago, IL, August 11, 2003.
56. Bose B. Anterior cervical instrumentation enhances fusion rates in multilevel reconstruction in smokers. *J Spinal Disord* 2001;14(1):3–9.
57. Hilibrand AS, Fye MA, Emery SE, et al. Impact of smoking on the outcome of anterior cervical arthrodesis with interbody or strut-grafting. *J Bone Joint Surg Am* 2001;83-A(5):668–673.
58. Samartzis D, Lyon C, Phillips M, et al. Comparison of non-plating to plating in one-level anterior cervical discectomy and fusion. Cervical Spine Research Society, Miami, FL, December 5, 2002.
59. Aebi M, Zuber K, Marchesi D. Treatment of cervical spine injuries with anterior plating. *Spine* 1991;16(3S):538–545.
60. Stauffer ES, Kelly DG. Fracture-dislocations of the cervical spine. *J Bone Joint Surg* 1977;59A:45.
61. Cloward RD. Treatment of acute fractures and fracture dislocations of the cervical spine by vertebral body fusion. A report of 11 cases. *J Neurosurg* 1961;18:205–209.
62. Vaccaro AR, Balderston RA. Anterior plate instrumentation for disorders of the subaxial cervical spine. *Clin Orthop* 1997;(335):112–121.
63. Schulte K, Clark CR, Goel VK. Kinematics of the cervical spine following discectomy and stabilization. *Spine* 1989;14(10):1116–1121.

64. Koh Y, Lim TH, You JW, et al. A biomechanical comparison of modern anterior and posterior plate fixation of the cervical spine. *Spine* 2001;26(1):15–21.
65. Richman JD, Daniel TE, Anderson DD, et al. Biomechanical evaluation of cervical spine stabilization methods using a porcine model. *Spine* 1995;20(20):2192–2197.
66. Spivak JM, Bharam S, Chen D, et al. Internal fixation of cervical trauma following corpectomy and reconstruction. The effects of posterior element injury. *Bull Hosp Jt Dis* 2000;59(1):47–51.
67. Casper W, Barbier DD, Klara PM. Anterior cervical fusion and Caspar plate stabilization for cervical trauma. *Neurosurgery* 1989;25:491–502.
68. Goffin J, van Loon J, Van Calenbergh F, et al. Long-term results after anterior cervical fusion and osteosynthetic stabilization for fractures and/or dislocations of the cervical spine. *J Spinal Disord* 1995;8(6):500–508.
69. Garvey TA, Eismont FJ, Roberti LJ. Anterior decompression, structural bone grafting and Caspar plate stabilization for unstable cervical spine fractures and/or dislocations. *Spine* 1992;17:5431–5435.
70. Bohler J, Gaudernak T. Anterior plate stabilization for fracture-dislocations of the lower cervical spine. *J Trauma* 1980;20:203–205.
71. Bremer AM, Nguyen TQ. Internal metal plate fixation combined with anterior interbody fusion in cases of cervical spine injury. *Neurosurgery* 1983;12:649–653.
72. DeOliviera JC. Anterior plate fixation of traumatic lesions of the lower cervical spine. *Spine* 1987;12:324–329.
73. Cabanela ME, Ebersold MJ. Anterior plate stabilization for bursting teardrop fractures of the cervical spine. *Spine* 1988;13:888–891.
74. Randle MJ, Wolf A, Levi L, et al. The use of anterior Caspar plate fixation in acute cervical spine injury. *Surg Neurol* 1991;36:181–189.
75. Ripa DR, Kowall MG, Meyer PR, et al. Series of ninety-two traumatic cervical spine injuries stabilized with anterior ASIF plate fusion technique. *Spine* 1991;16(3):S46–S55.
76. Bohlman HH, Anderson PA. Anterior decompression and arthrodesis of the cervical spine: long-term motor improvement. Part I—Improvement in incomplete traumatic quadriparesis. *J Bone Joint Surg Am* 1992;74(5):671–682.
77. Fisher CG, Dvorak MF, Leith J, et al. Comparison of outcomes for unstable lower cervical flexion teardrop fractures managed with halo thoracic vest versus anterior corpectomy and plating. *Spine* 2002;27(2):160–166.
78. Brodke DS, Harris M. Subaxial cervical trauma: evaluation and management options. *Semin Spine Surg* 2001;13:128–141.
79. An HS. Cervical spine trauma. *Spine* 1998;23:2713–2729.
80. Northrup BE, Vaccaro AR, Rosen JE, et al. Occurrence of infection in anterior cervical fusion for spinal cord injury after tracheostomy. *Spine* 1995;20(22):2449–2453.
81. Constans J, de Divitiis E, Donzelli R, et al. Spinal metastases with neurological manifestations. Review of 600 cases. *J Neurosurg* 1983;59:111–118.
82. Hammerberg K. Surgical treatment of metastatic spine disease. *Spine* 1992;17:1148–1153.
83. Rao S, Badini K, Schildhauer T, et al. Metastatic malignancy of the cervical spine. A nonoperative history. *Spine* 1992;17S:407–412.
84. Schaberg J, Gainor B. A profile of metastatic carcinoma of the spine. *Spine* 1985;10:19–20.
85. Rao S, Davis R. Cervical spine metastases. In: Clark C, ed. *The cervical spine*, 3rd ed. The Cervical Spine Research Society. Philadelphia: Lippincott–Raven Publishers, 1998:603–619.
86. Siegal T, Siegal T. Current considerations in the management of neoplastic spinal cord compression. *Spine* 1989;14:223–228.
87. Tomita T, Galicich J, Sundaresan N. Radiation therapy for spinal epidural metastases with complete block. *Acta Radiol Oncol* 1983;22:135–143.
88. Weissman D. Glucocorticoid treatment for brain metastases and epidural spinal cord compression. A review. *J Clin Oncol* 1988;3:543–551.
89. Bouchard J, Koka A, Bensauan M, et al. Effect of irradiation on posterior spinal fusions. A rabbit model. *Spine* 1994;19:1836–1841.
90. Emery S, Brazinski M, Koka A, et al. The biological and biomechanical effects of irradiation on anterior spinal bone grafts in a canine model. *J Bone Joint Surg* 1994;76A:540–548.
91. Mardjetko S, DeWald C. Management of metastatic spinal disease. In: *Spine: state of the art reviews*. Vol. 10. Philadelphia: Hanley and Belfus, Inc., 1996:89–95.
92. Jenis LG, An HS. Cervical spine metastasis. In: Herkowitz HN, ed. *Cervical Spine Research Society's The cervical spine*. In Press.
93. Atanasiu J, Badatcgeff F, Pidhorz L. Metastatic lesions of the cervical spine. *Spine* 1993;18:1279–1284.
94. Kostuik J, Weinstein J. Differential diagnosis and surgical treatment of metastatic spine tumors. In: Frymoyer J, ed. *The adult spine: principles and practice*. New York: Raven Press, 1991:861–888.
95. DeWald R, Bridwell K, Prodromas C, et al. Reconstructive spinal surgery as palliation for metastatic malignancies of the spine. *Spine* 1985;10:21–26.
96. King G, Kostuik J, McBroom R, et al. Surgical management of metastatic renal cell carcinoma of the spine. *Spine* 1991;16:265–271.
97. Gellad F, Sadato N, Numaguchi Y, et al. Vascular metastatic lesions of the spine: preoperative embolization. *Radiol* 1990;176:683–686.
98. Roscoe M, McBroom R, St. Louis E, et al. Preoperative embolization in the treatment of osseous metastases from renal cell carcinoma. *Clin Orthop* 1989;238:302–307.
99. Hall D, Webb J. Anterior plate fixation in spine tumor surgery. *Spine* 1991;16S:80–83.
100. Caspar W, Pitzen T, Papavero L, et al. Anterior cervical plating for the treatment of neoplasms in the cervical vertebrae. *J Neurosurg* 1999;90[1 Suppl]:27–34.
101. Dunn E. The role of methyl methacrylate in the stabilization and replacement of tumors of the cervical spine. *Spine* 1977;2:15–24.
102. Sherk H, Nolan J, Mooar P. Treatment of tumors of the cervical spine. *Clin Orthop* 1988;233:163–167.
103. Clark C, Keggi K, Panjabi M. Methylmethacrylate stabilization of the cervical spine. *J Bone Joint Surg* 1984;66A:40–46.
104. Sundaresan N, Galicich J, Lane J, et al. Treatment of neoplastic epidural cord compression by vertebral body resection and stabilization. *J Neurosurg* 1985;63:676–684.
105. Harrington K. The use of methylmethacrylate for vertebral-body replacement and anterior stabilization of pathological fracture-dislocations of the spine due to metastatic malignant disease. *J Bone Joint Surg* 1981;63A:36–46.
106. Siegal T, Tiqva P, Siegal T. Vertebral body resection for epidural compression by malignant tumors. Results of forty-seven consecutive operative procedures. *J Bone Joint Surg* 1985;67A:375–382.
107. Nicholls P, Jarecky T. The value of posterior decompression by laminectomy for malignant tumors of the spine. *Clin Orthop* 1985;201:210–213.
108. Coric D, Branch CL Jr, Jenkins JD. Revision of anterior cervical pseudoarthrosis with anterior allograft fusion and plating. *J Neurosurg* 1997;86(6):969–974.
109. Tribus CB, Corteen DP, Zdeblick TA. The efficacy of anterior cervical plating in the management of symptomatic pseudoarthrosis of the cervical spine. *Spine* 1999;24(9):860–864.
110. Lowery GL, Swank ML, McDonough RF. Surgical revision for failed anterior cervical fusions. Articular pillar plating or anterior revision? *Spine* 1995;20(22):2436–2441.
111. Riew KD, Hilibrand AS, Palumbo MA, et al. Anterior cervical corpectomy in patients previously managed with a laminectomy: short-term complications. *J Bone Joint Surg Am* 1999;81(7):950–957.
112. Herman JM, Sonntag VK. Cervical corpectomy and plate fixation for postlamincectomy kyphosis. *J Neurosurgery* 1994;80:963–970.
113. Reference deleted.
114. Geisler FH, Caspar W, Pitzen T, et al. Reoperation in patients after anterior cervical plate stabilization in degenerative disease. *Spine* 1998;23(8):911–920.
115. Chen IH. Biomechanical evaluation of subcortical versus bicortical screw purchase in anterior cervical plating. *Acta Neurochir (Wien)* 1996;138(2):167–173.
116. Maiman DJ, Pintar FA, Yoganandan N, et al. Pull-out strength of Caspar cervical screws. *Neurosurgery* 1992;31(6):1097–1101, discussion, 1101.
117. Richter M, Wilke HJ, Kluger P, et al. Biomechanical evaluation of a newly developed monocortical expansion screw for use in anterior internal fixation of the cervical spine. *In vitro* comparison with two established internal fixation systems. *Spine* 1999;24(3):207–212.
118. Spivak JM, Chen D, Kummer FJ. The effect of locking fixation screws on the stability of anterior cervical plating. *Spine* 1999;24(4):334–338.

119. Pitzen T, Wilke HJ, Caspar W, et al. Evaluation of a new monocortical screw for anterior cervical fusion and plating by a combined biomechanical and clinical study. *Eur Spine J* 1999;8(5):382–387.
120. Ebraheim NA, Fow J, Xu R, et al. The vertebral body depths of the cervical spine and its relation to anterior plate-screw fixation. *Spine* 1998;23(21):2299–2302.
121. Xu R, Rezcallah AT, Huntoon M, et al. Computed tomographic evaluation of length of screw paths for anterior cervical plating. *Am J Orthop* 2000;29(8):622–625.
122. Rapoff AJ, O'Brien TJ, Ghanayem AJ, et al. Anterior cervical graft and plate load sharing. *J Spinal Disord* 1999;12(1):45–49.
123. Isomi T, Panjabi MM, Wang JL, et al. Stabilizing potential of anterior cervical plates in multilevel corpectomies. *Spine* 1999;24(21):2219–2223.
124. Panjabi MM, Isomi T, Wang JL. Loosening at the screw-vertebra junction in multilevel anterior cervical plate constructs. *Spine* 1999;24(22):2383–2388.
125. DiAngelo DJ, Foley KT, Vossel KA, et al. Anterior cervical plating reverses load transfer through multilevel strut-grafts. *Spine* 2000;25(7):783–795.
126. Wang JL, Panjabi MM, Isomi T. The role of bone graft force in stabilizing the multilevel anterior cervical spine plate system. *Spine* 2000;25(13):1649–1654.
127. Lowery GL, McDonough RF. The significance of hardware failure in anterior cervical plate fixation. Patients with 2- to 7-year follow-up. *Spine* 1998;23(2):181–186.
128. DiAngelo D, Foley KT, Liu W, et al. *In vitro* comparison of translational anterior cervical plate with a constrained anterior cervical plate. North American Spine Society Proceedings, 16th annual meeting. Washington State Convention and Trade center, Seattle, WA, October 31–November 3, 2001, pp. 129–130.
129. Kirkpatrick JS, Levy JA, Carillo J, et al. Reconstruction after multilevel corpectomy in the cervical spine. A sagittal plane biomechanical study. *Spine* 1999;24(12):1186–1190.
130. Foley KT, DiAngelo DJ, Rampersaud YR, et al. The in vitro effects of instrumentation on multilevel cervical strut-graft mechanics. *Spine* 1999;24(22):2366–2376.
131. Vaccaro AR, Balderston RA. Anterior plate instrumentation for disorders of the subaxial cervical spine. *Clin Orthop* 1997;(335):112–121.
132. Sutterlin CE III, McAfee PC, Warden KE, et al. A biomechanical evaluation of cervical spine stabilization methods in a bovine model. Static and cyclic loading. *Spine* 1988;13:775–780.
133. Coe JD, Warden KE, Sutterlin CE III, et al. Biomechanical evaluation of cervical spine stabilization methods in a human cadaveric model. Spine 1989;14:1122–1131.
134. Kalff R, Ulrich C, Claes L, et al. Comparative experimental biomechanical study of different types of stabilization methods of the lower cervical spine. *Neurosurgery Rev* 1992;15:259–264.
135. Hacker RJ. A randomized prospective study of an anterior cervical interbody fusion device with a minimum of 2 years of follow-up results. *J Neurosurg* 2000;93[2 Suppl]:222–226.
136. Riew KD, Rhee JM. The use of titanium mesh cages in the cervical spine. *Clin Orthop* 2002, 394:47–54.
137. Majd ME, Vadhva M, Holt RT. Anterior cervical reconstruction using titanium cages with anterior plating. *Spine* 1999;24(15):1604–1610.
138. Kandziora F, Pflugmacher R, Schafer J, et al. Biomechanical comparison of cervical spine interbody fusion cages. *Spine* 2001;26(17):1850–1857.
139. Greene DL, Crandall D, Chamberlain RH, et al. Biomechanical comparison of cervical interbody cage verus structural bone graft. North American Spine Society Proceedings, 16th annual meeting. Washington State Convention and Trade center, Seattle, WA, October 31–November 3, 2001, pp. 134–135.
140. Biyani A, Natarajan RN, Monteiro SK, et al. The stability of anterior cervical interbody fusion constructs using cage vs bone graft: a finite element model analysis. Submitted for presentation. 30th CSRS annual meeting. Miami Beach, FL, December 5–7, 2002.
141. Kettler A, Wilke HJ, Claes L. Effects of neck movements on stability and subsidence in cervical interbody fusion: an *in vitro* study. *J Neurosurg* 2001;94[1 Suppl]:97–107.
142. Shimamoto N, Cunningham BW, Dmitriev AE, et al. Biomechanical evaluation of stand-alone interbody fusion cages in the cervical spine. *Spine* 2001;26(19):E432–E436.
143. ElSaghir H, Bohm H. Anterior versus posterior plating in cervical corpectomy. *Arch Orthop Trauma Surg* 2000;120(10):549–554.
144. Paramore CG, Dickman CA, Sonntag CKH. Mechanisms of Caspar plate failure. *J Neurosurg* 1995;82:3611.
145. Gaudinez RF, English GM, Gebhard JS, et al. Esophageal perforations after anterior cervical surgery. *J Spinal Disord* 2000;13(1):77–84.
146. Geyer TE, Foy MA. Oral extrusion of a screw after anterior cervical spine plating. *Spine* 2001;26(16):1814–1816.
147. Fujibayashi S, Shikata J, Kamiya N, et al. Missing anterior cervical plate and screws: a case report. *Spine* 2000;25(17):2258–2261.
148. Epstein NE, Hollingsworth R, Nardi D, et al. Can airway complications following multilevel anterior cervical surgery be avoided? *J Neurosurg* 2001;94[2 Suppl]:185–188.
149. Sagi HC, Beutler W, Carroll E, et al. Airway complications associated with surgery on the anterior cervical spine. *Spine* 2002;27(9): 949–953.
150. Capen DA, Garland DE, Waters RL. Surgical stabilization of the cervical spine. A comparative analysis of anterior and posterior spine fusions. *Clin Orthop* 1985;196:229–237.
151. Hilibrand AS, Carlson GD, Palumbo MA, et al. Radiculopathy and myelopathy at segments adjacent to the site of previous anterior cervical arthrodesis. *J Bone Joint Surg* 1999;81A:519–528.
152. Gore DR, Sepic SB. Anterior cervical fusion for degenerated or protruded discs. *Spine* 1986;9:667–671.
153. Lunsford LD, Bissonette DJ, Jannetta PJ, et al. Anterior surgery for cervical disc disease. Part 1: Treatment of lateral cervical disc herniation in 253 cases. *J Neurosurg* 1980;53(1):1–11.
154. Henderson CM, Hennessey RG, Shuey HM Jr, et al. Posterior lateral foraminotomy as an exclusive operative technique for cervical radiculopathy; a review of 846 consecutively operated cases. *Neurosurgery* 1983;13:504–512.
155. Hilibrand AS, Yoo JU, Carlson GD, et al. The success of anterior cervical arthrodesis adjacent to a previous fusion. *Spine* 1997;22 (14):1574–1579.
156. Cauthen JC, Kinard RE, Vogler JB, et al. Outcome analysis of noninstrumented anterior cervical discectomy and interbody fusion in 348 patients. *Spine* 1998;23(2):188–192.
157. McLaughlin MR, Purighalla V, Pizzi FJ. Cost advantages of two-level anterior cervical fusion with rigid internal fixation for radiculopathy and degenerative disease. *Surg Neurol* 1997;48(6):560–565.
158. Castro FP Jr, Holt RT, Majd M, et al. A cost analysis of two anterior cervical fusion procedures *J Spinal Disord* 2000;13(6):511–514.

CHAPTER 40

Internal Fixation of the Cervical Spine

C. Posterior Instrumentation of the Lower Cervical Spine

John Gaylord Heller and Paul Jeffords

The techniques of posterior cervical spine instrumentation have evolved considerably over the last 25 years. Traditional posterior wiring techniques now are one of many options available to a surgeon who can select devices that meet the unique circumstances of a given patient. Advances in segmental fixation techniques have paralleled advances in understanding the anatomy and biomechanics of the posterior cervical region. Surgical implants are increasingly available and adaptable to regional anatomic variations far better than more traditional techniques, often reducing the need for external postoperative immobilization. As the methods of instrumentation have become more sophisticated, the surgeon is required to have a greater understanding of the regional anatomy, as the margins for error may often be quite narrow. Indeed, some anatomic variations may preclude the use of these methods.

This chapter presents a quantitative approach to applied posterior cervical anatomy as the basis for selecting the appropriate instrumentation, as well as understanding anatomic limits. The spectrum of posterior fixation techniques for the lower cervical spine is explored, from the occiput to the upper thoracic spine. These techniques are primarily used to impart segmental stability and promote fusion healing, not as a substitute for osseous fusion. It remains essential for the exposure, decortication, and bone grafting to be done with careful attention to detail. Failure to achieve a fusion results in implant loosening or failure at some point in time. There are exceptions in which fusion is not the ultimate goal, such as oncologic reconstructions in patients with limited life expectancy. In such instances, contemporary fixation methods are better suited to providing brace-free activity for the patients' life span.

APPLIED ANATOMY

Traditionally, the cervical spine has been divided into two qualitatively distinct regions: the upper and lower cervical spine. The division was morphologically descriptive and based on the similarities of the vertebrae from C-3 to C-7 compared to the oddly shaped vertebrae above. The proliferation of quantitative cervical anatomic data during the 1990s and the concomitant evolution in surgical methods invites reconsideration of this dichotomy. From a surgical perspective, it appears more useful to classify the cervical spine into three distinct regions based on the surgical anatomy and implications for spinal instrumentation techniques: the cervicocranium (occiput to C-2), the "true" subaxial region (C3-6), and the cervicothoracic junction (C-7 to T-2). This chapter focuses on the latter two regions, but includes the axis vertebra (C-2) as an anchor point for certain circumstances.

Cervicocranium

The axis is the component of the cervicocranium, which may be an important proximal anchor for segmental fixation of the poste-

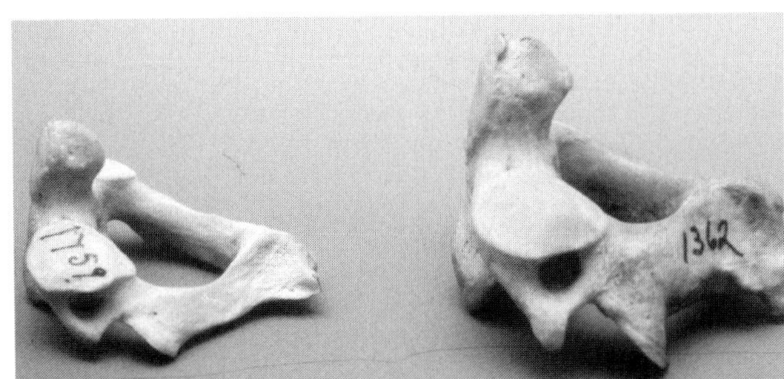

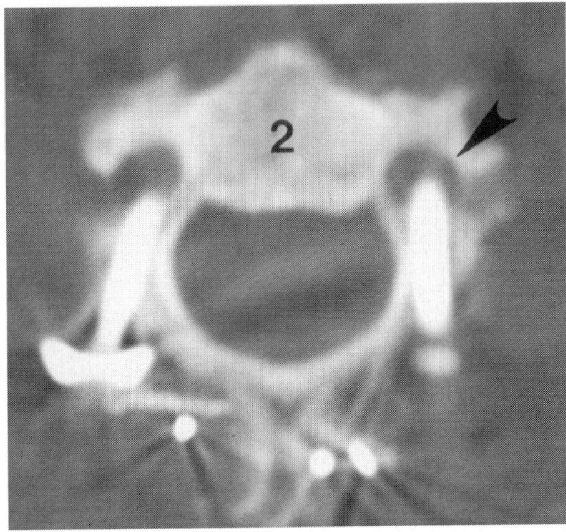

A B

FIG. 1. A: Photograph of axis vertebrae illustrating the range of size that might be encountered clinically. While planning a given fixation procedure, one should take note of the relevant osseous dimensions, as well as local anatomic variations (e.g., the size and locations of the foramina transversaria containing the vertebral arteries). **B:** A postoperative axial computed tomography scan indicating the potential for compromise of a vertebral artery if too long a screw were inserted (*arrow*). In this instance, the artery was not injured.

rior subaxial cervical spine. The axis vertebra (C-2) is easily recognized due to the vertical prominence of the odontoid process. Its posterior arch has a well-developed spinous process that can be engaged with wires or cables. The lamina of C-2 may also be engaged with hooks, wires, and cables when indicated. The pedicles of C-2 are especially suited to screw insertion owing to their easy surgical accessibility, as well as their size and orientation. The size and position of the foramina transversaria should be noted, however, so that the intended path of any screw avoids injury to the vertebral arteries. Other important anatomic variations exist, including the size of C-2 itself (Fig. 1).

Subaxial Spine

Vertebral Body

The transverse dimensions of the vertebral bodies, including end-plate width, depth, and cross-sectional area, increase from rostral to caudal in the cervical and thoracic spine (1). The most apparent increases occur at the cervicothoracic transition levels (C-6 to T-1). There is a steady flattening of the vertebral bodies as measured by the width to depth ratio. The vertebral height remains constant from C-3 to C-5 and then decreases slightly at C-6 before increasing rapidly at C-7. The normal lordosis from C-2 to C-7 is 35 degrees, divided in equal 7-degree segments (2). At T-1, the lower end-plate inclination suddenly reverses. This results in a slightly kyphotic bony wedge at each level, which initiates the normal thoracic kyphosis.

The spinal canal width, determined by the bordering pedicles and lateral masses, remains fairly constant throughout the cervical spine because as the vertebral body widens, the pedicle angles narrow. The canal depth and cross-sectional area are greatest at C-1 and C-2, but decrease precipitously at C-3 (3). The difference between the cross-sectional area of the spinal cord and that of the spinal canal itself defines the space available for the spinal cord. Under normal circumstances, the space is very generous in the cervicocranial region, but it is notably reduced below C-2, particularly in the presence of congenital stenosis. In stenotic patients who need posterior cervical instrumentation, the risk for further compromise of the space available for the spinal cord should be accounted for when selecting among instrumentation techniques. For example, iatrogenic spinal cord injury could result from inappropriate use of sublaminar devices.

Posterior Elements

Thorough preoperative assessment of regional bone anatomy precedes any instrumentation procedure. In the case of posterior cervical instrumentation, most of the attention is directed to the posterior elements, pedicles, spinous processes, and lateral masses. These structures must be assessed for each operative level. As there can be significant asymmetry in certain values between the right and left sides, these individual variations must also be considered (Fig. 2).

Pedicle

The pedicle is surrounded by essential structures on all sides. The vertebral artery and its associated venous plexus abut laterally. The dura and spinal cord lie medially. The nerve roots abut superiorly and are separated only slightly from the pedicle margin inferiorly. Numerous investigators have shown the outer pedicle dimensions (i.e., height, width, and cross-sectional area) are largest at C-2 and decrease significantly from C-3 to C-6 (1,4). The height stays fairly constant while the width slowly increases from C-7 downward. Due to the pedicle's oval shape, it is its width that is the limiting dimension for pedicle screw fixation. Panjabi reported that external pedicle dimensions consistently exceed 4.0 mm (1). Subsequent studies have demonstrated the outer pedicle width is frequently 4 mm or less, however, particularly at C-3 or C-4. The inner pedicle dimensions, the important determinants of safe pedicle fixation, are

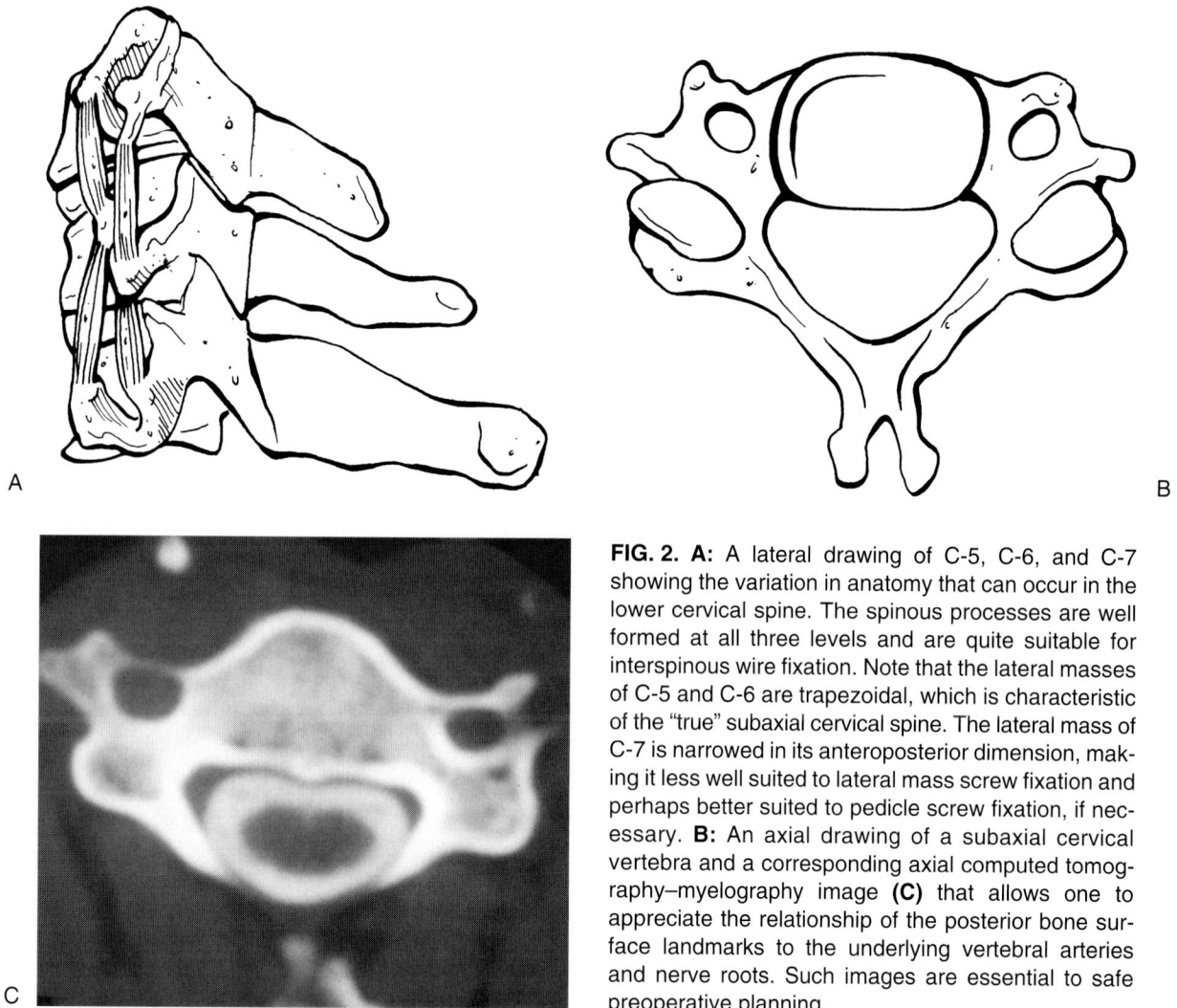

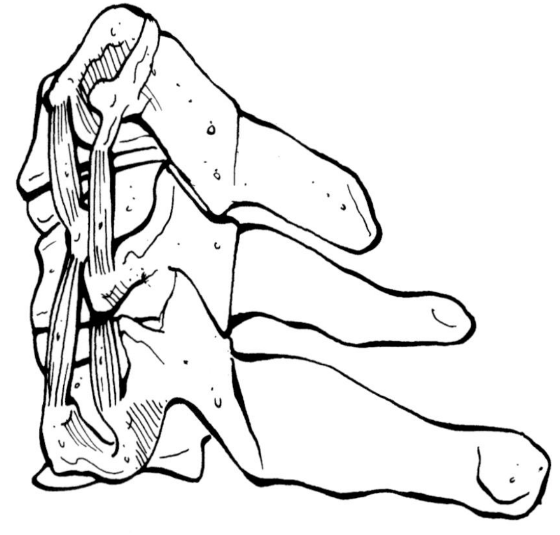

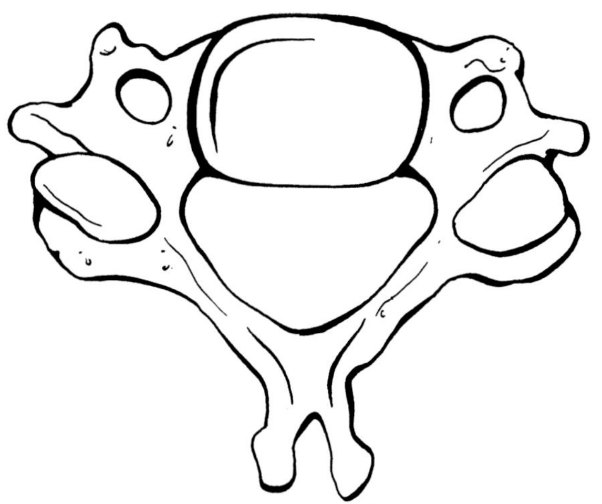

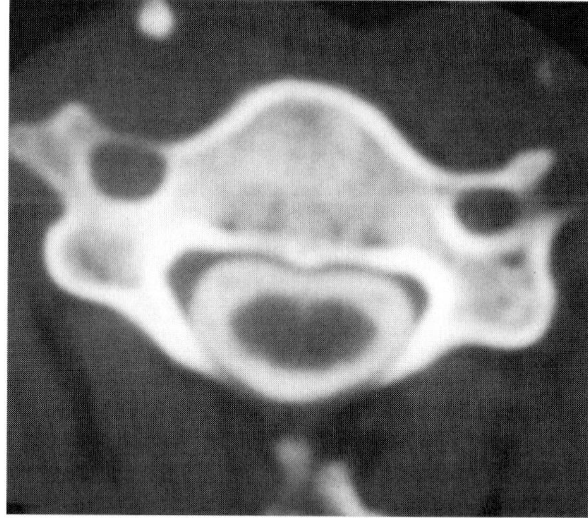

FIG. 2. A: A lateral drawing of C-5, C-6, and C-7 showing the variation in anatomy that can occur in the lower cervical spine. The spinous processes are well formed at all three levels and are quite suitable for interspinous wire fixation. Note that the lateral masses of C-5 and C-6 are trapezoidal, which is characteristic of the "true" subaxial cervical spine. The lateral mass of C-7 is narrowed in its anteroposterior dimension, making it less well suited to lateral mass screw fixation and perhaps better suited to pedicle screw fixation, if necessary. **B:** An axial drawing of a subaxial cervical vertebra and a corresponding axial computed tomography–myelography image **(C)** that allows one to appreciate the relationship of the posterior bone surface landmarks to the underlying vertebral arteries and nerve roots. Such images are essential to safe preoperative planning.

usually adequate at C-2 and C-7 but often less than 2 mm at C-3 through C-6, with the thinnest cortex along the lateral wall throughout the cervical spine (4). The pedicle at T-1 is larger in both dimensions than that of C-7 and is similar in size to that of C-2.

The axial or transverse plane (medial) angle of the pedicle is lowest (i.e., has the most sagittal orientation) at C-2 (10 to 15 degrees), then increases significantly at C-3 (mean, 44 degrees) and slowly decreases to C-7 (mean, 37 degrees) (5). The projection of the pedicle axis on the dorsal surface of the lateral mass has been localized with respect to vertical and horizontal reference lines. The inferior edge of the superior facet is the standard horizontal reference line, but some studies have used the inferior facet or the midline of the transverse process. The outermost margin of the articular mass provides the most reproducible vertical line. For clinical purposes, the horizontal pedicle offset at C-2 is best measured from the lateral extent of the spinal canal at the junction of the lateral mass and lamina (mean, 7.2 mm) so as to avoid excessive lateral dissection (6). When measured from the lateral wall of the articular process, the horizontal offset increases from a mean of 4.9 mm at C-3 to a mean of 6.2 mm at C-6 corresponding to the changes in transverse plane angle described previously (7). At C-7, the mean horizontal offset is only 2.7 mm, corresponding to the decrease in transverse plane angle reported by Xu (8). The use of such topographic landmarks for pedicle screw insertion has proven rather unreliable in comparison to other methods, however (9–11).

Transverse Processes

The transverse processes project anterolateral from the pedicle and decrease in length from C-2 to C-6, whereas the vertebral body width increases, keeping the transverse process band constant. At C-7, the transverse process length increases significantly along with the vertebral body, causing an increase in overall width. They provide a convenient radiographic reference point on a "true lateral" view of the subaxial vertebrae but have no practical role as points of purchase during instrumentation.

Lateral Masses

The dimensions of the facet joint surfaces remain constant throughout the cervical and upper thoracic spine with the exception of the C-2 superior articular facet, which is approximately 50% larger (12). The mean C-2 superior facet transverse and sagittal plane angles are 37.1 and 116.0 degrees, respectively. This makes it nearly horizontal in comparison to the remaining joints. The facets become less coronal and more vertical in orientation from C-6 to T-4, with the most rapid changes seen in the cervicothoracic transition zone (13).

The depth of the lateral mass as measured from the midpoint of its posterior surface to its junction with the transverse process at the nerve root groove decreases slowly from C-3 (mean, 8.9 mm) to C-6 (mean, 8.0 mm) and then drops sharply at C-7 (mean, 6.4 mm) (14). In the absence of well-formed spinous processes, the lateral masses have become the principal points of purchase for screws in the posterior subaxial region.

Lamina

The lamina of C-2 is quite thick. The laminae from C-3 to C-6 are much thinner and shingled, with the inferior edge of the upper lamina often overlapping the superior edge of the lower lamina. The lamina at C-7 is once again quite stout, with a rapid increase in height and especially thickness reflecting the muscle forces applied here as well as the force transmission through the posterior elements at this transitional region (5,15). In the upper thoracic region, the laminar height and thickness remain constant, whereas the length of the lamina decreases, corresponding to the more sagittal pedicle angle (5,16).

Spinous Process

The spinous processes at C-2 and C-7 are consistently well developed with strong, dense bone. The other spinous processes are far more variable in their development, typically increasing in size and strength as one descends from C-3 to C-6. Their individual size and strength determine whether they are amenable to interspinous wire fixation methods. They may also be structurally inadequate points of fixation due to trauma, surgical removal, or poor bone quality.

Nerve Root

Each cervical nerve exits the spinal canal through an intervertebral foramen and lies in a nerve root groove, which extends from the superior edge of the subjacent pedicle along the superior surface of the transverse process to its tip (14). The foraminal dimensions steadily increase in size from C3-4 to C-7 to T-1. As it enters the foramen, the root runs posterior to the inferolateral corner of the upper vertebral body, which forms the upper one-half of the anterior foraminal wall. The rootlets then cross the midportion of the foramen at the level of the intervertebral disc to the superior lateral border of the lower pedicle. Here, they come to lie in the medial zone of the nerve root groove, which comprises the narrower, inferior one-half of the foramen with its edges defined by the underlying pedicle and its length corresponding to the pedicle width. The width of the groove is proportionally smaller than that of the foramen and smallest at C-4, similar to patterns of foraminal dimensions. The medial zone, the narrowest portion of the intervertebral foramen, is bordered anteriorly by the uncinate process and posteriorly by the anteromedial edge of the superior articular process. Spondylosis can cause symptoms of nerve root compression here from osteophytic overgrowth of the uncinate processes, the facet joints, or a combination of the two.

In the middle zone, the dorsal rootlets coalesce into the dorsal root ganglion, which lies in the posterior and caudal aspects of the groove in a sulcus that crosses the anterior surface of the superior articular process at the inferior one-third of the articular mass. The ventral rootlets join to form the more anterior and cranial ventral root lying directly posterior to the vertebral artery and its transverse foramen, which defines this zone (17).

The dorsal root emerges from the dorsal root ganglion and then combines with the ventral root to form the spinal root in the lateral zone. The lateral zone is quite variable in dimensions, with an average width of 6.0 mm and average length of 4.8 mm. The lateral zone is bordered by anterior and posterior ridges that expand to form tubercles at the end of the transverse process. The nerve exits the groove at the anterolateral portion of the superior facet and branches into ventral, dorsal, and communicating rami. The ventral ramus is referred to as the *spinal nerve* (18).

Vertebral Artery

The vertebral artery enters the cervical spine above the transverse sulcus at C-7 and ascends in a slightly posteromedial course from C-6 to C-3 within the foramina transversaria of the transverse processes in the middle zone of the nerve root groove. The vertebral artery foramen (also known as *foramen transversarium*) is circular, and its dimensions are uniform from C-6 up to C-3 with an average diameter of 5.2 mm (19). The position is slightly more lateral at C-6 than in the upper levels, whereas the apex of the lateral mass is slightly more medial (20). The transverse foramen becomes more medial with decreasing interforaminal distance as it ascends to C-3. With rare exceptions, the foramen lies lateral to the vertebral body at its posterior one-third and is adjacent to the lateral wall of the pedicle at all levels. From C-6 to C-3, the foramen moves progressively more posterior with respect to the vertebral body (21). Depending on arterial dominance patterns, there may be a significant difference in the size of the foramen from right to left. Before performing a posterior lateral mass or pedicle screw fixation procedure, the surgeon's preoperative planning should include an assessment of the size and location of the vertebral arteries. An abnormal size or location of the foramina transversaria may indicate an arterial dominance pattern, which places the patient at greater risk for harm if an artery is injured. Certain levels may also be deemed unsuitable for screw fixation due to the artery's location.

The artery continues in its posteromedial ascent from C-3 to the base of C-2, where it passes the anteromedial corner of the C2-3 facet and enters an oblique and slightly enlarged vertebral artery foramen. This foramen lies even more posterior with respect to the vertebral body than at the subaxial levels, with its margin overlapping the posterior vertebral body cortex (21). In contrast, the C-2 foramen reverses the medial migration of the C3-5 foramina to lie more laterally with an interforaminal distance similar to C-6. The artery assumes the path of the foramen, which is angled 45 degrees laterally and slightly anterior, crossing the inferior aspect of the anterolateral mass wall. On exiting the foramen, it turns rostral and continues slightly ventral, crossing the anterolateral border of the C-2 isthmus. As it crosses the C1-2 facet joint, the artery turns from a slightly anterolateral course to a posteromedial angle into the C-1 foramen, which is angled in this direction. This vertebral foramen lies directly lateral to the lateral mass of C-1. Because this articular process is more anterior than in the lower levels, however, the transverse foramen is still more anterior than at C-2. The artery exits the foramen and turns sharply to a horizontal posterolateral path. After passing the lateral mass, the artery continues posteromedially in a shallow extension of the same groove that lies along the superior surface of the C-1 arch halfway to the midline. Here, it turns anteromedially, sometimes through an accessory foramen, and ascends along the clivus to merge with the artery from the contralateral side, forming the basilar artery.

POSTERIOR INSTRUMENTATION TECHNIQUES

Subaxial Spine

Interspinous Wiring

Interspinous wiring remains the mainstay of treatment for subaxial posterior ligamentous instability. Posterior wire constructs act as tension bands to resist distraction and flexion around an anterior axis of rotation. Overtightening must be avoided, because the induced hyperextension can lead to spinal canal or neuroforaminal stenosis. Use of a properly fashioned posterior interspinous buttress, such as a corticocancellous graft of proper height, can resist such hyperextension and posterior translation forces. Resistance of shear and torsion forces in most of the wiring methods depends on facet joint integrity. These methods should not be used in the presence of anterior column injuries that have compromised vertical load bearing, because they are incapable of resisting vertical settling or kyphosis.

The original technique described by Rogers involved extraosseous open-loop fixation around adjacent spinous processes with onlay bone grafting (22,23). This method does not block extension, and wire slippage is possible. Extension can be prevented by inserting a tailored interspinous buttress graft.

The Bohlman triple-wire technique and its modifications involve a double loop through the burr hole at each vertebral level to increase wire cutout resistance, reinforced with two structural corticocancellous bone graft buttresses (24). The latter are fastened across the midline using separate upper and lower wires through the same spinous process drill holes. This technique avoids sublaminar wire passage, provides biomechanically stronger fixation, and yields higher fusion rates (5,25). This technique should probably not be used for more than three levels of fixation because of the risk of hyperlordosis or inadequate fixation. As with any transspinous fixation method, its applicability is limited by the size and strength of the spinous processes at the levels to be instrumented.

Rotational ligamentous instability from facet dislocation with or without articular process fractures can be treated using an oblique wiring configuration (26). Before midline interspinous wiring is performed, a separate strand is passed through a drill hole in the inferior articular process of the damaged facet. The wire is threaded through a burr hole in the base of the subjacent spinous process. Separate wires are then used to complete the midline wiring.

Multilevel Facet Buttress Wiring

Originally conceived by Southwick and reported by Callahan et al., the articular process wiring method had been clinically useful in the era preceding lateral mass screw fixation (Fig. 3) (27). It was particularly applicable when fusions were deemed necessary after multilevel cervical laminectomies. Wires are passed through drill holes in the inferior articular masses of each level to be included in the fusion. The inferiormost level of fixation necessitates sublaminar wire passage to avoid an iatrogenic arthrosis or an additional fusion level due to the presence of the wire within the facet joint. The buttress element used initially consisted of rib grafts or iliac crest struts. Later adaptations used morcellized autograft with contoured smooth or threaded Steinmann pins and other variations on that theme. Substantial external bracing was still required, often a halo vest. These methods have been largely replaced by screw fixation procedures.

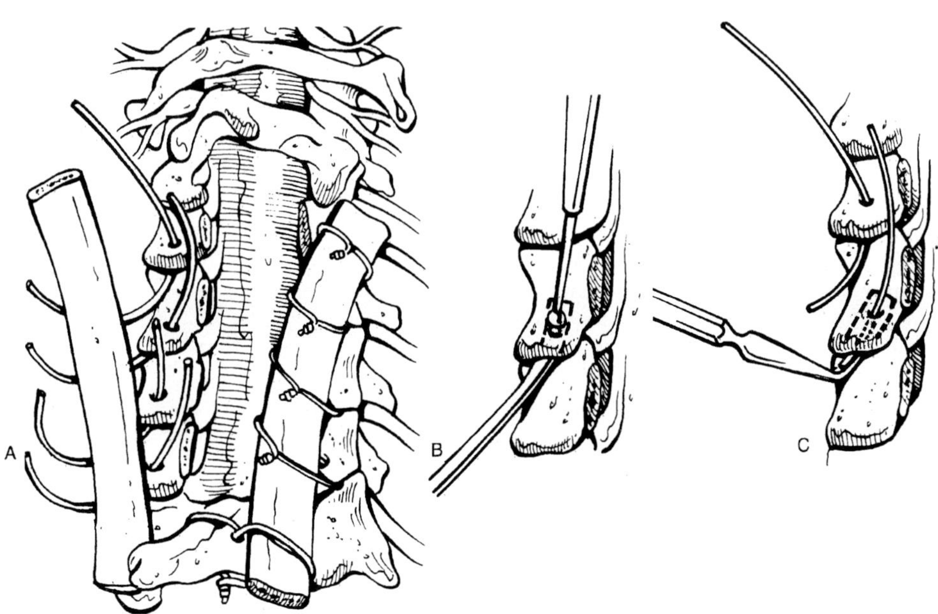

FIG. 3. A schematic illustration of the posterior facet buttress wiring method. In this instance **(A)**, a rib graft has been used to impart some degree of intersegmental immobilization. One might also use contoured metal rods. **B** and **C** illustrate a method of wire or cable passage through the inferior articular process.

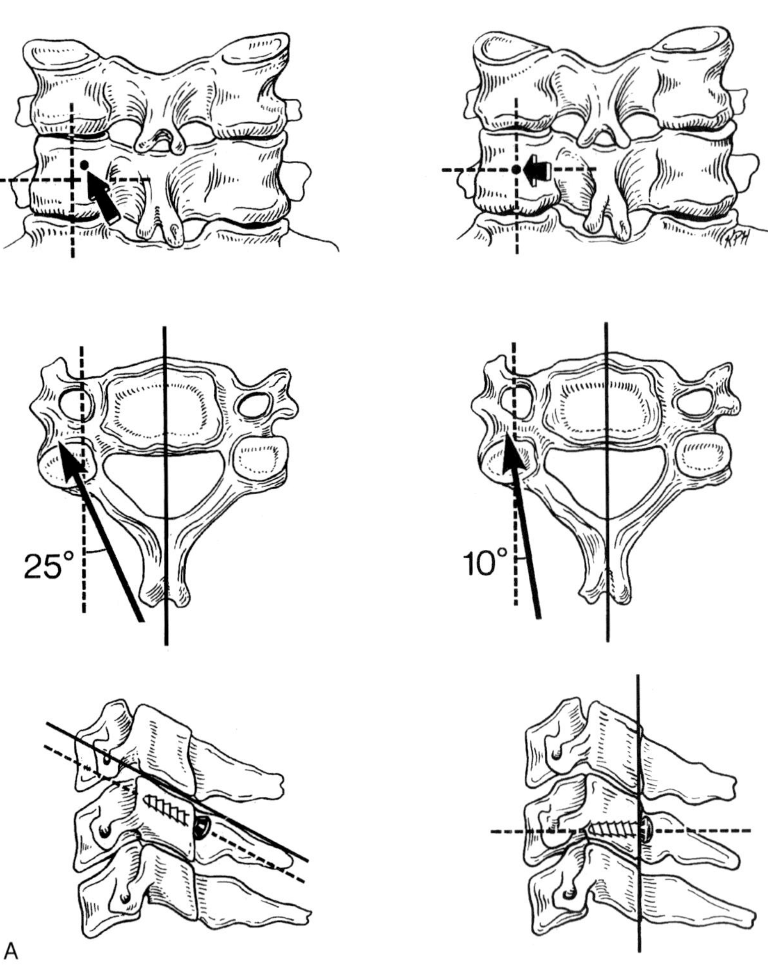

FIG. 4. A schematic comparison of the **(A)** Magerl and **(B)** Roy-Camille techniques of lateral mass screw insertion. These were the first two methods described and differed in their chosen starting points and screw trajectories. Other methods would later be described. As mentioned in the text, however, the point of screw exit, if the ventral (second) cortex is penetrated for extra purchase, determines the possibility of nerve root, facet joint, or vertebral artery injury.

Subaxial Cervical Screws

Rigid internal fixation of the posterior cervical spine can be achieved with lateral mass, transpedicular, or transarticular screws through various types of plates or plate-rods to provide single-level or multilevel stabilization. Cervical plating can be applied despite posterior element deficiencies without extending the construct to normal motion segments.

Originally, two conceptually distinct techniques of lateral mass screw fixation for the lower cervical spine were described by Roy-Camille (28) and Magerl (28a) (Fig. 4). Roy-Camille pioneered lateral mass screw fixation techniques using an anterior/posterior trajectory that trades intraosseous screw working length for simplicity and safety (28). The entry point is at the center of the rectangular posterior face of the lateral mass or can be measured 5 mm medial to the lateral edge and midway between the facet joints. The drill is directed perpendicular to the posterior wall of the vertebral body with a 10-degree lateral angle. This trajectory yields an exit point slightly lateral to the vertebral artery and below the exiting nerve root (19,20). The lateral mass depth from C-3 to C-6 ranges from 6 to 14 mm in men (average, 8.7 mm) and 6 to 11 mm in women (average, 7.9 mm). An adjustable drill guide set to a depth of 10 to 12 mm is used to prevent penetration beyond the anterior cortex. The depth can then be gradually and safely increased as the local anatomy permits. If the additional 20% of pullout strength with bicortical fixation is desired, then the exit point should be at the junction of the lateral mass and transverse process (18). Lateral fluoroscopic imaging makes it easier to choose the optimum trajectory and avoid penetration of the subjacent facet joint, which is especially important at the caudal level of fixation because this joint should not be included in the fusion.

The Magerl technique uses an entry point that is 1 mm medial and rostral to the center point of the posterior surface of the lateral mass (28a). It is oriented at a 45- to 60-degree rostral angle, parallel to the adjacent facet joint articular surface, and at a 25-degree lateral angle. This path yields a potential exit point lateral to the vertebral artery and above the exiting nerve root while engaging the lateral portion of the ventral cortex of the superior articular facet. The proper trajectory for this technique is more difficult to achieve than the Roy-Camille technique. The prominence of the thorax can impede proper alignment of drill and guide, risking injury to the nerve root if the second cortex is penetrated. The depth of penetration at this angle is approximately 18 mm compared to 14 mm for the Roy-Camille technique, which has some implications for purchase strength and mode of screw failure *in vitro* (29–31).

The incremental 20% of pullout resistance provided with bicortical fixation must be balanced against the increased risk of morbidity associated with anterior cortical penetration (32). Among young healthy trauma victims, the bone integrity may be enough without incurring the incremental morbidity risk.

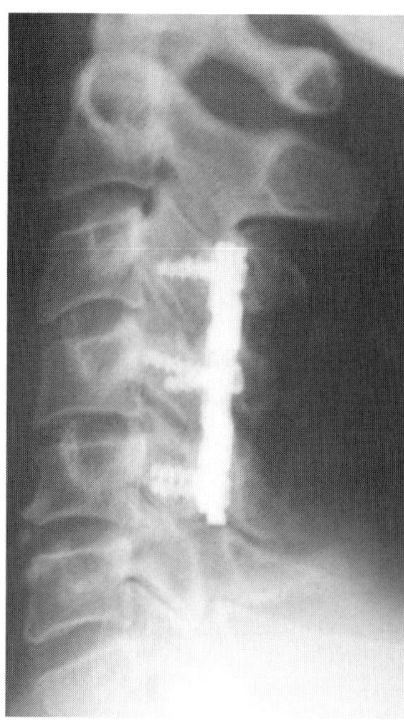

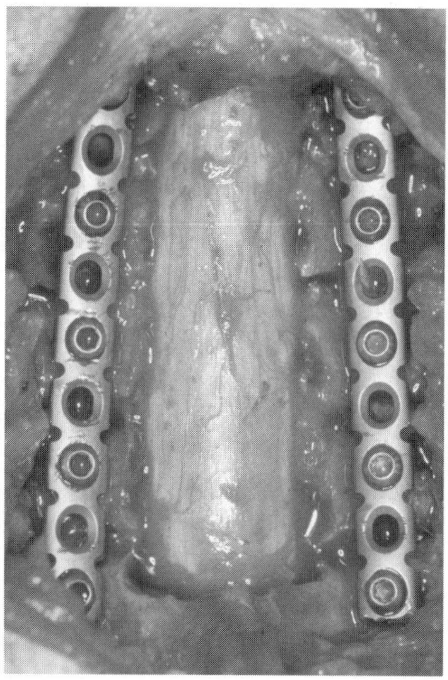

A,B

FIG. 5. A: A lateral postoperative radiograph of a patient who has undergone lateral mass plating and bone grafting from C-3 to C-5. The technique used was essentially that of Roy-Camille. **B:** An intraoperative photograph of a lateral mass plating from C-3 to C-7 after a multilevel laminectomy.

Factors that might favor bicortical fixation include osteopenia, especially in patients with steroid-dependent rheumatoid and metastatic disease, and those with anterior column compromise as well as conditions that require longer fixation constructs, especially at the cranial and caudal levels. Heller et al. demonstrated that the pullout strength of lateral mass screws is maximal in the midcervical region and then tapers significantly in either direction (32). The bone of the lateral masses is relatively spared in osteopenia compared to the significant reductions in bone mass affecting the vertebral body trabecular bone. Thus, posterior segmental screw fixation is particularly helpful in such difficult hosts.

An et al. demonstrated the optimal position at C3-6 to be an even greater lateral trajectory, requiring an entry point 1 mm medial to the center of the lateral mass with a 33-degree lateral angle and a compromise between the previously described techniques with a 17-degree cephalad angle (18). Anderson proposed another compromise trajectory, with starting point 1 mm medial to the midpoint of the lateral mass angled 30 to 40 degrees cranial and 10 degrees lateral (33). This orients the screw for the safest anterior cortical fixation point at the lateral ventral surface of the superior articular facet lateral to the vertebral artery and above the exiting nerve root. This can be used for bicortical fixation and may be most appropriate in the upper levels or in cases in which the vertebral foramen is more medial as documented by preoperative computed tomography (CT) scan.

The common theme running through each of the various screw insertion methods described to date is anatomic safety. Thus, it is not really the point of entry or trajectory of the screw that threatens the patient: It is the point of exit of the drill bit or screw tip that can cause injury. Armed with this understanding, the wary surgeon can readily appreciate how to safely adapt the fixation methods to the unique circumstances of each level in each patient. It is also for this reason that the authors prefer to use true lateral fluoroscopic views of each level to be instrumented, as long as the patient's body habitus allows such imaging.

Lateral Mass Plating

Lateral mass plating is indicated in cases of posterior element fracture, facet fracture with rotational instability, burst fractures, postlaminectomy instability or kyphosis, certain tumors, and fixation to the cervicothoracic junction (Fig. 5). It is better suited to multilevel fusions than wire because it provides translational stability without hyperextension, provides enhanced torsional stiffness, and resists axial shortening. As long as the facets remain intact to act as a buttress, even moderate anterior osteoligamentous injuries, such as burst fractures and flexible kyphotic deformities, can be stabilized by lateral mass plates.

Hook Plates

Hook plates use a combination of sublaminar and interference fixation. This construct increases flexion and torsional stiffness, prevents anterior translation, and provides compression. This procedure requires intact inferior lamina. Axial compression is also provided by the upward angle of the Magerl screw used in this construct, which pulls the hook cephalad. Hook plate constructs cause extension and posterior translation of the upper vertebral level, which can result in hyperlordosis unless blocked by an interspinous buttress graft. With advances in implant designs, this method has become rather uncommon.

Cervical Rod Systems

Cervical rod systems are modular tension band systems for posterior fixation of the occipitocervical spine, upper and lower cervical spine, and upper thoracic spine. A choice of clamps and hooks are fixed on small-diameter rods, typically 3.5 mm, by means of set screws or by engaging small polyaxial screw heads. The bone screws can be optimally positioned through the clamps

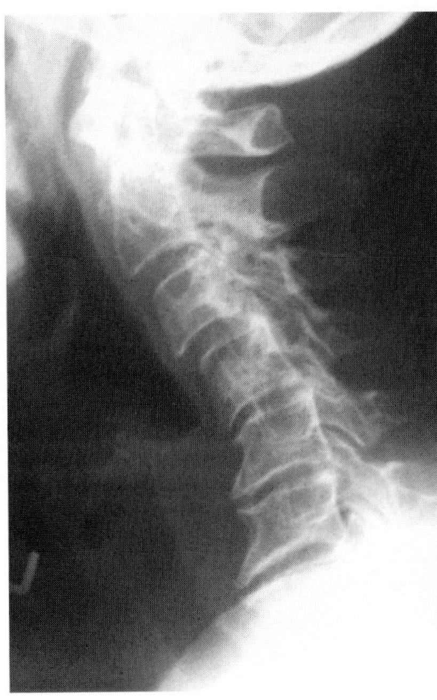
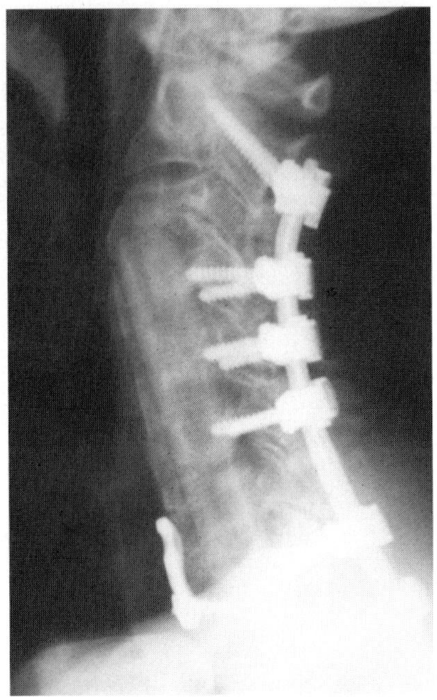

A,B

FIG. 6. Preoperative lateral radiograph **(A)** of an adult spastic diplegic patient who had developed progressive cervical myelopathy. He was treated with a multilevel anterior corpectomy and fusion **(B)**, followed by posterior segmental instrumentation and fusion with a modular rod-screw system from C-2 to T-2. Pedicle fixation was used at C-2, T-1, and T-2. Lateral mass screws were inserted at C-4, C-5, and C-6. The posterior fusion was extended to these levels to maximize screw purchase, given the superior pullout resistance of pedicle fixation.

in any desired direction and on each motion segment. For fixation to the occiput, rods with one end shaped like a reconstruction plate have been designed. Cross-linking devices can also be used to connect the rods and provide optimum torsional rigidity. These systems may also be extended down into the thoracic region via tapered rods or connectors to larger-diameter rods (Fig. 6). Although much more costly than lateral mass plates, these systems are by far the most adaptable and mechanically stable of the posterior cervical instrumentation constructs available.

Pedicle Screw Fixation

At C-2, no true lateral mass is available for fixation. A medial and superior trajectory is available into the relatively spacious pedicles at this level, providing a longer and safer path for improved fixation. C-2 pedicle screws can even be used with a lag technique to reduce and fix traumatic spondylolisthesis of the axis. When such a C-2 traumatic spondylolisthesis is associated with an inferior facet fracture, facet dislocation, C-2 teardrop fracture, or C2-3 instability, segmental fixation can be achieved with a two-hole plate using a C-2 pedicle and C-3 lateral mass screws.

To guide screw placement, Roy-Camille described direct visualization and palpation of the medial and superior walls of the C-2 pedicle through the C1-2 interlaminar interval, where the space available for the cord is greatest. He recommended using the superomedial quadrant of the C-2 lateral mass for the entry point, to keep the screw rostral and medial within the pedicle. The trajectory of the screw should have a 10- to 15-degree upward inclination and medial angulation and a length of 20 to 30 mm. Magerl recommended a more lateral and caudal entry point 2 mm below the midpoint with a shallow and inward trajectory 25 degrees cranial and medial. The authors prefer a combination of local anatomic landmarks and intraoperative lateral fluoroscopy to guide the trajectory of the drill bit and depth of penetration. As with the Magerl technique described previously, the principal risk to the patient would be inadvertent injury to the vertebral artery.

Subaxial pedicle fixation may be indicated in the face of bone deficiencies, such as hypoplastic or malformed lateral masses, bone destruction due to infection or tumors, facet fracture, partial facetectomy, bilateral C-2 pedicle fracture with traumatic spondylolisthesis of the axis, or articular mass fracture separation. Pedicle fixation is the only posterior technique that can provide three-column fixation of the cervical spine. This added stability might be desirable in extremely unstable situations, such as osteoligamentous injuries, or insufficiency with loss of axial stability, such as rheumatoid arthritis, kyphotic deformity, severe fracture, or diffuse tumor involvement. Greater pullout strength than that obtained with lateral mass screws makes this technique desirable for long constructs with greater moments at their upper and lower ends (34,35).

In single-level posterior ligamentous and circumferential discoligamentous injuries, pedicle screws provide no significant advantage over lateral mass plating, triple wiring, or a combination of the two techniques. In multilevel involvement of these same instability patterns, pedicle fixation produces a significant increase in torsional and extension stiffness over the three other techniques. Screw loosening with pseudarthrosis or loss of deformity reduction can be expected in some patients instrumented with lateral mass screws, but it has not been reported with pedicle fixation (33,36,37).

Abumi has used transpedicular screw plate fixation in the subaxial spine for traumatic and nontraumatic lesions (38–42). Among trauma victims, he reported 100% solid fusion with no loss of reduction and no implant or skeletal failure. No complications involving the spinal cord, nerve root, or vertebral artery were clinically evident. Three medial and one inferior cortical penetrations were documented. In 45 cases of nontraumatic lesions, Abumi achieved 100% fusion with good correction and maintenance of alignment. Postoperative magnetic resonance

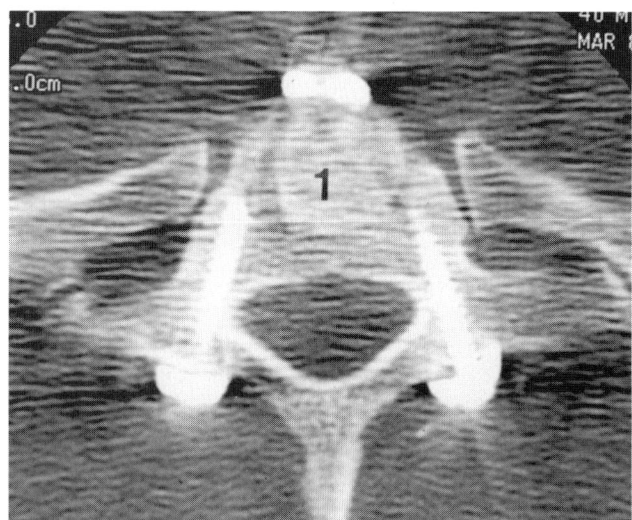

FIG. 7. An axial computed tomography scan through the T-1 level of a patient treated with plate-screw fixation across the cervicothoracic junction. Note the trajectory of the screws in the axial plane is opposite to that for lateral mass screws, which made the use of this method much more difficult until the advent of modular rod-screw systems.

imaging and CT scan documented no malposition in the 24 C-2 pedicle screws, but there was 6.9% risk of penetration in the subaxial pedicles. Different methods of cervical pedicle screw insertion have been evaluated *in vitro* (9–11,43). The use of topographic landmarks alone was not capable of providing accurate and safe insertion. Frameless stereotactic navigation and the fluoroscopically assisted method of Abumi resulted in similar and modest rates of screw insertion error. The low rate of clinical complications described by Abumi speaks more to the tolerance of the local anatomy to modest errors, rather than to absolute accuracy of any method of pedicle screw insertion. Finally, one should note the observation of Ludwig et al. with respect to error rates and minimum pedicle diameters (10). Cervical pedicle screws ought not to be attempted in pedicles smaller than 4.5 mm at their narrowest point, especially if there is not a distinctive cancellous center within the pedicle.

Jeanneret recommended pedicle fixation using progressively increasing screw lengths at more caudal levels (44). He measured the distance from the lateral mass posterior cortex to the vertebral body and anterior cortex and subtracted 6 mm to calculate the optimal screw length as 26 mm for C3-4, 28 mm for C-5, and 30 mm for C-6. At C-7, the total depth measured was 41 mm, with the increase primarily in the vertebral body segment of the screw path, which is not used for fixation (7). At this level, Jeanneret recommended a 32-mm screw; however, other anatomic studies suggest that a 30-mm screw may be safer (8). Although 3.5- to 4.0-mm screws are most commonly used in the cervical spine, smaller screws (e.g., 2.7 mm) should be considered if indicated by preoperative CT scan findings, especially at the upper subaxial cervical levels.

The upper thoracic spine is usually well suited to pedicle screw fixation (Fig. 7). As pointed out by An and others, the size and orientation of the pedicles can typically accommodate 3.5- to 4.0-mm screws (18,30,45–49). If the pedicles are too small or the appropriate starting point and trajectory cannot be achieved through the plate, then placing bicortical screws into the base of the upper thoracic transverse processes should be considered. There is no neurologic risk and the rib head usually protects the pleura. Shuster et al. found that the mean pullout strength of pedicle screws inserted from T-1 to T-4 is greater than that of those inserted into the transverse processes (47). However, the loads to failure for the transverse process screw were comparable to those measured by Heller et al. for lateral mass screws in the subaxial region. Therefore, the transverse process technique remains a safe, albeit biomechanically inferior, alternative to thoracic pedicle screw fixation (Fig. 8).

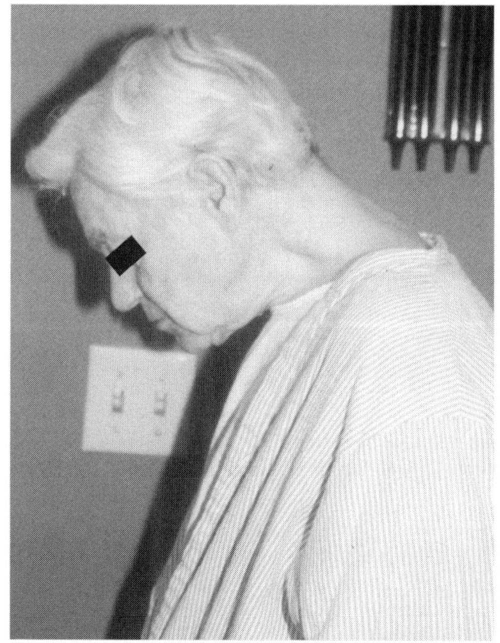

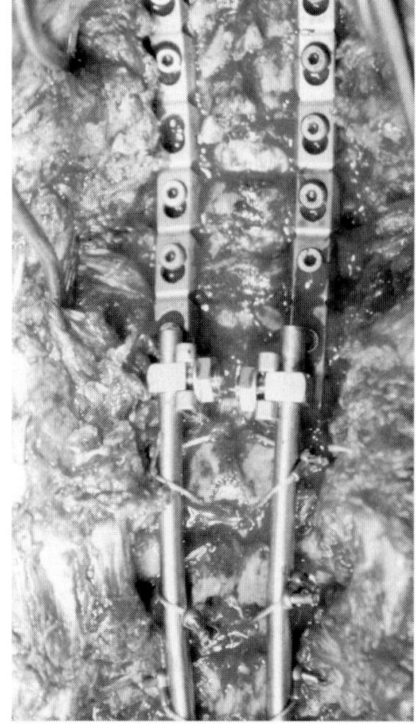

A,B

FIG. 8. A: Preoperative lateral photograph of a patient with neuromuscular cervicothoracic kyphosis due to advanced Parkinson's disease. **B:** The deformity was reduced with preoperative traction, then instrumented and fused posteriorly. In this case, lateral mass screws were used in the cervical region. The special plates were then connected to rods in the thoracic spine. Sublaminar cables were used for multilevel thoracic fixation due to their minimal profile in the setting of very atrophic paravertebral muscles. This should only be done when the surgeon has verified that sufficient subarachnoid space exists to execute the technique safely.

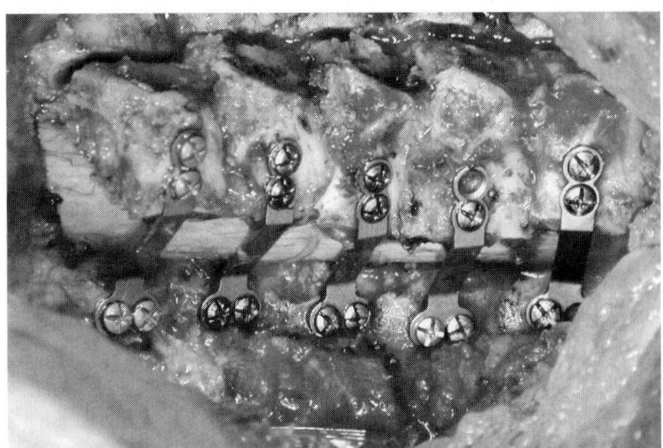

FIG. 9. An intraoperative photograph after an open-door laminoplasty. Specially designed plates have been used to achieve intrasegmental fixation of the laminae in their new position until their bone hinges heal permanently. This technique has given the authors greater confidence in pursuing early active range of motion postoperatively, eliminating the need for external immobilization.

Intrasegmental Fixation

Under certain circumstances, it may be desirable to secure the posterior elements at a given vertebral level(s), rather than across motion segments. Such intrasegmental fixation can be used when reconstructing the posterior cervical lamina after resection of intradural tumors to reduce the likelihood of kyphosis in growing children, or after laminoplasty in adults. Most commonly, the posterior arches and their associated ligaments may be wired or sutured back *in situ* through small burr holes in the lamina and cut edges of the lateral masses. This is most commonly done in growing children due to their uniquely high risk for postlaminectomy kyphosis.

In the case of open-door laminoplasty, a myriad of methods has been described to maintain the laminae in their new position while the bone hinges heal (50–53). Classically, as described by Hirabayashi, the laminae were tethered open with sutures passed between the spinous processes or interspinous ligaments and the lateral soft tissues, such as the facet capsules or paravertebral muscles (54). The "door" may also be propped open with spacers of different sorts, such as bone grafts, ceramic or plastic devices, and so forth. These are typically wired or sutured in place through small drill holes.

O'Brien et al. first described the use of mini-plates for screw fixation of the open side (51). Since that time, the concept has increased in popularity, especially as the benefits of early active range of motion have piqued the interest of spinal surgeons in their attempt to minimize postoperative axial pain and preserve maximal range of motion. Recently, plates adapted to this purpose have become available. Their principal benefit over other contoured fracture plates is their ease of insertion (Fig. 9).

CONCLUSION

Spine surgeons need no longer rely on only wire fixation techniques and external immobilization to surgically stabilize the cervical spine. Better appreciation for the osseous anatomy of the occiput, posterior cervical, and thoracic elements, as well as their associated neural and vascular structures, has allowed for the development of screw-based fixation techniques. When appropriate, such contemporary instrumentation techniques may impart greater rigidity, promote higher union rates, and/or reduce postoperative bracing requirements. As these methods narrow the margins for error, however, they must not be applied indiscriminately. Often, the traditional methods of posterior wiring may be easier, less expensive, and less prone to anatomic complications. In such cases, one would be wise to select the method most likely to accomplish the task at hand while engendering the lowest risk profile. Familiarity with all of these methods and the relevant applied anatomy enables surgeons to adapt any given method to best suit the particular circumstances of their patient.

REFERENCES

1. Panjabi MM, Duranceau J, Goel V, et al. Cervical human vertebrae: quantitative three-dimensional anatomy of the middle and lower regions. *Spine* 1991;16:861–869.
2. Harrison DD, Janik TJ, Troyanovich SJ, et al. Comparisons of lordotic cervical spine curvatures to a theoretical ideal model of the static sagittal cervical spine. *Spine* 1996;21:667–675.
3. White AA III. Clinical biomechanics of cervical spine implants. *Spine* 1989;14:1040–1045.
4. Karaikovic EE, Daubs MD, Madsen RW, et al. Morphological characteristics of human cervical pedicles. *Spine* 1997;22:493–500.
5. Sutterlin CE III, McAfee PC, Warden KE, et al. A biomechanical evaluation of cervical spinal stabilization methods in a bovine model: static and cyclical loading. *Spine* 1988;13:795–802.
6. Ebraheim N, Rollins JR, Xu R, et al. Anatomic consideration of C2 pedicle screw placement. *Spine* 1996;21:691–695.
7. Ebraheim NA, Xu R, Knight T, et al. Morphometric evaluation of lower cervical pedicle and its projections. *Spine* 1997;22:1–6.
8. Xu R, Ebraheim NA, Yeasting R, et al. Anatomy of C7 lateral mass and projection of pedicle axis on its posterior aspect. *J Spinal Disord* 1995;8:116–120.
9. Ludwig SC, Kramer DL, Balderston RA, et al. Placement of pedicle screws in the human cadaveric cervical spine: comparative accuracy of three techniques. *Spine* 2000;25:1655–1667.
10. Ludwig SC, Kowalski JM, Edwards CC Jr, et al. Cervical pedicle screws: comparative accuracy of two insertion techniques. *Spine* 2000;25:2675–2681.
11. Ludwig DJ, Kramer DL, Vaccaro AR, et al. Trans-pedicle screw fixation of the cervical spine. *Clin Orthop* 1999;359:77–88.
12. Panjabi MM, Oxland T, Takata K, et al. Articular facets of the human spine: quantitative three-dimensional anatomy. *Spine* 1991;16:888–901.
13. Boyle JJ, Singer KP, Milne N. Morphologic survey of the cervicothoracic junctional region. *Spine* 1996;21:544–548.
14. Ebraheim NA, An HS, Xu R, et al. The quantitative anatomy of the cervical nerve root groove and the intervertebral foramen. *Spine* 1996;21:1619–1623.
15. Pal GP, Sherk HH. The vertical stability of the cervical spine. *Spine* 1988;13:447–449.
16. Bailey AS, Stanescu S, Yeasting RA, et al. Anatomic relationships of the cervicothoracic junction. *Spine* 1995;20:1431–1439.
17. Yabuki S, Kikuchi S. Positions of dorsal root ganglia in the cervical spine: an anatomic and clinical study. *Spine* 1996;21:1513–1517.
18. An HS, Gordin R, Renner K. Anatomic considerations for plate-screw fixation of the cervical spine. *Spine* 1991;16:S548–S551.
19. Ebraheim NA, Xu R, Yeasting RA. The location of the vertebral artery foramen and its relation to posterior lateral mass screw fixation. *Spine* 1996;21:1291–1295.
20. Xu R, Ebraheim NA, Naudad MC, et al. The location of the cervical nerve roots on the posterior aspect of the cervical spine. *Spine* 1995;20:2267–2271.

21. Vaccaro AR, Ring D, Scuderi G, et al. Vertebral artery location in relation to the vertebral body as determined by two-dimensional computed tomography evaluation. *Spine* 1994;19:2637–2641.
22. Rogers WA. Treatment of fracture-dislocation of the cervical spine. *J Bone Joint Surg* 1942;24:245–258.
23. Rogers WA. Fractures and dislocations of the cervical spine. *J Bone Joint Surg [Am]* 1957;39A:341–375.
24. McAfee PC, Bohlman HH, et al. The triple wire fixation technique for stabilization of acute cervical fracture-dislocations: a biomechanical analysis. *J Bone Joint Surg Orthop Trans* 1985;9A:142.
25. Montesano PX, Juach EC, Anderson PA, et al. Biomechanics of cervical spine internal fixation. *Spine* 1991;16:S10–S16.
26. Cahill DW, Bellegarrigue R, Ducker TB. Bilateral facet to spinous process fusion: a new technique for posterior spinal fusion after trauma. *Neurosurgery* 1983;13:1–4.
27. Callahan RA, Johnson RM, Margolis RN, et al. Cervical facet fusion for control of instability following laminectomy *J Bone Joint Surg [Am]* 1977;59(8):991–1002.
28. Roy-Camille R, Saillant G, Mazel C. Internal fixation of the unstable cervical spine by posterior osteosynthesis with plates and screws. In: Sherk HH, ed. *The cervical spine*, 2nd ed. Philadelphia: JB Lippincott, 1989:390–403.
28a. Magerl F, Seeman P. Stable posterior fusion of the atlas and axis by transarticular screw fixation. In: Kehr P, Weidner A, eds. *Cervical spine I*. Vienna: Springer-Verlag, 1985:322–327.
29. Heller JG, Carlson GD, Abitbol JJ, et al. Anatomic comparison of the Roy-Camille and Magerl techniques for screw placement in the lower cervical spine. *Spine* 1991;16:S552–S557.
30. Stanescu S, Ebraheim NA, Yeasting R, et al. Morphometric evaluation of the cervico-thoracic junction: practical considerations for posterior fixation of the spine. *Spine* 1994;19:2082–2088.
31. Montesano PX, Juach EC, Jonsson H Jr. Anatomic and biomechanical study of posterior cervical spine plate arthrodesis: an evaluation of two different techniques of screw placement. *J Spinal Disord* 1992;5:301–305.
32. Heller JG, Estes BT, Zaouali M, et al. Biomechanical study of screws in the lateral masses: variables affecting pullout resistance. *J Bone Joint Surg [Am]* 1996;78A:1315–1321.
33. Anderson PA, Henley MB, Grady MS, et al. Posterior cervical arthrodesis with AO reconstruction plates and bone graft. *Spine* 1991;16:S72–S79.
34. Jones E, Heller JG, Silcox DH III, et al. Cervical pedicle screws versus lateral mass screws: anatomic feasibility and biomechanical comparison. *Spine* 1997;22:977–982.
35. Kotani Y, Cunningham BW, Abumi K, et al. Biomechanical analysis of cervical stabilization systems. An assessment of transpedicular screw fixation in the cervical spine. *Spine* 1994;19:2529–2539.
36. Fehlings MG, Cooper PR, Errico TJ. Posterior plates in the management of cervical instability: long-term results in 44 patients. *J Neurosurg* 1994;81:341–349.
37. Heller JG, Silcox DH III, Sutterlin CE. Complications of posterior cervical plating. *Spine* 1995;20:2442–2448.
38. Abumi K, Itoh H, Taneichi H, et al. Transpedicular screw fixation for traumatic lesions of the middle and lower cervical spine: description of the techniques and preliminary report. *J Spinal Disord* 1994;7:19–28.
39. Abumi K, Kaneda K, Shono Y, et al. One-stage posterior decompression and reconstruction of the cervical spine by using pedicle screw fixation systems. *J Neurosurg* 1999;90:19–26.
40. Abumi K, Shono Y, Ito M, et al. Complications of pedicle screw fixation in reconstructive surgery of the cervical spine. *Spine* 2000;25:962–969.
41. Abumi K, Takada T, Shono Y, et al. Posterior occipitocervical reconstruction using cervical pedicle screws and plate-rod systems. *Spine* 1999;24:1425–1434.
42. Abumi K, Kaneda K. Pedicle screw fixation for non-traumatic lesions of the cervical spine. Presented in part at the 62nd Annual Meeting of the American Academy of Orthopaedic Surgeons, February 16–21, 1995.
43. Lamb DJ, Silcox DH III, Heller JG, et al. Different methods of fixation for atlantoaxial instability. Presented at the 65th Annual AAOS Meeting, New Orleans, LA, 1998.
44. Jeanneret B, Gebhard JS, Magerl F. Transpedicular screw fixation of articular mass fracture-separation: results of an anatomic study and operative technique. *J Spinal Disord* 1994;7:222–229.
45. An HS, Vaccaro AR, Cotler J, et al. Spinal disorders at the cervicothoracic junction. *Spine* 1994;19:2257–2264.
46. Heller JG, Estes BT. Biomechanical comparison of posterior screw fixation techniques at the cervicothoracic junction [abstract]. Presented at the 61st Annual AAOS Meeting, New Orleans, LA, February, 1994.
47. Heller JG, Shuster JK, Hutton WC. Pedicle and transverse process screws of the upper thoracic spine: biomechanical comparison of loads to failure. *Spine* 1999;24:654–658.
48. Thanapipatsiri S, Chan DP. Safety of thoracic transverse process fixation: an anatomical study. *J Spinal Disord* 1996;9:294–298.
49. Vaccaro AR, Rizzolo SJ, Addardyce TJ, et al. Placement of pedicle screws in the thoracic spine. *J Bone Joint Surg [Am]* 1995;77A: 1193–1206.
50. Deutsch D, Mummaneni PV, Rodts GE, et al. Posterior cervical laminoplasty using a new plating system: technical note. *J Spinal Disord Tech* 2003 (*in press*).
51. O'Brien MF, Peterson D, Casey AT, et al. A novel technique for laminoplasty augmentation of spinal canal area using titanium miniplate stabilization. A computerized morphometric analysis. *Spine* 1996;21:474–483; discussion 484.
52. Wang JM, Roh KJ, Kim DJ, et al. A new method of stabilising the elevated laminae in open-door laminaplasty using an anchor system. *J Bone Joint Surg [Br]* 1998;80:1005–1008.
53. Yonoenobu, K, Heller JG, Oda T. Posterior decompression for myelopathy: laminoplasty. In: Herkowitz HN, ed. *Cervical Spine Research Society: Atlas of surgical techniques*, 2nd ed. Philadelphia: Lippincott, 2003.
54. Hirabayashi K, Satomi K. Operative procedure and results of expansive open-door laminaplasty. *Spine* 1988;13:870–876.

IV

Thoracolumbar Spine

Editor

Robert F. McLain

CHAPTER 41

Thoracolumbar Fractures: Evaluation, Classification, and Treatment

Kai-Uwe Lewandrowski and Robert F. McLain

Fractures of the thoracic and lumbar spine are the most common nonosteoporotic spine fractures. When compared to the cervical and lumbar regions, motion in this area of the spine is quite limited by the thoracic rib cage. In turn, a high-energy injury is required to disrupt the spinal column in this transition zone (Fig. 1). Therefore, severely traumatized patients with suspected spine fractures must be expeditiously treated for life-threatening injuries, receive initial supportive care, and complete appropriate diagnostic studies—all the while, the neural elements must be protected until definitive treatment can be provided. Whether initiated by a team of trauma specialists or a lone surgeon in the emergency department, an orderly, stepwise approach to assessment and management of these patients improves overall outcome and ensures that serious injuries are not overlooked.

DEVELOPMENT OF OPERATIVE TREATMENT

Since the early 1980s, operative treatment has moved to the forefront of fracture management in the spine. Technologies and implants have evolved to provide better results with decreased morbidity and mortality, and current operative management more rapidly returns the patient to work and satisfactory function (1–9). Changes in health care management and patient expectations have made prolonged bed rest or immobilization unacceptable (10). Improved imaging, a better understanding of fracture and implant biomechanics, and the introduction of a variety of new anterior and posterior fixation devices permit surgeons to plan definitive stabilizing procedures for any fracture pattern, allowing rapid mobilization and return to function. Hence, patients who cannot be mobilized in a cast or brace within a few days of their injury are often more reasonably

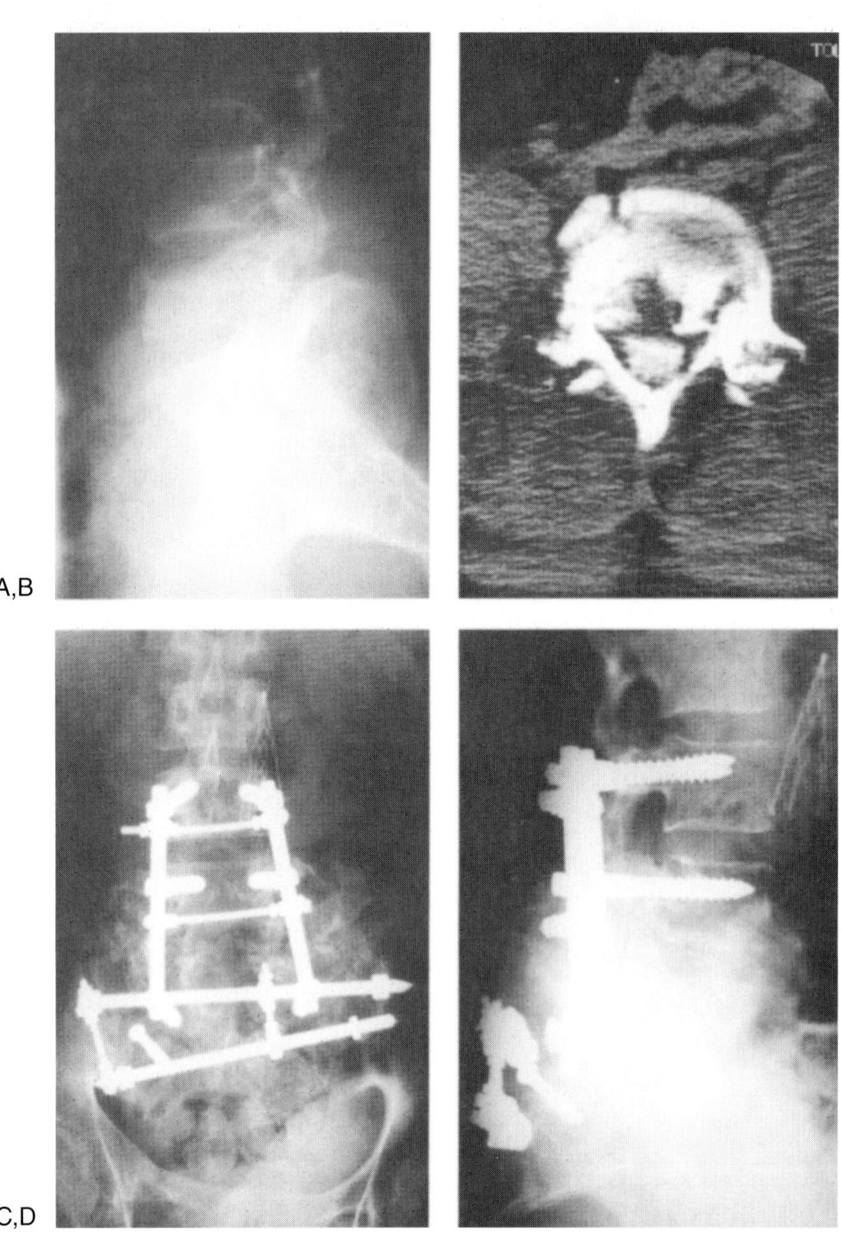

FIG. 1. Spinal trauma—a high-energy injury. **A:** Lateral radiograph of an 18-year-old man crushed under a wall, which forced him into extreme hyperflexion. He had massive thoracic injuries, a splenic laceration, and a progressive cauda equine injury. Radiograph demonstrates a L-5 burst fracture. Pelvic radiograph also demonstrates ipsilateral sacroiliac fracture-dislocations. **B:** The computed tomography (CT) scan shows a comminuted lumbar fracture with retropulsed vertebral body fragment abutting the volar surface of the laminae. **C,D:** Anteroposterior and lateral radiographs after emergent stabilization and resuscitation. The patient underwent multiple procedures under the initial anesthetic, including splenectomy, chest tube placement, L-5 vertebrectomy, cauda equina decompression, posterior spinal stabilization, L-4 to sacrum placement of vena caval filter, and posterior stabilization of the pelvic disruption. The aggressive approach provided enough spinal column stability to allow early mobilization with aggressive pulmonary toilet. Four years after this massive injury, the patient was ambulatory with an ankle-foot orthosis. He had mild back pain, and he had returned to college. (From *Chapman's operative orthopaedics,* 2nd ed. Philadelphia: JB Lippincott Co., 2001, with permission.)

treated with surgery. The goal of treatment—operative or otherwise—remains to protect neural elements, restore or maintain neurologic function, prevent or correct segmental collapse and deformity, prevent spinal instability and pain, permit early ambulation and return to function, and restore normal spinal mechanics.

POLYTRAUMATIZED PATIENT

Unstable thoracic and lumbar spine fractures are usually high-energy injuries. Anywhere from 40 to 80% of the injuries result from motor vehicle accidents involving drivers and passengers of automobiles, riders of motorcycles, and pedestrians (11–18). Other causes of spine fractures include falls from height, penetrating trauma, and crush injuries, such as those sustained by a worker caught beneath a collapsing structure. Patients with unstable thoracolumbar fractures suffer an average of two or more major injuries in addition to their spinal fracture (15).

Common injuries associated with thoracolumbar and thoracic fracture reflect the forces of blunt trauma and rapid deceleration. Pneumothorax and hemothorax associated with rib fractures and/or bronchial disruption, myocardial or pulmonary contusion, great vessel injury, hemopericardium and cardiac tamponade, diaphragmatic rupture and acute hiatal hernia have been reported (19–21). In seat belt injuries, indicated by the presence of lap belt abrasions with the classic flexion-distraction fracture, intraabdominal injuries are highly likely (22,23). Because this fracture occurs as the body is flexed forward over the lap belt, visceral injuries are found in 40 to 60% of patients (24–27). Solid viscera may be injured directly when they are compressed between the body wall and the lap belt, or they may be torn from their attachments when the body is suddenly and rapidly decelerated. Hollow viscera may be ruptured, perforated, or torn from their mesenteries. A rigid abdomen, falling hematocrit, and abdominal pain or tenderness are clear signs of intraabdominal injuries (23,28–33). Additional skeletal injuries involving the long bones are also common (17), which, in the case of multiple long-bone fractures, can result in shock (10).

As many as 25% of patients with thoracic and lumbar spine fractures have associated vertebral fractures somewhere in the spinal column, often involving the cervical spine. The unconscious, obtunded, or intoxicated patient, who cannot provide a dependable history or reliably report pain or numbness, should be protected as though a cervical injury existed until proven otherwise (6,34,35). Although plain radiographs demonstrate the majority of bone injuries, they may not reveal soft-tissue disruptions. Retropharyngeal hematoma is indicative of significant soft-tissue injury and mandates a formal cervical workup (36). Patients with head injuries may be evaluated by magnetic resonance imaging (MRI) or computed tomography (CT) scan before anesthesia if surgery is needed, or they may be held under observation if otherwise stable.

Neurogenic shock may ensue and will manifest itself with hypotension and tachycardia because of loss of normal vasomotor tone. Although patients in neurogenic shock may be warm with well-perfused skin and peripheral tissues, they may not respond to fluid bolus, and vasopressors may be needed. In addition, shock may result from any condition that reduces cardiac output, including cardiac tamponade, tension pneumothorax, myocardial injury, or myocardial infarction. In every case, rapid vascular access and fluid resuscitation are the vital initial treatments for spinal trauma patients.

FRACTURE CLASSIFICATION SYSTEMS

Holdsworth first characterized spinal fractures according to a two-column anterior and posterior model of the spinal column (37,38). This model has since given way to the three-column model of Denis, which considers the vertebral body, annulus, and posterior longitudinal ligament to be the middle column—a discrete unit separate from the anterior and posterior stabilizer (39–41) (Fig. 2). The classic description of burst fractures was provided by Denis in 1983 (39), and Denis further subclassified the types of burst fractures in 1984 (42). The Denis classification takes into account the location of fracture, comminution in the vertebral body, and any deformity.

According to the Denis criteria, fractures may be classified as stable or unstable. Unstable injuries include the following: (a) any three-column disruption, (b) greater than 50% collapse of anterior cortex, (c) greater than 25 degrees of focal kyphosis, and (d) any extent of neurologic deficit. Although all stable injuries may be treated nonoperatively, not all unstable injuries need to be treated operatively. A simple algorithm for treatment is indicated in Figure 3. As indicated in Table 1, the Denis fracture classification depends on information about the fracture pattern, the mechanism of injury, and the deforming forces that caused the fracture. The differences between severe burst fractures and rotational fracture-dislocations and severe seat belt injuries and flexion-distraction fracture dislocations are subtle and of limited importance. These severe injuries are all clearly unstable, and all require operative treatment.

Magerl introduced another comprehensive classification system based on pathomorphologic criteria in 1994 (43). The classification reflects a progressive scale of morphologic damage with increasing instability, which is expressed by its ranking within the classification system. The 3-3-3 scheme of the AO fracture classification was used in grouping the injuries into A, B, and C types. Every type has three groups, each of which contains three subgroups with specifications. The types are reflective of common injury patterns as determined by compression, distraction, and axial torque forces. Type A injuries are vertebral body compression fractures. Type B injuries result from distraction of the anterior and posterior elements. Axial torque forces produce type C injuries, where the anterior and posterior elements are disrupted with rotation. Type C lesions commonly coexist with either type A or type B lesions. Magerl's classification system uses additional morphologic criteria for further subdivision of the injuries. Severity progresses from type A through type C as well as within the types, groups, and further subdivisions. Of the 1,445 cases that were analyzed in Magerl's study, 66.1% of the patients had type A fractures. Type B fractures were found in 14.5% of patients, and type C fractures were

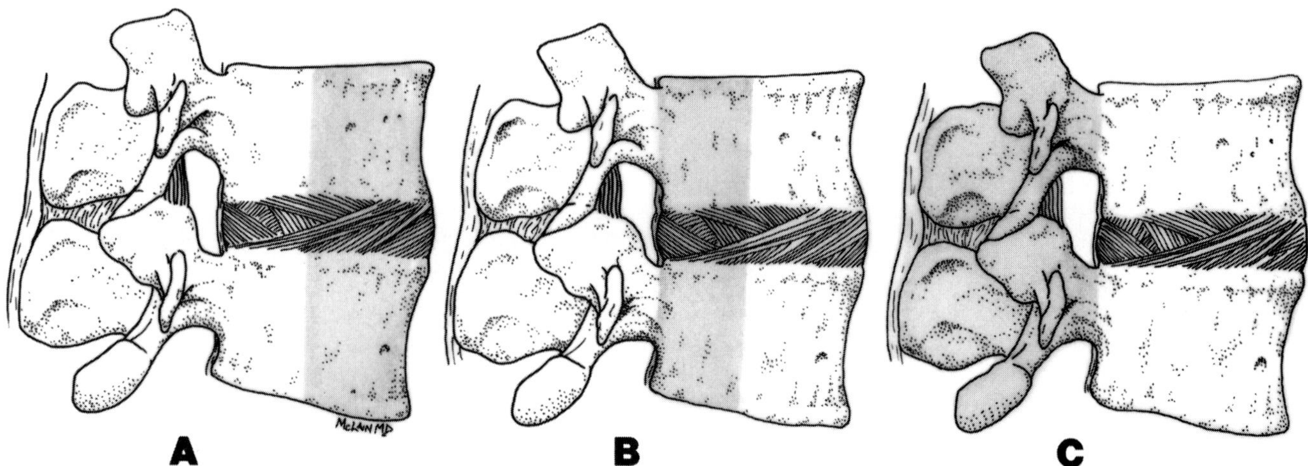

FIG. 2. Three-column model of Denis. **A:** Anterior column. **B:** Middle column. **C:** Posterior column.

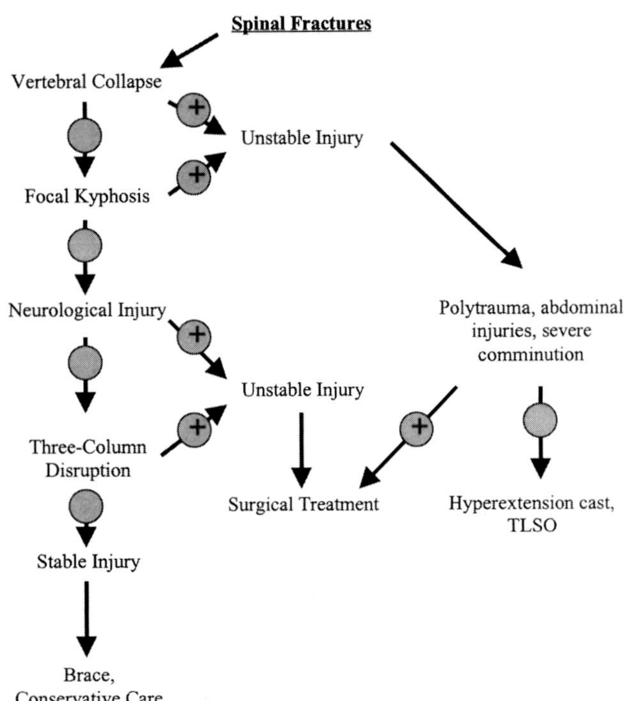

FIG. 3. Treatment algorithm for thoracolumbar fractures. TLSO, thoracolumbar spinal orthosis. (From *Chapman's operative orthopaedics,* 2nd ed. Philadelphia: JB Lippincott Co., 2001, with permission.)

found in 19.4% of the patients. Stable type A1 fractures accounted for 34.7% of the total. Magerl noted that certain injury patterns were typical of certain sections of the thoracolumbar spine and others for age groups and found the classification scheme prognostic of clinical outcomes.

Leibl et al. investigated whether the assessment of spinal fracture stability according to the Magerl classification permits a better therapeutic decision than using the Denis three-column model (44). The authors compared x-ray and CT images of 99 consecutive patients treated for thoracolumbar spine fractures and classified them accordingly. Using the three-column model, the involvement of two or more columns was considered unstable, whereas the fracture types A3.2, A3.3, B, and C of the Magerl classification were defined as unstable. The stability evaluation was compared with the therapeutic decision and outcome. According to the three-column model, 23 of 53 fractures that were classified as unstable were treated surgically. Only five of the 30 (16%) conservatively treated unstable fractures showed a reduced healing process. All of the 46 stable fractures were treated conservatively with good results. Using the Magerl classification, there were 28 unstable fractures, 21 of which were treated surgically. Four of the remaining seven unstable cases (57%) showed a reduced healing process. Of the 71 stable fractures, only two were treated surgically, and in one patient, minimal neurologic symptoms occurred. The authors concluded the Magerl classification enables a more exact differentiation of stable from unstable spinal fractures.

McCormack et al. described a "load-sharing" classification system to quantify the degree of vertebral body comminution and potential mechanical instability (45). The authors followed 28 patients who had three-column spinal fractures surgically stabilized by short-segment instrumentation with first generation variable screw placement (Steffee) screws and plates and autograft fusion. The follow-up radiographs revealed 10 patients (35%) with broken screws. A retrospective examination of preoperative radiographs and CT axial and sagittal reconstruction images demonstrated that the screw fractures all occurred in patients with a disproportionately greater amount of injury to the vertebral body. The author's load-sharing classification grades comminution as follows: (a) the amount of damaged vertebral body, (b) the spread of the fragments in the fracture site, and (c) the amount of corrected traumatic kyphosis. This point system can be used preoperatively to select spinal fractures for anterior plate with strut graft, short-segment–type reconstruction. Although this classification system was specifically designed to guide the need for anterior column reconstruction after posterior short-segment pedicle screw stabilization, it is a useful guide to the magnitude of comminution and potential mechanical insufficiency.

Oner et al. attempted to correlate the MRI appearance of fractures of the thoracolumbar spine with immediate and long-term mechanical stability (46). The state of the anterior longitudinal ligament, posterior longitudinal ligament, posterior ligamentous

TABLE 1. *Denis fracture classification*

Fracture type	Subtype	Deforming forces	Columns injured	Stability
Compression	—	Axial loading	1: Anterior	Stable
Burst fracture	Type A	Axial loading	2: Anterior + middle	Unstable
	Type B	Flexion, axial loading	2: Anterior + middle	Possibly unstable
	Type C	Flexion, axial loading	2: Anterior + middle	Possibly unstable
	Type D	Axial loading, rotation	3: Anterior + middle + posterior	Unstable
	Type E	Lateral compression	2–3: Anterior + middle + posterior	Possibly unstable
Seat belt	—	Flexion-distraction	2: Posterior + middle	Unstable
Fracture-dislocation	Flexion-rotation	Hyperflexion-rotation	3: Anterior + middle + posterior	Unstable
	Shear	Extension, translation	3: Anterior + middle + posterior	Unstable
	Flexion-distraction	Hyperflexion-distraction	3: Anterior + middle + posterior	Unstable

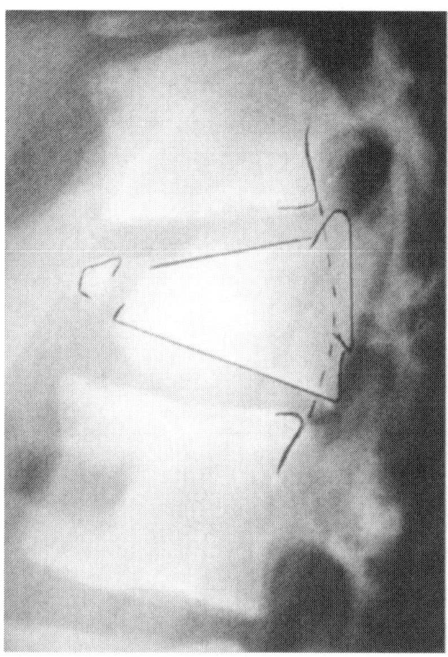
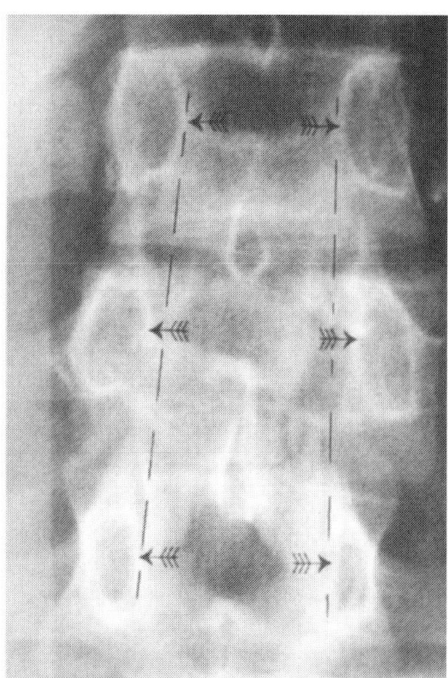

A,B

FIG. 4. Radiographic characteristics of burst fractures. **A:** Lateral view demonstrates fracture of anterior cortex and superior end-plate, with resulting focal kyphosis. The posterosuperior portion of the vertebral body can be seen retropulsed into the spinal canal, with loss of normal concave contour of the posterior vertebral body. **B:** Anteroposterior radiograph demonstrates the increased intrapedicular distance associated with a burst fracture; the distance between the L-1 pedicles is significantly greater than in the levels above or below, indicating a complete disruption of anterior, middle, and posterior columns. (From *Chapman's operative orthopaedics,* 2nd ed. Philadelphia: JB Lippincott Co., 2001, with permission.)

complex, cranial and caudal end-plates, cranial and caudal discs, and the vertebral body were defined using clinical, experimental, and radiologic data. The state of these structures was reported for each fracture on the MRI examinations, and the different MRI features appropriate for different fracture classes were defined. Wide variations on MRI appearance were seen, and specific patterns that would lead to a clinical classification scheme could not be defined. However, the author recommended that MRI findings be integrated into future classification schemes of thoracolumbar spine fractures.

Although these classification systems are comprehensive, many combinations of thoracic and thoracolumbar fractures exist, requiring careful assessment and analysis of the mechanical failure that has occurred in the injury complex.

SPECIFIC FRACTURE TYPES

Compression Fractures

Compression fractures are common injuries, occurring with moderate trauma in young patients and minimal to no trauma in elderly, osteoporotic patients. The anterior column collapses under an axial or flexion load, with fracture of one or both end-plates, but the middle and posterior columns are undamaged. These stable injuries are appropriately treated with a removable brace and symptomatic care. Physicians should observe patients with advanced osteoporosis for progressive collapse; severe compression fractures may warrant an MRI examination to rule out a burst component (33). Patients with persistent pain or advanced osteoporosis may benefit from kyphoplasty.

Burst Fractures

Burst fractures occur when the vertebral body is subjected to higher axial or flexural loads at a high loading rate, commonly the result of motor vehicle accidents, falls from height, or crush injuries (Fig. 4). The anterior cortex fails in compression, and one or both end-plates are fractured. The middle column also fractures, and a portion of the body is typically retropulsed backward into the canal (47). The posterior elements may be fractured as well. The need for surgery depends on the extent of vertebral comminution, the extent of canal compromise, and the status of the posterior column structures (15). Burst fractures may be subdivided by fracture pattern as follows (Fig. 5):

- Type A: Occurs with axial loading; fractures both upper and lower end-plates
- Type B: Most common (50%); fractures only the upper end-plate
- Type C: Uncommon; disruption of only the lower end-plate
- Type D: Rotational displacement of one body relative to the other
- Type E: Lateral compression injury; occurs with traumatic scoliosis

Canal compromise is estimated from the CT scan, comparing the anteroposterior (AP) spinal canal diameter at an adjacent level to the reduced diameter at the injured level (48) (Fig. 6). The greatest compromise occurs at the level of the pedicles and upper vertebral body. In type A and B burst fractures, the posterior cortex and vertebral body are driven back into the canal between the two pedicles, which then traps the fragment and prevents it from reducing. Because of the differing volumes of neural tissues at different levels of the spinal canal, a 50% compromise may produce symptoms at the thoracolumbar junction, whereas compromise of 85% or more may be well tolerated at the lumbosacral junction (48–50).

Flexion-Distraction Fractures

Flexion-distraction, or seat belt fractures, may be one- or two-level injuries (22,39,51,52). The classic one-level injury occurs transversely through bone and is the Chance fracture.

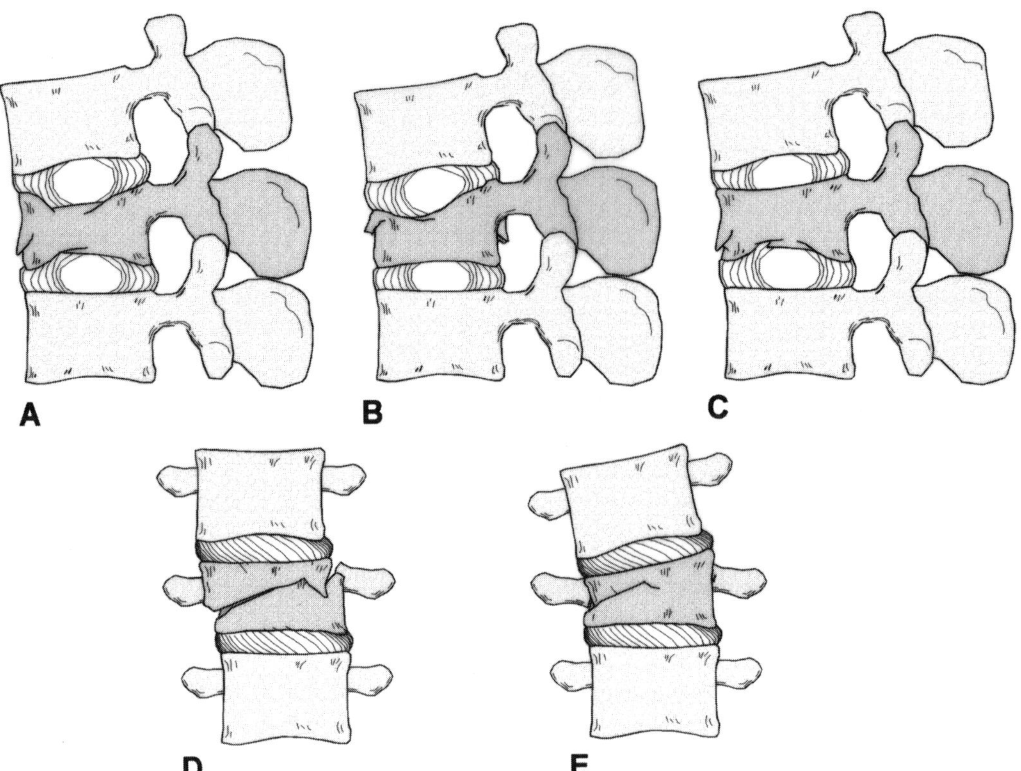

FIG. 5. A–E: Burst fracture patterns.

The mechanism of injury involves the patient's being thrown forward across an intact lap belt, resulting in a hyperflexion force acting around a center of rotation anterior to the spinal column at the belt itself. This results in distraction forces at all three columns of the spine: (a) The posterior elements are torn apart through the facet joints or the bone itself, (b) the middle column is torn apart through the posterior disc or the posterior vertebral body, and (c) the anterior column is disrupted (in severe injuries) or left as a hinge that cannot resist flexion or rotational displacement. Plain radiographs demonstrate the gap between the spinous processes and the disruption of the pedicle in most cases but may show minimal displacement when the patient is supine, because the fracture tends to reduce in this position (Fig. 7). CT may miss the transverse injuries if the fracture plane parallels the image plane. An MRI shows the injury clearly.

The violent compression of viscera between the spinal column and the lap belt can rupture hollow viscera, lacerate solid viscera (liver and spleen), and avulse major vascular pedicles. Unrecognized, any of these injuries can prove rapidly fatal; it is

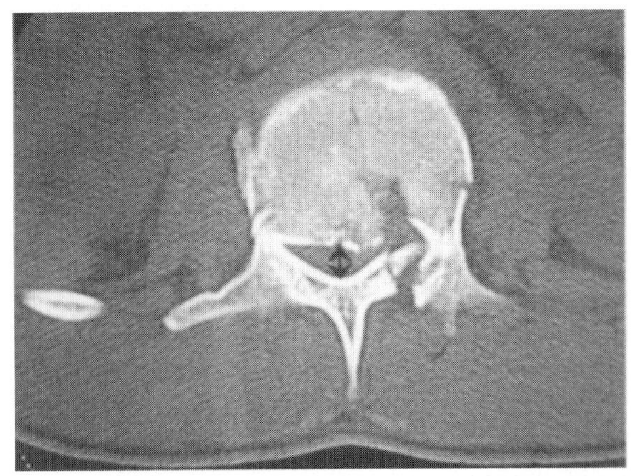

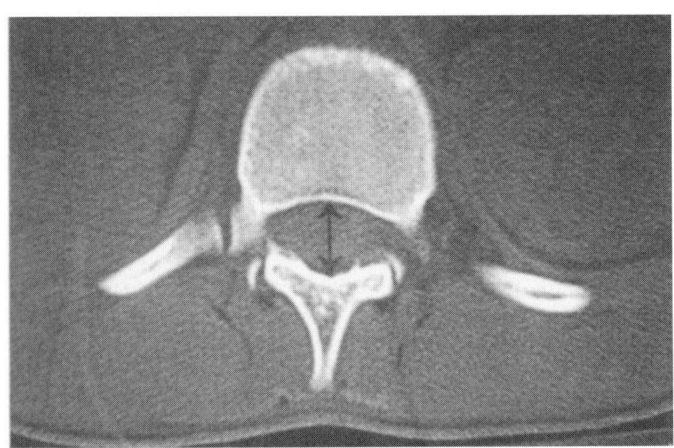

FIG. 6. Canal dimension at injured level **(A)** is compared to adjacent normal level **(B)** to determine percent canal compromise. (From *Chapman's operative orthopaedics,* 2nd ed. Philadelphia: JB Lippincott Co., 2001, with permission.)

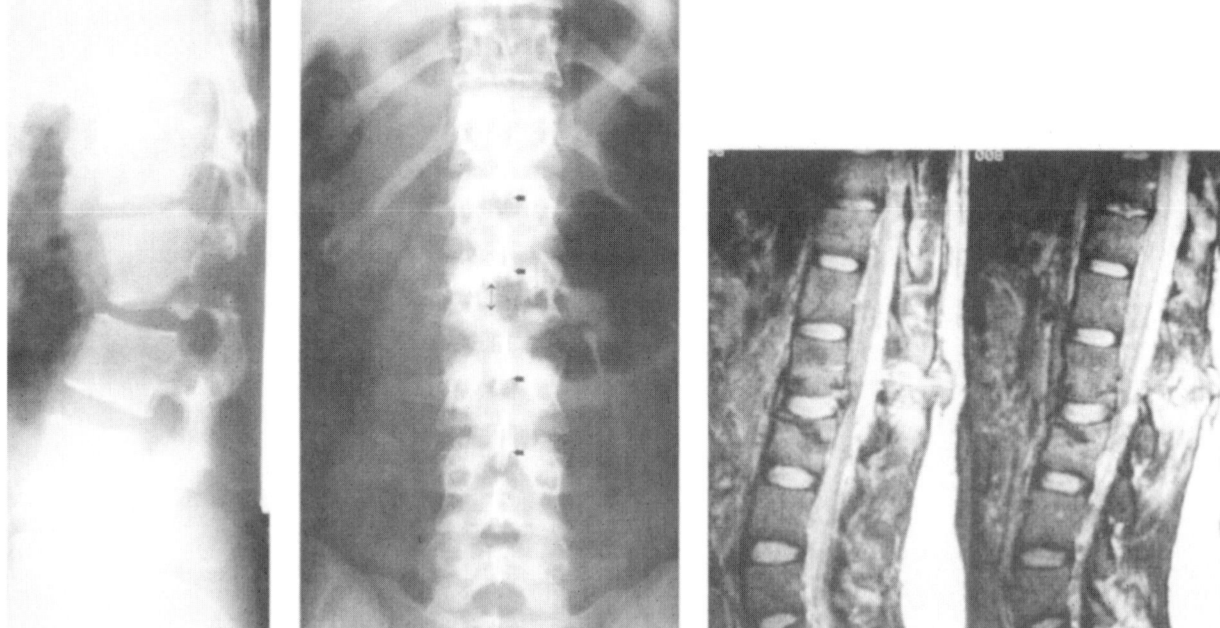

FIG. 7. Radiographic characteristics of seat belt fractures. **A:** Lateral radiograph of a severe flexion-distraction injury, taken in sitting position. The patient was admitted after a head-on motor vehicle accident and treated for abdominal contusions, splenic rupture, and rupture of the colon. Injury was not apparent on supine radiographs. **B:** Anteroposterior radiograph shows wide spacing between spinous processes at the level of injury. **C:** Magnetic resonance imaging confirms extensive soft-issue disruption, including rupture of the lumbodorsal fascia. (From *Chapman's operative orthopaedics,* 2nd ed. Philadelphia: JB Lippincott Co., 2001, with permission.)

therefore necessary that any patient with a seat belt injury be carefully assessed by a general surgeon for acute or occult intra-abdominal injury.

Single-level injuries pass through the posterior ligamentous structures and the underlying disc at the same level, or through the posterior lamina, pedicle, and vertebral body in the same transverse plane (Fig. 8). These injuries disrupt only a single motion segment. Two-level injuries begin posteriorly at one level of lamina or facet joint, then proceed anteriorly in an oblique fashion so that the injury passes out of the vertebral body into an adjacent disc or through the disc into an adjacent body. In these injuries, two adjacent motion segments are disrupted, and stabilization requires addressing both levels of injury.

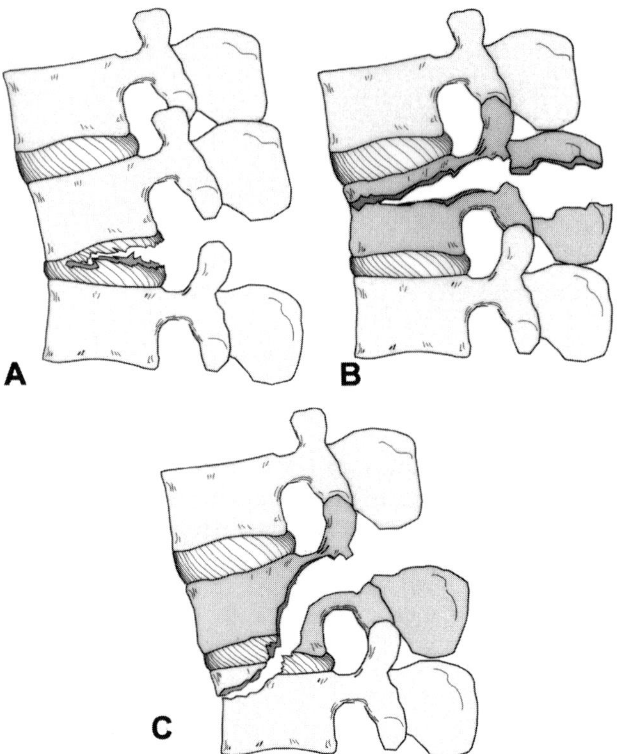

FIG. 8. Seat belt fractures. **A:** Injury to soft tissues only. **B:** Bony chance fracture. **C:** Mixed injury.

Fracture-Dislocations

Fracture-dislocations are, by definition, three-column injuries. They are highly unstable, usually associated with neurologic injury, and often associated with other musculoskeletal and visceral injuries. The neurologically intact patient must be carefully protected during any necessary testing or emergent operative procedures, and the spine is to be stabilized at the first reasonable opportunity, to allow early mobilization and prevent paralysis. In the patient with neurologic deficit, postural reduction may improve alignment and reduce neural compression, and longitudinal traction may allow manual reduction of a dis-

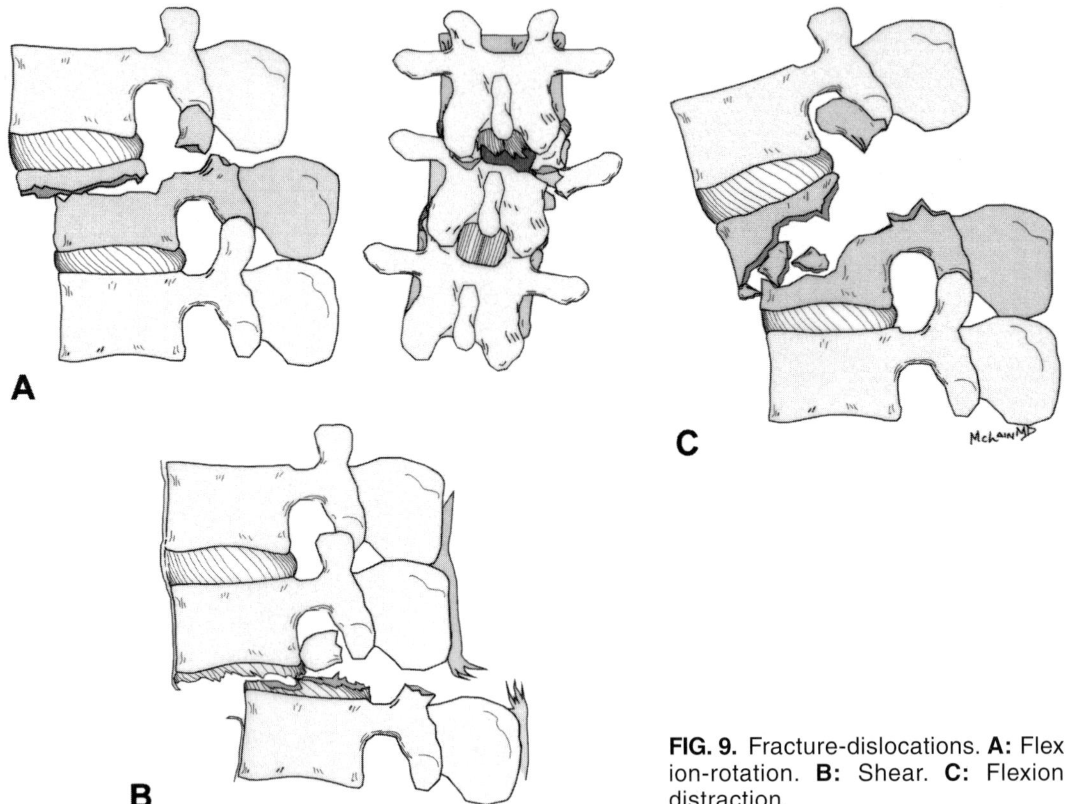

FIG. 9. Fracture-dislocations. **A:** Flexion-rotation. **B:** Shear. **C:** Flexion-distraction.

placed dislocation. Neither reduce neural compression by retropulsed vertebral fragments, however, and direct decompression is indicated for those patients with an incomplete injury and hopes of improvement.

Flexion-rotation fracture-dislocations are caused by hyperflexion and rotation forces, such as may be seen when a patient is ejected from a vehicle traveling at high speed (Fig. 9). Vertebral body fractures may be indistinguishable from severe type D burst fractures. Shear fractures are more uncommon and occur in the absence of axial loading or flexion-extension forces. Translational forces—occurring when the subject is struck squarely from the side, front, or back—act to shift one vertebral body relative to the next by shearing through bony articulations and ligamentous structures. Flexion-distraction fracture-dislocations occur when all three columns fail in hyperflexion. These injuries are often not distinguishable from severe seat belt injuries.

A key consideration in fracture-dislocations is that all three columns are unstable in both axial loading and in longitudinal traction. Instrumentation systems that depend on distraction forces to secure hook purchase cannot be safely applied in these injuries, and any system incorrectly applied may overdistract the fracture and stretch the neurologic elements, precipitating or worsening the neurologic injury.

INITIAL SPINAL EVALUATION

With the patient hemodynamically and mechanically stabilized, the extent of any spinal injury should be further assessed. A complete history should be obtained, paying close attention to reports of transient paresthesias, acute back or neck pain, or temporary weakness or paralysis at the time of injury. The location and radiation of pain symptoms, as well as any radicular symptoms should be recorded. Moreover, any history of previous injury, fracture, or pain symptoms should be noted. A global examination of motor and sensory function should rapidly focus on any areas of deficit. If the patient cannot cooperate with the examination, the physician needs to carefully observe and note spontaneous movements and withdrawal responses. A rectal examination should be done to assess rectal tone, voluntary rectal control, and the bulbocavernosus reflex. If the patient is neurologically normal, a log-roll to one side should be performed so that the spine can be palpated for step-offs, tenderness, or kyphosis. The condition of the skin over the symptomatic area should be noted. If a neurologic deficit exists, radiographs of the symptomatic level should be obtained before moving the patient.

If a spinal cord injury is identified, some literature suggests the patient should be started on high-dose steroids to attempt to facilitate recovery (53,54). Steroids have been shown to improve spinal cord recovery relative to placebo and naloxone therapy and are thought to combat abnormal biochemical processes brought on by thromboxanes and prostaglandins released at the site of injury. Such improvement is relatively modest in terms of function. However, steroids should be given within 3 to 8 hours of injury to have any beneficial effect. Patients treated with high-dose steroids may be exposed to an increased risk of gastrointestinal hemorrhage or infection. Current recommendations are that patients seen before 8 hours from injury be given a bolus dose of 30 mg per kg methylprednisolone, followed by 5.4 mg per kg methylprednisolone per hour for maintenance.

The maintenance dose should be discontinued at 24 hours if the initial dose was given within 3 hours of injury. Maintenance steroids should be discontinued at 48 hours if the first dose was given between 3 and 8 hours of injury. Patients started on steroid therapy more than 8 hours after injury have not done as well as patients treated with placebo and should not be started on a methylprednisolone protocol.

In high-energy injuries, it is often difficult to determine exactly what forces acted on the spine to produce fracture, but knowledge of the injury mechanism can help to identify associated injuries and provide clues to the level of stability to be expected. A lap-belted patient in a motor vehicle accident may present with a straightforward flexion-distraction injury, whereas a patient ejected from the vehicle or from a motorcycle frequently presents with a more complex fracture pattern consistent with the combination of torsional and axial forces experienced when striking the ground (55). If the forces involved in the fracture were rather low, an underlying pathologic process must be considered. If the forces involved were very high and multiple injuries are present, the risk of prolonged recumbency to the patient's life must be considered in timing a surgical procedure.

If the patient can recall the event, it is important to note any history of transient paresthesias or paralysis from time of injury. Even if the patient's symptoms resolve quickly, these symptoms imply a nerve root or cord trauma has occurred at the time of the injury; therefore, spinal fracture must be assumed to be unstable until proven otherwise. If the patient cannot recall the details of the event, careful scrutiny of the emergency technicians' field notes may provide important clues to as whether the patient had abnormal findings at the accident site. These notes are gross evaluations only, however, and a patient with cord or cauda equina injury may still be able to move all four extremities.

RADIOGRAPHIC STUDIES

Plain radiographs should include AP and lateral views of the thoracic spine or the lumbosacral spine, depending on the symptomatic level (56). On occasion, standard thoracic films will be cut off at T-12 to L-1, and lumbosacral films will start at L-1, giving an inadequate view of the most frequently injured level. If fracture of the thoracolumbar junction is suspected, repeat AP and lateral radiographs should be centered at the T-12 level. In stable fractures (compression fractures, mild burst fractures, and mild flexion-distraction injuries), plain radiographs are sufficient to allow definitive treatment, and no further diagnostic studies are needed (56–58). In unstable spine fractures, however, additional imaging studies are often indicated (32,59–62). Unstable fractures (severe burst fractures, fracture-dislocations, significant flexion-distraction injuries, and any fracture with a neurologic deficit) require further study to assess the extent of bony disruption, spinal cord impingement, canal compromise, or cord injury (59–62). A CT scan provides the most definitive information on bony characteristics, such as fracture pattern and comminution (56,63–65). The axial cuts of the CT scan can completely miss flexion-distraction injuries, however. An MRI is superior for soft-tissue details, such as cord injury, cord compression, disc herniation, and ligamentous disruption (61). The MRI has the added benefit of scanning the entire thoracolumbar spine, and it can pick up noncontiguous fractures, cord injury, and epidural hematoma at levels other than that of the primary fracture. Longitudinal MRI cuts show the soft-tissue disruption and bony separation of flexion-distraction injuries well.

Myelography, the gold standard for assessing neural compromise just a decade ago, has been replaced by MRI in all but a few cases. When an MRI is contraindicated (e.g., intraocular fragments, cardiac valves), CT-myelography is an appropriate but more invasive alternative. An MRI or myelography should be ordered in the acutely injured patient (a) if there is progressive neurologic deficit and (b) if the neurologic level does not coincide with the recognized injury (patient requires further evaluation for an unrecognized fracture or disc disruption).

Plain tomography is sometimes useful for evaluating the cervicothoracic junction when a CT scan cannot be obtained immediately. Flexion-extension studies or nuclear medicine scans have little role in acute trauma. There is no role for electrodiagnostic testing in the acute management of spine trauma patients.

NEUROLOGIC EXAMINATION

The physical examination for the spinal-injured patient centers on a careful, complete neurologic assessment. Having examined the musculoskeletal system in the emergency room, the extremities should be carefully reexamined for tenderness and pain.

A complete motor and sensory examination is documented. Each motor group is tested for the lumbar and sacral plexuses independently and compared to the contralateral group (Fig. 10). Motor strength is recorded on six-point scale:

5 Full strength adequate to powerfully resist the examiner
4 Power to resist but not overcome the examiner
3 Power to overcome gravity
2 Power to move the joint but not to overcome gravity
1 Capacity to contract the muscle without functional power
0 No motor function

The sensory examination begins at the chest wall and seeks a level of anesthesia, root-by-root, down to the sacrum. Patients with thoracic cord injuries will have an anesthetic level at or just below their fracture. If the anesthetic level and the recognized fracture do not coincide, an MRI should be obtained to determine

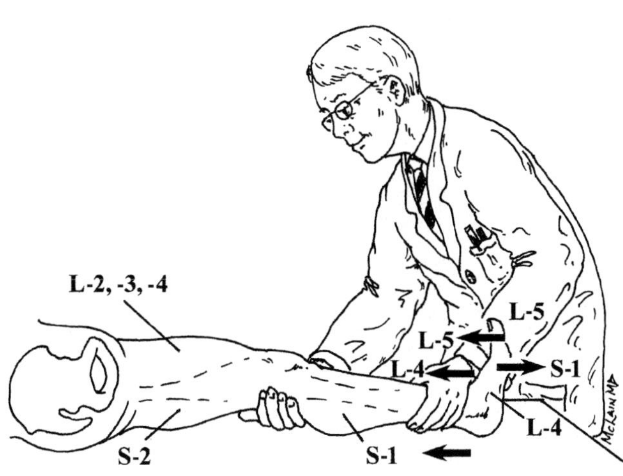

FIG. 10. Motor testing.

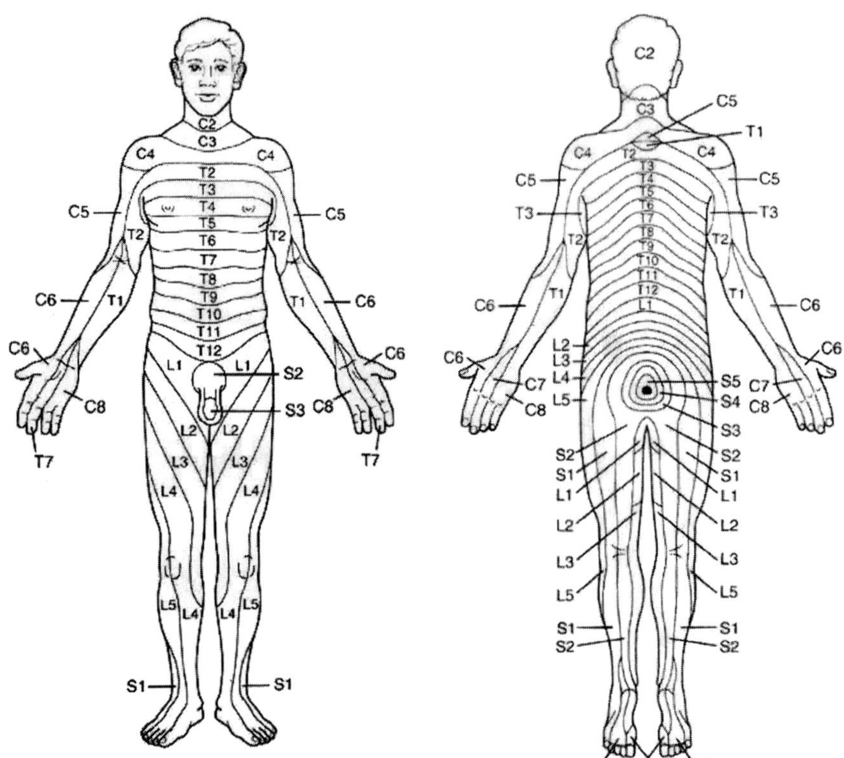

FIG. 11. Dermatomal patterns. (From *Chapman's operative orthopaedics,* 2nd ed. Philadelphia: JB Lippincott Co., 2001, with permission.)

the actual cause of the cord impairment. Sensation in the lower extremities follows a dermatomal pattern; each dermatome should be tested for light-touch and pin-prick sensation (Fig. 11).

The superficial abdominal reflex should be checked above the umbilicus (T7-10) and below the umbilicus (T-11 through L-1). Reflexes at both the knees (L3-4) and the ankles (S-1) should be checked. The bulbocavernosus reflex, an involuntary contraction of the rectal sphincter, can be triggered by gently squeezing the glans penis or glans clitoris or by gently tugging on the Foley catheter. If this reflex is absent, the patient is in spinal shock or has suffered an injury to the caudal segments of the conus medullaris (S3-4). Hyperactive reflexes suggest disinhibition due to a cord-level injury, whereas absent reflexes in an isolated distribution suggest an incomplete injury or root lesion. Complete absence of reflexes may be due to spinal cord shock or a complete cauda equina injury. Spinal cord shock occurs at the time of injury and may persist for 72 hours. During this time, the neurologic examination remains unreliable, and an incomplete injury may appear complete due to the overriding effects of cord shock. Once shock resolves and caudal reflexes return, the examination provides clear prognostic information: Incomplete injuries have potential for improvement, whereas complete injuries have almost none. The bulbocavernosus reflex is the most reliable level for testing reflex return because it tests the most caudal segment of the spinal cord.

The rectal examination deserves special comment. The most caudal motor and sensory unit in the body is the rectum, the function of which is crucial to independent social activity. An independent examination of rectal tone, sensation, and reflex activity should be conducted. Emergency department records should not be relied on if there is any concern of neurologic injury. Resting tone, voluntary contraction, perianal sensation, and bulbocavernosus reflex should be documented.

GRADING OF NEUROLOGIC DEFICITS

In patients with no neurologic injury, treatment is based primarily on issues of mechanical stability, alignment, and canal compromise. In the thoracic region, sagittal deformities are correlated with longitudinal distraction, which may also indirectly pull some retropulsed vertebral fragments from the canal. In the lumbar region, forceful distraction tends to reduce lumbar lordosis, introducing sagittal imbalance and a flat back. Forceful distraction in a patient with a three-column injury may inadvertently lengthen the column and stretch the spinal cord, causing neurologic injury.

Canal compromise becomes a concern only when a high degree of compromise is recognized. Residual compromise greater than 50% of the cross-sectional area is worrisome at the T-12 to L-1 level, where the conus medullaris and cauda equina fill the spinal canal. Further small increments of axial or sagittal collapse can compromise neurologic elements, and anterior decompression and stabilization should be considered for both mechanical and neurologic reasons. On the other hand, 80 to 85% canal compromise may be well tolerated in the lower lumbar spine, where only a few roots remain in the otherwise capacious canal (50). Retropulsed bony fragments reabsorb and remodel over time and do not need to be removed (66). Sagittal collapse and kyphosis of a moderate degree are usually well tolerated in the thoracic region and do not require aggressive reconstruction. Lower lumbar burst fractures are also well toler-

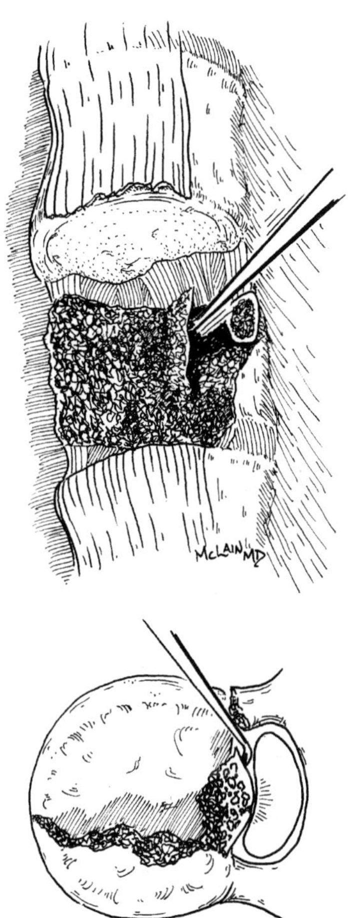

FIG. 12. Reduction of retropulsed fragments. (From *Chapman's operative orthopaedics,* 2nd ed. Philadelphia: JB Lippincott Co., 2001, with permission.)

ated and most have a satisfactory outcome without reconstruction. Retropulsion of middle-column bone fragments represents the major risk to the neural structures in thoracolumbar burst fractures (Fig. 12). As the cord ends at L-1 and the cauda equina roots cascade off the cord over many segments closely approximated to the distal end of the cord, a variety of neurologic structures may be damaged, with a variety of neurologic abnormalities (Fig. 13).

Cord injuries can be complete (total loss of cord function) or incomplete. Another way of classifying cord injury is by the anatomic localization of the involved tracts (i.e., anterior, central, Brown-Séquard, and posterior cord syndrome). In the anterior cord syndrome, the dorsal columns remain intact. Hence, proprioception, vibration, and light touch are preserved. Protective pain sensation is frequently absent. In thoracolumbar spine fractures, a preferential upper lumbar neurologic deficit with relative sparing of the lower sacral roots is frequently observed because of the anatomic distribution of the long tracts, where the lumbar tracts are more central and the sacral tracts are more peripheral.

The certainty of outcome of neural function does not exist for cauda equina injuries, where the roots behave more like peripheral nerves with potential for later recovery. Severe neural injuries above L-1 damage the lower spinal cord, resulting in an upper motor neuron picture of spastic paralysis. Similar severe neural injuries below L-1 may result in a lower motor neuron flaccid paralysis. Neural injuries between these two extremes may result in complex patterns of injury further complicated when lesions are incomplete. An interesting variation, usually associated with L-1 injuries, is the conus paraplegic. Injury to the tip of the cord, the conus, results in paralysis of the sacral segment. Loss of bladder and bowel control occurs, yet the patient's cauda equina roots originating proximal to the conus may be spared, giving near normal lower limb function. These differing patterns of neural injury mandate meticulous neurologic evaluation at initial assessment. Some have advocated that the classification of complete spinal cord injuries be limited to the upper thoracic spine and cervical spine only because of the potential for recovery of the differing neural tissues in injuries at the thoracolumbar junction (67–69).

RETURN OF NEUROLOGIC FUNCTION

Cord injury consists of the primary contusion, secondary injury due to cellular changes at the injury site, and the effects of ongoing neural compression. The first mechanism is amenable only to preventative treatment. Intensive investigation for effective agents is underway that may modify the secondary injury response. The use of methylprednisolone in the immediate postinjury phase has been shown to marginally improve outcomes in the National Acute Spinal Cord Injury Study investigations (53), but this improvement has not been substantiated in other studies, and its role remains controversial (54).

The role of surgery for any ongoing compression remains controversial. It is intuitively attractive to consider that decompression of damaged and compressed neural structures could reduce cellular and neuronal deformity, decompress vascular structures, and decompress cells and neurones in the cord. Clinical studies have suggested that effective cord decompression after injury is associated with improved outcomes (3,42,60,67,70–80). A number of authors have suggested that anterior decompression results in better neural recovery than nonoperative treatment or posterior decompression (71,72,74,76–84). Gertzbein summarized these data by suggesting that although nonoperative treatment is associated with improved neural function, anterior decompression is associated with more rapid and better neurologic recovery (85); however, a review of these studies reveals that the methodology does not stand up to the vigorous evaluation required for evidence-based practice.

Equally effective neural recovery has been demonstrated by Katoh et al. with conservative management of these injuries (86), and critical literature reviews have cast doubt about the real benefit of surgical decompression (87). In reality, the role of surgical decompression is likely to remain unclear, and the ever-present call for randomized prospective studies remains unfulfilled. What is clear is that late decompression, once natural recovery has ended, is associated with further improvement in neural function (88). The role of active decompression is also supported by animal studies, where a meticulously controlled experimental environment can be

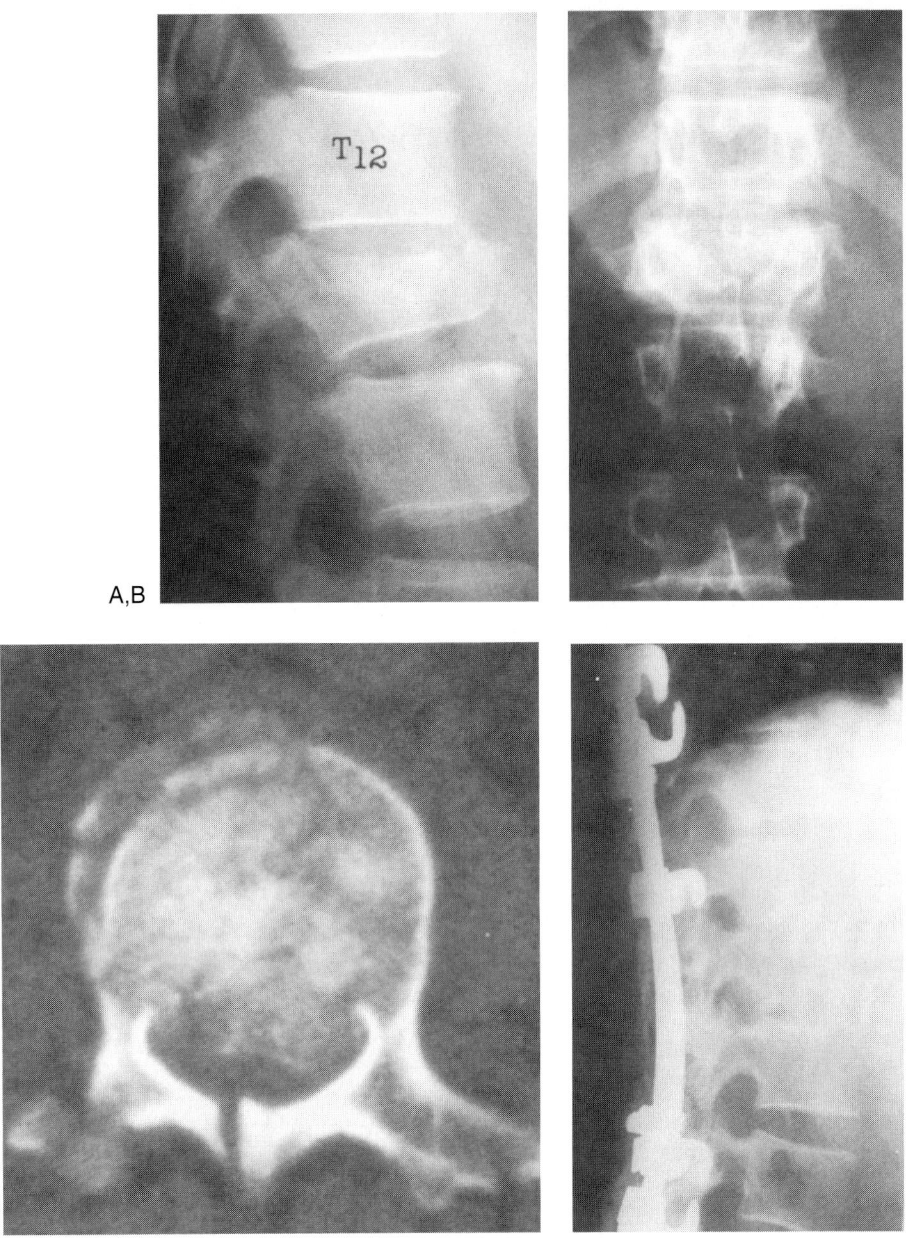

FIG. 13. Burst fracture. A 32-year-old man fell 35 ft., sustaining a severe L-1 burst fracture (Denis type B) and an open tibial shaft fracture. A,B: Lateral and anteroposterior radiographs demonstrate loss of vertebral height and widening of the pedicles, with little kyphosis. Cortical retropulsion is difficult to appreciate on plain radiograph. C: Computed tomography demonstrates severe comminution and canal compromise. A fracture of the lamina is seen. Although the patient was neurologically intact, the 75% compromise at the L-1 level seen here was considered too severe, and the spine was unstable. D: Anterior vertebrectomy was followed by strut graft reconstruction, restoring anterior column support and thoracolumbar alignment. Posterior segmental instrumentation stabilizes the spine; the intermediate, downgoing hook compresses and entraps the anterior strut graft. The patient had a full recovery and returned to work and sports with restrictions. (From *Chapman's operative orthopaedics,* 2nd ed. Philadelphia: JB Lippincott Co., 2001, with permission.)

developed (89–91). Such studies have shown benefit of early and late decompression.

Incomplete neurologic deficit remains a relative indication for anterior decompression. Because functional outcome is more clearly related to the residual neurologic deficit than to any other parameter, the need to maximize early neurologic recovery should be emphasized. This entails early recognition, rapid resuscitation, corticosteroid therapy, and surgical decompression when the patient is hemodynamically stable (10,71,92). It should be recognized, however, that canal compromise can be improved through indirect reduction, and that bony remodeling improves canal diameter over time irrespective of treatment (9,66,93,94). Still, persistent neural compression can inhibit neurologic recovery, and anterior decompression can provide dramatic neurologic improvement in many patients (64,78,84,94).

NONOPERATIVE TREATMENT

Only 20 to 30% of spine fractures require surgery. The remainder can be treated nonoperatively with a brace, molded orthosis, or hyperextension cast. Bed rest has also been effective, even in severe fractures, but prolonged immobilization carries risks of its own. With rigorous skin care and deep vein thrombosis prophylaxis, bed rest can provide good outcomes without surgery (95). Single-column injuries (e.g., compression fractures, laminar fracture, and spinous process fracture) are treated with an off-the-shelf brace that encourages normal spinal alignment and limits extreme motion (Fig. 14). Ohana et al. even showed that thoracolumbar fractures with compression as great as 30% of vertebral body height can be treated with early ambulation and no external support. However, close clinical

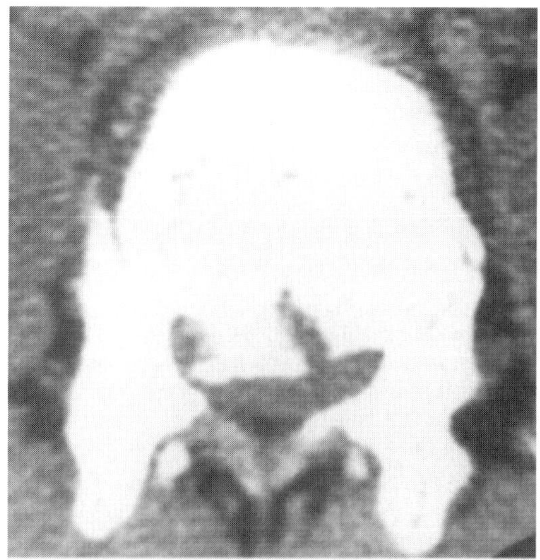

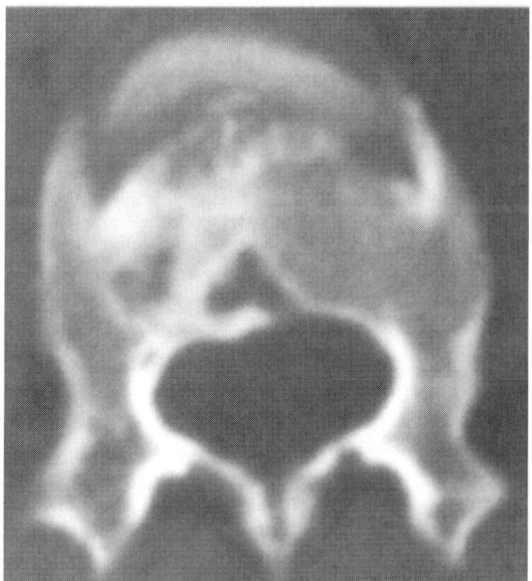

FIG. 14. Fracture remodeling. **A:** Thoracic level 11 fracture. With nonoperative treatment, normal remodeling mechanisms tend to restore canal diameter compromised by retropulsed bony fragments. **B:** Resorption of the retropulsed vertebral body results in a "heart-shaped" canal with near-normal anteroposterior diameter 1 year later. (Courtesy of John Mumford, M.D. Topeka, KS.)

and radiographic follow-up was deemed essential (96). More significant compression fractures may be treated in a molded orthosis. Two-column injuries, including severe compression fractures, mild to moderate burst fractures, and bony Chance fractures, are too unstable to be braced but may well be reduced and maintained by bed rest or in a hyperextension cast. Previous studies have shown that even severe burst fractures can be treated with a regimen of bed rest, postural reduction, and casting (66,95,97) (Fig. 15). Bony remodeling reduces residual canal compromise by more than 50% over the course of 1 year, making surgical treatment unnecessary in many patients, including those with retropulsed fragments in the spinal canal (94,98) (Fig. 14A).

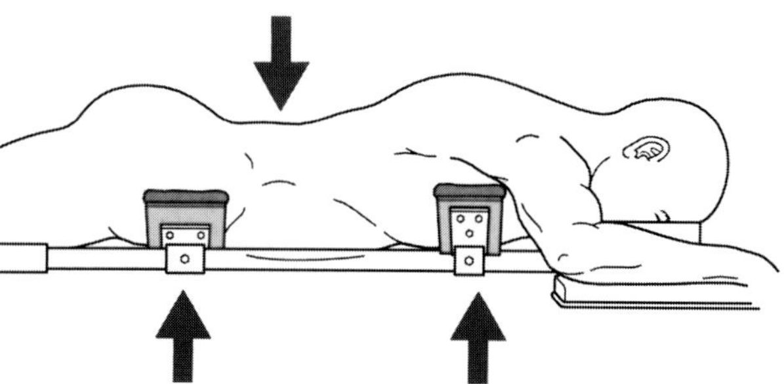

FIG. 15. Postural reduction of burst and distraction injuries. Normal thoracolumbar lordosis can be restored by placing the patient on a spinal frame supporting the thorax and pelvis and allowing the abdomen to hang free. Furthermore, elevating the thighs increases the lordosis in segments adjacent to the fracture, which helps in restoring normal alignment. (From *Chapman's operative orthopaedics,* 2nd ed. Philadelphia: JB Lippincott Co., 2001, with permission.)

Hyperextension casting allows immediate mobilization and early return to independent function. A hyperextension cast can be used in many patients with severe compression fractures or burst fractures (Fig. 14). If the posterior elements are intact, axial loads transferred posteriorly through the facet joints allow immediate weight bearing and good restoration of sagittal alignment and vertebral body height. In Chance fractures, hyperextension closes the posterior defect and approximates the fracture margins. The cast cannot be placed until any abdominal injury is resolved and any ileus or distention has subsided. However, the use of a cast in polytrauma patients is limited. Patients with abdominal trauma, prolonged ileus, chest trauma, or multiple extremity fractures may not be suitable for casting for some time after admission. Once a well-molded cast is applied, the patient may begin transfer and ambulation. Braces and removable orthoses cannot generate the hyperextension forces necessary to maintain sagittal alignment and should not be considered substitutes for a well-molded hyperextension cast.

OPERATIVE TREATMENT

Operative treatment offers significant advantages over casting or recumbency (12,51,75,99–101). First, immediate spinal stability is provided for patients who cannot tolerate a cast or prolonged recumbency. Prompt surgical stabilization allows the patient to sit upright, transfer, and start rehabilitation earlier, with fewer complications (67,73,102). Second, surgical treatment restores sagittal alignment, corrects translational deformities, and restores canal dimensions more reliably than does cast treatment. Finally, surgical decompression more reliably restores neurologic function and decreases rehabilitation time (66,70,71,75).

TREATMENT OF SPECIFIC FRACTURES

Compression Fractures

Compression fractures are single-column injuries, are typically stable, and rarely cause neurologic injury. In most cases, the anterior column fails in axial load, applied in combination with flexion or lateral bending, resulting in a stable fracture pattern. Therefore, most of these cases can be treated with a hyperextension orthosis or a chair-back brace, allowing ambulation and return to limited activity. Fractures with more than 50% collapse of the anterior vertebral body or with more than 20 degrees of sagittal angulation are considered potentially unstable. A CT scan may be necessary to distinguish these injuries from a burst fracture. Severe compression fractures can usually be treated with a hyperextension cast, but some may require posterior instrumentation and fusion. Fractures occurring in osteoporotic bone may respond favorably to kyphoplasty (103). More aggressive surgical treatment may be indicated if contiguous fractures are present and the cumulative angulatory and compression deformities exceed criteria for nonoperative treatment. Ultimately, the decision depends on the patient's general health, the bone quality, and whether the patient can tolerate the procedure.

Compression fractures that occur in young, healthy individuals after a high-energy injury may mask more severe spinal injuries. Seat belt–type injuries or a flexion-distraction injury can be misdiagnosed (39,104). Careful evaluation of axial imaging studies is necessary to look for "naked facets" (105). Therefore, thin 1-mm or 2-mm CT sections or MRI imaging through the area of injury are recommended.

Another phenomenon in the elderly with osteoporotic compression fractures is worth mentioning. Heggeness reported that in this patient population, these fractures may progress to burst fractures with increasing kyphosis and middle column extrusion over time (106). This should be suspected if elderly patients with compression fractures continue to complain about back pain or are unable to maintain their ambulatory function. A follow-up CT or MRI study readily reveals the problem if it exists.

Burst Fractures

In burst fractures, disruption of the medial column always occurs, and the posterior column may be involved as well. Retropulsion of bony fragments typically occurs and can be reliably seen on axial CT images. Unstable fractures may demonstrate the following:

- Greater than 50% axial compression
- Greater than 20 degrees of angular deformity
- Three-column injuries and dislocations
- Multiple contiguous fractures
- Neurologic injury (complete or incomplete)
- Patients with extensive associated injuries

Stable burst fractures (two-column injuries) may be treated in a hyperextension cast if the patient has no abdominal or thoracic injuries and no neurologic deficit (107). Nonoperative care can be limited to 2 weeks of bed rest followed by bracing and mobilization. There is often slight settling of the fracture with the development of a mild kyphosis, but this does not correlate with inferior clinical results and seldom results in any clinically detectable deformity. Long-term outcome of fractures treated primarily with bed rest can be excellent, as demonstrated by Weinstein et al., who followed patients over 20 years and found 88% of all patients were working (108). The average residual kyphosis was 26.5 degrees, and most patients had mild back pain but were not taking any narcotics.

Unstable injuries typically require operative reduction and stabilization (Fig. 16). Although the degree of canal compromise correlates poorly with neurologic deficit, at least in part because most of the injury may occur at the time of impact (70,104,109,110), many practitioners use the evidence from late decompression (71,72,76–78,109) or from animal studies (89,111) to justify early decompression in spinal cord or cauda equina injuries. As noted above, the evidence suggests that anterior decompression will be more effective for anterior neural compression, such as occurs in a burst fracture. The disadvantages of posterior approaches to achieve anterior decompression include the need to resect major portions of the neural arch, which often are uninjured, to obtain access to the middle column. The surgeon is working around already compromised neural structures, risking further neural damage to them, and anterior decompression will be less effective as compared with that achievable by anterior approaches. Finally, it is difficult to reconstruct the anterior and middle columns after a posterior approach has been used to decompress a burst fracture, and there is a significant risk of construct failure if the anterior column is not restored (15).

Posterior surgery with short-segment pedicle screw fixation stabilizes the fracture and allows early mobilization. If posterior surgery is performed alone, modest recurrence of deformity is common, even when transpedicular bone grafting is performed, as the anterior column remains deficient (47,82,83,112,113).

Anterior surgery with corpectomy and reconstruction should be considered when neural injury does occur in association with a burst fracture, as incomplete neural injury may recover better with effective decompression. The advantages of anterior surgery include direct atraumatic decompression of the spinal canal when neural injury has occurred and the ability to reconstruct the anterior column deficiency. Relative indications for anterior surgery also include severe comminution, fragmentation, segmental kyphosis, and AP malalignment (Denis type D injuries). In patients with medical comorbidities, the posterior approach may be preferred to address thoracolumbar burst fractures with significant neurologic deficit, realizing that the patient may not tolerate a thoracotomy. Disadvantages of anterior surgery include the more extensive approach required, lack of familiarity by many spinal surgeons, increased hemorrhage in acute fractures, the potential for thoracotomy pain, and the potential for pulmonary complications.

Seat Belt Injury

The initial report by Chance in 1948 described pure bony injury as a horizontal fracture through the upper half of the spinous process, parallel to disc spaces and extending anteriorly through the pedicles into the superior aspect of the vertebral body (114). Later, the seat belt has been appreciated as the fulcrum around which the fracture occurred due to flexion (22,24–27,39,40,52,57,115–121). This fracture type may be confused with a compression or burst component, and the posterior element disruption may easily be missed on initial evaluation

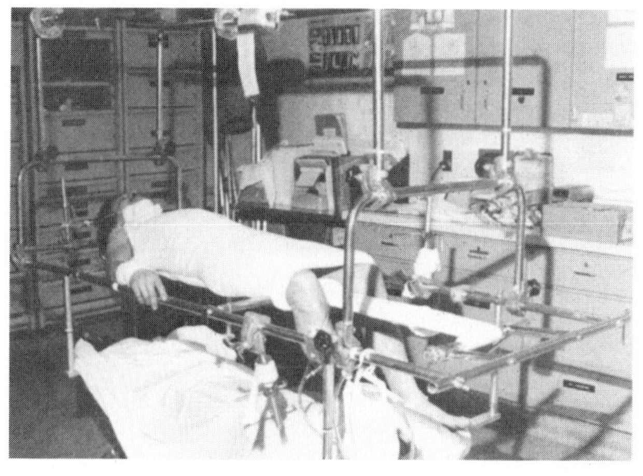

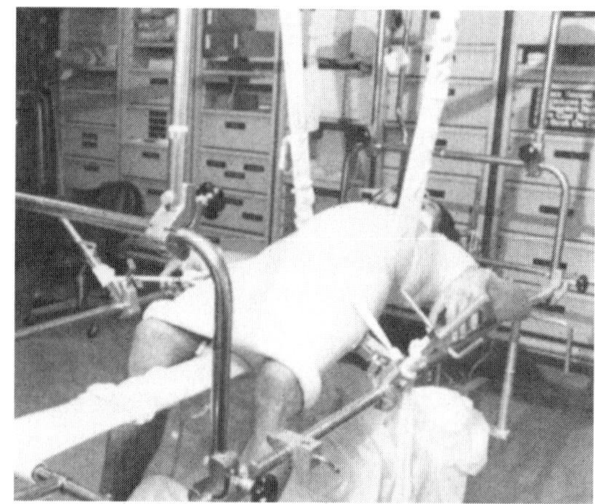

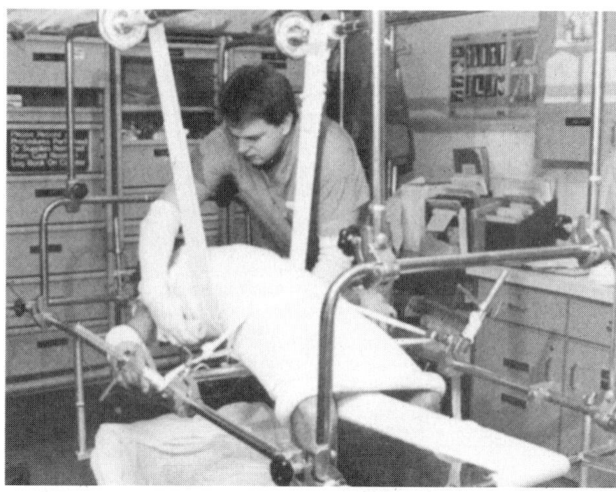

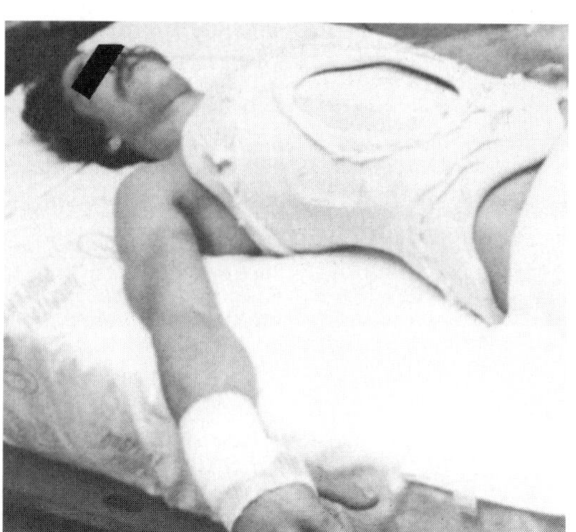

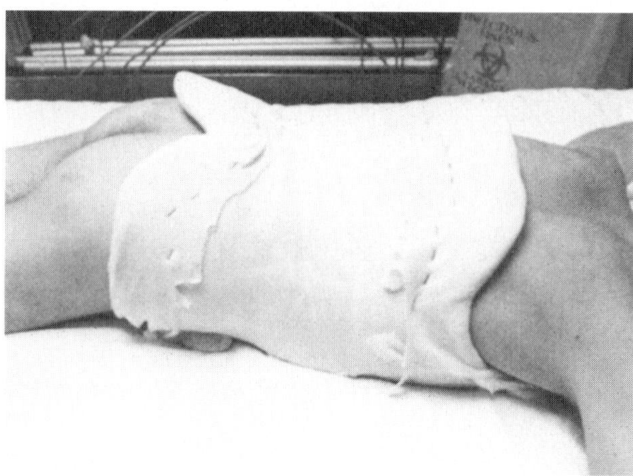

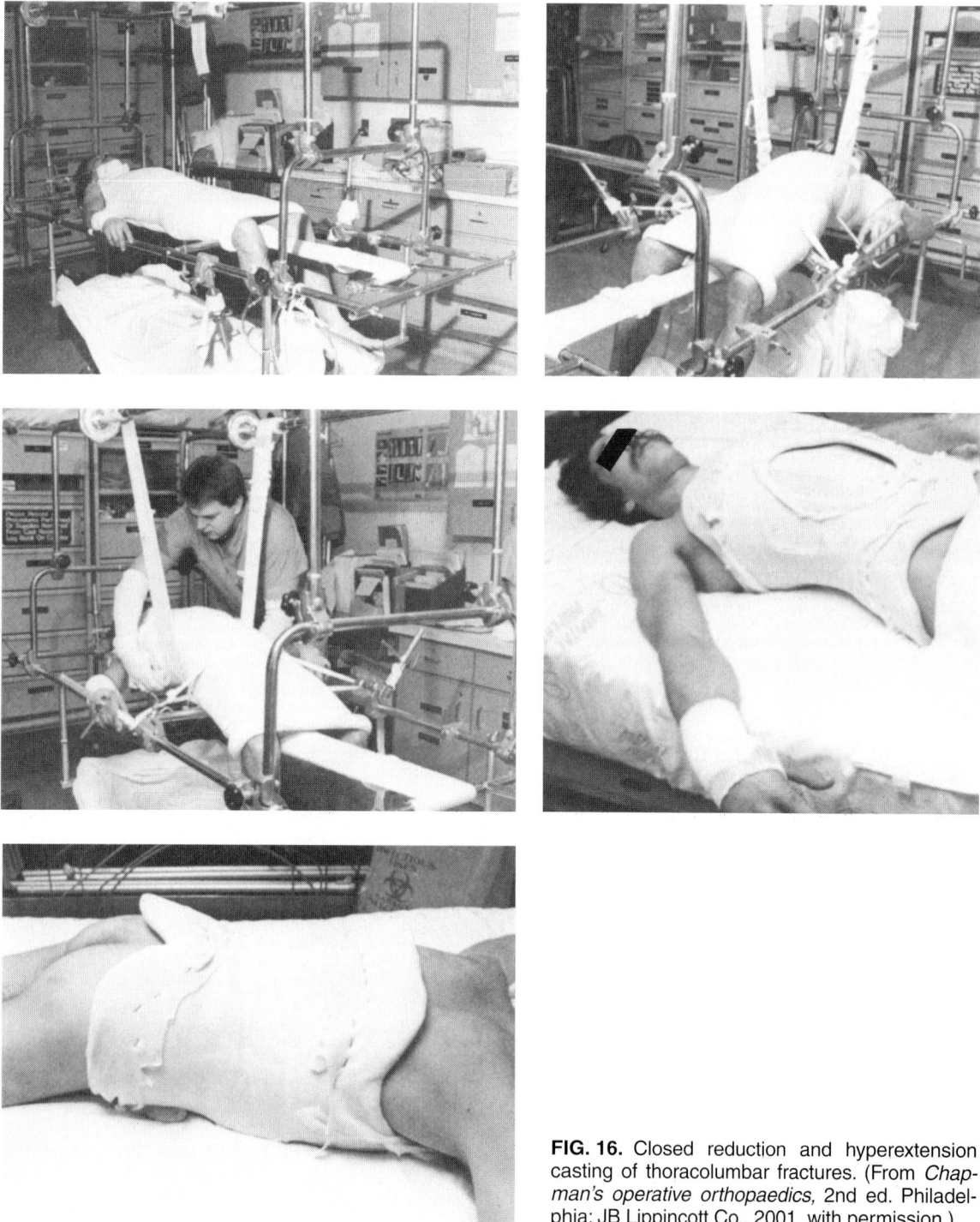

FIG. 16. Closed reduction and hyperextension casting of thoracolumbar fractures. (From *Chapman's operative orthopaedics,* 2nd ed. Philadelphia: JB Lippincott Co., 2001, with permission.)

(122). Radiographic criteria suggestive of a seat belt injury are widening of the spinous processes or the interlaminar space. In addition, subtle facet subluxation may be present. Thin 1-mm or 2-mm axial CT cuts may reveal the diagnosis, particularly if the "naked facet" sign is found (105). This occurs because the posterior distraction forces disrupted the interspinous ligaments, the facet capsules, and the ligamentum flavum. MRI demonstrates this injury clearly, revealing both bone and soft-tissue disruption.

Flexion-Distraction Injuries

Flexion-distraction injuries may occur through bone or soft tissue and may involve one or multiple motion segments (39,40,47,51,123). McAfee (104) classified these fractures as anterior compression and posterior distraction injuries with the middle column being the fulcrum. Two-column injuries may well be treated in a hyperextension cast, because bone heals reliably. Ligamentous injuries, however, do not heal reliably and

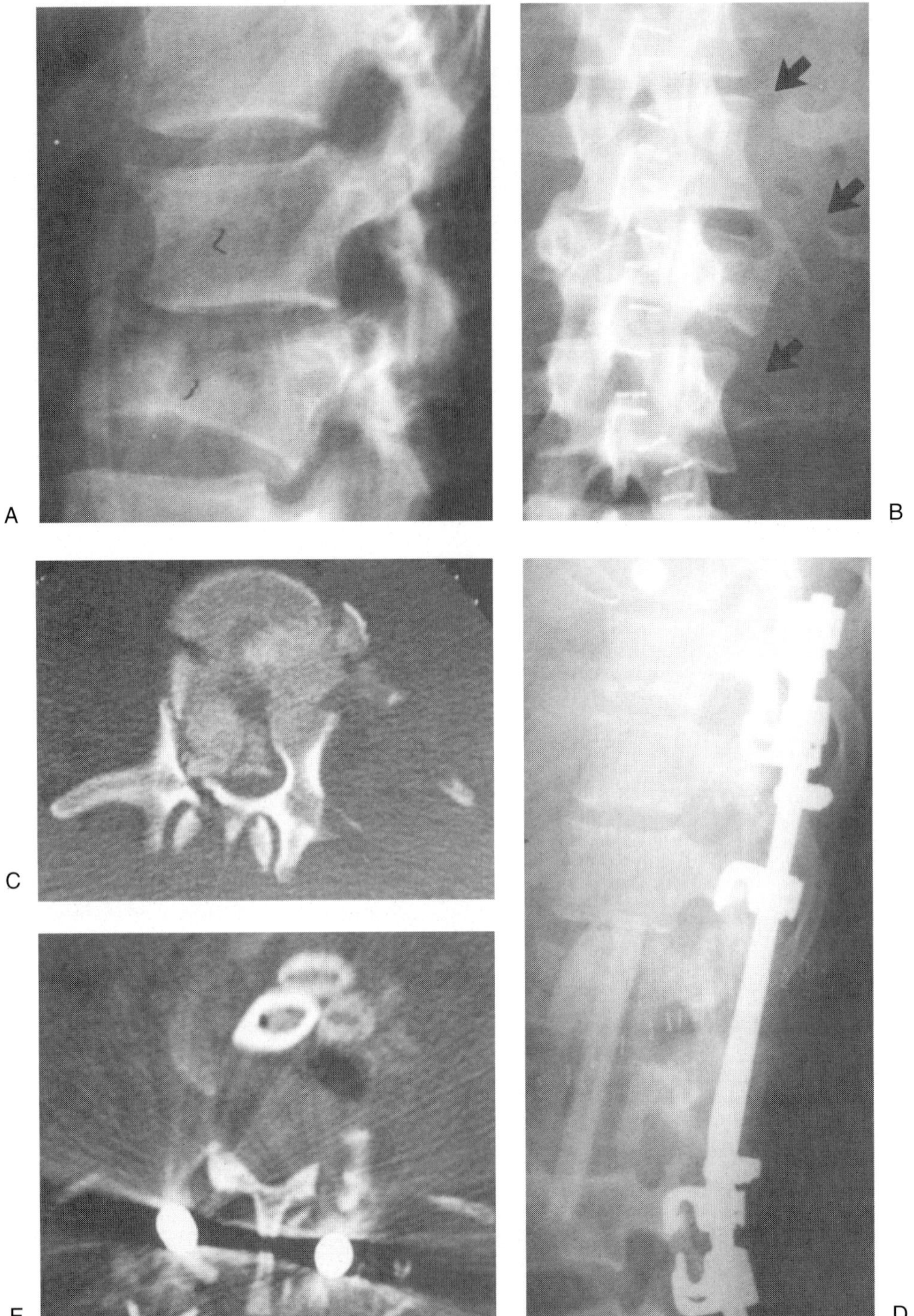

FIG. 17. Burst fracture—contiguous levels. An 18-year-old man, status post–motor vehicle accident, sustained L-2 and L-3 burst fractures with incomplete cauda equine injury. **A,B:** Lateral and anteroposterior radiographs. Multiple transverse process fractures suggest extent of soft-tissue trauma. **C:** Computed tomography (CT) of L-3 demonstrates greater than 80% canal compromise, laminar fractures, and extensive comminution. L-2 was less disrupted but unable to support an anterior strut. **D:** Lateral radiograph after L-2 partial and L-3 total vertebrectomy, followed by fibular autograft reconstruction. Construct was stopped at L-4 to spare the adjacent discs. At 4-year follow-up, the patient had normal neurologic function and minimal, intermittent back pain. **E:** Postoperative CT of patient after anterior decompression and reconstruction with autograft fibula and rib. The entire vertebral body has been removed from pedicle to pedicle, and all fragments have been removed from the canal. The patient had full neurologic recovery. (From *Chapman's operative orthopaedics,* 2nd ed. Philadelphia: JB Lippincott Co., 2001, with permission.)

more often result in residual instability and pain. Because these fractures may easily be confused with stable burst fractures, a careful evaluation of the radiographic studies should be done to rule out any posterior column disruption that could allow progressive kyphosis to occur. For this reason, this injury is best treated acutely with a short compression construct and posterior fusion to restore lordosis (Fig. 17). Patients with abdominal injuries who cannot tolerate a cast are also candidates for surgical treatment. Three-column flexion-distraction injuries are highly unstable. The risk of spinal cord injury is high, as is the frequency of intraabdominal injury, necessitating a more aggressive surgical approach. Pedicle instrumentation or extended segmental constructs are often needed to stabilize these fractures.

Fracture-Dislocations

Fracture-dislocations are the result of high-energy trauma (motor vehicle accidents and falls from height) and are typically associated with severe neurologic damage and multiple associated injuries (16,41,124). This translational shear injury represents a compromise of the neural canal with complete three-column ligamentous disruption due to combined shear, rotational, and hyperflexion forces. Complete spinal cord lesions do not improve with surgery, but mortality and morbidity are both reduced by early mobilization and rehabilitation. Cauda equina lesions are less predictable than thoracic lesions (some improvement may be seen), and restoration of spinal alignment is indicated to stabilize the spine and to decompress entrapped and compressed roots. This is best done with posterior reduction, instrumentation, and fusion. Depending on the fracture pattern, some fracture dislocations may regain anterior column load-bearing capacity once the dislocation is reduced. Anterior procedures may only be necessary for late reconstruction of kyphotic deformities.

INSTRUMENTATION OPTIONS

Because the decision to intervene surgically is usually predicated on the presence of spinal instability, instrumentation is almost always incorporated into the surgical plan. The type of instrumentation used depends on the injured level, the fracture pattern, the need for anterior stabilization or decompression, and the surgeon's level of experience and training.

Options for instrumentation include

Posterior instrumentation (Fig. 18)

- Nonsegmental rod/hook systems (Harrington rod) and hybrid systems (Luque; Harrington rod with sublaminar wires)
- Segmental systems
  - Rod/hook constructs
  - Extended pedicle screw constructs
  - Short-segment pedicle screw constructs
  - Compression instrumentation

Anterior instrumentation

- Anterior screw/plate or screw/rod instrumentation
- Anterior struts and vertebral body replacements

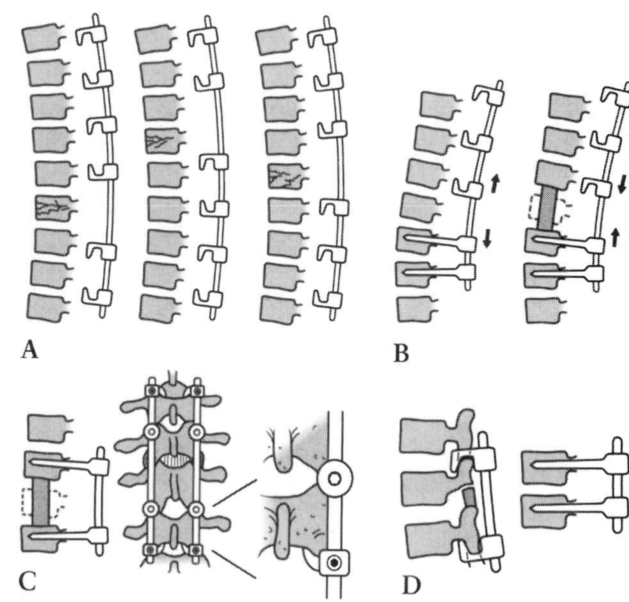

FIG. 18. Construct patterns for posterior instrumentation. Four basic construct patterns have been applied in thoracic, thoracolumbar, and lumbar fractures, with or without anterior reconstruction. **A:** Upper and lower hook patterns used primarily in the thoracic segments but sometimes in the thoracolumbar segments. These consist of claw configurations above and below the fractured level, with supplemental hooks applied as an additional claw above the fracture in lower thoracic fractures, below the fracture in upper thoracic fractures, and across the fracture in the midthoracic region. **B:** Extended pedicle screw patterns used at the thoracolumbar junction. Pedicle screws placed below the fractured level are supported by offset laminar hooks or additional screw fixation at the level below. Proximal fixation is provided by a claw construct carried to the lower thoracic segment. A supplemental hook is placed above the fracture, providing distraction against the lumbar screws when an indirect reduction is desired and compressing the anterior graft when a direct decompression has been performed. **C:** Short-segment pedicle instrumentation (SSPI) patterns used in thoracolumbar and lumbar fractures to limit fusion. Specifically designed constructs are available, or SSPI constructs can be designed from standard instrumentation sets. If the anterior column is unstable, protect posterior screws with an anterior strut or with offset hooks applied above and below the screws. **D:** Compression construct patterns. Flexion distraction injuries are generally treatable with a simple posterior compression construct. If a fracture dislocation has occurred, pedicle screw instrumentation may be required to combat translational and rotational displacements. (From *Chapman's operative orthopaedics,* 2nd ed. Philadelphia: JB Lippincott Co., 2001, with permission.)

Nonsegmental and Hybrid Constructs

Harrington rods can still play a role in fracture stabilization, primarily in the thoracic spine (Fig. 19). Applied properly, Harrington distraction rods can reduce angular deformity, restore vertebral body height, and provide adequate stiffness to allow early mobilization (75,125–127). Fixation is dependent on strong distraction

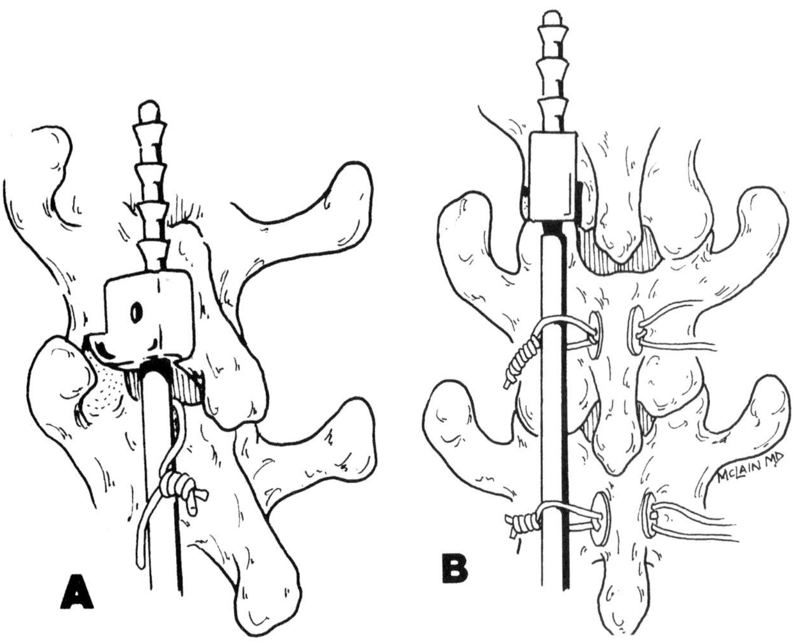

FIG. 19. Harrington rod fixation for thoracic fractures **(A)**. Harrington rods, supplemented with sublaminar wires and interspinous wires **(B)**, provide sufficient rigidity and allow surgeons to treat many thoracic level fractures and fracture dislocations. (From *Chapman's operative orthopaedics,* 2nd ed. Philadelphia: JB Lippincott Co., 2001, with permission.)

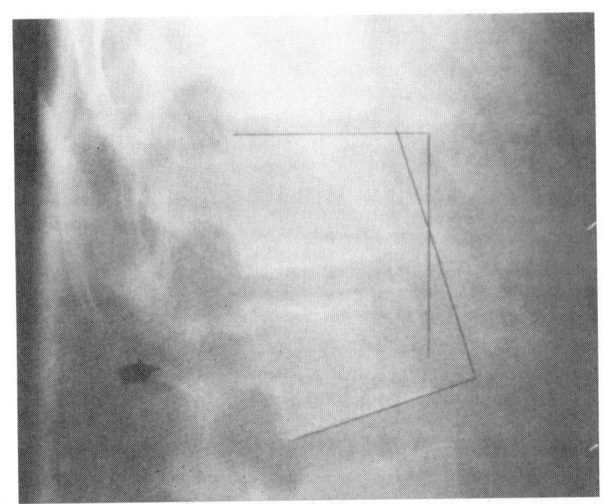

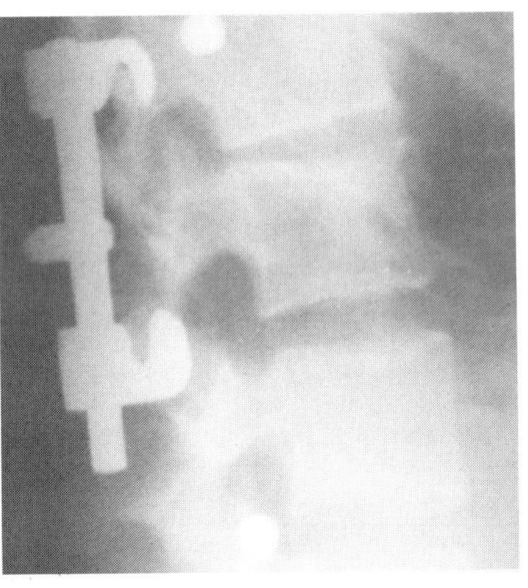

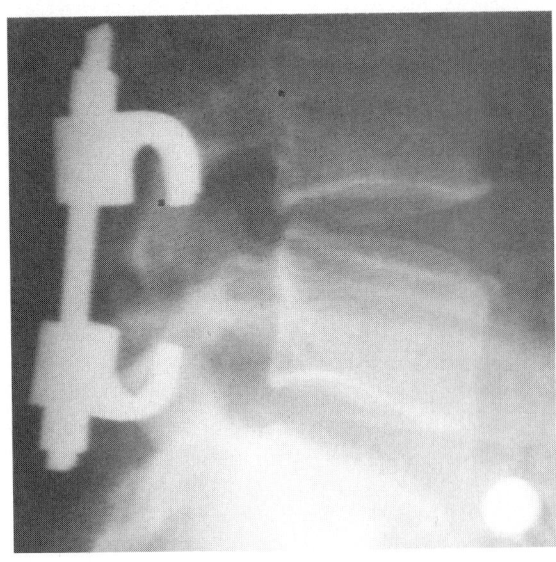

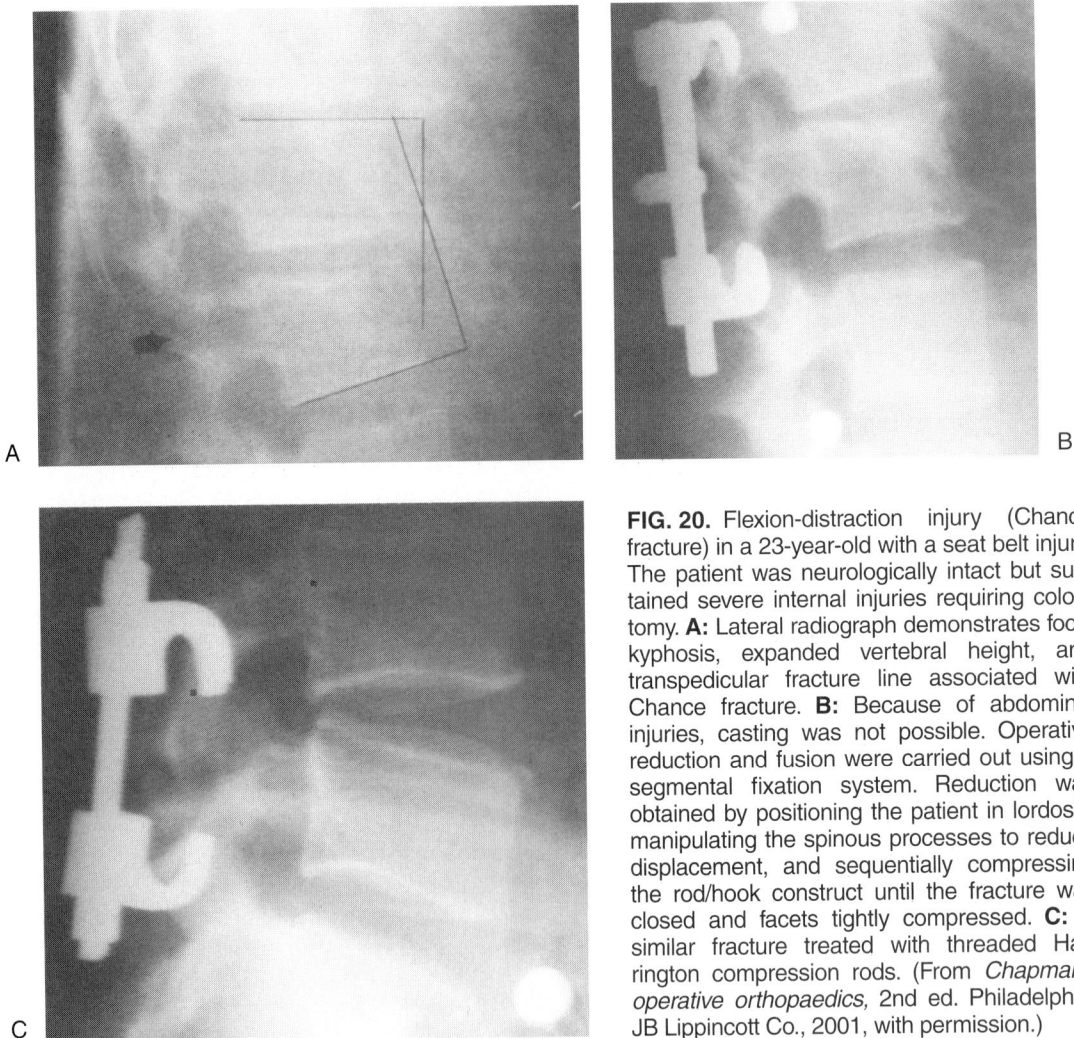

FIG. 20. Flexion-distraction injury (Chance fracture) in a 23-year-old with a seat belt injury. The patient was neurologically intact but sustained severe internal injuries requiring colostomy. **A:** Lateral radiograph demonstrates focal kyphosis, expanded vertebral height, and transpedicular fracture line associated with Chance fracture. **B:** Because of abdominal injuries, casting was not possible. Operative reduction and fusion were carried out using a segmental fixation system. Reduction was obtained by positioning the patient in lordosis, manipulating the spinous processes to reduce displacement, and sequentially compressing the rod/hook construct until the fracture was closed and facets tightly compressed. **C:** A similar fracture treated with threaded Harrington compression rods. (From *Chapman's operative orthopaedics,* 2nd ed. Philadelphia: JB Lippincott Co., 2001, with permission.)

forces between the superior and inferior hooks, however, and constructs must span a number of vertebrae to provide optimal corrective forces. Constructs that span three levels above and two below the injury are biomechanically superior to shorter constructs. Three-column spinal injuries cannot resist the distraction forces of the Harrington rod, however, and rods placed in these injuries will overdistract the spinal column or will not be firmly fixed.

Because there are only two points of fixation on each rod, forces tend to concentrate at those points, and lamina fracture or hook dislodgement is frequent, leading to complete loss of fixation (12,128,129). Harrington rods also break in 7 to 10% of cases, usually at the junction of the ratchet and the main rod body (130).

Sublaminar or spinous process wires significantly improve fixation of rod constructs and limit the risk of hook displacement (131). Spinous process wires are less likely to pull sublaminar hooks into the canal, but well-fitted hooks are unlikely to displace with either technique (Fig. 20). These constructs are best suited to fractures of the midthoracic spine, where extended fusions are relatively well tolerated. Although the addition of sublaminar segmental wires has improved the sagittal and torsional stiffness of Harrington constructs, it has not eliminated rod breakage (132–136). Luque instrumentation may prove useful in some thoracic fractures but does not provide sufficient axial stability to treat burst fractures.

Segmental Spinal Instrumentation

Segmental spinal instrumentation (SSI) has improved treatment results for a variety of spinal disorders (Fig. 21). Originally intended for scoliosis patients, segmental hook and rod systems have now been used to successfully treat trauma, infections, tumors, and degenerative disorders (17,137,138). Clinical series have documented the efficacy and technical demands of segmental systems in scoliosis, kyphosis, and congenital deformities, and have provided the clinician with enough information to develop rational and reliable treatment plans for trauma patients.

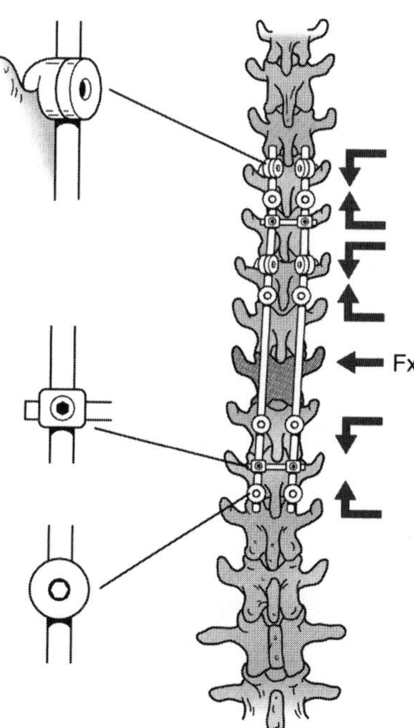

FIG. 21. Segmental fixation allows the surgeon to neutralize the overall length of the spinal segment, preventing distraction, and segmentally distract within the construct to either decompress the fracture or to compress an anterior graft. (From *Chapman's operative orthopaedics,* 2nd ed. Philadelphia: JB Lippincott Co., 2001, with permission.)

SSI is being used with increasing frequency for thoracic and thoracolumbar spine fractures, but only a handful of clinical studies have been published to support this application (13,52,139). McBride reported good results in thoracic and thoracolumbar fractures treated with longer hook and rod constructs, and SSI constructs have been endorsed for treatment of lumbar fractures (7,11,13,14). However, enthusiasm for SSI has been tempered somewhat by recent studies identifying a high rate of screw failure in unstable fractures (15,140–142).

Segmental rod/hook constructs take advantage of three-point bending mechanics to reduce and maintain thoracic kyphosis and prevent translation of disrupted vertebral segments. The success of this strategy has been documented in nonsegmental systems (Harrington rods), and a number of construct patterns have been presented for segmental systems (13,14,120). Although they use the same basic reduction strategy as the Harrington rod, segmental rod/hook systems offer several unique advantage over first-generation instrumentation systems (13,14,120,143,144).

Pedicle Screw Fixation

Pedicle screws allow the surgeon to directly instrument vertebrae with absent or fractured laminae. They provide three-column fixation in unstable injuries and limit the length of fusion in the lumbar spine (145). Pedicle screws may be used exclusively or in combination with hook constructs to address a wide variety of fracture patterns. Combined (or "extended") constructs are particularly useful at the thoracolumbar junction. Here, the thoracic spine is relatively immobile and has little functional consequence in fusion. Extending the construct into these segments incurs little mechanical cost and provides more extensive fixation. This improved proximal fixation allows the surgeon to apply enough corrective force to restore sagittal alignment—an imperative at the thoracolumbar junction (Fig. 22). Pedicle screws are then applied in the upper lumbar segment to limit the length of the construct, minimizing interference with lumbar motion segments. Extending fusion into the lower lumbar spine does alter mechanics and predisposes patients to junctional pain and subsequent motion segment degeneration.

The extended construct may incorporate an intermediate hook applied just above the fracture and just below the upper claw, directed cranially or caudally, depending on the situation. In most constructs, a narrow-width hook is placed up-going under the lamina of the vertebra two levels above the fracture. With the upper and lower fixation points locked in place to neutralize the construct length, this hook allows segmental distraction of the fracture to improve vertebral height and decompress the spinal canal indirectly, without overdistracting the spine. In combined anterior-posterior reconstructions, this additional

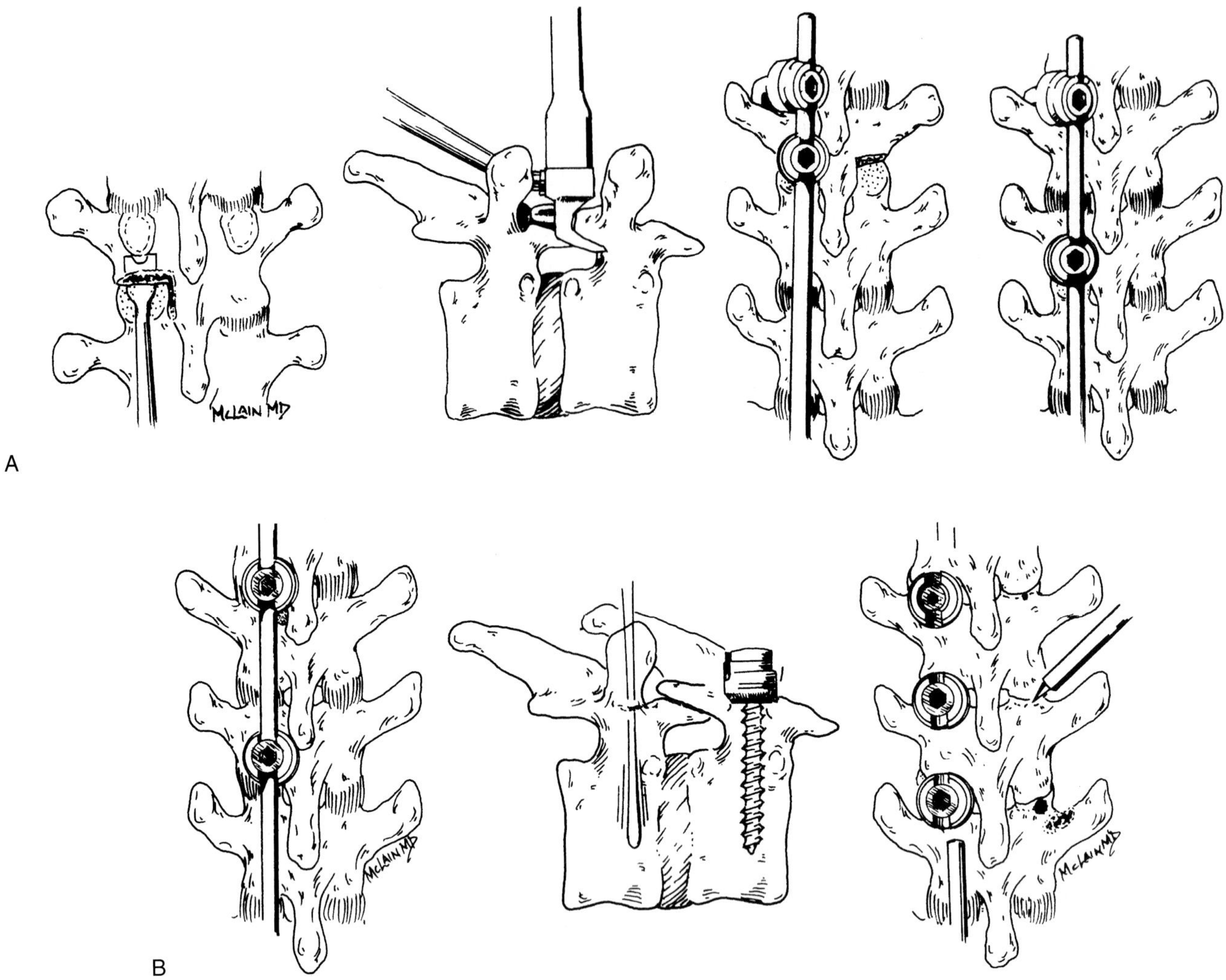

FIG. 22. Proximal fixation patterns. **A:** Proximal transversopedicular claw constructs mirror those applied in adult deformities. **B:** In osteoporotic bone, or when the transverse process has been broken, a lamino-laminar claw can be substituted. (From *Chapman's operative orthopaedics,* 2nd ed. Philadelphia: JB Lippincott Co., 2001, with permission.)

hook may be directed downward to compress and capture the anterior strut graft.

Short-segment constructs allow rigid fixation of short segments of the lumbar spine and provide sagittal, axial, and torsional stability superior to rod/hook constructs or sublaminar wiring (145,146). Fixation is not dependent on intact lamina, so there is no need to extend the fusion in patients with laminar fracture or who require a laminectomy. Because distraction is unnecessary to correct the axial deformity, the risk of overdistracting the disrupted segment or producing a flatback syndrome is lessened. Both the surgical and mechanical disturbances to the adjacent lumbar segments are minimized. Nevertheless, SSI is limited in its ability to maintain sagittal correction in severe burst fractures (11,15,142). If the anterior and middle spinal columns cannot share axial loads, the bending movements generated at the pedicle screw hub result in a high rate of instrument bending failure or fracture. Once initial bending has occurred, progressive collapse is more likely, accompanied by progressive loss of lordosis in some patients. The choice of the anterior or posterior approach for short-segment instrumentation has also been based on grading comminution by use of the load-sharing classification published in 1994 by McCormack et al. (45,147).

Anterior Bone Grafts, Cages, Plates, and Screws

Corpectomy reconstruction options must provide support to the anterior and middle columns. Options include autogenous bone graft, long-bone allograft in conjunction with anterior plates and screws, and titanium or carbon fiber mesh cages. Autologous bone graft options include iliac crest, fibula, or rib. All of these have problems with donor site morbidity and nonoptimum shape for reconstruction. The narrow shape of the rib and fibula make these constructs more prone to subside through the adjacent end-plates. Despite these limitations, one large series

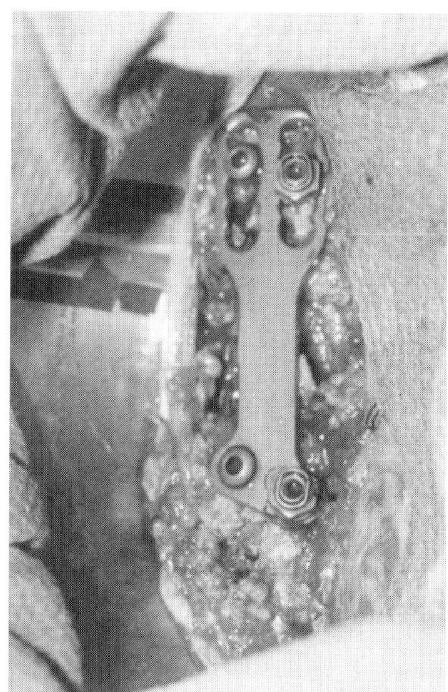

FIG. 23. Anterior instrumentation for burst fracture treatment. (From *Chapman's operative orthopaedics,* 2nd ed. Philadelphia: JB Lippincott Co., 2001, with permission.)

reported autologous strut grafting to be a safe and reliable option after anterior decompression (148).

A number of anterior fixation systems have been developed over the past 10 years, based on the principle of anterolateral screw fixation coupled with longitudinal plates or rods (Fig. 23). These devices can span multiple segments and can be applied from the midthoracic region down to the L-5 vertebral body. They are intended to augment anterior column reconstruction, providing torsional and translational stability while sharing axial loads with a strut graft or cage. When posterior soft tissues and structures are intact, an anterior reconstruction and instrumentation may be adequate to stabilize the spine. If the posterior elements are disrupted, however, the anterior construct is more likely to fail unless posterior instrumentation is performed to restore that tension band.

Long-bone allograft segments, packed with autograft, are a useful alternative to segmental autograft harvested from the iliac crest or fibula (149). Alternatively, titanium mesh cages have provided biomechanical support for the anterior column, along with cancellous autograft packed into the center of the cage. This attractive option allows easy contouring of the cage to fit the corpectomy site and the use of the cancellous bone resected from the fracture site, with no graft site morbidity. The cylindrical cages fit around the strong peripheral rim of the vertebral

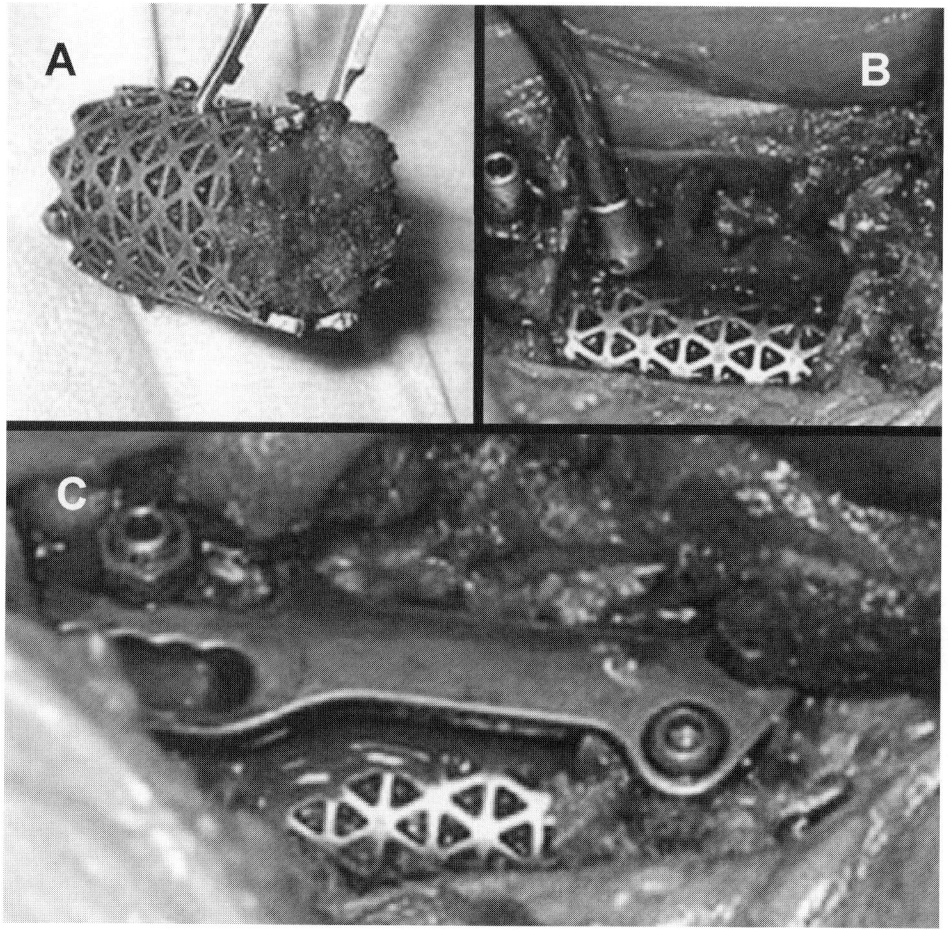

FIG. 24. A: Titanium mesh cage packed with autogenous cancellous bone that can be resected from the fracture site. **B:** The cage was placed at the corpectomy site. Bolts for the lateral stabilizing plate are *in situ* at the vertebra above and below. **C:** The cage was secured with lateral plate.

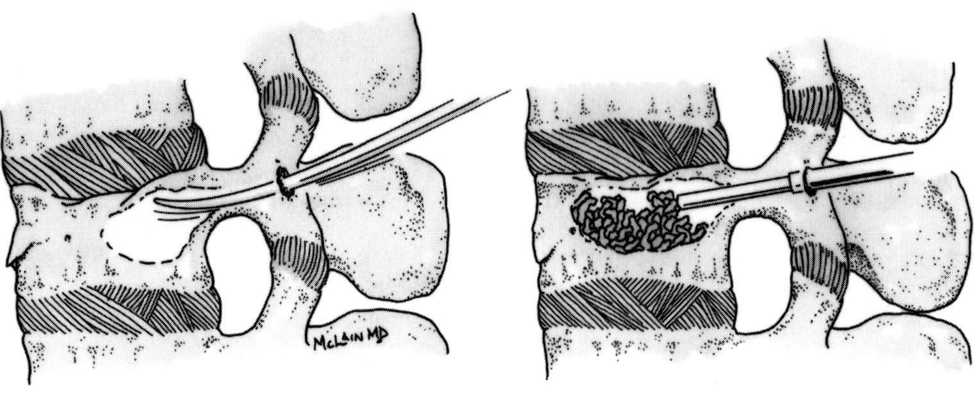

FIG. 25. Transpedicular bone graft. Anterior instrumentation for burst fracture treatment.

body end-plate, and because of their shape, they are resistant to translation or toggle (150).

Titanium cages appear a reliable option for corpectomy reconstruction. Kyphosis can be reliably corrected when necessary, and any significant kyphosis recurrence or implant settling into adjacent vertebrae is usually minimal. Once cages have been placed, a lateral stabilizing plate or a screw and double rod system provides additional stability (Fig. 24). These devices are placed with screws, achieving bicortical fixation and sparing the discs above and below the proximal and distal vertebrae. Such constructs minimize the reconstruction length and the length of the fused segment.

SPECIFIC POINTS ON SURGICAL TECHNIQUES

Instrumentation provides little benefit unless the spinal alignment is corrected at the time of fixation. Failure to correct sagittal alignment results in a fixed kyphotic deformity, predisposing the patient to dysfunction, pain, and instrumentation failure and often necessitating late revision and reconstruction. Failure to correct translational deformity results in a residual stenosis at the level of offset and may predispose the patient to nonunion and treatment failure.

Postural Reduction of Fracture

The residual deformity in compression, burst, and many dislocation injuries is kyphosis. If this deformity is allowed to persist, it will become fixed and irreducible, whereas immediately after fracture, fragments are typically mobile and amenable to indirect reduction.

Fractures at the thoracolumbar junction are most problematic for the following reasons: (a) The injured segments are junctional between the rigid thoracic spine and the well-supported lumbosacral vertebrae; (b) the neural elements at risk include the conus medullaris and entire cauda equina; and (c) residual deformity is poorly tolerated, and mechanical imbalance predisposes the patient to pain and construct failure.

Open Reduction of Fracture

To complete reduction of a burst fracture, it may be necessary to manipulate the spine intraoperatively. *In situ* contouring of the implants may be performed to restore lordosis to segments that are not completely restored passively. For this purpose, one may carefully contour standard rod and screw or plate constructs *in situ* to restore sagittal balance or contour the rod before placement and then insert and rotate into sagittal orientation to increase lordosis. Care must be taken not to overpower and damage the implants. Supplement pedicle screws by offset laminar hooks before attempting vigorous contouring. Implants designed specifically for fracture reduction are available; they are designed to neutralize and correct spinal column length and at the same time allow manipulation to correct sagittal collapse (11,151–153).

Transpedicular Bone Graft

Another option for reduction of vertebral collapse is transpedicular bone grafting directly through a posterolateral approach. Using this method, the surgeon elevates the depressed end-plate through a transpedicular approach and reinforces the fracture site with a transpedicular bone graft (Fig. 25). Irreducible facet dislocations may require an operative reduction to restore align-

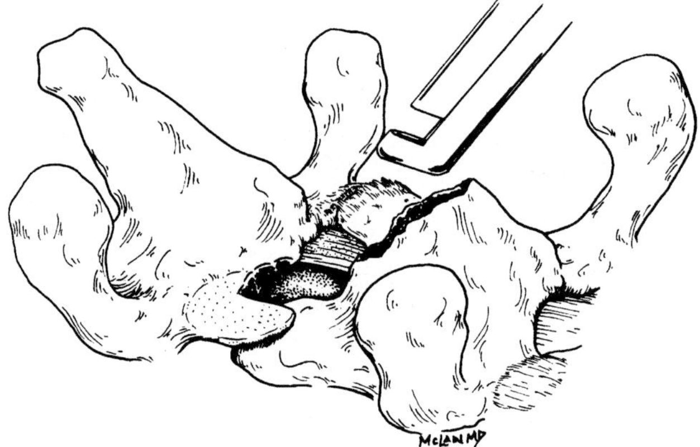

FIG. 26. Reduction of fracture-dislocation. When simple distraction cannot easily reduce a dislocated facet in a neurologically intact patient, resection of the overlapping articulation with a Kerrison rongeur or burr allows gentle reduction. (From *Chapman's operative orthopaedics,* 2nd ed. Philadelphia: JB Lippincott Co., 2001, with permission.)

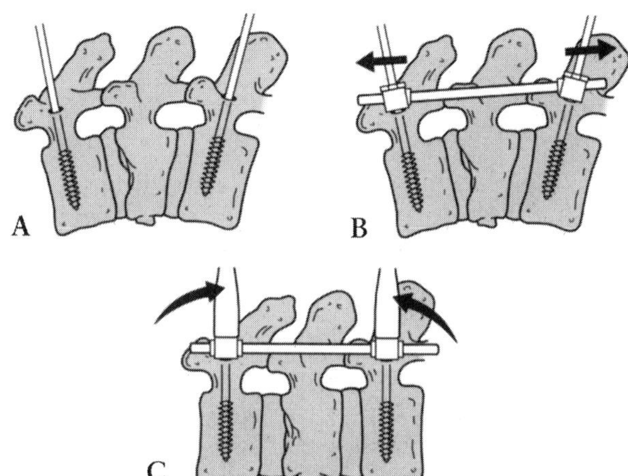

FIG. 27. A–C: Short-segment pedicle instrumentation. (From *Chapman's operative orthopaedics,* 2nd ed. Philadelphia: JB Lippincott Co., 2001, with permission.)

ment. Fracture dislocations are usually easily reduced because the soft tissues are completely disrupted. If part of the facet capsule or posterior longitudinal ligament is intact, manual reduction is more difficult. In such a case, in a neurologically intact patient, a burr is used to take down the locked facet, which allows a gentle reduction without overdistracting the spine (Fig. 26).

Fusion Technique

Because segmental instrumentation allows the surgeon to instrument only those segments intended for fusion, it is routine to fuse all instrumented segments. Long rod and short fusion constructs have been only marginally successful at protecting lumbar segments in fracture patients, and newer systems allow surgeons to avoid instrumenting the lower lumbar spine altogether (132). This technique eliminates the need for a second surgery to remove the hardware and avoids concerns about degenerative changes seen in immobilized, unfused facet joints (92,154).

Anterior reconstruction is often warranted in addition to posterior fusion if the anterior and middle columns cannot withstand axial loads. If the anterior column is not restored, a large bending movement is generated in the pedicle screw hub, resulting in a high rate of instrument bending failure. Acute bending failure occurs before a solid arthrodesis has been achieved and before anterior column structures have regained enough strength to share compressive loads. Failure during this period allows progressive collapse of the fractured segment, with progressive kyphosis and clinical symptoms. Ebelke et al. found transpedicular bone grafting eliminated pedicle screw failure in their series (see Transpedicular Bone Graft), and similarly, patients with an intact or restored anterior column do not experience screw-bending failure (15,155).

If care is taken to protect pedicle screws in patients with anterior column instability, short-segment pedicle instrumentation (SSPI) is still an ideal approach for selected patients (Figs. 27 and 28). If the anterior column is intact, screws alone provide reliable rigid fixation. The SSPI construct limits fixation to the fewest possible motion segments and is ideal for lumbar spine fractures where larger screws can be safely placed. *In situ* contouring of the rod should not be attempted unless offset laminar hooks are applied to supplement screw fixation. These hooks provide improved clinical results (140,144) and have been shown to improve construct stiffness and to reduce screw bending

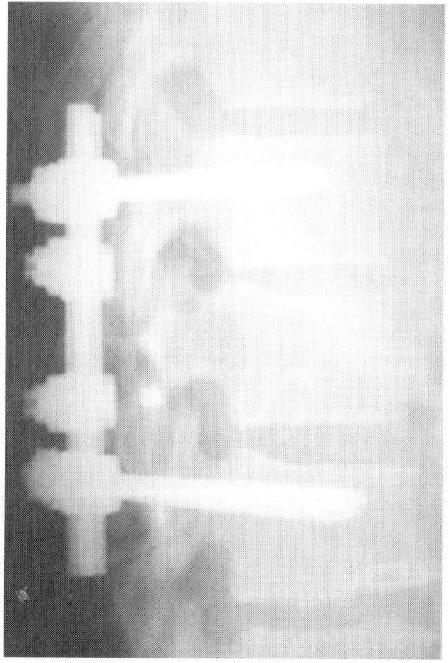

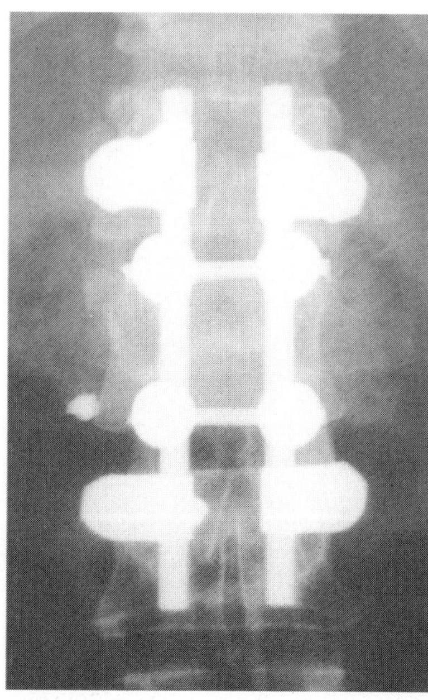

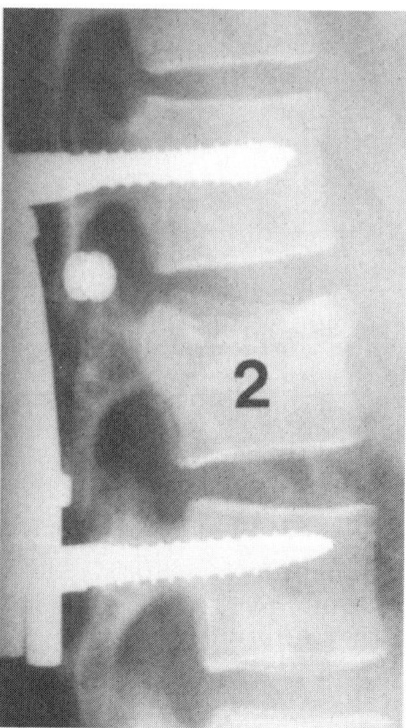

A–C

FIG. 28. Short-segment pedicle instrumentation. **A,B:** Lateral and anteroposterior views of a 38-year-old patient with an L-1 burst fracture and marked sagittal collapse. Synthes Universal System fracture module was applied to correct kyphosis and anterior vertebral collapse. **C:** Similar fracture pattern treated with Cotrel-Dubousset segmental instrumentation. Because anterior column disruption was not severe, offset hooks were not applied. (From *Chapman's operative orthopaedics,* 2nd ed. Philadelphia: JB Lippincott Co., 2001, with permission.)

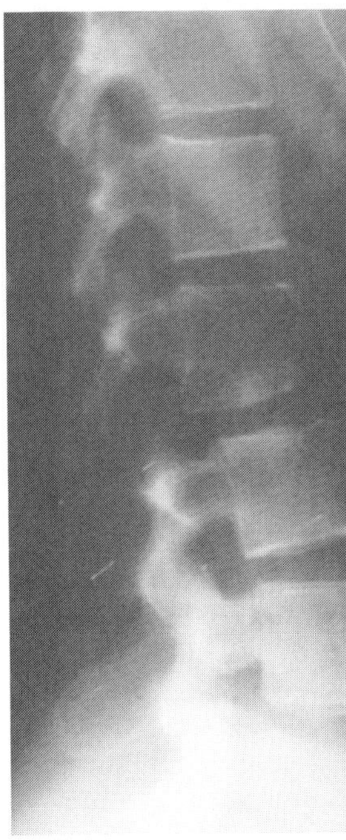
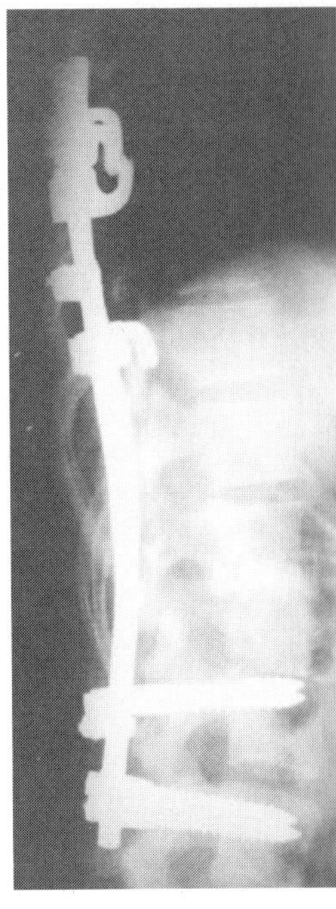
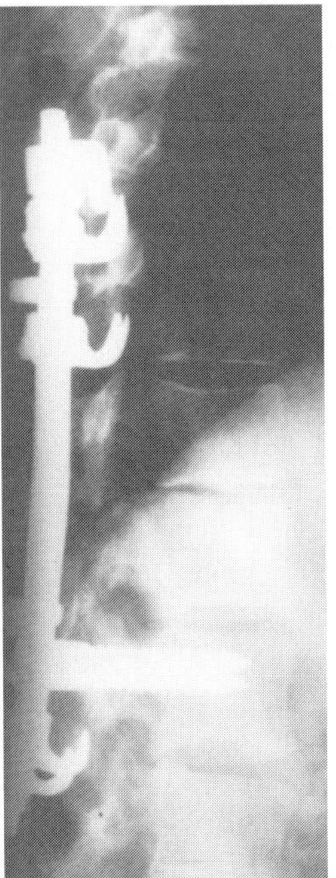

A–C

FIG. 29. Extended pedicle screw constructs. **A:** Lateral view of an 18-year-old patient with L1-2 fracture-dislocation and incomplete cauda equina syndrome. **B:** Extended construct using pedicle screws at L-2 and L-3 to stabilize the spinal column, with a down-going supplemental hook to compress the anterior strut graft. **C:** Extended pattern using supplemental offset hooks to protect pedicle screws. Intermediate hooks are directed cranially to decompress the fracture site indirectly. (From *Chapman's operative orthopaedics,* 2nd ed. Philadelphia: JB Lippincott Co., 2001, with permission.)

moments significantly both in sagittal loading and during *in situ* contouring (18,156). Extended pedicle screw constructs are intended to address thoracolumbar fractures by extending proximal fixation into the thoracic segments with as little alteration of lumbar spinal mechanics as possible (Fig. 29).

The weak link in the extended construct, as in the short-segment construct, is the pedicle screw itself. Unless they are supplemented with an offset laminar hook, additional levels of fixation, or an anterior reconstruction, the pedicle screws are exposed to large cantilever bending loads (48,157). These forces are concentrated just distal to the screw hub, a natural stress riser, and the contact point between the screw and the lamina at the midpoint of the pedicle itself (15,156,158,159). Bending failure that occurs before the fracture has consolidated results in progressive material failure and sagittal collapse and can occur even in braced patients (7,112,160). Screw breakage that occurs after healing is complete is often asymptomatic (161). Patients treated with supplemental offset hooks or with an anterior reconstruction rarely develop segmental collapse.

REFERENCES

1. Aebi M, Etter C, Kehl T, et al. The internal skeletal fixation system. A new treatment of thoracolumbar fractures and other spinal disorders. *Clin Orthop* 1988;227:30–43.
2. Bernard TN Jr, Whitecloud TS III, Rodriguez RP, et al. Segmental spinal instrumentation in the management of fractures of the thoracic and lumbar spine. *South Med J* 1983;76:1232–1236.
3. Bohlman HH, Freehafer A, Dejak J. The results of treatment of acute injuries of the upper thoracic spine with paralysis. *J Bone Joint Surg* 1985;67:360–369.
4. Bosch A, Stauffer ES, Nickel VL. Incomplete traumatic quadriplegia. A ten-year review. *JAMA* 1971;216:473–478.
5. Bradford DS, Thompson RC. Fractures and dislocations of the spine. Indications for surgical intervention. *Minn Med* 1976;59: 711–720.
6. Bohlman HH. Treatment of fractures and dislocations of the thoracic and lumbar spine. *J Bone Joint Surg* 1985;67:165–169.
7. Carl AL, Tromanhauser SG, Roger DJ. Pedicle screw instrumentation for thoracolumbar burst fractures and fracture-dislocations. *Spine* 1992;17:S317–S324.
8. McLain RF, Benson DR, Burkus JK. Segmental instrumentation for thoracic and thoracolumbar fractures: prospective analysis of construct survival and five-year follow-up. *Spine J* 2001;1:310–323.
9. Wenger DR, Carollo JJ. The mechanics of thoracolumbar fractures stabilized by segmental fixation. *Clin Orthop* 1984;89–96.
10. Bone L. Management of polytrauma. *Chapman's operative orthopaedics,* 2nd ed. Philadelphia: JB Lippincott Co., 1993:299.
11. Benson DR, Burkus JK, Montesano PX, et al. Unstable thoracolumbar and lumbar burst fractures treated with the AO Fixateur Interne. *J Spinal Disord* 1992;5:335–343.
12. Dickson JH, Harrington PR, Erwin WD. Results of reduction and stabilization of the severely fractured thoracic and lumbar spine. *J Bone Joint Surg* 1978;60:799–805.
13. McBride GG. Cotrel-Dubousset rods in spinal fractures. *Paraplegia* 1989;27:440–449.
14. McBride GG. Cotrel-Dubousset rods in surgical stabilization of spinal fractures. *Spine* 1993;18:466–473.
15. McLain RF, Sparling E, Benson DR. Early failure of short-segment pedicle instrumentation for thoracolumbar fractures. A preliminary report. *J Bone Joint Surg* 1993;75:162–167.
16. Place HM, Donaldson DH, Brown CW, et al. Stabilization of thoracic spine fractures resulting in complete paraplegia. A long-term retrospective analysis. *Spine* 1994;19:1726–1730.
17. Saboe LA, Reid DC, Davis LA, et al. Spine trauma and associated injuries. *J Trauma* 1991;31:43–48.
18. Tasdemiroglu E, Tibbs PA. Long-term follow-up results of thoracolumbar fractures after posterior instrumentation. *Spine* 1995;20:1704–1708.
19. Dennis LN, Rogers LF. Superior mediastinal widening from spine fractures mimicking aortic rupture on chest radiographs. *AJR Am J Roentgenol* 1989;152:27–30.
20. Woodring JH, Dillon ML. Radiographic manifestations of mediastinal hemorrhage from blunt chest trauma. *Ann Thorac Surg* 1984;37:171–178.
21. Woodring JH, Lee C, Jenkins K. Spinal fractures in blunt chest trauma. *J Trauma* 1988;28:789–793.
22. Gumley G, Taylor TK, Ryan MD. Distraction fractures of the lumbar spine. *J Bone Joint Surg* 1982;64:520–525.
23. Inaba K, Kirkpatrick AW, Finkelstein J, et al. Blunt abdominal aortic trauma in association with thoracolumbar spine fractures. *Injury* 2001;32:201–207.

24. Ritchie WP Jr, Ersek RA, Bunch WL, et al. Combined visceral and vertebral injuries from lap type seat belts. *Surg Gynecol Obstet* 1970;131:431–435.
25. Snyder CJ. Bowel injuries from automobile seat belts. *Am J Surg* 1972;123:312–316.
26. Stevenson JH. Severe thoracic intra-abdominal and vertebral injury occurring in combination in a patient wearing a seat belt. *Injury* 1979;10:321–323.
27. Zacheis HG, Condon RE. Seat belts and intra-abdominal trauma: report of two unusual cases. *J Trauma* 1972;12:85–90.
28. Brown BM, Brant-Zawadzki M, Cann CE. Dynamic CT scanning of spinal column trauma. *AJR Am J Roentgenol* 1982;139:1177–1181.
29. Daffner RH, Daffner SD. Vertebral injuries: detection and implications. *Eur J Radiol* 2002;42:100–116.
30. Dalinka MK, Boorstein JM, Zlatkin MB. Computed tomography of musculoskeletal trauma. *Radiol Clin North Am* 1989;27:933–944.
31. Moll R, Schindler G, Weckbach A. [Evaluation of ventral stabilization techniques for thoracolumbar fractures by helical computer tomography]. *Rofo Fortschr Geb Rontgenstr Neuen Bildgeb Verfahr* 2002;174:880–886.
32. Post MJ, Green BA, Quencer RM, et al. The value of computed tomography in spinal trauma. *Spine* 1982;7:417–431.
33. Trafton PG, Boyd CA Jr. Computed tomography of thoracic and lumbar spine injuries. *J Trauma* 1984;24:506–515.
34. McLain RF, Benson DR. Missed cervical dissociation—recognizing and avoiding potential disaster. *J Emerg Med* 1998;16:179–183.
35. Reid DC, Henderson R, Saboe L, et al. Etiology and clinical course of missed spine fractures. *J Trauma* 1987;27:980–986.
36. Vandemark RM. Radiology of the cervical spine in trauma patients: practice pitfalls and recommendations for improving efficiency and communication. *AJR Am J Roentgenol* 1990;155:465–472.
37. Holdsworth F. Fractures, dislocations, and fracture-dislocations of the spine. *J Bone Joint Surg* 1970;52:1534–1551.
38. Holdsworth FW. Diagnosis and treatment of fractures of the spine. *Manit Med Rev* 1968;48:13–15.
39. Denis F. The three-column spine and its significance in the classification of acute thoracolumbar spinal injuries. *Spine* 1983;8:817–831.
40. Denis F. Spinal instability as defined by the three-column spine concept in acute spinal trauma. *Clin Orthop* 1984;65–76.
41. Panjabi MM, Oxland TR, Kifune M, et al. Validity of the three-column theory of thoracolumbar fractures. A biomechanic investigation. *Spine* 1995;20:1122–1127.
42. Denis F, Armstrong GW, Searls K, et al. Acute thoracolumbar burst fractures in the absence of neurologic deficit. A comparison between operative and nonoperative treatment. *Clin Orthop* 1984;142–149.
43. Sasso RC, Jeanneret B, Fischer K, et al. Occipitocervical fusion with posterior plate and screw instrumentation. A long-term follow-up study. *Spine* 1994;19:2364–2368.
44. Leibl T, Funke M, Dresing K, et al. [Instability of spinal fractures—therapeutic relevance of different classifications]. *Rofo Fortschr Geb Rontgenstr Neuen Bildgeb Verfahr* 1999;170:174–180.
45. McCormack T, Karaikovic E, Gaines RW. The load sharing classification of spine fractures. *Spine* 1994;19:1741–1744.
46. Oner FC, van Gils AP, Dhert WJ, et al. MRI findings of thoracolumbar spine fractures: a categorisation based on MRI examinations of 100 fractures. *Skeletal Radiol* 1999;28:433–443.
47. Slosar PJ Jr, Patwardhan AG, Lorenz M, et al. Instability of the lumbar burst fracture and limitations of transpedicular instrumentation. *Spine* 1995;20:1452–1461.
48. Shuman WP, Rogers JV, Sickler ME, et al. Thoracolumbar burst fractures: CT dimensions of the spinal canal relative to postsurgical improvement. *AJR Am J Roentgenol* 1985;145:337–341.
49. Guerra J Jr, Garfin SR, Resnick D. Vertebral burst fractures: CT analysis of the retropulsed fragment. *Radiology* 1984;153:769–772.
50. Finn CA, Stauffer ES. Burst fracture of the fifth lumbar vertebra. *J Bone Joint Surg* 1992;74:398–403.
51. Gertzbein SD, Court-Brown CM. Rationale for the management of flexion-distraction injuries of the thoracolumbar spine based on a new classification. *J Spinal Disord* 1989;2:176–183.
52. Smith WS, Kaufer H. Patterns and mechanisms of lumbar injuries associated with lap seat belts. *J Bone Joint Surg* 1969;51:239–254.
53. Bracken MB, Shepard MJ, Collins WF, et al. A randomized, controlled trial of methylprednisolone or naloxone in the treatment of acute spinal-cord injury. Results of the Second National Acute Spinal Cord Injury Study. *N Engl J Med* 1990;322:1405–1411.
54. Ducker TB. Treatment of spinal-cord injury. *N Engl J Med* 1990; 322:1459–1461.
55. Ball ST, Vaccaro AR, Albert TJ, et al. Injuries of the thoracolumbar spine associated with restraint use in head-on motor vehicle accidents. *J Spinal Disord* 2000;13:297–304.
56. Keene JS. Radiographic evaluation of thoracolumbar fractures. *Clin Orthop* 1984;58–64.
57. Dalinka MK, Kessler H, Weiss M. The radiographic evaluation of spinal trauma. *Emerg Med Clin North Am* 1985;3:475–490.
58. Murphey MD, Batnitzky S, Bramble JM. Diagnostic imaging of spinal trauma. *Radiol Clin North Am* 1989;27:855–872.
59. Blumenkopf B, Juneau PA III. Magnetic resonance imaging (MRI) of thoracolumbar fractures. *J Spinal Disord* 1988;1:144–150.
60. Bondurant FJ, Cotler HB, Kulkarni MV, et al. Acute spinal cord injury. A study using physical examination and magnetic resonance imaging. *Spine* 1990;15:161–168.
61. Tarr RW, Drolshagen LF, Kerner TC, et al. MR imaging of recent spinal trauma. *J Comput Assist Tomogr* 1987;11:412–417.
62. Tracy PT, Wright RM, Hanigan WC. Magnetic resonance imaging of spinal injury. *Spine* 1989;14:292–301.
63. el Khoury GY, Kathol MH, Daniel WW. Imaging of acute injuries of the cervical spine: value of plain radiography, CT, and MR imaging. *AJR Am J Roentgenol* 1995;164:43–50.
64. Golimbu C, Firooznia H, Rafii M, et al. Computed tomography of thoracic and lumbar spine fractures that have been treated with Harrington instrumentation. *Radiology* 1984;151:731–733.
65. Keene JS, Goletz TH, Lilleas F, et al. Diagnosis of vertebral fractures. A comparison of conventional radiography, conventional tomography, and computed axial tomography. *J Bone Joint Surg* 1982;64:586–594.
66. Mumford J, Weinstein JN, Spratt KF, et al. Thoracolumbar burst fractures. The clinical efficacy and outcome of nonoperative management. *Spine* 1993;18:955–970.
67. Bostman OM, Myllynen PJ, Riska EB. Unstable fractures of the thoracic and lumbar spine: the audit of an 8-year series with early reduction using Harrington instrumentation. *Injury* 1987;18:190–195.
68. Chadha M, Bahadur R. Steffee variable screw placement system in the management of unstable thoracolumbar fractures: a Third World experience. *Injury* 1998;29:737–742.
69. Gaebler C, Maier R, Kukla C, et al. Long-term results of pedicle stabilized thoracolumbar fractures in relation to the neurological deficit. *Injury* 1997;28:661–666.
70. Bradford DS, McBride GG. Surgical management of thoracolumbar spine fractures with incomplete neurologic deficits. *Clin Orthop* 1987;201–216.
71. Clohisy JC, Akbarnia BA, Bucholz RD, et al. Neurologic recovery associated with anterior decompression of spine fractures at the thoracolumbar junction (T12-L1). *Spine* 1992;17:S325–S330.
72. Dunn HK. Anterior spine stabilization and decompression for thoracolumbar injuries. *Orthop Clin North Am* 1986;17:113–119.
73. Fletcher DJ, Taddonio RF, Byrne DW, et al. Incidence of acute care complications in vertebral column fracture patients with and without spinal cord injury. *Spine* 1995;20:1136–1146.
74. Ghanayem AJ, Zdeblick TA. Anterior instrumentation in the management of thoracolumbar burst fractures. *Clin Orthop* 1997;89–100.
75. Jacobs RR, Asher MA, Snider RK. Thoracolumbar spinal injuries. A comparative study of recumbent and operative treatment in 100 patients. *Spine* 1980;5:463–477.
76. Kaneda K, Abumi K, Fujiya M. Burst fractures with neurologic deficits of the thoracolumbar-lumbar spine. Results of anterior decompression and stabilization with anterior instrumentation. *Spine* 1984;9:788–795.
77. Kostuik JP. Anterior spinal cord decompression for lesions of the thoracic and lumbar spine, techniques, new methods of internal fixation results. *Spine* 1983;8:512–531.
78. Kostuik JP. Anterior fixation for burst fractures of the thoracic and lumbar spine with or without neurological involvement. *Spine* 1988;13:286–293.
79. McGuire RA Jr. The role of anterior surgery in the treatment of thoracolumbar fractures. *Orthopedics* 1997;20:959–962.

80. Stancic MF, Gregorovic E, Nozica E, et al. Anterior decompression and fixation versus posterior reposition and semirigid fixation in the treatment of unstable burst thoracolumbar fracture: prospective clinical trial. *Croat Med J* 2001;42:49–53.
81. Knop C, Bastian L, Lange U, et al. [Transpedicular fusion of the thoraco-lumbar junction. Clinical, radiographic and CT results]. *Orthopade* 1999;28:703–713.
82. Knop C, Fabian HF, Bastian L, et al. Late results of thoracolumbar fractures after posterior instrumentation and transpedicular bone grafting. *Spine* 2001;26:88–99.
83. Knop C, Fabian HF, Bastian L, et al. Fate of the transpedicular intervertebral bone graft after posterior stabilisation of thoracolumbar fractures. *Eur Spine J* 2002;11:251–257.
84. McAfee PC, Bohlman HH, Yuan HA. Anterior decompression of traumatic thoracolumbar fractures with incomplete neurological deficit using a retroperitoneal approach. *J Bone Joint Surg* 1985;67:89–104.
85. Triantafyllou SJ, Gertzbein SD. Flexion distraction injuries of the thoracolumbar spine: a review. *Orthopedics* 1992;15:357–364.
86. Yokoyama T, Inoue S, Imamura J, et al. Sphenoethmoidal mucoceles with intracranial extension—three case reports. *Neurol Med Chir (Tokyo)* 1996;36:822–828.
87. Boerger TO, Limb D, Dickson RA. Does "canal clearance" affect neurological outcome after thoracolumbar burst fractures? *J Bone Joint Surg* 2000;82:629–635.
88. Bohlman HH, Kirkpatrick JS, Delamarter RB, et al. Anterior decompression for late pain and paralysis after fractures of the thoracolumbar spine. *Clin Orthop* 1994;24–29.
89. Delamarter RB, Bohlman HH, Dodge LD, et al. Experimental lumbar spinal stenosis. Analysis of the cortical evoked potentials, microvasculature, and histopathology. *J Bone Joint Surg* 1990;72:110–120.
90. Fehlings MG, Rao SC, Tator CH, et al. The optimal radiologic method for assessing spinal canal compromise and cord compression in patients with cervical spinal cord injury. Part II: Results of a multicenter study. *Spine* 1999;24:605–613.
91. Fehlings MG, Tator CH. An evidence-based review of decompressive surgery in acute spinal cord injury: rationale, indications, and timing based on experimental and clinical studies. *J Neurosurg* 1999;91:1–11.
92. Casey VIP, Jacobs RR, Asher MA. The rod-long-short technique in treatment of thoracolumbar, lumbar spine fractures. 1984.
93. Sasso RC, Cotler HB. Posterior instrumentation and fusion for unstable fractures and fracture-dislocations of the thoracic and lumbar spine. A comparative study of three fixation devices in 70 patients. *Spine* 1993;18:450–460.
94. McLain RF, Benson DR. Urgent surgical stabilization of spinal fractures in polytrauma patients. *Spine* 1999;24:1646–1654.
95. Rechtine GR, Cahill D, Chrin AM. Treatment of thoracolumbar trauma: comparison of complications of operative versus nonoperative treatment. *J Spinal Disord* 1999;12:406–409.
96. Ohana N, Sheinis D, Rath E, et al. Is there a need for lumbar orthosis in mild compression fractures of the thoracolumbar spine? A retrospective study comparing the radiographic results between early ambulation with and without lumbar orthosis. *J Spinal Disord* 2000;13:305–308.
97. Frankel HL, Hancock DO, Hyslop G, et al. The value of postural reduction in the initial management of closed injuries of the spine with paraplegia and tetraplegia. I. *Paraplegia* 1969;7:179–192.
98. Wessberg P, Wang Y, Irstam L, et al. The effect of surgery and remodelling on spinal canal measurements after thoracolumbar burst fractures. *Eur Spine J* 2001;10:55–63.
99. Broom MJ, Jacobs RR. Update 1988. Current status of internal fixation of thoracolumbar fractures. *J Orthop Trauma* 1989;3:148–155.
100. Gaines RW, Humphreys WG. A plea for judgment in management of thoracolumbar fractures and fracture-dislocations. A reassessment of surgical indications. *Clin Orthop* 1984;36–42.
101. Jacobs RR, Casey MP. Surgical management of thoracolumbar spinal injuries. General principles and controversial considerations. *Clin Orthop* 1984;22–35.
102. Dickman CA, Yahiro MA, Lu HT, et al. Surgical treatment alternatives for fixation of unstable fractures of the thoracic and lumbar spine. A meta-analysis. *Spine* 1994;19:2266S–2273S.
103. Lieberman IH, Dudeney S, Reinhardt MK, et al. Initial outcome and efficacy of "kyphoplasty" in the treatment of painful osteoporotic vertebral compression fractures. *Spine* 2001;26:1631–1638.
104. McAfee PC, Yuan HA, Fredrickson BE, et al. The value of computed tomography in thoracolumbar fractures. An analysis of one hundred consecutive cases and a new classification. *J Bone Joint Surg* 1983;65:461–473.
105. O'Callaghan JP, Ullrich CG, Yuan HA, et al. CT of facet distraction in flexion injuries of the thoracolumbar spine: the "naked" facet. *AJR Am J Roentgenol* 1980;134:563–568.
106. Heggeness MH. Spine fracture with neurological deficit in osteoporosis. *Osteop Int* 1993;3:215–221.
107. Jones RF, Snowdon E, Coan J, et al. Bracing of thoracic and lumbar spine fractures. *Paraplegia* 1987;25:386–393.
108. Weinstein JN, Collalto P, Lehmann TR. Thoracolumbar "burst" fractures treated conservatively: a long-term follow-up. *Spine* 1988;13:33–38.
109. Dall BE, Stauffer ES. Neurologic injury and recovery patterns in burst fractures at the T12 or L1 motion segment. *Clin Orthop* 1988;171–176.
110. Weinstein JN, Collalto P, Lehmann TR. Long-term follow-up of nonoperatively treated thoracolumbar spine fractures. *J Orthop Trauma* 1987;1:152–159.
111. Ducker TB, Hamit HF. Experimental treatments of acute spinal cord injury. *J Neurosurg* 1969;30:693–697.
112. Kramer DL, Rodgers WB, Mansfield FL. Transpedicular instrumentation and short-segment fusion of thoracolumbar fractures: a prospective study using a single instrumentation system. *J Orthop Trauma* 1995;9:499–506.
113. Leferink VJ, Zimmerman KW, Veldhuis EF, ten Vergert EM, et al. Thoracolumbar spinal fractures: radiological results of transpedicular fixation combined with transpedicular cancellous bone graft and posterior fusion in 183 patients. *Eur Spine J* 2001;10:517–523.
114. Chance. Note on a type of flexion fracture of the spine. *Br J Radiol* 1948;21:452–453.
115. Bannister J, Taylor TK, Nade SM. Proceedings: seat belt fractures of the spine. *J Bone Joint Surg* 1975;57:252.
116. Burke DC. Spinal cord injuries and seat belts. *Med J Aust* 1973; 2:801–806.
117. Christian MS. Non-fatal injuries sustained by back seat passengers. *Br Med J* 1975;1:320–322.
118. Dooley BJ. Proceedings: the effect of compulsory seat belt wearing on the mortality and pattern of injury to car occupants. *J Bone Joint Surg* 1975;57:252.
119. Holt BW. Spines and seat belts: mechanisms of spinal injury in motor vehicle crashes. *Med J Aust* 1976;2:411–413.
120. Smith WS, Kaufer H. Patterns and mechanisms of lumbar injuries associated with lap seat belts. *J Bone Joint Surg* 1969;51:239–254.
121. Trinca GW, Dooley BJ. The effects of seat belt legislation on road traffic injuries. *Aust N Z J Surg* 1977;47:150–155.
122. Gertzbein SD, Court-Brown CM. Flexion-distraction injuries of the lumbar spine. Mechanisms of injury and classification. *Clin Orthop* 1988;227:52–60.
123. Davis AG. Fractures of the spine. *J Bone Joint Surg Am* 1929;11: 133–152.
124. McEvoy RD, Bradford DS. The management of burst fractures of the thoracic and lumbar spine. Experience in 53 patients. *Spine* 1985;10:631–637.
125. Ashman RB, Birch JG, Bone LB, et al. Mechanical testing of spinal instrumentation. *Clin Orthop* 1988;227:113–125.
126. Flesch JR, Leider LL, Erickson DL, et al. Harrington instrumentation and spine fusion for unstable fractures and fracture-dislocations of the thoracic and lumbar spine. *J Bone Joint Surg* 1977;59:143–153.
127. Jacobs RR, Nordwall A, Nachemson A. Reduction, stability, and strength provided by internal fixation systems for thoracolumbar spinal injuries. *Clin Orthop* 1982;300–308.
128. Erwin WD, Dickson JH, Harrington PR. Clinical review of patients with broken Harrington rods. *J Bone Joint Surg* 1980;62:1302–1307.
129. Sullivan JA. Sublaminar wiring of Harrington distraction rods for unstable thoracolumbar spine fractures. *Clin Orthop* 1984;178–185.
130. McAfee PC, Bohlman HH. Complications following Harrington instrumentation for fractures of the thoracolumbar spine. *J Bone Joint Surg* 1985;67:672–686.
131. Johnston CE, Ashman RB, Sherman MC, et al. Mechanical consequences of rod contouring and residual scoliosis in sublaminar segmental instrumentation. *J Orthop Res* 1987;5:206–216.
132. Akbarnia BA, Fogarty JP, Tayob AA. Contoured Harrington instrumentation in the treatment of unstable spinal fractures. The effect of supplementary sublaminar wires. *Clin Orthop* 1984;186–194.

133. Bryant CE, Sullivan JA. Management of thoracic and lumbar spine fractures with Harrington distraction rods supplemented with segmental wiring. *Spine* 1983;8:532–537.
134. McAfee PC, Werner FW, Glisson RR. A biomechanical analysis of spinal instrumentation systems in thoracolumbar fractures. Comparison of traditional Harrington distraction instrumentation with segmental spinal instrumentation. *Spine* 1985;10:204–217.
135. Stambough JL. Cotrel-Dubousset instrumentation and thoracolumbar spine trauma: a review of 55 cases. *J Spinal Disord* 1994;7:461–469.
136. Weinstein JN, Collalto P, Lehmann TR. Thoracolumbar "burst" fractures treated conservatively: a long-term follow-up. *Spine* 1988;13:33–38.
137. Gurr KR, McAfee PC. Cotrel-Dubousset instrumentation in adults. A preliminary report. *Spine* 1988;13:510–520.
138. Graziano GP. Cotrel-Dubousset hook and screw combination for spine fractures. *J Spinal Disord* 1993;6:380–385.
139. Markel DC, Graziano GP. A comparison study of treatment of thoracolumbar fractures using the ACE Posterior Segmental Fixator and Cotrel–Dubousset instrumentation. *Orthopedics* 1995;18:679–686.
140. Argenson C, Lover J, de Peretti F. The treatment of spinal fractures with Cotrel Dubousset Instrumentation. Results of the first 85 cases. Scoliosis Research Society/European Spine Meeting. *Orthop Trans* 14, 776. 90.
141. Benzel EC. Short-segment compression instrumentation for selected thoracic and lumbar spine fractures: the short-rod/two-claw technique. *J Neurosurg*. 1993;79:335–340.
142. McKinley LM, Obenchain TG, Roth KR. *Loss of correction: late kyphosis in short segment pedicle fixation in cases of posterior transpeduncular decompression*. Montpellier, France: Sauramps Medical, 1989.
143. Benli IT, Tandogan NR, Kis M, et al. Cotrel-Dubousset instrumentation in the treatment of unstable thoracic and lumbar spine fractures. *Arch Orthop Trauma Surg* 1994;113:86–92.
144. Farcy JP, Weidenbaum M, Michelsen CB, et al. A comparative biomechanical study of spinal fixation using Cotrel-Dubousset instrumentation. *Spine* 1987;12:877–881.
145. Gurr KR, McAfee PC, Shih CM. Biomechanical analysis of anterior and posterior instrumentation systems after corpectomy. A calf-spine model. *J Bone Joint Surg* 1988;70:1182–1191.
146. Gurr KR, McAfee PC, Shih CM. Biomechanical analysis of posterior instrumentation systems after decompressive laminectomy. An unstable calf-spine model. *J Bone Joint Surg* 1988;70:680–691.
147. Parker JW, Lane JR, Karaikovic EE, et al. Successful short-segment instrumentation and fusion for thoracolumbar spine fractures: a consecutive 4 1/2-year series. *Spine* 2000;25:1157–1170.
148. Dimar JR, Wilde PH, Glassman SD, et al. Thoracolumbar burst fractures treated with combined anterior and posterior surgery. *Am J Orthop* 1996;25:159–165.
149. Finkelstein JA, Chapman JR, Mirza S. Anterior cortical allograft in thoracolumbar fractures. *J Spinal Disord* 1999;12:424–429.
150. Grant JP, Oxland TR, Dvorak MF. Mapping the structural properties of the lumbosacral vertebral endplates. *Spine* 2001;26:889–896.
151. Dick W. The "fixateur interne" as a versatile implant for spine surgery. *Spine* 1987;12:882–900.
152. Esses SI, Botsford DJ, Kostuik JP. Evaluation of surgical treatment for burst fractures. *Spine* 1990;15:667–673.
153. Esses SI, Botsford DJ, Wright T, et al. Operative treatment of spinal fractures with the AO internal fixator. *Spine* 1991;16:S146–S150.
154. Kahanovitz N, Bullough P, Jacobs RR. The effect of internal fixation without arthrodesis on human facet joint cartilage. *Clin Orthop* 1984;204–208.
155. Ebelke DK, Asher MA, Neff JR, et al. Survivorship analysis of VSP spine instrumentation in the treatment of thoracolumbar and lumbar burst fractures. *Spine* 1991;16:S428–S432.
156. Chiba M, McLain RF, Yerby SA, et al. Short-segment pedicle instrumentation. Biomechanical analysis of supplemental hook fixation. *Spine* 1996;21:288–294.
157. Osebold WR, Weinstein SL, Sprague BL. Thoracolumbar spine fractures. Results of treatment. *Spine* 1981;6:13–34.
158. Davis AG. Fractures of the spine. *J Bone Joint Surg Am* 1929;11:133.
159. McKinley TO, McLain RF, Yerby SA, et al. The effect of pedicle morphometry on pedicle screw loading. A synthetic model. *Spine* 1997;22:246–252.
160. Devito DP, Tsahakis PJ. *Cotrel-Duboursset instrumentation in traumatic spine injuries*. France: Sauramps Medical, 1989.
161. McAfee PC, Weiland DJ, Carlow JJ. Survivorship analysis of pedicle spinal instrumentation. *Spine* 1991;16:S422–S427.

CHAPTER 42

Late Sequelae of Thoracolumbar Trauma

Drew A. Bednar

Thoracolumbar trauma represents a wide spectrum of pathologies. A comminuted bursting fracture/dislocation of the junction incurred in a high-energy motor vehicle crash is totally different from an osteoporotic compression fracture occurring spontaneously in a geriatric patient. This chapter focuses on the late sequelae of major *trauma*. Osteoporosis is covered in Chapters 8 and 61.

Ideally, a chapter such as this is a comprehensive summary of leading-edge data defining the current state of the spine care art. Often that "leading edge" is contained in clinical series and research projects that have yet to pass peer review. Using the gold standard of peer-reviewed published material, the information may seem somewhat dated. Moreover, the published literature is relatively scant regarding the long-term sequelae of thoracolumbar fusion. For example, a PubMed search using the key word "thoracolumbar fractures" in 2002 produced 59 citations. Of these, only twenty-one references (1–21) were clinical series, and of these only three (19–21) presented any comparative data. One compared the results of surgical to nonsurgical care (19), one compared the results of anterior to posterior approaches (20), and one compared instrumentations with and without bone grafting (21).

Of those twenty-one clinical series, eight were clearly studies of burst fracture care (2,3,8,14,17,19–21), whereas one reviewed flexion/distraction injuries. The remaining 12 series did not describe fracture type other than by the anatomic siting designation "thoracolumbar." In all these, fracture classification schemes were referenced only twice (7,8; different ones each time), and comprehensive outcome tools were reported only four times (17,19–21; again, different ones every time). The conceptually very important load-sharing classification (Fig. 1) of McCormack et al. (22) was mentioned only once (3). This review underscores the compelling need for a designated injury classification scheme and a consistent outcomes measurement tool.

There are additional problems in the current literature. It is often difficult to decide in surgical cohort studies if treatment has been only instrumentation, or instrumentation and fusion. Usually, studies using the anterior approaches are straightforward, and the types of fusion used are generally obvious. Reports of transpedicular anterior column support, such as Daniaux (23), are also clear, whereas studies involving pedicle screw are often very unclear on the type of fusion. Some might be intertransverse fusions, some interlaminar. Instrumentation, other than in some palliative cases, should always be accompanied by arthrodesis; however, the mechanics of the hardware (e.g., plate vs. rod, large vs. small-diameter rods, etc.) and associated outcomes may differ significantly between trauma and reconstructive applications (24). Moreover, hardware is usually removed routinely in Asia and Europe (18), and in the United States and Canada much less often (25). Finally, significant questions remain about the definition of instability (26,27).

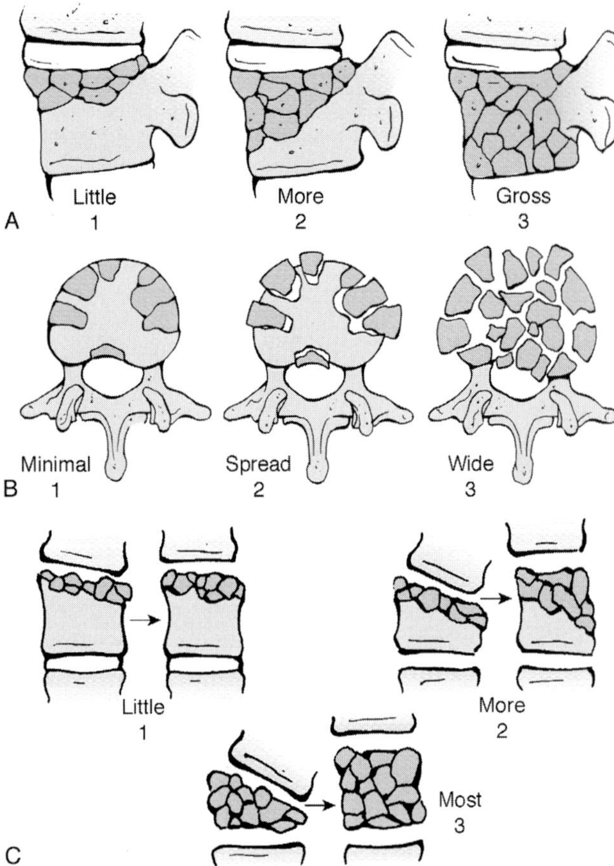

FIG. 1. The load-sharing classification of McCormack was conceived as a method of predicting which "stable" or "pure" burst fractures (i.e., those burst fractures without obvious disruption of the posterior column) would require anterior column support by quantifying fracture displacement. **A:** Comminution/involvement. Little (*1*) = <30% comminution on sagittal plane section computed tomography (CT). More (*2*) = 30 to 60% comminution. Gross (*3*) = >60% comminution. **B:** Apposition of fragments. Minimal (*1*) = minimal displacement on axial CT cut. Spread (*2*) = at least 2-mm displacement of <50% cross-section of body. Wade (*3*) = at least 2-mm displacement of >50% cross-section of body. **C:** Deformity correction. Little (*1*) = kyphotic correction ≤3 degrees on lateral plain films. More (*2*) = kyphotic correction 4 to 9 degrees. Most (*3*) equals kyphotic correction ≥10 degrees. Cases scoring over 6 points uniformly went on to implant failure. Cases scoring 6 points or less had no implant breakage.

Amidst all of these unresolved issues are important models for advancing knowledge, such as McCormack et al.'s classification based on load sharing (22) and the carefully detailed prospective clinical outcome analysis. That study shared excellent results of surgical repair of thoracic spine injuries with properly applied modern segmental instrumentation systems, suggesting *thoracic* spine injury may be a solved problem when appropriate reconstructive principles are followed. The *late sequelae* of injuries are more controversial at the thoracolumbar junction, however, which is the more frequently injured. This chapter focuses more on this anatomic area.

DEMOGRAPHICS OF THORACOLUMBAR SPINAL INJURY

The demographics of thoracolumbar fracture are largely the demographics of trauma, and trauma is largely a disease of young men. The incidence of thoracolumbar fracture with (28) or without (29) spinal cord injury (SCI) peaks early in the fourth decade of life (26,30,31).

The importance of effective treatment of these injuries is amplified by the fact that these injuries so often involve young men with families and children to support. Disability support cost is extended by the decades of life that follow these injuries. Socioeconomic consequences affect not only the patient but also their spouses and children.

ALIGNMENT

Kyphosis—Acute

The thoracolumbar junction represents a transition in alignment between the normal lumbar lordosis and the kyphotic thoracic spine, and in general, it is straight in both planes (i.e., neutrally aligned) (32). Rarely, spinal dysplasias or Scheuermann's disease may create kyphosis in younger individuals, whereas in older populations, degenerative disc disease and resultant anterior column shortening may create some kyphosis (32). Acute kyphosis in spine trauma is, of course, a major factor in decision making.

In assessing posttraumatic kyphosis, the literature clearly shows optimum consistency when measurements are made comparing the orientation of the upper end-plate of the uninjured vertebra above the injury to the lower vertebral end-plate of the intact bone below (33,34).

If the vertebra is not badly crushed, kyphotic angulations may reflect splay in the posterior elements with disruption of the dorsal tension band and resultant spinal instability. If the vertebra is crushed badly enough to create significant angulation without disruption of the posterior elements, will the resultant pathologic biomechanics promote continued angulation? How much kyphosis is acceptable? In considering static deformity, the literature (31,35,36) has shown patients with 30 degrees or more of focal thoracolumbar kyphosis are at risk for chronic pain and should be realigned. The thoracic spine, at least proximally, may tolerate this degree of angulation well but the thoracolumbar junction cannot. This is part of the reason for the commonly accepted threshold surgical indication of 30 degrees acute kyphosis in managing thoracolumbar junctional injury (9). Additionally, *progression* of kyphosis beyond the 5-degree margin of error in measurement accepted in the literature is another accepted indication for surgical care (33). Anterior column support procedures may be required in these circumstances.

Historically, progressive kyphosis treated with posterior-only instrumentation procedures has been considered a rare event (4,31,35,36). It is not. Data from McLain (25) and the author (37) suggest that between 28 and 67% of thoracolumbar injuries treated with only posterior instrumentation have sagittal collapse of 10 degrees or more at 1 year. The tendency is for the initial impressive improvement in alignment obtained surgically to gradually, but progressively, deteriorate over the ensuing 1 to 2 years, returning eventually to the preoperative position (18,19). Attempted anterior column support via transpedicular bone graft-

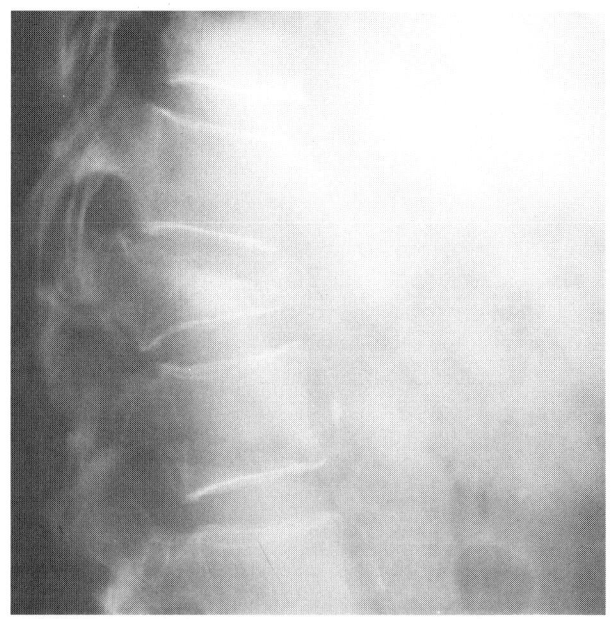
A

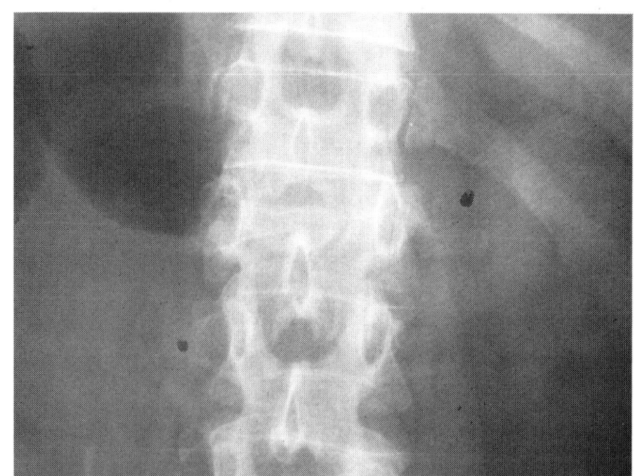
B

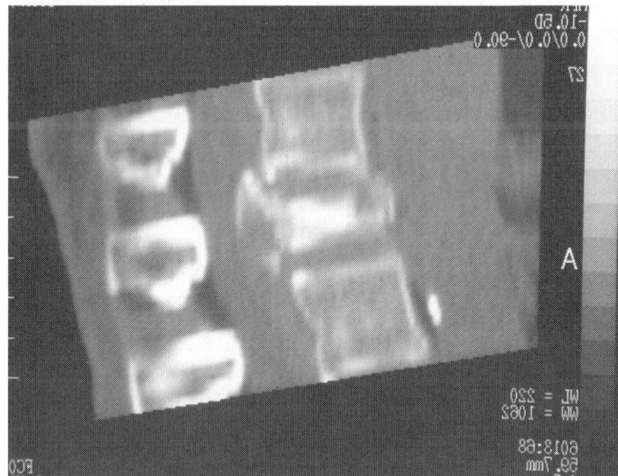
C

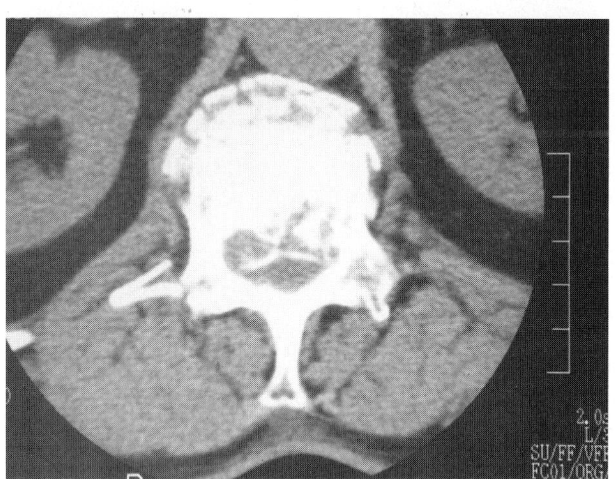
D

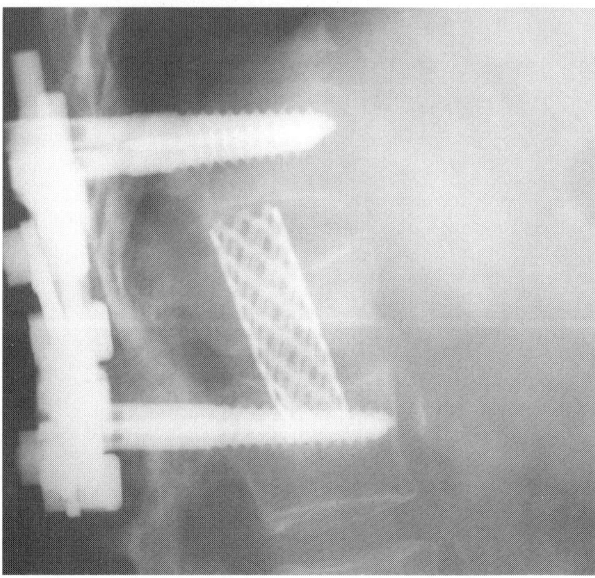
E

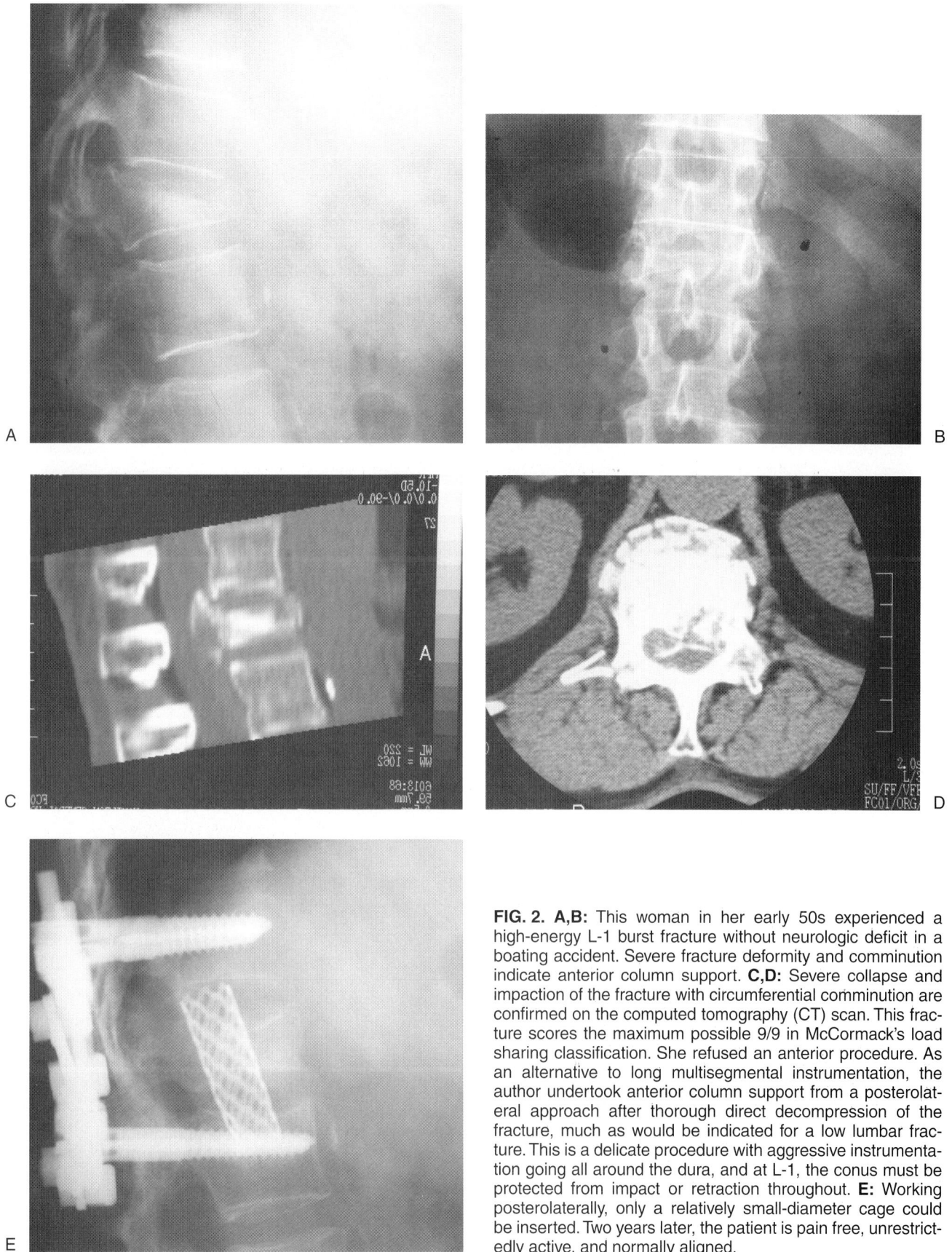

FIG. 2. A,B: This woman in her early 50s experienced a high-energy L-1 burst fracture without neurologic deficit in a boating accident. Severe fracture deformity and comminution indicate anterior column support. **C,D:** Severe collapse and impaction of the fracture with circumferential comminution are confirmed on the computed tomography (CT) scan. This fracture scores the maximum possible 9/9 in McCormack's load sharing classification. She refused an anterior procedure. As an alternative to long multisegmental instrumentation, the author undertook anterior column support from a posterolateral approach after thorough direct decompression of the fracture, much as would be indicated for a low lumbar fracture. This is a delicate procedure with aggressive instrumentation going all around the dura, and at L-1, the conus must be protected from impact or retraction throughout. **E:** Working posterolaterally, only a relatively small-diameter cage could be inserted. Two years later, the patient is pain free, unrestrictedly active, and normally aligned.

ing (8,18,21) has not been entirely successful in preventing this later collapse seen in thoracolumbar fractures.

In contrast, fractures of the thoracic spine are stabilized by the rib cage and can be addressed successfully with long posterior constructs. In the thoracolumbar and lumbar spine, primary anterior column reconstruction of cases presenting with 30 degrees or more of acute posttraumatic kyphosis is indicated, particularly in highly comminuted fractures (22,38). At the thoracolumbar junction, this may best be achieved through an anterolateral approach.

In the lower lumbar spine, the prevertebral vascular structures may make anterior surgery more difficult, and posterolateral procedures are relatively indicated (Fig. 2) to prevent late collapse.

Kyphosis—Late

The problem of how to manage *late* posttraumatic kyphosis, after the fracture is healed, increasingly confronts us as a result of failed reconstruction when isolated posterior procedure was the primary treatment. Early reconstruction incorporating anterior column reconstruction of failed cases is indicated to prevent this deformity.

With lesser degrees of deformity (i.e., 30 degrees or less), the problem of shortening in the anterior column may be best addressed with anterior column reconstruction. If the deformity is rigid, reconstruction may require a multistage procedure with primary posterior release and removal of old instrumentation preceding anterior column reconstruction. A third-stage posterior reinstrumentation and fusion may be required to reconstruct the dorsal tension band of the spine.

After anterior release and decompression, reconstruction can be accomplished with a number of alternatives, including autograft, allograft, cages, and screw/plate and screw/rod systems in various combinations (12,13,38–42). The clinical results of such procedures are generally excellent, even if completely anatomic realignment can sometimes not be achieved (5,43,44).

The concept of compensatory posterior column shortening through pedicle subtraction osteotomy has also been applied to the acute treatment of thoracolumbar fractures, with excellent preliminary results in a series of six cases (3).

In cases in which the degree of malalignment is great (i.e., more than 30 degrees), posterior column shortening via single-stage posterior pedicle-subtraction osteotomy with aggressive multilevel segmental instrumentation and fusion (Fig. 3) may be indicated (39), and the results are good (5,45).

Scoliosis

The coronal orientation of the normal thoracolumbar junction is, again, straight. Significant posttraumatic scoliosis can be caused by eccentric or "lateral compression" burst fractures, or fracture-subluxations.

This is a sufficiently rare condition to have escaped direct citation in the 2002 PubMed search, as well as the contemporary review article on posttraumatic spinal deformity by Silber and Vaccaro (9) and the AO manual (46). Accordingly, an acceptable amount of posttraumatic scoliosis is difficult to define.

In static imaging, a deformity beyond 5 to 10 degrees is worrisome because it implies disruption of normal dorsal stabilizing structures and therefore might warrant consideration of surgical stabilization. Certainly, any *progression* of posttraumatic scoliotic deformity beyond the accepted measurement error of 5 degrees confirms that the spine is unstable and surgery is indi-

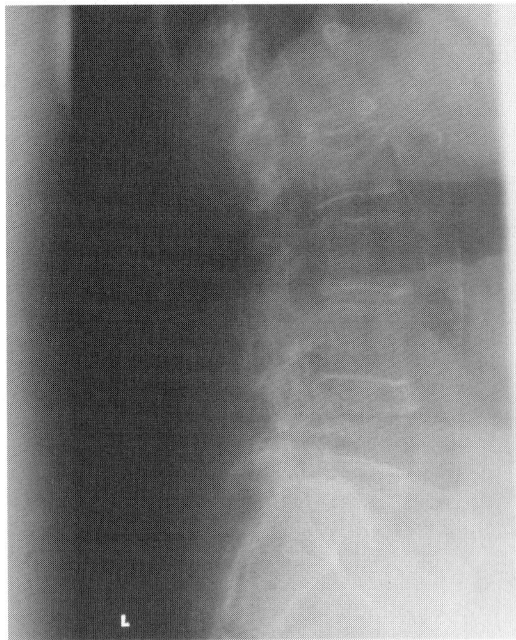

A

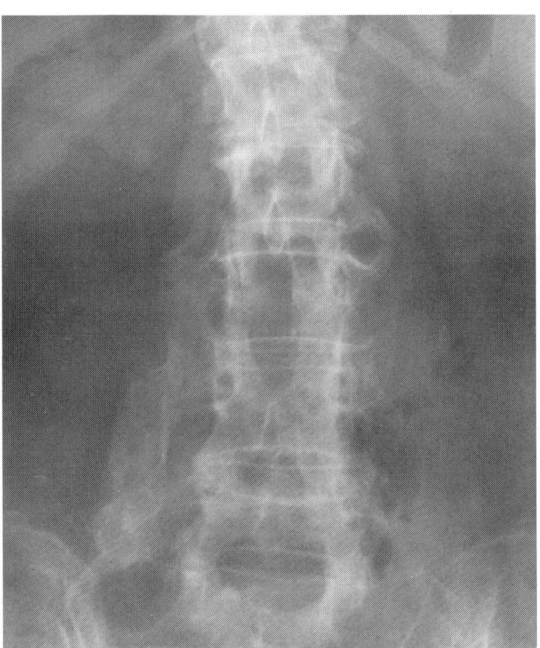

B

FIG. 3. A,B: This 76-year-old woman had lumbar decompression and fusion from L-2 to the sacrum more than a decade previously. Painful instrumentation was removed approximately 5 years after the surgery. At the hardware removal procedure, the fusion was explored and found to be solid. (*continued*)

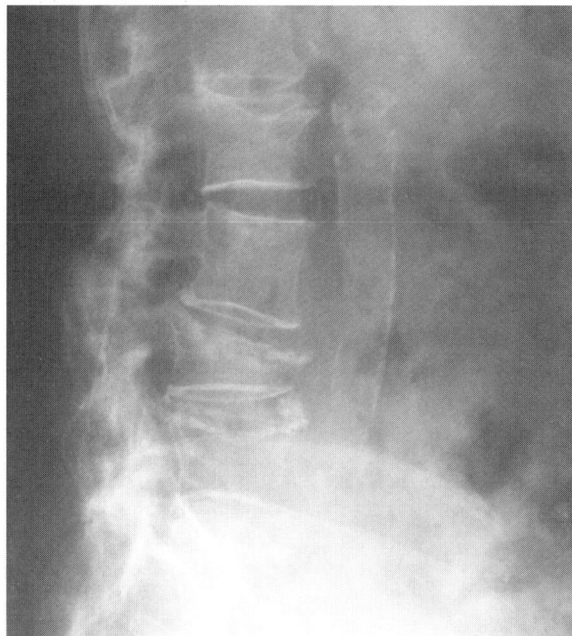
C

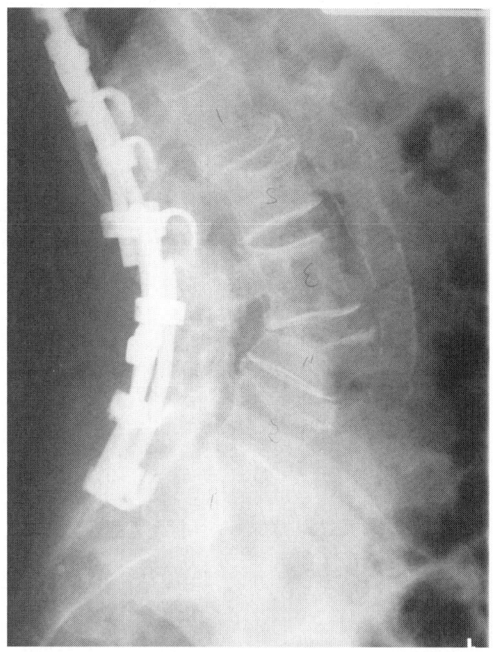
D

FIG. 3. *Continued.* She was pain free until 3 years later, when she presented with progressive back pain, newly stooped posture, and difficulty walking several months after a heavy fall wherein she landed on her buttocks **(C,D)**. X-rays showed an anterior column compression fracture at L-4 under her intact, but very osteoporotic fusion mass. The deformity was confirmed to be progressive over serial films. Magnetic resonance imaging confirmed an isolated anterior column fracture with no compression of the thecal sac. Anterior column reconstruction at L-4 would be difficult at the best of times. Here, heavy aortic calcification and severe osteoporosis of the spine in this geriatric patient precluded the attempt. Alternatively, she was treated with posterior column shortening via pedicle subtraction osteotomy (the old fusion mass was intact—it had undergone plastic deformation with the loss of anterior column support), which relieved pain and abnormal posture immediately.

cated (45). When indicated, stabilization can generally be accomplished by posterior approaches with segmental instrumentation. Pedicle screws help minimize the required number of instrumented motion segments, as they do in treating kyphotic fracture deformity (47).

Flatback

Flatback relates to loss of *lumbar* lordosis, causing kyphotic decompensation of the spine. Although this deformity can have a degenerative etiology, it was historically first recognized as secondary to the use of distractive instrumentation systems in lumbar reconstruction (48) and thoracolumbar fractures. It has been treated by corrective osteotomy (48,49), similar to the techniques for a fixed kyphosis. The primary indication for surgical treatment in these cases is pain. Rarely, progressive deformity or neurologic symptoms may ensue.

Since the advent of modern segmental spinal instrumentation systems allowing reconstruction of the spine without distraction, this problem should soon become relatively infrequent, although careful attention to sagittal alignment in fracture repair is always required. However, segmental instrumentation alone is not the solution to posttraumatic kyphosis. Only careful and exacting surgical technique can prevent this complication.

PAIN

Late back and/or leg pain after spinal fracture can originate in the damaged structural elements of the spine, in soft tissue through malalignment or spinal imbalance; from the neural elements through compression, syrinx, or tethering (50); or at the donor site of bone graft harvested for reconstruction (51).

The exact source of pain can sometimes be difficult to determine. The differential diagnosis includes nonunion, infection, loose implants, ongoing compression of the thecal sac, syrinx, cord tethering, neurotropic spine, and sagittal spinal imbalance. A detailed history and physical examination are always the most important primary diagnostic tools. Imaging studies should generally complement, being directed by and undertaken to confirm the clinical diagnostic impression.

The frequency of problematic posttraumatic back pain is not well defined (26). At a mean follow-up of 52 months, McLain found that 58% of his surgical patients were pain free, 17% had mild pain, and 25% had moderate to severe pain (25). Of note, two of four patients with more than 10 degrees progression of kyphosis had moderate to severe leg and back pain symptoms of a magnitude to indicate a realignment and/or decompressive procedure.

In patients with SCI, problem pain is more frequent. Summary literature reveals that approximately two-thirds of SCI

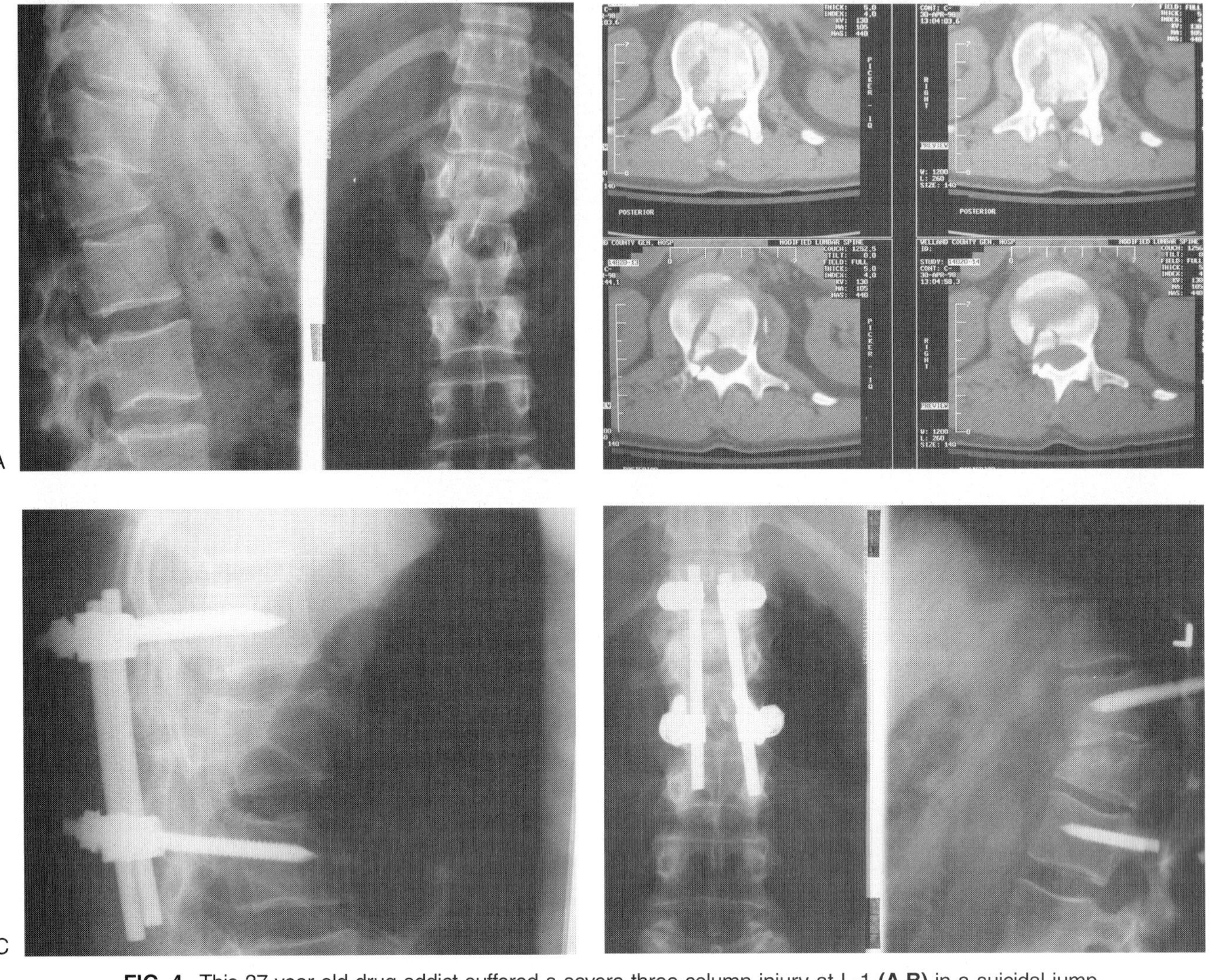

FIG. 4. This 37-year-old drug addict suffered a severe three-column injury at L-1 **(A,B)** in a suicidal jump from considerable height. She was neurologically intact. This is much more than just a burst fracture. Translation is seen in the anteroposterior and lateral projections, the posterior elements are splayed at T-12/L-1, and the computed tomography scan shows an obvious subluxed facet. **C:** A colleague undertook her reconstruction with posterior short-segmental instrumentation and transpedicular grafting of the anterior column at T-12/L-1. An excellent morphologic reduction was achieved. After 3 months in a Jewett orthosis, the patient was weaned, rehabilitated, and discharged from active care at 1 year **(D)**. She did well until almost 4 years later, when she presented with a painful gibbus that developed over several months. X-rays confirmed screw breakage with recurrent kyphosis. After workup for sepsis was negative, she was reconstructed in two stages. First, after the old hardware was removed she had PSO at L-1 and repeat segmental instrumentation with iliac-autografted intertransverse fusion. Next, after residual corpectomy at L-1 the anterior column was reconstructed with a titanium mesh cage and rib graft. At 2 years, she is pain free and fully active.

patients report chronic pain and of that, 50% is severe (50). Treatment options are multiple and protocol complex.

Late iliac wing bone graft donor site pain is as yet poorly understood and often impossible to treat effectively. Whereas significant donor-site pain occurs in one-third or more of elective lumbar reconstructive cases (51), the frequency in trauma is fortunately much lower (52–54).

Pseudarthrosis after spinal fracture repair is rare enough to have escaped the PubMed search. This condition can be subtle and difficult to diagnose, and when missed, it can evolve to catastrophic structural failure even many years after the index trauma (Fig. 4). The approximate frequency of nonunion in pedicle screw–instrumented fusions generally ranges from 5 to 15% (55–57).

FUNCTIONAL STATUS

Pain may or may not cause disability. Again, the probability of posttraumatic disability after thoracolumbar spine fracture is historically not well defined (26). The literature to date focuses largely on the issue of return to work after fracture and lacks a comprehensive late follow-up report.

McLain reviewed 30 cases, at a mean of 52 months (25). Seven were disabled by neurologic injury and might be excluded from considerations focused on pain. Of the remaining 23, 11 patients (48%) had returned to their previous work, seven (30%) took lighter full-time work, and two more (9%) were physically unrestricted but unemployed. Only three (13%) were permanently disabled by back or leg pain.

At a mean of 3 years, Knop et al. reviewed a group of 56 patients and found that the probability of return to heavy work was only 50% (11 of 22), that disability doubled (four cases preoperatively, eight at review) and only one-half (21 of 42) of those participating in sports before injury were able to return to them (18).

Bednar et al. found that 58% of their patients were pain free and fully 68% were working (58% at their preinjury jobs, 10% in lighter work) at a mean of 42 months (39).

Belmont et al. reviewed 30 U.S. Army aviators experiencing thoracolumbar fractures in the course of military duty (10). This may represent a prognostically "optimal" group of highly educated and motivated patients. Some 10% suffered neurologic injury that would presumably preclude them from flying. At a mean of 6.5 years, fully 77% of this group, or 23 of 27 (85%) who were not paralyzed, returned to aviation duties.

Burnham et al. reviewed 479 spine fracture patients and confirmed that fully 54% were employed at 1 year after injury (30).

NEUROLOGIC STATUS

Neurologic prognosis after SCI depends largely on the initial degree and completeness of deficit. This can be difficult to determine with accuracy in the trauma suite or intensive care unit perioperatively. The prognosticating examination is probably best performed not before 72 hours after injury (57,58), and perhaps optimally at 1 month (59,60).

A complete neurologic deficit is best defined as the complete absence of sensory and motor function in the lowest sacral segment (61). Any sparing at all makes the injury incomplete, with correspondingly improved prognosis. Neurologic, sensory, and motor levels and motor strength are defined according to the criteria of the American Spinal Injury Association (62).

In specifically addressing the late neurologic prognosis of thoracolumbar trauma, it is impossible to present comprehensive data applicable to all patients. The SCI literature usually has analyzed the outcomes of paraplegia, which is less useful for thoracolumbar lesions (see later; also references 57–62). Neurologic deficit incurred at the thoracolumbar junction anatomically represents a mix of lesions of the low thoracic spinal cord, the conus medullaris, and the proximal cauda equina. Lower motor neuron lesions of the conus and cauda equina are well recognized to do better, that is to be "less complete," than upper motor neuron injuries of the spinal cord itself. Accordingly, the data on paraplegia summarized later in this chapter may in fact be somewhat pessimistic.

MOTOR RECOVERY—COMPLETE PARAPLEGIA

Waters reported on 148 patients and found that 73% who were thought to be motor-complete paraplegics at 1 month were unchanged in neurologic level at 1 year, 70% of muscles initially graded 1 to 2 on a scale of 5 improved to 3 or greater at 1 year, and 3 to 7% of those initially grade 0 improved to grade 3 at 1 year (59). The majority of neural recovery occurred in the first 6 to 9 months, with no improvement beyond 12 to 18 months. Four percent of his patients initially assessed as complete converted "late" to incomplete status. Of these six cases, four regained continence and two became ambulatory with a reciprocal gait.

In contrast, those with incomplete paraplegia had the following results: 85% of muscles graded 1 to 2 on a scale of 5 at 1 month improved to 3 or greater at 1 year, and of muscles graded 0/5 at 1 month fully 55% regained some volitional control and 26% regained useful motor function (60).

Ambulation

Community ambulation requires motor useful function of the hip flexors on one side and the quadriceps on the other side. Waters found that only 5% of complete paraplegics became community ambulators with conventional orthoses and crutches (59), but fully 76% of incomplete paraplegics eventually became community ambulators (60).

Continence

Normal voiding and elimination are often not regained after paraplegia. Most patients can regain social continence with appropriate rehabilitative training, urologic care, and surveillance (63).

Sexual and Reproductive Function

Fully 75% of male SCI patients are found to be impotent (64), and less than 50% of females can achieve orgasm (65). Whereas ovulation and fertility in women are not impaired by paraplegia (66), most males are infertile (67) and spontaneous procreation without medical intervention is rare in these men (68).

LATE NEUROLOGIC DETERIORATION

Late neurologic deterioration in the thoracolumbar fracture patient may present with deterioration of preserved neurologic function or increasing pain, or both. It can result from one or more of multiple possible causes, including fracture fragments in the spinal canal, osteophyte overgrowth, instability with progressive malalignment, syrinx formation, or cord tethering.

Oner et al. have demonstrated that some cases of late neurologic deterioration in association with progressive kyphosis might have been predicted with early magnetic resonance imaging (MRI) examination to better define the extent of end-plate involvement and vertebral body comminution (40). This may be analogous to the morphologic prognosis as determined from the load-sharing classification of McCormack et al. (22).

In cases in which late neurologic deterioration is detected, urgent evaluation of the relevant bony and soft-tissue anatomy with plane x-rays and ideally computed tomography (CT) and MRI scans is indicated. When ferrous metal implants are present, the CT scan may be augmented by myelographic enhancement.

Late decompression of incomplete lesions where there is ongoing spinal cord compression has been demonstrated to have excellent results. Bohlmann achieved significant improvement in 90% of patients treated at a mean of 4.5 years after the initial injury (69).

Lee et al. treated 53 patients for neurologic deterioration developing at a mean of 11 years after injury as a result of a syrinx with or without cord tethering (70). Treatment involved detethering where indicated, cyst shunting, and expansile duraplasty. They found improvement in 73% (33 of 45) of their patients evaluated at a mean of 22.5 months after these procedures.

MANAGEMENT OF ASYMPTOMATIC STENOSIS OF THE SPINAL CANAL AFTER FRACTURE

Given the sometimes progressive nature of degenerative stenosis of the lumbar and cervical spinal canals, there has historically been concern that patients with residual canal stenosis after thoracolumbar fracture, particularly burst fractures, might be at risk for late neurologic deterioration and should be decompressed. The literature suggests otherwise in consistently demonstrating late *decompressive* remodeling of the spinal canal of a variable degree. Generally, higher degrees of residual stenosis are found to remodel more extensively than minor bony intrusions to the spinal canal. Mohanty and Venkatram studied 45 patients with thoracolumbar or lumbar fractures treated nonoperatively (2). Remodeling of posttraumatic canal stenosis averaged 51.7% in patients who made neurologic recovery and 46.1% in those who did not.

Alanay et al. reviewed 21 patients with thoracolumbar fractures at 50 months after injury (8). Mean canal compromise of 38.5% on initial presentation improved to 22.1% after surgery but further improved to a mean of only 2.5% at late evaluation.

Dai reported on 31 patients followed from 3 to 7 years and found that canal stenosis decreased from a mean of 26.2% (ranging up to 74.5%) to only 19.2% (with a maximum of only 46.5%) (17).

Wessberg et al. reported on 157 patients treated surgically for thoracolumbar fractures at a minimum follow-up of 5 years (14). Average preoperative canal diameter was reduced to 1.4 cm^2, or 49% of normal. This was improved to 2.0 cm^2, or 72% of normal after surgery, but further improved to 2.6 cm^2, or 87% of normal at late review.

Shen et al., in a prospective clinical trial, found that initial mean retropulsion of 34% decreased to 15% in their 47 nonoperative patients at 2 years (19).

Classically, Mumford et al. reported in 1993 that there was consistent decompressive remodeling of the canal in their study of nonoperative cases, and suggested that nonoperative management might be proposed as a standard of care (71).

LATE COMPLICATIONS OF SURGICAL CARE

Implant Failure

Implant failure is predictably frequent in posterior-only constructs when instrumentation is not accompanied by arthrodesis. Leferink et al. found 10.9% of their series of 183 cases of low thoracic, thoracolumbar, and mid-lumbar fractures had broken pedicle screws when coming to elective hardware removal at a mean of only months (7). Alanay et al. found fully 45% of their cases had broken screws at slightly later review (21). Presumably this frequency would only increase with longer follow-up, and one might consider that instrumentation without arthrodesis for fracture might best be avoided (Fig. 4).

When arthrodesis accompanies implants, the reported frequency of failure after posterior-only procedures is much more inconsistent. The author found seven cases of implant failure in our series of 67 thoracolumbar and lumbar fractures reviewed at a mean of 42 months (37). Esses et al. found a 5% probability of screw failure in 120 cases reviewed at a mean of 17 months in their multicenter study (38). Shen et al. found screw fracture in 2 of 33 operative cases (6%) at 2 years (19). McLain found 24 of 94 screws (25%) bent or broken at a mean of 52 months despite solid fusion in a number of cases (25).

Some of this inconsistency may be explained by the degree of vertebral disruption at injury. The more comminuted the fracture, the more load on the implant after fracture reduction and (it seems) the greater the risk of implant failure. McCormack et al. have suggested that analysis of preoperative x-rays and CT scan morphology according to their load-sharing classification be used to predict the requirement for primary anterior column reconstruction to prevent this (22), and Oner et al. have suggested that careful preoperative analysis of preoperative MRI data may be of similar benefit (40).

With additional anterior column support procedures done from an anterior approach, implant failure can be essentially eliminated as reported by McLain (25), Sar and Bilen (4), and McCormack et al. (22).

Infection

The late presentation of infection after spine instrumentation is an unusual event (72). The real frequency is unknown, with risk presumably increased in patients with neurologic compromise who experience increased risk of urosepsis and skin breakdown.

Management is according to the principles of treating any orthopedic implant–related infection. Infected hardware is removed. Any abscess cavity is débrided, drained, and redébrided serially until clean. Large cavities may require closure/coverage with a tissue flap. Culture-specific antibiotics are administered until infection is eradicated and all wounds fully healed. If necessary, stability should be reconstituted through an alternative approach working through noninfected tissue planes.

Reoperation for Prominent or Painful Hardware

Implants used to repair fractures of the spine, like any fracture stabilization device, can occasionally cause pain and require elective removal. The frequency of this phenomenon is again not well described. The practice in many centers, particularly in Europe (7,11,21), is to undertake routine implant removal at relatively short-term. Although this might avoid the problem, it may result in unnecessary operations.

In elective lumbar reconstruction, Lonstein's review of data on almost 1,000 cases suggests approximately 20% of pedicle screw implants eventually become painful and require removal (73).

In thoracolumbar trauma, Carl et al. had to remove 3% of their implants for reasons of pain (74), whereas McLain et al. found that 6% of their implants became painful and required removal (25).

Neurotropic Spine

In the paraplegic patient, the spine may be effectively denervated and Charcot-type arthropathy can develop. This may be analogous to the problematic feet of diabetic patients with peripheral neuropathy, but it seems much more rare. The literature to date cannot provide an exact frequency. This condition often presents perhaps unexpectedly in the denervated paraplegic patient, with poorly localized pain and disability that can progress to include sitting imbalance, gibbus, and ulceration secondary to progressive deformity of the spine. Imaging shows a massively destructive hypertrophic spondylosis. The differential diagnosis should include osteomyelitis.

This condition was once thought to be caused by the concentration of mechanical stresses below a long fracture implant construct, but it has been observed to occur remote to any surgical site and in patients who have not had surgical fracture repair.

Treatment is complicated by the extreme biomechanical forces and unprotected loading that these spines experience, unprotected by active muscular balance or pain inhibition of extremes of motion. Also, disuse osteopenia in the paraplegic spine may compromise implant fixation. Stabilization should include rigid segmental fixation with a long, circumferential fusion and is ideally supplemented by external support (75). Consideration may be given to extending fusion to the pelvis to prevent recurrence or "transitional syndrome," but the ensuing loss of lumbopelvic mobility has implications to sitting balance and transfer capability that may be equally profound (76).

Spondylosis

Any possibly accelerated probability of degenerative spondylosis after spine fracture is to date not reported in the literature.

Furderer et al. studied the MRI morphology of discs adjacent to fractured end-plates after elective implant removal at 10 months and found no consistent deterioration, arguing against routine interbody fusion (11). The inference here is that premature spondylosis (i.e., disc degeneration) was not consistently detectable at 10 months.

REFERENCES

1. El-Awad AA, Othman W, Al-Moutaery KR. Treatment of thoracolumbar fractures. *Saudi Med J* 2002;23(6):689–694.
2. Mohanty SP, Venkatram N. Does neurological recovery in thoracolumbar and lumbar burst fractures depend on the extent of canal compromise? *Spinal Cord* 2002;40(6):295–299.
3. Reyes-Sanchez A, Rosales LM, Miramontes VP, et al. Treatment of thoracolumbar burst fractures by vertebral shortening. *Eur Spine J* 2002;11(1):8–12.
4. Sar C, Bilen FE. Thoracolumbar flexion-distraction injuries combined with vertebral body fractures. *Am J Orthop* 2002;31(3):147–151.
5. Illes T, de Jonge T, Doman I, et al. Surgical correction of the late consequences of posttraumatic spinal disorders. *J Spinal Disord Tech* 2002;15(2):127–132.
6. Yu X, Liang G, Chai Y. Diagnosis and treatment of spinal fractures combined with paraplegia and diaphragm injury. *Chin J Traumatol* 2001;4(3):168–171.
7. Leferink VJ, Zimmerman KW, Veldhuis EF, et al. Thoracolumbar spinal fractures: radiological results of transpedicular fixation combined with transpedicular cancellous bone graft and posterior fusion in 183 patients. *Eur Spine J* 2001;10(6):517–523.
8. Alanay A, Acaroglu E, Yacizi M, et al. The effect of transpedicular intracorporeal grafting in the treatment of thoracolumbar burst fractures on canal remodeling. *Eur Spine J* 2001;10(6):512–516.
9. Vaccaro AR, Silber JS. Post-traumatic spinal deformity. *Spine* 2001;26[24 Suppl]:S111–S118.
10. Belmont PJ Jr, Taylor KF, Mason KT, et al. Incidence, epidemiology, and occupational outcomes of thoracolumbar fractures among U.S. Army aviators. *J Trauma* 2001;50(5):855–861.
11. Furderer S, Wenda K, Thiem N, et al. Traumatic intervertebral disc lesion—magnetic resonance imaging as a criterion for or against intervertebral fusion. *Eur Spine J* 2001;10(2):154–163.
12. Nakamura H, Yamano Y, Seki M, et al. Use of folded vascularized rib graft in anterior fusion after treatment of thoracic and upper lumbar lesions. Technical note. *J Neurosurg* 2001:94[2Suppl]:323–327.
13. Vanderschot P, Caluwe G, Lateur L, et al. The use of "hybrid" allografts in the treatment of fractures of the thoracolumbar spine: first experience. *Eur Spine J* 2001;10(1):64–68.
14. Wessberg P, Wang Y, Irstam L, et al. The effect of surgery and remodeling on spinal canal measurements after thoracolumbar burst fractures. *Eur Spine J* 2001;10(1):55–63.
15. Inaba K, Kirkpatrick AW, Finkelstein J, et al. Blunt abdominal aortic trauma in association with thoracolumbar spine fractures. *Injury* 2001;32(3):201–207.
16. Vaccaro AR, Nachwalter RS, Klein GR, et al. The significance of thoracolumbar spinal canal size in spinal cord injury patients. *Spine* 2001;26(4):371–376.
17. Dai LY. Remodeling of the spinal canal after thoracolumbar burst fractures. *Clin Orthop* 2001;(382):119–123.
18. Knop C, Fabian HF, Bastian L, et al. Late results of thoracolumbar fractures after posterior instrumentation and transpedicular bone grafting. *Spine* 2001;26(1):88–99.
19. Shen WJ, Liu TJ, Shen YS. Nonoperative treatment versus posterior fixation for thoracolumbar junction burst fractures without neurological deficit. *Spine* 2001;26(9):1038–1045.
20. Stancic MF, Gregorovic E, Nozica E, et al. Anterior decompression and fixation versus posterior reposition and semirigid fixation in the treatment on unstable burst thoracolumbar fracture: prospective clinical trial. *Croat Med J* 2001;42(1):49–53.
21. Alanay A, Acaroglu E, Yazici M, et al. Short-segment pedicle instrumentation of thoracolumbar burst fractures: does transpedicular intracorporeal grafting prevent early failure? *Spine* 2001;26(2):213–217.
22. McCormack T, Karaikovic E, Gaines RW. The load sharing classification of spine fractures. *Spine* 1994;19(15):1741–1744.
23. Daniaux H, Seykora P, Genelin A, et al. Application of posterior plating and modifications in thoracolumbar spine injuries. Indications, techniques, results. *Spine* 1991;16[3 Suppl]:S125–S133.
24. Bednar DA, Ali P, Berumen E. Comparative survivorship of the AO internal fixator and Rogozinski constructs in elective adult spinal reconstruction. Canadian Orthopaedic Association. Minutes of the 49th Annual Meeting, Winnipeg, Manitoba, 1994:122.
25. McLain RF, Burkus JK, Benson DR. Segmental instrumentation for thoracic and thoracolumbar fractures: prospective analysis of construct survival and five-year follow-up. *Spine J* 2001;1:310–323.
26. Bolesta MJ, Bohlmann HH. Late sequelae of thoracolumbar fractures and fracture-dislocations: surgical treatment. In: Frymoyer JW, et al., eds, *The adult spine: principles and practice.* Philadelphia: Lippincott–Raven, 1997:1513–1533.
27. White AA III, Panjabi MM. The problem of clinical instability in the human spine: a systematic approach. In: White AA III et al., eds. *Clinical biomechanics of the spine*, 2nd ed. Philadelphia: JB Lippincott, 1990:277–278.
28. DeVivo MJ, Kartus PL, Rutt RD, et al. The influence of age at time of spinal cord injury on rehabilitation outcome. *Arch Neurol* 1990;47:687–691.
29. Denis F, Armstrong GW, Serls K, et al. Acute thoracolumbar burst fractures in the absence of neurologic deficit: a comparison between operative and non-operative treatment. *Clin Orthop* 1984:189;142–149.
30. Burnham RS, Warren SA, Saboe LA, et al. Factors predicting employment 1 year after traumatic spine fracture. *Spine* 1996;21(9):1066–1071.
31. Gertzbein SD. Scoliosis Research Society: multicenter spine fracture study. *Spine* 1992;17:528–540.
32. Sledge JB, Allen D, Hyman J. Use of magnetic resonance imaging in evaluating injuries to the pediatric thoracolumbar spine. *J Paediatric Orthop* 2001;21(3):288–293.
33. Banse X, Devogelter JP, Munting E, et al. Inhomogeneity of human vertebral cancellous bone: systematic density and structure patterns inside the vertebral body. *Bone* 2001;28(5):563–571.

34. Bernhardt M, Bridwell KH. Segmental analysis of the sagittal plane alignment of the normal thoracic and lumbar spines and the thoracolumbar junction. *Spine* 1989:14:717–721.
35. Kuklo TR, Polly DW, Owens BD, et al. Measurement of thoracic and lumbar fracture kyphosis: evaluation of intraobserver, interobserver, and technique variability. *Spine* 2001;26(1):61–65.
36. Polly DW Jr, Klemme WR, Shawen S. Management options for the treatment of posttraumatic thoracolumbar kyphosis. *Semin Spine Surg* 2000;12:110–116.
37. Bednar DA, Berumen E, Ali P, et al. The AO internal fixator for fractures: alternative techniques of reduction and bone grafting. North American Spine Society. Minutes of the 9th Annual Meeting, Minneapolis, MN, 1994:172.
38. Esses SI, Botsford DJ, Wright T, et al. Operative treatment of spinal fractures with the AO internal fixator. *Spine* 1991;16[3 Suppl]:S146–S150.
39. Bednar DA. Experience with the "Fixateur Interne": initial clinical results. *J Spinal Disord* 1992;5(1):93–96.
40. Oner FC, van Gils AP, Faber JA, et al. Some complications of common treatment schemes of thoracolumbar spine fractures can be predicted with magnetic resonance imaging: prospective study of 53 patients with 71 fractures. *Spine* 2002;27(5):543–548.
41. Butterman GR, Glazer PA, Hu SS, et al. Anterior and posterior allografts in symptomatic thoracolumbar deformity. *J Spinal Disord* 2001;14(1):54–66.
42. Knop C, Lange U, Bastian L, et al. Biomechanical compression tests with a new implant for thoracolumbar vertebral body replacement. *Eur Spine J* 2001;10(1):30–37.
43. Vaccaro AR, Cirello J. The use of autograft bone and cages in fractures of the cervical, thoracic and lumbar spine. *Clin Orthop* 2002;394:19–26.
44. Polly DW Jr, Klemme WR, Shawen S. Management options for the treatment of posttraumatic thoracolumbar kyphosis. *Semin Spine Surg* 2000;12:110–116.
45. Malcolm BW, Bradford DS, Winter RB, et al. Posttraumatic kyphosis: a review of forty-eight surgically treated patients. *J Bone Joint Surg* 1981;63(A):891–899.
46. Robertson JR, Whitesides TE Jr. Surgical reconstruction of late posttraumatic thoracolumbar kyphosis. *Spine* 1985;10:307–312.
47. Shufflebarger HL, Clarke CE. Thoracolumbar osteotomy for postsurgical sagittal imbalance. *Spine* 1992;17[suppl]:287–290.
48. O'Dowd J. Spine. In: Rüedi TP, Murray WM, eds. *AO principles of fracture management*. New York: Thieme, 2000.
49. McLain RF, Sparling E, Benson DR. Early failure of short-segment pedicle instrumentation for thoracolumbar fractures. A preliminary report. *J Bone Joint Surg* 1993;75(2):162–167.
50. Lagrone MO, Bradford DS, Moe JH, et al. Treatment of symptomatic flatback after spinal fusion. *J Bone Joint Surg* 1988;70(A):569–580.
51. Kostuik JP, Maurais GR, Richardson WJ, et al. Combined single-stage anterior and posterior osteotomy for correction of iatrogenic lumbar kyphosis. *Spine* 1988;13:257–266.
52. Burchiel KJ, Hsu FPK. Pain and spasticity after spinal cord injury: mechanisms and treatment. *Spine* 2001;26[24 Suppl]:S146–S160.
53. Colterjohn N, Bednar DA. Procurement of bone graft from the iliac crest: an operative approach with decreased morbidity. *J Bone Joint Surg* 1997;79(A):756–760.
53a. Goulet JA, Senunas LE, DeSilva GL, et al. Autogenous iliac crest bone graft. Complications and functional assessment. *Clin Orthop* 1997;339:76–81.
53b. Robertson PA, Wray AC. Natural history of posterior iliac crest bone graft donation for spinal surgery: a prospective analysis of morbidity. *Spine* 2001;6(13):1473–1476.
54. Frymoyer JW, Howe J, Kuhlmann D. The long term effects of spinal fusion on the sacroiliac joint and the ileum. *Clin Orthop* 1978;134:196–201.
55. Yahiro MA. Comprehensive literature review. Pedicle screw fixation devices. *Spine* 1994;19(S20):S2274–S2278.
56. Yuan HA, Garfin SR, Dickman CA, et al. A historical cohort study of pedicle screw fixation in thoracic, lumbar and sacral spinal fusions. *Spine* 1994;19(S20):S2279–S2296.
57. Brown PJ, Marino RJ, Herbison GJ, et al. The 72-hour examination as a predictor of recovery in motor complete quadriplegia. *Arch Phys Med Rehabil* 1991;72:546–548.
58. Burns AS, Ditunno JF. Establishing prognosis and maximizing functional outcomes after spinal cord injury. *Spine* 2001;26[24 Suppl]:S137–S145.
59. Waters RL, Yakura JS, Adkins RH, et al. Recovery following complete paraplegia. *Arch Phys Med Rehabil* 1992;73:784–789.
60. Waters RL, Adkins RH, Yakura JS, et al. Motor and sensory recovery following incomplete paraplegia. *Arch Phys Med Rehabil* 1994;75:67–72.
61. Waters RL, Adkins RH, Yakura JS. Definition of complete spinal injury. *Paraplegia* 1991;29;573–581.
62. *International standards for neurological classification of spinal cord injury*. Chicago: American Spinal Injury Association, 2000.
63. Burns AS, Rivas DA, DiTunno JF. The management of neurogenic bladder and sexual dysfunction after spinal cord injury. *Spine* 2001;26[24 Suppl]:S129–S136.
64. Stone AR. The sexual needs of the inured spinal cord patient. *Probl Urol* 1987;3:529–536.
65. Sipski ML, Alexander CJ, Rosen R. Sexual arousal and orgasm in women: effects of spinal cord injury. *Ann Neurol* 2001;49:35–44.
66. Burns AB, Jackson AB. Gynaecologic and reproductive issues in women with spinal cord injury. *Phys Med Rehabil Clin North Am* 2001:12:183–199.
67. Ohl DA, McCabe M, Sonksen J, et al. Management of infertility in spinal cord injury. *Top Spinal Cord Injury Rehabil* 1996;1:65–75.
68. Sonksen J, Biering-Sorenson F. Fertility in men with spinal cord or cauda equina lesions. *Semin Neurol* 1992;12:106–114.
69. Bohlmann HH, Kirkpatrick JS, Delamarter RB, et al. Anterior decompression for late paralysis after fractures of the thoracolumbar spine. *Clin Orthop* 1994;300:24–29.
70. Lee TT, Alameda GJ, Camilo E, et al. Surgical treatment of post traumatic myelopathy associated with syringomyelia. *Spine* 2001;26[24 Suppl]:S119–S127.
71. Mumford J, Weinstein JN, Spratt KF, et al. Thoracolumbar burst fractures. The clinical efficacy and outcome of nonoperative management. *Spine* 1993;18(8):955–970.
72. Clark CE, Shufflebarger HC. Late developing infection in instrumented idiopathic scoliosis. *Spine* 1999;24:1909.
73. Lonstein JE, Denis F, Perra JH, et al. Complications associated with pedicle screws. *J Bone Joint Surg* 1999;81(A);11:1519–1528.
74. Carl AL, Tromanhauser SG, Roger DJ. Pedicle screw instrumentation for thoracolumbar burst fractures and fracture-dislocations. *Spine* 1992;17[8 Suppl]:S317–S324.
75. Sobel JW, Bohlmann HH, Freehaufer AA. Charcot's arthropathy of the spine following spinal cord injury: a report of 5 cases. *J Bone Joint Surg* 1985;76(A):771–776.
76. Brown CW, Jones B, Donaldson DH, et al. Neuropathic (Charcot) arthropathy of the spine after traumatic spinal paraplegia. *Spine* 1992;17(6S):S103–S108.

CHAPTER 43

Thoracic Disc Disease and Myelopathy

Theodore A. Belanger and Sanford E. Emery

Thoracic disc disease is an uncommon clinical manifestation of a common degenerative process that presents as axial back pain, radiculopathy, or myelopathy. Heightened awareness and improved imaging technology have aided in more accurate and timely diagnosis, although it remains a clinical challenge. Thoracic myelopathy may present in the context of an isolated thoracic disc herniation; degenerative stenosis of the thoracic spinal canal; or from other pathologic entities, including congenital, infectious, neoplastic, and traumatic processes. This chapter focuses on thoracic disc disease and thoracic spinal stenosis as causes of myelopathy.

Treatment of thoracic myelopathy is generally surgical, with approaches directed at complete decompression of neural impingement and strict avoidance of any manipulation of the spinal cord to reduce the risk of iatrogenic paralysis. Treatment of thoracic disc disease and thoracic stenosis can yield excellent results, although it is associated with some risk to the patient.

HISTORICAL BACKGROUND

The first case report of thoracic disc disease associated with myelopathy was published in 1838 by Key (1). In 1911, Middleton and Teacher described a patient who died of complications related to paraplegia resulting from a large, central disc herniation at the thoracolumbar junction (2). The first surgery for herniated thoracic disc was performed in 1922 by Adson and later reported in 1931 by Elsberg (3). Adson performed a laminectomy and discectomy with improvement of the patient's symptoms. Since then, many publications have noted a high frequency of surgical complications, particularly paraplegia and death associated with laminectomy (4–6). Benjamin reviewed 206 patients with thoracic radiculopathy (23 patients) or myelopathy (183 patients) treated with a posterior laminectomy approach. Approximately one-half of the patients were improved after surgery, but one-sixth of patients were no better off and one-third were made worse (4).

Because of the dismal results of the laminectomy for thoracic discectomy, numerous anterior, lateral, and posterolateral approaches to the thoracic intervertebral disc have been developed. In 1960, Hulme reported six cases of thoracic disc herniation treated with a costotransversectomy approach—originally described by Menard for treatment of Pott's disease. In this small series, the outcomes were superior to laminectomy, (7) and later this experience was been shared by other authors (8–12). Larson described a lateral extracavitary approach that is akin to the costotransversectomy method (11–13). Crafoord et al. described the first transthoracic discectomy in 1959 (14). The transthoracic approach was used by Perot and Munro (15), as well as Ransohoff and associates (16). They simultaneously reported their experiences in 1969, establishing that approach as an alternative to costotransversectomy for anterior thoracic spinal cord decompression. Another method was the transpedicular approach, originally described in 1978 by Patterson and Arbit, as well as other variations on the posterolateral approach (17–20). Numerous specialized surgical approaches were then designed to access the upper thoracic spine (21). Bohlman and Zdeblick reported good and excellent results in 16 of 19 thoracic disc patients treated with various anterior exposures for decompression. They recommended the thoracotomy approach over costotransversectomy owing to improved visualization. Also, postoperative neurologic complications occurred in two patients who had costotransversectomy approaches (8). In 1993, Mack et al. reported the use of video-assisted thoracoscopy (VATS) for removal of intervertebral discs (22). Other authors have since validated this technique (23,24).

In 1998, Fessler and Sturgill compared the various surgical approaches for thoracic discectomy and concluded that all of the described surgical approaches to the thoracic disc are viable with the exception of laminectomy, which is associated with an unacceptably high risk of neurologic injury (25). Similarly, Mulier and Dubois compared the various surgical approaches, and concluded that the severity and rates of morbidity were similar among the various posterolateral, lateral, and anterior approaches to the thoracic spine. However, the anterior transthoracic approach was associated with the highest rate of postoperative neurologic improvement (93% vs. 80 to 87% in 331 reported cases) (26). Both papers concluded mortality had been essentially eliminated after abandonment of the laminectomy approach. Neither of these papers addressed the emerging technique of VATS discectomy, however.

In comparison to thoracic disc herniation, the literature concerning thoracic stenosis consists mainly of case reports and small series, with only a few long-term follow-up studies of patients treated surgically (27). Marzluff et al. were the first to report on thoracic stenosis secondary to facet joint arthrosis in 1979 (28). They described four patients with thoracic myelopathy successfully treated surgically with a posterior decompression. Barnett et al. described six patients treated for thoracic stenosis with laminectomy and partial medial facetectomy in 1987 (29). Most recently, Palumbo et al. reported 12 patients treated surgically, anteriorly or posteriorly depending on the location of greatest neurologic compression (30). Eight patients were treated with laminectomy, and four were treated with anterior discectomy by various approaches. Satisfactory early results were achieved, though several patients went on to require further spinal surgery for various late problems, such as recurrence of stenosis and instability. Also in 2001, Chang et al. reported 28 cases of thoracic spinal stenosis with myelopathy (31). Most of their patients had ossification of the ligamentum flavum or posterior longitudinal ligament, which was not a prevalent finding in the other case reports that did not involve an Asian population.

INCIDENCE AND PREVALENCE

The true incidence and prevalence of thoracic disc disease complicated by radiculopathy or myelopathy (or both) is unknown. Asymptomatic thoracic disc herniation may be as prevalent as 15 to 37% (32,33). Love and Kiefer suggested thoracic disc herniation was the cause of symptoms in 2 per 1,000 patients with back pain (34). Surgery for thoracic disc herniations has been estimated to comprise approximately 0.15 to 1.80% of all disc excisions (8,35), meaning that a surgeon would expect to perform approximately 55 to 650 cervical and lumbar discectomies for every thoracic discectomy performed.

Thoracic stenosis is even less frequently encountered. Strict prevalence data are not available, but the paucity of case reports in the literature speaks to the rarity of thoracic stenosis in clinical practice. Palumbo et al.'s series reported only 12 cases over a 14-year period (30). Only four of these patients had isolated thoracic spinal stenosis; the remainder had concurrent lumbar stenosis in continuity with their stenotic lower thoracic spine. In Barnett et al.'s series, six patients were encountered over a 2-year period at two major centers (29).

ETIOLOGY

Most authors favor a degenerative process as the cause of thoracic disc herniation (Fig. 1). This is supported by their predominant occurrence at the same levels that degenerative changes are most often found (i.e., the thoracolumbar junction). Case reports of thoracic disc disease coexisting in patients with Scheuermann's kyphosis exist, but the pathophysiology of that relationship is unclear (36,37). Trauma is often a part of the history given by the patient, but it is often difficult to confirm as the cause of the herniation or symptoms (4,9,34,38).

Spinal stenosis in the thoracic region is certainly much less common than in the cervical and lumbar spine. It has been recognized in the context of various generalized disorders, including achondroplasia, osteochondrodystrophy, Paget's disease, diffuse idiopathic skeletal hyperostosis (39), and renal osteodystrophy (30). It has also been reported in association with localized spinal conditions including degenerative spondylosis (Figs. 2 and 3), ossification of the posterior longitudinal ligament (31,40), and ossification of the ligamentum flavum (41,42). Thoracic stenosis likely has a degenerative etiology similar to lumbar stenosis, supported by the common coexistence of the two (43). Barnett et al. suggested a congenital con-

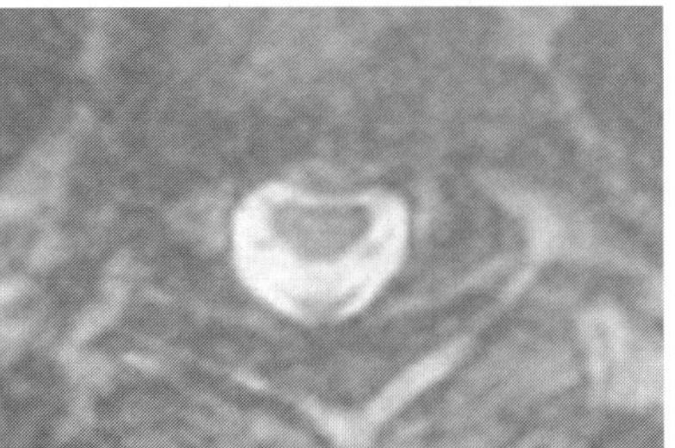

A

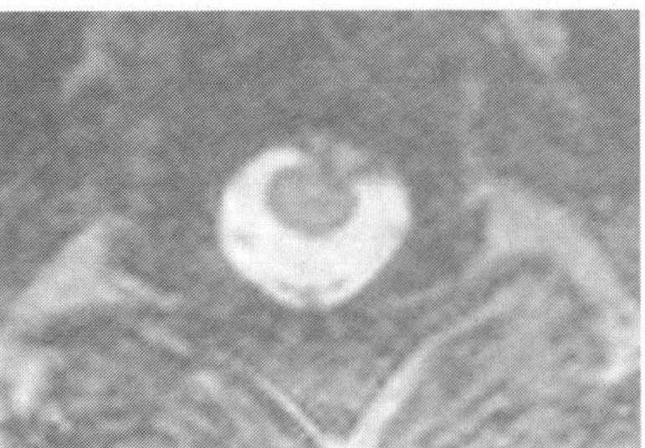

B

FIG. 1. A: Magnetic resonance imaging (MRI) scan showing a centrally herniated intervertebral disc at T7-8 causing spinal cord deformation. **B:** MRI scan showing a left paracentrally herniated intervertebral disc at T8-9 with deformation of the spinal cord. These images are from the same patient, who presented with a 4-year history of thoracic radiculopathy from these adjacent-level herniated thoracic discs. He had no clinical evidence of myelopathy.

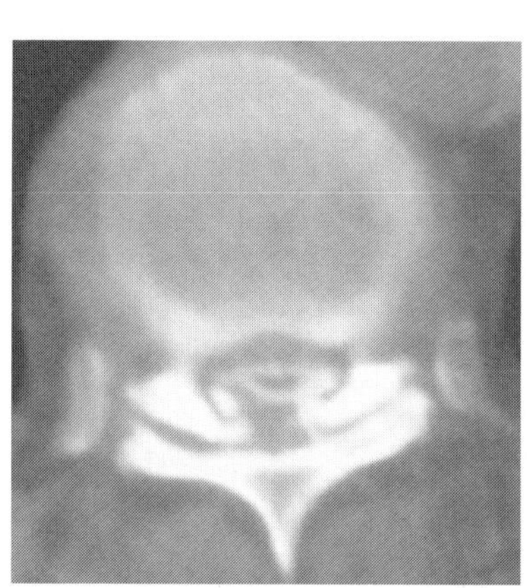
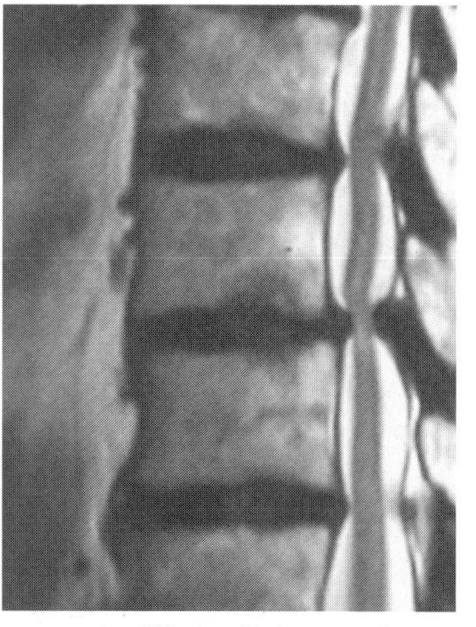
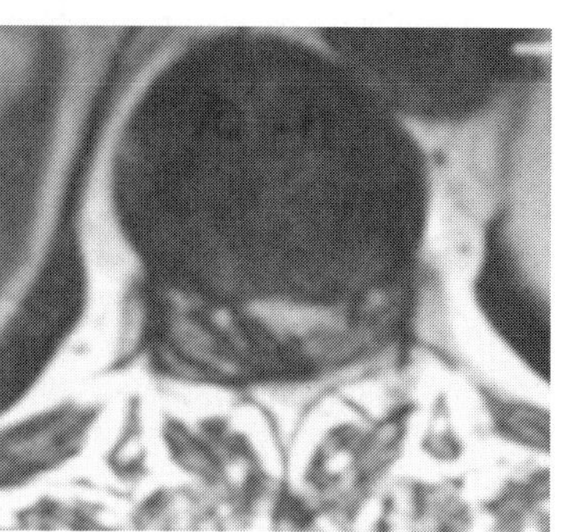

A–C

FIG. 2. Post-myelogram computed tomography **(A)**, sagittal magnetic resonance imaging (MRI) **(B)**, and axial MRI views **(C)** of a thoracic segment showing moderate ligamentum flavum and bilateral facet hypertrophy, disc bulging, and spinal cord deformation in a patient with myelopathy from thoracic spinal stenosis. Note the circumferential pathoanatomy that encroaches on the spinal cord.

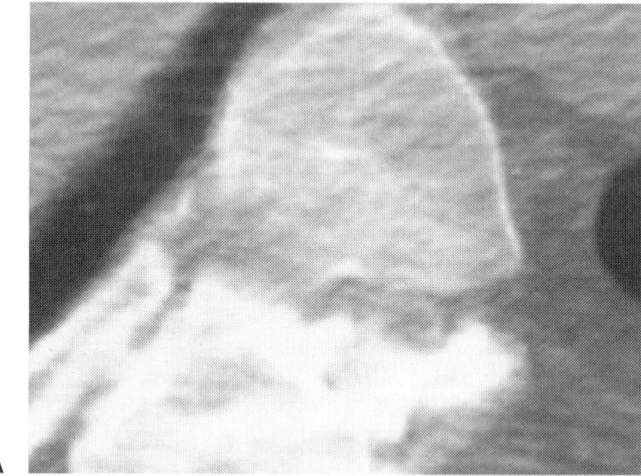

A

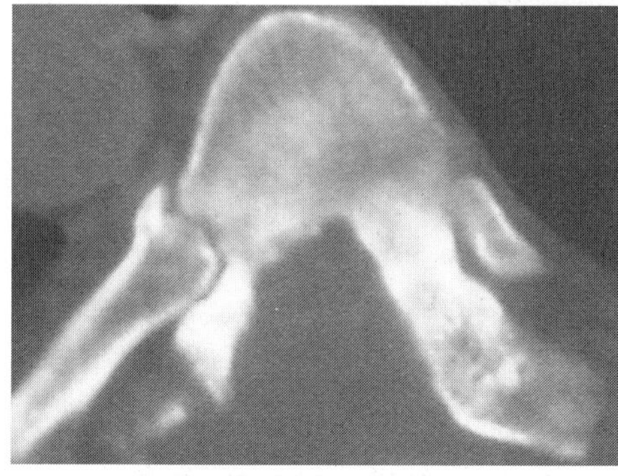

B

FIG. 3. A: Post-myelogram computed tomography (CT) scan of the ninth thoracic vertebra showing severe displacement and compression of the spinal cord from profound, asymmetric facet hypertrophy. This patient presented with radicular flank pain, paraparesis, and a sensory deficit up to T-8. Because compression of the spinal cord was mainly from posterior structures, this patient was decompressed posteriorly with wide laminectomies and partial facetectomies at each involved level. **B:** Postoperative CT scan showing wide decompression of previously severely stenotic thoracic segment.

tribution to thoracic stenosis, which may make some patients more susceptible to neurologic compression by degenerative posterolateral structures (29).

PATHOPHYSIOLOGY

Direct pressure on the spinal cord by thoracic disc herniation can cause local vascular compromise, which can result in impairment of nerve tissue function. Several anatomic features of the thoracic spine may predispose the spinal cord to compromise by a disc herniation. These features include the watershed nature of the blood supply to the midthoracic spinal cord (44), tethering of the spinal cord by the dentate ligaments, physiologic kyphosis of the thoracic spine with draping of the spinal cord over the vertebral bodies and discs, and the relative size of the spinal cord in relation to the spinal canal in the thoracic region, leaving little room for intrusive disc fragments. The contribution of local vascular compromise is supported clinically by the observance of neurologic dysfunction several levels above the area of compression in many case reports, as well as the failure of some patients to improve after adequate decompression (45).

Experimental support for the vascular theory of spinal cord dysfunction has been provided by Doppman and Girton. They performed posterior decompression in animals with experimentally induced spinal cord compression and observed their neurologic recovery and blood flow dynamics. They showed reversal of neurologic deficit despite significant cord distortion in animals with restored normal arteriovenous hemodynamics, and paraplegia in those animals that failed to recover venous or arterial flow (46). Kikuchi et al. described 20 patients with neurogenic claudication secondary to thoracic or cervical spinal stenosis. In their series, they performed selective angiography on nine patients with myelopathy, all of whom demonstrated immediate relief of claudication symptoms. Neurologic improvement lasted from 2 weeks to 6 months after angiography (47).

There are some differences between herniated intervertebral discs in the thoracic spine and those of the cervical and lumbar regions that need to be considered by the treating physician. Thoracic discs tend to herniate more centrally than lumbar or cervical discs. This may dictate the surgeon's choice of surgical approach (i.e., posterolateral approach for a more laterally positioned disc herniation, versus thoracotomy for a central herniation). Thoracic disc herniations are also known to calcify more frequently (48). They can also be adherent to, or even penetrate through, the dura mater. This event is uncommon, however, accounting for 1 to 4% of cases (49–51). There is a relative tethering of the spinal cord and a small amount of space available around the spinal cord in the thoracic spine. The lack of any "forgiveness" of the thoracic dura, combined with a prolonged time period between herniation and surgical treatment, may result in erosion through the dura. When present, it may alter the surgeon's choice of surgical approach (i.e., thoracotomy) to provide improved visualization of the dura and the disc fragment.

NATURAL HISTORY

It is unknown how often an asymptomatic thoracic disc herniation progresses to causing symptoms. Wood et al. described 20 asymptomatic patients with thoracic disc protrusions of various sizes who were re-evaluated an average of 26 months later. All patients remained asymptomatic, and most of the disc herniations were smaller or unchanged on repeat magnetic resonance imaging (MRI) (40 of 48 disc herniations) (32). Patients with thoracic disc herniation and radiculopathy, without spinal cord dysfunction, may stabilize or resolve their symptoms without specific treatment. Brown et al. reported that only 15 of 55 patients with a total of 72 thoracic disc herniations required surgical intervention. Only two patients in their series had myelopathy, both of whom were treated surgically (38). It is generally felt that patients with established myelopathy secondary to disc herniation are not likely to spontaneously improve; occasionally progression can occur rapidly, but typically patients who progress do so over a long period of time.

The natural history of thoracic stenosis has not been extensively investigated. It is reasonable to assume that a patient with myelopathy from thoracic stenosis is no more likely to spontaneously improve with conservative treatment than a patient with cervical myelopathy or thoracic myelopathy from another cause. Therefore, surgical treatment is justified once the diagnosis is established if frank myelopathy is present.

CLINICAL PRESENTATION

Thoracic disc herniation can occur at virtually any age, but it is most common in the fourth through sixth decades. There is a slight male predominance. There is wide variation in the clinical presentation, and complaints are often vague. The hallmark symptom is back pain. This pain can be severe and is classically described as pain that "bores right through the chest" (4,52). Some patients point to their sternum or epigastrium, stating that the pain "goes right through," from back to front. Others describe a band-like pain that radiates along their chest wall or flank, in an intercostal nerve distribution. Involvement at lower thoracic levels may produce flank, abdominal, or groin pain. Coughing or positional changes (i.e., spinal extension) may exacerbate axial or radicular pain (53).

There is wide variation in the neurologic presentation, including pain, sensory disturbance/dysesthesias, motor disturbance, and, finally, bowel or bladder dysfunction (or both). The occasional patient has very little back or radicular pain but has lower-extremity sensory and/or motor deficit. Gait disturbance and upper-motor neuron deficits are found in the lower extremities in myelopathic patients. The upper extremities should be neurologically normal and asymptomatic. Because of the often vague description of pain in the chest, epigastrium, or flank, and the rarity of thoracic disc herniations, patients often have been diagnosed with—or even treated for—gallbladder disease, gastritis, gastric ulcers, angina, renal calculi, lumbar stenosis, lumbar herniated disc, pericardial cysts, multiple sclerosis, testicular disorders, and hip arthritis (8,54–57).

Seventy-five percent of herniated thoracic discs occur between T-8 and L-1 (8), but they have been reported at every thoracic level (8,52,58,59). Roughly 70% are central or centrolateral disc herniations (59), in contradistinction to cervical or lumbar disc herniations, which are more commonly posterolateral or foraminal. Herniation of discs above the conus medullaris may cause myelopathy. Lesions between T-11 and L-1 can compress the conus and cauda equina, potentially causing lower-extremity radiculopathy and sphincter disturbance. Disc herniations that are intradural have been reported but are a small subset of these patients (49–51). Multilevel disc herniations are not uncommon, representing 5 to 33% of surgically treated patients in some series (8,10,23,32,38,48,60).

Patients with thoracic stenosis present with neurogenic claudication, limited walking tolerance, back pain, and leg pain, much like lumbar stenosis patients. Radiculopathy from thoracic root impingement may produce radiating pain in the thorax, abdomen, flank, or groin. Symptoms may be asymmetric and may worsen with spinal extension. Bowel and/or bladder dysfunction—retention, frequency, incomplete evacuation, or incontinence—may be present as a result of compression of the conus medullaris between T-11 and L-2. Myelopathy with long-tract signs, gait disturbance, and weakness or spasticity (or both) in the lower extremities can occur when stenosis is present above the level of the conus medullaris. As noted previously, thoracic stenosis patients commonly also have clinically significant lumbar stenosis, which confounds the clinical picture.

DIAGNOSIS

The evaluation of thoracic disc herniation or stenosis includes correlating the clinical symptoms with a neurologic examination and neuroradiologic imaging, if indicated. When myelopathy is found, upper extremity or cervical involvement should be sought to rule out cervical disease as the underlying cause. In the absence of long-tract signs, it is easy to conclude that the patient has only a degenerative lumbar process to blame for their pain. Allowing patients to localize and describe their back pain in detail may guide the clinician to the correct diagnosis under these circumstances.

MRI is the key radiologic study to confirm the diagnosis and localize the level of pathology in patients suspected to have thoracic disc herniation (61) (Fig. 1) or stenosis (Figs. 2–4). MRI can differentiate between congenital, infectious, neoplastic, and

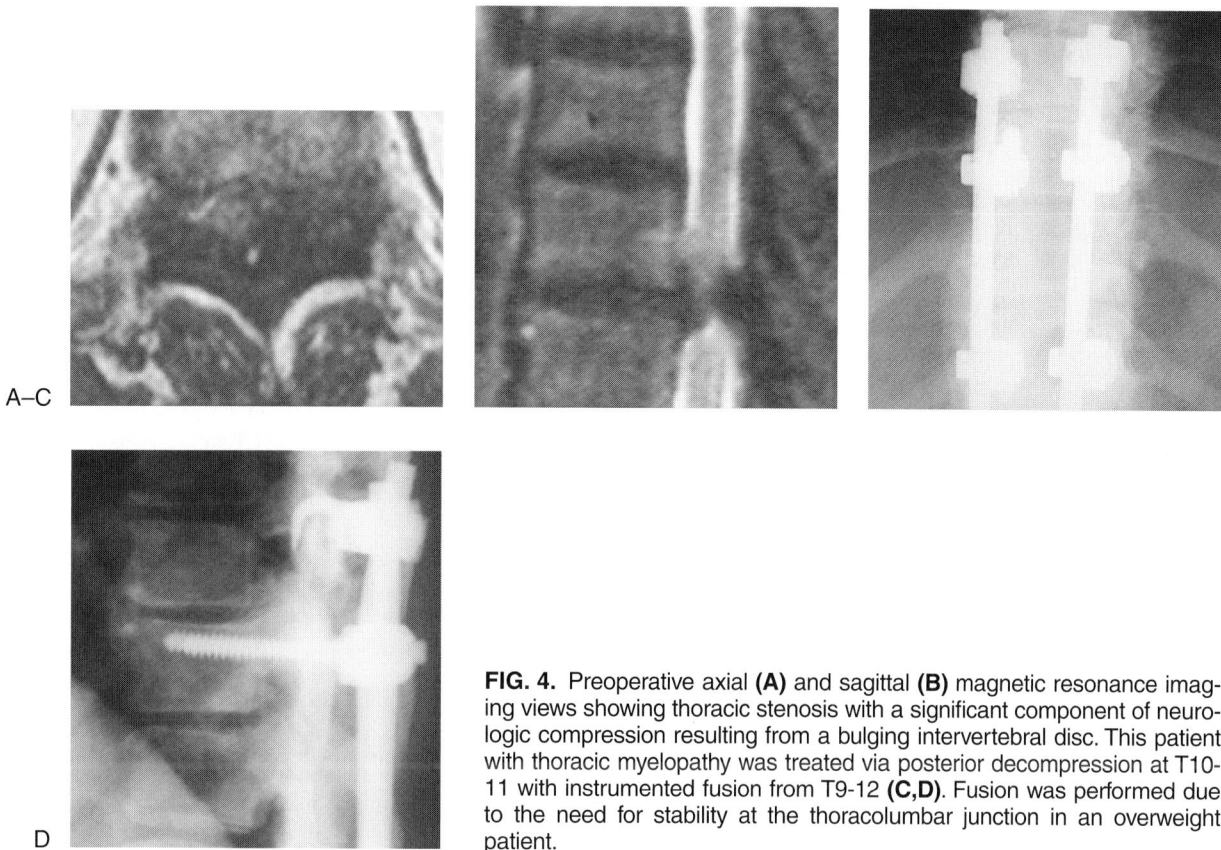

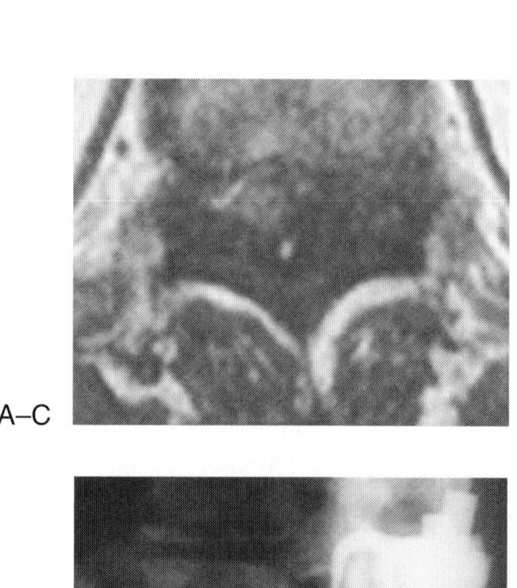
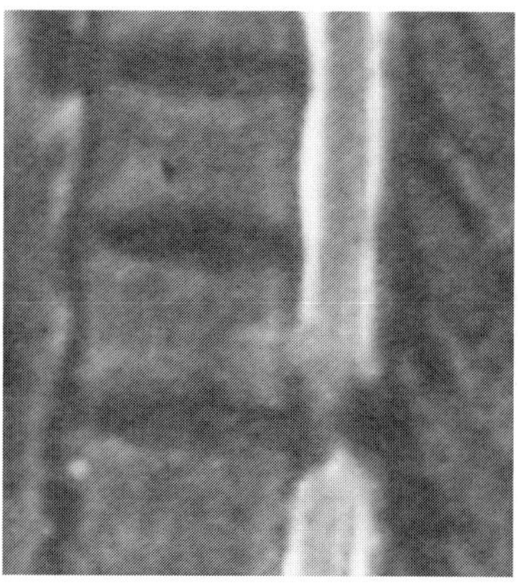
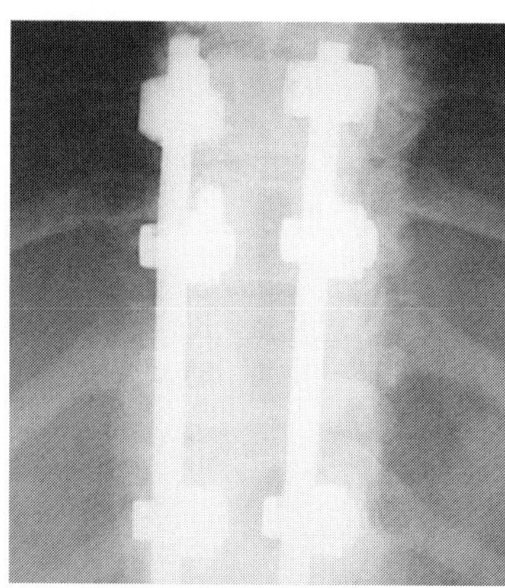

A–C

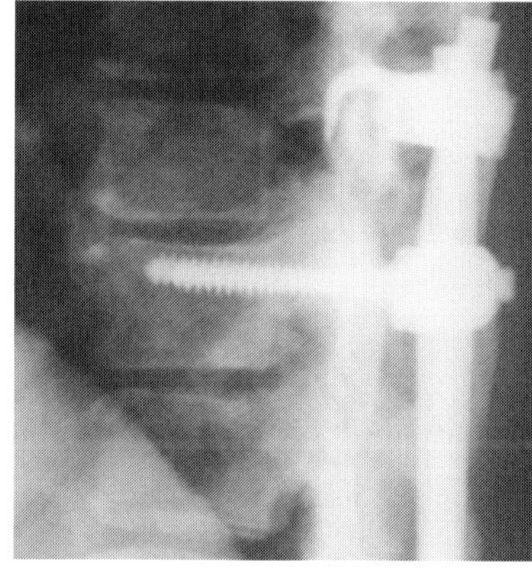

D

FIG. 4. Preoperative axial **(A)** and sagittal **(B)** magnetic resonance imaging views showing thoracic stenosis with a significant component of neurologic compression resulting from a bulging intervertebral disc. This patient with thoracic myelopathy was treated via posterior decompression at T10-11 with instrumented fusion from T9-12 **(C,D)**. Fusion was performed due to the need for stability at the thoracolumbar junction in an overweight patient.

degenerative processes. Intradural extension should be sought on MRI. Distortion of the thoracic spinal cord on MRI should also be sought, as this correlates best with a symptomatic disc herniation. A disc bulge without neurologic compression on MRI may be an incidental finding. Computed tomography–myelography is often helpful in delineating the degree of compression better than MRI. It can detail ossification of the posterior longitudinal ligament or ligamentum flavum, and it helps clarify if cord compression is more anterior (i.e., from disc or spondylophyte) or circumferential (i.e., from stenosis). The precise pathoanatomy is important in determining which surgical approach is most appropriate for treatment, and it is often useful to obtain an MRI and a computed tomography–myelogram for patients who are candidates for surgical treatment.

TREATMENT

In the absence of myelopathy, most patients with herniated thoracic discs can be treated conservatively (32,38). This is true for patients with back pain only and for those with mild radiculopathy. Options include intercostal nerve blocks; exercise therapy; and drug therapy with antiinflammatory, narcotic, or third-generation pain medicines, such as tricyclics, serotonin-reuptake inhibitors, and antiepileptics. Most surgeons take an operative approach to treatment when myelopathy or unremitting pain is present (8,52). When surgery is undertaken, it should be directed at the level(s) with confirmed deformation of the spinal cord on MRI.

As previously discussed, numerous surgical approaches have been used for thoracic discectomy (Table 1). A direct posterior laminectomy for discectomy is generally regarded as a poor option secondary to a dismally high rate of unimproved or worsened neurologic status in patients treated by this approach (i.e., 50%). Transthoracic, costotransversectomy, and transpedicular approaches can achieve the goal of discectomy without manipulation of the spinal cord. These approaches each carry their own risks and benefits, and they have not eliminated the risk of iatrogenic spinal cord injury from thoracic disc surgery. The transthoracic approach may be the most straightforward approach, with the highest likelihood of achieving neurologic benefit and a low frequency of serious complications (8). This is the preferred approach of the authors.

Excellent exposure across the entire disc space and wide decompression without manipulation of the spinal cord can be achieved with the anterior approach via a thoracotomy described in 1969 by Perot and Munro, and again in 1988 by Bohlman and Zdeblick (Fig. 5). A standard thoracotomy is performed, entering the chest one or two ribs above the level of the herniation. The rib head overlying the disc space of interest is resected, followed by removal of the base of the pedicle to visualize the dura. The dorsal one-half of each adjacent end-plate is removed with a burr all the way across the midline, leaving a shell of posterior cortex and protruding disc fragment up against the dura mater. The thin shell of posterior cortex and disc is then curetted downward into the cavity created in the vertebral bodies. Thus, careful and thorough decompression of the spinal canal can be achieved without manipulating the spinal cord. Also, by not entering the canal

TABLE 1. *Surgical approaches for thoracic disc excision*

Type of approach	Advantages	Disadvantages
Transthoracic	Best visualization completely across the spinal canal Easiest for bone graft placement if desired Multiple levels accessible	Morbidity of an open thoracotomy
Costotransversectomy	Avoids open thoracotomy Can address multiple levels	Difficult to visualize opposite side of canal; satisfactory for pathology located to one side of the midline If facet removed, ?need to fuse
Transpedicular	Avoids open thoracotomy	Cannot visualize middle or opposite side of canal; satisfactory approach for true posterolateral pathology Need to fuse in thoracolumbar region
Video-assisted thoracoscopic approach	Excellent visualization Smaller incisions than open thoracotomy	Steep learning curve Small number of myelopathy patients in literature

through the neuroforamen, the surgeon avoids violating the collateral blood flow to the spinal cord that can be found there. Only two patients in the series of nineteen had poor results, both due to postoperative paraparesis, and both of whom had costotransversectomies. They advocated the transthoracic approach with end-plate, posterior cortex, and disc resection, outlined previously (8). Currier et al. advocated the transthoracic approach for more central herniations, but supported the costotransversectomy approach for more laterally positioned lesions (62).

If considerable bone is removed, or if the lesion involves thoracolumbar junction, arthrodesis can be performed to prevent instability using rib or iliac crest strut grafting (63). The limited bony resection and the stabilizing effect of the rib cage often obviate the need for arthrodesis in the mid- and upper thoracic spine (8). Some surgeons believe fusion may help relieve axial back pain (62), but no study to better define the need for arthrodesis has been performed. When performing strut grafting, the authors' preferred method of postoperative treatment is with a thoracolumbosacral orthosis for 8 weeks to promote fusion. Instrumentation has not been found to be necessary in patients with normal sagittal alignment and without a laminectomy defect (63).

Intradural disc herniations are also best approached by a thoracotomy, as this provides the best visualization of the anterior dura. The surgical approach and extradural decompression are identical to that described previously for a dural defect, which needs to be addressed. At surgery a small rent in the anterior dura may be encountered, which can be extended to allow adequate exposure of the intruding disc fragment if necessary. Depending on the size of the resulting dural defect, it may be repaired primarily with suture or patched with a fascial graft. Adjuncts to dural repair, such as a lumbar subarachnoid drain, muscle or fat patch, Gelfoam, or fibrin glue, may be useful depending on the nature of the defect and the quality of the repair. The authors recommend strict bed rest for approximately 5 days to promote healing of the defect; persistent leakage empties into the chest cavity and may not be as obvious as in lumbar cases.

The costotransversectomy approach should also be in the armamentarium of the spine surgeon, as it may be preferable under certain circumstances, such as posterolateral disc herniations. Some patients may be medically unfit candidates for an open thoracotomy, whereas others may be undergoing a posterior procedure at the same time, making simultaneous anterior access from a posterior incision desirable. These approaches may also be preferred for the upper thoracic spine (T1-5), which is more difficult to expose anteriorly. A posterior curvilinear incision is made off of the midline on the side of the disc herniation. A plane is developed between the periscapular (trapezius, latissimus dorsi, rhomboids) and the erector spinae muscles. One to three rib heads are removed to allow wide visualization of the disc space of interest. Removal of one or more transverse processes may be necessary, thus making it a costotransversectomy. Intercostal neurovascular bundles are preserved, if practical. At times, they need to be sacrificed to facilitate exposure. The decompression/discectomy portion of the procedure is identical to that previously described for the thoracotomy approach, including pediculectomy, partial corpectomy, and so forth. The advantages of this approach are avoidance of an open thoracotomy, access to every level of the thoracolumbar spine, and the potential ability to perform a combined posterior procedure through the same incision. These approaches are not as useful as open thoracotomy for patients with central or intradural disc herniations, due to the inferior visualization across the entire canal.

A transpedicular approach is another choice for thoracic discectomy. It provides much more limited exposure than the anterior or lateral approaches described previously and is only suitable for posterolateral or foraminal herniations. Its main advantages include avoidance of thoracotomy, limited rib resection, ability to perform a simultaneous posterior procedure, and utility along the entire length of the thoracolumbar spine. Its disadvantages include limited access to the intervertebral disc and anterior dura and violation of the facet joint and neuroforamen.

Several series have appeared in the literature supporting the use of VATS for removal of thoracic disc herniations. Most of the experience reported is when there is an associated deformity or thoracic disc herniation in the absence of myelopathy (23). Anand et al. recently described their experience with VATS for thoracic disc disease in 100 patients (23). In their patient population of mainly nonmyelopathic individuals, they were able to achieve results with thoracoscopic discectomy that

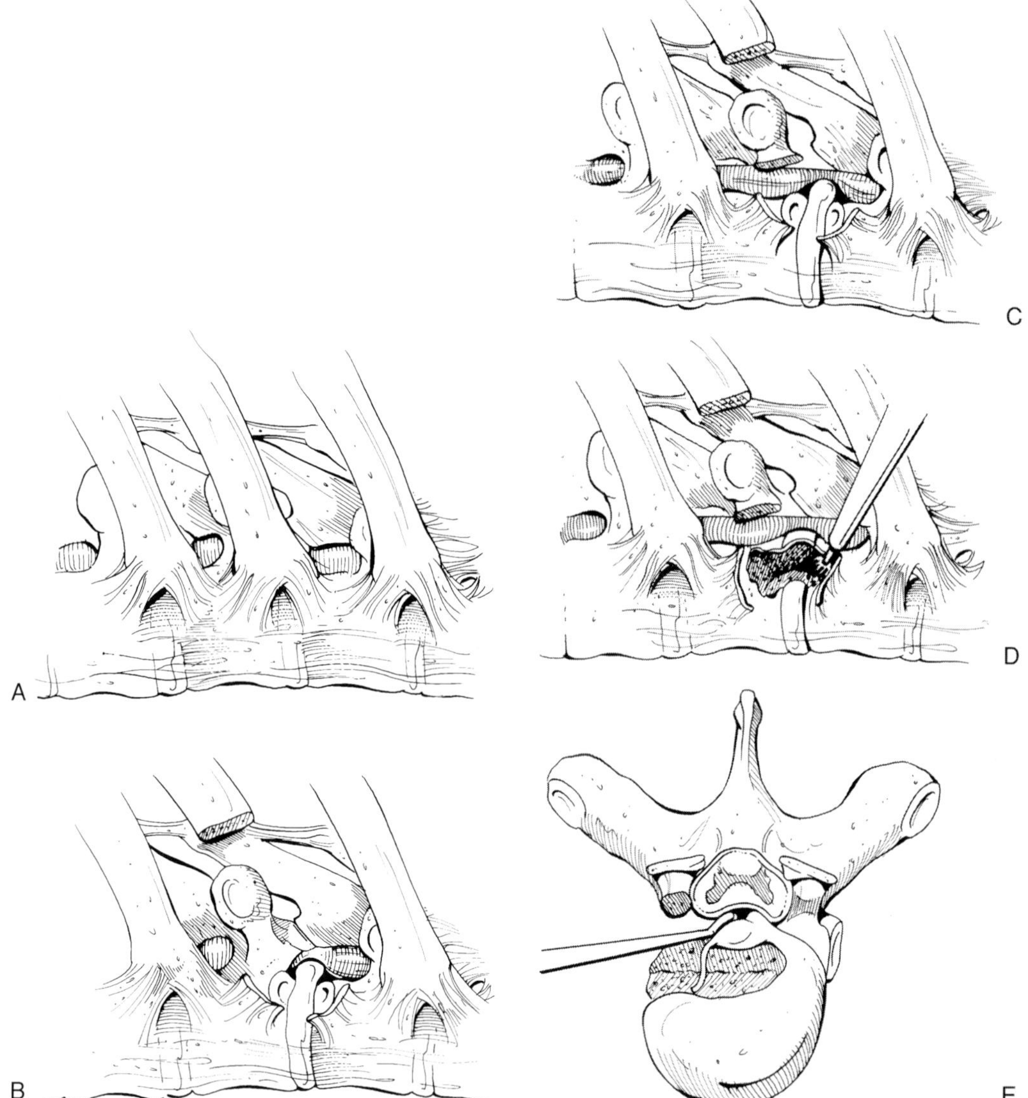

FIG. 5. Surgical technique for anterior thoracic spinal cord decompression as described by Zdeblick and Bohlman. Surgical exposure is via transthoracic, lateral extracavitary, or costotransversectomy approach **(A)**. When working above T-11, the rib heads lie over the intervertebral disc spaces, and must be subperiosteally dissected. The rib head is then removed, and the underlying pedicle is identified, projecting posterosuperiorly from the vertebral body, partially concealing the disc and spinal canal **(B)**. This is followed by excision of the pedicle, allowing clear visualization of the spinal canal and its relationship to the posterior vertebral cortices, disc, and offending disc fragment **(C)**. Next, a portion of the posterior vertebral bodies, end-plates, and discs are carefully removed, leaving a thin shell of posterior cortex, end-plate, and annulus anterior to the spinal cord **(D)**. This thin shell is then carefully and completely removed, curetting it into the cavity created in the previous step **(E)**. When decompression is carried out all the way to the opposite side, the contralateral pedicle can be palpated with an instrument.

were comparable to open thoracotomy techniques. The major advantage of this approach is avoidance of a larger open thoracotomy, which is associated with chest wall pain, shoulder dysfunction from shoulder girdle muscle transection, and longer hospitalization (64). Disadvantages of VATS include the need for significant experience with thoracoscopy before thorough visualization and decompression of the area of interest can be achieved reproducibly and reliably. This "learning curve" may result in prolonged operative times, as well as occasional conversion to formal open thoracotomy in a surgeon's early experience with this technique (23,24). A direct comparison of VATS and open thoracotomy for thoracic disc herniation associated with myelopathy has not been performed. As long as strict adherence to the major goals of complete neurologic decompression without spinal cord manipulation is observed, VATS treatment of thoracic disc herniation with associated myelopathy could prove to be a viable alternative to more surgically invasive techniques in appropriate hands.

SURGICAL TREATMENT OF THORACIC STENOSIS

Surgical treatment of degenerative thoracic stenosis may be anterior or posterior. In contrast to herniated thoracic discs, most patients with thoracic stenosis may be successfully treated via decompressive laminectomy (Fig. 3). An anterior decompression can be useful when most of the neurologic compression is occurring anterior to the spinal cord. A combined approach is rarely necessary, even in the face of severe circumferential compression. Such cases are best treated with laminectomy. In Palumbo et al.'s series, eight of twelve patients were treated with decompressive laminectomy, which included partial medial facetectomy (30). Of the remaining four, one patient had transthoracic discectomy, one had transthoracic two-level partial corpectomy, one had an anterolateral extrapleural discectomy, and one had a retroperitoneal discectomy at T-12 to L-1. All four who had anterior approaches were decompressed using the technique described by Bohlman and Zdeblick for excision of herniated thoracic discs. Using this algorithm, 8 of 10 patients with motor deficit improved in muscle strength, 7 of 11 patients with gait disturbance had improvement in ambulation, and 8 of 12 improved with respect to pain. In Barnett et al.'s series, all six patients were treated with posterior decompression (29). All six showed improvement of lower-extremity paresthesias, three of three had improvement in walking tolerance, three of three had improvement in weakness, and two of two had significant relief of pain (45). In Chang et al.'s series, 23 patients were treated by laminectomy, four by anterior approach, and one by a combined approach. Symptomatic improvement occurred in 22 of 28 patients, whereas two patients were unchanged and four patients were neurologically worse postoperatively. All of those who did not improve or were worse postoperatively had extensive ossification of the posterior longitudinal ligament or ligamentum flavum (31). Posterior fusion with or without instrumentation is not necessary after laminectomies for stenosis under most circumstances. Some situations that may warrant stronger consideration for arthrodesis include laminectomies at the thoracolumbar junction, areas of excessive kyphosis, or adjacent to a long previous fusion to prevent late instability or kyphosis (Fig. 4) (63).

PROGNOSIS

Surgeons can expect satisfactory results with some version of anterior or lateral herniated disc excision and dismal results with laminectomy for herniated thoracic discs. Appropriate surgical treatment provides motor improvement and gait improvement, and pain relief occurs in approximately 80 to 90% of patients. Coexistent neurologic disease, advanced age, long duration of illness, and severe myelopathy are associated with less postoperative improvement than in the typical patient (8–10,20,23,35,48,52,62,63,65,66). VATS techniques have demonstrated substantial improvement in 70% of patients with myelopathy, axial back pain, or leg pain, but less success in patients with radicular pain (23). More studies with larger numbers of patients are needed to determine the efficacy of thoracoscopic discectomies for patients with frank cord compression and myelopathy.

Thoracic stenosis with resultant myelopathy can often be treated successfully with posterior or anterior decompression, but delayed complications, such as instability, deformity or recurrence, can occur, requiring further treatment. Eight of twelve patients in Palumbo et al.'s series had improvement in pain, eight of ten with a preoperative motor deficit were improved after surgery, and seven of eleven who were nonambulatory preoperatively became ambulatory after decompressive surgery. During the 2- to 9-year period of follow-up, deterioration of postoperative results occurred in 5 of 12 patients. Four patients underwent eight further surgeries, including thoracic laminectomy for ossification of the ligamentum flavum in one patient; revision decompression with fusion for recurrent stenosis with instability in two patients; lumbar extension osteotomy for fixed sagittal imbalance in one patient; and further extensive thoracic laminectomy for stenosis, a cervical laminectomy for stenosis, and two anterior thoracic arthrodesis procedures for instability in one patient with rheumatoid arthritis (30). Early results in Barnett et al.'s series were excellent, but no long-term follow-up was reported. All six patients experienced some measure of improvement with respect to pain, paresthesias, walking tolerance, spasticity, gait disturbance, and weakness (29). Chang and colleague's series suggests overall favorable short-term results, although less satisfactory in the setting of diffuse ossification of the posterior longitudinal ligament or ligamentum flavum in the thoracic spine (31).

CONCLUSION

Thoracic disc herniation remains a challenging clinical entity, due to its rarity and often nonspecific clinical presentation. Diagnosis is frequently delayed, and some patients receive inappropriate treatment for other diagnoses that later prove false. Treatment is nonoperative unless pain is refractory or there is neurologic compromise. A posterior laminectomy approach for disc excision is associated with an unacceptably high incidence of failure and neurologic injury. A transthoracic, transpedicular, or costotransversectomy approach allows decompression without manipulation of the spinal cord. These approaches are not without risk, and have similar overall complication rates. The authors favor the transthoracic approach because it offers the best visualization completely across the canal, ensuring complete decompression of the spinal cord. For posterolateral disc herniations, however, a costotransversectomy approach is quite satisfactory and safe. VATS has emerged as a viable alternative to formal open thoracotomy in appropriate hands. Thoughtful preoperative planning and careful surgical decompression of the spinal cord are necessary regardless of the chosen approach, and they can result in a gratifying outcome for the surgeon and the patient.

Several conclusions regarding thoracic stenosis can be drawn from the literature. First, a surgeon can expect satisfactory early results from surgical decompression in the majority of patients. Second, unlike thoracic disc herniation, thoracic stenosis can often be successfully treated by posterior decompression, including laminectomy, partial medial facetectomy, and removal of hypertrophic ligamentum flavum and facet joint capsule. Third, deterioration of long-term results can be expected due to adjacent level disease, recurrence, or development of instability or deformity as a consequence of decompressive surgery. Fourth, ossification of the ligamentum flavum or posterior longitudinal ligament portends a more difficult surgical procedure and, often, less satisfactory clinical result. The challenge remains in identifying those patients that would benefit from surgery, and planning an operation that optimizes the likelihood of a positive and lasting outcome.

REFERENCES

1. Key CA. On paraplegia depending on disease of the ligaments of the spine. *Guys Hosp Rep* 1838;3:17–34.
2. Middleton GS, Teacher JH. Injury of the spinal cord due to rupture of an intervertebral disc during muscular effort. *Glasgow Med J* 1911;76:1–6.
3. Elsberg CA. The extradural ventral chondromas (eccondroses), their favorite sites, the spinal cord and root symptoms they produce, and their surgical treatment. *Bull Neurol Inst N Y* 1931;1:350–388.
4. Benjamin V. Diagnosis and management of thoracic disc disease. *Clin Neurosurg* 1983;30:577–605.
5. Epstein JA. The syndrome of herniation of the lower thoracic intervertebral discs with nerve root and spinal cord compression: a presentation of four cases with a review of the literature, methods of diagnosis and treatment. *J Neurosurg* 1954;11:525–538.
6. Russell T. Thoracic intervertebral disc protrusion: experience of 67 cases and review of the literature. *Br J Neurosurg* 1989;3:153–160.
7. Hulme A. The surgical approach to thoracic intervertebral disc protrusions. *J Neurol Neurosurg Psych* 1960;23:133–137.
8. Bohlman HH, Zdeblick TA. Anterior excision of herniated thoracic discs. *J Bone Joint Surg* 1988;70-A(7):1038–1047.
9. Otani K, Yoshida M, Fujii E, et al. Thoracic disc herniation: surgical treatment in 23 patients. *Spine* 1988;13(11):1262–1267.
10. Simpson JM, Silveri CP, Simeone FA, et al. Thoracic disc herniation: re-evaluation of the posterior approach using a modified costotransversectomy. *Spine* 1993;18(13):1872–1877.
11. Benzel EC. The lateral extracavitary approach to the spine using the three-quarter prone position. *J Neurosurg* 1989;71:837–841.
12. Delfini R, Di Lorenzo N, Ciappetta P, et al. Surgical treatment of thoracic disc herniation: a reappraisal of Larson's lateral extracavitary approach. *Surg Neurol* 1996;45:517–523.
13. Maiman DJ, Larson SJ, Luck E, et al. Lateral extracavitary approach to the spine for thoracic disc herniation: report of 23 cases. *Neurosurgery* 1984;14:178–182.
14. Crafoord C, Hiertonn T, Lindblom K, et al. Spinal cord compression caused by a protruded thoracic disc: report of a case treated with anterolateral fenestration of the disc. *Acta Orthop Scand* 1959;28:103–107.
15. Perot PL Jr, Munro DD. Transthoracic removal of midline thoracic disc protrusions causing spinal cord compression. *J Neurosurg* 1969;31:452–458.
16. Ransohoff J, Spencer F, Siew F, et al. Transthoracic removal of thoracic disc: report of three cases. *J Neurosurg* 1969;31:459–461.
17. Patterson RH, Arbit E. A surgical approach through the pedicle to protruded thoracic discs. *J Neurosurg* 1978;48:768–772.
18. Le Roux PD, Haglund MM, Harris AB. Thoracic disc disease: experience with the transpedicular approach in twenty consecutive patients. *Neurosurgery* 1993;33:58–66.
19. Ahlgren BD, Herkowitz HN. A modified posterolateral approach to the thoracic spine. *J Spinal Dis* 1995;8(1):69–75.
20. Fujimura Y, Nakamura M, Matsumoto M. Anterior decompression and fusion via the extrapleural approach for thoracic disc herniation causing myelopathy. *Keio J Med* 1997;46(4):173–176.
21. Sharan AD, Przybylski GJ, Tartaglino L. Approaching the upper thoracic vertebrae without sternotomy or thoracotomy: a radiographic analysis with clinical application. *Spine* 2000;25(8):910–916.
22. Mack MJ, Regan JJ, Bobechko WP, et al. Application of thoracoscopy for diseases of the spine. *Ann Thorac Surg* 1993;56:736–738.
23. Anand N, MchOrth, Regan JJ. Video-assisted thoracoscopic surgery for thoracic disc disease. *Spine* 2002;27(8):871–879.
24. McAfee PC, Regan JR, Zdeblick TA, et al. The incidence of complications in endoscopic anterior thoracolumbar spinal reconstructive surgery: a prospective multicenter study comprising the first 100 consecutive cases. *Spine* 1995;20:1624–1632.
25. Fessler RG, Surgill M. Complications of surgery for thoracic disc disease. *Surg Neurol* 1998;49:609–618.
26. Mulier S, Debois V. Thoracic disc herniations: transthoracic, lateral, or posterolateral approach? A review. *Surg Neurol* 1998;49:599–606.
27. Ungersbock K, Perneczky A, Korn A. Thoracic vertebrostenosis combined with thoracic disc herniation: case report and review of the literature. *Spine* 1987;12(6):612–615.
28. Marzluff JM, Hungerford GD, Kempe LG. Thoracic myelopathy caused by osteophytes of the articular processes. Thoracic spondylosis. *J Neurosurg* 1979;50:779–783.
29. Barnett GH, Hardy RW, Little JR, et al. Thoracic spinal canal stenosis. *J Neurosurg* 1987;66:338–344.
30. Palumbo MA, Hilibrand AS, Hart RA, et al. Surgical treatment of thoracic spinal stenosis. *Spine* 2001;26(5):558–566.
31. Chang UK, Choe WJ, Chung CK, et al. Surgical treatment for thoracic spinal stenosis. *Spinal Cord* 2001;39:362–369.
32. Wood KB, Blair JM, Aepple DM, et al. The natural history of asymptomatic thoracic disc herniations. *Spine* 1997;22(5):525–530.
33. Awwad EE, Martin DS, Smith KR, et al. Asymptomatic versus symptomatic herniated thoracic discs: their frequency and characteristics as detected by computed tomography after myelography. *Neurosurgery* 1991;28(2):180–186.
34. Love JG, Kiefer EJ. Root pain and paraplegia due to protrusions of thoracic intervertebral discs. *J Neurosurg* 1950;7:62–69.
35. Otani K, Nakai S, Fujimura Y, et al. Surgical treatment of thoracic disc herniation using the anterior approach. *J Bone Joint Surg* 1982; 64-B(3):340–343.
36. Lesoin F, Leys D, Rousseaux M, et al. Thoracic disk herniation and Scheuermann's disease. *Eur Neurol* 1987;26:145–152.
37. Bhojraj SY, Dandawate AV. Progressive cord compression secondary to thoracic disc lesions in Scheuermann's kyphosis managed by posterolateral decompression, interbody fusion and pedicular fixation. *Eur Spine J* 1994;3:66–69.
38. Brown CW, Deffer PA, Akmakjian J, et al. The natural history of thoracic disc herniation. *Spine* 1992;17(6S):S97–S102.
39. Belanger TA, Rowe DE. Diffuse idiopathic skeletal hyperostosis: musculoskeletal manifestations. *J Am Acad Orthop Surg* 2001;9(4):258–267.
40. Fujimura Y, Nishi Y, Nakamura M, et al. Long-term follow-up study of anterior decompression and fusion for thoracic myelopathy resulting from ossification of the posterior longitudinal ligament. *Spine* 1997;22(3):305–311.
41. Okada K, Oka S, Tohge K, et al. Thoracic myelopathy caused by ossification of the ligamentum flavum: clinicopathologic study and surgical treatment. *Spine* 1991;16:280–287.
42. Omojola MF, Cardoso ER, Fox AJ. Thoracic myelopathy secondary to ossified ligamentum flavum. *J Neurosurg* 1982;56:448–450.
43. Epstein NE, Schwall G. Thoracic spinal stenosis: diagnostic and treatment challenges. *J Spinal Dis* 1994;7:259–269.
44. Dommisse GF. The blood supply of the spinal cord: a critical vascular zone in spinal surgery. *J Bone Joint Surg* 1974;56-B:225–235.
45. Bennett MH, McCallum JE. Experimental decompression of spinal cord. *Surg Neurol* 1977;8:63–67.
46. Doppman JL, Girton M. Angiographic study of the effect of laminectomy in the presence of acute anterior epidural masses. *J Neurosurg* 1976;45:195–202.
47. Kikuchi S, Watanabe E, Hasue M. Spinal intermittent claudication due to cervical and thoracic degenerative spine disease. *Spine* 1996; 21:331–318.
48. Severi P, Ruelle A, Andrioli G. Multiple calcified thoracic disc herniations: a case report. *Spine* 1992;17(4):449–451.
49. Stone JL, Lichtor T, Banerjee S. Intradural thoracic disc herniation. *Spine* 1994;19(11):1281–1284.
50. Epstein NE, Syrquin MS, Epstein JA, et al. Intradural disc herniations in the cervical, thoracic, and lumbar spine: report of three cases and review of the literature. *J Spinal Dis* 1990;3(4):396–403.
51. Yildishan A, Pasaoglu A, Okten T, et al. Intradural disc herniations: pathogenesis, clinical picture, diagnosis and treatment. *Neurochir* 1991;160–165.
52. Vanichkachorn JS, Vaccaro AR. Thoracic disk disease: diagnosis and treatment. *J Am Acad Orthop Surg* 2000;8(3).
53. Morgenlander JC, Massey EW. Neurogenic claudication with positional weakness from a thoracic disk herniation. *Neurology* 1989;39: 1133–1134.
54. Lyu RK, Chang HS, Tang LM, et al. Thoracic disc herniation mimicking acute lumbar disc disease. *Spine* 1999;24(4):416–418.
55. Eleraky MA, Apostolides PJ, Dickman CA, et al. Herniated thoracic discs mimic cardiac disease: three case reports. *Acta Neurochir* 1991;111:22–32.
56. Whitcomb DC, Martin SP, Schoen RE, et al. Chronic abdominal pain caused by thoracic disc herniation. *Am J Gastroenterol* 1995;90:835–837.
57. Benson MKD, Byrnes DP. The clinical syndromes and surgical

treatment of thoracic intervertebral disc prolapse. *J Bone Joint Surg* 1975;57-B:471–477.
58. Morgan H, Abood C. Disc herniation at T1-2: report of four cases and literature review. *J Neurosurg* 1998;88:148–150.
59. Stillerman CB, Chen TC, Couldwell WT, et al. Experience in the surgical management of 82 symptomatic herniated thoracic discs and review of the literature. *J Neurosurg* 1998;88:623–633.
60. Turgut M. Spinal cord compression due to multilevel thoracic disc herniation: surgical decompression using a "combined" approach. *J Neurosurg Sci* 2000;44:53–59.
61. Blumenkopf B. Thoracic intervertebral disc herniations: diagnostic value of magnetic resonance imaging. *Neurosurgery* 1988;23:36–40.
62. Currier BL, Eismont FJ, Green BA. Transthoracic disc excision and fusion for herniated thoracic discs. *Spine* 1994;19(3):323–328.
63. Korovessis PG, Stamatakis M, Michael A, et al. Three-level thoracic disc herniation: case report and review of the literature. *Eur Spine J* 1997;6:74–76.
64. Landreneau RJ, Hazelrigg SR, Mack MJ, et al. Postoperative pain-related morbidity: video-assisted thoracic surgery versus thoracotomy. *Ann Thorac Surg* 1998;56:1285–1289.
65. Sekhar LN, Jannetta PJ. Thoracic disc herniation: operative approaches and results. *Neurosurgery* 1983;12(3):303–305.
66. El-Kalliny M, Tew JM, van Loveren H, et al. Surgical approaches to thoracic disc herniations. *Acta Neurochir* 1991;111:22–32.

CHAPTER 44

Differential Diagnosis of Low Back Pain

Eugene J. Carragee

Low back pain (LBP) has been recorded as a common human complaint since the time of Hippocrates. Back pain has been variously attributed to local structures (i.e., lumbago) or generalized malady (i.e., arthritis) (1). Determining the "cause" of LBP in most instances is unimportant, however, because the symptoms are most often transient and do not seriously interfere with function. Even severe episodes are most often self-limited in duration. Although LBP may be the second most common cause of visits to a physician in the United States, evidence available suggests many more episodes of LBP are never evaluated by a health professional and no formal "diagnosis" is considered.

This chapter concerns the differential diagnosis of LBP in clinical practice. Particular emphasis is placed on chronic, nonspecific back pain and the role of discography in diagnosis. There is, however, no practical list of "differential diagnoses" that apply in all LBP. In fact, applying a generalized approach to diagnosing all LBP has resulted in much of the confusion seen in the field. In the initial stages of an evaluation, the goal of differential diagnosis is to identify or exclude serious conditions (i.e., tumors, infection, neurologic injury, visceral disease, etc.). The physician can then direct specific treatment, if those potentially catastrophic causes of LBP are found, or initiate nonspecific supportive treatment if no specific pathologic process is identified. This is fundamentally different than the evaluation of chronic LBP illness. When a practitioner sees a patient with persistent LBP that is functionally debilitating, the "practical" differential diagnosis becomes a more complex affair. In that situation, a precise diagnosis is important if possible because a more invasive or morbid treatment may be considered.

This chapter discusses the practical approaches to the diagnosis of LBP complaints in the acute and chronic phases. Significant limitations in the data that estimate the incidence of specific causes of LBP and the tests used to establish a diagnosis are also discussed. Particular emphasis is given to discography, which is commonly used to define the cause of chronic LBP. The goal of this chapter is to place the strengths and limitations of diagnostic strategies in perspective for acute and chronic back pain assessments.

DIAGNOSES

Historically, LBP has been attributed to a variety of causes. It is interesting to note that throughout history, most LBP was not associated with trauma or "injury." Rather, LBP was thought to have a "humoral" or "rheumatic" cause. It has been only in the past century that LBP as an "injury" has become a popular supposition. The reality is that few patients with acute or chronic

TABLE 1. *Differential diagnosis of low back pain complaints*

Generalized disease
- Viral illnesses (e.g., viral myalgia of viral hepatitis, mononucleosis)
- Psychological disease (e.g., somatization disorder)

Generalized disease with spinal pathology
- Bacterial sepsis with spinal infection
- Metastatic disease
- Rheumatic/immunologic disease (e.g., rheumatoid arthritis, psoriatic arthritis)
- Congenital diseases of connective tissue (e.g., Marfan's syndrome)
- Sickle cell disease (e.g., bone infarction)
- Metabolic disorders (e.g., rickets, senile osteoporosis)
- Degenerative arthritis/osteoarthritis

Spinal pathology
- Primary spinal neoplasm
  - Benign
  - Malignant
- Spinal infection without generalized sepsis
- Noninfectious inflammatory disease
- Acute traumatic bone or soft tissue injury to the spine
- Deformity (e.g., kyphosis, scoliosis)
- Instability (e.g., spondylolisthesis)

Nonspinal pathology
- Vascular disease (e.g., aortic aneurysm)
- Retroperitoneal disease (e.g., pancreatic disease)
- Urologic disease (e.g., prostatic infection, renal calculi)
- Gynecologic/obstetric disease (e.g., endometriosis, ectopic pregnancy)

Multifactorial

LBP symptoms have experienced serious trauma; however, low-intensity, repetitive movements and forces are postulated to produce traumatic injuries over time (1).

A comprehensive differential diagnosis (Table 1) of LBP lists many causes, the majority of which are associated with systematic disease. However, an exhaustive listing of diseases associated with LBP is of little practical value to the clinician attempting to make a diagnosis. To be useful in practice, the practical differential diagnosis should help direct the evaluation and weigh the implications of various treatments. To be meaningful, a practical approach to the diagnosis of LBP must be epidemiologically and therapeutically balanced. Table 1 gives a listing of potential anatomic sites from which nociceptor stimulation may be centrally interpreted as LBP. The perception of LBP, regardless of the nociceptive site, is modulated by local, regional, central, and systemic factors (Fig. 1). The following factors are important in understanding the clinical expression of LBP syndromes:

Adjacent tissue injury. Significant injury to nearby structures may increase the perception of pain in a hyperalgesic effect. This is a well-known phenomenon that may amplify pain perception by increased local inflammatory processes or neurologic sensitization (2,3).

Local anesthetic. Local anesthetic or antiinflammatory (steroid) injections may decrease the perception of pain. Interesting work on local anesthetic blocks has shown that percutaneous injection to areas of referred pain, but not the true pain generator, can provide pain relief. It has been also shown that local anesthetics applied distal to a lesion can modulate pain perception. The mechanisms of these remote actions to mitigate pain sensation are not clear but affect the fundamental premise of diagnostic blocks as used in practice.

Nearby tissue injury. Tissue injury having the same or adjacent sclerotomal afferents as lower spinal elements may increase LBP sensitivity. This effect is thought to be due to physiologic or histologic changes at the level of the dorsal root ganglion or spinal cord ascending tracts (5).

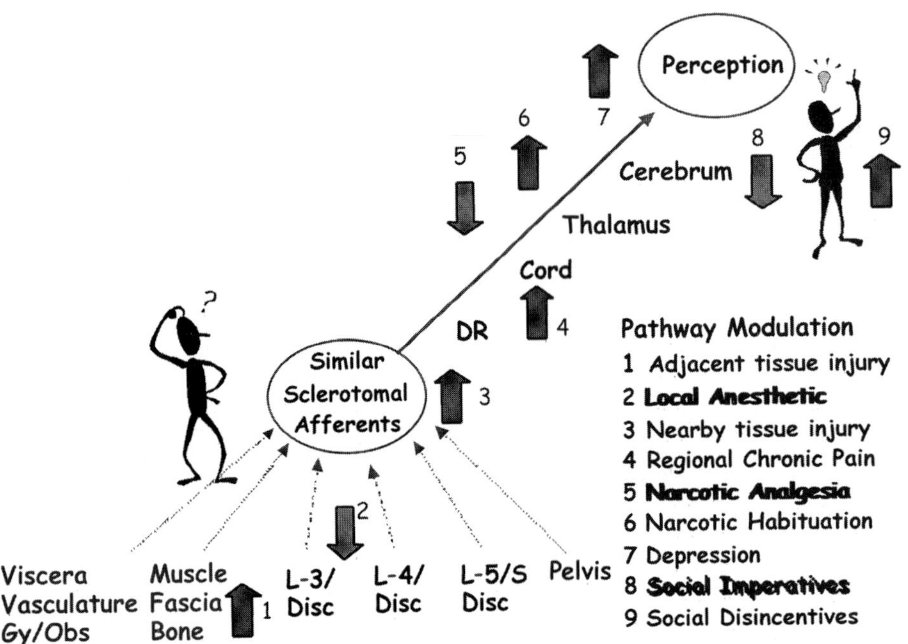

FIG. 1. Low back pain pathways. DR, dorsal root; Gy/Obs, gynecologic/obstetric.

Chronic regional pain syndromes. Chronic pain processes from regional pathology may increase pain sensitivity at lower spinal elements. This effect may be regional or global and may be related to physiologic changes at multiple levels, including the spinal cord and brain (3).

Narcotic analgesia. Narcotic medications can decrease the sensitivity and affective response to spinal pain. This effect is also likely at multiple levels of the neural axis (3,6,7).

Narcotic habituation. Chronic narcotic habituation decreases endogenous abilities to modulate peripheral nociceptive input and may exacerbate clinical depression. This effect is multifactorial (3,6,7).

Depression/anxiety. Clinical depression and anxiety disorders may increase the perception of pain intensity and amplify the affective response to pain. These effects likely are due to central neurochemical changes and systemic effects (1,3,6–12).

Social imperatives. Overriding social imperatives or incentives may result in a decreased pain perception. This decreased pain response or behavior can be seen in those experiencing some short-term stressful events, such as accident victims and soldiers in combat, or in certain training environments. Similarly, social incentives and supports can decrease the pain behavior over extended timeframes in some groups (1,8,9,13–15).

Social disincentives. When the intensity of pain is correlated with a perceived social benefit or monetary compensation, the measurable pain perception may be increased (1,8,9,11,13,14,16–28).

For a particular individual with local pathology, there may be a variable pain response, depending on the absence, presence, or degree of these variables in modulating pain perception and reaction. Because these variable associative factors exist in many cases, the apparent clinical syndrome associated with local pathologic diagnosis may vary widely.

Epidemiology and the Practical Diagnosis of Low Back Pain

Epidemiologic studies demonstrate that definitive clinical causation of LBP is relatively rare in population studies. Back pain in a population may be seen to exist at different levels of personal impact and social relevance, such as the following:

1. LBP associated with no functional limitations and not presenting for medical evaluation or treatment.
2. LBP associated with some functional limitations and yet not presenting for medical evaluation or treatment.
3. LBP that presents for medical evaluation but resolves before any diagnosis is confirmed.
4. LBP that is medically evaluated in detail and diagnoses excluded or confirmed.

Depending on which of these subgroups is studied, the perception of what "commonly" causes LBP is correspondingly biased. Investigators examining the prevalence of any degree of LBP in subjects not seeking medical treatment construct a different set of likely diagnoses than, for instance, an oncologist, a discographer, or a spinal surgeon who sees patients with back pain.

Outside of the medical arena, many persons have back pain that is commonly borne without the perception of significant illness. In a survey of nearly 1,000 subjects seen for other musculoskeletal complaints, it was found that 60% had experienced LBP, which they described as mild. The most common syndrome in this study was minor low back discomfort with no functional impairment in subjects who indicated they would not seek medical treatment for this problem despite at least 2 years of some low back symptoms (18). Other investigations have shown that even relatively severe back pain may exist outside any medical setting in subjects with no functional impairment (15,29). Finally, there are some select populations in whom significant back pain at very high intensity levels is the occupational and social norm. In soldiers undergoing very strenuous training involving the continuous carrying of heavy loads (>25 kg), significant back pain is nearly universal (15).

"Pseudodiagnosis" in Acute Low Back Pain

A "pseudodiagnosis" may be thought of as a specific "diagnosis" given to a patient as a practical and economical means of labeling the problem in the absence of any confirmation (8). Patients are routinely told they have a "lumbar sprain" in the absence of significant trauma or a "slipped disc" in the absence of sciatica. These "pseudodiagnoses" are applied for the patient, his or her family, and possibly their insurance or employer. The author believes that in most cases these diagnoses are made in good faith to assuage fear, encourage mobilization, and avoid unnecessary testing. Although this practice has dubious scientific merit, the author believes that this is an innocuous practice without a serious downside. Others, however, believe that labeling may reinforce illness behavior and lead to unnecessary fear or avoidance of physical activity.

The reason "pseudodiagnosis" is an attractive practice to use in those patients seeking medical care for acute LBP is because a specific diagnosis is usually neither required nor obtained. In patients presenting for assessment from general medical practitioners, imaging studies, laboratory analysis, and specialty investigations are generally not recommended during the first 4 to 8 weeks of symptoms as long as there are no collateral signs or symptoms of neurologic impairment, infection, tumor, serious disease, or major injury (Table 2). First-line treatment of back pain in this population is usually based in over-the-counter analgesics, reassurance, and encouragement of continued activity.

TABLE 2. *Practical differential diagnosis of acute low back pain*

Acute serious trauma
Neurologic injury
No neurologic injury
Minor trauma
Risk factor for pathologic fracture or instability
Risk factor for infection, tumor, or inflammatory disease
Risk factor for psychological or social instability
No risk factors
No trauma
Risk factor for infection, tumor, or inflammatory disease
Risk factor for psychological or social decompensation
No risk factors

In common practice, it is assumed, if not articulated, that there is no sign of infection, cauda equina compression, or malignancy and no history consistent with fracture, etc. Despite this being the truth of the encounter, a "pseudodiagnosis" is often made without evidence. These "diagnoses" include "lumbar strain," "lumbar sprain," "sacroiliac dysfunction," "facet capsule impingement," and others.

Application of these diagnostic labels is not meant to be critical of the enormously difficult job presented to the primary care physician who takes care of the overwhelming majority of life's aches and pains in a fog of uncertainty and social need. When the clinician makes an affirmative show of certainty in giving a diagnostic label (e.g., "lumbar strain"), this alone may help in reassuring the patient and facilitating recovery. However, the label given in this situation, "lumbar strain," has little to due with the bona fide pathologic diagnosis of disruption of muscular tissue by trauma. In most cases, the experienced clinician also is concomitantly inferring a low level of risk of serious underlying pathology based on history and examination. The "pseudodiagnosis" expresses this low risk as a positive, specific, and usually benign diagnosis. A paradigm for the thinking of diagnostic groups to facilitate evaluation and treatment is given in Table 2.

Persistent or Chronic Low Back Pain

Some patients continue to have LBP. Some have persistent pain without functional impairment or illness behavior. Others may develop a chronic LBP illness with serious personal, social, and economic effects. Determining a pathoanatomic diagnosis in chronic LBP is important and difficult. The patient who has not recovered, or who has recurrent serious episodes of back pain, seeks explanation and treatment. By this point, the readily identifiable diagnoses have usually been made, the patient has demonstrated an inability to accommodate to the LBP illness they experience, and a number of "pseudodiagnoses" may have been applied without confirmation.

Much of the data presented in this chapter on the diagnosis of LBP comes from this subset of patients who fail to recover from or accommodate to back pain. In a minority of these patients, serious pathologic conditions are still found, such as metastatic disease, spinal abscesses, and gross spinal instability and deformity, and others have neurologic symptoms. More often, however, such specific and accepted diagnoses are not found. The only spinal "pathology" encountered by imaging studies may be within the range of the common degenerative changes seen with aging.

Degenerative spinal changes have been known for centuries to occur with aging. However, serious persistent disability in people who have a primary complaint of back pain is a more recent health problem. Early in the twentieth century, work loss due to back complaints was rare, but as the century progressed, 2 to 5% of the potential working population in the United States became so disabled (1,9,11). Exactly what causes this severe LBP illness is unclear.

Many factors appear to be associated with persistent severe back pain complaints. Among these are low education or class status, poor job satisfaction, heavy machinery operation, heavy labor, cigarette smoking, emotional troubles, lumbar spondylosis, and workers' compensation or personal injury claims (1,9,11,13,14,30). Severe anatomic pathology, such as infection, tumor, deformity, fracture, or gross instability, is usually excluded early in the course of evaluating patients with LBP. The sensitivity of magnetic resonance imaging (MRI) and advanced computed tomographic imaging for such serious pathology as spinal infection, malignancy, and fracture is such that missing such diagnoses is rare (31,32). Nonetheless, as in major trauma, a "secondary survey" of patients with persistent and clinically severe LBP is probably justified when the initial period of observation and treatment appears to fail.

Yet, for the patient in whom the first and second evaluation for serious disease has failed to reveal unequivocal pathologic finding, there has been considerable speculation on what anatomic structures may cause such significant clinical distress. There is debate as to whether specific local degenerative changes in the spine, which may cause pain, are sufficient to cause the extreme morbidity associated with chronic back pain illness. Some argue that without compounding social or neuropsychological factors, common degenerative spine changes do not cause serious functional impairments.

DIAGNOSING THE CAUSE OF LOW BACK PAIN IN THE ABSENCE OF SERIOUS PATHOLOGY

There are two schools of thought regarding the diagnosis of persistent disabling LBP illness in the absence of serious pathology (Table 3). One school believes that specific local pathology exists

TABLE 3. *Theoretical causes of chronic low back pain illness*

Structural failure of the spine as primary cause of chronic LBP illness (Fig. 2A)
The spinal lesion alone causes serious disabling illness.
The spinal lesion is rarely, if ever, found in people without serious LBP problems.
The elimination of the spinal lesions should reliably relieve LBP.
Psychosocial failure to accommodate normal spinal nociception (Fig. 2B)
The local spinal lesions are not specific to the illness.
The severity of the illness is primarily related to a failure to accommodate to common spinal nociceptor input.
Failure to accommodate to common spinal discomfort is primarily a psychological or social event.
Neurophysiologic failure to modulate LBP (Fig. 2C)
The local spinal lesions are insufficient alone to cause serious LBP illness.
The psychological and social variables alone do not explain the severity of the illness.
There is a failure at the neurophysiologic level to modulate relatively minor local nociceptive input resulting in the perception of severe pain.
The psychological and social deterioration is secondary to chronic LBP states.
Combination of abnormal spinal pain, abnormal modulation, and abnormal accommodation processes.

LBP, low back pain.

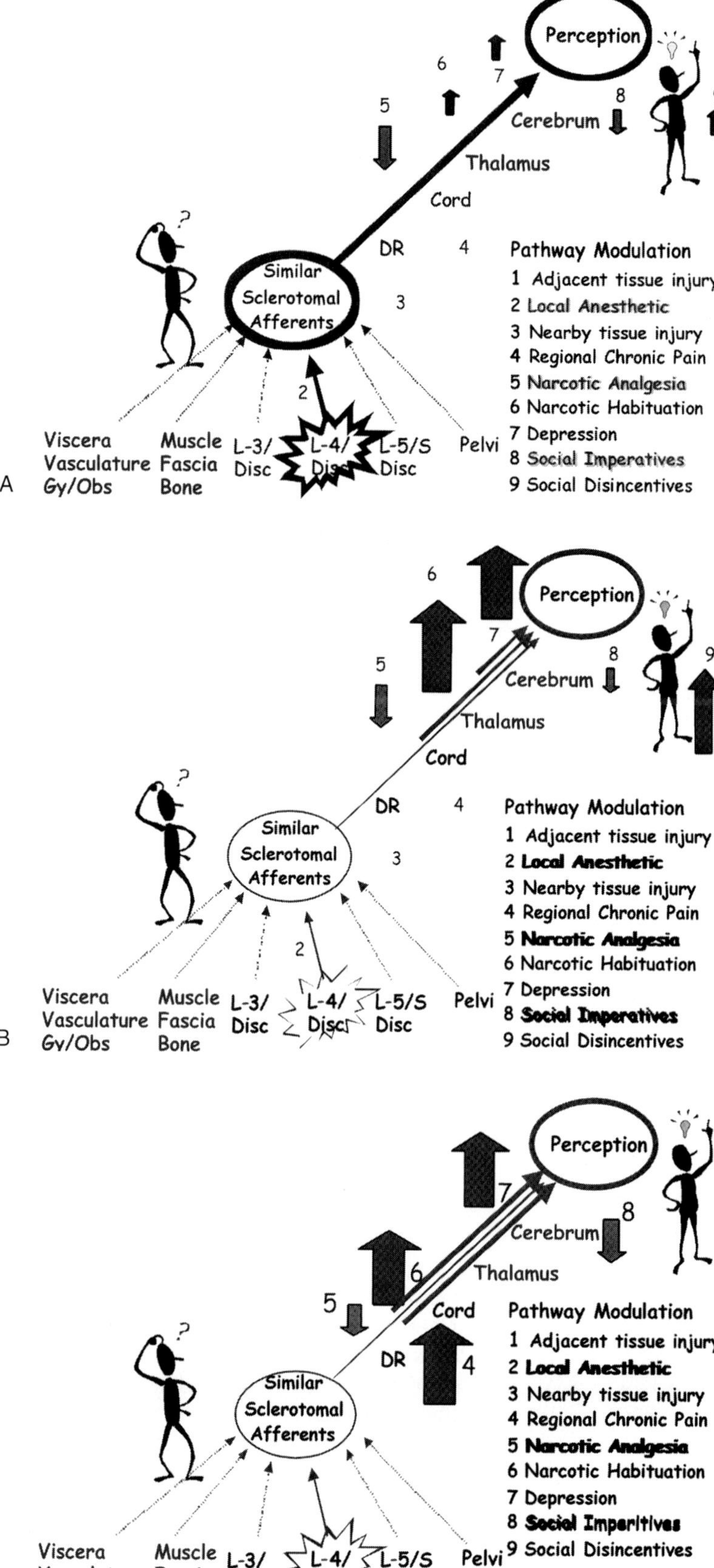

FIG. 2. **A:** Structural failure of the spine as primary cause of chronic low back pain illness. **B:** Psychosocial failure to accommodate normal spinal nociception. **C:** Neurophysiologic failure to modulate low back pain. DR, dorsal root; Gy/Obs, gynecologic lobstetric.

in the spine (i.e., an annular fissure, a facet subluxation, subtle segmental instability) that alone is sufficient to cause serious LBP. In this theory, there are spinal lesions that, when present, are universally crippling to anyone with this lesion, regardless of concomitant factors (e.g., social factors, physical conditioning, motivation, psychological reserves, and so forth). Therefore, the diagnostic goal is to identify the spinal lesion causing this illness. There are a number of potential flaws in this conceptual model.

The presence of significant "concomitant factors" is much greater in patients in whom serious pathology is not found. In patients with serious spinal disease and chronic pain (e.g., infection or unstable spondylolisthesis), the rate of abnormal psychological testing is only slightly more than in the general population despite chronic pain (11). However, in patients diagnosed with "primary discogenic pain" on the basis of discography, 80% have been shown to have abnormal psychological profiles, with approximately 20% being severely distressed psychologically. Likewise, in large series of patients being evaluated for "discogenic" pain, 70 to 80% of these patients have claims for workers' compensation or personal injury litigation (33,34). Despite these confounding factors, many believe the clinical picture of severe illness is due primarily to a specific spinal lesion alone.

The opposing school of thought believes the clinical dysfunction seen in chronic LBP cannot be accounted for by any common degenerative finding. In this model, the severe functional limitations and pain behaviors seen are usually the result of a failure to accommodate the common low back discomforts of daily life. Therefore, in this model, the diagnostic goal is to identify the social, emotional, or neurologic failures to modulate common backache.

In the schematic shown in Figure 2A, a single, severe pain generator at the L4-5 disc is perceived as severe pain. In Figures 2B and 2C, relatively minor nociceptor input is perceived as severe pain because of failures of normal neuromodulation or psychosocial reserve to accommodate common low back discomfort.

The evaluation of the patient with findings of a "degenerative" spine to determine the cause of chronic LBP illness is an extraordinarily difficult clinical task. The findings of x-rays, computed tomographic scanning, and MRI have been shown to be too nonspecific to differentiate patients with chronic LBP from those with no back pain at all or clinically insignificant back pain. Studies of MRI findings in asymptomatic subjects have shown 30 to 40% have pathologic degenerative changes (35,36), and these increase with age (37). Even among symptomatic subjects, MRI findings of mild to moderate neurologic compression, disc degeneration or bulging, and central stenosis were not found to correlate with severity of symptoms (38). Whereas sciatica is related to disc morphology/degeneration on MRI, local LBP is not found to correlate with the MRI findings of degeneration (39). Other investigations have shown only a weak association between LBP development and even progressive degenerative changes seen on MRI over a 5-year period (40).

Because standard imaging techniques are inadequate to differentiate symptomatic from asymptomatic patients on the basis of degenerative changes, other strategies have been developed. Implicit in these strategies is the notion that there commonly exists a definable spinal lesion (the "pain generator") that can account for persistent, severe, incapacitating LBP. The diagnostic tests purported to identify these "pain generators" are diagnostic blocks and provocative disc injections (i.e., discography).

DIAGNOSTIC ANESTHETIC INJECTIONS

Diagnostic anesthetic blockade of a suspected "pain generator" site is another method recommended to establish a diagnosis in persistent LBP syndromes. This method is used primarily for suspected facet and sacroiliac (SI) joint pain. Occasionally, anesthetic injections may be used to evaluate isthmic spondylolysis. A pathologic diagnosis is assumed if the anesthetic injection of a suspected structure results in some arbitrary degree of pain relief (i.e., 50%, 75%, 100%, etc.). Based on diagnostic methods, prevalence of facet joint pain ranges from 15 to 40% in select groups (4). Once again these estimates are conjectural, as there is no gold standard test to establish the validity of these injection blocks in making a diagnosis. Neurophysiologic studies also indicate that anesthetic blockade at one site may affect distal or proximal pain sites, or even distant or regional pain perception (3,4). Simply stated, you do not have to block the painful site itself to have subjective relief, even in the absence of a placebo effect.

Facet Joint Pain

Stimulation of facet joint, synovium, and capsules results in low back discomfort in asymptomatic volunteers and patients undergoing diagnostic injections. There is modest predictability in the location and character of referred pain with saline injections into the facet joints in asymptomatic volunteers (41), but no predictable pattern of referral in LBP patients (42,43). This finding appears to confirm that the pain "wiring" and perception is altered in symptomatic persons in ways that are poorly understood.

The experimental pain associated with facet capsule distension appears to be usually blocked by local anesthetic at the medial branches of the primary dorsal rami above and below a facet (44). Whether this would apply to arthritic or subchondral pain associated with spondylosis is unknown.

When clinical features of LBP patients are compared against the response to facet joint blockade, no clinical presentation typical of "facet syndrome" (as defined by the results of injection studies) could be appreciated (34). From a statistical standpoint, older patients with pain unaffected by flexion and extension but reportedly relieved by recumbency or made worse with coughing or Valsalva's maneuver have been found to respond more frequently to injections. However, 25 to 75% of nonresponders to facet anesthetic injections had one or more of these characteristics, making the predictive value of these associated clinical features low (45). In addition, the positive response of pain relief to anesthetic facet injections does not appear to correlate with radiographic evidence of facet arthrosis (46).

The failure to identify any reliable clinical syndrome or radiologic finding associated with pain relief by facet block is interesting. It may indicate that the painful lesion being locally anesthetized is simply not detectable by imaging studies and is protean in symptom manifestation. On the other hand, it may indicate that the test does not identify a true clinical entity of any sort, and the response is related to the anesthetic effects on collateral or central pain pathways/perception.

An effort to lower the possibility of placebo or collateral effects and increase the reliability of result reproducibility has been made by some authors. Some have advocated additional "controls" on the blocks, including the routine and random use of placebo injections, and short- versus long-acting anesthetic agents to differentiate true responders from false-positive results. Others have stressed the careful placement on very small anesthetic doses on the posterior primary ramus (median branch) innervating the facet joint. Whether these carefully placed injections with controls are actually isolating facet joint pain or acting more widely along the neural pathways effecting pain perception is unknown. Even highly reproducible results may not be due to the simple "numbing" of a painful structure.

It may be possible to support a diagnostic method, such as anesthetic facet injections, if a certain treatment method were reliably effective. There have been numerous trials using steroid injections and a smaller series of local nerve ablation in subjects diagnosed by these injection techniques.

There is little evidence from the best-controlled trials of steroid injections that a therapeutic effect exists. Therefore, treatment outcomes in these series cannot confirm diagnostic accuracy (47). These trials used relatively old diagnostic injections, however, if any.

Ablation procedures have shown more promise. The study by van Kleef et al. showed some effect of facet denervation within subjects responding (50% pain relief) to a single injection of lidocaine to the median branch above and below the facet. In this small, randomized controlled trial, 67% of the treatment group was judged as successful at 8 weeks, compared to 38% of the sham denervation group. It is noteworthy that subjects with advanced spondylosis and those with any other pain syndrome were excluded from this study (48).

Leclaire et al., using single intraarticular injections without a placebo control for diagnosis, found little effect of radiofrequency denervation on clinical outcome (49). Others reported on a trial of median branch ablation when the diagnosis of "chronic zygapophysial joint pain" was made using differential blocks of short- and long-acting anesthetics. In this study, a greater than 80% pain relief for longer than 1 hour after a lidocaine injection and longer than 2 hours after bupivacaine injection was used to determine a positive response to median branch block. It is interesting to note that lidocaine (short-acting) and bupivacaine (long-acting) anesthetic injections produced the same duration of relief (approximately 4 to 5 hours). For patients meeting these criteria, the results were reported as highly successful in pain relief and improved function (50). Increasingly elaborate methods are reported to accurately diagnose this syndrome. However, no method exists to confirm that facet pathology is truly the primary source of a patient's illness, as opposed to other spinal structures or the central effects of neurophysiologic or psychosocial factors.

Sacroiliac Pain

The diagnosis of SI pain is sometimes straightforward, such as when there has been a Malgaigne-type fracture, or when associated with infectious or inflammatory arthritis. The diagnosis is usually made in the absence of these specific conditions, however, and is based on manual diagnostic techniques or SI joint injections. The physical examination maneuvers thought to establish SI joint pain do not correlate with the results of SI joint anesthetic blocks, however.

As with the facet joint, asymptomatic subjects can report pain with SI joint stimulation (51). Also, as with suspected facet joint pain, anesthetic blocks have been postulated to diagnose SI joint pain when pain is relieved by the injection. However, none of 12 common or esoteric signs on physical examination appeared to correlate with response to SI joint blocks (52).

The sensitivity and specificity of these blocks is unknown. No study has looked at the response to anesthetic injections of clearly pathologic SI joint pain (e.g., in fracture malunion or spondyloarthropathy), nor has sensitivity been analyzed in subjects who are known to be without SI joint disease.

Indirect evidence regarding the incidence of SI joint–related LBP has been gathered from the reported relief of low back symptoms with SI joint injection. Single injection of a short-acting anesthetic gave some relief of discomfort in 30% of a small cohort of subjects with maximal pain below the L-5 to S-1 level (33). No association with any particular clinical pattern was associated with the responders compared to nonresponders. In another study, approximately 20% of select LBP patients (with unilateral low back and buttock pain, SI joint area tenderness, and a failure of facet and epidural injections) were found to respond to differential SI joint anesthetic blocks with short- and long-acting agents (7). Again, no physical examination sign or provocative maneuver correlated with response to these differential blocks. Another report indicated that a small group of patients with positive technetium-99m bone scans for abnormal SI joint uptake had relief of their usual pain with SI joint blocks; however, most patients responding to SI joint blocks do not have abnormal bone scans (53).

In summary, patients who respond to SI joint injections with pain relief do not have a characteristic history or response to physical examination maneuvers. It is not clear if the injection responder group represents patients with particular SI joint pathology, or whether they are a diverse group with various local, regional, or complex pain sites. It appears clear that no specific pathology found on imaging studies correlates with response to SI joint anesthetic injections.

DISCOGRAPHY IN CHRONIC LOW BACK PAIN ILLNESS

Discography was first reported on by Lindblom and Hirsch in 1948 as a method to identify herniated discs in the lumbar spine. As a secondary attractive feature of the test, it was noted that a reproduction of the patient's usual sciatica sometimes occurred during injection of the contrast material. With subsequent use, it was often noted that familiar back pain was sometimes reproduced during the test. This finding caused some to begin using the test to evaluate lumbar discs as the origin of patients' chronic LBP. From the early use of discography, it has been unclear what a painful injection means. What is the specificity of the test? It is unknown if a disc that is painful when injected can be reliably diagnosed as the cause of clinically significant LBP illness.

Technique

Discography is performed by the injection of a nonirritating radiopaque dye, under fluoroscopic guidance, into several intervertebral discs. The central portion of the disc is percutaneously penetrated by a fine-gauge needle. This can be done from a posterior-lateral approach in most cases. At the L-5 to S-1 level, successful introduction may sometimes require bending of the needle or an introducer. In skilled hands, needle placement with a local anesthetic at the skin puncture should be quickly and atraumatically performed. The dye is then slowly injected into the nucleus of several lumbar discs with the patient blinded to the timing and site of injection. The distribution of the dye in the disc is noted, as is the patient's response to injection. The patient is asked whether each injection seems painful and is asked to rate the pain against some standardized scale (e.g., 0 to 5, 0 to 10, "none" to "unbearable").

A completely intact disc without any degenerative or developmental changes always retains the dye in a central globular or bilobed pattern (5). Even at pressures of 100 psi, these injections are usually not very uncomfortable. In more advanced disc degeneration, individuals may experience varying degrees of discomfort and pain as the dye is injected. Pain is more commonly associated with disc degeneration and fissuring extending into the annulus (5–7).

If the injection is painful, the discomfort provoked by the injection is rated as similar (concordant) or dissimilar to the patient's usual LBP. A similar or exact pain reproduction (i.e., concordant pain response) and a significant pain rating (usually meaning at 6 of 10 or greater) is considered to be a positive disc injection. Painless and minimally painful disc injections or disc injections causing dissimilar pain to the patient's usual symptoms are considered negative injections (54).

Criteria for Positive Test

In an effort to improve the specificity of discography in diagnosing so-called "discogenic pain," some investigators have used additional criteria beyond pain reproduction on injection. The criteria for establishing a positive discogram are controversial. The primary criteria for a "positive" disc injection are pain of "significant" intensity on disc injections and a reported similarity of that pain to the patient's usual, clinical discomfort.

The experimental work by Walsh et al. in 1990 proposed that "significant pain" be defined as 3 out of 5 (or 6 out of 10) on an arbitrary pain thermometer. The word used as the descriptor for 3 of 5 pain on that thermometer was "bad pain" and of greater intensity than "moderate pain" (2 out of 5). The Walsh et al. group did not stringently define concordance of pain reproduction (54).

Nonetheless, some spine specialists believe that a patient having chronic back pain, no other clearly identifiable spinal or regional pathology, and a reproduction of the back pain by a disc injection establishes disc pathology. Specifically, it is degenerative or traumatic fissuring through the innervated outer annulus of the disc that is the perceived significant pathology.

Some investigators have held more complex, stringent, and sometimes idiosyncratic criteria for positive injections, as follows:

Negative control disc: Most clinicians require that at least one additional disc, a "control" disc, be examined. This control disc injection should ideally be "negative" to confirm a positive study. It is not clear whether this means an adjacent "control" disc injection must be "painless," or just not significantly painful in intensity. It is also not clear whether a painful but discordant disc satisfies the "negative control" requirement. Although a reasonable concept, there are no data to confirm that having documented a negative control disc increases the validity of the test.

Concordant pain: Most discographers have required that a painful injection be considered negative if the sensation is clearly unfamiliar. On the other hand, it is not clear how "exact" a reproduction is required for a "positive test." Some prominent investigators have advocated that only an "exact" reproduction be accepted (55), whereas others have not (54,56,57). The requirement of "exact" reproduction is probably unrealistic. The author's experience with pain descriptors in a clinical setting is that a patient only occasionally repeats exactly his or her own description of the "usual" pain from one visit to the next.

Dye penetration on injection: Some have maintained that dye penetration must extend to or through the outer annulus for scoring a "true" positive injection (55). That is, painful injections, even those with concordant pain reproduction, are not in some investigators' schemes and are not a true positive injection unless the dye tracts to the outer annulus.

Demonstration of pain behavior: Others have indicated that the patient must also exhibit "behavioral" signs of pain during the injection for a positive test: guarding, withdrawal, grimacing, and so forth. For example, a patient who claims an 8 out of 10 pain severity without concomitant "pain behavior" would not be viewed to have a true positive injection by this standard (54).

Maximum pressure on injection: Some have argued that only pain elicited during low pressure injections be considered positive. Some data suggest high-pressure injections (>80 to 100 psi) may cause deflection of the vertebral end-plates or the rupture of membranes over sealed and presumably asymptomatic fissures (56,58).

Only one or two positive discs: More recently, some have suggested that multiple painful injections, despite one "control disc," is still an equivocal study (N. Bogduk, *personal communication*). The assumption is that a generalized hyperalgesic effect may lead to multiple positive discs around a single pain generator.

Validity

The validity of a test usually matches the test result against some criterion standard, such as a pathologic specimen examination. Validity may be expressed as sensitivity or the likelihood that a positive test will occur in an individual with the condition, and specificity or the likelihood a test will be negative in an individual without the condition (see Chapter 2).

Discography purports to diagnose the presence or absence of a disc lesion responsible for the syndrome of chronic LBP illness caused by primary discogenic pain. There is no established gold standard criterion for this condition. However, some authors believe it is the most common single cause of chronic LBP illness.

Specificity of Positive Discography: Testing on Asymptomatic Subjects

Careful technique and the standardization of the study are felt by some practitioners of discography to have lowered the false-positive rate to a negligible level in experienced hands. In 1990, Walsh and colleagues performed a carefully controlled set of discographic lumbar injections in ten paid volunteers, all asymp-

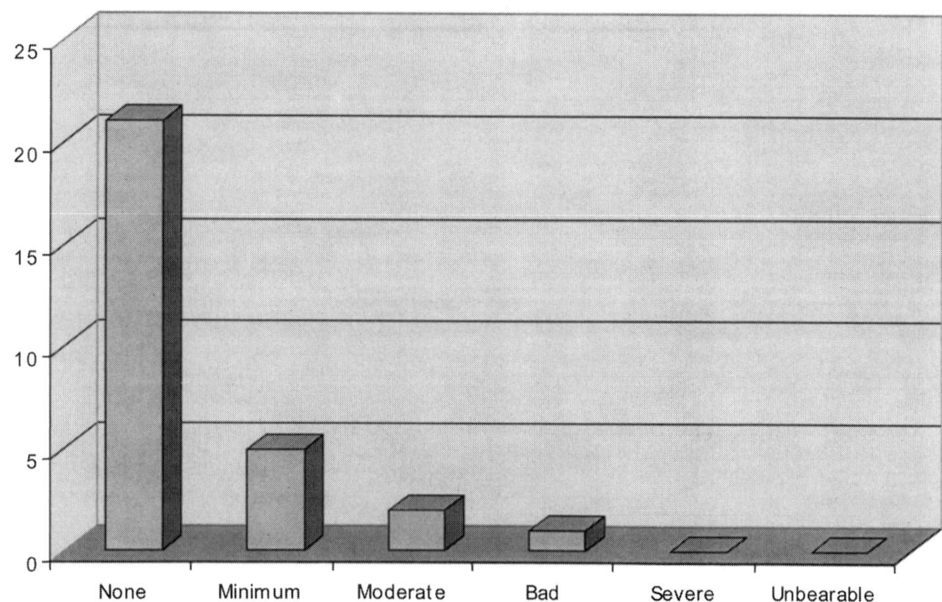

FIG. 3. Pain intensity during disc injection in ten asymptomatic young men with minimal disc degeneration.

tomatic young men (mean age, 22 years). Of 30 discs injected in this asymptomatic group, five produced "minimum" pain (16.7%), two "moderate" pain (6.7%), and one "bad" pain (3.3%) (Fig. 3). During injections, the subjects' reactions were videotaped and scored according to behavioral signs of discomfort. In this group with no preexisting chronic painful illness, the pain behavior scores were also low: three disc injections of 30 produced one pain behavior sign (10%), and one produced two pain behavior signs (3.3%) (54). From these data, the authors felt the risk of false-positive injections was very low. This paper is frequently cited to confirm a zero-percent false-positive rate (8–14).

In clinical practice however, the false-positive rate appeared to be higher. In 1997, the author's group reported a review of discography experience and found cases that appeared to be clinically apparent false-positives (16). These injections were felt to meet a strict criteria for discogenic pain but on follow-up revealed other causes of the patient's back pain illness, including spinal tumor, SI joint disease, and emotional problems. Block et al. reported psychological influences perhaps causing false-positive results (59), and Ohnmeiss et al. related pain drawings with "nonorganic" features being associated with possible false-positive injections as well (60).

With these results in mind, the author's group undertook a series of clinical experiments in an attempt to systematically analyze the validity of the two major criteria for a positive test in provocative discography: the pain intensity on injection and the reproduction pain by quality and location (concordance). To examine these criteria a select group of subjects was studied, without discogenic LBP but with other clinical and demographic features commonly seen in those patients with intractable back pain syndromes. Compared to the study by Walsh et al., the group was interested in older subjects with age-related changes in the lumbar spine, some with chronic pain syndromes unrelated to the spine, some with emotional and behavioral problems, and some with compensation issues.

In the first of the experimental series, 30 volunteer subjects with no history of LBP were recruited to undergo a protocol physical examination, MRI imaging, psychometric testing, and provocative discography. Of these, 10 had previous cervical spine surgery with excellent results (pain-free group), 10 had undergone the same surgery with poor results (chronic pain group), and six had no previous spine surgery but had a clinical diagnosis of somatization disorder (22).

The results showed that little pain was elicited by injection of any anatomically normal disc. In discs with advanced degenerative fissuring of the annulus so that the dye leaked to the outer (innervated) margins, the injections were more commonly painful. The intensity of the pain reported by the subjects was predicted by the presence of chronic nonlumbar pain and abnormal psychological scores. Compared to the healthy young men in the Walsh et al. study, it is clear that this group reported much more pain (Fig. 4). Whereas only 10% of the pain-free group had a positive disc injection by the Walsh et al. criteria, 40% of the chronic pain group and 80% of the somatization group had at least one positive disc.

From these data it appears that in a group of subjects without back pain but otherwise more closely resembling those patients coming to discography in clinical practice, disc injections are frequently painful. In approximately 20% of these subjects, at least one injection was very painful. Whereas many subjects had degenerative disc changes, the presence of chronic pain and perhaps generalized pain sensitization was associated with higher pain intensity reported with disc injections. Psychological factors, such as depression and increased somatic awareness, were strongly associated with greater reported pain intensity after injection (22).

Disability and Compensation Claims versus Discography Response

The interaction of compensation claims and discographic pain was also significant in this select group of volunteers (22). At the time of the study, only 7 of the 26 patients completing an injec-

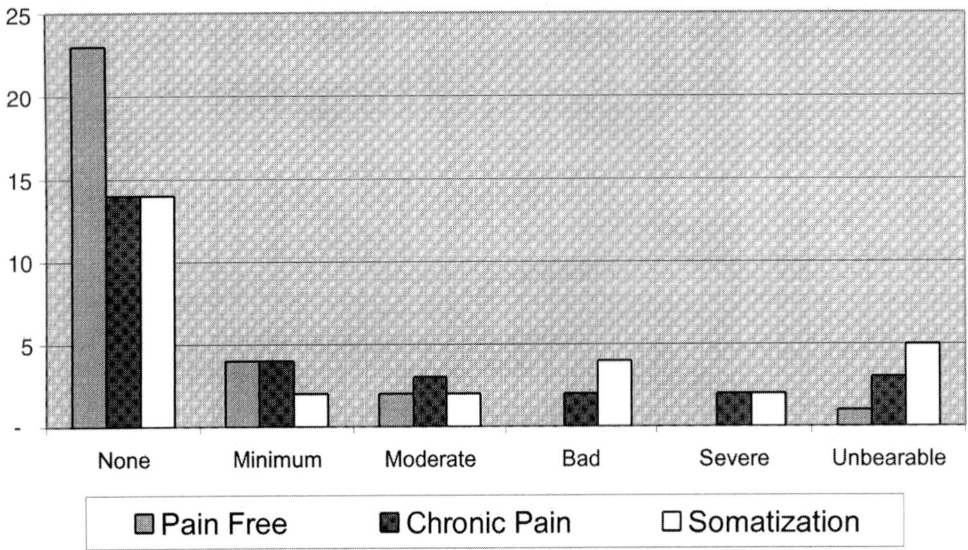

FIG. 4. Discographic pain intensity in asymptomatic subjects with characteristics of low back pain patients.

tion in this study were disabled from employment. However, even in this group without LBP, six of these seven (86%) had positive pain with injection. This rate of positive injection was much more frequent than in nondisabled patients ($p = .0004$).

A similar trend was found regarding active compensation claims. Of the ten subjects with positive injections, eight had active workers' compensation or personal injury claims with ongoing litigation. Conversely, of nine subjects with active litigation claims, eight had positive injections ($p < .0001$). It was not found, however, that all subjects involved in previous work injury claims had similar rates of positive disc injection. A history of a closed claim from the past compensation injury and no pending legal action did not predict significant pain on disc injection. The five subjects whose original neck trouble was attributed to a work injury but who had no ongoing claim all had negative injections (22).

Given that no subject in this study stood to have any secondary gain from a positive injection in discography, the increased pain reporting in subjects with unrelated but contested compensation claims is intriguing. It is possible that the effect of the prolonged social turmoil associated with a litigation dispute has the effect of diminishing one's resilience to irritative stimuli. Another explanation could be that persons with abnormally low pain tolerance are more likely to have a legal dispute regarding the significance and damages associated with minor injury.

Discographic Injections in Previously Operated Discs

Provocative discography is frequently used to evaluate persistent or recurrent LBP syndromes in patients who have undergone posterior discectomy. The validity of interpreting painful injections after herniation and discectomy is unknown despite its common usage. Heggeness et al. have reported the most extensive review of patients undergoing discography after lumbar discectomy and laminectomy (61). Of 83 patients retrospectively reviewed, 72% had a positive concordant pain response on injection of the previously operated disc. They also found this to be associated with dye penetration posteriorly. Heggeness et al. did not, however, address the possibility of false-positive injections. All positive injections were assumed to be true positive for identifying the source of the patient's pain.

Following the same methodology developed by Walsh et al., the author's group again performed experimental discography in a large study of asymptomatic patients after discectomy for sciatica (20). In this case, patients without any persistent symptoms after lumbar discectomy were recruited to participate, undergoing disc injection using the standard discography protocol. These results were compared against the results of discography in symptomatic patients being evaluated for fusion for persistent symptoms after discectomy (Fig. 5).

Painful disc injections were frequently seen in the asymptomatic postdiscectomy group. The asymptomatic group had 40% positive injections of previously operated discs, compared with 63% positive injections in the symptomatic group. If the psychological profiles were normal, however, the rate of positive disc injections was the same in symptomatic and asymptomatic groups—namely, the higher rate of positive injections in the symptomatic group appeared to be due predominantly to psychological variables, as opposed to structural findings. Injections of previously operated discs had a mean pain score of 2.1 of 5.0 in the asymptomatic group, 2.1 in the symptomatic group with normal psychometric scores, and 3.4 in the symptomatic group with abnormal psychometric scores. It appears that the validity of diagnostic disc injections using current techniques in previously operated discs may be limited. One would expect the test would evoke a similar pain intensity response in symptomatic and asymptomatic discs on which surgery has been performed.

High-Intensity Zone and Discography

Annular fissures with high signal intensity on MRI have been purported to be a reliable marker of active and clinically significant annular disc disruption. Aprill and Bogduk have reported that the finding of a high-intensity zone (HIZ) on MRI has a very high positive predictive value for discogenic pain as the cause of chronic LBP illness. This theory was based on the finding that discography was very frequently painful in patients with chronic LBP illness when an HIZ was present. The rate of pos-

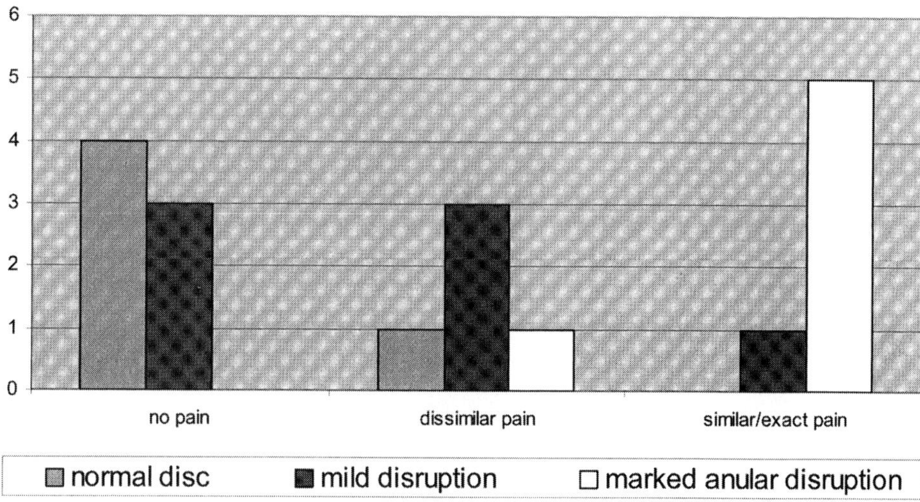

FIG. 5. Concordance of pain with disc injection in subjects after bone graft harvesting.

itive injections appeared to be much more frequently encountered in HIZ discs than in discs without HIZ (62). However, the theory that HIZ was a pathognomonic marker for severely symptomatic LBP was developed without a clear knowledge of the incidence of HIZ in the population without clinically significant back pain (36,63–67).

In an effort to establish a baseline of HIZ prevalence in subjects without LBP but with lumbar disc degeneration, the author's group selected subjects with a known propensity to lumbar disc degeneration but who were completely asymptomatic for LBP (21). Comprehensive clinical, psychometric, radiographic, and MRI evaluations were done, followed by provocative discography. The incidence of annular disruption, HIZ, and positive pain response with discography were reported and compared to LBP patients undergoing clinical evaluations for LBP. To standardize the HIZ finding in this study, the group defined the signal intensity of the HIZ relative to the adjacent cerebrospinal fluid on the T2-weighted images. A posterior or posterolateral bright annular signal within 10% of the cerebrospinal fluid signal was arbitrarily defined as an HIZ.

The prevalence of an HIZ in the LBP patient populations was 59%. However, 24% of the asymptomatic subjects were also found to have HIZ. In the symptomatic group, approximately 70% of the discs with an HIZ were positive on discography. This was indeed higher than the rate of positive injections (40%) in the discs without an HIZ. In the asymptomatic group, however, 70% of the discs with an HIZ were also positive on discography for significant pain on injection, whereas only 10% of discs without an HIZ were positive. As in previous studies, the group found that nonanatomic variables strongly predict pain on disc injections. In the patients with normal psychometric testing, 50% of the discs with an HIZ were positive on discography, compared to 100% positive discography in those patients with abnormal psychometric testing or chronic pain (or both).

It may be concluded that a disc with an HIZ, when injected, frequently has contrast dye extension to the outer annulus. It appears that this finding is likely to be associated with a painful disc injection regardless of whether a subject is usually symptomatic. Although the HIZ was found more frequently in patients with chronic LBP illness (60%) than in asymptomatic subjects (25%), the relatively frequent finding in asymptomatic subjects is much too high for the finding to prove useful as a reliable marker for chronic LBP illness.

Because the HIZ disc very frequently is painful on injection, the potential for false-positive diagnoses, especially in pain-sensitive individuals, may be very high. Therefore, discography may not be helpful in discriminating the symptomatic patient with an HIZ from one in whom the HIZ is a serendipitous finding.

Concordance

From these recent discography studies the following can be assumed:

- The discographic pain response can be of significant intensity in discs not actually causing the patient's primary pain.
- Certain "asymptomatic" discs, with particular structural findings, are more likely to be painful on injection, such as discs with annular fissures or discs after previous surgery, and so forth.
- Individuals with certain psychosocial characteristics are more likely to report high pain intensity levels with disc injections than others, such as those with psychological stressors, chronic pain states, litigation involvements, and so forth.

Provocative discography is only considered positive, however, when pain reproducing the patient's usual pain in quality and location is also elicited on injection. The reliability of the test would be substantially supported if patients could identify the quality of pain coming from a particular disc and differentially compare that sensation to their usual pain.

The ability to accurately locate a pain source by its quality and location may be quite good on undamaged skin or distal extremity joints. Whether that same degree of qualitative specificity of pain reproduction in stimulating an intervertebral disc in the presence of chronic regional pain has not been proven in discography. Data from the evaluation of other provocative tests would indicate that caution should be used in interpreting the "concordant" pain response. In the presence of chronic pain, there is a known increased responsiveness to normally innocuous stimuli generally. Furthermore, there may be hyperalgesia

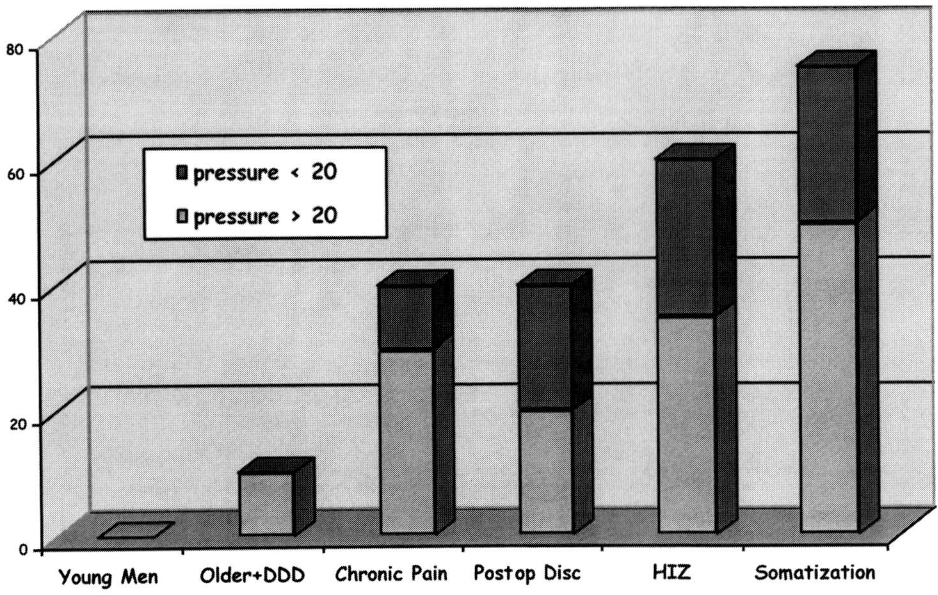

FIG. 6. Positive pain responses as a function of the pressure of injection. DDD, degenerative disc disease; HIZ, high-intensity zone demonstrated on magnetic resonance imaging; Post-op Disc, patients with prior discectomy.

of uninjured tissue in the area surrounding an injury. It is also known that stimulation of structures proximal to a lesion may mimic the quality and affective component of the patient's usual pain (68,69). Even primarily psychogenic pain may be simulated by provocative testing at a specific anatomic stimulation (15,16).

It has been shown that some patients with LBP syndromes may report reproduction of their pain by stimulation of anatomic parts unrelated to the spine. A classic example is the Waddell sign, which includes such distraction or sham tests on physical examination. In these tests, a patient's LBP may be provoked by maneuvers at distant sites without true stress to the spine. When gentle tapping on a patient's head acutely and severely exacerbates one's usual LBP, the inference is not that the cranium is the spinal "pain generator" but, rather, that the patient's illness may be related to social emotional stressors.

It has not been clear to what extent similar neurologic and behavioral factors may be influencing the results in provocative discography. It is possible that the disc stimulation in discography may also provoke a "concordant" pain response without actually having located a true pain source. In earlier work, the author's group reported cases of individuals who underwent discography and were diagnosed as having discogenic pain as the source of their illness on the basis of positive concordant disc injections but who were subsequently shown to have nonspinal sources for their pain (17). Among the nonspinal sources of pain in this group were two patients with pathology at the SI joint and one with a posterior element neoplasm. In these cases, the treatment of the nondisc pathology relieved the pain.

The neurophysiologic literature and these clinical observations in discography may lead one to believe that the concordance rating a patient gives at discography may not be a reliable indicator of the location of a clinical pain source. That is, a patient's impression may be that the quality of pain on discography reproduced their usual pain, but the usual pain may be unrelated or only in small part related to the disc being injected. To test this hypothesis, the author's group determined the response to disc injection in an experimental setting of patients with known nonspinal back pain (23). Volunteer subjects were tested with no history of back pain but who were scheduled to undergo posterior iliac crest bone graft harvesting for nonspinal problems, mainly fracture nonunions or bone tumors. Most patients experience low back and buttock pain for some months after posterior iliac crest bone graft, and this pain is in a similar distribution to what is normally considered discogenic lumbar pain. The areas have similar sclerotomal origins and referred pain distributions. Presumably sensory afferent pathways are similar. Discography was then performed some months after the bone graft harvesting and subjects were asked to compare the quality and location of disc injection pain to their usual iliac crest pain.

Twenty-four discs were injected in eight volunteer subjects, and the same protocol as the Walsh et al. study was used. Of the 14 disc injections causing some pain response, five were felt to be "different" (nonconcordant) pains (35.7%), seven were "similar" (50.0%), and two were "exact" pain reproductions (14.3%) (Fig. 5). An interesting finding was that disc injection in one patient "reproduced" leg pain due to a fracture nonunion. With pressurization of a disc, the patient described buttock and thigh pain and described the thigh pain as "exactly" reproducing his thigh pain associated with a femoral nonunion.

The presence of annular disruption predicted concordant pain reproduction ($p < .05$). Of ten discs with annular tears, injection of seven elicited "similar" or "exact" pain reproduction to the iliac crest bone graft harvest site pain (Fig. 5). By the strict criteria for positive discography, four of the eight patients (50%) would have been classified as positive. In these subjects, the pain on a single disc injection was "bad" or "very bad," and the pain quality was noted to be exact or similar to the usual discomfort. All subjects had a negative control disc. All positive disc injections had annular fissures. One-half of the positive disc injections occurred at low pressures (<20 psi).

Judging from these data, it is not clear what should be inferred from a report of concordant pain on discography. Sensory input from the lumbar and pelvic regions may not have sufficiently detailed sensory cortical representation for a patient to reliably distinguish discogenic from nondiscogenic pain. By extension, adjacent discs should be expected to have very similar cortical sensory perception; one may not be able to distinguish a "typical" L4-5 sensation from that at L3-4 or L-5 to S-1. A patient with central or neuropathic pain associated with spinal cord or thalamic changes may not be able to distinguish the quality of his or her usual pain from the pain of disc injection. The same may be true for visceral pain from intrapelvic pathology, or gastrointestinal or vascular lesions. Psychogenic pain syndromes or somatization disorder patients may also find peripherally stimulated disc pain to be similar to their usual but predominantly nonspinal pain.

The failure to confirm a highly reliable concordance in these experimental tests should lead us to reexamine the discography literature to date. There has been little serious discussion in clinical practice or in numerous clinical series with the consideration that if a patient with appropriate control injections claims the pain to be concordant on injection that the injected disc is the source of the problem (8,10–12,14,18–24). As there has never been a gold standard by which to confirm the diagnosis of discogenic pain, the various series reporting the results and correlations of positive discography with various clinical presentations and responses to treatment may be without scientific foundation.

Discography in Subjects with Minimal Low Back Symptoms

Earlier in this chapter, it was discussed that 60% of adults report some mild backache that is generally without clinical implications (18). The cause of this common benign backache is not known, but it is reasonable to assume there are multiple causes, ranging from muscle ache to spinal arthritic pain. Experimental discography was performed in 25 volunteer subjects who had persistent low back ache unassociated with any physical restrictions and who indicated they would not seek medical care for this discomfort (18). All of these subjects had normal psychological profiles. In 36% of these subjects, discographic injection of one or more discs was significantly painful and concordant. All positive discs had annular disruption and all had negative control discs; that is, by the usual criteria, these were fully positive. Low pressure–sensitive discs were found in 28% of subjects, which was not significantly different from chronic LBP controls or the percent seen by Derby et al. in their original description of "chemically sensitive" discs (25).

As in the author's previous studies on discography in asymptomatic subjects, annular disruption and preexisting pain syndrome distant from the lumbar spine predicted increased pain with disc injection.

Pressure-Sensitive Injections

In some cases, very little dye at low pressures may cause severe pain. Derby and his colleagues have called these "chemically" sensitive discs as opposed to discs that are only painful on injection with high pressures (56). These authors have theorized that "chemically" sensitive discs are painful due to the exposure of annular nerve endings or nearby neural structures to the leakage of irritating substances. It is postulated that this pain is incited by chemical leakage from the disc during daily activities. This leakage is thought to be simulated by the disc injections. Low pressure–positive discs are arbitrarily defined as those found to be painful at pressures less than 15 to 22 psi above opening pressures (25,26). Derby et al. have further postulated that disc injections eliciting pain at higher pressures (>50 psi), called "mechanically" sensitive discs, physically distend the annulus and simulate a mechanical loading. In these discs, it is presumed that a mechanical deformation of the annulus is the inciting painful event in daily activities.

The use of pressure measurements has been postulated as a means to decrease the risk of false-positive injections. This would be true if injections were rarely, if ever, positive at low pressures in subjects without true LBP illness.

Discographic injections have been performed with pressure measurements in asymptomatic or minimally symptomatic volunteers. Table 4 shows the rate of painful injections at low pressures in volunteers and cohorts of clinical patients with chronic LBP illness. It appears from these data that low-pressure injections are more likely positive in subjects with some type of chronic pain state and, presumably, a generalized sensitization to irritable stimuli (18,20–23,56) (Fig. 6). This increased perception of pain at low-pressure injections appears to exist regardless of whether the pain state was referable to the low back.

Evidence That Primary Discogenic Pain Can Cause Chronic Low Back Pain Illness

In summary, recent experimental work on discography has shown frequently positive disc injections in asymptomatic subjects, subjects with pelvic pain due to iliac crest harvesting, and frequent

TABLE 4. *Low-pressure positive disc injections in volunteer subjects with chronic low back pain illness*[a]

Subject characteristics	Study	N	Injections
No LBP, no chronic pain states	Carragee et al. (2000)	10	0% low pressure
No LBP and chronic nonlumbar pain	Carragee et al. (2000)	16	31% low pressure
No LBP after limited discectomy	Carragee et al. (2000)	20	30% low pressure
Experimental pelvic pain, no LBP	Carragee et al. (1999)	8	25% low pressure (concordant)
Mild persistent backache	Carragee et al. (2002)	25	28% low pressure positive (concordant)
Chronic LBP illness	Derby et al. (1999)	109	33% low pressure positive (concordant)
Chronic LBP illness	Carragee et al. (2002)	52	27% low pressure positive (concordant)

LBP, low back pain.
[a]Pain response ≥3/5 at 20 ppi or less over opening pressure.

fully concordant injections in subjects with clinically irrelevant backache. These findings may appear to support the school of thought claiming there is no primary chronic LBP illness without concomitant social or neuropsychologic amplification of symptoms. Certainly, that may explain the high rates of failure in the surgical treatment of this difficult clinical problem. It is not clear that discography results improve the results of surgical treatment. In one study, the results of discography appeared to modestly predict better outcomes with surgery (70); in another, no difference was seen between a group of spinal fusion patients who had had discography and another who did not (71). Nonetheless, clinical experience has shown that some patients appear to be cured of LBP by spinal fusion, possibly removing a pain generator detected by discography.

The author's group examined a highly select group of patients operated on for a presumed diagnosis of primary discogenic pain and tried to exclude all concomitant social or neuropsychological factors that may have amplified the pain process. The group of 30 highly selected patients with 6 to 18 months of severe LBP had normal psychological testing, no previous or concomitant pain syndromes, and no workers' compensation or personal injury claims. All were positive at one level only on discography, at low pressures (<20 psi). All had been working full time before their back problem. No patient was taking daily narcotic medications. All 30 had an anterior spinal fusion with posterior instrumentation and fusion.

Two years after surgery, eight patients (27%) met a stringent criteria for success: full return to work, full return to recreational activities, pain scores on visual analogue scale <2, Oswestry Disability Index <15, and no daily medications for back pain—namely, only 8 of 30 patients, with the least risk factors for failure, were symptomatically and functionally cured. Similar outstanding results in a minority of operated patients (14%) have been reported by Fritzell et al. in a controlled trial (72).

It is highly likely that this small group of "cured" patients had a primary structural cause of disability and chronic LBP illness, probably discogenic in origin. These data indicate that there are probably primary lesions of the lumbar spine that alone do cause such severe illness without any apparent amplification on a neurophysiologic, social, or psychological basis (Table 3, Fig. 2A). There does not, however, appear to be a reliable diagnostic technique to identify this small subgroup and distinguish these from the many patients with no primary spinal lesion accountable for their illness. Therefore, a validated approach to even this most thoroughly investigated diagnosis of chronic LBP illness has not been developed.

CONCLUSION

Assessing the results of these studies on LBP diagnosis indicates a complex picture. Physical signs and imaging studies occasionally reveal unequivocal pathology. However, most patients have imaging studies reflecting only common degenerative changes. Discography is a primary tool used to try to identify the "true pain generator" in these patients. A high specificity of this test was not found in the author's recent series of experimental work (16,18–23,29). Because the reliability of patient response is fundamental to discography, interpretation of the test in different settings must be carefully considered.

At one end of the spectrum, the injection of discs with no degenerative pathology, no annular disruption, performed under low pressures does not cause much pain at all (22,54). Even subjects with serious emotional or chronic pain behaviors report little pain with these injections. In the presence of an annular tear or a previously operated disc, however, the disc may be quite painful with injection whether there is a back pain problem or not. The risk of a false-positive result appears to increase with emotional distress, chronic pain behavior, and ongoing compensation issues. In subjects with none of these issues, the pain intensity rating during provocative discography, as an index of symptomatic disc disease, may be reliable.

Table 5 presents a variety of possible LBP scenarios in which discography may be used. In one of these, the true cause of the LBP illness is primary discogenic pain without any confounding factors. The other scenarios presented indicate situations in which discography may be performed and the risks associated with a false-positive result are given.

The best usage for the test may be in the patient with clear pathology (e.g., spondylolisthesis or scoliosis) in whom the extent of the proposed fusion is uncertain and the integrity of the adjacent segments is important to establish. In that case, a negative result—with a normal disc structure and painless injection—may be helpful clinically. A positive test may be more problematic.

Similarly, in the patient with a single arthritic or disrupted lumbar segment, without emotional troubles, with a stable family and occupational support, no history of chronic or unexplained pain syndromes, and no compensation issues, discography may be helpful in confirming that the disrupted segment does hurt while the adjacent segments do not.

In general, however, this is not the usual profile of a patient coming to discography. Chronic pain, emotional troubles, poor job satisfaction, alcohol or narcotic abuse, and compensation issues are the main confounding problems in patients with chronic disabling back pain as a whole (1,9,11). In some series, 75% of patients coming to discography have active compensation claims (33,55). In the author's group's review, only 20% of patients coming to discography for possible discogenic pain had normal psychological testing on screening depression and somatic awareness questionnaires (29).

The poorest indication may be in the disturbed patient in search of an anatomic diagnosis of a chronic pain illness. Similarly, the use of discography in the patient with litigation or a contested compensation claim seeking validation of injury or causation is completely unproven, and the author's data indicate the test would be very unreliable. Finally, discography is not likely to be helpful in patients with multiple reasons for regional pain (e.g., multiple previous failed spinal surgeries, painful hip graft sites, concomitant pain syndromes in referable other areas) or generalized pain intolerance (e.g., drug and alcohol abuses, narcotic dependence, depression or somatization disorders) (Table 5).

Obviously, this leaves a considerable gray area. Until good controlled studies may show a clear positive impact of discography on patient care and outcomes, the procedure remains controversial and at present does not have basic experimental support. In the end, the discogram and other spinal diagnostic tests are tools, and these tools have certain clear limitations. Clinical judgment starts with understanding the patient's life and circumstances. Knowing the patient cannot be replaced by knowing the pain drawing, the discography results, or the visual analogue scale scores, as it appears one may strongly determine the other.

TABLE 5. *True and false positive discography: neurophysiologic mechanisms of positive painful and concordant disc injections at low pressures*

Cause of LBP illness	Pain pathway	False-positive risk factors
Primary discogenic LBP illness from the injected disc	Injected disc is the site of a pain generator, possibly an annular fissure or reaction to fissuring, which causes severe local pain. This lesion, regardless of pain tolerance, social, and emotional factors causes a crippling illness.	True positive.
Primary discogenic LBP illness from a neighboring disc, not the injected disc	Injected disc alone would not normally cause significant illness. Adjacent disc is actually the primary pain generator and injected disc manifests a hyperalgesic response.	Some annular disruption required allow dye to penetrate annulus. Multilevel degenerative disc disease on magnetic resonance imaging. Previous discectomy surgery.
Regional/spinal pathology (nondiscogenic)	Injected disc alone would not normally cause significant illness. Adjacent structures are diseased (e.g., sacroiliac disease, bone tumor, etc.), and the injected disc manifests a hyperalgesic response.	Annular disruption. Pelvic or spinal pathology. Failed spinal surgery. Previous iliac crest bone graft harvesting.
Primary neurophysiologic impairment	Injected disc alone would not normally cause significant illness. Concomitant chronic pain syndromes (e.g., "fibromyalgia," "irritable bowel disease," etc.) have altered pain perception and a relatively small nociceptive input.	Annular disruption. History of chronic pain syndrome or unexplained prolonged convalescence. Somatization disorder or somatic distress on psychometric testing. Narcotic or alcohol dependency/abuse.
Primary psychologic/social illness	Injected disc alone would not normally cause significant illness. Amplification of minor peripheral nociception due to psychological or social processes.	Annular disruption. Psychologic distress on psychometric testing. Clinical depression, somatization, or anxiety disorders. Fear avoidance maladaptive behavior. Chaotic or absent social supports. Compensation claim with disincentive to usual discomfort accommodation.
Combined disorders	Injected disc alone would not normally cause significant illness. Multiple pain amplifiers: local, regional, and constitutional. Social and emotional processes acting against usual accommodations to LBP.	All of the above risk factors may apply.

LBP, low back pain.

REFERENCES

1. Allan DB, Waddell G. An historical perspective on low back pain and disability. *Acta Orthop Scand* 1989;234:1–23.
2. North R, Kidd D, Zahurak M, et al. Specificity of diagnostic nerve blocks: a prospective, randomized study of sciatica due to lumbosacral spine disease. *Pain* 1996;65:77–85.
3. Siddle P, Cousins M. Spinal pain mechanisms. *Spine* 1997;22:98–104.
4. Kibler R, Nathan P. Relief of pain and paraesthesiae by nerve block distal to a lesion. *J Neurol Neurosurg Psychiatry* 1960;23:91–98.
5. Kawakami MT, Hashizume H, Weinstein JN, et al. The role of phospholipase a2 and nitric oxide in pain-related behavior produced by an allograft of intervertebral disc material to the sciatic nerve of the rat. *Spine* 1997;22:1074–1079.
6. Gracely R, Dubner R, McGrath P. Narcotic analgesia: Fentanyl reduces the intensity but not the unpleasantness of painful tooth pulp stimulation. *Science* 1979;203:1261–1263.
7. Mersky H, Bogduk N. *Classification of chronic pain syndromes and definition of pain terms*. Seattle: IASP Press, 1994:180–181.
8. Barbour A. Caring for patients. A critique of the medical model. Stanford, CA: Stanford University Press, 1995.
9. Burton AK, Tillotson KM, Main CJ. Psychosocial predictors of outcome in acute and subchronic low back trouble. *Spine* 1995;20:2738–2745.

10. Gaskin ME, Greene AF, Robinson ME, et al. Negative affect and the experience of chronic pain. *J Psychosomatic Res* 1992;36:707–713.
11. Pincus T, Burton AK, Vogel S, et al. A systematic review of psychological factors as predictors of chronicity/disability in prospective cohorts of low back pain. *Spine* 2002;27:E109–E120.
12. Trief P, Grant W, Fredrickson B. A prospective study of psychological predictors of lumbar surgery outcome. *Spine* 2000;25:2616–2621.
13. Bigos S, Battie M, Spengler D, et al. A prospective study of work perceptions and psychosocial factors affecting the report of back injury. *Spine* 1991;16:1–6.
14. Bigos S, Battie M, Spengler D, et al. A longitudinal, prospective study of industrial back injury reporting. *Clin Orthopaed Rel Res* 1992;279:21–34.
15. Carragee E, McCormack M, Schilling P, et al. Resilience in occupational low back disability: back pain, disability and stress in soldiers undergoing heavy physical training. *Proceedings of the International Society for the Study of the Lumbar Spine*. Edinburgh, UK, 2001.
16. Carragee E, Tanner C, Vittum D, et al. Positive provocative discography as a misleading finding in the evaluation of low back pain. *NASS Proceedings* 1997:388.
17. Carragee EJ. Psychological screening in the surgical treatment of lumbar disc herniation. *Clin J Pain* 2001;17:215–219.
18. Carragee EJ, Alamin TF, Miller J, et al. 2001 Outstanding paper award. Provocative discography in volunteer subjects with mild persistent low back pain. *Spine J* 2002;2:25–34.
19. Carragee EJ, Chen Y, Tanner CM, et al. Can discography cause long-term back symptoms in previously asymptomatic subjects? *Spine* 2000;25:1803–1808.
20. Carragee EJ, Chen Y, Tanner CM, et al. Provocative discography in patients after limited lumbar discectomy: a controlled, randomized study of pain response in symptomatic and asymptomatic subjects. *Spine* 2000;25:3065–3071.
21. Carragee EJ, Paragioudakis SJ, Khurana S. 2000 Volvo Award winner in clinical studies: lumbar high-intensity zone and discography in subjects without low back problems. *Spine* 2000;25:2987–2992.
22. Carragee EJ, Tanner CM, Khurana S, et al. The rates of false-positive lumbar discography in select patients without low back symptoms. *Spine* 2000;25:1373–1380, discussion, 1381.
23. Carragee EJ, Tanner CM, Yang B, et al. False-positive findings on lumbar discography. Reliability of subjective concordance assessment during provocative disc injection. *Spine* 1999;24:2542–2547.
24. Carragee EJ, Vittum D, Truong TP, et al. Pain control and cultural norms and expectations after closed femoral shaft fractures. *Am J Orthoped* 1999;28:97–102.
25. Cassisi JE, Sypert GW, Lagana L, et al. Pain, disability, and psychological functioning in chronic low back pain subgroups: myofascial versus herniated disc syndrome. *Neurosurgery* 1993;33:379–385, discussion, 385–386.
26. Klenerman L, Slade P, Stanley I, et al. The prediction of chronicity in patients with acute attack of low back pain in a general practice setting. *Spine* 1995;20:478–484.
27. Simmonds MJ, Olson SL, Jones S, et al. Psychometric characteristics and clinical usefulness of physical performance tests in patients with low back pain. *Spine* 1998;23:2412–2421.
28. Swimmer GI, Robinson ME, Geisser ME. Relationship of MMPI cluster type, pain coping strategy, and treatment outcome. *Clin J Pain* 1992;8:131–137.
29. Carragee E. Psychological and functional profiles in select subjects with low back pain. *Spine J* 2001;1:198–204.
30. Burton A. Spine update: back injury and work loss: biomechanical and psychosocial influences. *Spine* 1997;22:2575–2580.
31. Carragee EJ. Pyogenic vertebral osteomyelitis [see comments]. *J Bone Joint Surg (Am)* 1997;79:874–880.
32. Carragee EJ. The clinical use of magnetic resonance imaging in pyogenic vertebral osteomyelitis. *Spine* 1997;22:780–785.
33. Schwarzer A, Aprill C, Bogduk N. The sacroiliac joint in chronic low back pain. *Spine* 1995;20:31–37.
34. Schwarzer AC, Wang SC, Bogduk N, et al. Prevalence and clinical features of lumbar zygapophysial joint pain: a study in an Australian population with chronic low back pain. *Ann Rheum Dis* 1995;54:100–106.
35. Jarvik JJM, Hollingworth W, Heagerty P, et al. The Longitudinal Assessment of Imaging and Disability of the Back (LAIDBack) study—baseline data. *Spine* 2001;26:1158–1166.
36. Jensen M, Brant-Zawadzki M, Obuchowski N, et al. Magnetic resonance imaging of the lumbar spine in people without back pain. *N Engl J Med* 1994;331:69–73.
37. Boden S, Davis D, Dina T, et al. Abnormal magnetic resonance scans of the lumbar spine in asymptomatic subjects: a prospective investigation. *J Bone Joint Surg (Am)* 1990;72-A:403–408.
38. Beattie P, Meyers S, Stratford P, et al. Associations between patient report of symptoms and anatomic impairment visible on lumbar MR imaging. *Spine* 2000;25:819–828.
39. Luoma K, Riihimäki H, Luukkonen R, et al. Low back pain in relation to lumbar disc degeneration. *Spine* 2000;25:487–492.
40. Elfering ADP, Semmer N, Birkhofer D, et al. Young Investigator Award 2001 Winner: Risk factors for lumbar disc degeneration—a 5-year prospective MRI study in asymptomatic individuals. *Spine* 2002;27:125–134.
41. McCall I, Park W, O'Brien J. Induced pain referral from posterior lumbar elements in normal subjects. *Spine* 1979;4:441–446.
42. Fukui S, Shiotani M, et al. Distribution of referred pain from the lumbar zygapophyseal joints and dorsal rami. *Clin J Pain* 1997;13:303–307.
43. Marks R, Thulbourne T. Facet joint injection and facet nerve block: a randomised comparison in 86 patients with chronic low back pain. *Pain* 1992;49:325–328.
44. Kaplan M, Dreyfuss P, Halbrook B, et al. The ability of lumbar medial branch blocks to anesthetize the zygapophysial joint: a physiologic challenge. *Spine* 1998;23:1847–1852.
45. Revel M, Poiraudeau S, Auleley G, et al. Capacity of the clinical picture to characterize low back pain relieved by facet joint anesthesia: proposed criteria to identify patients with painful facet joints. *Spine* 1998;23.
46. Schwarzer A, Wang SC, O'Driscoll D, et al. The ability of computed tomography to identify a painful zygapophysial joint in patients with chronic low back pain. *Spine* 1995;20:907–912.
47. Nelemans P, deBie R, deVet H, et al. Injection therapy for subacute and chronic benign low back pain. *Spine* 2001;26:501–515.
48. van Kleef M, Barendse G, Kessels A, et al. Denervation for chronic low back pain. *Spine* 1999;23:1937.
49. Leclaire R, Fortin L, Lambert R, et al. Radiofrequency facet joint denervation in the treatment of low back pain: a placebo-controlled clinical trial to assess efficacy. *Spine* 2001;26:1411–1416.
50. Dreyfus P, Halbrook B, Pauza K, et al. Efficacy and validity of radiofrequency neurotomy for chronic lumbar zygapophysial joint pain. *Spine* 2000;25:1270–1277.
51. Fortin J, Dwyer A, West S, et al. Sacroiliac joint: pain referral maps upon applying a new injection/arthrography technique. Part I: asymptomatic volunteers. *Spine* 1994;19:1475–1482.
52. Dreyfus P, Michaelson M, Pauza K, et al. The value of medical history and physical examination in diagnosing sacroiliac joint pain. *Spine* 1996;21:2594–2602.
53. Slipman C, Sterenfeld E, Chou L, et al. The value of radionuclide imaging in the diagnosis of sacroiliac joint syndrome. *Spine* 1996;21:2251–2254.
54. Walsh T, Weinstein J, Spratt K, et al. Lumbar discography in normal subjects: a controlled prospective study. *J Bone Joint Surg* 1990;72-A:1081–1088.
55. Schwarzer A, Aprill C, Derby R, et al. The prevalence and clinical features of internal disc disruption in patients with chronic LBP. *Spine* 1995;20:1878–1883.
56. Derby R, Howard MW, Grant JM, et al. The ability of pressure-controlled discography to predict surgical and nonsurgical outcomes. *Spine* 1999;24:364–371, discussion, 371–372.
57. Guyer R, Ohnmeiss D. Lumbar discography. Position statement from the North American Spine Society Diagnostic and Therapeutic Committee. *Spine* 1995;20:2048–2059.
58. O'Neill C, Kaiser J, Derby R, et al. Pain thresholds on discography: an examination of the distension pressure clustering across intervertebral discs. Proceedings of the International Society for the Study of the Lumbar Spine, 29th annual meeting. 2002:150.
59. Block A, Vanharanta H, Ohnmeiss D, et al. Discographic pain report: influence of psychological factors. *Spine* 1996;21:334–338.
60. Ohnmeiss DD, Vanharanta H, Guyer RD. The association between pain drawings and computed tomographic/discographic pain responses. *Spine* 1995;20:729–733.

61. Heggeness MH, Watters WC 3rd, Gray PM Jr. Discography of lumbar discs after surgical treatment for disc herniation. *Spine* 1997;22:1606–1609.
62. Aprill C, Bogduk N. High-intensity zone: a diagnostic sign of painful lumbar disc on magnetic resonance imaging. *Br J Radiol* 1992;65:361–369.
63. Ito M, Incorvaia KM, Yu SF, et al. Predictive signs of discogenic lumbar pain on magnetic resonance imaging with discography correlation. *Spine* 1998;23:1252–1258, discussion, 1259–1260.
64. Kaiser J. Point of view. *Spine* 1996;21:86.
65. Kaiser J. Point of view. *Spine* 1999;24:1920.
66. Ricketson R, Simmons JW, Hauser BO. The prolapsed intervertebral disc. The high-intensity zone with discography correlation [see comments]. *Spine* 1996;21:2758–2762.
67. Schellhas KP, Pollei SR, Gundry CR, et al. Lumbar disc high-intensity zone. Correlation of magnetic resonance imaging and discography. *Spine* 1996;21:79–86.
68. Lenz FA, Gracely RH, Hope EJ, et al. The sensation of angina can be evoked by stimulation of the human thalamus. *Pain* 1994;59: 119–125.
69. Lenz F, Gracely R, Romanoski A, et al. Simulation in the somatosensory thalamus can reproduce both the affective and sensory dimensions of previously experienced pain. *Nat Med* 1995;1:910–913.
70. Colhoun E, McCall IW, Williams L, et al. Provocation discography as a guide to planning operations on the spine. *J Bone Joint Surg (Br)* 1988;70:267–271.
71. Madan SG, Harley JM, Boeree NR, et al. Does provocative discography screening of discogenic back pain improve surgical outcome? *J Spinal Dis Tech* 2002;15:245–251.
72. Fritzell P, Hägg O, Wessberg P, et al. 2001 Volvo Award Winner in Clinical Studies. Lumbar fusion versus nonsurgical treatment for chronic low back pain—a multicenter randomized controlled trial from the Swedish Lumbar Spine Study Group. *Spine* 2001;26: 2521–2532.

CHAPTER 45

Nonoperative Treatment of Low Back Pain

Daniel Mazanec

The vast majority of patients with low back pain are successfully managed nonoperatively. A wide array of nonsurgical treatments are available and are used by a diverse group of practitioners. Considerable variability in treatment protocol exists, driven in part by the specialty and training of the clinician directing care—"who you see is what you get" (1). Comparative evaluation of treatment in the literature is confounded by the lack of consistent diagnostic terminology for back disorders, even within the same medical specialty (2). This chapter reviews nonoperative and noninterventional management of acute and chronic nonspecific low back pain, emphasizing, when available, evidenced-based treatment principles with the dual objectives of pain relief and functional restoration.

ISSUES IN DIAGNOSIS AND TREATMENT

Ideally, the nonoperative treatment of low back pain should be based on a clear understanding of the etiology of the symptoms, knowledge of the natural history of the untreated condition, and evidence-based treatment principles. In reality, however, in most patients with acute or chronic back pain, a specific pain generator cannot be isolated (3–5). Aggressive use of interventional diagnostic procedures, such as discography or facet joint blocks, may identify a putative pathoanatomic etiology in some patients who previously might have been categorized as having nonspecific back pain (6,7). The inability to identify a consistent set of clinical features associated with diagnoses such as facet syndrome or internal disc disruption limits the application of these techniques. There is a lack of randomized prospective trials that evaluate nonoperative and operative treatment whose diagnosis is based on discography or facet injection, which further limits their utility in the precise location of a pain generator. The search for a precise anatomic cause of the patient's pain is further complicated by poor correlation between abnormal imaging findings on computed tomography or magnetic resonance scans and the presence or absence of symptoms (8–11). Attribution of symptoms to radiographic findings without careful clinical correlation may result in unnecessary and inappropriate treatment.

The Quebec classification of activity-related spinal disorders remains useful in patients in whom a precise anatomic source of pain cannot be identified (12) (Table 1). This approach categorizes patients into those with primarily back pain versus those with dominant leg (radicular) symptoms. In addition, patients are further subclassified based on duration of symptoms. Although variable definitions exist, acute low back pain is usually viewed as less than 4 weeks in duration. Subacute back pain is an appropriate designation for pain of 1 to 3 months of duration. Pain persisting beyond 3 months is termed *chronic*. However, most studies of patients with back pain often overlap acute and subacute or subacute and chronic patients.

The search for a diagnosis in the patient with low back pain cannot ignore the psychosocial dimension. Particularly in patients with chronic low back pain, so-called nonorganic issues may

TABLE 1. *Classification of nonspecific low back pain*

Back pain is categorized on the basis of location and duration of symptoms.	
I. Location of pain	
Low back without radiation	Most common pattern; nonradicular, typically mechanical
Low back with proximal radiation (above the knee)	Referred spinal pain; possibly neurogenic
Low back with distal radiation (below the knee)	Radicular or pseudosciatic
Low back with distal radiation and neurologic signs	Radicular
II. Duration of symptoms	
Acute	<4 wk
Subacute	4–12 wk
Chronic	>12 wk

Modified from the Spitzer WO, LeBlanc FE, Dupuis M, et al. Scientific approach to assessment and mangement of activity-related spine disorders. A monograph for clinicians. Report of the Quebec Task Force on Spinal Disorders. *Spine* 1987;12[Supp1]:S17–S21.

dwarf any underlying identifiable structural source of pain. For many patients with chronic back pain, psychosocial issues antedate the onset of symptoms. More than 90% of patients with substance abuse or anxiety disorders experienced these problems before the onset of back pain (13). Burton et al. prospectively evaluated 252 patients with acute low back pain for 1 year and found that persisting disability at 12 months depended primarily on the psychosocial domain (14). Andersson has suggested that chronic low back pain may be a "diagnosis of convenience" for persons whose actual reason for disability is socioeconomic, work-related, or psychological (15). Failure to recognize these psychosocial issues in patients with low back pain will frustrate the most well-conceived nonoperative or surgical treatment approach.

Studies of the natural history of acute nonspecific back pain suggest that most patients are significantly improved within 2 or 3 weeks, but up to one-third of patients report significant symptoms at 1-year follow-up (16–18). Although acute episodes usually resolve quickly, recurrences occur in up to 75% of patients within 1 year (19,20). Given this natural history, treatment strategies should address not only improvement in acute symptoms but risk of recurrence and long-term satisfaction as well.

As is evident in the discussion that follows, many of the treatments commonly used in patients with low back pain are inadequately studied. Diagnostic ambiguity and variable terminology often result in studies of heterogeneous populations of patients. For some treatment modalities, blinded trials with true controls are difficult to perform (e.g., acupuncture or manipulation). Only relatively recently have validated outcome parameters for assessing pain and function been widely adopted in back pain trials. Despite these shortcomings, there is remarkable consensus on appropriate management of acute back pain in a primary care setting, as evidenced in a review of clinical guidelines for low back pain treatment from 11 different countries (21). Because the short-term prognosis for recovery is excellent for most patients with acute nonspecific low back pain, activity advice complemented by simple medications or manipulation is often all that is required.

Optimal treatment of chronic nonspecific low back pain beyond general recommendations for exercise is much more controversial. Considerable variability exists among providers of different specialties in management approaches. Critical evaluation of limited evidence of efficacy of some of these therapies has been increasingly attempted in the form of systematic reviews and metaanalyses, such as by the Cochrane Collaboration. Although certainly a step in the right direction, a number of shortcomings of this approach have been described, including use of somewhat arbitrary rating criteria in evaluating studies, almost exclusive reliance on randomized controlled trials as acceptable evidence of efficacy, and concerns regarding impartiality of reviewers (22).

THERAPEUTIC OPTIONS FOR LOW BACK PAIN

Education

Providing patients with information about back anatomy, causes and natural history of back pain, and advice about activity and exercise are important aspects of management. Education is helpful in setting realistic expectations for treatment outcome, particularly in chronic back pain. Information may be provided via individual face-to-face contact with a physician or nurse, in an informational booklet, or in group sessions, commonly referred to as *back schools*. In patients with acute low back pain, these educational efforts have at least short-term impact on outcomes, including pain and function. Little et al. found the use of an educational booklet or advice to take regular exercise in 311 patients with acute low back pain improved pain and function scores at 1 week in comparison to patients given neither the booklet nor advice (23). These differences disappeared at 3-week follow-up. In this study, patient satisfaction with care also improved with these interventions. Surprisingly, providing both the booklet and exercise advice was counterproductive. In a comparison of usual care with an educational booklet or a 15-minute encounter with a clinic nurse including the booklet, Cherkin et al. found the nurse intervention improved patient satisfaction and perceived knowledge about back pain, as well as improved participation with recommended exercises (24). However, no significant differences among the three groups in pain or functional status were found. A recent randomized trial found that providing an educational leaflet to patients with acute low back pain produced improved knowledge of proper sitting posture and actual behavioral change, which was sustained at 3-month follow-up (25).

It has been difficult to demonstrate that group back education in the form of back schools produces tangible improvements in outcomes of patients with acute and chronic low back pain. A systematic review of 13 trials of group interventions in acute and chronic back pain concluded that evidence was insufficient to recommend this approach for persons with low back pain (26). The back school approach has been used as a preventive strategy, particularly in the workplace. However, a large-scale, randomized controlled trial of an educational program to prevent work-related injuries in more than 2,500 postal workers was unable to demonstrate any benefit of training (27).

Rest

In most patients with acute low back pain, bed rest for more than 1 or 2 days should not be recommended. The primary negative consequence of inappropriate bed rest is delay in return to normal activities (i.e., recovery). Deyo et al. compared recommendations for 2 days of bed rest with 7 days in 203 patients, most of whom had acute mechanical back pain. The only difference in outcome was 45% fewer missed work days by patients advised to rest for only 2 days (28). In a comparison of bed rest for 4 days with isometric exercise or usual care in patients with acute low back pain, Gilbert et al. reported similar findings, noting that patients randomized to bed rest took 42% longer to return to normal activity level (29). A more recent randomized study in patients with acute occupational nonspecific back pain compared bed rest for 2 days, back-mobilizing exercises, and continuation of ordinary activities as tolerated (16). Patients randomized to bed rest incurred almost twice as many sick days as persons advised to continue activities as tolerated. Rozenberg et al. compared 4 days of bed rest with continued normal daily activity in patients with back pain of less than 72 hours' duration (30). At 1- and 3-month follow-up, no difference in pain intensity or functional disability was noted. A higher proportion of patients in the bed rest group had an initial period of work absence. Finally, a recent systematic review of advice to stay active as a single treatment in patients with back pain and sciatica concluded that although this advice had little beneficial effect in itself, prolonged bed rest was potentially harmful and should be avoided (31).

In addition to delay in recovery, other potential adverse consequences of bed rest include rapid loss of muscular strength at a rate of approximately 5% per week, bone loss at a rate of nearly 1% per week, general deconditioning, and increased social isolation and depression (32,33). Probably as a result of excessive rest and disuse, muscular function and cross-sectional area in patients with chronic low back pain is decreased (34). Studies assessing aerobic fitness in persons with chronic low back pain are conflicting, although the hypothesis that inactivity promotes deconditioning, which contributes to chronicity of pain, is frequently cited (35–38).

Physical Therapy

Physical therapy is frequently recommended for persons with low back pain. In its broadest sense, physical therapy encompasses patient education regarding activity, passive modalities, and active exercise of several varieties. Although physical therapy is frequently considered the cornerstone of nonoperative management, well-designed prospective randomized controlled trials demonstrating efficacy of many commonly prescribed treatments are lacking. In the past decade, however, several careful analyses of available studies have been able to begin to clarify the role of selected forms of therapy in patients with acute or chronic back pain (39–43). These reviews found no evidence that passive modalities, such as ultrasound or mechanical traction, improve short-term or long-term outcomes in patients with acute, subacute, or chronic nonspecific back pain. There is reasonable evidence, however, that active exercise-oriented therapy programs may have a role in management of patients with subacute and chronic symptoms, as well as in prevention of recurrent episodes of nonspecific back pain.

Exercise

Acute Low Back Pain

Although commonly recommended, there is little evidence that formal physical therapy referral for therapeutic exercises is beneficial in acute nonspecific low back pain. For most patients, advice to continue normal activities as tolerated produces superior outcomes. In fact, in a randomized trial with 270 patients with acute low back pain, Gilbert et al. found that an individualized isometric flexion exercise program and education had a negative effect on several functional outcome measures in comparison to controls (29). A McKenzie-based extension exercise program that included postural correction was superior to a single back education session in 100 patients with acute low back pain at 1 year follow-up in parameters such as return to work rate, recurrences, and days of sick leave during the initial episode (44). No control group was included in this study, however. In addition, 5 years later, differences between the treatment groups were considerably less (45). Likewise, in another more recent trial comparing the McKenzie approach with chiropractic manipulation and a simple educational booklet in 321 patients with acute low back pain, Cherkin et al. reported only marginally better outcomes in actively treated patients (46). In a randomized trial comparing placebo ultrasound therapy with an individualized physical therapy exercise program incorporating flexion exercises, stretching, and isometric abdominal strengthening in 473 patients with acute low back pain, Fass et al. found no difference in outcome between the two groups at 3 months (47). In a direct comparison of flexion and extension exercises with no exercise in 149 soldiers with acute low back pain, no significant differences in outcome were present at 8-week follow-up (48). Of interest, patients in the "no exercise" group noted greater improvement in spinal flexion and extension than the exercise groups. Similarly, a more recent trial comparing back-mobilizing exercises with continuation of ordinary activities as tolerated found superior results in the latter group (16). The duration of pain was significantly greater in patients randomized to the exercise group. Clearly, these studies suggest that no particular exercise approach is more effective than placebo or no treatment in patients with nonspecific acute low back pain. A recent systematic review of this literature by the Cochrane Collaboration Back Review Group concluded, "exercise therapy is not more effective than inactive or active treatments with which it has been compared" (39). In the acute setting, patient education and advice to continue activities as tolerated produces equal or superior outcomes.

Chronic Low Back Pain

For persons with nonspecific chronic low back pain (duration of symptoms greater than 12 weeks), exercise therapy is central to treatment. Typical programs include aerobic conditioning, the

McKenzie approach, intensive dynamic back extensor strengthening (DYN), stretching, or flexion (William's) exercises. Combinations of these various approaches are often used. Currently available studies do not adequately compare efficacy of the different exercise programs (41).

The rationale for recommending an active exercise program in patients with chronic back pain is based on the observations that they may have reduced muscle strength, increased muscle fatigability, and abnormality in muscular function (49–52). Aerobic conditioning, isometric strengthening, and muscle reconditioning using training devices have all been shown to improve isometric trunk muscle strength and improve back muscle endurance in patients with chronic low back pain (53,54). Improvement in muscle strength and endurance in this cohort of patients with chronic back pain was associated with improvement in pain intensity and pain frequency (55). In addition, patients demonstrating improved lumbar strength also reported improved psychosocial functioning. However, 3 months of active therapy did not produce significant changes in spinal muscle mass as assessed by magnetic resonance imaging or alteration in muscle fiber type (56).

Aerobic Exercise. Aerobic exercise, typically low impact in quality, is frequently included in comprehensive treatment programs for patients with low back pain. Generally, clinical trials have demonstrated active treatment (including aerobic conditioning) is superior to control groups, including usual care (57–59). Few studies have assessed the effect of aerobic conditioning in isolation in patients with low back pain. Recently, a retrospective review of an aerobic fitness program in patients with chronic low back pain demonstrated a statistically significant increase in aerobic capacity that correlated with statistically significant improvements in pain and disability scores (60). In this study, however, other concurrent treatment modalities, including manipulation and medication, may have contributed to the improved outcomes. Aerobic conditioning exercises appear at least as effective as alternative exercise programs in patients with chronic back pain. Mannion et al. reported a randomized comparison of a 1-hour low-impact aerobics class twice weekly for 3 months with active physiotherapy and muscle reconditioning on training devices in 148 patients with chronic low back pain (55). Comparable improvement in pain intensity and frequency was seen in all treatment groups, but improvement in disability was noted only in the aerobics and devices groups. Whether a combination of different exercise programs (e.g., aerobic conditioning and isometric strengthening) is more effective than one approach alone remains unclear.

Stretching Exercise. Because many patients with chronic back pain describe muscle spasms and stiffness, muscle stretching exercises have been incorporated in many treatment programs. Kraus pioneered a 6-week exercise program used at YMCAs across the country and reported that 80% of nearly 12,000 participants reported decreased back discomfort (61). This program included primarily stretching exercises with some strengthening as well. This prospective cohort study did not include a control group. Deyo et al. compared transcutaneous electrical nerve stimulation (TENS) with a stretching exercise program based on Kraus' program in 145 patients with chronic low back pain (62). Patients in the exercise group experienced significant improvement in pain scores and improved activity compared to nonexercisers. However, within 2 months, most patients had stopped exercising, and these gains were lost.

Dynamic Back Extensor Strengthening Exercises. Active exercises to strengthen spinal extensor muscles have been proposed as treatment to address the diminished strength and endurance of spinal musculature present in some patients with chronic back pain (63). Exercises representative of this approach include trunk-lifting in the prone position and leg lifts in the prone position. Some programs emphasize extensor strengthening using isotonic resistive exercise equipment. Studies comparing this approach with modality-oriented physical therapy and a strengthening program reduced to 20% of the full schedule ("low-dose") demonstrated significant improvement in the DYN treatment group in an index measuring pain, disability, and physical impairment (64,65). The patient population studied was nonhomogeneous, and the benefits of DYN persisted at 1 year only in patients who continued exercising at least once weekly. Hansen et al. found that DYN exercises were more effective in women than in men and in persons with sedentary or light occupations (66). Using exercise equipment to provide dynamic, progressive resistance exercise to strengthen spinal extensor musculature in patients with back pain in whom surgery had been recommended, Nelson et al. found that surgery was avoided in 35 of 38 persons completing the program who were available for follow-up (67). Of these individuals, 90% had failed previous exercise programs. Comparisons of dynamic extensor strengthening exercises with other exercise programs used in the treatment of chronic back pain are few, but a recent randomized trial compared DYN with the McKenzie method in 260 patients with back pain of at least 8 weeks' duration (68). At 8-month follow-up, both methods were equally effective in reducing measures of pain and disability. No control group was included in this trial. In summary, available evidence suggests that extensor strengthening may be effective in treatment of chronic nonspecific back pain, but evidence demonstrating superiority to other active exercise regimes is lacking. As with other exercise programs, continued benefit requires continued exercise. Likewise, some patients, particularly the frail elderly, may have difficulty performing some of these exercises without active therapist assistance.

McKenzie Approach. Initially based on empiric observations made by Robin McKenzie in the 1950s, this technique uses repetitive spinal movements to end-range in various directions to categorize patients with back pain into three different syndromes. The critical observation is whether the pain can be centralized (i.e., moved from the periphery to the midline with specific repeated movements). For most (but not all) patients, the direction of lumbar movement that results in centralization of pain is extension (69). This has led some to incorrectly equate the McKenzie approach with an extension exercise program. In fact, some patients centralize with lateral movements called *side-glides* or, more rarely, *flexion* (70). The therapist develops home exercise recommendations for the patient based on the movements, which centralized the pain. The centralization phenomenon has been attributed to displacement of the nucleus pulposus within the intact annulus. In essence, the most common syndrome described by McKenzie is "derangement," based on the concept of a discogenic source of pain. In most cases, he believes back (and leg) symptoms are the result of pathologic posterior nuclear migration mechanically stimulating the annulus or nerve root (69,71). Therapeutically repeated movements, which produce a force on the nucleus moving it toward a more central location, should alleviate symptoms. Identification of a directional preference, which reduces and centralizes symptoms, is the core of this approach. Conceptually, this explanation for centralization requires a competent annulus with a functional intradiscal hydrostatic mechanism. In support of this model, Donelson et al. have demonstrated that 74% of patients with low back pain who centralized their symptoms with the McKenzie assessment had positive discograms, of which 91% had an intact annulus (69). Conversely, although 69% of patients with chronic low back pain who peripheralized (did not centralize) had positive discography, only 54% had an intact annulus. In patients whose pain did not respond at all to test movements, only 12.5% had positive discography.

How commonly is the centralization phenomenon observed in patients with chronic low back pain? In the Donelson study, 50% of 63 patients with back pain of at least 3 months' duration (mean, 15.3 months) were centralizers (69). In a study of 223 patients with chronic low back pain with or without leg symptoms, Long found that 105 (43%) were classified as centralizers based on a McKenzie protocol (72). Although the patient groups in both of these studies were nonhomogeneous and included patients with radicular features, these data suggest that the disc may be the source of symptoms in a substantial fraction of patients with chronic low back pain.

Identification of a derangement in a patient with chronic low back pain (i.e., a directional preference identified and centralization observed) is associated with a better prognosis for response to exercise-oriented treatment. Long compared outcomes in 223 patients (105 centralizers and 118 noncentralizers) treated in an interdisciplinary work-hardening program (72). Centralizers had superior improvement in pain scores and a higher return-to-work rate. Donelson et al. reported that 77% of patients with chronic back pain of at least 12 weeks' duration whose symptoms centralized had a good to excellent response to McKenzie-based exercise treatment (73).

McKenzie identified two additional syndromes in which pain is not present with movement or does not centralize. The so-called *postural syndrome* is a consequence of prolonged sitting in slouched position at end-range flexion and without proper lumbar lordosis. Pain is not seen with movement, and treatment emphasizes education regarding proper posture. The dysfunction syndrome is attributed to repeated healed soft tissue trauma with shortening or contracture of these tissues. Pain is noted at end-range and does not centralize. Treatment of this syndrome emphasizes frequent stretching.

Few comparative studies of the effectiveness of the McKenzie approach in patients with chronic low back pain are available. As noted earlier, a recent comparison of a dynamic extensor strengthening program with a McKenzie-based approach in 260 patients with back pain of at least 8 weeks' duration found no differences in outcome (68). Another trial compared a flexion-oriented program (William's approach) with extension exercises based on the McKenzie method in 56 patients with chronic low back pain (74). Reduction of pain severity index (by approximately one-third) was similar in both groups. However, the extension-treated patients were not formally assessed using a McKenzie approach.

The McKenzie approach provides a useful construct to assess the contribution of disc pathology to symptoms in patients with chronic low back pain. In appropriate patients (i.e., centralizers), it may be useful in guiding the development of a customized exercise approach. This approach emphasizes patient self treatment and responsibility for management and requires a motivated patient. Noncentralizers, on the other hand, are unlikely to respond to the McKenzie approach, and an alternative exercise program should be considered. The requirement for frequent repetition of therapeutic exercises may be a barrier to compliance in some. Integration of the McKenzie approach with other exercise regimens (e.g., dynamic extensor strengthening) may be appropriate in some patients.

Flexion Exercises. Williams popularized the concept that abdominal muscle weakness resulting in increased lumbar lordosis and redistribution of forces to the posterior aspect of the lumbar disc might produce disc injury and pain (75). Based on this thesis, an exercise approach emphasizing flexion-oriented abdominal strengthening with passive stretching of lumbar extensors and reduction in lumbar lordosis was recommended (76). Despite widespread use, data available regarding the efficacy of this approach in patients with chronic back pain are sparse and conflicting. Kendell et al. compared flexion with extension exercises as well as spinal mobilization in patients with chronic back pain and concluded that flexion exercises were superior (77). However, a later trial found no significant difference in reduction in back pain severity in patients treated with flexion or extension exercises (74). Helewa et al. were unable to demonstrate that an abdominal strengthening exercise program reduced the risk of future back pain episodes in comparison to back education only (78). Conceptually, in patients with existing disc protrusion, an exercise program emphasizing flexion might increase intradiscal pressure, aggravating the herniation.

Manipulation

Spinal manipulation or spinal adjustment refers to the "application of a force to specific body tissues with therapeutic intent" (79). Although chiropractors provide more than 90% of manipulative therapy in the United States, osteopathic physicians and physical therapists also commonly use the procedure (80). Practiced since the days of Hippocrates and Galen, the role of manipulation in the management of back pain continues to expand, as evidenced by a tripling of chiropractic use in the United States since 1980 (79). In the mid-1990s, widely disseminated clinical practice guidelines in the United States and Great Britain recommended manipulation as effective treatment for low back pain (81,82). Since the 1970s, chiropractic services, including manipulation, have been covered by Medicare, all state workers' compensation plans, and most health management organizations and private insurance plans (79). Despite these developments, the efficacy, safety, and cost-effectiveness of manipulation, as well as its appropriate role in back pain management, remain controversial (79,83–85).

Manipulative technique varies considerably depending on the training and experience of the practitioner. Long-lever, low-velocity manipulation, usually associated with osteopathy, uses a long bone, typically the femur, to increase the force applied manually by the clinician to one or more joints in a nonspecific fashion (86). Short-lever, high-velocity manipulation, more typical of chiropractic, is more discretely focused on a specific vertebral contact point. This manual thrust is designed to move the joint slightly beyond the passive end-range of motion but not beyond its anatomic range (86,87). This movement is typically associated with an audible "pop," possibly a result of a transient vacuum phenomenon produced in the facet joint. Another variation of manipulative treatment is referred to as *spinal mobilization*. In this technique, low-velocity force is applied to the spinal joint, moving it within its passive range (87).

Although the earliest rationale for chiropractic manipulation was based on the premise that nerve impingement was the mechanism of most illness, current hypotheses for the efficacy of manipulation are based primarily on correction of facet joint dysfunction (79). However, in patients with chronic low back pain, demonstration of abnormal findings on an examination correlating with such a lesion may not reproducible, even with experienced examiners (86). Manipulation of the suspect joint has been theorized to improve joint mobility by releasing entrapped synovial folds, relaxing paraspinal muscle spasm, disrupting joint adhesions, or "unbuckling" abnormal motion segments (87,88). In addition to mechanical effects on the facet, it has been proposed that manipulation may have specific neurologic effects resulting in inhibition of excessive reflex activity in the spinal muscles (89). The hands-on nature of manipulative therapy has also raised the possibility that the therapeutic benefits of this treatment may be related to the therapist-patient interaction itself (90). Chiropractors and the patients seeking their care typically share similar beliefs about the etiology of back pain and the benefits of manipulation (91). This congruence of belief may be an important element in the favorable outcome of manipulative therapy (92).

Manipulation is one of the most frequently studied nonoperative treatment modalities for low back pain. However, the quality of the literature is extremely variable, and the results are often conflicting. Several recent reviews have attempted a meta-analysis of this extensive literature. Shekelle et al. reviewed 58 studies, 25 of which were controlled. The authors concluded that for persons with acute uncomplicated low back pain, manipulation increased the probability of recovery at 3 weeks from 50% to 67% (80). Data were deemed insufficient to assess efficacy of manipulation in chronic low back pain. Koes et al. analyzed 35 randomized controlled trials of manipulation versus other therapies in persons with low back pain (93). Study quality was scored on the basis of study population, interventions, measurement of effect, and data analysis. Only 5 of 35 studies were deemed of good or reasonable quality. The authors concluded that the efficacy of manipulation for acute or chronic back pain could not be assessed based on the available studies. Van Tulder et al. reviewed 16 randomized controlled trials of manipulation in acute low back pain, only two of which were of high quality, and concluded that there was limited evidence that manipulation was more effective than placebo (94). There was no evidence that manipulation was superior to alternatives such as physical therapy or drug therapy. For chronic low back pain, the evidence was deemed strong that manipulation was superior to placebo. Based on a review of nine randomized controlled trials in which it was possible to isolate the contribution of spinal manipulation to the overall treatment effect in patients with acute low back pain, Bronfort concluded there was moderate evidence of short-term efficacy (88). Treatment was more successful in the subgroup of patients with symptoms of 2 to 4 weeks' duration in two trials of moderate to high quality (95,96). For chronic low back pain, Bronfort found 11 studies isolating the effects of manipulation and concluded that there was moderate evidence of efficacy in comparison to placebo and routine medical management. Meeker et al. found 43 randomized trials of spinal manipulation for treatment of acute, subacute, and chronic low back pain, 30 of which favored manipulation over the comparison treatment in at least a subgroup of patients (79). They concluded that the "positive effect sizes (of manipulation) appear to be clinically and statistically significant but not dramatic" (79). A recent randomized controlled trial compared osteopathic manipulation with "standard medical therapies" in 155 patients with acute and subacute back pain (97). No difference in primary outcomes was observed, and 90% of patients in both groups were satisfied with their care. Patients treated with manipulation used fewer medications. The study design did not permit an actual cost of care comparison. Another recent comparison of chiropractic manipulation, physical therapy exercises using the McKenzie approach, and minimal intervention (providing an educational booklet) in 321 patients with acute low back pain found only minimal differences in clinical outcomes but large differences in expense (46). The cost of chiropractic care or physical therapy was nearly three times the cost of the minimal intervention. Chiropractic care often provides other physical modalities, such as ultrasound or diathermy, in addition to manipulation in patients with back pain. A recent randomized controlled trial found no evidence that the addition of such modalities improved long-term outcome (98).

Adverse effects of lumbar spinal manipulation are frequent but typically mild and brief. A prospective survey of 4,712 chiropractic manipulative procedures in more than 1,000 patients found "unpleasant" side effects in 55% of patients (99). This study included cervical and lumbar treatment. The most common adverse reactions were local discomfort (53%), headache (12%), tiredness (11%), and radiating discomfort (10%). Adverse reactions were categorized as mild or moderate in 85% of instances. Most appeared within 4 hours of treatment and disappeared within 24 hours. Serious adverse reactions of lumbar spinal manipulation are rare. Cauda equina syndrome represents the most feared adverse consequence of lumbar manipulation. The occurrence of this complication has been estimated at less than one per 100 million manipulations (80). Although a concern, no data are available regarding the risk of manipulation-related vertebral fracture in older patients with osteoporosis.

Manipulation therapy may have an adjunctive role in the short-term management of selected patients with acute and chronic nonspecific low back pain. Patient satisfaction is higher with manipulation than other traditional medical therapy. Available studies demonstrate comparable efficacy to alternatives such as exercise-oriented physical therapy in acute patients. In such patients, however, limited data suggest that simple education may produce similar results and is more cost-effective.

Massage Therapy

Massage therapy in various forms has been widely used in the treatment of acute and chronic back pain for many years. Massage therapists represent one of the most popular alternative health care providers in the United States (100). Massage therapy takes many forms, including classical Swedish massage, deep-tissue massage, acupuncture massage, friction massage, myofascial release, and other variations. As with manipulation, the diversity of techniques as well as the difficulty in conducting placebo or sham trials confounds assessment of the efficacy of this therapy.

However, a number of studies comparing massage therapy with other modalities suggest some efficacy in patients with acute and chronic back pain. Long-term benefits are not well established, and the role of massage therapy as a component of a comprehensive treatment approach has not been evaluated. Likewise, inadequate data exist comparing various techniques of therapeutic massage to recommend a particular form of therapy.

Comparison of massage therapy with exercise-oriented physical therapy in patients with chronic back pain has not been extensively studied. However, at least one recent trial found massage therapy superior to a remedial exercise program (101). However, the massage treatment group was also instructed to exercise aerobically and perform a stretching program. Furlan et al. performed a systematic review of massage therapy in nonspecific back pain and identified eight randomized trials, most comparing massage with other treatments and concluded that massage might be of benefit for patients with subacute and chronic back pain, particularly if combined with exercises and education (102). Cherkin et al. found massage therapy superior to acupuncture and self-care education in a study of 262 patients with 1-year follow-up (103). At 1 year, massage and education produced comparable results, both superior to acupuncture. Patients treated with massage used the least amount of medications and had the lowest cost of care. Studies comparing massage and manipulation have found similar effects on pain reduction but better functional outcomes in manipulation-treated patients (104,105).

Transcutaneous Electrical Nerve Stimulation

TENS has been used for pain relief for more than 30 years. As originally conceived, TENS was a noninvasive technique of peripheral nerve stimulation based on the premise that counterstimulation of the appropriate nerve fibers could alter pain perception. The gate-control theory of pain provided the initial theoretical framework for TENS development. As suggested in animal models, high-frequency, low-intensity TENS was believed to stimulate large afferent nerve fibers that activate inhibitory neurons at the local dermatomal spinal cord level, resulting in inhibition of smaller sensory nociceptive fiber input (106,107). More recently, evidence suggests an alternative explanation for TENS-induced analgesia based on nonsegmental, supraspinal inhibitory influences or central endorphin release as low-frequency, high-intensity TENS stimulates both small and large sensory fibers nonselectively (108,109). Regardless of these elegant hypotheses, demonstration of the efficacy of TENS in low back pain has proven difficult. However, perhaps because of its safety and noninvasive nature, TENS remains a widely used treatment in patients with back pain.

At least three major reviews of TENS in back pain have concluded that there is insufficient evidence of efficacy to recommend its use (42,43,106). In the most recent and rigorous attempt to assess the available studies of TENS in back pain, Brousseu et al. reviewed five randomized controlled trials of TENS for the treatment of chronic low back pain (106). Their metaanalysis included 170 patients treated with sham TENS and 251 receiving active TENS, including 98 who received "acupuncture-like" TENS. They concluded that there were no statistically significant differences in outcome between the active TENS-treated patients and the placebo group. However, TENS-treated patients consistently reported better functional status and less pain and were more likely to desire continued TENS therapy. Because of inadequate numbers, the analysis could not compare different TENS methodologies or techniques.

Several trials have compared TENS to other treatment modalities for back pain. In a randomized, sham-controlled trial, Deyo et al. found a uniform set of 12 exercises more effective than TENS in patients with chronic low back pain (62). These authors also addressed the difficulty of performing a valid placebo or "sham" TENS trial (110). In this study, 84% of the sham group believed they had functioning TENS units and clinicians guessed the treatment group correctly 61% of the time. A later randomized trial compared exercise-oriented rehabilitation with and without TENS using a sham TENS group in persons with occupational low back pain (111). The addition of TENS to the exercise program did not improve outcomes of functional status or return to work.

A number of trials have compared TENS with needle-based techniques, including acupuncture and neuromuscular electrical stimulation (NMES) [e.g., percutaneous electrical nerve stimulation (PENS)]. Acupuncture and TENS produced similar beneficial results in pain and functional scores in patients older than age 60 with chronic back pain (112). This study did not include a placebo group and could not exclude the possibility that both treatments were themselves placebos. In a small, randomized, placebo-controlled comparison of TENS and NMES in patients with chronic back pain, both modalities produced significant short-term pain reduction (113). Combined TENS and NMES was more effective than either treatment alone. Another more recent comparison of NMES with TENS as well as exercise therapy and a sham group in 60 patients with chronic back pain found PENS to be significantly more effective than TENS or exercises in providing short-term pain relief and improved function (114). The PENS-treated patients had a significant reduction in use of nonopioid analgesic medications.

As with other modalities frequently used in the management of back pain, solid evidence of efficacy for TENS is lacking. Virtually all available data are in studies of chronic pain only. As suggested by a recent metaanalysis, new trials are required that clearly delineate and compare the types of devices, the sites of application, duration, frequency, and intensity of treatments while using standardized outcome measures (106).

Acupuncture

Acupuncture is a centuries-old therapy, rooted in East Asian medicine, which has been increasingly adopted and adapted by Western practitioners. More than 1 million Americans are treated with acupuncture annually for a variety of musculoskeletal conditions, including fibromyalgia and low back pain (115,116). Recent surveys report that 57% of rheumatologists and 69% of pain specialists have made referrals to practitioners of acupuncture (117,118). Like other complementary and alternative therapies, the role of acupuncture in the management of back pain remains controversial. However, a recent National Institutes of Health consensus conference concluded that "ample clinical experience supported by some research data suggests that acupuncture may be a reasonable option for a number of clinical conditions. Examples are postoperative pain, myofascial pain, and low back pain" (116).

Acupuncture involves stimulation of precisely localized points on the body typically by insertion of solid needle. Variations of the technique include moxibustion—burning powdered moxa herb at the point of stimulation—as well as electrical acupuncture with an electrical stimulator attached to the needle (119). Stimulation by hand, a technique known as acupressure, represents another variation of the procedure. In traditional Chinese medicine, acupuncture is believed to correct disharmony or imbalance in yin and yang forces in the body and their connecting "energy" or *qi* (115). East Asian medical theory is based on the concept that this energy circulates along 14 meridians in the body. Needling of acupuncture points located along these meridians is believed to restore balance in the body, thereby alleviating symptoms.

Varying physiologic effects of acupuncture have also been proposed to explain its purported therapeutic benefits. These include stimulation of endogenous opioid production (endorphins and enkephalins) as well as serotonin and adrenocorticotrophic hormones (115,120). Supporting this concept, acupuncture anesthesia may be reversible with naloxone (121). Other proposed mechanisms have been based on the gate-control theory of pain modulation as well as effects on immune function (116,122). These physiologic changes may not be specific to acupuncture, as they have been observed with needling of sham acupuncture points as well as after nonspecific painful stimuli (116). This clearly complicates development and interpretation of sham-controlled clinical trials of acupuncture.

Studies of the effectiveness of acupuncture in patients with back pain experience the usual problems in the alternative medicine and back pain literature. Poorly described patient populations, insufficient sample size, nonstandardized outcome parameters, and lack of long-term follow-up are not unique to the acupuncture literature. In addition, effects of patient expectation on treatment results and heterogeneity of practitioner methodology complicate analysis of results of the available randomized controlled trials (115,123). For example, a study assessing acupuncture technique in chronic back pain found only 14% concordance in choice of acupuncture points by at least two of seven therapists (124). A recent metaanalysis found 12 randomized controlled trials of acupuncture for back pain and pooled data from nine studies (377 patients) (125). Generally, acupuncture was superior to the various control treatments in the different studies, but insufficient evidence was found to demonstrate superiority to placebo. Another systematic review of the efficacy for acupuncture for low back pain identified 11 randomized controlled trials, only two of which were rated as high quality (122). No study selectively evaluated acupuncture for acute low back pain. The reviewers concluded that there was insufficient evidence to recommend acupuncture for management of back pain. There was moderate evidence that acupuncture was no more effective than TENS or trigger point injection, suggesting either similar placebo effect or that cutaneous stimulation itself—regardless of localization—produced similar biologic effects. A subsequent 4-week randomized controlled trial comparing TENS and acupuncture in patients aged 60 years and older with chronic back pain produced similar findings (126). A recent comparison of massage therapy with traditional Chinese acupuncture and self-care education in persons with chronic back pain found massage superior to acupuncture at 10 weeks and 1 year follow-up (127). Acupuncture was no better than self-care.

Adverse effects of acupuncture are rare. Concerns include transmission of infectious disease, needle breakage, minor hemorrhage, pain, and even organ puncture (115).

Convincing evidence supporting a unique role for acupuncture in the management of back pain is lacking. Efficacy is comparable to other alternative therapies such as TENS. Any therapeutic benefit may represent a nonspecific biologic response to cutaneous stimulation or a placebo effect.

Nonopioid Analgesics and Nonsteroidal Antiinflammatory Drugs

Acetaminophen and nonsteroidal antiinflammatory drugs (NSAIDs) are widely used as initial pharmacologic therapy in the management of acute and chronic back pain. In most primary care clinical practice guidelines for back pain, NSAIDs are recommended if nonprescription analgesics are inadequate (128,129). However, clinical studies of NSAIDs in the management of back pain are surprisingly limited. Conceptually, NSAIDs are used because of their combined analgesic and antiinflammatory properties, but whether they are more efficacious in back pain than pure analgesics remains controversial. In patients with chronic back pain, particularly the elderly, a major concern is NSAID toxicity—gastrointestinal, renal, and cardiovascular—with prolonged use. The newer class of NSAIDs that are selective inhibitors of cyclooxygenase 2 (COX-2) appears to offer the advantage of lowered risk of gastrointestinal toxicity but may be associated with increased risk of adverse cardiovascular events (130).

Efficacy in Acute and Chronic Back Pain

Two recent metaanalyses of NSAIDs in back pain concluded there was sufficient evidence demonstrating that NSAIDs are more effective than placebo for short-term relief of acute low back pain (131,132). Comparison of relative effectiveness of different NSAIDs was not possible based on the available studies. Adequate trials were not found to demonstrate NSAID efficacy in chronic back pain or in patients with radicular pain. The fact that most studies of NSAID therapy in back pain included mixed populations of patients with acute, subacute, and chronic symptoms confounded analysis.

Comparison of NSAIDs with pure analgesics such as acetaminophen yields conflicting results in persons with low back pain (132). In persons with osteoarthritis of the knee, a comparison of ibuprofen and acetaminophen found no difference in pain or functional outcomes (133). However, a more recent study found diclofenac more efficacious than high-dose acetaminophen in patients with osteoarthritis, particularly in persons with more severe disease (134). Clearly, further study of NSAID efficacy in patients with back pain is required. Such studies must include clearly delineated patient populations, well-defined outcomes, and long-term follow-up.

Nonsteroidal Antiinflammatory Drug Toxicity

Because compelling evidence of superior efficacy of NSAIDs compared to simple analgesics such as acetaminophen is lacking in persons with acute and chronic back pain, the choice of first-line therapeutic agent may be guided by risk of adverse effects, particularly in the older patient. Gastrointestinal symptoms develop in 15 to 20% of persons taking long-term NSAID therapy (135,136). Approximately 2 to 4% of NSAID-treated patients develop symptomatic ulcers. Of these, 1 to 2% develop complications, including perforation or bleeding. Risk factors for NSAID gastropathy include older age (older than 60 years), history of peptic ulcer disease, concomitant use of glucocorticoids, and higher-dose therapy (137,138). Early detection of serious NSAID-induced gastrointestinal lesions is problematic; fewer than one-third of such patients experience even dyspepsia as a warning sign (136). Therefore, if efficacy is comparable, acetaminophen is generally preferred to an NSAID as initial treatment in patients at high risk for gastropathy. However, recent data suggest that even acetaminophen is associated with risk of gastrointestinal adverse effects in elderly patients treated with higher doses (greater than 2,000 mg/day) (139–141).

NSAID gastropathy is primarily a result of inhibition of cyclooxygenase 1 (COX-1) and interference with production of gastroprotective prostaglandins. By the early 1990s, two distinct forms of the enzyme COX were described. COX-1 is found in virtually all tissues and is believed to function constitutively in the gastric mucosa, kidney, and platelets. In contrast, COX-2 is inducible and found in large quantities in areas of inflammation. COX-2 is induced by a variety of proinflammatory mediators including interleukin-1, tumor necrosis factor alpha, lipopolysaccharide, and other growth factors (142). These observations led to the so-called *COX hypothesis*—selective inhibition of COX-2 would produce antiinflammatory therapeutic effects without the adverse consequences of nonselective COX-1 and COX-2 inhibition. Development of selective COX-2 inhibitors (coxibs) followed. Two large trials comparing available coxibs with nonselective NSAIDs have demonstrated a 50% reduction in ulcers and ulcer complications (143,144).

Renal adverse effects of NSAIDs include acute renal failure, sodium and water retention, and hypertension; these effects are related to inhibition of renal prostaglandin synthesis. In patients with known cardiovascular disease, particularly those on diuretic therapy, NSAID therapy significantly increases the risk of congestive heart failure (145–147). Similar renal adverse effects occur with both older NSAIDs and selective COX-2 inhibitors (coxibs) (148–150).

COX-2–inhibiting NSAIDs decrease vascular prostacyclin synthesis. Prostacyclin inhibits platelet aggregation and induces vasodilation. COX-1 inhibition decreases the thromboxane A_2 synthesis that plays an essential role in platelet aggregation. Unlike nonselective older NSAIDs, which produce a balanced effect on these mechanisms, COX-2 inhibitors may shift the balance between prothrombotic and thrombotic mediators toward a prothrombotic state. Analysis of a large trial of rofecoxib versus naproxen in more than 8,000 patients found increased cardiovascular events (myocardial infarction, unstable angina, cardiac thrombus, sudden death, and ischemic stroke) in rofecoxib-treated patients compared with naproxen (relative risk, 2.38) (130,140). Other studies have suggested that COX-2 inhibition does not increase the risk of myocardial infarction and that the results reported above reflect a cardioprotective effect of naproxen (151–155). Based on currently available data, clinicians should remain cautious that coxib agents may increase cardiovascular events, particularly in high-risk patients. Cotherapy with low-dose aspirin may balance the prothrombotic effect and reduce cardiovascular risk. However, the reduced risk of gastrointestinal toxicity associated with coxib therapy may be jeopardized with the addition of aspirin.

Analgesics and Nonsteroidal Antiinflammatory Drugs: Clinical Guidelines

In acute back pain, acetaminophen and NSAIDs appear to have comparable efficacy. Because anticipated use is less than 1 month, risk of toxicity is limited. Choice of NSAID may be guided by cost (generic available), convenience of dosing [once or twice daily (e.g., naproxen, diclofenac)], time to onset of action [more rapidly acting, shorter-acting agents (e.g., ibuprofen)], and previous patient experience with a particular drug. Considerable variation in response to various NSAIDs in the same individual is a common observation. As a result, it is reasonable to try more than one NSAID in a given patient before abandoning this class of drug.

For long-term use in chronic back pain, unless there is a compelling reason for an antiinflammatory agent (e.g., ankylosing spondylitis), pure analgesics—beginning with acetaminophen—are preferred. In very high-risk patients—particularly the elderly, persons with known cardiovascular or renal disease, and patients with a previous history of ulcer disease—NSAIDs should be avoided. Because coxibs are no more efficacious than other NSAIDs, their use is based on risk of gastrointestinal toxicity. With long-term use of NSAIDs, regular monitoring for blood loss (complete blood cell count) and renal dysfunction (creatinine) is required. Serious gastrointestinal complications may present without antecedent symptoms.

Opioid Analgesics

Opioids are not required or recommended in the management of most patients with acute back pain. Although still controversial, long-term opioid therapy is gaining acceptance for carefully selected and monitored patients with chronic low back pain (156,157). Impediments to the use of opioids for chronic back pain have included fear of inducing addiction, potential adverse effects (particularly on cognitive function), fear of drug diversion, and fear of regulatory action (156,158). Furthermore, anecdotal evidence suggests that in some patients, pain improves on withdrawal of opioid therapy (159); randomized, blind clinical trials of opioid therapy with well-delineated outcomes in patients with chronic low back pain are few. However, as noted in the 1997 consensus statement of the American Pain Society and the American Academy of Pain Medicine on the use of opioids in the treatment of chronic pain, "current information and experience suggest that many commonly held assumptions (regarding addiction, side effects, tolerance, and diversion) need modification" (160). The most recent clinical practice guideline of the American Geriatric Society on management of pain in older persons endorses opioid analgesics for selected patients with moderate to severe persistent nonmalignant pain (161).

Opioid Efficacy in Back Pain

Since Portenoy and Foley's landmark paper in 1986, multiple trials have suggested that opioids effectively relieve pain in persons with nonmalignant pain, including back pain (162). Much less clear, however, is whether improvement in social or physical function—employment, recreational activities, or even self-care—parallels pain relief. Available clinical trials of opioids in chronic back pain are significantly flawed. Most studies mixed spinal and nonspinal nonmalignant pain. Furthermore, the patients with back pain are poorly described. Most trials are uncontrolled, nonrandomized, and unblinded. Standardized outcome parameters are usually not used. In a retrospective analysis of 112 patients, 45% of whom had chronic back pain and were treated with opioids for a mean of 2 years, 83% reported improved pain. Functional status was not assessed (163). In a subsequent report, the same group reported a randomized open trial of sustained-release morphine versus naproxen and oxycodone in 36 patients with chronic low back pain. Although opioid-treated patients demonstrated superior pain relief and less emotional distress, no difference was found in activity level or hours of sleep (164). Similarly, a randomized, double-blind crossover study of long-acting morphine in 46 patients with regional myofascial pain syndromes, including back pain, found significant improvement in pain control in opioid-treated patients but no improvement in physical or psychosocial function as assessed by the Sickness Impact Profile instrument (165). Conversely, an open trial of sustained-release therapy in 100 patients with neuropathic pain or back pain reported significant functional improvement in patients who experienced at least a 50% reduction in pain (166). A recent double-blind, placebo-controlled comparison of controlled-release oxycodone or fixed-combination oxycodone plus acetaminophen in osteoarthritis patients—49% of whom had back or neck as the primary site of involvement—demonstrated significant improvement in pain intensity and quality of sleep in both opioid treatment groups (167).

Clinical Pharmacology

In addition to more potent analgesia, opioids offer other potential clinical advantages over nonopioid agents, including NSAIDs. No end-organ toxicity—renal, hepatic, or otherwise—occurs with long-term opioid treatment (156,158). With opioid analgesics, no ceiling dose exists. The drug dose is titrated upward until adequate pain control is achieved or unacceptable toxicity occurs. For analgesic combination products containing acetaminophen, however, the total dose is limited by the nonopioid component. Neuropathic pain, however, may be relatively opioid resistant—not responsive progressively to increasing dosage (161). As with NSAIDs, considerable variability in analgesic effect and toxicity is observed with different opioids in the same patient.

Orally administered opioids reach peak plasma concentration in 60 to 90 minutes. Following hepatic conjugation, 95% of metabolites are renally excreted. Metabolic pathways are nonsaturable. The effective half-life of codeine, oxycodone, hydrocodone, morphine, and hydromorphone is approximately 3 to 4 hours. Steady state is reached with four or five half-lives, or approximately 1 day. Sustained-release preparations are released over 12 to 24 hours and must not be crushed or chewed. Methadone has a much longer and more variable half-life and should be prescribed by an experienced therapist. Meperidine is poorly absorbed orally and is metabolized to normeperidine, a toxin responsible for psychotomimetic adverse effects, including seizures (158). Propoxyphene is a poor analgesic with similar risk of toxic metabolite accumulation at higher doses, particularly in the elderly (161). Mixed opioid agonist-antagonists, such as pentazocine and butorphanol, may precipitate withdrawal symptoms in patients already on pure opioid agonists.

Potential Adverse Consequences of Opioid Analgesics

Fear of addiction has been a major barrier to opioid use in chronic back pain, particularly for physicians who may confuse physical dependence on opioids with true addictive behavior. Physical dependence occurs in most opioid-treated patients after a few weeks and is characterized by withdrawal symptoms in the absence of drug. In contrast, addiction refers to compulsive use of the drug despite physical, psychosocial, or occupational adverse consequences of continued use. True addiction may be further confused with pseudoaddictive drug seeking by patients with poorly managed chronic pain (158). True addiction is probably uncommon in patients with chronic pain treated with opioids who do not have a history of substance abuse (168). The risk of opioid abuse is much greater in persons with a history of substance abuse, particularly in persons without a support system, such as Alcoholics Anonymous (169).

Tolerance, defined as *the need to increase drug dose to maintain the same therapeutic effect*, has not been well studied in patients with chronic back pain on long-term opioid therapy. Anecdotal clinical experience suggests that tolerance is not a significant clinical problem in these patients (156,170). If dosage escalation is required in a patient on a previously stable opioid dose, disease progression or development of new pathology should be considered.

Impaired cognition related to opioid therapy might affect driving ability, predispose to falls (particularly in the older patient), and affect work ability. Recent studies suggest, however, that chronic opioid use may actually improve psychomotor function and attention span while reducing anxiety and hostility (171). Although mild sedation and impaired cognitive function may occur when opioid therapy is initiated or the dosage increased, tolerance to these affects usually develops rapidly. Further study of the effect of opioids on the driving ability of back pain patients is necessary, but the oncology and palliative medicine literature suggests driving ability is not negatively affected after the first several days of therapy (172).

Although tolerance to most opioid side effects—including fatigue, sedation, nausea, vomiting, or dysphoria—develops within a few days of initiation of treatment, drug-related constipation persists and should be managed expectantly. A prophylactic bowel regimen including adequate fluid intake, exercise, and a stimulant laxative (e.g., senna) should be recommended (161). Headache, pruritus, flushing, diaphoresis, hypotension, or pedal edema may occur with opioid administration as result of histamine and vasoactive substance release from mast cells (158). Tolerance to these reactions may not occur.

Guidelines for Opioid Use in Back Pain

Opioids are indicated in only a very small fraction of patients with chronic back pain. Most patients are successfully managed with nonpharmacologic treatments and nonopioid agents. Currently available studies are insufficient to clearly delineate subsets of patients most likely to respond well to opioid therapy with improvement in pain as well as functional status. Current consensus would suggest the following guidelines for selection of chronic back patients for opioid analgesic therapy:

1. Patients should have moderate to severe pain, be unresponsive to nonopioid analgesics and nonpharmacologic modalities, and have a well-defined structural source of the pain.
2. Opioids should be avoided in patients with significant psychosocial disorders. These include personality disorders, major depression, and current or previous substance abuse (158,173,174).
3. Patients with current or previous substance abuse should be considered for opioid therapy only rarely and after careful psychological assessment and with meticulous follow-up. In these patients, an opioid contract is mandatory.
4. Opioids should be used with caution and dosage modification in patients with significant renal disease, chronic obstructive lung disease with impaired respiratory drive, and severe hepatic disease.

For patients with fairly continuous chronic back pain, long-acting opioids given regularly should be used. This approach avoids daily miniwithdrawal episodes and, when titration is complete, achieves consistent analgesia (158). When the back pain is intermittent, activity-related, and predictable (incident pain), shorter-acting opioids with more rapid onset of action may be effective when used intermittently and taken before the triggering activity (161). For the reasons described above, meperidine, propoxyphene, pentazocine, and butorphanol should not be used in patients with chronic back pain, particularly the elderly. Opioid dose should be titrated to efficacy—pain reduction and improved functional ability—with increments of 25% of dose approximately every five half-lives (the time required to achieve a new steady-state level) (171).

Management of patients on opioids requires frequent regular visits for careful assessment of pain control and improvement in functional status. Regular use of validated tools for assessment of back-related disability, such as the Roland Morris or Oswestry index, is mandatory (174,175). If pain relief is unassociated with improvement in functional or activity parameters, opioid therapy should be discontinued. In addition to monitoring clinical response, regular assessment for adverse effects and aberrant drug taking is required.

Muscle Relaxants

Although the precise anatomic source of acute back pain is frequently undefined, muscle sprain or strain is believed to be responsible in many patients. Alternatively, muscle spasm in reaction to underlying spinal pathology may occur as a secondary phenomenon and augment the patient's symptoms. Surface electromyography clearly demonstrates abnormal patterns of muscular activation in patients with acute and chronic back pain (176–178). As a result of these considerations, muscle relaxants are commonly prescribed for patients with acute and chronic back pain. Furthermore, available agents, including baclofen, cyclobenzaprine, carisoprodol, and tizanidine, are centrally acting and typically produce some degree of sedation, potentially improving sleep.

Studies of centrally acting muscle relaxants in back pain are typically flawed by inconsistent description of patients and variable outcome parameters. A metaanalysis of the best-studied agent, cyclobenzaprine, concluded that the drug produces moderate improvement in local pain, muscle spasm, tenderness, range of motion, and activities of daily living in persons with acute low back pain in comparison to placebo-treated patients (179). Of the 14 studies included in the analysis, only three addressed chronic back pain. Treatment efficacy was best in the first week and declined thereafter. However, even at 14 days, there was evidence of improvement. Fifty-three percent of patients treated with 30 mg of cyclobenzaprine daily experienced an adverse effect, most commonly drowsiness. Similarly, baclofen has been demonstrated to be superior to placebo in patients with severe acute back pain, but 68% of treated patients experienced at least one adverse effect (180). Smaller randomized trials of carisoprodol and tizanidine produced similar findings (181–183). A recent review of conservative treatments of back pain, including muscle relaxants, found evidence for benefit as a class of agents but no evidence for differences in efficacy between the various drugs (43). Studies assessing the effectiveness of a combination of an NSAID and a muscle relaxant in back pain are limited but suggest the possibility of modest short-term additive benefit, particularly for relief of muscle spasm and tenderness in acute pain (184,185).

Although deficient, the literature suggests that muscle relaxants are effective in acute back pain within the first 2 weeks, alone or in combination with antiinflammatory agents. Side effects, particularly sedation and dry mouth, are common. Because of the risk of habituation with some agents (e.g., carisoprodol), use beyond 2 weeks is not advisable. Evidence of efficacy of muscle relaxants in chronic low back pain is lacking.

Antidepressants

Antidepressants are often used in the treatment of chronic musculoskeletal pain—including back pain, as well as in neuropathic pain syndromes. A useful approach is a combination of an antidepressant as an adjuvant analgesic with a pure analgesic or NSAID. Originally, it was suggested that the therapeutic efficacy of these agents as analgesics was related to their antidepressant properties in persons with pain and depression (186). Alternatively, inhibition of serotonin and norepinephrine uptake by the antidepressant drugs may explain their clinical effects in pain syndromes (187,188). The latter mechanism is supported by clinical studies demonstrating efficacy of antidepressants in patients with back pain without depression, particularly for agents that inhibit reuptake of both serotonin and norepinephrine (189–191). Finally, sedating antidepressants may affect pain perception by augmenting non–rapid eye movement phase IV sleep, a mechanism believed to contribute to the efficacy of tricyclic antidepressants in patients with fibromyalgia (192). Particularly in patients with coexisting depression or sleep disruption, antidepressants may serve as useful adjuvant analgesics.

The efficacy of antidepressants in patients with chronic low back pain is reasonably well established. There are no data supporting use in acute pain. A metaanalysis by Salerno et al. of antidepressants in chronic back pain found nine randomized trials, seven of which included patients with major depression (193). In the 504 patients included in the analysis, antidepressant therapy produced a small to moderate improvement in pain severity in comparison to placebo-treated patients, but no difference was found in activities of daily living. Four of six studies demonstrated significant improvement in clinical depression. However, in one trial comparing nortriptyline with placebo in 78 patients with chronic low back pain, persons with depression were specifically excluded (189). In this trial, nortriptyline-treated patients demonstrated significant reductions in pain (22%) versus placebo (9%). However, reduction in disability only marginally favored nortriptyline.

Most evidence for efficacy favors older tricyclic antidepressants (e.g., amitriptyline, imipramine, doxepin, nortriptyline, and trazodone) over newer selective serotonin reuptake inhibitors (e.g., paroxetine) (187,189,194).

Side effects of antidepressants were noted in 22% of patients in the metaanalysis reported by Salerno et al. Common side effects of these agents include drowsiness, dry mouth, dizziness, constipation, urinary retention, orthostatic hypotension, weight gain, sexual dysfunction, and cardiac conduction changes (193). Considerable variability exists in the risk of these adverse effects, depending on the pharmacology of the particular drug. Anticholinergic side effects are common with amitriptyline and doxepin but are not seen with fluoxetine or trazodone (195). Sedation is more common with amitriptyline, doxepin, and trazodone. These agents should be the first choice in patients with sleep difficulty. Tricyclic antidepressants should be avoided if possible in patients with significant cardiac disease, particularly the elderly.

SUMMARY: A RATIONAL APPROACH TO NONOPERATIVE MANAGEMENT OF LOW BACK PAIN

Acute Low Back Pain (0 to 4 Weeks)

Based on the evidence presented, acute nonspecific back pain is best managed with an approach that emphasizes symptomatic relief with NSAIDs or acetaminophen and activity advice recommending return to normal activities as soon as tolerable. In a few cases, short-term opioid use is necessary to permit movement and resumption of daily activities. Particularly in patients with significant muscle spasm, addition of a muscle relaxant for as long as 1 to 2 weeks is appropriate. Patients must be cautioned regarding the sedation associated with these drugs.

Massage therapy or manipulation may be of limited benefit in patients with acute nonspecific back pain. Because the natural history of an acute episode of pain is for resolution of symptoms in most patients within 2 weeks, only a limited number of such treatments should be required. There is no significant role for TENS, traction, corsets, or acupuncture in patients with acute back pain.

The importance of education of the patient regarding the generally favorable natural history of the problem and the appropriateness of reasonable activity (including the hazards of inactivity or bed rest) deserves emphasis. Correcting misconceptions about etiology and the need for radiographic imaging as well as addressing concerns about long-term prognosis may be required. General health maintenance education, including the role of exercise, weight reduction, and smoking cessation, may be appropriate for some patients in this setting and may play a role in prevention of recurrent episodes of back pain. Finally, reevaluation of patients whose pain is not responding to treatment as expected is mandatory.

Subacute Low Back Pain (4 to 12 Weeks)

Patients with nonspecific low back pain who remain significantly symptomatic more than 4 weeks after onset merit reevaluation. Although in most such patients a precise anatomic source of pain is not identified, the possibility of an infectious, malignant, visceral, or inflammatory cause should be reconsidered, particularly in the older patient. If indicated, appropriate laboratory and imaging studies may be required. In patients with persistent or escalating symptoms more than 4 weeks after onset, the possibility of overriding, complicating nonorganic or so-called *psychosocial* issues also should be assessed. These factors may represent the most important reasons for delay in recovery of patients with nonspecific acute low back pain (14). Finally, the previous treatment should be reevaluated. Clearly, excessive emphasis on bed rest delays recovery. Malmivaara et al. reported that patients with acute low back pain had prolonged pain if they were treated with active physical therapy exercises in comparison to patients simply advised to pursue activities as tolerated (16). In this subacute stage, however, active exercise-oriented physical therapy is recommended both for its reconditioning and educational benefits.

Chronic Low Back Pain (More than 12 Weeks)

In a subset of patients with chronic nonspecific back pain, interventional investigation may identify a potential precise pain generator. The size of this subset is controversial. Some have suggested the incidence of discogenic pain in such patients is as high as 35% (6). Another study estimated the incidence of facet syndrome at 15% (7). However, these findings are based on response to diagnostic injections without clinical correlation or validation by positive response to treatment. The actual frequency of both these diagnoses in patients with chronic back pain is probably much less. For most patients with chronic back pain, the etiology remains ambiguous. As noted previously, the presence of complicating psychosocial issues should be sought in patients with disability out of proportion to clinical findings.

Exercise improves pain intensity and functional status in persons with chronic back pain and is the cornerstone of management. Current evidence does not favor any particular exercise approach over others. Pure analgesics are often safer than NSAIDs—particularly for long-term use—and are usually as effective. In carefully selected patients, opioid analgesics may be appropriate. There is no role for muscle relaxants in chronic back pain. Tricyclic antidepressants may be useful as adjuvant analgesics in patients without contraindications.

Manipulation, acupuncture, or massage may be of some benefit as adjunctive treatment in selected patients with chronic back pain. Limited comparative trials, however, demonstrate similar efficacy to minimal intervention or education at significantly greater cost. Further study is needed to identify possible subsets of patients who might be more responsive to a particular therapeutic modality.

REFERENCES

1. Cherkin DC, Deyo RA, Wheeler K, et al. Physician variation in diagnostic testing for low back pain. Who you see is what you get. *Arthritis Rheum* 1994;37:15–22.

2. Fardon D, Pinkerton S, Balderston R, et al. Terms used for diagnosis by English speaking spine surgeons. *Spine* 1993;18:274–277.
3. Deyo RA, Weinstein JN. Primary care: low back pain. *N Engl J Med* 2001;344:363–370.
4. Fast A. Low back disorders: conservative management. *Arch Phys Med Rehabil* 1988;69:880–891.
5. Deyo RA. Diagnostic evaluation of LBP. Reaching a specific diagnosis is often impossible. *Arch Intern Med* 2002;162:1444–1447.
6. Schwartzer AC, Aprill CN, Derby R, et al. The prevalence and clinical features of internal disc disruption in patients with chronic low back pain. *Spine* 1995;20:1878–1883.
7. Schwartzer AC, Aprill CN, Derby R, et al. Clinical features of patients with pain stemming from the lumbar zygapophyseal joints. Is the lumbar facet syndrome a clinical entity? *Spine* 1994;19:1132–1137.
8. Boden SD, Davis DO, Dina TS, et al. Abnormal magnetic resonance scans of the lumbar spine in asymptomatic subjects. *J Bone Joint Surg* 1990;72A:403–408.
9. Jensen MC, Brant-Zawadski N, Obuchowski N, et al. Magnetic resonance imaging of the lumbar spine in people without back pain. *N Engl J Med* 1994;331:69–73.
10. Wiesel SW, Tsourmas N, Fefer HL, et al. A study of computer-assisted tomography I. The incidence of positive CAT scans in an asymptomatic group of patients. *Spine* 1984;9:549–551.
11. Weishaupt D, Zanetti M, Hodler J, et al. MR imaging of the lumbar spine: prevalence of intervertebral disk extrusion and sequestration, nerve root compression, end plate abnormalities, and osteoarthritis of the facet joint in asymptomatic volunteers. *Radiology* 1998;209:661–666.
12. Spitzer WO, LeBlanc FE, Dupuis M, et al. Scientific approach to assessment and management of activity-related spine disorders. A monograph for clinicians. Report of the Quebec Task Force on Spinal Disorders. *Spine* 1987;12[Suppl1]:S17–S21.
13. Polatin PB, Kinney RK, Gatchel RJ, et al. Psychiatric illness and chronic low back pain. The mind and the spine—which goes first? *Spine* 1993;18:66–71.
14. Burton AK, Tillotson KM, Main CJ, et al. Psychosocial predictors of outcome in acute and subacute low back trouble. *Spine* 1995;20:722–728.
15. Andersson GBJ. Epidemiological features of chronic low back pain. *Lancet* 1999; 354:581–585.
16. Malmivaara A, Hakkinen U, Aro T, et al. The treatment of acute low back pain—bed rest, exercises, or ordinary activity? *N Engl J Med* 1995;332:351–355.
17. Von Korff M, Saunders K. The course of back pain in primary care. *Spine* 1996; 21:2833–2839.
18. Carey TS, Garrett JM, Jackman A, et al. Recurrence and care seeking after acute back pain. Results of a long-term follow-up study. *Med Care* 1999;37:157–164.
19. Van der Hoogen HJ, Koes BW, van Eijk JT, et al. On the course of low back pain in general practice: a one-year follow up study. *Ann Rheum Dis* 1998;57:13–19.
20. Wahlgren DR, Atkinson JH, Epping-Jordan JE, et al. One-year follow up of first onset low back pain. *Pain* 1997;73:213–221.
21. Koes BW, van Tulder MW, Ostelo R, et al. Clinical guidelines for the management of low back pain in primary care. An international comparison. *Spine* 2001;26:2504–2514.
22. Gatchel RJ, McGeary D. Cochrane collaboration-based reviews of health-care interventions: are they unequivocal and valid scientifically or simply nihilistic? *Spine J* 2002;2:315–319.
23. Little P, Roberts L, Blowers H, et al. Should we give detailed advice and information booklets to patients with back pain? A randomized controlled factorial trial of a self-management booklet and doctor advice to take exercise for back pain. *Spine* 2001;26:2065–2072.
24. Cherkin DC, Deyo R, Street JH, et al. Pitfalls of patient education. Limited success of a program for back pain in primary care. *Spine* 1996;21:345–355.
25. Roberts L, Little P, Chapman J, et al. The Back Home trial. General practitioner-supported leaflets may change back pain behavior. *Spine* 2002;27:1821–1828.
26. Cohen JE, Goel V, Frank JW, et al. Group education interventions for people with low back pain. An overview of the literature. *Spine* 1994;19:1214–1222.
27. Daltroy LJ, Iversen MD, Larson MG, et al. A controlled trial of an educational program to prevent low back injuries. *N Engl J Med* 1997;337:322–328.
28. Deyo RA, Diehl AK, Rosenthal M. How many days of bedrest for acute low back pain? A randomized clinical trial. *N Engl J Med* 1986;315:1064–1070.
29. Gilbert JR, Taylor DW, Hildebrand A, et al. Clinical trial of common treatments for low back pain in family practice. *BMJ* 1985;291:791–794.
30. Rozenberg S, Delval C, Rezvani Y, et al. Bed rest or normal activity for patients with acute low back pain. A randomized controlled trial. *Spine* 2002;27:1487–1493.
31. Hagen KB, Hilde G, Jamtvedt G, et al. The Cochrane review of advice to stay active as a single treatment for low back pain and sciatica. *Spine* 2002;27:1736–1741.
32. Muller EA. Influence of training and of inactivity on muscle strength. *Arch Phys Med Rehabil* 1970;51:449–462.
33. Krolner B, Toft B. Vertebral bone loss: an unheeded side effect of therapeutic bed rest. *Clin Sci* 1983;64:537–540.
34. Hultman G, Nordin M, Saraste H, et al. Body composition, endurance strength, cross-sectional area, and density of MM erector spinae in men with and without low back pain. *J Spinal Disord* 1993;6:114–123.
35. Wittink H, Michel TH, Wagner A, et al. Deconditioning in patients with chronic low back pain. Fact or fiction? *Spine* 2000;25:2221–2228.
36. Hurri H, Mellin G, Korhonen O, et al. Aerobic capacity among chronic low back pain patients. *J Spine Disord* 1991;4:34–38.
37. McQuade K, Turner J, Buchner DM. Physical fitness and chronic low back pain. An analysis of the relationship among fitness, functional limitations, and depression. *Clin Orthop* 1988;233:198–204.
38. Davis V, Fillingim R, Doleys D, et al. Assessment of aerobic power in chronic pain patients before and after a multidisciplinary treatment program. *Arch Phys Med Rehab* 1992;73:726–729.
39. van Tulder M, Malmivaara A, Esmail R, et al. Exercise therapy for low back pain. A systematic review within the framework of the Cochrane Collaboration Back Review Group. *Spine* 2000;25:2784–2796.
40. Faas A. Exercises: Which ones are worth trying, for which patients, and when? *Spine* 1996;21:2874–2879.
41. Nordin M, Campello M. Physical therapy. Exercises and the modalities: when, what, and why? *Neurol Clin North Am* 1999;17:75–89.
42. Philadelphia Panel. Philadelphia Panel evidence-based clinical practice guidelines on selected rehabilitation interventions for low back pain. *Physical Therapy* 2001; 81:1641–1674.
43. Van Tulder MW, Koes BW, Bouter LM. Conservative treatment of acute and chronic nonspecific low back pain. A systematic review of randomized controlled trials of the most common interventions. *Spine* 1997;22:2128–2156.
44. Stankovic R, Johnell O. Conservative treatment of acute low back pain. A prospective randomized trial: McKenzie method of treatment versus patient education in "Mini Back School." *Spine* 1990;15:120–123.
45. Stankovic R, Johnell O. Conservative treatment of acute low back pain. A 5-year follow-up study of two methods of treatment. *Spine* 1995;20:469–472.
46. Cherkin DC, Deyo RA, Battie M, et al. A comparison of physical therapy, chiropractic manipulation, and provision of an educational booklet for the treatment of patients with low back pain. *N Engl J Med* 1998;339:1021–1029.
47. Fass A, Chavannes AW, van Eijk JTM, et al. A randomized, placebo-controlled trial of exercise therapy in patients with acute low back pain. *Spine* 1993;18:1388–1395.
48. Dettori JR, Bullock SH, Sutlive TG, et al. The effects of spinal flexion and extension exercises and their associated postures in patients with acute low back pain. *Spine* 1995;20:2303–2312.
49. Shirado O, Ito T, Kaneda K, et al. Flexion-relaxation phenomenon in the back muscles: a comparative study between healthy subjects and patients with chronic low back pain. *Am J Phys Med Rehabil* 1995;74:139–144.
50. Mooney V, Gulick J, Perlman M, et al. Relationship between myoelectric activity, strength, and MRI of lumbar extension muscles in back pain patients and normal subjects. *J Spinal Dis* 1997;10:348–356.
51. Nicolaisen T, Jorgensten K. Trunk strength, back muscle endurance and low-back trouble. *Scand J Rehabil Med* 1985;17:121–127.
52. Lee JH, Ooi Y, Nakamura K. Measurement of muscle strength of the trunk and the lower extremities in subjects with history of low back pain. *Spine* 1995;20:1994–1996.

53. Mannion AF, Taimela S, Muntener M, et al. Active therapy for chronic back pain. Part 1. Effects on back muscle activation, fatigability, and strength. *Spine* 2001;26:897–908.
54. Risch SV, Norvell NK, Pollock ML, et al. Lumbar strengthening in chronic low back pain patients. Physiologic and psychological benefits. *Spine* 1993;18:232–238.
55. Mannion AF, Muntener M, Taimela S, et al. Comparison of three active therapies for chronic low back pain: results of a randomized clinical trial with one-year follow up. *Rheumatology* 2001;40:772–778.
56. Kaser L, Mannion AF, Rhyner A, et al. Active therapy for chronic low back pain. Part 2. Effects on paraspinal muscle cross-sectional area, fiber type size, and distribution. *Spine* 2001;26:909–919.
57. Lindstrom I, Ohlund C, Eek C, et al. Mobility, strength, and fitness after a graded activity program for patients with subacute low back pain. A randomized prospective clinical study with a behavioral therapy approach. *Spine* 1992;17:641–652.
58. Frost H, Lamb SE, Moffett JAK, et al. A fitness program for patients with chronic low back pain: 2-year follow-up of a randomized controlled trial. *Pain* 1998;75:273–279.
59. Moffett JK, Torgerson D, Bell-Byer S, et al. Randomized controlled trial of exercise for low back pain: clinical outcomes, costs, and preferences. *BMJ* 1999;319:279–283.
60. Van der Velde G, Mierau D. The effect of exercise on percentile rank aerobic capacity, and self-rated disability in patients with chronic low-back pain: a retrospective chart review. *Arch Phys Med Rehabil* 2000;81:1457–1463.
61. Kraus H, Nagler W, Melleby A. Evaluation of an exercise program for back pain. *Am Fam Phys* 1983;28(3):153–158.
62. Deyo RA, Walsh NE, Martin DC, et al. A controlled trial of transcutaneous electrical nerve stimulation (TENS) and exercise for chronic low back pain. *N Engl J Med* 1990; 322:1627–1634.
63. Plum P, Rehfeld JF. Muscular training for acute and chronic back pain. *Lancet* 1985;1:453–454.
64. Manniche C, Hesselsoe G, Bentzen L, et al. Clinical trial of intensive muscle training for chronic low back pain. *Lancet* 1988;2:1473–1476.
65. Manniche C, Lundberg E, Christensen I, et al. Intensive dynamic back exercises for chronic back pain. A clinical trial. *Pain* 1991; 47:53–63.
66. Hansen FR, Bendix T, Skov P, et al. Intensive, dynamic back-muscle exercises, conventional physiotherapy, or placebo-control treatment of low-back pain. A randomized, observer-blind trial. *Spine* 1993;18:98–107.
67. Nelson BW, Carpenter DM, Dreisinger TE, et al. Can spinal surgery be prevented by aggressive strengthening exercises? A prospective study of cervical and lumbar patients. *Arch Phys Med Rehabil* 1999;80:20–25.
68. Peterson T, Krkyger P, Ekdahl C, et al. The effect of McKenzie therapy as compared with that of intensive strengthening training for the treatment of patients with subacute or chronic low back pain. *Spine* 2002;27:1702–1709.
69. Donelson R, Aprill C, Medcalf R, et al. A prospective study of centralization of lumbar and referred pain. A predictor of symptomatic discs and anular competence. *Spine* 1997;22:1115–1122.
70. Donelson R, Grant W, Kamps C, et al. Pain response to sagittal endrange spinal motion: a multi-centered, prospective randomized trial. *Spine* 1991;16:S206–212.
71. Taylor M. The McKenzie method: a general practice interpretation. The lumbar spine. *Aust Fam Phys* 1995;24:1–7.
72. Long AL. The centralization phenomenon. Its usefulness as a predictor of outcome in conservative treatment of chronic low back pain. (A pilot study). *Spine* 1995;20:2513–2521.
73. Donelson RG, Silva G, Murphy K. The centralization phenomenon: its usefulness in evaluating and treating referred pain. *Spine* 1990;15:211–213.
74. Elnaggar I, Nordin M, Sheikhzadeh A, et al. Effects of spinal flexion and extension exercises on low back pain and spinal mobility in chronic mechanical low-back pain patients. *Spine* 1991;16:967–972.
75. Williams PC. Examination and conservative treatment for disc lesions of the lower spine. *Clin Orthop* 1955;5:28–40.
76. Ponte DJ, Jensen GJ, Kent BE. A preliminary report on the use of the McKenzie protocol versus Williams protocol in the treatment of low back pain. *Orthop Sports Phys Ther* 1984;6:130–139.
77. Kendell PH, Jenkins JM. Exercises for backache: a double blind controlled trial. *Physiotherapy* 1968;54:154–157.
78. Helewa A, Goldsmith CH, Lee P, et al. Does strengthening the abdominal muscles prevent low back pain—a randomized controlled trial. *J Rheumatol* 1999;26:1808–1815.
79. Meeker WC, Haldeman S. Chiropractic: a profession at the crossroads of mainstream and alternative medicine. *Ann Intern Med* 2002;136:216–217.
80. Shekelle PG, Adams AH, Chassin MR, et al. Spinal manipulation for low back pain. *Ann Intern Med* 1992;117:590–598.
81. Bigos SJ, Bowyer OR, Braen GR, et al. *Acute low back problems in adults: clinical practice guideline* no. 14. AHCPR publication no. 95-0642. Rockville, MD: Agency for Health Care Policy and Research, December 1994.
82. Royal College of General Practitioners. Clinical guidelines for the management of acute low back pain. London: Royal College of General Practitioners, 1996.
83. Ernst E, Assendelft WJJ. Chiropractic for low back pain: we don't know whether it does more good than harm. *BMJ* 1998;317:160.
84. Shekelle PG. What role for chiropractic in health care? *N Engl J Med* 1998;339:1074–1075.
85. Waddell G. Chiropractic for low back pain: evidence for manipulation is stronger than that for most orthodox medical treatments. *BMJ* 1999;318:262.
86. French SD, Green S, Forbes A. Reliability of chiropractic methods commonly used to detect manipulable lesions in patients with chronic low back pain. *J Manipulative Physiol Ther* 2000;23:231–238.
87. Shekelle PG. Spine update. Spinal manipulation. *Spine* 1994;19:858–861.
88. Bronfort G. Spinal manipulation. Current state of research and its indications. *Neurol Clin* 1999;17:91–111.
89. Bolton PS. Reflex effects of subluxation. The peripheral nervous system: an update. *J Manipulative Physiol Ther* 2000;23:101–103.
90. Cherkin DC, MacCornack FA. Patient evaluations of low back pain care from family physicians and chiropractors. *West J Med* 1989;150:351–355.
91. Coulter ID, Hurwitz EL, Adams AH, et al. Patients using chiropractors in North America. Who are they, and why are they in chiropractic care? *Spine* 2002;27:291–298.
92. Bass MJ. The physician's actions and the outcome of illness in family practice. *J Fam Prac* 1986;23:43–47.
93. Koes BW, Assendelft WJJ, Geert JMG, et al. Spinal manipulation for low back pain. An updated systematic review of randomized clinical trials. *Spine* 1996;21:2860–2873.
94. Van Tulder MW, Koes BW, Bouter LM. Conservative treatment of acute and chronic nonspecific low back pain. A systematic review of randomized controlled trials of the most common interventions. *Spine* 1997;22:2128–2156.
95. Hadler NM, Curtis P, Gillings DB, et al. A benefit of spinal manipulation as adjunctive therapy for acute low back pain: a stratified controlled trial. *Spine* 1987;12:702–706.
96. MacDonald RS, Bell CM. An open controlled assessment of osteopathic manipulation in nonspecific low back pain. *Spine* 1990;15:364–370.
97. Andersson GBJ, Lucente T, Davis AM, et al. A comparison of osteopathic spinal manipulation with standard care for patients with low back pain. *N Engl J Med* 1999;341:1426–1431.
98. Hurwitz EL, Morgenstern H, Harber P, et al. The effectiveness of physical modalities among patients with low back pain randomized to chiropractic care: findings from the UCLA low back pain study. *J Manipulative Physiol Ther* 2002;25:10–20.
99. Senstad O, Leboeuf-Yde C, Borchgrevink C. Frequency and characteristics of side effects of spinal manipulative therapy. *Spine* 1997;22:435–441.
100. Eisenberg DM, Davis RB, Ettner SL, et al. Trends in alternative medicine uses in the United States, 1990–1997: results of a follow up national survey. *JAMA* 1998;280: 1569–1575.
101. Preyde M. Effectiveness of massage therapy for subacute low back pain: a randomized controlled trial. *Can Med Assoc J* 2000;162:1815–1820.
102. Furlan AD, Brosseau L, Imamura M, et al. Massage for low back pain: a systematic review within the framework of the Cochrane Collaboration Back Review Group. *Spine* 2002;27:1896–1910.

103. Cherkin DC, Eisenberg D, Sherman KJ, et al. Randomized trial comparing traditional Chinese medical acupuncture, therapeutic massage, and self-care education for chronic low back pain. *Arch Intern Med* 2001;161:1081–1088.
104. Pope MH, Phillips RB, Haugh LD, et al. A prospective randomized three-week trial of spinal manipulation, transcutaneous muscle stimulation, massage and corset in the treatment of subacute low back pain. *Spine* 1994;19:2571–2577.
105. Hseich CY, Phillips RB, Adams AH, et al. Functional outcomes of low back pain: comparison of four treatment groups in a randomized controlled trial. *J Manipulative Physiol Ther* 1992;15:4–9.
106. Brosseau L, Milne S, Robinson V, et al. Efficacy of the transcutaneous electrical nerve stimulation for the treatment of chronic low back pain. A meta-analysis. *Spine* 2002; 27:596–603.
107. Woolf CJ, Wall PD. Chronic peripheral nerve section diminishes the primary afferent A-fibre mediated inhibition of rat dorsal horn neurones. *Brain Res* 1982;242:77–85.
108. DeBroucker T, Cesaro P, Willer JC, et al. Diffuse noxious inhibitory controls in man: involvement of the spinoreticular tract. *Brain* 1990;113:1223–1234.
109. Han JS, Chen XH, Sun SL. Effect of low and high frequency TENS on metenkephalin-Arg-Phe and dynorphin: an immunoreactivity in human lumbar CSF. *Pain* 1991;47:295–298.
110. Deyo RA, Walsh NE, Schoenfeld LS, et al. Can trials of physical treatments be blinded? The example of transcutaneous electrical nerve stimulation for chronic pain. *Am J Phys Med Rehabil* 1990;69:1–10.
111. Herman E, Williams R, Stratford P, et al. A randomized controlled trial of transcutaneous electrical nerve stimulation (CODETRON) to determine its benefits in a rehabilitation program for acute occupational low back pain. *Spine* 1994;19:561–568.
112. Grant DJ, Bishop-Miller J, Winchester DM, et al. A randomized comparative trial of acupuncture versus transcutaneous electrical nerve stimulation for chronic back pain in the elderly. *Pain* 1999;82:9–13.
113. Moore SR, Shurman J. Combined neuromuscular electrical stimulation and transcutaneous electrical nerve stimulation for treatment of chronic back pain: a double-blind, repeated measures comparison. *Arch Phys Med Rehabil* 1997;78:55–60.
114. Ghoname EA, Craig WF, White PF, et al. Percutaneous electrical nerve stimulation for low back pain: a randomized crossover study. *JAMA* 1999;281:818–823.
115. Kaptchuk TJ. Acupuncture: theory, efficacy, and practice. *Ann Intern Med* 2002;136:374–383.
116. NIH Consensus Conference. Acupuncture. *JAMA* 1998;1518–1524.
117. Berman BM, Bausell RB, Lee WL. Use and referral patterns for 22 complementary and alternative medical therapies by members of the American College of Rheumatology. Results of a national survey. *Arch Intern Med* 2002;162:766–770.
118. Berman BM, Bausell RB. The use of non-pharmacological therapies by pain specialists. *Pain* 2000;85:313–316.
119. Lao L. Acupuncture techniques and devices. *J Altern Complement Med* 1996;2:23–25.
120. Pomeranz B, Stux G, eds. *Scientific basis of acupuncture*. New York: Springer-Verlag, 1989.
121. Cheng RS, Pomeranz BH. Electroacupuncture analgesia is mediated by stereospecific opiate receptors and is reversed by antagonists of type I receptors. *Life Sci* 1980; 26:631–638.
122. Van Tulder MW, Cherkin DW, Berman B. The effectiveness of acupuncture in the management of acute and chronic low back pain. A systematic review within the framework of the Cochrane Collaboration Back Review Group. *Spine* 1999;24:1113–1123.
123. Kalauokalani D, Cherkin DC, Sherman KJ, et al. Lessons from a trial of acupuncture and massage for low back pain. Patient expectations and treatment effects. *Spine* 2001;26:1418–1424.
124. Kalauokalani D, Sherman KJ, Cherkin DC. Acupuncture for chronic low back pain: diagnosis and treatment patterns among acupuncturists evaluating the same patient. *South Med J* 2001;94:486–492.
125. Ernst E, White AR. Acupuncture for back pain: a meta-analysis of randomized controlled trials. *Arch Intern Med* 1998;158:2235–2341.
126. Grant DJ, Bishop-Miller J, Winchester DM, et al. A randomized comparative trial of acupuncture versus transcutaneous electrical stimulation for chronic back pain in the elderly. *Pain* 1999;82:9–13.
127. Cherkin DC, Eisenberg D, Sherman KJ, et al. Randomized trial comparing traditional Chinese acupuncture, therapeutic massage, and self-care education for chronic low back pain. *Arch Intern Med* 2001;161:1081–1088.
128. Bigos SJ, Bowyer OR, Braen GR, et al. *Acute low back problems in adults: clinical practice guideline* no. 14. AHCPR publication no. 95-0642. Rockville, MD: Agency for Health Care Policy and Research, December 1994.
129. Waddell G, McIntosh A, Lewis M, et al. *Low back pain evidence review*. London: Royal College of General Practitioners, 1996.
130. Mukherjee D, Nissen S, Topol E. Risk of cardiovascular events associated with selective COX-2 inhibitors. *JAMA* 2001;286:954–959.
131. Koes BW, Scholten RJPM, Mens JMA, et al. Efficacy of non-steroidal anti-inflammatory drugs for low back pain: a systematic review of randomized clinical trials. *Ann Rheum Dis* 1997;56:214–223.
132. Van Tulder MW, Scholten RJPM, Koes BW, et al. Nonsteroidal anti-inflammatory drugs for low back pain. *Spine* 2000;25:2501–2513.
133. Bradley JD, Brandt KD, Katz BP, et al. Comparison of an antiinflammatory dose of ibuprofen, an analgesic dose of ibuprofen, and acetaminophen in the treatment of patients with osteoarthritis of the knee. *N Engl J Med* 1991;325:87–91.
134. Pincus T, Koch GG, Sokka T, et al. A randomized, double-blind, crossover clinical trial of diclofenac plus misoprostol versus acetaminophen in patients with osteoarthritis of the hip and knee. *Arthritis Rheum* 2001;44:1587–1598.
135. Singh G, Ramey DR, Morfeld D, et al. Gastrointestinal tract complications of nonsteroidal antiinflammatory drug treatment in rheumatoid arthritis. *Arch Intern Med* 1996;156:1530–1536.
136. Wolfe MM, Lichtenstein DR, Singh G. Medical progress: gastrointestinal toxicity of nonsteroidal antiinflammatory drugs. *N Engl J Med* 1999;340:1888–1899.
137. Simon LS, Goodman T. NSAID-induced gastrointestinal toxicity. *Bull Rheum Dis* 1995;44:1–5.
138. Hernandez-Diaz S, Rodriguez LAG. Association between nonsteroidal anti-inflammatory drugs and upper gastrointestinal tract bleeding/perforation. *Arch Intern Med* 2000;160:2093–2099.
139. Garcia Rodriguez LA, Hernandez-Diaz S. Risk of upper gastrointestinal complications among users of acetaminophen and nonsteroidal antiinflamatory drugs. *Epidemiology* 2001;12:570–576.
140. Rahme E, Pettit D, LeLorier J. Determinants and sequelae associated with utilization of acetaminophen versus traditional nonsteroidal antiinflammatory drugs in an elderly population. *Arthritis Rheum* 2002;46:3046–3054.
141. Abramson SB, et al. Acetaminophen. *Arthritis Rheum* 2002;46:2831–2835.
142. Lipsky PE, Brooks P, Crofford LJ, et al. Unresolved issues in the role of cyclooxygenase-2 in normal physiologic processes and disease. *Arch Intern Med* 2000;160:913–920.
143. Bombardier C, Laine L, Reicin A, et al. Comparison of upper gastrointestinal toxicity of rofecoxib and naproxen in patients with rheumatoid arthritis. *N Engl J Med* 2000;343:1520–1528.
144. Silverstein FE, Faich G, Goldstein JL, et al. Gastrointestinal toxicity with celecoxib vs nonsteroidal antiinflammatory drugs for osteoarthritis and rheumatoid arthritis. *JAMA* 2000;284:1247–1255.
145. Page J, Henry D. Consumption of NSAIDs and the development of congestive heart failure in elderly patients. An underrecognized public health problem. *Arch Intern Med* 2000;160:777–784.
146. Heerdink ER, Leufkens HG, Hering RMC, et al. NSAIDs associated with increased risk of congestive heart failure in elderly patients taking diuretics. *Arch Intern Med* 1998;158:1108–1112.
147. Fenstra J, Heerdink ER, Grobbee DE, et al. Association of nonsteroidal antiinflammatory drugs with first occurrence of heart failure and with relapsing heart failure. *Arch Intern Med* 2002;162:265–270.
148. Swan SK, Rudy DW, Lasseter KC, et al. Effect of cyclooxygenase-2 inhibition on renal function in elderly persons receiving a low-salt diet. *Ann Intern Med* 2000;133:1–9.
149. Whelton A, Schulman G, Wallemark C, et al. Effects of celecoxib and naproxen on renal function in the elderly. *Arch Intern Med* 2000;160:1465–1470.
150. Fitzgerald GA, Patrono C. The coxibs, selective inhibitors of cyclooxygenase-2. *N Engl J Med* 2001;345:433–442.

151. White WB, Faich G, Whelton A, et al. Comparison of thromboembolic events in patients treated with celecoxib, a cyclooxygenase-2 specific inhibitor, versus ibuprofen or diclofenac. *Am J Cardiol* 2002;89:425–430.
152. Watson DJ, Rhodes T, Cai B. Lower risk of thromboembolic cardiovascular events with naproxen among patients with rheumatoid arthritis. *Arch Intern Med* 2002;162:1105–1110.
153. Rahme E, Pilote L, LeLorier J. Association between naproxen use and protection against acute myocardial infarction. *Arch Intern Med* 2002;162:1111–1115.
154. Solomon DH, Glynn RJ, Leven R, et al. Nonsteroidal antiinflammatory drug use and acute myocardial infarction. *Arch Intern Med* 2002;162:1099–1104.
155. Dalen JE. Selective COX-2 inhibitors, NSAIDs, aspirin, and myocardial infarction. *Arch Intern Med* 2002;162:1091–1092.
156. Schofferman J. Long-term use of opioid analgesics for the treatment of chronic pain of nonmalignant origin. *J Pain Symptom Manage* 1993;8:279–288.
157. Molloy AR, Nicholas MK, Cousins MJ. Role of opioids in chronic non-cancer pain. *Med J Aust* 1997;167:9–10.
158. Pappagallo M, Heinberg LJ. Ethical issues in the management of chronic nonmalignant pain. *Semin Neurol* 1997:17:203–211.
159. Taylor CMB, Zutnick SI, Corley MJ, et al. The effects of detoxification, relaxation, and brief supportive therapy on chronic pain. *Pain* 1980;8:319–329.
160. American Academy of Pain Medicine and the American Pain Society. *The use of opioids for the treatment of chronic pain.* 1997.
161. AGS Panel on Persistent Pain in Older Persons. The management of persistent pain in older persons. *J Am Geriatr Soc* 2002;50:1–20.
162. Portenoy RK, Foley KM. Chronic use of opioid analgesics in nonmalignant pain: report of 38 cases. *Pain* 1986;25:171–186.
163. Jamison RN, Anderson KO, Peters-Asdourian C, et al. Survey of opioid use in chronic nonmalignant pain patients. *Reg Anesth* 1994; 19:225–230.
164. Jamison RN, Raymond SA, Slawsby EA, et al. Opioid therapy for chronic non-cancer back pain. A randomized prospective study. *Spine* 1998;23:2591–2600.
165. Moulin DE, Iezzi A, Amireh R, et al. Randomized trial of oral morphine for chronic non-cancer pain. *Lancet* 1996;347:143–147.
166. Zenz M, Strumpf M, Tryba M. Long-term oral opioid therapy in patients with chronic nonmalignant pain. *J Pain Symptom Manage* 1992;7:69–77.
167. Caldwell JR, Hale ME, Boyd RE, et al. Treatment of osteoarthritis pain with controlled release oxycodone or fixed combination oxycodone plus acetaminophen added to nonsteroidal antiinflammatory drugs: a double blind, randomized multicenter, placebo controlled trial. *J Rheumatol* 1999;26:862–869.
168. Porter J, Jick H. Addiction rare in patients treated with narcotics. *N Engl J Med* 1980;302:123.
169. Dunbar SA, Katz NP. Chronic opioid therapy for nonmalignant pain in patients with a history of substance abuse: report of 20 cases. *J Pain Symptom Manage* 1996;11:163–171.
170. Conigliaro DA. Opioids for chronic non-malignant pain. *J Fla Med Assoc* 1996;83:708–711.
171. Haythornthwaite JA, Menefee LA, Quatrano-Piacentini AL, et al. Outcome of chronic opioid therapy for non-cancer pain. *J Pain Symptom Manage* 1998;15:185–194.
172. Zacny JP. Should people taking opioids for medical reasons be allowed to work and drive? *Addiction* 1996;11:1581–1684.
173. Elliott TE. Chronic noncancer pain management. *Minn Med* 2002;84:28–34.
174. Brown RL, Fleming MF, Patterson JJ. Chronic opioid analgesic therapy for low back pain. *J Am Board Fam Pract* 1996;9:191–204.
175. McQuay H. Opioids in pain management. *Lancet* 1999;353:2229–2232.
176. Roy SH, De Luca CJ, Emley, et al. Classification of back muscle impairment based on surface electromyographic signal. *J Rehabil Res Dev* 1997;34:405–414.
177. Oddsson LIE, Giphart JE, Bjijs RJC, et al. Development of new protocols and analysis procedures for the assessment of LBP by surface EMG techniques. *J Rehabil Res Dev* 1997;34:415–426.
178. Mannion AF, Connolly B, Wood K, et al. The use of surface EMG power spectral analysis in the evaluation of back muscle function. *J Rehabil Res Dev* 1997;34:427–439.
179. Browning R, Jackson JL, O'Malley PG. Cyclobenzaprine and back pain: a meta-analysis. *Arch Intern Med* 2001;161:1613–1620.
180. Dapas F, Hartman SF, Martinez L, et al. Baclofen for the treatment of acute low back pain syndrome: a double blind comparison with placebo. *Spine* 1985;10:345–349.
181. Hindle TH. Comparison of carisoprodol, butabarbital, and placebo in treatment of low back pain syndrome. *Calif Med* 1972;117:7.
182. Berry H, Hutchinson DR. A multicentre placebo-controlled study in general practice to evaluate the efficacy and safety of tizanidine I acute low back pain. *J Int Med Res* 1988;16:75.
183. Berry H, Hutchinson DR. Tizanidine and ibuprofen in acute low back pain: results of a double blind multicentre study in general practice. *J Int Med Res* 1988;16:83.
184. Basmajian JV. Acute back pain and spasm: a controlled multicenter trial of combined analgesic and antispasm agents. *Spine* 1989;14: 438–439.
185. Borenstein DG. Cyclobenzaprine and naproxen versus naproxen alone in the treatment of acute low back pain and muscle spasm. *Clin Ther* 1990;12:125–131.
186. France RD, Houpt JL, Ellinwood EH. Therapeutic effects of antidepressants in chronic pain. *Gen Hosp Psychiatry* 1984;6:55–63.
187. Ward NG. Tricyclic antidepressants for chronic low back pain. Mechanisms of action and predictors of response. *Spine* 1986;11: 661–665.
188. Magni G. The use of antidepressants in the treatment of chronic pain. A review of the current evidence. *Drugs* 1991;42:730–748.
189. Atkinson JH, Slater MA, Williams RA, et al. A placebo controlled randomized clinical trial of nortriptyline for chronic low back pain. *Pain* 1998;76:287–296.
190. Fishbain D. Evidence-based data on pain relief with antidepressants. *Ann Med* 2000;32:305–316.
191. Carette S, Bell MJ, Reynolds WJ, et al. Comparison of amitriptyline, cyclobenzaprine, and placebo in the treatment of fibromyalgia. *Arthritis Rheum* 1994;37:32–40.
192. Salerno SM, Browning R, Jackson JL. The effect of antidepressant treatment on chronic back pain. *Arch Intern Med* 2002;162:19–24.
193. Goodkin K, Gullion CM, Agras WS. A randomized double blind placebo-controlled trial of trazodone hydrochloride in chronic low back pain syndrome. *J Clin Psychopharmacol* 1990;10:269–278.
194. Atkinson JH, Slater MA, Wahlgren DR, et al. Effects of noradrenergic and serotonergic antidepressants on chronic low back pain intensity. *Pain* 1999;83:137–145.
195. Potter WZ, Rudorfer MV, Husseini M. The pharmacologic treatment of depression. *N Engl J Med* 1991;325:633–642.

CHAPTER 46

Lumbar Disc Disease

A. Pathophysiology of Lumbar Spondylosis and Discogenic Back Pain

J. Kenneth Burkus and Thomas A. Zdeblick

Spondylosis is a generalized process that affects all levels of the axial skeleton. The development of spondylosis with the lumbar vertebral motion segments involves a sequence of degenerative changes that first occur on the biochemical and cellular levels and are ultimately manifested by commonly seen clinical changes on the biomechanical and morphologic levels. The initiating factor in degenerative cascade may be an injury to annulus fibrosus, an alteration in matrix composition of the nucleus pulposus, or a change in the vascularity and permeability of the vertebral end-plate. However, the primary causative agent in lumbar disc degeneration is rarely identified. The process of disc degeneration is multifactorial: Its clinical presentation and the diagnostic modalities used to identify and categorize this process vary. The symptoms, physical findings, and imaging studies must also vary and are largely dependent on how far along in this degenerative process the patient's condition has progressed.

PATHOPHYSIOLOGY OF LUMBAR SPONDYLOSIS

The lumbar spinal motion segment is a three-joint complex that includes the intervertebral disc, the facet joints, the ligamentous structures, and the vertebral bodies. Each undergoes unique changes with aging and exhibits morphologic changes characteristic of degeneration.

Lumbar Spinal Motion Segment

Intervertebral Disc

The intervertebral disc is a hydrostatic, load-bearing structure between the vertebral bodies. In conjunction with the facet joints, the disc carries the compressive loads of the trunk and is subject to a variety of forces and moments. It is composed of two primary components: the nucleus pulposus and the annulus fibrosus. The nucleus is centrally located and comprises approximately 50% of the total disc cross-sectional area in the lumbar spine. The nucleus is composed of type II collagen strands that lie in a mucoprotein gel containing various mucopolysaccharides. These fine collagenous fibrous stands are surrounded by hydrophilic proteoglycans that imbibe water. The water content of the disc varies with the age of the disc and in the normal disc ranges from 70 to 90% (1). The nucleus acts as a confined fluid within the annulus. The nucleus converts loads into tensile strain on the annular fibers and the vertebral end-plates. Chondrocytes, which manufacture the matrix components of the nucleus pulposus, are the only cells present within the normal adult nucleus.

The annulus fibrosus forms the outer boundary of the disc. It is a histologic structure distinct from the nucleus. It is composed of more than 60 distinct, concentric layers of overlapping lamellae of type I collagen fibers. These fibers are oriented at 30-degree angles to the disc space and at 120 degrees to each other. They are all configured in a helicoid pattern, which aids in resisting tensile, torsional, and radial stresses. The annulus attaches to the cartilaginous and bony end-plates at the periphery of the vertebra.

Vertebral End-Plates

The vertebral end-plates are composed of cartilaginous and osseous components. In the adult spine, the disc has no blood supply. In fact, the L4-5 disc space is the largest avascular structure in the body. Nutritional support for the nucleus is obtained by passive diffusion from the rich blood supply in the vertebral end-plates.

Facet Joints

Facet joints are synovial joints that are richly innervated with sensory nerve fibers. They are subject to the same pathologic processes as other larger synovial joints. The mechanical load sharing between the facets and the disc is rather complex; however, it has been estimated that they carry approximately 18% of the load of the lumbar spine.

Morphologic, Cellular, and Biochemical Changes of Lumbar Spondylosis

The degenerative process of the intervertebral disc begins early in life and may be due to environmental factors and genetic predisposition, as well as to normal aging. A variety of biochemical and structural changes take place during the process of degeneration. The response to biomechanical stresses within the spinal motion segment is, in part, determined by the extent of degeneration of soft tissue and bony elements. Progressive morphologic changes commonly occur in the third through fifth decades of life.

Intervertebral Disc

Degenerative disc changes begin with early disc desiccation as indicated by decreased proteoglycan water binding (2). As the nucleus ages, the collagen content of the disc increases. In addition to the decreased proteoglycan aggregates within the nucleus, there is a loss of negatively charged proteoglycan side chains. Both of these chemical processes lead to water loss within the nucleus pulposus, resulting in a decrease in the hydrostatic properties of the disc (3) and often a loss of disc space height. As the nucleus loses its ability to imbibe water, stresses are distributed unevenly on the annulus.

One of the earliest and most common morphologic findings in disc degeneration is bulging of the annulus fibrosus often associated with the presence of radial tears within the overlapping lamellae of the annulus. Radial annular tears can accelerate the degenerative process. The subsequent in-growth of granulation tissue in the annulus represents an attempt to heal these tears. Overall, the cellular population within the nucleus decreases as cellular necrosis occurs. There is a loss of the distinct border between the nucleus and the annulus, and focal extrusion of disc material may occur.

Degeneration in the annulus results in a decreased number of cells and an enlargement of the collagen fibril with a shift to more type II collagen (4,5). With time, there is an alteration in the distribution of type I and type II collagen, which alters the mechanical loading characteristics of the annulus (6). Disruption of the annular fibers occurs. These isolated defects in the lamellae can extend through adjacent annular layers and develop into distinct clefts and fissures that extend radially through the entire annulus. Fissuring, granulation tissue, and regenerating chondrocytes can be seen in the disc end-plate and annulus fibrosus (6,7).

As the aging process continues, the nucleus is no longer present as a distinct structure. Eventually, the disc becomes progressively more fibrous and disorganized. At the end stage of its degenerative change, it is replaced by an amorphous fibrocartilage with no clear distinction between nucleus and annulus fibrosus (8). Gas formation may occur with full desiccation of the disc space, resulting in the "vacuum disc sign" on plain radiographs (9).

Vertebral End-Plates

With aging, the cartilaginous end-plates become thinner and more hyalinized. The permeability of the end-plate decreases (10). The decreased permeability of the end-plate compromises the disc's nutrition, and it may affect nuclear metabolism and cause cell necrosis. In turn, these cellular changes can lead to alteration in the composition of the nucleus with increases in collagen content and reduction in matrix.

With time, continued narrowing of the disc occurs with osteophyte formation at the end-plate–annular junction. With increased axial loading, marrow changes occur in the end-plate trabecular bone of the vertebral body (8). Eventually, end-plate eburnation results (11). Subluxation and other instability patterns can occur independently of these bony changes.

Facet Joints

With a reduction in disc space height, the facet joints settle and their joint capsules become lax. Loss of normal disc space height can also result in an increasing load being transferred to the facet joints, which may, in turn, accelerate their degeneration (10). Joint subluxation can occur, and joint hypertrophy and osteophyte formation commonly occur.

Biomechanical Changes of Spondylosis

Experimental evidence supports the view that primary degeneration of the disc results in secondary changes in the posterior facet joints and soft-tissue elements (2,12,13). In addition, animal models demonstrate that peripheral injuries to the annulus lead to degenerative changes in the disc space (14). Desiccation of the disc alters the load-bearing capabilities of the disc. As the spine ages or is injured, the fluid-binding capabilities of the nucleus are reduced, and it is unable to produce sufficient fluid pressure to load the central part of the spinal motion segment. As a result, the loads are distributed to the periphery of the disc space and the stresses on the annulus are increased (15). The increasing unequal distribution of stresses leads to reactive bony changes (e.g., radial osteophyte formation) and degeneration of the annulus (e.g., radial tears and fissuring).

As degeneration progresses, slackening of the annulus, posterior joint capsules, and ligaments can result in motion segment instability in certain circumstances. It is also clear that instability is not always the end result of these pathologic and biomechanical changes. The prototype is degenerative spondylolisthesis typically involving the L4-5 interspace, more commonly in women. The additional factors that allow forward displacement are uncertain. It is proposed that abnormal orientation of the affected facet joints and biomechanical stresses affecting particularly the L4-5 motion segment may be causative. Because the condition is more common in diabetics, endocrine changes affecting connective tissue are a consideration. Some think that the condition is part of a more generalized osteoarthritis based on the common finding of an associated osteoarthritis of the hip.

These progressive degenerative changes may also result in complete loss of the disc space with bone-on-bone contact of the vertebral end-plates. Despite this contact, autofusion rarely occurs, although some have proposed that a physiologic fibrous union occurs from connective tissue ingrowth. In this situation, magnetic resonance imaging (MRI) may reveal Modic III changes.

DISCOGENIC BACK PAIN

Discogenic Pain Syndromes

Degenerative disorders of the lumbar spine are usually first identified in patients in their fourth decade of life and occur with equal frequency in men and women. The most common clinical manifestation is the complaint of persistent low back pain. It has been estimated that 80% of the population of the United States experiences low back pain at some time in their lives (16). In the industrialized nations, low back pain is one of the most common causes of disability. How many of these symptoms are due to spinal degeneration is unknown. Significant back pain has been reported in 53% of persons engaged in light physical activity and 64% of those involved in heavier labor. Impairments of the back and spine are the most frequent cause of activity limitation in persons younger than 45 years, and from 45 to 65 years of age, low back pain ranks third after heart conditions and generalized arthritis as a cause of disability (17,18). In men, the prevalence of low back pain increases up to the age of 50 years and then begins to decline. In women, the prevalence of backache continues to increase even after age 50, reaching a peak at age 60 years (18).

In most patients, low back pain is self-limiting and requires no treatment. Only 7% of patients with low back pain episodes have symptoms that persist beyond 2 weeks (16), and only 1% of those patients require prolonged treatment. Even fewer eventually require a surgical intervention.

Only 15% of patients who are initially examined for low back pain can be given a pathoanatomic diagnosis (19). Short-term, self-limited episodes of low back pain are probably muscular in origin; these transient complaints of low backache account for the majority of new episodes of low back pain.

Patients with degenerative disc disease (DDD) syndromes have a markedly different presentation. These patients describe daily, persistent pain that lasts 3 months or longer. They may also report buttock pain or sporadic episodes of radicular leg pain. Their symptoms are usually made worse with activities and are somewhat relieved with rest. Sitting and rising from a chair also are uncomfortable. In many instances, a diagnosis can be surmised based on the history, physical examination, and plain radiographs. Additional diagnostic methods most commonly used to verify the diagnosis include flexion-extension radiographs, MRI scanning, computed tomographic (CT)–myelography, provocative discography, CT-discography, facet injections, and selective nerve root blocks. Many of the symptoms, signs, and radiographic changes are nonspecific, however. For example, many patients with chronic back pain have difficulty getting in and out of a chair. Plain radiographs often show disc space narrowing in the absence of symptoms. Similarly, degenerative changes such as annular bulging and facet arthropathy are commonly seen on CT and MRI. For these reasons, provocative discography is often used to establish a diagnosis.

Discogenic pain syndromes are a continuum of diagnostic categories all related to specific degenerative patterns involving the intervertebral disc. Although these degenerative processes occur in the majority of people as a consequence of aging, it is unclear why some patients become symptomatic. There are certain behavioral and biologic factors that predispose some patients to having painful degenerative changes, whereas in others in others they remain asymptomatic (20).

Discogenic pain syndromes fall into three distinct diagnostic categories: (a) internal disc disruption (IDD), (b) DDD, and (c) segmental instability. IDD often incorporates other diagnostic terms, such as annular tear, internal disc derangement, and "dark disc disease." These conditions have plain radiographic findings that are unremarkable but can be detected on MRI and painful symptoms that can be reproduced with discography. The category of DDD includes lumbar spondylosis and isolated disc resorption. It encompasses conditions that involve changes, such as disc narrowing, end-plate sclerosis, and radial osteophyte formation, which can be seen on plain radiographs.

Segmental instability refers to excessive translational or rotational segmental motion at the intervertebral level. This diagnostic category includes spondylolisthesis, lateral listhesis, rotatory subluxation, and scoliosis. The resultant deformities often may be seen on static radiographs but require dynamic stress radiographs for identification. Segmental instability is also used to refer to conditions in patients who have had multiple discectomies. Iatrogenic instability is also identified in patients who have had an extensive facet or pars resection. However, most instabilities require some type of translational shift or excessive sagittal rotation visible on dynamic radiographic studies to be included in this diagnostic group. No radiographic criteria have been established for sagittal plain or rotational instability (19,21).

Internal Disc Disruption

In 1970, Henry Crock coined the term *internal disc disruption* (IDD) based on a retrospective analysis of patients who had continued to complain of disabling back and leg pain after operations for lumbar disc prolapse (22). IDD was defined as a condition marked by alterations in the internal structure and metabolic functions of the lumbar disc that usually followed significant trauma (23). The clinical manifestation of the syndrome included diffuse aching leg pain and symptoms that were exacerbated by physical activity, particularly those activities that increased the compressive forces on the spine.

Tears in the annulus can serve as the initiating event of IDD (24). Loss of annular continuity through a radial tear allows for the release of certain proteins that are noxious to the surrounding regional nerves that are present in the cartilaginous end-plate and the disc tissue but are usually contained within the disc space (25). It is theorized that spinal nerves may be irritated by the noxious chemicals released from the degenerating disc, escaping through annular fissures adjacent to the route. Usually imaging does not reveal direct compression by the adjacent disc or from bone overgrowth at the facets (20).

IDD is a diagnostic category that is distinct from the category that includes disc protrusions, disc bulges, and disc herniations. A radial disc bulge alone seen on CT scan or MRI is most commonly a normal finding in the aging spine and has no clinical significance (26). A bulging disc represents desiccation of the disc with reduction in disc space height. Similarly, disc herniations, which include protrusions, extrusions, and free fragments, are not considered IDD (27). These disc conditions are associated with focal extrusions of disc material that extend outside the confines of the annulus, sometimes associated with sciatica or some form of radiculopathy.

IDD is a clinical syndrome distinct from advanced DDD. In general, patients with IDD have essentially normal radiographs (22,23). There is minimal, if any, narrowing; there is no end-plate sclerosis or osteophyte formation; and, in general, the facet joints have maintained their cartilaginous surfaces and are without osteophytes.

Clinical Presentation

IDD syndrome usually follows significant trauma to the lower back. Patients can often identify a distinct mechanism or injury. They may describe a sudden and unexpected weightlifting episode, a fall with a landing on the legs or buttocks, or a sudden twisting motion. In most cases, some amount of axial compressive force or rotation can be surmised to have occurred during the incident. Most patients report a deep-seated midline lower backache. Pain often does not resolve with rest, and it usually increases in intensity and duration over a period of several months. Activities such as bending, stooping, and lifting aggravate the pain. Patients commonly report having difficulty arising from or sitting down on a chair and may describe a climbing movement with the hands on the thighs as a means of arising from a chair. Physical therapy and rehabilitation exercises often exacerbate the patient's pain, particularly if the exercise causes axial compression or flexion and extension. Ill-defined leg pain develops slowly, usually weeks or months after the initial injury. Patients often describe the pain as being centrally located within the limb, and it does not follow a dermatomal pattern. They may also describe heaviness or cramps in the buttocks and legs, but paresthesia and sensory loss are uncommon.

Physical Findings

Usually, the examination of the patient with IDD is nonspecific. Point tenderness of the lumbar spine or paraspinal muscles is absent, but paraspinal muscle spasms may be present. Flexion-extension, rotation, and lateral bending motions are often painful, and the range of motion is limited by pain. Nerve root tension signs are negative. The neurological examination is usually normal without motor weakness, sensory loss, or reflex changes.

Diagnostic Evaluation

Radiographic Studies. Plain radiographs are unremarkable for any pronounced deformity or suggestion of instability. There is no evidence of facet narrowing, disc space narrowing, osteophyte formation, or end-plate sclerosis (28). Flexion and extension radiographs are of no value in making the diagnosis unless an occult instability pattern is observed. Similarly, myelography and CT scanning of the lumbar spine are of no diagnostic value and may reveal nothing or annular bulging.

Magnetic Resonance Imaging. MRI plays an important role in the diagnosis of IDD. Changes in disc morphology and hydration can represent the earliest stages in the cascade of DDD (29,30). These result in early MRI changes that often reflect the normal physiologic process of aging, independent of any disease process (31–34) (Fig. 1). Approximately 30% of asymptomatic individuals have abnormal signal intensity in one of their lumbar discs (24,35–37). Other MRI abnormalities, such as dark discs, bulges, and herniations, have been found in 57% of asymptomatic volunteers (38). These MRI changes are, in part, age related. Degenerative changes in at least one lumbar level were found in 35% of subjects between the ages of 20 and 39 years and in almost all patients older than 60 years (26).

In a patient with persistent lumbar pain and normal radiographs, an MRI scan can be used as a screening tool (Fig. 2). Although the diagnosis of IDD can be made with a normal MRI scan, it is distinctly rare. Zucherman reported on three patients with positive discograms after normal MRIs who eventually underwent surgical fusions (39). Another study showed that IDD was ruled out in 95% of patients who had normal signal intensity and an absence of annular tears on MRI scan (40). MRIs that showed no evidence of disruption of the posterior annulus and normal signal intensity from within the nucleus were unlikely to be painful on provocative discograms in 95% of the patients in that study (40).

MRI does not have the capability of being the sole diagnostic modality in establishing the diagnosis of IDD, particularly in older patients. When the physician evaluates a patient with IDD for further treatment, age is a strong consideration. Signal changes of the disc on MRI are a normal part of the aging process. It is the younger patient with a history of trauma, persistent pain, and isolated disc changes in whom MRI proves useful to the physician in determining which patients can benefit from further treatment. Patients who have a single dark disc and an annular tear identified on MRI have a much higher frequency of positive discography confirming IDD (40).

Discography in Patients with Internal Disc Disruption. Intervertebral discography is the single most important test in the diagnosis of IDD (Fig. 3). Researchers found that the frequency of positive discography in asymptomatic volunteers was low, with high specificity and sensitivity in patients suspected of IDD when proper techniques were followed (41,42). Gresham and Miller noted in a cadaver study that 90% of the discs in subjects between the ages of 14 and 34 years were normal by morphologic criteria

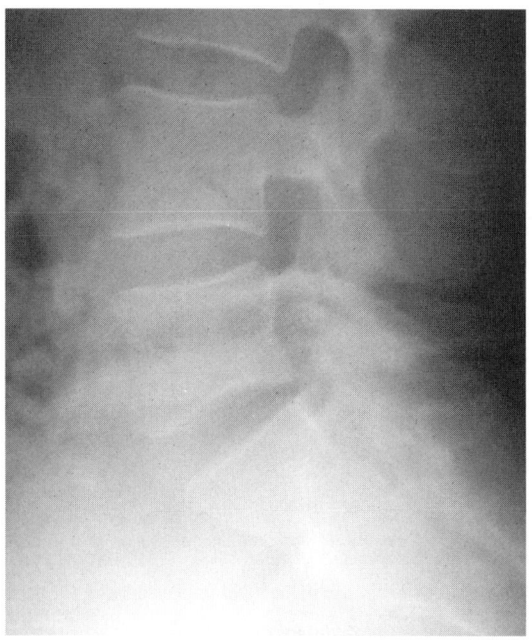

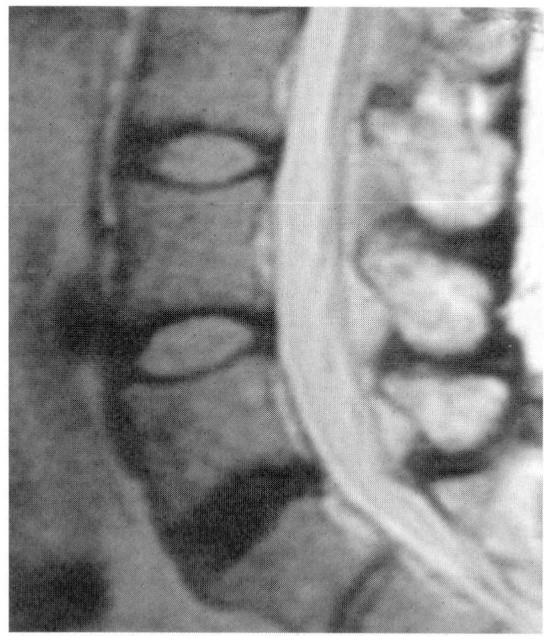

FIG. 1. A: Lateral standing radiograph of a 35-year-old man with a 4-week history of backache shows good maintenance of disc space height and no evidence of any translational instability. **B:** Sagittal magnetic resonance imaging shows isolated desiccation of the disc at L-5 to S-1. There is no radial disc bulge, and no defects in the annulus were identified. Adjacent discs at L3-4 and L4-5 are well hydrated.

(43). In contrast, by age 60 years, 95% of the discs had abnormal morphology. Similar to the findings on MRI, it is clear that proper clinical correlation is needed when discography results are examined (44). In the older patient with multilevel annular tears and degenerative changes, discography plays a much less important role in the diagnosis of painful conditions. When appropriately performed with negative controls and a correlative MRI scan, discography has a high degree of sensitivity in the diagnosis of IDD.

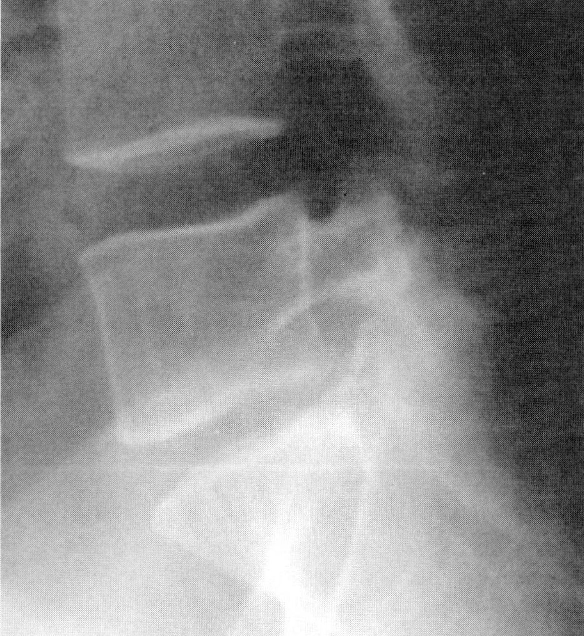

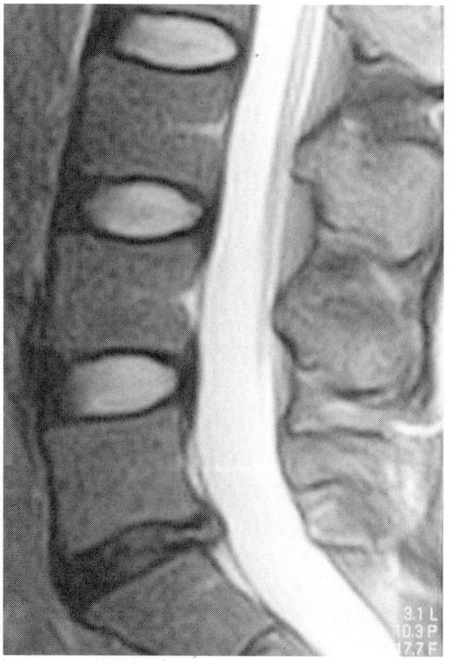

FIG. 2. A: Lateral standing radiograph of a 40-year-old man with persistent back and referred leg pain shows early disc space narrowing at the L-5 to S-1 disc with good preservation of disc space heights at L3-4 and L4-5. There are no radial osteophytes or evidence of instability. **B:** Sagittal magnetic resonance imaging shows desiccation of the disc with a radial disc protrusion extending outside the borders of the vertebral bodies. No disc herniation is seen.

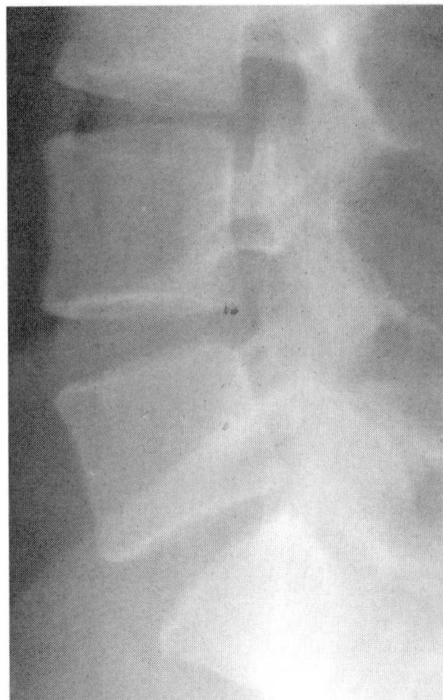
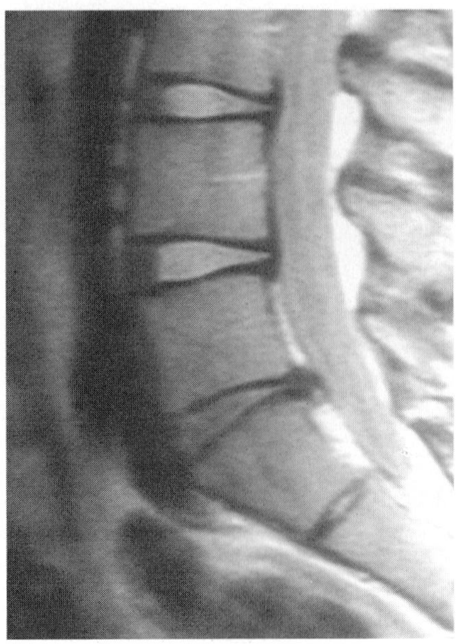
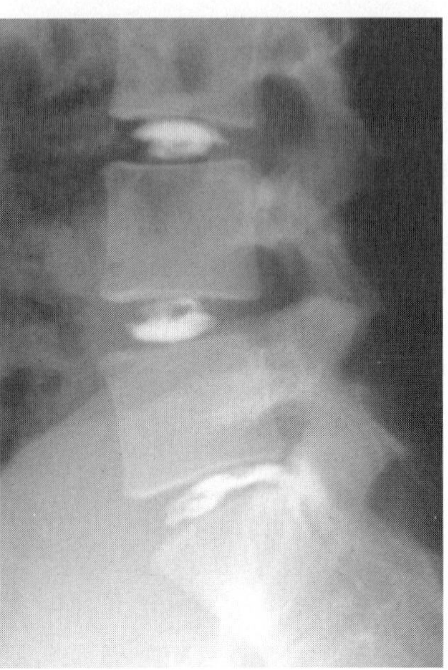

A–C

FIG. 3. A: Standing lateral radiograph of a 42-year-old man with a 6-month history of back and leg pain shows good preservation of disc space height and slight retrolisthesis at L-5 to S-1. **B:** Sagittal magnetic resonance imaging shows isolated desiccation of the L-5 to S-1 disc and an associated radial disc bulge. **C:** Provocative discography confirmed the presence of a concordant pain response on injection at the L-5 to S-1 disc space. Discography also confirmed the presence of an annular tear at L-5 to S-1 with dye leakage into the epidural space. The adjacent discs are normal.

An appropriately performed discogram produces four important pieces of information: the morphology of the discs being injected; the disc pressure or volume of fluid accepted by the disc, or both; the subjective pain response of the patient to injection; and the lack of pain response at adjacent disc levels injected (normal control) (44–46). All four of these criteria must be used to evaluate an appropriately performed discogram. In a well-performed discogram, multiple discs must be injected for intrapatient controls. Fluoroscopic guidance and radiopaque dye injection are necessary to preclude annular or epidural injections. In a morphologically normal disc, there is pooling of the dye in a tight, globular pattern within the centrum of the nucleus (47,48). In an abnormal disc, there is leakage of the dye through concentric annular tears or leakage into the epidural space through a complete annular tear (47,49). Not all abnormal morphology is painful. End-plate lesions such as limbus vertebrae or Schmorl's nodes are rarely symptomatic. In contrast, contained radial fissures that are visible on discography are almost always painful (45). In these discograms, contrast material can be seen extending from the nucleus through the annulus into the outermost rings of the annulus.

The use of discography followed by CT scanning has been reported to increase the ability to diagnose radial tears of the annulus (50–52). The greatest use of post-discography CT, however, is to diagnose far lateral disc herniation, particularly in patients who have a recurrence of disc herniation.

Discography is a provocative test. The patient must be awake during the procedure and must be able to report to the physician conducting the procedure the quality and intensity of the pain. It is only through an understanding of the patient's pain response that the physician can correlate the radiographic finding on fluoroscopy and CT scan.

Degenerative Disc Disease

The etiology of symptomatic DDD is not fully understood. The radiographic changes that result from the biochemical, biomechanical, and morphologic events affecting the spinal motion segments often occur in patients with no symptoms and thus are a normal part of the aging process (51). Disc space narrowing, vertebral end-plate sclerosis, osteophyte formation, and vacuum signs often affecting many levels of the lumbar spine are common, particularly in the population older than 50 years. These changes are uncommon in patients younger than 40 years. Crock coined the term *isolated disc resorption* to describe young patients with single-level advanced degeneration, manifested in all the radiographic changes listed previously. He thought this diagnosis had quite different clinical symptoms and signs to differentiate it from IDD, or multilevel DDD. The following discussion considers isolated disc resorption as simply one part of the spectrum of DDD.

The etiology of symptomatic degenerative disc disease (DDD) is not fully understood. In some patients, the syndrome of IDD may lead in later years to degenerative disc disease. Often, there is a remote history of sciatica or documented trauma. Degenerative disc disease also occurs after disc herniation or discectomy surgery. Chymopapain chemonucleolysis may be a predecessor to degenerative disc disease (53). However, many patients diagnosed with degenerative disc disease have a gradual onset of increasing midline lower back pain. Often, back pain begins after a rather trivial work injury. It is unknown what role, if any, these injuries have in precipitating symptomatic episodes or in accelerating degenerative changes.

Occupational and leisure time physical loading conditions, in particular, heavy material handling, postural loading, and vehicular vibration, have been more extensively studied and identi-

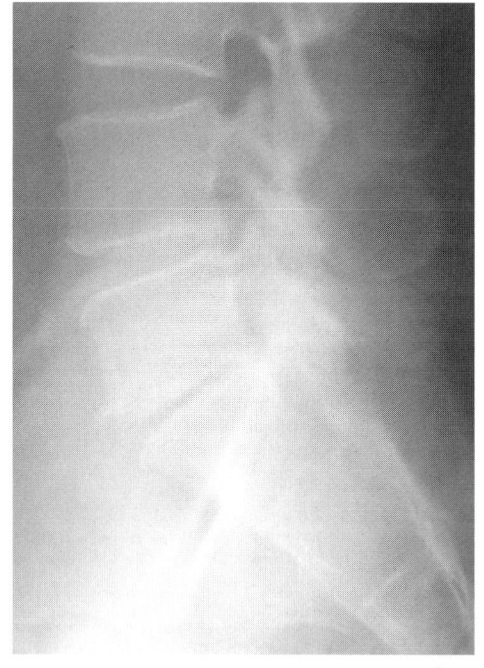
A

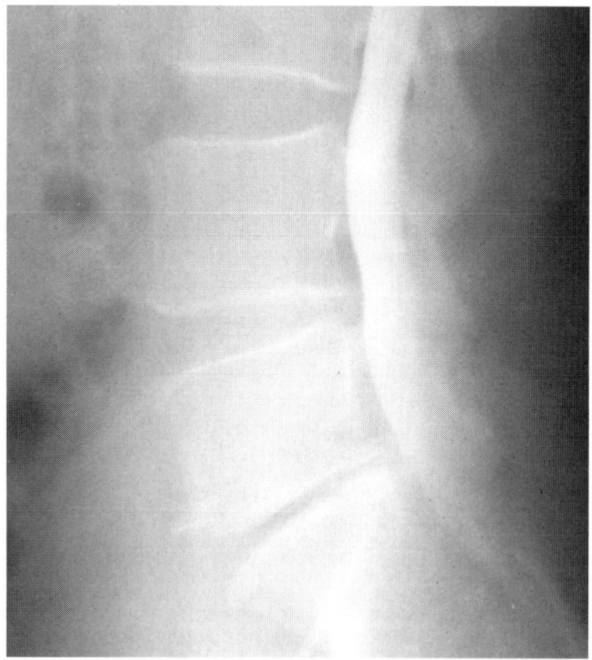
B

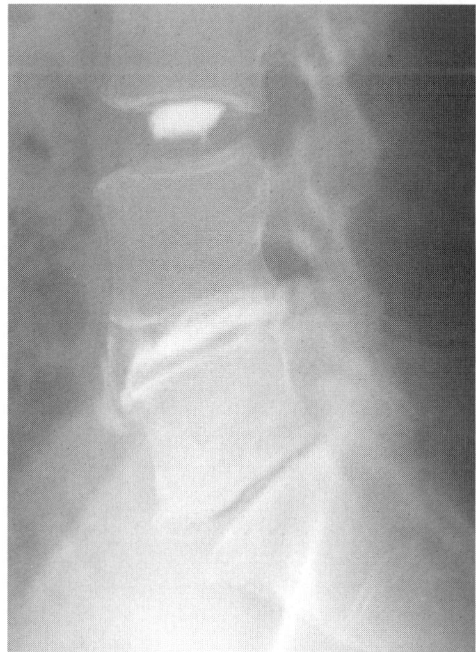
C

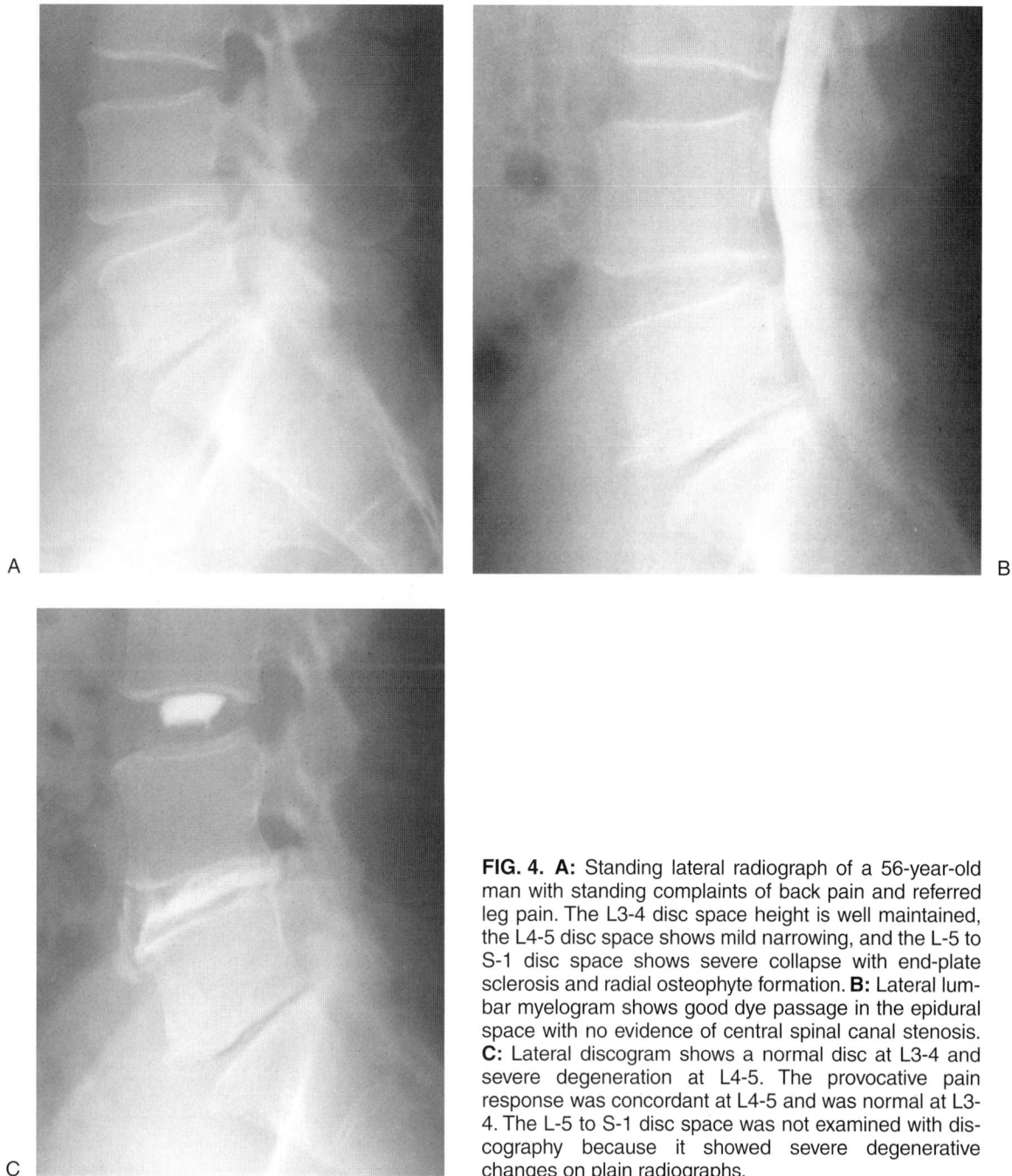

FIG. 4. A: Standing lateral radiograph of a 56-year-old man with standing complaints of back pain and referred leg pain. The L3-4 disc space height is well maintained, the L4-5 disc space shows mild narrowing, and the L-5 to S-1 disc space shows severe collapse with end-plate sclerosis and radial osteophyte formation. **B:** Lateral lumbar myelogram shows good dye passage in the epidural space with no evidence of central spinal canal stenosis. **C:** Lateral discogram shows a normal disc at L3-4 and severe degeneration at L4-5. The provocative pain response was concordant at L4-5 and was normal at L3-4. The L-5 to S-1 disc space was not examined with discography because it showed severe degenerative changes on plain radiographs.

fied as the cause of abnormal symptomatic disc degeneration than normal age-related changes (18,54–60). In some studies, prolonged cigarette smoking has been shown to be a risk factor for disc degeneration (61).

In 1995, Battie et al. published a large retrospective cohort study of identical twins to investigate the effects of lifetime exposure to commonly suspected risk factors for disc degeneration (62). They found that genetic influences had the greatest effect on predicting degenerative disc changes. Although heavier occupational and leisure physical loading was associated with disc degeneration in the upper lumbar levels, this association was not identified in the lower lumbar levels. Specifically, they did not find that heavy work, occupational driving, or cigarette smoking significantly increased the prevalence of degenerative disc disease in this cohort.

Clinical Presentation

Midline back pain with referred pain over the sacroiliac joints, iliac crests, and posterior aspect of the thighs are the most typical symptoms. Aching of the buttock and posterior thigh with ambulation is common. With continued disc space collapse, neural foraminal narrowing can occur, resulting in root stenosis. At the L-5 to S-1 level, this leads to buttock pain with mild L-5 radiculopathy or at the L4-5 level, lateral and anterior thigh pain with L-4 radiculopathy.

Physical Findings

The physical examination of patients with degenerative disc disease is often nonspecific. Point tenderness of the lumbar spinous processes is unusual. An aching sensation with palpation over the sacral iliac joints is common. Sciatic notch tenderness or positive sciatic stretch tests are absent. Range of motion of the lumbar spine is often restricted because of pain. Extension, in particular, often exacerbates a patient's symptoms and is usually limited to less than 30 degrees. Extension may precipitate buttock pain or leg heaviness. The neurologic examination is usually normal in patients with degenerative disc disease. Examination of motor strength, sensation, and reflexes reveal no abnormalities.

Diagnostic Evaluation

Plain Radiographs. The plain radiograph is the initial diagnostic test of choice. As mentioned previously, a radiograph usually shows a single level disc (most commonly, L-5 to S-1 or L4-5) that has undergone narrowing, end-plate osteophyte formation, end-plate sclerosis, and, possibly, gas formation within the disc space (32,63). In general, surrounding discs maintain their normal architecture. Flexion and extension radiographs do occasionally show increased translation or angulation or retrolisthesis (21,64). Often, however, segmental motion may be diminished on dynamic radiographs (19).

Computed Tomography–Myelography. A CT-myelogram only occasionally confirms the diagnosis of DDD. Myelography may show root-sleeve blunting in the foramen secondary to foraminal stenosis. CT scans may show marginal osteophytes causing mild to moderate lateral recess and foraminal stenosis. They can also demonstrate end-plate sclerosis and disc space vacuum signs.

Magnetic Resonance Imaging. MRI is capable of detecting the initial changes of dehydration within the nucleus pulposus associated with early degeneration. Within a severely degenerated disc, there is overall signal intensity loss. There may be linear areas of high signal intensity on T2-weighted spin echo axial images that represent free fluid within cracks or fissures of the degenerated complex (29,65,66).

Modic and associates described three signal-intensity patterns in the vertebral body marrow adjacent to the end-plates of degenerative discs (36). Type I changes are a decreased signal intensity on T1 images and an increased signal intensity on T2 images. These changes have been identified in approximately 4% of patients with low back pain. In patients who have been previously treated with chymopapain, 30% have type I marrow space changes (24,53).

Type II Modic changes are represented by an increased signal intensity on T1 images and an isointense signal on T2, and they occur in approximately 16% of patients with degenerative disc disease. These changes are always associated with degenerative disc changes on plain radiographs. Discs with type II changes show evidence of end-plate disruption with yellow marrow replacement in the adjacent vertebral body. This increase in lipid content within the marrow spaces has been suggested to be an inflammatory response suggestive of a painful disc.

Type III Modic changes show decreased signal intensity on T1 and T2 images. These MRI findings correlate with extensive bony sclerosis on plain radiographs and reflect the relative absence of marrow elements within the end-plate as advancing bony sclerosis takes over.

Discography. Discography has a limited role in the diagnosis and treatment of patients with DDD. An accurate diagnosis of DDD can be made on the basis of plain radiographs and MRI alone. Discography is used more in a confirmatory role and to evaluate adjacent level disc degeneration (67). In this instance in which the adjacent disc may have loss of signal intensity but otherwise normal radiographic findings (the "dark disc"), provocative discography is indicated to determine whether the disc should be included in a planned fusion (Fig. 4). Surgery can then be based on the results of provocative discography (66,68).

Treatment

Identifying patients with a symptomatic degenerative disc who will benefit from interventional treatment is challenging for the physician. Approximately 30% of asymptomatic younger subjects have degenerative changes on plain radiographic studies (51), and the frequency increases with aging. The selection of appropriate treatment modalities is dependent on the patient's symptoms, physical findings, and diagnostic testing.

NATURAL HISTORY

Low back pain has a benign natural history. Symptoms are most often self-limiting and resolve spontaneously. Most episodes of acute low back pain last less than 2 weeks. Seven percent of patients who complain of acute low back pain go on to develop chronic symptoms. Of those complaining of pain for more than 3 months, only one-third develop significant disabling symptoms that warrant further diagnostic evaluation. The majority of patients with complaints of backache and normal plain radiographs never receive a specific diagnosis (69). Smith and coworkers studied the outcomes of patients with documented IDD to examine the natural history of their condition (70). Over a period of 5 years, clinical improvement occurred in 68% of their patients. In 24% of them, low back pain worsened along with the associated disability. Patients who did show improvement were older by an average age of 45 years versus 33 years in those who did not.

NONOPERATIVE TREATMENT

Nonoperative treatment of low back pain includes bed rest, exercise, traction, acupuncture, bracing, drug therapy, and manipulation. In general, bed rest should be used sparingly, if at all, in the treatment of discogenic pain syndromes (71). Avoidance of pain reproducing activities may be more efficacious than avoidance of all activity.

Several clinical trials of conventional traction have failed to show any significant benefit of traction over any control treatment (16,72). The control treatments have included sham traction, bed rest, heat, and massage. The Quebec Task Force on Spinal Disorders concluded that there is no scientific evidence to support the use of spinal traction in the diagnosis or the treatment of low back pain (16). Acupuncture has received similar scrutiny in the literature (73). There have been at least nine comparative studies using acupuncture to treat discogenic pain syndromes (74). No consensus exists that acupuncture offers any substantial advantage in the treatment of discogenic pain syndromes.

The use of bracing in the treatment of discogenic pain syndrome has been studied in at least three clinical trials. Although compliance in the blinding of the review is difficult to assess, none of the studies showed any benefit of a corset or a brace in the treatment of low back pain (75). Similarly, the Quebec Task Force concluded that there was not sufficient scientific evidence to demonstrate efficacy of a lumbar corset or support (16). Crock believes that in internal disc derangement syndrome, the use of a lumbar brace is contraindicated as it often worsens the patient's pain (22,23).

Chiropractic manipulation has been found to be effective in the treatment of low back pain of short duration (76). Although the exact mechanism by which spinal manipulation relieves back pain is not clear, several comparative studies have found it to be effective (16,77). The data supporting the use of long-term manipulation for chronic back pain are less convincing. Most patients with a diagnosis of internal disc disruption or degenerative disc disease can benefit from a trial of manipulation for a 3- to 4-week period. After this trial period, it should be discontinued if unsuccessful.

Medication to treat discogenic pain syndromes has a long and varied history. Three studies have compared nonsteroidal antiinflammatory medications to placebo in the treatment of acute low back pain (74,78,79). These drugs were found to be efficacious. Muscle-relaxing drugs have also received a similar level of scrutiny and have also been found effective. The use of nonnarcotic antiinflammatory medications and muscle relaxants is indicated for short-term relief of acute discogenic pain. However, the use of narcotic pain medication for the control of chronic discogenic pain is not recommended.

The results of exercise regimens in the treatment of low back disorders vary markedly based on the patient's diagnosis and the exercise ordered (74,80–83). In patients with internal disc derangement, compressive or aerobic exercises that include flexion, extension, and rotational trunk activities are often poorly tolerated. Nonimpact aerobic exercise, such as swimming or warm water hydrotherapy, is well tolerated by these patients. In addition, isometric trunk stabilization strengthening exercises have proven beneficial. They consist of a series of rigorous abdominal and paraspinal isometric exercises that are performed without much trunk mobilization. Patients with discogenic pain syndromes should undergo at least 3 months of nonoperative care that includes the use of nonsteroidal antiinflammatory medications, muscle relaxants, and a supervised physical rehabilitation program before surgery is considered.

SURGICAL TREATMENT

Surgical treatment for axial pain from a disrupted or degenerated disc most commonly involves a spinal fusion. At this time, the choices for spinal fusion are posterolateral fusion with or without instrumentation, posterior lumbar interbody fusion (PLIF), anterior lumbar interbody fusion (ALIF), and combined anterior and posterior fusion. The surgical approach for the arthrodesis should be based on the diagnosis, clinical complaints, and physical findings.

In patients with segmental instability and evidence of nerve-root compression, such as degenerative spondylolisthesis and stenosis, the fusion procedure must be combined with a decompressive procedure (25,84–86). For this reason, most surgical approaches are posterior. However, in patients with discogenic pain syndromes (i.e., IDD and DDD), the success of the fusion procedure depends exclusively on its ability to eliminate the pain focus within the disc. The pain generator can be successfully eliminated through one of two mechanisms—complete disc ablation or elimination of all motion at the affected interspace.

Posterolateral fusion reduces stress and motion across a degenerated and painful spinal motion segment. A successful posterolateral arthrodesis, however, has not always been directly associated with a successful clinical outcome (87). Zucherman et al. reported the results in a series of patients who underwent posterolateral pedicle screw fusions for degenerative disc disease (88). Although they had an 89% successful fusion rate, they found clinical success in only 60% of their patients. The results reported by Jackson and associates were similar (89). Again, although they had a fusion rate of 87%, only 58% of their patients with DDD had pain relief after a posterolateral fusion with pedicle screws. Wetzel and coworkers examined 48 patients who had positive discography and posterolateral lumbar arthrodeses and found that only 46% of their patients had a satisfactory clinical result at final follow-up (90). In 1993, Zdeblick published a prospective randomized study of fusions with and without pedicle screw instrumentation (91). Within this group of patients, there was a subset of patients who had degenerative disc disease. In this group, 93% achieved successful radiographic fusion, but only 64% achieved good or excellent results clinically. Posterolateral fusion alone may benefit those who have sedentary lifestyles, lower activity-related job demands, and the elderly.

The successful treatment of patients with DDD syndromes requires complete immobilization of the spinal motion segment, which often cannot be achieved through a posterolateral fusion (92). In laboratory investigations, a posterolateral fusion has been found to increase the stiffness of a spinal motion segment by 40% (93). It is important to note that an anterior interbody fusion increased the stiffness 80% and eliminated virtually all motion through the disc space. Zdeblick et al. showed in a biomechanical study that the most effective means of eliminating motion within a spinal motion segment is through the disc space rather than through the facets, transverse processes, or spinous processes (94). In a clinical study, Weatherly reported on five patients who had successful posterolateral fusions but continued to have low back pain. These patients had positive discography anterior to the fusion, and their pain was subsequently relieved by an anterior interbody fusion (95).

In clinical studies, an interbody fusion increased the clinical success rate for patients with discogenic pain syndromes (96–99). Lee et al. performed PLIF for internal disc disruption in 62 patients and reported a 94% successful fusion rate and a 96% clinical success rate at relieving back pain (100). Other surgeons, however, have not been as successful with the PLIF procedure (101). Using their PLIF and plate operation, Brantigan and associates found only a 56% fusion success rate and a 60% clinical success rate (102,103).

An unavoidable complication inherent in the posterior approach to spinal disorders is the disruption of the posterior musculature. To perform a posterolateral fusion or a posterior interbody fusion, the posterior paraspinal muscles must be detached from the bony elements. This muscle stripping and retraction during surgery can lead to ischemia, as well as to postoperative fibrosis of this muscle.

The anterior approach to the spine completely avoids injury to the posterior paravertebral muscles, retains all posterior-stabilizing structures and avoids epidural scarring and perineural fibrosis. This approach also allows the surgeon to reestablish the disc space height and regain the normal anatomic alignment and relationships of the spinal motion segments in the lumbar spine. ALIF procedures enable the surgeon to insert bone grafts into the intervertebral space and place them under constant compression, which biomechanically encourages bone formation and fusion (104).

ALIF was recommended by Crock in his original description of internal disc disruption (22). An anterior interbody fusion achieves both objectives: to eliminate the pain source by complete discectomy and to eliminate motion between the adjacent vertebrae. Several clinical studies have reported high rates of success using anterior interbody fusion with bone grafting alone (105–108). Loguidice et al. found using ALIF with autogenous bone graft alone reported an 80% rate of successful fusion and an 80% clinical success rate (109). Blumenthal, in a similar study, found a 73% successful fusion rate and 74% clinical success rate (110). Calhoun and associates reported satisfactory clinical results in 88% of a nonconsecutive group of patients who had fusion for positive discography (111). Newman and Grinstead examined 36 patients with internal disc derangement, all of whom were treated with ALIF (112). They found that 86% of their patients had successful clinical results and solid fusions were obtained in 89%. A commonly reported complication from using bone graft alone to obtain an anterior interbody fusion is subsidence or collapse of the graft during the healing process (113).

In an attempt to prevent graft resorption, collapse, and pseudarthrosis, surgeons have used combined anterior-posterior surgery. Using pedicle screw instrumentation to prevent graft collapse, surgeons have achieved a high degree of success. Kozak and others examined 69 patients treated with concomitant anterior-posterior fusion for discogenic pain (114). After an average 2.5-year follow-up, they noted fusion rates of 91% in one- or two-level fusions. They found acceptable clinical results in 80% of their patients. Their success rate dropped, however, when three-level fusions were done. Linson and Williams followed their patients treated similarly with combined anterior-posterior fusions and noted an overall success rate of 80% (115). O'Brien et al. examined their results for 360-degree combined fusion in 150 patients with 5-year follow-up (116). They noted that 86% of their patients were improved and that 60% were improved from disabling low back pain. Slosar et al. found a 99% fusion rate with combined instrumented 360-degree fusion (117). However, they noted an 18% complication rate primarily related to the anterior approach or spinal hardware, or both. They noted 81% clinical improvement, but overall, only 38% of the surgically treated patients were able to return to work. Using combined 360-degree fusion surgical techniques may ensure increased fusion rates; however, the same disabilities related to posterior exposure of the lumbar spine are also encountered with this technique. The disabilities resulting from posterior surgery remain.

Interbody fusion cages offer the surgeon an alternative approach to fusion for discogenic pain syndromes. Stand-alone ALIF procedures using only autogenous bone grafts have been associated with

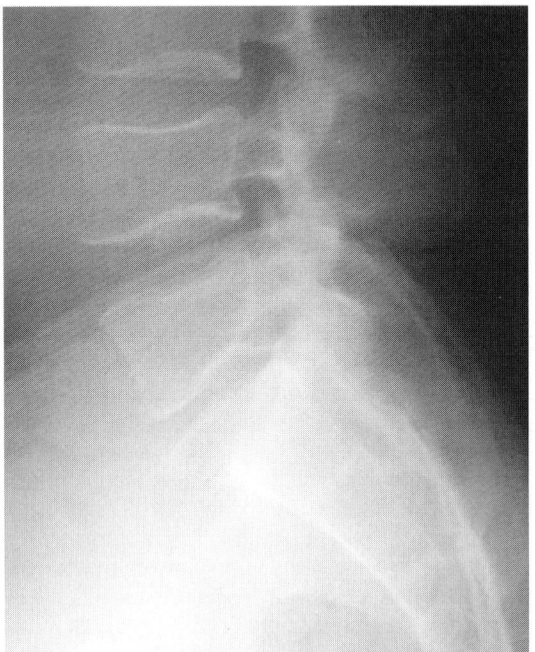

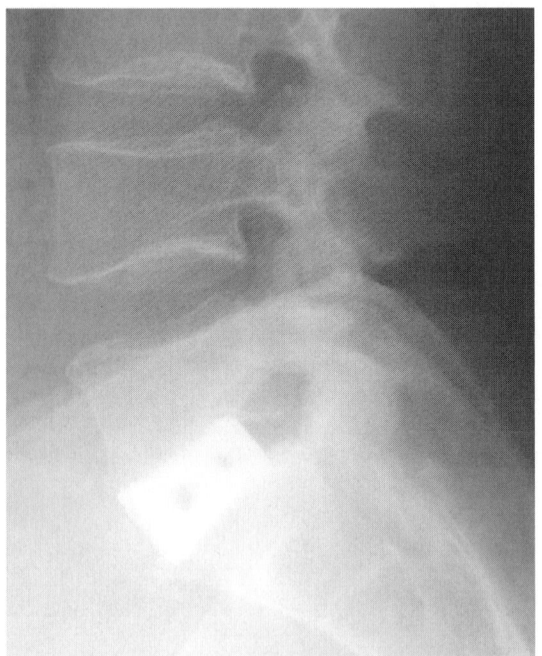

FIG. 5. A: Lateral standing radiograph in a 47-year-old man shows disc space collapse, end-plate sclerosis, and radial osteophyte formation at L-5 to S-1. **B:** A standing lateral radiograph taken 2 years after a stand-alone anterior interbody fusion with an interbody fusion device shows restoration of normal disc space height and segmental lordosis.

high rates of pseudarthrosis, graft subsidence, and graft extrusion (113). Recent advances in metallic interbody fusion devices have been introduced to stabilize intervertebral grafts and have been used to restore segmental lordosis, encourage fusion, and prevent disc space collapse during the healing process (Fig. 5). Their use has led to high rates of fusion and appears to be improving the clinical outcomes (118). However, the risk of retrograde ejaculation in male patients after surgery using anterior lumbosacral spinal exposure has deterred some surgeons from using this approach.

Stand-alone anterior interbody fusion using a tapered fusion device for the treatment of degenerative disc disease was assessed in a large multicenter clinical study (118). In a prospective study, clinical and radiographic outcomes of patients undergoing single-level ALIF were evaluated. Additionally, the outcomes at 24 months using iliac crest autograft were compared with those using recombinant human bone morphogenetic protein-2 (rhBMP-2). rhBMP-2 is an osteoinductive growth factor that stimulates pluripotential cells to form bone. At all postoperative intervals, the mean Oswestry Disability Index scores, back pain and leg pain scores, and neurologic status improved from preoperative scores in both treatment groups and were similar in both groups. At 24 months, the rhBMP-2 group's fusion rate of 94.5% remained higher than that of the autograft group at 88.7%. The group that received rhBMP-2 with the tapered cage device had a higher rate of fusion, reduced operative times, and decreased blood loss than the group who received autogenous bone graft with the tapered cage device. The rhBMP-2 group avoided the complications and morbidity arising from an iliac crest bone harvesting procedure. This group of patients has shown faster clinical improvements and higher rates of success when compared with other interbody devices. Complete outcomes measure evaluation has documented the success of treating back pain from disc degeneration by anterior interbody stand-alone cages.

SUMMARY

Discogenic pain syndromes can be classified as IDD, DDD, or segmental instability. The clinical presentation, diagnostic criteria, and treatment are different for IDD (i.e., dark disc disease, annular tears) and DDD (i.e., isolated disc resorption, lumbar spondylosis). The overriding concern for the treating physician is proper patient selection. The great majority of patients with discogenic pain do not require surgical treatment. Fusion surgery should be reserved only for those patients that are highly motivated, carefully selected, and without psychological magnification of their symptoms. ALIF surgery using stand-alone intervertebral fusion cages has been shown to be a promising method of facilitating intervertebral spinal fusion and in decreasing pain and improving clinical outcomes.

REFERENCES

1. Panagiotacopulos ND, Pope MH, Bloch R, et al. Water content in human intervertebral discs. Part II. Viscoelastic behavior. *Spine* 1987;12:918–924.
2. Lipson SJ, Muir H. Proteoglycans in experimental intervertebral disc degeneration. *Spine* 1981;6:194–210.
3. Wilder DG, Pope MH, Frymoyer JW. The biomechanics of lumbar disc herniation and the effect of overload and instability. *J Spinal Disord* 1988;1(1):16–32.
4. Pech P, Haughton VM. Lumbar intervertebral disc: correlative MR and anatomic study. *Radiology* 1985;156:699–701.
5. Tertti K, Paajanen K, Laato M, et al. Disc degeneration in magnetic resonance imaging: a comparative biochemical, histologic, and radiologic study in cadaver spines. *Spine* 1991;16:629–634.
6. Brown MD. The pathophysiology of disc disease. Symposium on disease of the intervertebral disc. *Orthop Clin North Am* 1971;2:359–370.
7. Park WM, McCall IW, O'Brien JP, et al. Fissuring of the posterior annulus fibrosus in the lumbar spine. *Br J Radiol* 1979;52:382–387.
8. Naylor A. Intervertebral disc prolapse and degeneration: the biomechanical and biophysical approach. *Spine* 1976;1:108–114.
9. Frymoyer JW, Newberg A, Pope MH, et al. Spine radiographs in patients with low back pain. An epidemiological study in men. *J Bone Joint Surg* 1984;66A:1048–1055.
10. Stokes IA, Frymoyer JW. Segmental motion and instability. *Spine* 1987;12:688–691.
11. Knutsson F. The instability associated with disc degeneration in the lumbar spine. *Acta Radiol* 1944;25:593–609.
12. Bradford DS, Oegama TR Jr, Cooper KM, et al. Chymopapain, chemonucleolysis, and nucleus pulposus regeneration: a biochemical and biomechanical study. *Spine* 1984;9:135–147.
13. Panjabi MM, Krag MH, Chung TQ. Effects of disc injury on mechanical behavior of the human spine. *Spine* 1984;9:707–713.
14. Osti OL, Vernon-Roberts B, Fraser RD. Anulus tears and intervertebral disc degeneration. An experimental study using an animal model. *Spine* 1990;15:762–767.
15. Shirazi-Adl SA, Shrivastava SC, Ahmed AM. Stress analysis of the lumbar disc-body unit in compression: a three-dimensional nonlinear finite element study. *Spine* 1984;9:120–134.
16. Quebec Task Force on Spinal Disorders. Scientific approach to the assessment and management of activity-related spinal disorders. A monograph for clinicians. *Spine* 1987;12 [7 Suppl]:S1–S59.
17. Miller JA, Schmatz C, Schultz AB. Lumbar disc degeneration: correlation with age, sex, and spine level in 600 autopsy specimens. *Spine* 1988;13:173–178.
18. Burdorf A. Exposure assessment of risk factors for disorders of the back in occupational epidemiology. *Scan J Work Environ Health* 1992;18:1–9.
19. Frymoyer JW, Selby DK. Segmental instability. Rationale for treatment. *Spine* 1985;10:280–286.
20. Bogduk N, Tynan W, Wilson AS. The nerve supply to the human lumbar intervertebral discs. *J Anat* 1981;132:39–56.
21. Stokes IA, Frymoyer JW. Segmental motion and instability. *Spine* 1987;12:688–691.
22. Crock HV. A reappraisal of intervertebral disc lesions. *Med J Aust* 1970;1:983–989.
23. Crock HV. Internal disc disruption. A challenge to disc prolapse fifty years on. *Spine* 1986;11:650–653.
24. Modic MT, Masaryk TJ, Ross JS. *Magnetic resonance imaging of the spine*. Chicago: Year-Book Medical, 1989:280.
25. Coppes MH, Marani E, Thomeer RT, et al. Innervation of annulus fibrosus in low back pain. *Lancet* 1990;336:189–190.
26. Boden SD, Davis DO, Dina TS, et al. Abnormal magnetic resonance scans of the lumbar spine in asymptomatic subjects. A prospective investigation. *J Bone Joint Surg* 1990;72A:403–408.
27. Mink JH. Imaging evaluation of the candidate for percutaneous lumbar discectomy. *Clin Orthop* 1989;238:83–91.
28. Dupuis PR, Yong-Hing K, Cassidy JD, et al. Radiologic diagnosis of degenerative lumbar instability. *Spine* 1985;10:262–276.
29. Tertti K, Paajanen K, Laato M, et al. Disc degeneration in magnetic resonance imaging: a comparative biochemical, histologic, and radiologic study in cadaver spines. *Spine* 1991;16:629–634.
30. Fischgrund JS, Montgomery DM. Diagnosis and treatment of discogenic low back pain. *Orthop Rev* 1993;22:311–318.
31. Haughton VM. Imaging of the spine. *Radiol* 1988;166:297–301.
32. Kornberg M. Discography and magnetic resonance imaging in the diagnosis of lumbar disc disruption. *Spine* 1989;14:1368–1372.
33. Nachemson A. Lumbar discography—where are we today? *Spine* 1989;14:555–557.
34. Ross JS, Modic MT. Current assessment of spinal degenerative disease with magnetic resonance imaging. *Clin Orthop* 1992;279:68–81.
35. Gibson MJ, Buckley J, Mawhinney R, et al. Magnetic resonance imaging and discography in the diagnosis of disc degeneration. A

comparative study of 50 discs. *J Bone Joint Surg* 1986;68B(3):369–373.
36. Modic MT, Steinberg PM, Ross JS, et al. Degenerative disc disease: assessment of changes in vertebral body marrow with MR imaging. *Radiology* 1988;166:193–199.
37. Powell MC, Szypryt P, Wilson K, et al. Prevalence of lumbar disc degeneration observed by MRI in symptomless women. *Lancet* 1986;2:1366–1367.
38. Evans W, Jobe W, Seibert C. A cross-sectional prevalence study of lumbar disc degeneration in a working population. *Spine* 1989;14:60–64.
39. Zucherman J, Derby F, Hsu K, et al. Normal magnetic resonance imaging with abnormal discography. *Spine* 1988;13(12):1355–1359.
40. Horton WC, Daftari TK. Which disc as visualized by magnetic resonance imaging is actually a source of pain? *Spine* 1992;17[6 Suppl]: S164–S171.
41. Walsh TR, Weinstein JN, Spratt KF, et al. Lumbar discography in normal subjects: a controlled prospective study. *J Bone Joint Surg* 1990;72A:1081–1088.
42. Weinstein J, Claverie W, Gibson S. The pain of discography. *Spine* 1988;13:1344–1348.
43. Gresham JL, Miller R. Evaluation of the lumbar spine by diskography and its use in selection of proper treatment of the herniated disk syndrome. *Clin Orthop* 1969;67:29–41.
44. North American Spine Society. Position statement on discography. *Spine* 1988;13:1343.
45. Aprill CN. Diagnostic disc injection. In: Frymoyer JW, ed. *The adult spine: principles and practice*. New York: Raven Press, 1991;403–442.
46. Panjabi M, Brown M, Lindahl S, et al. Intrinsic disc pressure as a measure of integrity of the lumbar spine. *Spine* 1988;13(8):913–917.
47. Adams MA, Dolan P, Hutton WC. The stages of disc degeneration as revealed by discogram. *J Bone Joint Surg* 1986;68B:36–41.
48. Birney TJ, White JJ Jr, Berens D, et al. Comparison of MRI and discography in the diagnosis of lumbar degenerative disc disease. *J Spinal Disord* 1992;5:417–423.
49. Collis JS Jr, Gardner WJ. Lumbar discography. An analysis of 1000 cases. *J Neurosurg* 1962;19:452–461.
50. Bernard TN. Lumbar discography followed by computed tomography. Refining the diagnosis of low back pain. *Spine* 1990;15:690–707.
51. Torgerson WR, Dotter WE. Comparative roentgenographic study of the asymptomatic and symptomatic lumbar spine. *J Bone Joint Surg* 1976;58A:850–853.
52. Vanharanta H, Guyer RD, Ohnmeiss DD, et al. Disc deterioration in low back syndromes. A prospective multicenter CT/discography study. *Spine* 1988;13:1349–1351.
53. Masatyk TJ, Boumphrey F, Modic MT, et al. Effects of chemonucleolysis demonstrated by MR imaging. *J Comput Assist Tomogr* 1986;10:917–923.
54. Frymoyer JW, Pope MH, Clements JH, et al. Risk factors in low back pain. An epidemiological survey. *J Bone Joint Surg* 1983;65A: 213–218.
55. Hulshof C, van Zanten BV. Whole body vibration and low back pain. A review of epidemiological studies. *Int Arch Occup Environ Health* 1987;59:205–220.
56. Pope MH, Hansson TH. Vibration of the spine and low back pain. *Clin Orthop* 1992;279:49–59.
57. Svensson HO, Andersson GB. Low back pain in 40- to 47-year old men: work history and work environment factors. *Spine* 1983;8: 272–276.
58. Granhed K, Morelli B. Low back pain among retired wrestlers and heavy weight lifters. *Am J Sports Med* 1988;16:530–533.
59. Mundt DJ, Kelsey JL, Golden AL, et al. An epidemiologic study of sports and weight lifting as possible risk factors for herniated lumbar and cervical discs. *Am J Sports Med* 1993;21:854–860.
60. Videman T, Sama S, Battie MC, et al. The long-term effects of physical loading and exercise lifestyles on back-related symptoms, disability, and spinal pathology among men. *Spine* 1995;20:699–709.
61. An HS, Silveri CP, Simpson JM, et al. Comparison of smoking habits between patients with surgically confirmed herniated lumbar and cervical disc disease and controls. *J Spinal Disord* 1994;7:369–373.
62. Battie MC, Videman T, Gibbons LE, et al. 1995 Volvo Award in Clinical Sciences. Determinants of lumbar disc degeneration. *Spine* 1995;20(24):2601–2612.
63. Jaffray D, O'Brien JP. Isolated intervertebral disc resorption. A source of mechanical and inflammatory back pain? *Spine* 1986; 11(4):397–401.
64. Knutsson F. The instability associated with disc degeneration in the lumbar spine. *Acta Radiol* 1944;25:593–609.
65. Aprill CN, Bogduk N. High-intensity zone: a diagnostic sign of painful lumbar disc on magnetic resonance imaging. *Br J Radiology* 1992;65:361–369.
66. Schneiderman G, Flannigan B, Kingston S, et al. Magnetic resonance imaging in the diagnosis of disc degeneration: correlation with discography. *Spine* 1987;12:276–281.
67. Vanharanta K, Sach BL, Ohnmeiss DD, et al. Pain provocation and disc deterioration by age. A CT/discographic study in a low back pain population. *Spine* 1989;14(4):420–423.
68. Simmons EH, Segil CM. An evaluation of discography in the localization of symptomatic levels in discogenic disease of the spine. *Clin Orthop* 1975;108:57–69.
69. Schwarzer AC, Aprill CN, Derby R, et al. The prevalence and clinical features of internal disc disruption in patients with chronic low back pain. *Spine* 1995;20(17):1878–1883.
70. Smith SE, Darden BV, Rhyne AL, et al. Outcome of unoperated discogram-positive low back pain. *Spine* 1995;20(18):1997–2001.
71. Deyo RA, Diehl AK, Rosenthal M. How many days of bed rest for acute low back pain? *N Engl J Med* 1986;315:1064–1070.
72. Mathews M, Mills SB, Jenkins VM, et al. Back pain and sciatica: controlled trials of manipulation, traction, sclerosant and epidural injections. *Br J Rheum* 1987;26:416–423.
73. Coan RM, Wong G, Ku SL, et al. The acupuncture treatment of low back pain: a randomized controlled study. *Am J Chin Med* 1980;8: 181–189.
74. Deyo RA. Conservative therapy for low back pain: distinguishing useful from useless therapy. *JAMA* 1983;250:1057–1062.
75. Million R, Nilsen KK, Jayson MI, et al. Evaluation of low back pain and assessment of lumbar corsets with and without back supports. *Ann Rheum Dis* 1981;40:449–454.
76. Brunarski DJ. Clinical trials of spinal manipulation: a critical appraisal and review of the literature. *J Manipulative Physiol Ther* 1984;7:243–249.
77. Wiesel SW, Cuckler JM, DeLuca F. Acute low back pain: an objective analysis of conservative therapy. *Spine* 1980;5:324–330.
78. Alcoff J, Jones E, Rust P, et al. Controlled trial of imipramine for chronic low back pain. *J Fam Pract* 1982;14:841–846.
79. Berry H, Bloom B, Hamilton EB, et al. Naproxen sodium, diflunisal, and placebo in the treatment of chronic low back pain. *Ann Rheum Dis* 1982;41:129–132.
80. Davies JE, Gibson T, Tester L. The value of exercises in the treatment of low back pain. *Rheumatol Rehabil* 1979;18:243–247.
81. DiMaggio A, Mooney V. The McKenzie program: exercise effective against low back pain. *J Musculoskel Med* 1987;December:63–74.
82. Kendall PH, Jenkins JM. Exercises for backache: a double-blind controlled trial. *Physiotherapy* 1968;54:154–157.
83. Nwuga GO, Nwuga VC. Relative therapeutic efficacy of the Williams and McKenzie protocols in back pain management. *Physiotherapy Practice* 1985;1:99–105.
84. Park WM, McCall IW, O'Brien JP, et al. Fissuring of the posterior annulus fibrosus in the lumbar spine. *Br J Radiol* 1979;52: 382–387.
85. MacNab I. Spondylolisthesis with an intact neural arch—the so-called pseudospondylolisthesis. *J Bone Joint Surg* 1950;32B:325–333.
86. West JL, Bradford DS, Ogilvie JW. Results of spinal arthrodesis with pedicle screw-plate fixation. *J Bone Joint Surg* 1991;73A:1179–1184.
87. Grubb SA, Lipscomb IFU. Results of lumbosacral fusion for degenerative disc disease with and without instrumentation: two to five year follow-up. *Spine* 1992;17(3):349–355.
88. Zucherman J, Hsu K, Picetti G, et al. Clinical efficacy of spinal instrumentation in lumbar degenerative disc disease. *Spine* 1992;17 (7):834–837.
89. Jackson RK, Boston DA, Edge AJ. Lateral mass fusion. A prospective study of a consecutive series with long-term follow-up. *Spine* 1985;10:828–832.

90. Wetzel FT, LaRocca SH, Lowery GL, et al. The treatment of lumbar spinal pain syndromes diagnosed by discography. Lumbar arthrodesis. *Spine* 1994;19(7):792–800.
91. Zdeblick TA. A prospective, randomized study of lumbar fusion: preliminary results. *Spine* 1993;18:983–991.
92. Rolander SD. Motion of the lumbar spine with special reference to stabilizing effect of posterior fusion. *Acta Orthop Scand Suppl* 1966;90:1–144.
93. Lee CK, Langrana NA. Lumbosacral spinal fusion: a biomechanical study. *Spine* 1984;9(6):574–581.
94. Zdeblick TA, Smith GR, Warden KE, et al. Two-point fixation of the lumbar spine. Differential stability in rotation. *Spine* 1991;16[6 Suppl]:S298–S301.
95. Weatherley CR, Prickett CF, O'Brien JP. Discogenic pain persisting despite solid posterior fusion. *J Bone Joint Surg* 1986;68B(1):142–143.
96. Cloward RB. Lesions of the intervertebral discs and their treatment by interbody fusion methods. *Clin Orthop* 1963;27:51–77.
97. Cloward RD. Posterior lumbar interbody fusion updated. *Clin Orthop* 1985;193:16–19.
98. Lin PK, Cautilli RA, Joyce W. Posterior lumbar interbody fusion. *Clin Orthop* 1983;180:165–168.
99. Ma GW. Posterior lumbar interbody fusion with specialized instruments. *Clin Orthop* 1985;195:57–63.
100. Lee CK, Vessa P, Lee JK. Chronic disabling low back pain syndrome caused by internal disc derangements. The results of disc excision and posterior lumbar interbody fusion. *Spine* 1995;20(3):356–361.
101. Gill K, Blumenthal SL. Posterior lumbar interbody fusion: a 2 year follow-up of 238 patients. *Acta Orthop Scand Suppl* 1993;251:108–110.
102. Brantigan JW. Pseudarthrosis rate after allograft posterior lumbar interbody fusion with pedicle screw and plate fixation. *Spine* 1994; 19(11):1271–1280.
103. Brantigan JW, Steffee AD. A carbon fiber implant to aid interbody lumbar fusion. Two-year clinical results in the first 26 patients. *Spine* 1993;18:2106–2107.
104. Bagby G. Arthrodesis by the distraction-compression methods using stainless steel implant. *Orthopedics* 1988;11:931–934.
105. Goldner JL, Urbaniak JR, McCollum DE. Anterior disc excision and interbody spinal fusion for chronic low back pain. *Orthop Clin North Am* 1971;2:544–568.
106. Kozak JA, Heilman AE, O'Brien JP. Anterior lumbar fusion options: technique and graft materials. *Clin Orthop* 1994;300:45–51.
107. Gill K, Blumenthal SL. Functional results after anterior lumbar fusion at L5-S1 in patients with normal and abnormal MRI scans. *Spine* 1992;17(8):940–942.
108. Knox BD, Chapman TM. Anterior lumbar interbody fusion for discogram concordant pain. *J Spinal Disord* 1993;6:242–244.
109. Loguidice VA, Johnson RG, Guyer RD, et al. Anterior lumbar interbody fusion. *Spine* 1988;13:366–369.
110. Blumenthal SL, Baker J, Dossett A, et al. The role of anterior lumbar fusion for internal disc disruption. *Spine* 1988;13:566–569.
111. Colhoun E, McCall IW, Williams L, et al. Provocation discography as a guide to planning operations on the spine. *J Bone Joint Surg* 1988;70B:267–271.
112. Newman MH, Grinstead GL. Anterior lumbar interbody fusion for internal disc disruption. *Spine* 1992;17(7):831–833.
113. Dennis S, Watkins R, Landaker S, et al. Comparison of disc space heights after anterior lumbar interbody fusion. *Spine* 1989;18(8): 876–878.
114. Kozak JA, O'Brien JP. Simultaneous combined anterior and posterior fusion: an independent analysis of a treatment for the disabled low back pain patient. *Spine* 1990;15(4):322–328.
115. Linson MA, Williams H. Anterior and combined anteroposterior fusion for lumbar disc pain: a preliminary study. *Spine* 1991;16: 143–145.
116. O'Brien JP, Dawson MH, Heard CW, et al. Simultaneous combined anterior and posterior fusion: a surgical solution for failed spinal surgery with a brief review of the first 150 patients. *Clin Orthop* 1986;203:191–195.
117. Slosar PJ, Reynolds JB, Schofferman J, et al. Patient satisfaction after circumferential lumbar fusion. *Spine* 2000;25:722–726.
118. Burkus JK, Gornet MF, Dickman CA, et al. Anterior lumbar interbody fusion using rhBMP-2 with tapered interbody cages. *J Spinal Disord Tech (in press).*

CHAPTER 46

Lumbar Disc Disease

B. Lumbar Disc Herniation and Radiculopathy

Mark Weidenbaum

INTERVERTEBRAL DISC STRUCTURE

Each lumbar spinal motion segment includes an intervertebral disc as well as two facet joints that create a three-joint complex augmented by extensive soft-tissue connections. The disc consists of three major substructures: annulus fibrosus (annulus), nucleus pulposus (nucleus), and cartilage end-plates (end-plate). The composition and structure of each component is quite distinct, suggesting unique mechanical roles. Because these structures are coupled, they share load distribution while facilitating motion. Therefore, injury or degeneration affecting any of these structures alters the mechanics and function for the others.

The structure of the intervertebral disc allows it to perform several vital functions, including providing a bond that allows restricted intervertebral motion; contribution to stability; resistance to axial, rotational, and bending loads; and preservation of anatomic relationships. The concentric, multilayered lamellae of the annulus fibrosus form the tough outer portion of the intervertebral disc and have many unique functions. These collagen fibers attach to the remnants of the vertebral ring apophysis along the periphery of the vertebral body and are arranged such that when torsion occurs, some fibers become lax while others become taut. They are extremely strong and are primarily responsible for the "bond" and for setting limitations on motion (i.e., maintaining stability). This function is not limited only to the disc but is shared with the facet joints, ligaments, and other soft-tissue stabilizers.

The disc is anatomically and physiologically unique, being largely avascular and populated by a relatively meager number of cells in an extensive extracellular matrix. Disc nutrition is very limited. It depends on passive diffusion mechanisms resulting in a low oxygen tension at the center of the disc and limited ability for tissue repair. The cartilaginous end-plate is a thin layer of hyaline cartilage that surrounds the cranial and caudal surfaces of the central region of the disc. The orientation of collagen fibers and chondrocytes in the end-plate varies considerably depending on the depth within the cartilage layer (1,2). Although some transudation may occur from adjacent osseous vasculature across the end-plate, there is essentially no vascular supply after the second decade, as the small traversing blood vessels existing in childhood are no longer present in adults. Consequently, there is minimal communication between the cancellous trabecular network within the vertebral body and the contents of the disc itself (3). The minimal cell population within the disc depends almost entirely on diffusion for nutrition. Hence, the annulus and nucleus must provide millions of cycles of load support in varying magnitudes and direction with minimal nutrition. The resiliency of these tissues is remarkable considering the tremendous mechanical loads and repetitive stresses applied across this weightbearing and mobile region.

The nucleus pulposus (nucleus) is anatomically confined within the annulus and has several crucial functions that relate to its structure and composition. The nucleus consists of proteoglycan macromolecules trapped in a complex array of collagen. The proteoglycans have a net negative charge, which makes them hydrophilic. The combination of proteoglycans and collagen is constrained within the limits of the annulus, which allows some variability with regard to shape and size, but ultimately is bounded by the annulus. The end-plates along the superior and inferior surface of each vertebra form the "roof" and "floor" of the disc. Thus, the hydrated disc contains incompressible fluid drawn in by charged proteoglycans that are themselves trapped along with the collagen network by the surrounding annulus and end-plate (4). This phenomenon accounts in part for the hydraulic qualities of the disc in maintaining height and resisting axial load.

Nondegenerate discs have a gelatinous and shiny nucleus that is easily delineated from the surrounding annulus. The annulus has discrete fibrous lamellae that are layered composites with adjacent layers varying at approximately ±30 degrees to the horizontal axis. This organization optimizes the ability of the peripherally supporting annulus to resist torsion, axial, and tensile loads. Load distribution is optimized when there is minimal coronal deformity but lumbar lordosis is preserved. When disc height is maintained, the affected soft tissues (i.e., ligaments, capsules) are maintained at their optimal length so that they can function appropriately. When disc height is lost, these structures may become slack, allowing abnormal motion and loss of load support. Localized irregularities in the lamellae may lead to dehydration and loss of pressurization, leading to loss of disc height. As this occurs, the angle of inclination of collagen fibers declines, and with it, the ability of the annulus to resist tensile forces (5). In addition, with loss of height comes narrowing of the intervertebral foramen with possible compression of the traversing nerve root within the foramen, particularly if there is any preexisting decrease in foramen size as seen in patients with spinal stenosis. Facet subluxation and hypertrophy may cause nerve root compression as well. Furthermore, loss of effective soft-tissue stabilization resulting from loss of disc height may lead to progression of preexisting spinal deformity.

The biochemical composition of the disc includes water (65 to 90% wet weight), collagen (15 to 65% dry weight), proteoglycan (10 to 60% dry weight), and other matrix proteins (15 to 45% dry weight) (6,7). Glycosaminoglycans identified in the disc include chondroitin-6 sulfate, chondroitin-4 sulfate, keratan sulfate, biglycan, decorin, versican, and hyaluronan (6–8). In addition, a highly heterogenous population of aggregating and nonaggregating proteoglycans exists within the disc. The collagen composition of the end-plate is almost exclusively type II and is similar in concentration and organization to that of articular cartilage (2,9). Differences in disc composition and structure distinguish its regions. Significant variation in composition from outer to inner regions has been reported, with water and proteoglycan content greatest in the nucleus and inner annulus, whereas collagen content is greatest in the outer annulus. The outer annulus is predominantly type I collagen, whereas the inner annulus is mostly type II, with a decreasing ratio of type I to type II from outer to inner annulus.

These findings are consistent with behavioral properties of different disc components. The disc functions as a hydraulic unit that accepts axial load. Hydration is supported by the high net negative charge of the proteoglycans in the nucleus. Maintaining disc height preserves anatomic relationships within the foramina, and keeps the annulus/ligaments out to length and foramen wide open. The end-plates control nutrition as well as fluid flow in and out, thereby helping to maintain pressurization (9).

In general, as discs degenerate, the nucleus changes to a more consolidated fibrous structure and is less clearly demarcated from the annulus. Degeneration and age-related changes in the biochemical composition and structure of each disc component have been widely reported (1,6,10,11). Changes in disc substructures with degeneration have also been noted as changes in geometry or signal intensity in magnetic resonance images (12,13). Mucinous material is deposited between the lamellae of the annulus, and focal defects become apparent in the end-plate. The severely degenerated disc is characterized by a loss of disc material and prevalent fissures and disruptions throughout the nucleus and annulus. With increasing degeneration, hydration decreases for the nucleus and annulus, accompanied by a decrease in proteoglycan content and significant alterations in proteoglycan structure. Although collagen content in the disc appears to remain relatively constant with degeneration, alterations in the distribution of collagen types I and II has been reported and low disc proteoglycan concentrations precede degeneration (6,7,14,15). With breakdown of the proteoglycans/collagen network, the ability of the disc to retain water diminishes, and with dehydration comes loss of height, annular laxity, and inefficiency in load transfer. This inefficiency leads to site-specific load variation, wherein the natural isotropic load distribution is lost, resulting in focal areas of greater stress and degeneration (16,17).

DISC BIOMECHANICS

Disc loads are higher in the sitting than the standing patient, as the lordotic posture in the standing subject allows axial load transfer to the facets so that the disc experiences a lower axial load (18). Added stresses due to torsion, prolonged sitting, and vibration may contribute (19). Although there are wide variations between studies because of different loading conditions, the overall results of biomechanical studies give evidence that torque and rotation applied to nondegenerate disc cause deformation of the annulus, whereas compressive forces are more related to deformation of the vertebral body, end-plates, and disc bulging. Motion segments involving aged or degenerated discs demonstrate increased deformability, decreased nucleus pressure, reduced magnitudes of stiffness and fatigue strength, altered failure properties, and changes in the viscoelastic effects of the motion segments compared to nondegenerate discs. These studies indicate disc degeneration may be involved in altered mechanics for the various motion segments and spine.

The nondegenerate nucleus appears to function predominantly as a biologic fluid under static loading conditions, generating large hydrostatic pressures in the disc. The disc is a hydraulic unit that accepts loads in compression (particularly flexion), while some of the load is distributed to the facets in extension. The end-plates help to maintain pressurization by controlling fluid flow in and out. The relatively high hydraulic permeability of the end-plate serves to transfer loads in a uniform manner across the annulus and nucleus. In addition, the swelling pressure mechanisms arising from a high concentration of negatively charged proteoglycans in this structure serve to maintain disc height and additionally contribute to the pressurization mechanism of load support and transfer.

The outer annulus, the region with the highest tensile modulus, is ideally suited for minimizing disc bulging generated during compression, bending, or torsional loading of the motion segment. Experimental surface measurements of the outer annulus indicate that the extension of the fibers and circumferential strains is relatively small (<5%), suggesting that the high tensile modulus of the outer annulus limits its deformation (20). In contrast, the lower modulus of the inner annulus permits larger deformation in response to applied loading rather than restricting deformation as occurs in the outer annulus. These greater deformations at the inner annulus give rise to viscoelastic dissipation through a flow-dependent mechanism likely to be the dominant mechanism for energy dissipation and "shock absorption" in the entire disc (21).

With age there is a decrease in the proteoglycan content of the nucleus pulposus, leading to loss of hydration. The nucleus loses its ability to absorb stress and increases the demands placed on the annulus fibrosus and other supporting structures. Repetitive axial and torsional stresses applied to the disc lead to tears of the annulus and subsequent herniation of the nucleus pulposus (22).

Thus, changes in the material behaviors of the substructures of the disc with aging or degeneration may predispose the disc to failure in the absence of any change in the type, frequency, or magnitude of loading. Kirkaldy-Willis suggested that the first of three "stages of clinical evolution" of disc degeneration included subtle alterations in the biochemistry and biomechanics of the motion segment, which predispose the entire motion segment to further degeneration (23). It appears that torsion is the most common mode of failure, leading to weakness and annulus tear/end-plate avulsion, whereas compression is less important. It is generally accepted that abnormal magnitudes or frequencies of externally applied loads relate to clinical failure of the disc *in vivo*. In this manner, these studies suggest another pathway in the etiology of disc degeneration or failure.

The alternative hypothesis suggested that the loss of hydrostatic pressurization in the nucleus and end-plate with degeneration has a deleterious effect on the entire disc. The loss of a uniform load transfer mechanism and an isotropic load support mechanism in the nucleus and end-plate is associated with increasing frequency of nonuniform stresses in the annulus with degeneration. This may result in the development of focal stress concentrations and resulting material failures.

PATHOPHYSIOLOGY

The characteristic pain that defines radiculopathy has long been thought to arise from nerve root compression (24,25). However, the natural history of the pain associated with radiculopathy is that resolution may occur despite continued nerve root compression. This finding raises the difficult question of how pain is generated. The herniated disc, particularly the nucleus pulposus, is not simply an inert structure that produces mechanical nerve root deformation but is a biologically active tissue that may induce pathologic processes. Inflammatory, biochemical, vascular, and compressive events probably all are contributory.

Inflammation clearly plays a central role in radiculopathy. In landmark studies, Olmarker showed epidural application of autologous nucleus pulposus without any pressure not only induced impairment in nerve function, but also caused axonal injury with significant primary cell damage (26,27). The mere epidural exposure of the root to nucleus pulposus induced histologic and functional changes of the exposed nerve roots. Because the nucleus is totally avascular, when it becomes exposed as a result of annulus disruption, it is perceived as an antigen, and an intense inflammatory response is induced. This takes place immediately adjacent to the nerve root, which is involved in the response as well. Application of annulus fibrosus did not induce reduction of nerve conduction velocity, but application of nucleus pulposus cells did. Because membranes of the nucleus pulposus cells had similar effects, it can be assumed that the effects are related to membrane-bound substances or structures (28). In a related study, brown deposits indicating antigen-antibody complexes were found in pericellular capsules of cells in herniated discs but not in control discs (29). These findings support the role of inflammatory mediation in disc herniation. Furthermore, evidence suggests that different types of disc herniation have different inflammatory properties (30). It has been noted that annular tears or nucleus herniations are initially associated with significant inflammation, accompanied by increased phospholipase A_2 levels and increased production of cytokines. These inflammatory markers may correlate with the clinical finding that rest, nonsteroidal antiinflammatory agents (NSAIDs), and epidural steroids often alleviate sciatica (31).

It is interesting that *in vitro* and postmortem degenerated nucleus pulposus induces a reduction of nerve conduction velocity similar to that of normal nucleus pulposus, whereas annulus does not induce any reduction in nerve conduction velocity (32). Because freezing of the nucleus pulposus probably kills the cells but does not affect other components, one may assume that the biologic effects induced by the nucleus pulposus may be related to its cell population (33). Furthermore, nucleus pulposus–induced nerve root injury reverses in 2 months and may be present without simultaneous nerve root compression. Previously described nucleus pulposus–induced nerve root changes may therefore be of clinical importance. Experimental study of these mechanisms is probably relevant for an expanded understanding of the pathophysiologic mechanism behind sciatica that is caused by disc herniation (34).

Patients with disc herniation and sciatica have increased concentrations of neurofilament protein and S-100 in their cerebrospinal fluid, indicating axonal and Schwann's cell damage in the affected nerve root (35,36). A specific substance, monoclonal antibody for tumor necrosis factor, has been linked to the nucleus pulposus–induced change in nerve root conduction velocity (37). The effects of this substance may be synergistic with those of other similar substances; the data of the current study may be of significant importance for the continued understanding of nucleus pulposus' biologic activity, and of possible potential use for future strategies in managing sciatica (38). It is interesting that early treatment with lidocaine may reduce nucleus pulposus–induced nerve root injury (39). Although nucleus pulposus in some way irritates or sensitizes nerve roots to produce ectopic discharges that may well be equivalent to radicular sciatic pain, the mechanisms mediating these biologic effects remain unproven.

Nucleus pulposus cells are capable of cytokine production, giving rise to the possibility that "inflammatory effects" may be induced directly by cytokines such as interleukin (IL)-6, IL-1, and tumor necrosis factor, from within nucleus pulposus cells. Accordingly, macrophage accumulation may result from the leukotactic properties of these cytokines, with unclear pathophysiologic significance (40). Because various cytokines have been identified as being involved in these events, speculation exists that there may be possible therapeutic opportunities to reduce the sciatic symptoms by pharmacologic inhibition of such cytokines (41).

It is known that pain severity in herniated discs is worse the closer the disc is to the dorsal root ganglion, suggesting the dorsal root ganglion may be a crucial mediator of pain and an important processor in "chemical radiculitis." Glutamate originating from degenerated disc proteoglycan may diffuse to the dorsal root ganglion and effect glutamate receptors (42). Neuron stimulation by noncompressing nucleus suggests that pathogenic factors in the nucleus pulposus may have a crucial role in the induction of hyperalgesia. This may help to elucidate the reason why severe pain is sometimes induced without a visually identified protrusion (43).

Furthermore, because pure mechanical compression alone is not sufficient to cause lumbar radiculopathy, the pathophysiology of lumbar radiculopathy most likely involves a biochemical process. Cells within a herniated lumbar disc are very active, making increased amounts of matrix metalloproteinases, nitric oxide, prostaglandin E_2, and IL-6. These products may be involved in the pathophysiology of radiculopathy, and their mere presence implicates biochemical processes in intervertebral disc degeneration (44,45). The biochemistry of acute inflammation is extremely complex. It is possible that cytokines and prostaglandins produced during the degenerative cycle of the disc before herniation may be involved in degradation of the intervertebral disc matrix. Such a mechanism has been shown for articular cartilage wherein IL-1, tumor necrosis factor, prostaglandin E_2, and IL-6 are involved in the possible regulatory mechanisms of proteoglycan synthesis (46). Intervertebral disc cells are biologically responsive and increase their production of matrix metalloproteinases, nitric oxide, IL-6, and prostaglandin E_2 when stimulated by IL-1. Endogenously produced nitric oxide appears to have a strong inhibitory effect on the production of IL-6, which suggests that autocrine mechanisms play an important role in the regulation of disc cell metabolism (47). Chemical mediators such as phospholipase A_2 and nitric oxide, induced by extruded or sequestrated intervertebral discs, are apparently involved in the mechanisms of painful radiculopathy in lumbar disc herniations (48).

In addition to the biochemical and inflammatory effects noted previously, mechanical nerve root compression may cause local damage and intraneural ischemia. Cornefjord found decreased nerve conduction velocity in compressed compared with noncompressed spinal nerve roots after 1 to 4 weeks, with induced nerve fiber damage, reduction in number of myelinated fibers, endoneurial hyperemia, bleeding, and inflammation at the compression zone (49). Chronically compressed nerve roots acquire a tolerance to acute compression, indicating a possible adaptation process in the compressed nerve tissue (50). Chronic double-level compression did not induce more changes than single-level compression, although recovery was less complete with double-level compression. This less-complete recovery may be a result of nerve root adaptation to the applied pressure (51). Of note, intramuscular administration of antiinflammatory agents reduced spinal nerve root dysfunction induced by compression in an experimental pig model (52).

Experimental data also indicate that mechanical compression is necessary for induction of pain involving nerve roots preconditioned by the nucleus pulposus, but that such effects can involve adjacent or even contralateral nerve roots. Such findings may explain why symptoms may be present from multiple levels even when radiologic evidence of herniation is limited to only one level (40).

Finally, vascular pathophysiologic mechanisms have been suggested as well. Experimental data suggest that nerve root injury adjacent to areas of nucleus pulposus leakage through annular tears might have a vascular pathophysiologic mechanism (53). These findings may underlie symptomatic sciatica without radiographic or surgical evidence of disc herniation. Application of nucleus pulposus to nerve root increased endoneurial fluid pressure and decreased blood flow in the dorsal root ganglia, prompting the suggestion that exposure to nucleus pulposus may establish a "compartment syndrome" in the dorsal root ganglia (54).

Clearly, numerous mechanisms are involved and their respective relationships are evolving.

CLINICAL ANATOMY

The semantics of disc herniation may be confusing and are generally defined by the relative location of displaced disc material with reference to the annulus and posterior longitudinal ligament (PLL). In the healthy disc, the end-plates and annulus constrain the nucleus pulposus and form a "retaining wall" that preserves the internal pressure within the disc. When there is disc injury or degeneration leading to radiculopathy, the events culminating in annular disruption can occur slowly over many years, earlier with fissuring and degeneration, or they may come on suddenly as with a traumatic event. Whether initiated by injury to the nucleus, annulus, or end-plate, the final common pathway is most often an annular defect, often starting at the inner annulus (21). Once the annulus has been damaged, disc biomechanics change drastically.

When the inner aspect of the annulus begins to fissure and allows intrusion of nucleus, disc bulging or protrusion may result. Although the outside annular remains intact (i.e., no disc material has escaped), the disc can bulge or protrude beyond its normal size limit, thereby possibly causing mechanical pressure on an adjacent nerve root (55). The most common location of herniation is posterolateral, possibly as a result of the combined forces of load, site-specific degeneration, and motion. Because no disc material has escaped from within the disc, this is also referred to as a *contained herniation*. Once fissuring and tears have extended through to the periphery of the annulus fibrosus, the annulus loses much of its "retaining wall" features. Depending on loading patterns, local anatomy, and defect location, the displacing disc material follows the "path of least resistance" wherein fragments of nucleus, annulus, and/or end-plate can displace into the outer one-third of the annulus. Such herniations are termed *noncontained* (56), as displaced nucleus has pushed through and exited from the annulus. The central position of the PLL tends to direct fragments laterally, where there is less resistance. Disc may remain trapped under the PLL (i.e., subligamentous) or less commonly may come through the PLL (i.e., transligamentous) into the canal. As long as the displaced disc material remains contiguous with the remaining nuclear material within the disc, this protruding material is referred to as *extruded*. When such fragments "pinch off" and become totally detached from their points of origin such that they are free within the canal they are *sequestered*. Once outside the annulus and PLL, disc material can migrate proximally, distally, medially, or laterally.

Anatomically the disc is closer to the more distal pedicle and nerve root at the affected level. The dorsal root ganglion lies within the foramen, just below the pedicle. Because the more cephalad nerve root exits the canal immediately below the proximal pedicle, posterolateral herniations usually affect caudal nerve roots. Proximal roots may be affected by displaced extruded or sequestered fragments, or where herniation occurs laterally. Displaced fragments that migrate cephalad and medial may lead to axillary fragments.

Lumbar disc herniations occur most commonly at L4-5 and L-5 to S-1. These two levels account for over 90% of cases, with a nearly even split between the two (57). Reasons for these levels being most commonly affected relate to their anatomy and physiology. Although L-5 to S-1 is the most caudal and therefore carries the greatest axial load, the L-5 to S-1 disc is somewhat protected from torsion by the stabilizing iliolumbar ligaments that attach to L-5. In addition, L-5 is also partially shielded from torsion due to its depth within the pelvis. Because iliolumbar ligaments do not stabilize L-4, there is a natural stress riser resulting from lordotic shear at L4-5. Therefore, L4-5 is more affected by torsion, and L-5 to S-1 by compression.

HISTORY

Symptoms of disc herniation may present acutely after a traumatic insult or may develop gradually without an inciting event, especially in the middle-aged or older patient. Lumbar disc herniation is most common in the third and fourth decades but may occur at any age, including adolescence. The chief complaint is usually pain, often described as radiating from the back or buttock into the leg, sometimes accompanied by numbness and weakness involving the lower extremity. It is important to obtain the exact distribution of the patient's symptoms. Complaints of bilateral leg pain or bowel and bladder symptoms should alert the clinician to the possibility of cauda equina compression syndrome. Pain is exacerbated with coughing or Valsalva maneuver because this increases intrathecal pressure and may increase contact between the irritated nerve root and its surrounding structures. Symptoms are often exacerbated in the sitting position, particularly with driving, because this position reduces lumbar lordosis. As the spine comes out of lordosis, load across the motion segment shifts from the facets posteriorly to the disc anteriorly, thereby increasing intradiscal pressure and pain.

It is fundamentally important to separate back pain from leg pain. Pain radiating to the leg, particularly below the knee, suggests irritation of the large ventral portion of the root exiting from the canal via the foramen and continuing distally into the leg. The term "sciatica" is often used to refer loosely to pain radiating down the leg for whatever reason, although it specifically refers to nerve root compression (most commonly L-5 or S-1) by a herniated nucleus pulposus. Pain radiating down the leg as a result of nerve root irritation is referred to as *radiculopathy*. Determining the dermatomal distribution of these symptoms within the leg is essential in identifying the specific nerve root involved. Patients with radicular pain often describe their pain as sharp and lancinating, usually starting in the buttock or "hip" and shooting/radiating down the leg posteriorly below the knee. Onset of leg pain may be insidious or sudden.

Back pain may result from irritation of the posterior primary ramus, the small branch coming posteriorly off the nerve root immediately after its exit from the foramen. This branch supplies the facet capsules and some of the local musculature. Ninety percent of patients eventually developing radicular symptoms have long-standing prior episodic low back pain (58). Such pain may arise from changes in disc loading and shape as biomechanics change with loss of viscoelasticity from degeneration. Pain may also be mediated by the sinuvertebral branch supplying the posterior annulus, which may be stimulated by events ongoing in the disc.

The quality of pain and any associated symptoms are also very important components. Is the pain a dull ache, or is it a sharp, stabbing pain? Is there "electricity, tingling, or numbness" shooting down the leg? Is there any associated weakness? Does anything make the pain better or worse? Ask patients to describe the condition in their own words. Does forward flexion exacerbate the pain while hyperextension relieves it? Some patients prefer to stand because they are more comfortable than when sitting. Whenever the patient prefers to stand in the examination room, consider disc disease at the top the list.

Sometimes patients state that their back pain abated when their leg pain developed. This finding may be due to relief of annular tensile stress as the displacing fragment finally exits the confining wall of annulus and exerts its effects on the nearby nerve root. Acute disc extrusions can also lead to isolated leg pain without any concomitant back pain. This pain can be so intense that the patient may lie in only one position for hours.

In evaluating patients with leg pain (particularly those older than 50 years of age), it is important to keep other diagnoses in mind. Vascular claudication is an important cause of leg pain and must be differentiated from neurogenic resulting from spinal stenosis. If there is any doubt regarding the diagnosis, vascular assessment and flow studies are indicated. Leg pain, dysesthesias, and paresthesias from stenosis are often not dermatomal, and result from mechanical compromise of the spinal canal and neural foramina. The combination of lordosis and axial load resulting from walking brings on the symptoms. Unlike the patient with a herniated disc, these patients typically become symptomatic while walking and gain relief by sitting. Maneuvers that reduce lordosis (e.g., walking while leaning on a shopping cart) increase central and foraminal canal dimensions and relieve symptoms. Calf pain must also be differentiated from thrombophlebitis. Metabolic or peripheral neuropathies (e.g., diabetes) manifesting with pain as well as motor and/or sensory loss must be kept in mind.

PHYSICAL EXAMINATION

Physical examination of the spine should begin with having the patient fully disrobe down to his or her underwear. Posterior inspection is then done with the patient standing in the upright position, if possible. Initially, one should also look for old scars, muscle spasm, or even unsuspected findings, such as cutaneous stigmata (e.g., café-au-lait spots, hairy patches). Spine alignment should be evaluated, particularly loss of lordosis owing to muscle spasm.

With acute sciatic pain, the patients instinctively lean or hold themselves in the position that minimizes root stretch or irritation. It is important to distinguish between lumbosacral list and lumbosacral scoliosis (58). Finneson hypothesized that disc location could be predicted from physical examination in that fragments lateral to the root resulted in deviation in the direction away from the fragment (59). Axillary herniations medial to the root may result in listing toward the side of the lesion. "Sciatic scoliosis" results from listing or leaning to one side to minimize root irritation. However, neither Porter nor Lorio confirmed that laterality of list indicated any relationship of the disc herniation to the nerve root (58,60). Suk also found no correlation with location of root compression other than it was related to the side of disc herniation (61).

After inspection, the spine should be palpated in a systematic fashion to identify areas of tenderness. It is often helpful to begin palpating in a pain-free area. Touching the patient without causing pain helps the patient gain confidence, reduces anxiety, and allows more accurate definition of areas of tenderness. Paraspinal tenderness and rigidity indicate spasm with loss of range of motion. Focused palpation is directed at specific regions including lumbar spine, sciatic notches, iliac crests, sacroiliac joints, and greater trochanters. Conditions affecting these areas may present with complaints of "back pain" that is not really coming from the back. Because injury to these areas can also result in limited radiation of pain to the leg, it is particularly important to physically localize them.

Increased sensitivity on palpation of the sciatic notch is suggestive of discogenic radiculopathy, but it may rarely also be due to local or nerve tumors. Midline tenderness is common but nonspecific and is usually accompanied by paraspinal spasm. Lumbar percussion may elicit local back pain or reproduce sciatica. Such findings are not diagnostic, as they may be caused by tumor, infection, pathologic fracture, or nonorganic disorders.

Physical examination should also include palpation of the costovertebral angles and the abdomen. Kidney pathology, stones, and retroperitoneal and intraabdominal abnormalities should be kept in mind, particularly when examining older patients. Pain in the area of the coccyx (i.e., coccydynia) is characterized by exquisite local tenderness. This pain may be better appreciated by palpating the anterior and posterior aspects of the coccyx during a rectal examination.

Patients should be asked to walk on their toes and heels to provide information as to the general strength of the lower extremities. Having the patients walk, preferably without knowing they are being observed, may reveal a spinal radiculopathy with associated leg pain and weakness or Trendelenburg signs. Gait may be very abnormal, as the painful leg is usually maintained flexed, often with the foot held in equinus in a reflexive effort to minimize root stretch and keep it relaxed. Antalgic gait is common as well, with hesitation to weight bear on the affected side.

For similar reasons, flexion in the lower spine leads to the reversal of lumbar lordosis and rotation of the pelvis. Commonly with lower spine injuries, muscle spasm prevents motion in the lumbar spine, and thus flexion is performed solely through rotation of the pelvis while maintaining lumbar lordosis. Limitation of forward flexion may also result from hamstring tightness. Evaluation of extension should be performed in the standing position. Limitation in spinal motion and loss of lumbar lordosis generally accompany disc herniation, as a result of local muscle spasm.

Extension places stress on the posterior elements, including the pars interarticularis and facet joints, and decreases the opening of the intervertebral foramen. This motion may exacerbate symptoms secondary to abnormality in these regions. Rotation and lateral bending can be best evaluated with the patient sitting on a chair securing the pelvis and lower extremities. Rotation and lateral bending should be symmetric. Lateral bending may compress the intervertebral foramen on the ipsilateral side, aggravating impingement of the spinal nerve in patients with radicular symptoms.

The examiner can easily separate out hip pathology even in the presence of radiculopathy (e.g., groin pain caused by flexing and rotating the hip, maneuvers that do not produce root tension). The Patrick's [FABER (*f*lexion, *ab*duction, *e*xternal *r*otation)] test is used to detect hip or sacroiliac abnormality. The patient lies supine on the examining table with the foot of the involved side placed on the opposite knee, which positions the hip in flexion, abduction, and external rotation. Downward force applied to the knee with the pelvis secure produces pressure on the sacroiliac joint. Pain radiating to the groin is suggestive of hip abnormality.

Evaluation of vascular status should include posterior tibialis and dorsalis pulses, as well as skin temperature and atrophic changes. When there is an index of suspicion, abdominal, rectal, and pelvic examinations may be indicated as well.

NEUROLOGIC EXAMINATION

Neurologic examination routinely focuses on motor, sensory, and reflex evaluation of the lumbar region (Table 1). Attention to individual dermatomes suggests common expected patterns defined by segmental innervation patterns (62). Of note, manual

TABLE 1. *Neurology of the lower extremity*

Root	Sensory	Motor	Reflex
L-1	Groin		—
L-2	Anterior thigh	Iliopsoas	—
L-3	Lateral thigh/knee	Quadriceps	—
L-4	Medial leg (posterolateral thigh, across patella, anteromedial leg)	Anterior tibialis, quadriceps	Patella
L-5	First dorsal web space; medial foot (posterior thigh, anterolateral leg, medial foot, and great toe)	Extensor hallucis longus; extensor digitorum longus and brevis, gluteus medius	None (posttibialis)
S-1	Lateral foot (posterior thigh and leg, posterolateral foot, lateral toes)	Gastrocnemius; peroneus longus and brevis, gluteus maximus	Achilles

From Hoppenfeld S. *Physical examination of the spine and extremities.* Norwalk, CT: Appleton-Century-Crofts, 1976, with permission.

strength testing by the examiner may fail to reveal relative leg weakness because an examiner's hands and arms may not be strong enough to overcome these muscle groups, even when they are partially weakened. Therefore, when possible, heel-toe walking and squatting and rising from full squat are important motor tests.

A careful neurologic examination may not always localize the compressed nerve root. Because the L4-5 and L-5 to S-1 levels affect nearly 90% of patients, these are the focus for most back examinations. Although involvement of more proximal levels is rare, familiarity with their examination is essential as well.

Barring other factors, classic posterolateral disc pathology affects the more distal root at a given level. Therefore, an L-5 to S-1 disc herniation would affect S-1, L4-5 would affect L-5, and so forth. When herniation is central or far lateral, however, or if there is associated foraminal stenosis or multilevel pathology, findings may be different. Multiple roots may be affected by central herniations. The more proximal root is affected in far lateral pathology as the root is compressed within the foramen. Accordingly, physical examination must be correlated with imaging studies to be sure that the picture fits anatomically.

Prolonged nerve root compression results in weakness and, later, muscular atrophy. A patient's awareness of motor deficit depends on several factors including which group of muscles is supplied by the same nerve, and the functions served. It is interesting that the patient may be unaware of weakness until there is profound loss.

Although distribution of sensory involvement with nerve root compression may be dermatomal, some patterns of sensory change may not necessarily correlate and may be nonspecific, because many things can impact this (e.g., number of levels involved, other conditions, anatomic variability, etc.).

Deep tendon reflexes are frequently affected by nerve root compression. Reflex absence must be asymmetric to be significant. It is essential to make every effort to relax the patient to have an accurate examination. In the seated patient, this can be improved by having him or her sit further back on the table so the entire thigh is supported up to the knee. Facilitation may enhance examination. It is best to revisit each reflex site several times to evaluate overall responses. The examiner must remember that symmetric reflex loss occurs commonly with advanced age without any underlying spine pathology.

Occasionally, isolated lower-extremity weakness may occur without other signs or symptoms. Painless paresis (i.e., painless foot drop) should raise suspicion of neuropathy or cord lesion, in addition to possible disc herniation.

If there is concern of cauda equina compression syndrome, evaluation of sacral innervation is imperative. This evaluation should include sensory testing around the anus and rectal tone evaluation.

Root Tension Signs

Clinical examination maneuvers that increase tension on the sciatic nerve or contributes to it are referred to as *root tension signs*. Less commonly, root tension signs are identified by a positive formal stretch test for hyper-level lumbar root involvement. These techniques mechanically pull the inflamed, hypersensitive nerve root up against the irritating disc or physically stretch the nerve longitudinally to exacerbate pain. The initial part of the maneuver takes up the slack before tension is applied to the nerve itself. These tests also depend on nerve mobility, specifically its glide excursion within the foramen. Greater excursion leads to greater test sensitivity. In the lower lumbar spine, the relative glide of each nerve decreases with proximal migration—that is, S-1 glides more than L-5, L-5 glides more than L-4, and so forth (63). Therefore, straight-leg raising tests (SLR) are useful for L-5 and S-1 root involvement, but much less so for lesions involving L-4.

SLR is considered positive if radicular, not low back, symptoms are reproduced when the straight leg is raised with the patient supine (Table 2). The lower the angle of inclination necessary to produce symptoms, the more predictive the test. Dorsiflexion of the ankle places greater tension on the nerve and should exacerbate the patient's symptoms. The Lasègue's test performed in the supine position also places tension on the sciatic nerve (64). With the hip and knee initially flexed to 90 degrees, the knee is slowly extended to elicit the radicular symptoms. SLR may be performed with the patient supine or seated. A useful approach is to ask about and examine the foot or ankle while extending the knee in the seated patient. This distracts the patient's attention. Typically, the first 30 degrees of elevation gather the slack. Stretching beyond approximately 60 degrees may run into hamstring muscle tightness. Therefore, the usual range wherein the test is positive is 30 to 60 degrees. Note if an attempt is made to extend the hip, as this protective behavior would be considered a positive finding. Radicular pain, not back pain, must be reproduced for the test to be positive. A positive contralateral SLR strongly indicates surgical pathology (65) and is a highly specific, but not sensitive test for lumbar disc herniation.

Like the Valsalva maneuver, the Milgram test is designed to increase the intrathecal pressure (66). In the supine position, the patient is asked to maintain both extended legs approximately 3 in. off the table for 30 seconds. If there is root impingement, the increase in intrathecal pressure may exacerbate radicular symptoms.

Radicular symptoms may be reproduced by performing femoral or sciatic nerve tension tests or by performing a Valsalva maneuver. The nerve tension tests must reproduce the patient's radicular symptoms to be considered significant. SLR in the sit-

TABLE 2. *Straight-leg raise (SLR) testing*

Test	Maneuver	Roots tested
SLR	Elevate painful leg while keeping it straight to see if radicular **leg pain** can be reproduced; exacerbate with passive ankle dorsiflexion (reproduction of **back pain is not** a positive finding)	L-5, S-1
Contralateral SLR	Elevate opposite leg (nonpainful)—may indicate presence of sequestered or extruded fragment	L-5, S-1
Femoral stretch reverse SLR	Place hip in extension (lateral decubitus or prone position) to stretch femoral nerve—reproduce L-3 or L-4 radiculopathy	L-3, L-4

ting position, along with a host of other clinical examinations, may help differentiate real abnormality from malingering.

More proximal lumbar roots (i.e., L-3, L-4) innervate the femoral nerve. To place these under tension and reproduce anterior/lateral groin, thigh, knee, and/or leg pain, the opposite maneuver is required—that is, hip extension and knee flexion (i.e., the femoral stretch test). Like the SLR, a contralateral femoral stretch sign may be present.

DIAGNOSTIC TESTS

Plain radiographs can indirectly suggest disc pathology such as decreased disc space, but do not directly show disc herniation. Without a history of trauma, lumbosacral spine radiographs are often unnecessary at the time of initial office visit. The favorable natural history of low back pain justifies waiting to perform routine radiography only if the patient fails to improve after an initial 4-week period of therapy (67). Suggested guidelines for urgency in ordering plain radiographs in patients with low back pain include patients older than 50 years, history of serious trauma, known cancer, night pain, pain at rest, unexplained weight loss, drug or alcohol abuse, treatment with corticosteroids, temperature above 38°C, or a clinical history and examination that raise a suspicion of a spondyloarthropathy or demonstrate a neuromotor deficit (68).

Magnetic resonance imaging (MRI) has become the imaging procedure of choice in evaluating disc pathology, neural structures, and musculoligamentous components. MRI is also useful in evaluating surrounding soft tissues for evidence of trauma, including edema and hematoma formation, and intrinsic cord abnormalities such as syringomyelia. MRI is not predictive of development or duration of pain (69). Nearly 30% of asymptomatic individuals have abnormal MRI scans (70), and 27% actually have protrusions (71). However, MRI gives excellent visualization of root anatomy, disc herniation, and fragments, including foraminal and far-lateral pathology. MRI is useful to distinguish between disc herniation and other conditions that may mimic it, such as synovial cyst, neurofibroma, or perineural cysts. Nerve root position also may vary depending on the pathology and patient's anatomy, and MRI is a useful guide for directing surgical technique to avoid root injury (72). Contrast material (e.g., gadolinium) is not indicated in primary cases but may be used to differentiate scar from disc in postsurgical patients. A recent study in postsurgical patients indicated little added diagnostic value to contrast enhancement, however (73).

Myelography, in conjunction with computed tomography, remains an excellent but invasive diagnostic technique for evaluating the spinal canal and exiting nerve roots. With the advent of MRI, the use of myelography has declined, but it remains a powerful diagnostic tool in certain settings, such as evaluating patients with severe deformities and revision surgery, or when patients cannot have MRI scans due to pacemakers, other metallic objects, or claustrophobia.

Much has been written about imaging in disc herniations. Perhaps the most important aspect of radiographic imaging is that it must make sense in the context of the clinical signs and symptoms and must fit anatomically. A scan showing a large disc herniation to the left at L4-5 when the patient presents with right-sided S-1 findings must be carefully reevaluated. Perhaps this was a preexisting condition that is now irrelevant. Decisions must be based on close coordination of all available information. When there is discrepancy between clinical and radiographic data, the clinical data take precedence.

Electrodiagnostic testing is not a routine part of the workup but may be useful to rule out other neurologic disorders or additional sites of nerve compression.

NONOPERATIVE TREATMENT

In view of the natural history, most patients with disc herniations and radiculopathy are successfully treated nonoperatively. At least 90% of people with a disc herniation improve with conservative care (74). This natural history correlates with the inflammatory process involving the nerve root resulting from the adjacent disc pathology. Despite abundant literature, there is still a controversy concerning the treatment (75).

In the absence of an acute neurologic deficit, the mainstays of management include short-term rest, NSAIDs, antispasmodic medications, analgesics, and exercise and physical therapy (76). If the pain is extreme, narcotics may be necessary. Antidepressants and oral steroids may be indicated in certain situations. Oral corticosteroids have been shown to improve herniated disc symptoms and signs, but long-term effects such as avascular necrosis should be considered.

Bed rest should be kept to less than 2 to 5 days, and controlled activity (i.e., therapy, rehabilitation) is initiated as soon as it is tolerable. It is important to remember that time spent without substantial physical activity can lead to muscle atrophy, joint stiffness, disuse osteoporosis, and psychologic effects. Many patients markedly improve within 10 days, but conservative treatment should continue for 6 weeks before other measures are attempted.

There is considerable debate regarding mechanisms for pain reduction through exercise. Although flexion exercises reduce nerve root compression by opening the foramen, this same maneuver increases disc pressure. Extension exercises theoretically induce a shift of nuclear material away from the posterior rim of the annulus and thereby decrease nociceptive input from the annulus fibrosus or reduce disc material that has already protruded through an annular tear (77); however, in clinical application this theory remains unproven (78). Successful pain relief with exercise undoubtedly centers in part on the protective effect of strong abdominal muscles to load share and partially shield the disc from excessive load. Rehabilitation must include stretching, strengthening, and modalities. Abdominal strengthening and lumbar extension exercises are beneficial. Therapy should be started early to prevent deconditioning. By itself, simply staying active without any other treatment has no effect on sciatica but is still advisable to avoid harmful effects of bed rest (79).

Although there is little evidence to scientifically prove efficacy of heat, cold, massage, ultrasonography, or other modalities, many patients find these helpful. Caution should be used with heat in the first 48 hours because it increases local blood flow and may increase inflammation and edema.

If leg pain persists beyond 4 weeks, a series of epidural steroid injections may be considered. Maximum benefit is usually within 2 weeks, with a maximum of three injections given per year. Responses vary greatly, with short-term improvement seen in roughly 40% of patients, but no significant long-term results have been demonstrated (80). Response to epidural steroid

TABLE 3. *Waddell's tests*

Nonanatomic superficial tenderness
Simulation rotation/compression tests
Flip test: (+) straight-leg raising supine, but (–) sitting
Nonanatomic weakness/sensory findings
Overreaction

injections is highly variable, with one study showing 82% relief for one day, 50% relief for two weeks, and 16% for 2 months (81). In another study, 77% of patients were able to avoid surgery after epidural steroid injections, with alleviation of radicular pain from lumbar herniated discs for up to 27 months (82). Carette, however, found that epidural injections added neither significant functional benefit nor reduction in need for surgery (83). Although epidural injections may play a role in patients with radicular syndromes not responding to therapy or in whom surgery is not an option, patients must understand that positive responses to the injections are usually only temporary. Local trigger-point injections are totally unproven and may share a mechanism similar to acupuncture.

As with many elective surgical decisions, evaluation of emotional stability and reaction to pain is important. Waddell's criteria are very useful in this regard (Table 3) (84). If there is any uncertainty regarding these issues, psychological and/or psychiatric consultation is essential.

INDICATIONS FOR SURGERY

As noted previously, acute sciatica is usually transient and self-limited, resolving satisfactorily regardless of treatment method. Surgery, however, seems to offer a better long-term prognosis as measured by residual sciatica and recurrent symptoms. Pain relief is the primary surgical indication in most patients. Urgent intervention for progressive neurologic deficit is much less common. Disc surgery is most successful for alleviating unilateral leg pain that is not accompanied by back pain. The ideal candidate for disc surgery is a patient whose history, physical examination, and radiographic findings are consistent with one other. When discrepancies exist, the clinical picture should serve as the principal guide.

MRI findings are not in themselves indications for surgery, as noncontained and extruded fragments can resorb if patients can tolerate the symptoms for several months (85,86). The resorption mechanism may be similar to that identified where autologous intervertebral disc material grafted into the epidural space. The lesion is penetrated by newly formed vessels from the epidural fat tissue and resolves as the result of inflammatory reaction (87).

Controversy surrounds the relative urgency of surgery in the face of motor weakness. Moderate motor weakness permits the usual period of observation because recovery of strength commonly occurs with or without surgery. Progressive weakness is an indication for surgical decompression, but this is not the usual situation.

Return of motor function can occur with or without surgery but may require 3 years to be complete (74). Mild to moderate weakness, which is compatible with adequate function, allows a period of observation. If the motor weakness is progressive or becomes functionally significant, however, some believe surgery becomes more urgent. Similarly, acute and profound motor loss accompanied by pain often requires prompt surgical decompression. A recent study found the degree of recovery of motor function to be inversely related to the preoperative severity and duration of muscle weakness (88). In the face of a progressing neurologic deficit, surgical intervention is strongly indicated, particularly when there is clear correlation between imaging studies and clinical findings. Absolute surgical indications include cauda equina compression syndrome. Surgical indications are divided into absolute and relative.

Cauda equina syndrome is an extreme type of massive central herniation that presents with a combination of acute urinary retention/incontinence, saddle anesthesia, back/buttock/leg pain, weakness, difficulty walking, and sensory loss usually affecting the perineal area. Symptoms can vary greatly, and some or all may be present. Although immediate surgery for this surgical emergency does not always correlate with neurologic recovery, it is indicated to minimize further neurologic injury even if neurologic recovery is not likely. Sudden severe paresis or paraplegia merits immediate imaging and prompt decompression. Presentation may not always be acute and may sometimes develop over several days to weeks. Lower lumbar levels are most commonly affected, but there are a disproportionately high number of upper lumbar herniations in this syndrome (54). Typically, there is a large midline herniation compressing several lumbar and sacral nerve roots that is easily visualized on MRI or myelography, as it produces a complete block. Such herniations represent only 0.2% of all disc herniations (89). A similar clinical picture may result from other pathology, such as an intraspinal tumor, and it is important that imaging extend proximally to the lower thoracic cord.

Patients without neurologic deficit who have not responded to conservative therapy may also be considered as elective candidates for surgical intervention if there is clear correlation between symptoms, physical findings, imaging, and if performed, electrodiagnostic (e.g., electromyography, somatosensory-evoked potential) testing. Successful return to vigorous athletic activity is usually possible after surgery, as more than 80% of athletes return to sports after discectomy (90).

Surgery provides better short-term results than those of nonoperative treatment of sciatica, but long-term results are no different (74,91). Therefore, there is little risk in waiting. A nonoperative approach often means loss of 4 months of work or longer (74,92). However, waiting too long in symptomatic patients can lead to worse outcomes. Furthermore, the head of a household who must provide for his/her family may not be able to wait for months to resume work.

Absence of back pain correlates with better surgical results from discectomy (91). Patients' self-reported health outcomes after lumbar laminectomy correlate with the excellent results previously seen using physician-driven outcome measures in an appropriately selected population with radiculopathy (93).

It is interesting to note that preoperative pain drawings in patients subsequently undergoing surgery showed correlation between pain radiating to the foot with disc sequestration, whereas bilateral back pain correlated with disc protrusion (94).

Statistically, the best predictive factors for successful surgery are (a) persistent leg pain that fails to respond to a 6-week trial of nonoperative care, (b) well-defined neurologic deficit, (c) a positive SLR test, and (d) positive imaging that correlates anatomically to clinical findings. If at least three of these factors are present, surgery has at least a 90% success rate. Patients with large extruded fragments and sciatica do very well (95). Other factors such as duration of sciatica, sick leave stress, depression, level of education, and work/disability claims play a significant role (96,97). For patients with moderate or severe sciatica, surgical treatment was associated with greater improvement than nonsurgical treatment at 1 (98) and 5 years (99).

SURGICAL TECHNIQUE

Planning

Open discectomy through a limited incision is the gold standard for surgical management of single-level disc herniation (30,55,93, 99,100). Other techniques, particularly minimal access techniques, are promising but as yet unproven. Every effort should be made to be sure that the patient has realistic expectations and understands the risks and benefits of surgery. Anticoagulants such as coumadin should be stopped under medical supervision, and NSAIDs discontinued several days before surgery.

Anesthesia

Although spinal, epidural, and local anesthesias have been used, general anesthesia is most often preferred because it minimizes intraoperative patient discomfort and/or accidental movement, and maximizes intraoperative airway and blood pressure control. These advantages are particularly useful if surgery is prolonged or if complications arise. Postepidural anesthesia stress ulcers have been reported in older patients (100).

Positioning

Although lumbar disc surgery may be performed in the lateral or semilateral position, it is most commonly performed in the prone position. This position maximizes surgical options and maintains surgical anatomic orientation. Numerous positioning arrangements allow the abdomen to hang free, thereby decreasing pressure on the vena cava and Batson's plexus, minimizing bleeding in the surgical field, particularly from epidural veins that become engorged when the abdomen is compressed. Certain positions, such as the knee-chest position, maximally flex the lumbar spine. Although this position opens up the posterior elements and facilitates surgical entry into the canal, it does not give an accurate assessment of foraminal dimensions and architecture when the patient is standing and the spine is loaded. Accordingly, the surgeon may not appreciate coexisting foraminal stenosis at the time of disc surgery, and may fail to adequately address this coexisting pathology.

Frames that maintain the spine in kyphosis should not be used if lumbar fusion is contemplated because they contribute to fusing the spine in suboptimal lordosis (101). Positioning the spine so lumbar lordosis is maintained makes canal entry more difficult but more accurately simulates the anatomic situation faced by the upright spine. Thus, a more realistic view of how and where nerve root compression occurs is presented and can therefore be addressed.

Meticulous attention to positioning and padding of the shoulders, arms, legs, neck, face, chest/breasts, and genitalia minimizes problems associated with these structures in the prone position. In general, joints should be gently flexed to avoid stretch, particularly the shoulder, in which abduction should be avoided to prevent brachial plexus injury. All bony prominences need to be well padded and without compression by tape or straps over any neural or vascular structures. Particular attention should be paid to the knees and elbows, to protect the peroneal and ulnar nerves, respectively. The neck should be in neutral to avoid hyperextension, with the face and eyes carefully protected.

Depending on expected length of surgery, a Foley catheter may be placed. It is easier to place the catheter preoperatively and remove it postoperatively than to have to try to place the catheter intraoperatively. Routine use of elastic leg wraps or intermittent compression stockings/boots decreases venous pooling and risk of deep vein thrombosis.

Preparation and Draping

Meticulous attention to detail in skin preparation with antiseptic agents, along with careful and complete sterile draping of the surgical field is essential to minimize postoperative wound infection or discitis. Prophylactic intravenous antibiotics directed at Gram-positive organisms are given before incision and continued for at least 24 hours postoperatively. Overhead equipment, such as the image intensifier or microscope, must be properly draped. Although the incision is usually only several centimeters long, it is subjected to significant retraction and heat (e.g., electrocautery, overhead lights, headlight), both of which are significant risk factors for infection. Postoperative infections can be minimized with attention to eliminating any preexisting preoperative infection (e.g., periodontal, urinary, skin, etc.), careful preparation and draping, antibiotic prophylaxis, attention to soft-tissue retraction, and wound closure.

Incision

It is best to localize the surgical approach directly over the target level to minimize incision size and surgical dissection. Initial level localization may be guided by comparing preoperative radiographs with palpated surface anatomy such as iliac crests and spinous processes once the patient is positioned. In addition, the skin can be marked as determined by a preincision lateral radiograph taken with a needle or marker placed in the spinous process. Alternatively, the first radiographic localization may be done after limited initial exposure.

Despite careful preincision assessment, it is still possible to inadvertently approach an adjacent level rather than that intended. This is particularly true in (a) large patients in whom there is a significant distance from the skin to the spine, (b) in the presence of shingling or overlapping of posterior elements, and (c) when the sagittal contour on the operating room table varies from that on preoperative radiographs. Overlapping spinous processes, hypertrophic facets, and transitional levels are several common anatomic variations that can lead to confusion. Vertebral levels may be initially estimated by assessing spinous process motion resulting from pulling cephalad with an instrument. The surgeon cannot always assume that a spinous process that does not move is the sacrum because there may be variations due to transitional vertebrae. Clear, localizing, intraoperative radiographs are essential to assure approach to the proper level. Although every effort should be made to optimize cosmesis, a slightly larger incision may sometimes result in a faster and safer procedure.

A midline incision is most commonly used, typically 2 to 5 cm in length, depending on patient size. Meticulous hemostasis is used with electrocautery and the fascia is exposed. After unilateral subperiosteal exposure of the appropriate spinous process, a clamp is placed on the spinous process for radiographic confirmation and to localize the interlaminar space and the facets (which are not exposed). After radiographic level confirmation, the target lamina along with the cephalad portion of the next caudal lamina are exposed. Paraspinal muscle retraction and exposure is facilitated with a variety of retraction methods, often involving a retractor placed lateral to the facet. This retractor may be self-retaining or may need to be secured. Because prolonged deep retraction may lead to muscle ischemia, retractors should be removed periodically to allow muscle revascularization.

Every effort is made to preserve soft-tissue structures, minimize bony resection, and maintain stability. Meticulous sparing of interspinous ligaments and facet capsules along with careful bone resection allows precise decompression without needless destabilizing. The use of a headlight and loupes is encouraged.

Discectomy

Because disc pathology is often lateral, a slightly lateral approach to the disc is preferred as this minimizes nerve root retraction (and therefore, risk of neural injury) necessary for visualization (Fig. 1). After laminar exposure, an angled curette may be used to detach the superficial ligamentum flavum from the caudal edge of the proximal lamina and allow placement of a Woodson-type elevator under the lamina. A laminotomy is generally necessary to allow adequate access to the underlying neural structures and disc. This limited resection is performed using a Kerrison rongeur, often in association with limited resection of the medial portion of the inferior facet. If the lamina and facet are thickened, as in many older patients, they must first be thinned down with a burr to allow use of the Kerrison. The superior facet of the inferior level then comes into view. Undercutting this facet medially significantly improves lateral visualization and reduces the need for nerve root retraction without leading to instability. It is best to leave at least one-half of the facet intact to maintain stability. Facet fracture can be avoided by staying medial with the bony resection, avoiding the pars, minimizing leverage, and recognizing the size and shape of the remaining facet. If a facet or pars fracture occurs, it is best to inform the patient postoperatively so the situation can be monitored. In patients without deformity or instability, complete facetectomy from pars fracture may be well tolerated, but in some cases it may lead to chronic pain. A formal foraminotomy may also be performed, if indicated, by further undercutting the facet while preserving as much of the dorsal part of the joint as possible. Although laminotomy extension proximally and laterally, along with medial facetectomy may not be needed for all discec-

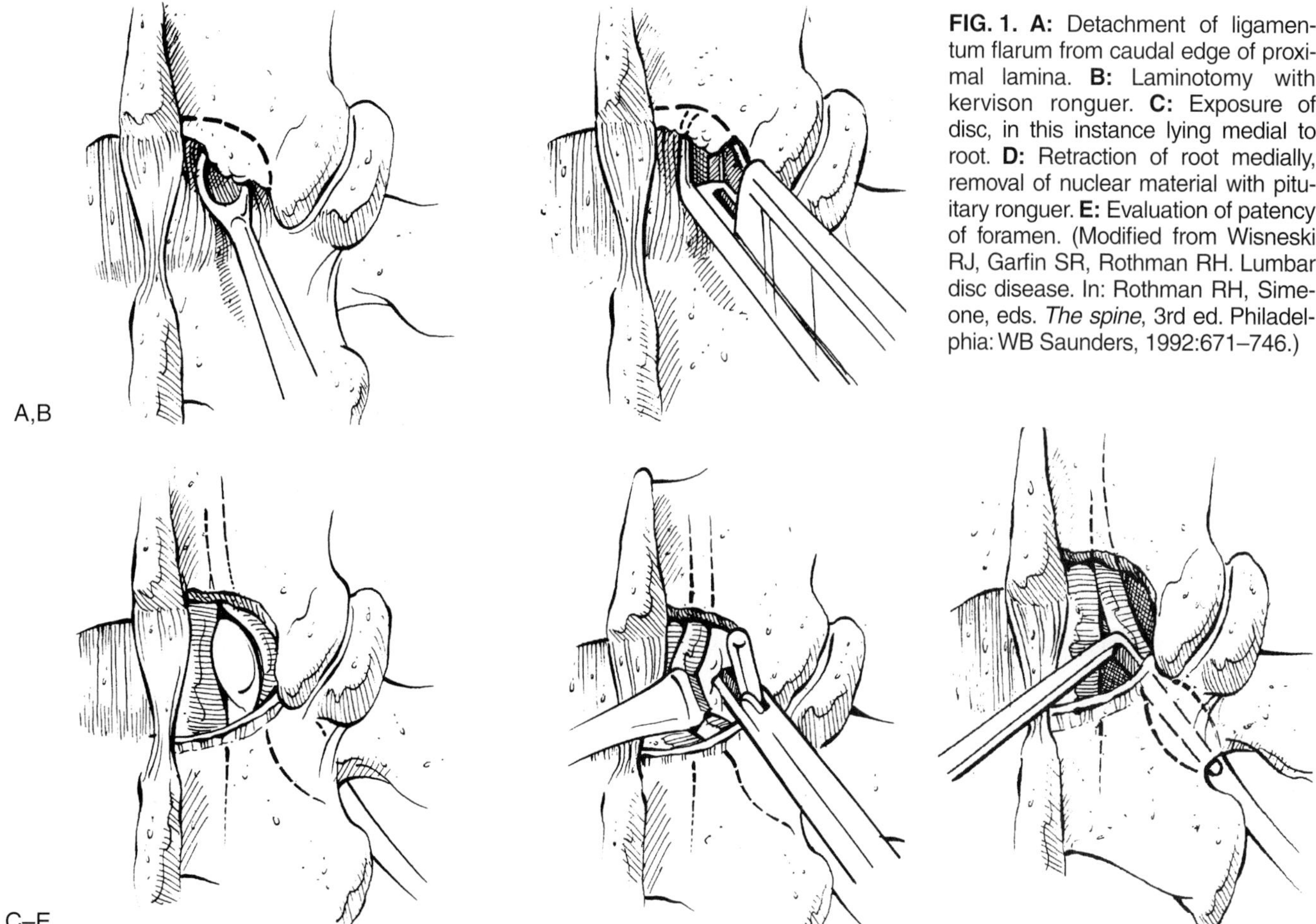

FIG. 1. A: Detachment of ligamentum flarum from caudal edge of proximal lamina. **B:** Laminotomy with kervison ronguer. **C:** Exposure of disc, in this instance lying medial to root. **D:** Retraction of root medially, removal of nuclear material with pituitary ronguer. **E:** Evaluation of patency of foramen. (Modified from Wisneski RJ, Garfin SR, Rothman RH. Lumbar disc disease. In: Rothman RH, Simeone, eds. *The spine*, 3rd ed. Philadelphia: WB Saunders, 1992:671–746.)

tomies, they should be kept in mind to facilitate exposure when needed.

After laminotomy and possible partial medial facet resection, the interlaminar interval comes clearly into view. The insertion of the ligamentum flavum to the distal lamina can then be detached and opened with a small-angled curette or a knife. Extreme caution is essential to avoid injury to the underlying dura and neural structures, which may have been pushed dorsally by displaced disc material. A cottonoid gently eased in under the ligamentum helps separate and protect the dura. The ligamentum can then be safely removed with a Kerrison. Removal of separate lateral bands of ligamentum may further improve visualization. Alternatively, if good visualization is obtained, much of the ligamentum may be spared and only small portions of lateral ligamentum are resected. If bony resection has been adequate, the dura and nerve root are well exposed and allow for the gentle retraction necessary to expose the underlying disc. In some situations (usually L-5 to S-1), the cephalad ligamentum attachments may be preserved, allowing the surgeon to "flip" the ligamentum proximally with a suture so it can be used to cover the dura at the end of the procedure (55). If there is any doubt or difficulty with exposure, however, it is better to remove the ligament.

With good exposure, it is possible to see and gently palpate the affected nerve root in order to assess whether or not it is under tension. Nerve root retraction must be gentle, without sudden movements. The entire root and nearby dural edge are protected, and must not be allowed to "sneak out" below the retractor with time. The importance of clear visualization with good light, gentle but adequate retraction, and hemostasis cannot be overemphasized. Intermittent relaxation of retraction reduces risk of root injury. Attempting to overcome inadequate exposure with excessive retraction causes operative complications. The potential instability resulting from excessive bone resection is far less of a problem than an irreversible neurologic injury resulting from poor exposure.

Direct visualization of the nerve root is mandatory to allow proper protection. Disc visualization usually begins with gentle medial nerve root retraction using a Penfield-type retractor. Initially, the floor of the spinal canal may be palpated before the disc is recognized. Adhesions commonly present between the inflamed root and the underlying disc or disc fragments may be gently teased away. Epidural bleeding is controlled with bipolar electrocautery or judicious placement of cottonoid patties and thrombin-soaked Gelfoam.

Extruded or sequestered fragments displace the root and distort the anatomy, so these fragments are best removed as early as possible to restore orientation and reduce root retraction. Before any such undertaking, however, the nerve root must be definitively and absolutely identified to avoid inadvertent root injury. With distorted anatomy, the root is not only displaced from where it should be but is also attenuated as it stretches around the displacing entity. As such, it may be more difficult to visualize initially. The departure of the nerve root from the dural sac may be a useful landmark. The pedicle is a constant anatomic landmark that is an excellent reference point. Once the displacing disc material is removed the root fills, returns to its normal position, and is easier to see. Extruded fragments are convenient in that they often lead you directly to the opening in the annulus from whence they came. When the anatomy is distorted by a large fragment, a useful technique involves gently grasping a small portion of the fragment with a pituitary rongeur and gently delivering it, then regrasping as it comes out to avoid pulling it apart and losing your grip. This obviously can only be done once you have confidence that the root and dural edge are protected. It is very reassuring to remove a large fragment that, on removal, leads to restoration of normal anatomy and distinct localization of where it came from. This hole in the annulus can then be used as an entry point for discectomy and removal of additional loose fragments. Extruded fragments are best removed in continuity. Furthermore, there may be multiple extruded fragments. Also, it should not be assumed that removal of a large fragment guarantees that there are not other significant fragments as well. Extruded fragments often contain a portion of end-plate that has dislodged or rotated, allowing the disc to extrude into the canal. This end-plate can be very tough at its remaining attachment points. Often, in a massive extrusion, there is little left within the disc space to remove.

Sequestered fragments, pieces that have completely exited the disc and have become completely separated, may be more difficult to find. The distinction between extruded and sequestered fragments can be difficult to make preoperatively, but the approximate location of these displaced fragments is provided by preoperative studies so that attention can be properly directed. Although most herniations occur lateral to the root, some may go into the axilla between the root and the dural sac. This is a particularly tricky area where it is not difficult to miss a fragment, but visualization may be limited by concerns about avoiding nerve root injury or dural leak.

Epidural bleeding can be brisk but is well controlled with bipolar cautery, thrombin-soaked Gelfoam or similar materials, and cottonoid sponges ("patties"). Gently packing and then revisiting the site often helps. Laterally placed cottonoids positioned proximal and distal to the disc may assist exposure by controlling hemostasis and providing medial root retraction more gently than with metal nerve root retractors.

In the absence of an extrusion, the white surface of the annulus comes into view after gently sweeping off overlying epidural veins and fat. Disc location may be confirmed by placing an 18- or 20-gauge spinal needle into it. A small, straight, blunt instrument, such as a tiny curette or Penfield elevator, may be used to explore the annulus for a defect. If none is found, a small blade (No. 15) may be used to open the annulus. A series of pituitary rongeurs can be carefully introduced into the disc for removal of nucleus pulposus, annulus, and/or cartilaginous end-plate. These rongeurs must be placed into the disc with the jaws closed to avoid injury to surrounding structures outside the disc. Once inside the disc, the jaws are opened to grasp and remove material. This maneuver is best done with two hands, one opening and closing the rongeur and the other controlling instrument depth, avoiding inadvertent too deep penetration. Sequential use of straight and then angled rongeurs allows safe access to different areas of the disc.

There is no absolute answer as to how much disc to remove. Fragments that are loose and easily reached should be removed to minimize reherniation or retained fragments. Aggressive end-plate curettage should be avoided. The goal of the surgery is not complete discectomy but removal of enough material to relieve symptoms and prevent recurrence.

After removal of disc, the inflamed nerve root may be erythematous but should move freely and easily with a very gentle retraction. This is the time to methodically inspect the epidural space medially around the root, anterior to the sac, distally to the level of the inferior pedicle, as well as proximally for other possible fragments. If the root is not free but no further fragments have been identified, consider a foraminotomy.

Careful review of preoperative images (e.g., MRI, computed tomography–myelography) localizes the pathology and focus areas to be searched. For example, an MRI showing disc at the level of the pedicle suggests that this is a displaced fragment because the disc is anatomically at the level of the facets, not the pedicle. But what if a search for disc material in this area is unrevealing? A note of caution is useful here. Keep in mind that "wrong-level" surgery occurs in approximately 1 to 2% of cases (102). On the other hand, some MRI scans appear to show large disc herniations that later prove difficult to find intraoperatively. Although a complete and thorough assessment at the proper anatomic level is essential, one should not search endlessly for something that is not there. If a reasonable search does not reveal the fragment, it is probably of marginal clinical importance. In these cases, it is better to leave well enough alone rather than risk injury with prolonged search. It is interesting that there is no association between nerve root thickening, nerve root enhancement, or nerve root displacement and clinical outcome (99).

The wound is irrigated, and exposed dura is covered with Gelfoam or fat graft to reduce perineural adhesions. There does not appear to be any long-term advantage to fat graft (103). Clinical outcome does not correlate with use or type of interposition membrane for preventing epidural fibrosis (104). Certain materials like Adcon-L may precipitate continued cerebrospinal fluid leakage if there is an unrecognized dural leak (105). The wound is closed without a drain. Twenty-four hours of IV antibiotic coverage is maintained, and ambulation begins as soon as possible. Muscular patients may benefit from muscle relaxants (e.g., diazepam) for 1 to 2 days as they may have spasm from muscle retraction. Same day or next day discharge is the norm.

Many patients note immediate reduction in radicular pain in the recovery room. A small percentage may experience transient worsening of their preoperative radiculopathy as a result of root manipulation and local inflammation. Most patients experience something in between, with clear reduction in magnitude of preoperative radiculopathy, but with some leg and back pain for weeks. NSAIDs and muscle relaxants are preferable to narcotics and analgesics, although a combination may be needed. In most situations, the need for medication drops off sharply within a few days to 2 weeks.

Activity as tolerated is encouraged, although sitting is avoided to minimize axial load on the disc. In particular, driving and riding in a car are discouraged to protect the disc from higher loads resulting from this position. Intensive physical therapy started 4 to 12 weeks after surgery is effective in reducing disability and pain (106,107).

RESULTS

Good to excellent clinical results in excess of 80 to 90% are widely reported (98–100,108,109). However, overall rates of unsatisfactory results after discectomy range between 5 and 20% (109–112). Factors contributing to these results include indications, comorbidities, nonmedical issues, and surgical technique.

Common causes of recurrent or persistent sciatic symptoms include recurrent herniation, retained fragments, nerve root trauma, epidural fibrosis, arachnoiditis, discitis, pseudomeningocele, and instability. Other causes of failure are surgery at the wrong level, inadequate decompression, unrecognized second disc herniation, tumor, and spondylolisthesis.

Direct correlation between postoperative MRI findings with symptomatic complaints does not exist. Although all postoperative patients have residual scar or fibrosis on follow-up MRI enhanced with gadolinium, many are asymptomatic. Why, then, are only certain patients symptomatic? The answer remains vague. In any case, perineural fibrosis and adhesions alter neural dynamics and may cause recurrent symptoms (113). Epidural fibrosis results from repeated insults external to the dura, as compared to arachnoiditis, which results from intradural injury (i.e., bleeding in the arachnoid). Fibrosis results in localized root tethering and subsequent traction when the nerve is stretched. Prevention of fibrosis is best accomplished by combining appropriate surgical indications, meticulous surgical technique, and minimizing of nerve root retraction. Twenty-three percent of surgical failures in one study were due to epidural fibrosis (110). In general, it is well established that nerve root injury may result from excessive retraction, compression, or contusion. These can often be avoided with better exposure, whether this means additional bone resection or a larger incision. Even "apparently innocent" materials, such as Gelfoam and cottonoids, can cause compression leading to nerve root injury, so these must be monitored closely as well (114).

When radiculopathy similar to that experienced preoperatively occurs after a period of improvement, the herniation of additional dura material should be suspected. When recurrent pain results from recurrent herniation, symptoms typically occur within the first 2 weeks postoperatively. This pain pattern must be distinguished from patients who never improve, who are more suggestive of retained fragments. Recurrence rates are significant, occurring in 5 to 11% of cases (115–117).

Despite a careful intraoperative search the surgeon may not remove all disc fragments, particularly if the disc is already fragmented at surgery. Most remaining fragments resorb, however, and pose little clinical problem. Furthermore, most patients experience some postoperative improvement even if it is short lived as a result of decompression and systemic endorphin release. Therefore, patients who are worse postoperatively or never enjoy even a transient period of postoperative pain relief must be suspected to harbor retained fragments. Retained fragments are present in 0.2% of cases (118).

Persistent and progressive low back pain occurring several weeks postoperatively should raise suspicion of discitis. This condition occurs in 1 to 5% of patients and is usually diagnosed at 2 to 8 weeks after an initial period of pain relief followed with pain out of proportion to physical findings (119–121). Physical back examination may (or may not) reveal low grade fever as well as severe para-vertebral spasm. Erythrocyte sedimentation rate and C-reactive protein are elevated more reliably than white blood cells. Radiographic changes may not be present on plain x-ray, and bone scan is of marginal value due to recent surgery. Gallium scanning is helpful, but biopsy-proven cultures are definitive. Incidence of postoperative discitis as well as wound infection drops to less than 1% when prophylactic antibiotics are used (122–124). Accordingly, prophylactic antibiotics are indicated in disc surgery.

Epidural abscess is a very rare complication from disc surgery. It usually presents in the first 2 to 4 weeks postoperatively with progressive back and leg pain. Neurologic deterioration calls for appropriate imaging (usually MRI) followed by immediate decompression.

Persistent post-discectomy low back pain is multifactorial. Severe residual low back pain has been reported in slightly less than 15% of patients (126,127). Pain does not correlate with loss of disc height, patient age, or length of time after surgery. Factors predisposing to disabling low back pain included workers' compensation, history of more than 15 pack-years of cigarette smoking, and an age older than 40 years (126).

Revision disc surgery raises many questions and should only be contemplated after sufficient postoperative care and diagnostic assessment. Additional surgery based on vague symptoms and without a clear surgical target likely results in more scar tissue and poor results. On the other hand, appropriately directed revision surgery can be very successful. Surgical results for recurrent lumbar disc herniation and for contralateral disc herniation compare favorably with those of primary discectomy (125,128,129). When disc herniation and radicular symptoms occur in the setting of back pain, deformity, or instability, however, complex decision making is the rule in sorting out other surgical issues such as indications for and length of fusion.

REFERENCES

1. Inoue H. Three-dimensional architecture of lumbar intervertebral discs. *Spine* 1981;6:139–146.
2. Roberts S, Menage J, Urban JP. Biochemical and structural properties of the cartilage end-plate and its relation to the intervertebral disc. *Spine* 1989;14:144–174.
3. Coventry MB, Ghormley RK, Kernohan JW. The intervertebral disc: its microscopic anatomy and pathology. Part 2. *J Bone Joint Surg [Am]* 1945;27:233–247.
4. Weidenbaum M, Iatridis JC, Setton LA, et al. Mechanical behavior of the intervertebral disc and the effects of degeneration. In: Weinstein JN, Gordon SL, eds. *Low back pain*. Rosemont, IL: American Academy of Orthopedic Surgeons, 1996:557–582.
5. Silveri CP, Simeone FA. Lumbar disc disease. In: An H, ed. *Principles and techniques in spine surgery*. Baltimore: Williams & Wilkins, 1998:425–441.
6. Eyre D, Benya P, Buckwalter J, et al. The intervertebral disc: basic science perspectives. In: Frymoyer JW, Gordon SL, eds. *New perspectives on low back pain*. Rosemont, IL: American Academy of Orthopedic Surgeons, 1989:147–207.
7. Pearce RH. Morphologic and chemical aspects of aging. In: Buckwalter JA, Goldberg VM, Woo SLY, eds. *Musculoskeletal soft-tissue aging: impact on mobility*. Rosemont, IL: American Academy of Orthopedic Surgeons, 1993:363–379.
8. Roberts S, Caterson B, Evans H, et al. Proteoglycan components of the intervertebral disc and cartilage endplate: an immunolocalization study of animal and human tissue. *Histochem J* 1994;26:402–411.
9. Setton LA, Zhu W, Weidenbaum M, et al. Compressive properties of the cartilaginous end plate of the baboon lumbar spine. *J Orthop Res* 1993;11:228–239.
10. Farfan HF, Huberdeau RM, Dubow HI. Lumbar intervertebral disc degeneration: the influence of geometrical features on the pattern of disc degeneration—a post mortem study. *J Bone Joint Surg* 1972;54A: 492–510.
11. Marchand F, Ahmed AM. Investigation of the laminate structure of lumbar disc annulus fibrosus. *Spine* 1990;15:402–410.
12. Pearce RH, Thompson JP, Bebault GM, et al. Magnetic resonance imaging reflects the chemical changes of aging degeneration in the human intervertebral disc. *J Rheumatol Suppl* 1991;27:42–43.
13. Schiebler ML, Camerino VJ, Fallon MD, et al. *In vivo* and *ex vivo* magnetic resonance imaging evaluation of early disc degeneration with histopathologic correlation. *Spine* 1991;16:635–640.
14. Lyons G, Eisenstein SM, Sweet MB. Biochemical changes in intervertebral disc degeneration. *Biochim Biophys Acta* 1981;673:443–453.
15. Pearce RH, Grimmer BJ, Adams ME. Degeneration and the chemical composition of the human lumbar intervertebral disc. *J Orthop Res* 1987;5:198–205.
16. Best BA, Guilak F, Setton LA, et al. Compressive mechanical properties of the human annulus fibrosus and their relationship to biochemical composition. *Spine* 1994;19:212–221.
17. Iatridis JC, Weidenbaum M, Setton LA, et al. Is the nucleus pulposus a solid or a fluid? Mechanical behaviors of the nucleus pulposus of the human intervertebral disc. *Spine* 1996;26:581–592.
18. Nachemson AL, Elfstrom G. Intravital dynamic pressure measurements in lumbar discs: a study of common movements, maneuvers, and exercises. *Scand J Rehabil Med* 1970;2[Suppl 1]:1
19. Ohshima H, Tsuji H, Hirano N. Water diffusion pathway, swelling pressure, and biomechanical properties of the intervertebral discs during compression load. *Spine* 1989;14:1234–1244.
20. Stokes IA Surface strain on human intervertebral disc. *J Orthop Res* 1987;5:348–355.
21. Skaggs DL, Iatridis JC, Gibbons JM, et al. Regional variations in the tensile properties and biochemical composition of single lamellae of human annulus fibrosus. *Spine* 1994;19:1310–1319.
22. Farfan HF, et al. The effects of torsion on the lumbar intervertebral joints: the role of torsion in the production of disc degeneration. *J Bone Joint Surg [Am]* 1970;52:468–497.
23. Kirkaldy Willis WH. *Managing low back pain*. New York: Churchill Livingstone, 1983.
24. Goldthwait JE. The lumbosacral articulation. An explanation of many cases of "lumbago," "sciatica," and paraplegia. *Boston Med Surg J* 1911;164:365–372.
25. Mixter WJ, Barr JS. Rupture of the intervertebral disc with involvement of the spinal canal. *N Engl J Med* 1934;211:210–215.
26. Olmarker K, Blomquist J, Stromberg J, et al. Inflammatogenic properties of nucleus pulposus. *Spine* 1995;20:665–669.
27. Olmarker K, Nordborg C, Larsson K, et al. Ultrastructural changes in spinal nerve roots induced by autologous nucleus pulposus. *Spine* 1996;21:411–414.
28. Kayama S, Olmarker K, Larsson K, et al. Cultured autologous nucleus pulposus cells induce functional changes in spinal nerve roots. *Spine* 1998;23:2155–2158.
29. Satoh K, Konno K, Nishiyama K, et al. Presence and distribution of antigen-antibody complexes in the herniated nucleus pulposus. *Spine* 1999;24:1980.
30. Nygaard OP, Mellgren SI, Osterud B. The inflammatory properties of contained and non-contained lumbar disc herniation. *Spine* 1997;22:2484–2488.
31. An H. *Synopsis of spine surgery*. Baltimore: Williams & Wilkins, 1998.
32. Iwabuchi M, Rydevik B, Kikuchi S, et al. Effects of annulus fibrosus and experimentally degenerated nucleus pulposus on nerve root conduction velocity. *Spine* 2001;26:1651–1655.
33. Olmarker K, Rydevik B, Nordborg C. Letter in response. *Spine* 1997;22:2194–2195.
34. Otani K, Arai I, Mao G-P, et al. Experimental disc herniation. Evaluation of the natural course. *Spine* 1997;22:2894–2899.
35. Brisby H, Olmarker K, Rosengren L, et al. Markers of nerve tissue injury in the cerebrospinal fluid in patients with lumbar disc herniation and sciatica. *Spine* 1999;24:742.
36. Skouen JS, Brisby H, Otani K, et al. Protein markers in cerebrospinal fluid in experimental nerve root injury. A study of slow-onset chronic compression effects or the biochemical effects of nucleus pulposus on sacral nerve roots. *Spine* 1999;24:2195.
37. Olmarker K, Rydevik B. Selective inhibition of tumor necrosis factor-alpha prevents nucleus pulposus-induced thrombus formation, intraneural edema, and reduction of nerve conduction velocity. *Spine* 2001;26: 863–869.
38. Olmarker K, Larsson K. Tumor necrosis factor and nucleus-pulposus-induced nerve root injury. *Spine* 1998;23:2538–2544.
39. Yabuki S, Kawaguchi Y, Nordborg C, et al. Effects of lidocaine on nucleus pulposus-induced nerve root injury. A neurophysiologic and histologic study of the pig cauda equina. *Spine* 1998;23:2383–2389.
40. Olmarker K. Point of view: A comparative immuno-histochemical study of inflammatory cells in acute-stage and chronic-stage disc herniations. *Spine* 1998;23:2166.
41. Olmarker K. Point of view. *Spine* 2001;26:2665.
42. Harrington JF, Messier AA, Bereiter D, et al. Herniated lumbar disc material as a source of free glutamate available to affect pain signals through the dorsal root ganglion. *Spine* 2000;25:929–936.
43. Anzai H, Hamba M, Onda A, et al. Epidural application of nucleus

pulposus enhances nociresponses of rat dorsal horn neurons. *Spine* 2002;27:E50–E55.
44. Kang J. Point of view: inflammatory cytokines in the herniated disc of the lumbar spine. *Spine* 1996;21:224.
45. Kang JD. Point of view: murine nucleus pulposus-derived cells secrete interleukins-1, -6, and -10 and granulocyte-macrophage colony-stimulating factor in cell culture. *Spine* 1997;22:2602.
46. Kang JD, Georgescu H, McIntyre-Larkin L, et al. Herniated lumbar intervertebral discs spontaneously produce matrix metalloproteinases, nitric oxide, interleukin-6, and prostaglandin E_2. *Spine* 1996;21:271–277.
47. Kang JD, Stefanovic-Racic M, McIntyre L, et al. Toward a biochemical understanding of human intervertebral disc degeneration and herniation. Contributions of nitric oxide, interleukins, prostaglandin E_2, and matrix metalloproteinases. *Spine* 1997;22:1065–1073.
48. Kawakami M, Tamaki T, Hayashi N, et al. Possible mechanism of painful radiculopathy in lumbar disc herniation. *Clin Orthop* 1998;351:241–251.
49. Cornefjord M, Sato K, Olmarker K, et al. A model for chronic nerve root compression studies. Presentation of a porcine model for controlled, slow-onset compression with analyses of anatomic aspects, compression onset rate, and morphologic and neurophysiologic effects. *Spine* 1997;22:946–957.
50. Kikuchi S, Konno S, Kayama S, et al. Increased resistance to acute compression injury in chronically compressed spinal nerve roots. An experimental study. *Spine* 1996;21:2544–2550.
51. Mao G-P, Konno S, Arai I, et al. Chronic double-level cauda equina compression. An experimental study on the dog cauda equina with analyses of nerve conduction velocity. *Spine* 1998;23:1641–1644.
52. Cornefjord M, Olmarker K, Otani K, et al. Effects of diclofenac and ketoprofen on nerve conduction velocity in experimental nerve root compression. *Spine* 2001;26:2193–2197.
53. Kayama S, Konno S, Olmarker K, et al. *Spine* 1996;21(22):2539–2543.
54. Yabuki S, Kikuchi S, Olmarker K, et al. Acute effects of nucleus pulposus on blood flow and endoneurial fluid pressure in rat dorsal root ganglia. *Spine* 1998;23:2517–2523.
55. Spangfort EV. The lumbar disc herniation. A computer-aided analysis of 2504 operations. *Acta Orthop Scand (Suppl)* 1972;142:1–95.
56. Hanley EN, Delamarter RB, McCulloch JA, et al. Surgical indications and techniques. In: Wiesel SW, Weinstein JN, Herkowitz H, et al., eds. *The lumbar spine*, 2nd ed, vol. 1. Philadelphia: WB Saunders, 1996:492–524.
57. Ljunggren AE. Natural history and clinical role of the herniated disc. In: Wiesel SW, Weinstein JN, Herkowitz H, et al., eds. *The lumbar spine*, 2nd ed, vol. 1. Philadelphia: WB Saunders, 1996:473–491.
58. Weber H. Lumbar disc herniation: a controlled prospective study with ten years of observation. *Spine* 1983;8:131–140.
59. Lorio MP, Bernstein AJ, Simmons EH. Sciatic spinal deformity—lumbosacral list: an "unusual" presentation with review of the literature. *J Spinal Disord* 1995;8:201–205.
60. Finneson BE. *Low back pain.* Philadelphia: Lippincott, 1973.
61. Porter RW, Miller CG. Back pain and trunk list. *Spine* 1986;11:596–600.
62. Suk K-S, Lee H-M, Moon S-H, et al. Lumbosacral scoliotic list by lumbar disc herniation. *Spine* 2001;26:667–671.
63. Hoppenfeld S. *Physical examination of the spine and extremities.* Norwalk, CT: Appleton-Century-Crofts, 1976.
64. Scham SM, Taylor TK. Tension signs in lumbar disc prolapse. *Clin Orthop* 1971;75:195.
65. Spangfort EV. Lasègue's sign in patients with lumbar disc herniation. *Acta Orthop Scand* 1971;42:459.
66. Jonsson B, Stromqvist B. Clinical appearance of contained and noncontained lumbar disc herniation. *J Spinal Disord* 1996;9:32–38.
67. Hazlett J. Kissing spines. *J Bone Joint Surg [Am]* 1964;46:1368–1369.
68. Liang M, Komaroff A. Roentgenograms in primary care patients with acute low back pain: a cost-effectiveness analysis. *Arch Intern Med* 1982;142:1108.
69. Deyo RA, Diehl AK. Lumbar spine films in primary care: current use and effects of selective ordering criteria. *J Gen Intern Med* 1986;1:20.
70. Borenstein DG, O'Mara JW, Boden SD, et al. The value of magnetic resonance imaging of the lumbar spine to predict low-back pain in asymptomatic subjects. A seven-year follow-up study. *J Bone Joint Surg* 2001;83A:1306–1311.
71. Boden SD, Davis DO, David DD, et al. Abnormal magnetic resonance imaging scans of the lumbar spine in asymptomatic subjects: a prospective investigation. *J Bone Joint Surg [Am]* 1990;72:403–408.
72. Jensen MC, Brant-Zawadzki MN, Obuchowski N, et al. Magnetic resonance imaging of the lumbar spine in people without back pain. *N Engl J Med* 1994;331:69–73.
73. Metellus P, Fuentes S, Dufour H, et al. An unusual presentation of a lumbar synovial cyst: case report. *Spine* 2002;27:E278–E280.
74. Mullin WJ, Heithoff KB, Gilbert TJ Jr, et al. Magnetic resonance evaluation of recurrent disc herniation: is gadolinium necessary? *Spine* 2000;25:1493–1499.
75. Weber H. Lumbar disc herniation: a controlled prospective study with ten years of observation. *Spine* 1983;8:131–140.
76. Benoist M. The natural history of lumbar disc herniation and radiculopathy. *Joint Bone Spine* 2002;69:155–160.
77. Waddell G. A new clinical model for the treatment of low back pain. *Spine* 1987;12:632–644.
78. Fennell AJ, Jones L, Hukins DWL. Migration of the nucleus pulposus within the intervertebral disc during flexion and extension of the spine. *Spine* 1996;21:2753–2757.
79. Korenko P, Boumphrey F, Bell G, et al. McKenzie extension exercises in the treatment of acute disc prolapse: a prospective study. *Orthop Trans* 1985;9:509.
80. Hagen KB, Hilde G, Jamtvet G, et al. The Cochrane review of advice to stay active as a single treatment for low back pain and sciatica. *Spine* 2002;27:1736–1741.
81. Wiesel SW, Boden SD. Diagnosis and management of cervical and lumbar disease. In: Weinstein JN, Rydevik BL, Sonntag VKH, eds. *Essential of the spine.* New York: Raven Press, 1995.
82. White AH. Injection techniques for the diagnosis and treatment of low back pain. *Orthop Clin North Am* 1983;14:553–567.
83. Wang JC, Lin E, Brodke DS, et al. Epidural injections for the treatment of symptomatic lumbar herniated discs. *J Spinal Disord Tech* 2002;15:269–272.
84. Carette S, Leclaire R, Marcoux S, et al. Epidural corticosteroid injections for sciatica due to herniated nucleus pulposus. *N Engl J Med* 1997;336:1634–1640.
85. Waddell G, McCullough JA, Kummel E, et al. Nonorganic physical signs in low-back pain. *Spine* 1980;5:117–125.
86. Ito T, Yamada M, Ikuta F, et al. Histologic evidence of absorption of sequestration-type herniated disc. *Spine* 1996;21:230–234.
87. Ito T, Takano Y, Yuasa N. Types of lumbar herniated disc and clinical course. *Spine* 2001;26:648–651.
88. Minamide A, Tamaki T, Hashizume H, et al. Effects of steroid and lipopolysaccharide on spontaneous resorption of herniated intervertebral discs. *Spine* 1998;23:870–876.
89. Postacchini F, Giannicola G, Cinotti G. Recovery of motor deficits after microdiscectomy for lumbar disc herniation. *J Bone Joint Surg [Br]* 2002;84:1040–1045.
90. Wisneski RJ, Garfin SR, Rothman RH. Lumbar disc disease. In: Rothman RH, Simeone FA, eds. *The spine*, 3rd ed. Philadelphia: WB Saunders, 1992:671–746.
91. Matsunaga S, Sakou T, Taketomi E, et al. Comparison of operative results of lumbar disc herniation in manual laborers and athletes. *Spine* 1993;18:2222–2226.
92. Postacchini F. Results of surgery compared with conservative management for lumbar disc herniations. *Spine* 1996;21:1383–1387.
93. Saal JA, Saal JS. Nonoperative treatment of herniated lumbar intervertebral disc with radiculopathy: an outcome study. *Spine* 1989;14:431–437.
94. Albert TJ, Mesa JJ, Eng K, et al. Health outcome assessment before and after lumbar laminectomy for radiculopathy. *Spine* 1996;21:960–962.
95. Vucetic N, Maatanen H, Svensson O. Pain and pathology in lumbar disc hernia. *Clin Orthop* 1995;32:65–72.
96. Carragee E. Indications for lumbar microdiskectomy. In: *AAOS Instructional course lectures*, vol 51. Rosemont, IL: American Academy of Orthopedic Surgeons, 2002:223–228.
97. Junge A, Dvorak J, Ahrens S. Predictors of bad and good outcomes of lumbar disc surgery. *Spine* 1995;20:460–468.
98. Nygaard OP, Jacobsen EA, Solberg T, et al. Nerve root signs on postoperative lumbar MR imaging. A prospective cohort study with contrast enhanced MRI in symptomatic and asymptomatic patients one year after microdiscectomy. *Acta Neurochir (Wien)* 1999;141(6):619–622.

99. Atlas SJ, Keller RB, Chang Y, et al. Surgical and nonsurgical management of sciatica secondary to a lumbar disc herniation: five-year outcomes from the Maine Lumbar Spine Study. *Spine* 2001;26:1179–1187.
100. Delamarter R. Lumbar microdiscectomy: microsurgical technique for treatment of lumbar herniated nucleus pulposus. In: *AAOS Instructional course lectures*, vol. 51. Rosemont, IL: American Academy of Orthopedic Surgeons, 2002:229–232.
101. McCulloch JA, Young PA. Microsurgery for lumbar disc herniations. In: *Essentials of spinal microsurgery*. Philadelphia: Lippincott–Raven, 1998:329–383.
102. Guanciale AF, Dinsay JM, Watkins RG. Lumbar lordosis in spinal fusion. A comparison of intraoperative results of patient positioning on two different operative table frame types. *Spine* 1996;21:964–969.
103. Marshall LF. Complications of surgery for degenerative cervical and lumbar disc disease. In: Garfin S, ed. *Complications of spine surgery*. Baltimore: Williams & Wilkins, 1989;Chapter 6:75–88.
104. Bernsmann K, Kramer J, Ziozios I, et al. Lumbar micro disc surgery with and without autologous fat graft. A prospective randomized trial evaluated with reference to clinical and social factors. *Arch Orthop Trauma Surg* 2001;121:476–480.
105. MacKay MA, Fischgrund JS, Herkowitz HN, et al. The effect of interposition membrane on the outcome of lumbar laminectomy and discectomy *Spine* 1995;20:1793–1796.
106. Kjellby-Wendt G, Styf J. Early active training after lumbar discectomy: a prospective, randomized, and controlled study. *Spine* 1998;23:2345–2351.
107. Danielsen JM, Johnsen R, Kibsgaard SK, et al. Early aggressive exercise for postoperative rehabilitation after discectomy. *Spine* 2000;25:1015–1020.
108. Aydin Y, Ziyal IM, Duman H, et al. Clinical and radiological results of lumbar microdiskectomy technique with preserving of ligamentum flavum compared to the standard microdiskectomy technique. *Surg Neurol* 2002;57:5–13.
109. Schoeggl A, Maier H, Saringer W, et al. Outcome after chronic sciatica as the only reason for lumbar microdiscectomy *J Spinal Disord Tech* 2002;15:415–419.
110. Crock HV. Observations on the management of failed spinal operations. *J Bone Joint Surg [Br]* 1976;58:193–199.
111. Ebeling U, Kalbarcyk H, Reulen HJ. Microsurgical reoperation following lumbar disc surgery. Timing, surgical findings, and outcome in 92 patients. *J Neurosurg* 1989;70(3):397–404.
112. Law JD, Lehman RW, Kirsch WM. Reoperation after lumbar intervertebral disc surgery. *J Neurosug* 1978;48:259–263.
113. Pheasant HC. Sources of failure in laminectomies. *Orthop Clin North Am* 1975;6:319–329.
114. Spencer DL. The anatomical basis of sciatica secondary to herniated lumbar disc: a review. *Neurol Res* 1999;[21 Suppl 1]:S33–S36.
115. Antonacci MD, Eismont FJ. Neurologic complications after lumbar spine surgery. *J Am Acad Orthop Surg* 2001;9:137–145.
116. Connolly ES. Surgery for recurrent lumbar disc herniations. *Clin Neurosurg* 1992;39:211–216.
117. O'Sullivan MG, Connolly AE, Buckley TF. Recurrent lumbar disc protrusion. *Br J Neurosurg* 1990;4:319–325.
118. Jonsson B, Stromqvist B. Clinical characteristics of recurrent sciatica after lumbar discectomy. *Spine* 1996;21:500–505.
119. Zeidman SM, Long DM. Failed back surgery syndrome. In: Menezes AH, Sonntag VKH. *Principles of spinal surgery*, vol. 1. New York: McGraw-Hill, 1996:657–679.
120. Piotrowski WP, Krombholz MA, Muhl B. Spondylodiscitis after lumbar disc surgery. *Neurosurg Rev* 1994;17:189–193.
121. Rhode, V, Meyer B, Schaller C, et al. Spondylodiscitis after lumbar discectomy: incidence and a proposal for prophylaxis. *Spine* 1998;23:615–620.
122. Dimick J, Lipsett PA, Kostuik JP. Antimicrobial prophylaxis in spine surgery: basic principles and recent advances. *Spine* 2002;25:2544–2548.
123. Horwitz NH, Curtin JA. Prophylactic antibiotics and wound infections following laminectomy for lumbar disc herniation. *J Neurosurg* 1975;43:727–731.
124. Rimoldi RL, Haye W. The use of antibiotics for wound prophylaxis in spinal surgery. *Orthop Clin North Am* 1996;27:47–52.
125. Weinstein MA, McCabe JP, Camissa FP. Postoperative spinal wound infection: a review of 2391 consecutive index procedures. *J Spinal Disord* 2000;13:422–426.
126. Hanley EN Jr, Shapiro DE. The development of low-back pain after excision of a lumbar disc. *J Bone Joint Surg [Am]* 1989;71:719–721.
127. Yorimitsu E, Chiba K, Toyama Y, et al. Long-term outcomes of standard discectomy for lumbar disc herniation: a follow-up study of more than 10 years. *Spine* 2001;26:652–657.
128. Cinotti G, Gumina S, Giannicola G, et al. Contralateral recurrent lumbar disc herniation results of discectomy compared with those in primary herniation. *Spine* 1999;24:800.
129. Suk K-S, Lee H-M, Moon S-H, et al. Recurrent lumbar disc herniation: results of operative management. *Spine* 2001;26:672–676.

CHAPTER 46

Lumbar Disc Disease

C. Lumbar Disc Disease in Children

Robert F. McLain

Children and adolescents account for approximately 2% of all patients presenting with disc herniation. Adolescent patients rarely present with neurologic signs but often do present with a positive straight-leg raising sign. As opposed to adult patients, 98% of children with disc herniation present primarily with back pain, some with and some without sciatica. Trauma is the precipitating cause in more than 50%, and associated anomalies, such as transitional vertebrae, spondylolisthesis, congenital spinal stenosis, and lateral recess stenosis, are common. As in adults, most herniations occur at the L4-5 or L-5 to S-1 levels (1). In contrast to adults, the classic herniated nucleus pulposus must be distinguished from the slipped vertebral apophysis in young patients. Apophyseal disruption frequently presents after acute trauma. Clinical signs and symptoms mimic disc herniation, but computed tomography (CT) and magnetic resonance imaging (MRI) studies demonstrate the displacement of the vertebral apophysis and a piece of adherent bone sitting within the canal. Differentiating a disc herniation from an apophyseal disruption is worthwhile, as surgical treatment may vary depending on the location and the size of the apophyseal fragment.

EPIDEMIOLOGY

Lumbar disc herniation is common in adults, producing severe leg pain symptoms in 1.6% of the adult population (2). In contrast, sciatica and disc herniation requiring surgical treatment is distinctly uncommon in children and adolescents. Large series of operative cases involving disc herniation report a prevalence of between 0.2% and 3.2% among patients younger than 16 years (3–6). Even then, most disc herniations among children and adolescents occur in the second decade, between the ages of 12 and 18 years. As in adults, men appear to be effected more often than women, by a ratio of 2:1 (7,8).

ETIOLOGY

Trauma

Most pediatric and adolescent disc herniations are associated in one way or another with trauma. Traumatic injuries may result in an acute disc herniation or ring apophysis disruption. Likewise, repetitive trauma and recurrent microtrauma have both been associated with herniated nucleus pulposus. Acute trauma may occur in injuries such as falls from height or motor vehicle accidents, whereas repetitive trauma is more commonly seen in athletic injuries occurring in gymnastics, football, or weightlifting, for instance.

Low back pain that is acutely associated with trauma should trigger a search for other causes of adolescent back pain, including fracture, spondylolysis, or previously asymptomatic spondylolisthesis.

The presence of disc degeneration at a specific level associated with acute back and leg pain may suggest the presence of instability due to an unrecognized spondylolisthesis, and full studies may be necessary to confirm the diagnosis. Rarely, an occult neoplasm or infection may become symptomatic after relatively minor trauma.

Individual Factors

Overall conditioning does play a role in determining the risk of disc herniation. Nutritional status, weight, and general conditioning may play a role in determining those patients at greatest risk. Postural habits and activity level may also relate to risk. At the same time, higher-demand athletes may be least tolerant of activity-related back and leg pain symptoms, and they may be most likely to seek a comprehensive evaluation to identify the pain generator.

Genetics

Roughly one-third of patients younger than 21 years with sciatic pain have been found to have a first-degree relative with sciatica (9); this compares to an incidence of only 7% among the general population. This strong genetic predisposition has been suggested by other studies (10,11). This predisposition occurs in adults as well, however, so it is not unique to younger patients (12,13). Younger patients may more fully express this predisposition, or a more virulent trait, as twin studies have shown very clear associations between heredity and precocious disc degeneration. Several authors have reported cases of monozygotic twins who have developed disc disease at the same age, including disc herniation (14–16). Other hereditary factors may predispose to symptom severity or impairment with herniated nucleus pulposus. It is likely that the presence of congenital stenosis, a familial trait, may predispose to more severe and intractable symptoms when disc herniation occurs. The lack of free space within the spinal canal ensures that mild to moderate disc protrusions have a greater impact on neural function than would be seen in "normal" individuals.

Congenital Malformation

Congenital anomalies or malformations of the lumbar spine are recognized in as many as 30% of young patients presenting with lumbar disc herniation (17–19). The existence of a transitional anomaly, such as a lumbarized S-1 vertebra or a complete or incomplete sacralization of the L-5 vertebra, may expose L4-5 and L-5 to S-1 discs to additional stress leading to herniation. Spina bifida may occur in as many as 15% of pediatric herniations, a prevalence considerably higher than seen in the general population. Congenital spinal stenosis may contribute to the clinical manifestation of sciatica associated with herniated nucleus pulposus or slipped vertebral apophysis (20,21). Although stenosis may not lead to a higher incidence of disc protrusion, the likelihood of a disc causing symptoms of intractable sciatica goes up as the space available for the nerve roots goes down.

Disc Degeneration

Disc desiccation and degeneration, as documented on MRI, is distinctly uncommon among asymptomatic teenagers. Among patients presenting with sciatic complaints, however, early disc degeneration and desiccation are often observed (22,23). Disc degeneration is often seen at the level of herniation but, more importantly, can be seen at multiple levels in the lumbar spine of patients who suffer a single-level herniation at L4-5 or L-5 to S-1 (22,24). Disc degeneration is seen at adjacent levels in up to two-thirds of patients who had a single-level herniation in the past.

PATHOANATOMY

The intervertebral disc consists of the nucleus pulpous, the annulus fibrosis, and the cartilaginous end-plates of the adjacent vertebrae. The end-plate of the immature spine is made up of hyaline cartilage adjacent to the nucleus pulpous, and a physeal cartilage ring adjacent to the bony vertebral body. The physeal cartilage is divided into a physeal plate, which is responsible for vertical growth of the spine, and a ring apophysis to which the outer layers of the annulus fibrosis and the longitudinal ligaments attached. The ring apophysis is a traction apophysis.

Between the ages of 10 and 14 years, the Sharpey fibers of the annulus insert into this structure, which forms a dense condensation of cartilage circumferentially around the outer rim of the end-plate. At the age of 14 years, the ring apophysis starts to ossify, and the Sharpey fibers become embedded in the bone on the outer rim of the vertebral body. At the age of 18 years, the ring apophysis fuses with the vertebral body as the epiphyseal plate ossifies and disappears. Up until the point where the ring apophysis ossifies with the vertebral body, the Sharpey fiber attachments of the annulus to the ring are stronger than the junction between the ring and the vertebral body through the epiphyseal plate. Because of this, the osteocartilaginous junction between the ring and the vertebral body is the weak point of the structure. Disc disruption occurring between the ages of 10 and 14 years, then, can occur through a disruption of the ring apophysis, in which the disc herniation forces not only the posterior annulus but also the attached osteocartilaginous ring back into the canal (Fig. 1). As this structure ossifies, an actual massive bone can be seen in the canal in addition to the disc material. This is best seen with CT scanning.

Herniation of the nucleus pulposus most often occurs through protrusion of the disc and annulus, in continuity, into the spinal canal compressing the nerve root or the thecal sac. A thin membrane formed by the annulus and the posterior longitudinal ligament typically covers the protruding disc, and true extruded fragments are uncommon. As in adult patients, the herniation is most commonly posterolateral, but there are instances in which the disc protrusion is central and subligamentous, producing generalized stenosis within the canal. These forms often produce more back pain symptoms than true sciatica, or may present with vague and nondermatomal leg pain symptoms in addition to back pain.

In addition to the mechanical factors involved in sciatica, the herniated disc produces a number of chemical mediators, which can trigger painful radiculopathy. Neuropeptides and cytokines generated by the degenerative nucleus pulposus can sensitize the nerve root and dorsal root ganglion, triggering pain and making the nerve root sensitive to otherwise normal stimuli that then also become painful. Because the herniation in children is most commonly subligamentous, it is unclear whether chemical mediators play the same role in adolescents as they may in adult patients with sciatica.

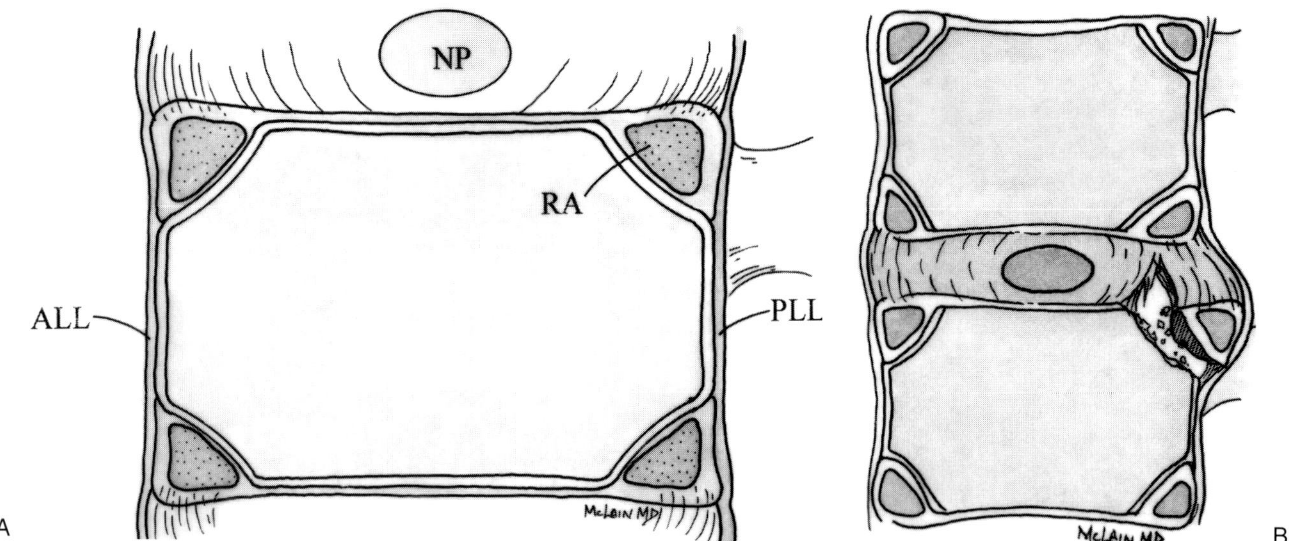

FIG. 1. A: The disc and end-plate of the immature spine. Between the ages of 10 and 14 years, the ring apophysis (RA) begins to ossify and becomes visible on radiographs. The Sharpey fibers that form the outer layers of the annulus insert into the ring apophysis. The apophysis remains separated from the vertebral body by the epiphyseal plate until approximately age 18 years. **B:** Slipped apophyseal ring injury. The posterior rim of the ring apophysis is displaced from the vertebral body, displacing dorsally into the canal. The outer layers of the annulus remain integrally attached to the ossifying ring. ALL, anterior longitudinal ligament; NP, nucleus pulposus; PLL, posterior longitudinal ligament.

CLINICAL PRESENTATION

Making the diagnosis of disc herniation in a child or adolescent patient is sometimes difficult, and the correct diagnosis is often delayed. Because the presentation of true sciatica is uncommon, and because children and adolescents frequently remain active despite their pain, clinicians are unlikely to obtain diagnostic studies early in the disease process. More often, the patient presents with a history of progressive back pain, stiffness, and pain with activity, which may be associated with unilateral or defuse leg pain symptoms. True neurologic deficits are uncommon; gait anomalous, antalgic scoliosis, pain with Valsalva's maneuver, and a positive straight-leg raising sign are all common findings. Adolescents often report an increase in pain with gym activities and may also experience increased pain and sciatica with prolonged sitting during class. Interference with school activities and classroom work is often a precipitating factor in seeking further medical evaluation.

DIAGNOSTIC STUDIES

Imaging studies have demonstrated an increased prevalence of apophyseal disruption beyond what has previously been recognized. Ring apophysis displacement accounts for between 19 and 32% of disc herniations in the 13- to 14-year-old subgroup (23,25). Associated lumbar anomalies, including spondylolysis and spinal stenosis, are also reliably identified through CT and MRI imaging. True herniated nucleus pulposus is easily seen on MRI, and the compression of the related nerve roots is best appreciated on this study. Plain radiographs are commonly normal but may demonstrate spondylolysis, spondylolisthesis, transitional vertebrae, or spinal bifida as associated anomalies in the patient with herniated nucleus pulposus. MRI also demonstrates the health or degeneration of adjacent level discs in children with a familial predisposition to herniation.

MRI also rules out most of the more ominous conditions that present in the differential diagnosis. These conditions include neoplasm, tethered cord, infection or discitis, and spondylolisthesis. Bone scan may be helpful in determining if a spondylolysis, which may be identified on plain x-rays or MRI, is an acute or chronic phenomenon.

TREATMENT

Conservative Care

Although some authors argue that conservative treatment is ineffective in children, this may be because patients with mild to moderate symptoms most often recover on their own and may not seek formal evaluation through a surgeon or spine specialist. The patients coming to full evaluation may, therefore, represent only the most severely involved. Among these patients, conservative therapy has been effective in as few as 25% of cases (1). Even when conservative measures are initially successful in reducing symptoms of sciatica, return to function often reaggravates the situation. Once the child tries to resume sports and other full activities at school, leg pain may reoccur. Another important factor predisposing to failure of conservative measures is the bony component of the ring apophysis disruption. Irrespective of conservative measures, bony fragments within the canal do not appreciably reabsorb or reduce in size with time or antiinflammatory medication.

Conservative measures that are most likely to benefit the adolescent patient include rest, antiinflammatory medications, and physiotherapy, including motion restoration and muscular strengthening exercises.

When acute sciatic symptoms present, the patient should be given an opportunity to rest from activities such as physical education and exercise, but he or she should also be restricted from other lifting and carrying activities, including carrying school books and heavy backpacks. Although 1 to 2 days of bed rest may prove beneficial in reducing acute symptoms, there is no evidence that prolonged bed rest benefits adolescent patients any more than it does adults.

Analgesic medications and muscle relaxants relieve spasm in the acute phase and permit activity during the most painful period. Antiinflammatory medications are beneficial after the initial period of pain, and epidural steroids may also provide some benefit. For patients with acute symptoms, a steroid "burst and taper" can sometimes provide excellent relief of neural symptoms but should not be repeated if symptoms recur.

In the early phase after disc herniation, light massage, local heat, or transcutaneous nerve stimulation may reduce muscle spasm and contraction. Passive modalities should give way to active modalities early on, however, and a program of muscle strengthening, stretching, and retraining of posture and daily active provide more benefit.

If symptoms persist at a level that impairs return to normal routine and physical activity, then conservative therapy may be considered a failure. At this point, operative treatment may become necessary.

Operative Intervention

Diagnostic studies must confirm the physical examination and patient complaints if the surgeon is to have confidence that disc excision will be successful. MRI and CT studies demonstrate whether the herniation is central or lateral, and whether there is a sequestered disc fragment or a ring apophysis fragment attached to annulus. These studies also demonstrate whether there is a component of spinal stenosis contributing to the patient's symptoms. Furthermore, preoperative studies confirm that the herniation is single level, and give the surgeon information about the health of adjacent-level discs.

The goal of surgical treatment is to remove pressure from the nerve root and thecal sac. When the patient has a focal herniation with discrete pressure on the nerve root, annulotomy and removal of the extruded nucleus pulposus fragment is likely to be successful by itself. Large, broad-based bulges, often seen in subligamentous herniations, may require more extensive discectomy. In these cases, enough material must be removed that the thecal sac is decompressed across the entire breadth of the extrusion. Removal of overlying lamina during the hemilaminotomy may further decompress the neural elements in these cases of more advanced degenerative disease. In cases of ring apophysis disruption, nuclear material may not be extruded into the canal or under the root. In these cases, excision of the avulsed fragment and its attached annulus may complete the decompression, and débridement of the nucleus pulposus may not be necessary.

Surgical excision is typically carried out through a microdiscectomy approach. Every attempt should be made to maintain normal structures to the best of the surgeon's ability, and a small surgical incision with limited dissection of the paraspinous muscles allows the most rapid and complete return to function after surgery. After identifying the proper level with a localizing x-ray, a small 2- to 3-cm incision is made over the interlaminal space. After elevating the paraspinous muscles and placing a small microsurgical retractor in the interval, the ligamentum flavum is released circumferentially and the lateral portion excised to allow exposure of the thecal sac. The operating microscope provides the surgeon binocular vision with excellent light during the decompression, even through a small incision. Once the thecal sac is mobilized medially, exposing the disc herniation, the annulus can be divided with a blunt probe in the craniocaudal direction, splitting the fibers as opposed to cutting them transversely. The extruded nuclear material can then be removed with a pituitary rongeur. If a broader-based extrusion is encountered, a wide annulotomy can be performed, removing redundant annular tissue along with the nuclear fragments. The avulsed ring apophysis may require sharp dissection and treatment before it can be removed completely to decompress the nerve root.

Cartilaginous fragments and pieces of bone should be fully removed from the canal. More so than in the adult, leaving fragments of displaced tissue in the canal may lead to ossification or fibrosis around the nerve roots in pediatric and adolescent patients.

Role of Spinal Fusion

Spinal fusion is rarely indicated at the time of discectomy. Only in a case of unstable spondylolisthesis should fusion be considered at the time of neural decompression, and most of these patients present with a long history of back pain and evidence of progressive slip as the primary indication for fusion. In these cases, discectomy and nerve root decompression may be carried out at the time of fusion. Recurrent disc herniation, occurring in 5% of adult patients, is very uncommon in adolescents. It would be rare to encounter this as an indication for fusion treatment.

Outcome

Surgical treatment of pediatric and adolescent patients with disc herniation is generally satisfactory. Eighty-five percent of patients in these age groups experience a good to excellent result after microdiscectomy and nerve root decompression. Radicular pain and back pain typically resolve soon after the operative procedure, and patients return to function rapidly. Long-term results tend to be good, but these patients experience degeneration and further problems because of their predisposition to disc degeneration and because of the normal progression of disc disease seen in the broader population. In Ebersold's study of patients, 21% underwent a second spine operation during a 34-year follow-up (26). Other authors have noted a 10% reoperation rate over a 3-year period of follow-up (27).

SUMMARY

Pediatric and adolescent patients presenting with persistent back and leg pain symptoms should be evaluated with CT and MRI to rule out more anomalous pathologies and to characterize the level of the extended disc disease or herniation. If a large disc extrusion or ring apophysis evolution is identified, the patient may require surgical treatment. Conservative therapy is still warranted as an initial intervention. If conservative therapy fails, surgical treatment can provide excellent relief of pain and return to function. Microdiscectomy is the most appropriate approach to these patients.

REFERENCES

1. DeLuca PF, Mason DE, Weiand R, et al. Excision of herniated nucleus pulposus in children and adolescents. *J Pediatr Orthop* 1994;14(3):318–322.
2. Deyo RA, Loeser J, Bigos S. Herniated lumbar intervertebral disc. *Ann Intern Med* 1986;315:1064.
3. Epstein JA, Lavine LS. Herniated lumbar intervertebral discs in teenage children. *J Neurosurg* 1964;21:1070–1075.
4. Giroux JC, Leclercq TA. Lumbar disc excision in the second decade. *Spine* 1982;7:168–170.
5. Raaf J. Some observations regarding 905 patients operated upon for protruded lumbar intervertebral disc. *Am J Surg* 1959;97:388–399.
6. Webb JH, Svien HJ, Kennedy RU. Protruded lumbar intervertebral discs in children. *JAMA* 1954;154:1153–1154.
7. Bradford DS, Garcia A. Lumbar intervertebral disc herniations in children and adolescents. *Orthop Gun North Am* 1971;2:583–592.
8. Clarke NMP, Cleak DK. Intervertebral lumbar disc prolapse in children and adolescents. *J Pediatr Orthop* 1983;3:202–206.
9. Varlotta GP, Brown MD, Kelsey JL, et al. Familial predisposition for herniation of a lumbar disc in patients who are less than twenty-one years old. *J Bone Joint Surg [Am]* 1991;73:124–128.
10. Matsui H, Terahata N, Tsuji H, et al. Familial predisposition and clustering for juvenile lumbar disc herniation. *Spine* 1992;17(11):1323–1328.
11. Nelson CI, Janecki CJ, Gildenberg PL, et al. Disc protrusions in the young. *CORR Gun Orthop* 1972;88:142–150.
12. Postaccini F, Lami R, Pugliese O. Familial predisposition to discogenic low back pain. An epidemiologic and immunogenetic study. *Spine* 1988;13:1403–1406.
13. Simmons ED Jr, Guntupalli M, Kowalski JM, et al. Familial predisposition for degenerative disc disease. A case control study. *Spine* 1996;21(13):1527–1529.
14. Gunzburg R, Fraser RD, Fraser GA. Lumbar intervertebral disc prolapse in teenage twins. *J Bone Joint Surg [Br]* 1990;72:914–916.
15. Matsui H, Tsuji H, Terahata N. Juvenile lumbar herniated nucleus pulposus in monozygotic twins. *Spine* 1990;15(11):1228–1230.
16. Obukhov SK, Hankenson L, Manka M, et al. Multilevel lumbar disc herniation in 12-year-old twins. *Child Nerv* Sys 1996;12(3):169–171.
17. Bradford DS, Garcia A. Herniations of the lumbar intervertebral disc in children and adolescents. *JAMA* 1969;210:2045–2051.
18. DeOrio JK, Bianco AJ Jr. Lumbar disc excision in children and adolescents. *J Bone Joint Surg [Am]* 1982;64:991–996.
19. O'Connell JEA. Intervertebral disc protrusions in children and adolescents. *Br J Surg* 1960;47:611–616.
20. Epstein JA, Epstein NE, Marc J, et al. Lumbar intervertebral disc herniation in teenage children: recognition and management of associated anomalies. *Spine* 1984;9:427–432.
21. Hasso AN, McKinney JM, Killeen J, et al. Computed tomography of children and adolescents with suspected spinal stenosis. *J Comput Assist Tomogr* 1987;11(4):609–611.
22. Gibson MJ, Szypryt EP, Buckley JH, et al. Magnetic resonance imaging of adolescent disc herniation. *J Bone Joint Surg [Br]* 1987;69(5):699–703.
23. Luukkonen M, Partanen K, Vapalahti M. Lumbar disc herniations in children: a long-term clinical and magnetic resonance imaging follow-up study. *Br J Neurosurg* 1997;11(4):280–285.
24. Poussa M, Schlenzka D, Maenpaa S, et al. Disc herniation in the lumbar spine during growth: long-term results of operative treatment in 18 patients. *Eur Spine J* 1997;6(6):390–392.
25. Banerian KG, Wang A, Saniberg LC, et al. Association of vertebral end plate fracture with pediatric lumbar intervertebral disk herniation: value of CT and MRI imaging. *Radiology* 1990;177:763–765.
26. Ebersold MJ, Quast LM, Bianco AJ Jr. Results of lumbar discectomy in the pediatric patient. *J Neurosurg* 1987;67(5):643–647.
27. Fisher RG, Saunders RL. Lumbar disc protrusion in children. *J Neurosurg* 1981;54(4):480–483.

CHAPTER 46

Lumbar Disc Disease

D. Algorithmic Approach to Low Back Pain

Brian R. McCall and Sam W. Wiesel

The patient who presents with a chief complaint of low back pain often does not receive a definitive diagnosis. It is the task of the treating physician to accurately assess the patient, use diagnostic tests properly, determine a logical diagnosis, and initiate appropriate treatment. To successfully return patients to optimal function in the shortest period of time possible, precise, timely, and accurate decisions are critical. In this endeavor, a standardized approach to patients with low back pain is useful. The low back pain algorithm presented here is a set of well-delineated rules designed to guide diagnosis and treatment. These rules are designed as a limited number of steps to final resolution of the problem; however, each step presents a decision-making point for the practitioner.

TREATMENT GOALS

There are four major goals to treatment in the algorithm. The first, and most important, goal is the early, expedient return of patients to their normal activities. Most patients are naturally eager to return to their normal function, and proper treatment can facilitate their goal. Complete relief of low back pain is not always achieved, however, and patients are reluctant to return to their normal activities. The natural history of lumbar degenerative disease must be explained, and the patient informed that mild low back pain is a normal pattern of aging and not a crippling disease. Emphasis on the benign nature of the disease process often assists patients' return to function and alleviates their concerns.

The second goal of the algorithmic approach is to avoid unnecessary surgery. The annual incidence of back surgery is 40% higher in the United States than any other industrialized nation, and two to five times higher than that of Canada and England, respectively (1). This incidence is increasing far faster than population growth, rising 55% during the period 1979–1990 (2). It is critical in this environment to maintain the strict indications for surgery, which multiple outcome studies show to be necessary for success. Poor patient selection has been identified as the most common cause of surgical failure. One recent review of surgical cases revealed less than one-half of the patients had appropriate indications for surgery (3).

When strict criteria are applied, however, surgical intervention can be very successful. In a review of 800 patients selected for lumbar spine surgery using the algorithmic indications presented here, 90 to 95% had good results, and others have duplicated these results (4,5). Strict reliance on objective criteria for surgical intervention cannot be overemphasized.

Conversely, when nonoperative management has failed to adequately treat a patient who meets the strict indications, surgery should not be unduly delayed. Little is gained from continued ineffective treatment, and surgery for disc herniation has been shown to be less effective when delayed longer than 3 to 4 months (6).

The third treatment goal of the algorithm is the efficient use of diagnostic tests. Increased patient awareness and familiarity with the diagnostic tests available to the physician, particularly magnetic resonance imaging (MRI), can make judicious use difficult. Patients too often insist on the latest technologic study, not realizing it may not contribute to proper diagnosis and may even cloud it. Abnormal findings are commonly seen in 24 to 38% of asymptomatic subjects screened with myelograms, computed tomography (CT), discograms, or MRI (7). Use of these studies should be restricted until clinically warranted.

The last goal is to provide appropriate care while minimizing societal cost. In the United States, the total annual cost of low back pain has been estimated to exceed $50 billion (2). Low back pain is nearly pandemic in modern society, and it is imperative that the treatment of low back pain be conducted in a fiscally responsible manner. With a careful approach to the low back pain patient, appropriate treatment should be available at an economy of societal and patient cost.

ALGORITHM CONCEPTS

An ideal algorithm is one that solves a problem in a limited number of steps. A decision is made at each step in the process, and the goal is effective treatment with a minimal number of steps. A decision point is encountered whenever consideration of a diagnostic study, treatment intervention, or patient assessment is made. The algorithm may be followed in a sequential manner (Fig. 1), or it may be used in tabular form (Table 1). At each decision point in the disease process, the appropriate med-

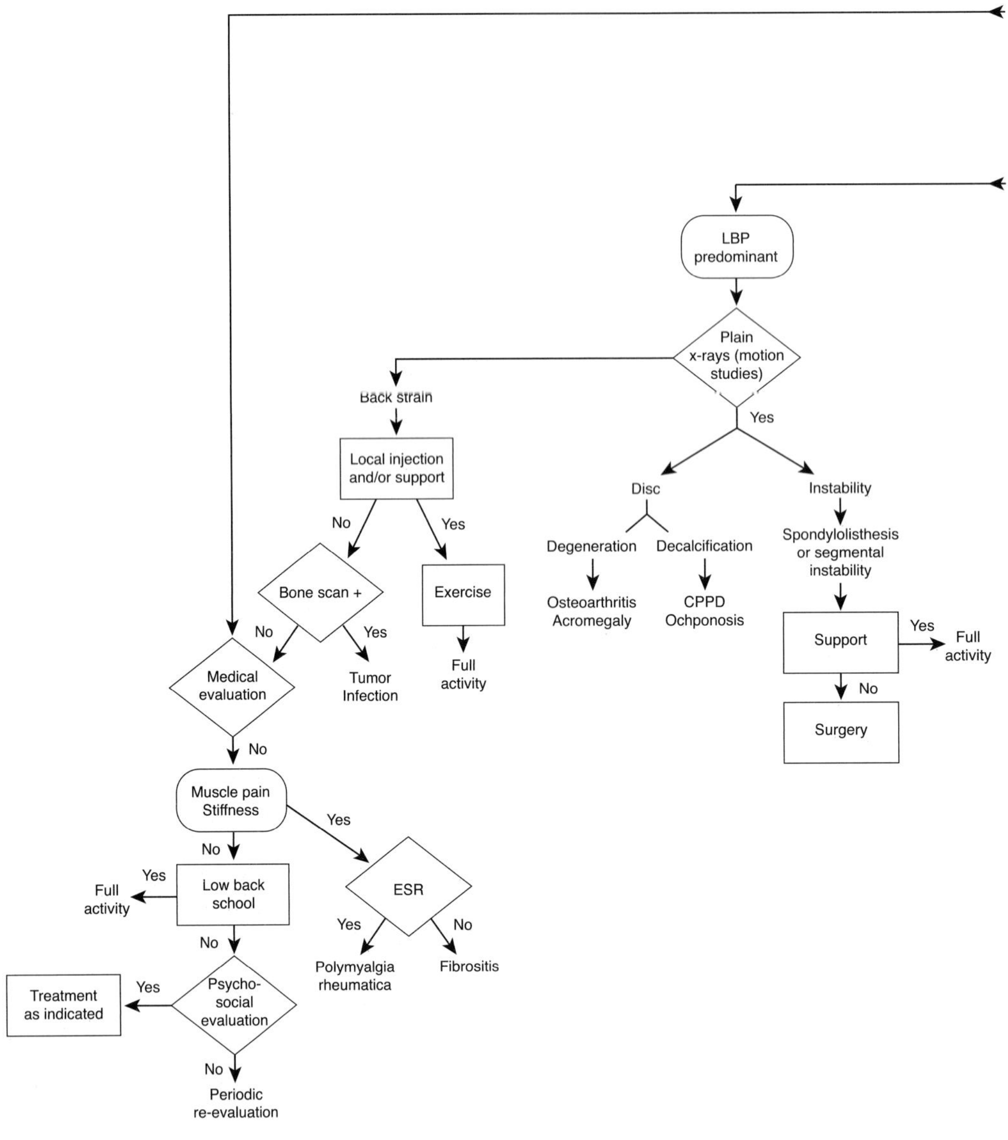

FIG. 1. Algorithm for the differential diagnosis of low back pain. CEC, cauda equina compression; CPPD, calcium pyrophosphate dihydrate; CT, computed tomography; EMG, electromyography; ESR, erythrocyte sedimentation rate; GTT, glucose tolerance test; HNP, herniated nucleus pulposus; IVP, intravenous pyelogram; LBP, low back pain; MRI, magnetic resonance imaging. (From Boden SD, Wiesel SW, Laws ER Jr, et al. *The aging spine*. Philadelphia: WB Saunders, 1991, with permission.) (*continued*)

ical literature is researched to delineate the correct pathway. When it is based on information derived from valid literature with sound methodology, statistics, and conclusions, an algorithm becomes a reasonable standard of diagnosis and treatment. It is estimated that when an algorithm is based on valid literature, it correctly includes 95% of the patients with a given set of symptoms for each decision point (8).

It is difficult, however, to create standards from the spine literature. Strict review reveals only a few definitive studies from which standards can be derived. The need for prospective, double-blinded, placebo-controlled studies on the natural history of back pain, as well as determining the efficacy interventions, is well recognized (9,10). Often, the literature has contradictory evidence on the effectiveness of many widely used nonoperative treatments. Barring high-quality primary trials that allow establishment of definitive, scientifically proven standards, the algorithm must be based on the consensus treatment guidelines derived from the literature. These guidelines allow less scientific data to be placed in

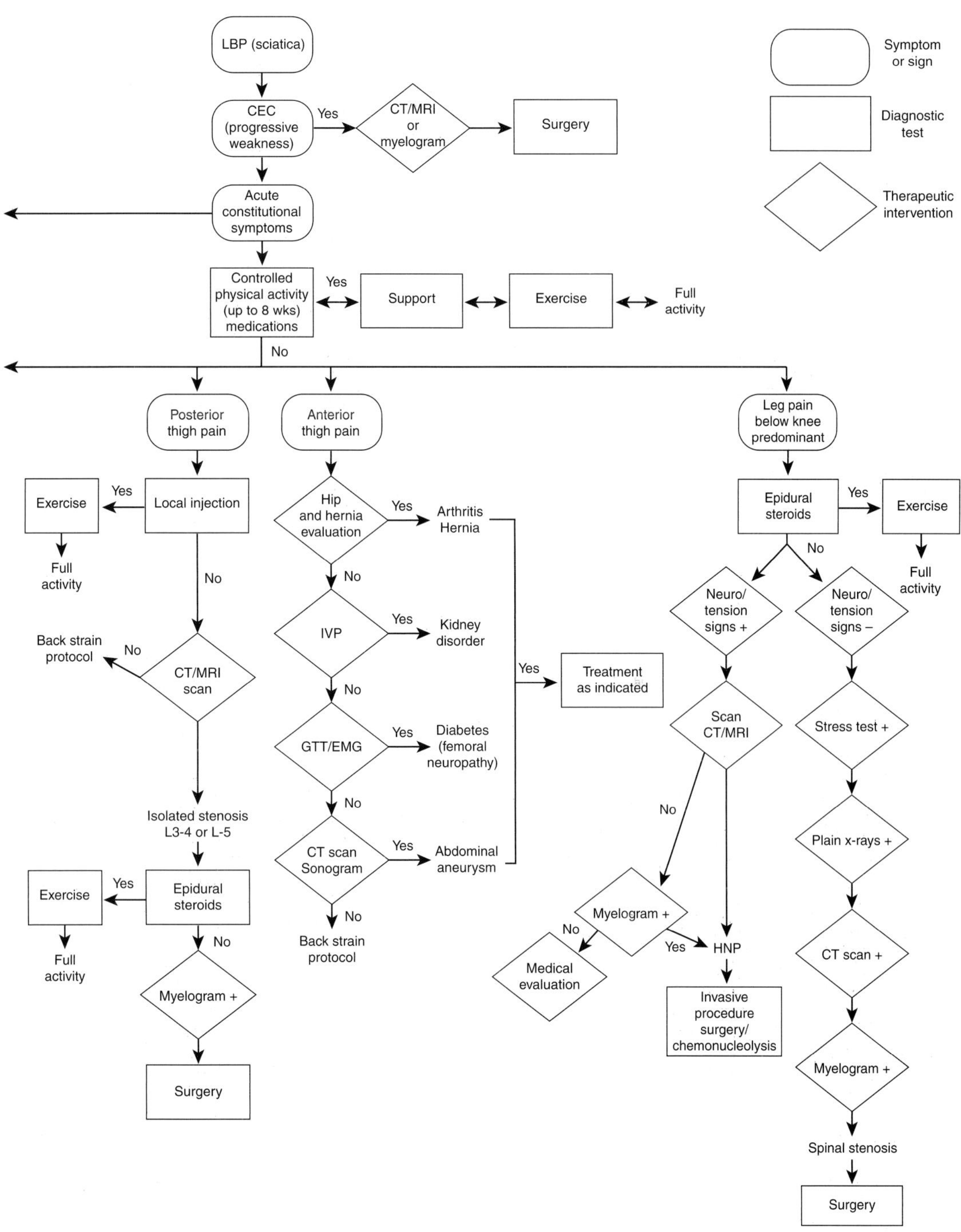

FIG. 1. *Continued.*

TABLE 1. *Differential diagnosis of low back pain*

Evaluation	Back strain	Herniated nucleus pulposus	Spinal stenosis	Spondylolisthesis/ instability	Spondyloarthropathy	Infection	Tumor	Metabolic	Hematologic	Visceral
Predominant pain (back vs. leg)	Back	Leg (below knee)	Back/leg	Back	Back	Back	Back	Back	Back	Back (buttock, thigh)
Constitutional symptoms					+	+	+	+	+	
Tension sign		+		±						
Neurologic examination		±	± after stress							
Plain x-rays			+	+	+	±	±	+	+	
Lateral motion x-rays				+						
CT/MRI		+	+			+	+			+
Myelogram		+	+							
Bone scan					+	+	+	+	+	
ESR					+	+	+		+	+
Serum chemistries							+	+	+	+

CT, computed tomography; ESR, erythrocyte sedimentation rate; MRI, magnetic resonance imaging.
From Borenstien DG, Wiesel SW. *Low back pain: medical diagnosis and comprehensive management*, 2nd ed. Philadelphia: WB Saunders, 1995, with permission.

the algorithm, and thus more deviation from the expected outcome may occur in patient care. Caution should be used to identify those who fall outside of the expected outcome in the algorithm and to alter care appropriately when needed. As further research becomes available, or as consensus guidelines change, it is necessary to update the decision points in the algorithm to reflect the new information. In fact, for an algorithm to be effective, it must be constantly updated based on new technology and research, as well as measuring outcomes from its use.

PATIENT EVALUATION

The information needed to use the algorithm is initially obtained through the history and physical examination of the patient. The history should allow the physician to focus on the subjective assessment of the patient's pain syndrome. Care should be taken to differentiate mechanical back pain from nonmechanical back pain; the latter is present at rest. The pain should be characterized in terms of location, radiation, type of pain (e.g., dull, aching, burning, dysesthetic), and whether there are ameliorating or exacerbating associations.

The patient should be asked about any recent trauma or changes in general health, as well as neurologic symptoms. Changes in bowel or bladder habits, progressive neurologic deficits, and symptoms of saddle anesthesia should be elicited. A thorough review of systems should be obtained, including constitutional symptoms, such as fever, chills, night sweats, or weight loss. These questions may point to systemic disease, infection, or neoplasm as the cause of back pain.

The physical examination is focused on gathering objective data about the patient's condition. The back posture, areas of tenderness, muscular spasm, neurologic findings, and nerve root tension signs are of chief importance. A complete examination should also include examination of the abdomen for masses or aneurysm and of the hips for arthritis and palpation of the peripheral pulses. Any suggestion of other medical problems should prompt complete examination of the involved organ system.

During the history and physical examination, attention should be given to any nonorganic signs demonstrated by the patient. These tests may help identify patients whose underlying psychosocial disorders may contribute to their symptoms and findings (11).

Cauda Equina Compression Syndrome

The first task incumbent on the physician is to identify any condition that necessitates immediate treatment. Cauda equina compression (CEC) syndrome is the major emergency entity possible for patients with low back pain. CEC is the result of central mechanical compression of the cauda equina. Classically, it presents in the third decade of life from an acute, massive herniation of the L4-5 disc, although more subtle presentations are reported.

The signs and symptoms of CEC are a mixture of low back pain, bilateral sciatica, saddle anesthesia, and even paraplegia with bowel and bladder dysfunction. Major progressive motor weakness should also generate suspicion. CEC may come from bone or soft-tissue pathology, but a large midline disc herniation is the most common cause.

When a patient presents with symptoms of CEC, immediate imaging of the spine with MRI or CT-myelogram should be obtained. If imaging is confirmatory, emergency surgical decompression should follow with a goal to stop the progression of neurologic loss. Successful recovery of neurologic function even after decompression is often poor (12). Although the frequency of CEC syndrome in the total population of patients is low, vigilance is warranted, as the consequence of missing the diagnosis can be disastrous to the patient.

Acute Medical Conditions

The next group of patients that needs to be identified has low back pain due to acute medical conditions. These patients often require urgent treatment for infection or neoplasms. These diagnoses should be considered in every new patient evaluation. Particular attention should be paid to young patients (younger than 15 years) and the elderly (older than 65 years). If constitutional signs and symptoms are present, a medical evaluation should be initiated. These patients should also be evaluated with plain radiographs and, possibly, bone scan and other imaging and laboratory tests to elucidate their pathology.

NONOPERATIVE CARE

The overwhelming majority of patients do not present with symptoms requiring immediate intervention. After excluding the emergent problems, the remainder of the algorithm is directed to the systematic evaluation and treatment of the other diagnostic possibilities. These patients, regardless of the specific diagnosis, are initially treated with a program of conservative, nonoperative therapy. At this stage, whether a patient has a herniated disc or a simple back strain is irrelevant because all diagnoses warrant the same initial treatment. Some of the patients eventually require an operation, but there is no means to differentiate between responders and nonresponders to conservative care.

Back Strain

The vast majority of patients in the initial group have nonradiating low back pain nonspecifically diagnosed as back strain or lumbago. The presumed etiology of back strain is varied. Possibilities include ligamentous or muscular strain, mechanical stress from poor posture, facet joint irritation, and a small tear in the annulus fibrosis. Patients report pain in the lower back, often localized to a small area. Physical examination demonstrates a decreased range of motion of the lumbar spine, tenderness to palpation over the involved area, and paraspinal muscle spasm. Plain radiographs are normal in most patients and are not needed initially. The exception to this rule are patients with a history of back trauma, known cancer, unexplained weight loss, fevers, and the very young or elderly patients. Radiographs should also be obtained in those who fail to respond to appropriate therapy to exclude other possible etiologic factors.

The early stage of the treatment of low back pain, with or without concomitant leg pain, is judicious waiting. The passage of time, use of antiinflammatory medication, and controlled physical activity are the mainstays of nonoperative treatment, and have been shown to be safe and efficacious in multiple studies (13–17). The vast majority of patients respond to this approach very quickly, usually within the first 10 days. Some patients do not respond as quickly, and the patients, family, and friends may advocate for more invasive procedures before they are warranted. It is critical to allow an adequate period of nonoperative treatment before proceeding further.

Activity Modification

Rest has traditionally been the first hallmark of therapy for the back. A brief period of rest allows injured tissues to heal, and often gives the patient substantial symptomatic relief. A brief period of bed rest up to 2 days may be considered but should not be prolonged, because there is no additive benefit (18–20). Patients should be encouraged to resume normal activity as their comfort allows but to avoid strenuous activity or prolonged sitting. Maintenance of normal activity level, within the confines of back comfort, has been shown to speed recovery (18,19). The speed at which a patient returns to activity should be monitored to guard against return of symptoms.

Drug Therapy

The judicious use of medication is an important adjunct to the treatment of low back pain. Antiinflammatory agents, analgesics, and muscle relaxants are the three mainstays of pharmacologic treatment (15,21).

Antiinflammatory medications are used based on the premise that inflammation of connective tissues is causing low back pain. Certainly, the herniated disc has a significant inflammatory component.

Many different antiinflammatory agents are available, and all appear to be equally efficacious for low back pain. For patients without gastrointestinal problems, aspirin and ibuprofen are effective and inexpensive. If the results are not satisfactory, other nonsteroidal antiinflammatory agents, such as naproxen or indomethacin, can be tried. For older patients or those with gastrointestinal problems, cyclooxygenase-2 inhibitors may be used. Any of the medications used should be employed in conjunction with controlled physical activity to relieve pain. Antiinflammatory medications may be used briefly in some patients, whereas others may find that a maintenance dose is required for a number of weeks to avoid recurrent back pain.

The use of narcotic medications in the treatment of low back pain should be avoided whenever possible. Occasionally, the patient's symptoms warrant narcotics. In these circumstances, the physician should maintain tight control of the patient's intake and access to refills. Narcotic medications are usually contraindicated in patients with chronic low back pain problems.

Muscle relaxants are not recommended for routine use in the treatment of low back pain. In most cases, spasm is related to an underlying primary problem, such as a herniated disc. When the pain from the herniated disc is controlled, the spasm often subsides. Occasionally, persistent spasm warrants the use of methocarbamol and carisoprodol. Diazepam or other central nervous system depressants are discouraged because they may exacerbate an underlying depression.

Braces and Corsets

As the patient responds to therapy, a lightweight, flexible corset may be used to assist mobilization. These devices are generally started when the patient has achieved significant symptomatic relief, and are used only briefly to speed the recovery of mobility. Nachemson has demonstrated a well-fitted lumbosacral corset can decrease intradiscal pressure in the lumbar region by 30% (22). Although effective in the acute care of low back pain, long-term use of a brace can lead to abdominal and lumbar muscle weakening, as well as contractures, and is not generally recommended. There are two exceptions in which long-term bracing seems reasonable. For the obese patient with weak abdominal muscles, a firm corset with flexible metal stays reinforces the deficient abdominal muscles. In the elderly patient with multilevel degenerative disease, exercise and strengthening is often not well tolerated, and a well-fitted brace may offer significant relief of pain. Most patients should be encouraged to strengthen the lumbar and abdominal muscles on the premise that they provide internal support to the spine.

Exercise

As patients increase their activity level, they are instructed to begin a program of exercise. This is one of the most common treatments used in patients recovering from low back pain episodes. Two regimens are commonly advocated: isometric flexion and hyperextension exercises. Both programs are designed to reduce the frequency and intensity of low back pain episodes, but there is no scientific evidence to support this contention. Several recent studies have found no significant effect of exercise therapy compared to placebo for acute back pain episodes (23–25). In other studies, however, recurrent back pain and work absenteeism were less in those who maintained regular exercise habits (26). Empirically, patients appear to have a positive psychological benefit from participation in exercise, and they like taking an active role in their treatment program.

Isometric flexion exercises were historically the most popular form of exercise for patients recovering from back pain. They are based on Williams' theory that a reduced lumbar lordosis causes back pain to decrease. This goal is achieved by strengthening the abdominal and the lumbar muscles, which are conceptualized to create a corset of muscles that supports the lumbar spine. Hyperextension exercises promulgated by McKenzie strengthen the paravertebral muscles. Generally, these exercises are begun after a patient has completed a full course of isometric flexion exercise. The strengthened paravertebral muscles can then be used as an internal support for the lumbar spine.

In the algorithm, the progression to exercise can be reversed if needed. If regression and exacerbation of symptoms occur, the patient can be stepped back to more conservative nonoperative treatment for a time. Most patients do not need this and proceed through the exercise portion of the protocol, returning to their normal life patterns within 6 weeks of the onset of symptoms.

Prognosis—Outcome

The vast majority of patients who present for low back pain are significantly improved within 10 days. Only 10% have symptoms that persist past 2 weeks, and with the normal nonoperative course, most return to normal activity by 6 weeks' time. If the initial management fails, the symptomatic patients are categorized into four subgroups. The first group consists of those in whom low back pain is the predominant complaint. The second group is composed of those who report mostly leg pain radiating below the knee, or sciatica. The third group of patients has anterior thigh pain, whereas the fourth group of patients has posterior thigh pain. A separate diagnostic approach is used for each group.

Refractory Low Back Pain

Patients who continue to report predominantly low back pain at 6 weeks should have plain radiographs carefully examined for abnormalities. Spondylolysis with or without spondylolisthesis is the most common structural abnormality to cause significant low back pain. Approximately 5% of the population has this defect, thought to be caused by a combination of genetic factors and repetitive stress (27). In spite of this defect, most of those affected are able to perform their normal activities with little or no discomfort. When symptoms are present, patients usually respond to nonoperative measures, such as education on the condition, a back support, and stabilizing exercise therapy (28). In a small percentage, conservative treatment fails, and a fusion of the involved spinal segment is necessary (29). This is one of the few indications for a primary fusion of the lumbar spine.

The vast majority of patients with refractory low back pain have normal plain radiographs. Without structural abnormality on radiographs, the diagnosis continues to be back strain. Before any additional investigation, a local trigger-point injection with lidocaine and steroid may be considered at the point of maximal tenderness. If there is a good response to injection, the patient may be progressed through increasing activity to strengthening exercise and return to normal activity. In some cases, when there are no objective findings, such a trigger-point injection can be considered as early as the third week of symptoms.

If the patient does not respond to local injection, other pathologic processes must be seriously considered and investigated, including tumors, infections, spondyloarthropathy, and referred pain from visceral disease. A medical evaluation should be obtained, and further radiographic evaluation should be pursued as well. A bone scan should be obtained to evaluate the possibility of neoplasm. A single-photon emission CT scan, which offers increased specificity with multiplanar views and superior detail, may be considered if available. MRI imaging is widely available, increasingly affordable, and sensitive and specific for many conditions affecting the lumbar spine. It is particularly important to obtain one of these imaging studies in the patient with nonmechanical back pain. If the pain is constant, unremitting, and unrelieved by postural adjustments, one must suspect an occult neoplasm or a metabolic disorder not readily apparent from other testing.

Medical consultation is important to evaluate these patients because as many as 3% of patients with low back pain who present to orthopedics have an extraspinal cause for their symptoms (29). A posterior penetrating gastric ulceration, pancreatitis, renal disease, and abdominal aneurysm are all medical issues that may first present as back pain and should be considered. Obviously, when one of these diagnoses is made, the patient should be treated appropriately as deemed by the medical team, and the orthopedic algorithm would no longer apply.

Patients with normal imaging and no other signs of medical disease as a cause of their back pain most likely have discogenic pain or facet joint pain syndrome. These patients are best treated by referral to low back school (30). The low back school concept is based on the belief that patients with low back pain can return to normal functional and productive lives when given proper education and understanding of their disease process. The proper and efficient use of the spine at work and in recreational activities is stressed, as is ergonomics. Back school may be as simple as a single educational session reviewing back problems and demonstrating exercise with patient participation, or it may be more involved. Even the single-session back schools have been shown to be effective. It is critical to properly screen patients before allocating them to this treatment, to avoid referral of a patient with a neoplasm or psychiatric disturbance.

Facet joint pain has been extensively studied with selective injections as a diagnostic and therapeutic role. Although selective injection with local anesthetic is thought to confirm the diagnosis in some cases, the role of therapeutic injections for facet joint pain remains highly controversial and cannot be included as part of the routine algorithm (31).

If the patient does not respond to back school, a thorough psychosocial evaluation should be obtained to evaluate the cause of treatment failure up to this point. This step is predicated on the understanding that a patient's disability is related not only to the pathologic anatomy but also to their perception of pain and the stability of the patient's social environment (32). The individual pain response is highly variable. It is common to see a stable patient with a large herniated disc continue to work, regarding the disability to be a minor problem, whereas a more unstable patient may be incapacitated with the slightest back discomfort.

Drug habituation, alcohol abuse, depression, and other psychiatric problems often contribute to the clinical presentation of low back pain. If an evaluation reveals any of these factors to be present, they should be addressed. An increasing number of ambulatory patients are recreational users or frank addicts of the medications commonly prescribed for back pain. Oxycodone, in the form of Percocet or OxyContin, and diazepam as well are some of the most popularly abused prescription medications nationally. When patients continue to need large quantities of these medications, one should be vigilant in considering that a secondary need or benefit may be prolonging their back symptoms. Care should also be used with diazepam, as it may exacerbate an underlying depression manifested as back pain.

Approximately 2% of patients who have low back pain fail to respond to treatment and elude any diagnosis (29). There is no evidence of any structural problem with the back and no criteria for underlying medical disease or psychiatric disorder. This is a difficult group of patients to manage. It is important to continue to work with these patients, as up to one-third eventually are found to have underlying medical causes for their back complaints. The continuing treatment of these patients is focused on discontinuing the use of narcotic pain medication, reassurance, and periodic reevaluation. These patients should be encouraged to continue as much physical activity as possible.

Refractory Patients with Sciatica

A chief complaint of pain radiating down the leg below the knee is characterized by the general term *sciatica*. These symptoms are produced by mechanical pressure and inflammation of a nerve root, which may be caused by soft tissue, such as a herniated nucleus pulposus, or by bone and osteophyte impingement. In patients who have had up to 6 weeks of appropriate controlled activity and medications but still have symptoms, it is appropriate to proceed with an imaging study to evaluate the pathology. MRI is the most commonly used study and provides excellent imaging while remaining safe and noninvasive. A CT-myelogram may be obtained if the patient cannot undergo or cannot tolerate MRI. These studies allow the physician to confirm the diagnosis and to validate the levels involved before proceeding further.

Epidural and nerve root injection should be considered as the next therapeutic step, and it can be accomplished safely and conveniently on an outpatient basis. Epidural injections have traditionally been the most popular technique, based on the concept of delivering strong antiinflammatory medication to the epidural space to reduce symptomatic inflammation. Multiple studies on the efficacy of this technique have been performed, with mixed results. Overall, one-half of the randomized clinical trials supports epidural steroids as being effective, whereas the other one-half does not. There is no relationship between the methodologic quality of these studies and their results (33). Nevertheless, an epidural injection of steroid may be a worthwhile treatment. One can expect approximately 40% success, with maximum benefit observed at about 2 weeks' time. The technique can be repeated two to three times, and ultimate patient response may lag 4 to 6 weeks behind treatment. Although success is not guaranteed, the technique carries low morbidity and may allow relief in patients who otherwise would be allocated to surgery.

Selective nerve root injections have become increasingly popular as another option for patients with sciatica not relieved by oral medication and activity modification. As with epidural steroids, selective nerve root injections deliver potent antiinflammatory medication to the epidural space with the added benefit of fluoroscopically targeted delivery to the effected level. The selective injection carries many potential benefits. First, the medication given is concentrated on the suspected pathology. Second, injection of fluid around the nerve root may break adhesions around the root and mechanically improve the environment. Finally, symptomatic relief from selective nerve root injection at a specific level can help confirm the pathology at that level as the cause of the pain. The efficacy of selective nerve root injections, like epidural injections, has been questioned. However, several studies have found selective nerve root injections to be cost effective, to decrease the rate of surgical intervention needed, and recommended in the nonoperative armamentarium for sciatica (34–37).

If injection therapy is successful in alleviating the patient's leg pain, a program of progressive activity and exercise is started. The patient is encouraged to resume normal activity as able; however, heavy labor and lifting is discouraged because of the risk of recurrent symptoms. This treatment regimen is usually completed in less than 3 months, and the majority of patients respond and do not need to undergo surgery.

If the injection therapy is not effective, the surgeon must consider surgery. The patient should be carefully reevaluated at this stage. If the patient continues to have symptoms and is found to have neurologic deficit and/or tension signs that correlate with unequivocal confirmatory pathology on MRI for the same level, surgery is indicated. If there is any question of the pathology on MRI, a CT-myelogram can be obtained.

Surgery has proven safe and effective in treating patients who have herniated discs when they fail to respond to conservative therapy. Successful results from surgery depend on rigid indications combining symptomatic pain, neurologic deficit and/or tension signs, and an abnormal imaging study to confirm nerve root compression. Patients without objective findings on physical examination should not be operated on based on abnormal imaging alone. The high rate of asymptomatic abnormalities on MRI and other studies, as discussed earlier, is well documented. When operative criteria are fulfilled, surgical success is reported with 80 to 90% good to excellent results over the short and medium follow-up periods, and equally good results after traditional or microdiscectomy techniques (5).

Spinal Stenosis

A second group of patients whose leg symptoms are based on mechanical pressure on the neural elements are those with spinal stenosis, a narrowing of the spinal canal due to hypertrophy and degenerative changes in the bone and soft tissue surrounding the thecal sac. This degeneration is a normal part of aging; however, it may become symptomatic as pressure builds around the nerve roots and may be quite pronounced in those who begin with a congenitally narrow canal. These patients may or may not have positive findings on neurologic examination or tension signs. If they are ambulated until their symptoms are reproduced, however, neurologic signs may often be elicited. Those who demonstrate this neurogenic claudication pattern are usually older than 60 years and are more frequently female.

The diagnosis of spinal stenosis can usually be made from plain radiographs that reveal facet degeneration, disc space narrowing, and decreased interpedicular and sagittal canal diameters. An MRI scan or CT-myelogram more clearly defines the pathologic anatomy and the levels of compression. Patients with spinal stenosis classically have a gradual decrease in function with periods of functional plateaus but without real improvement. If symptoms are severe and stenosis is apparent on imaging studies, surgical decompression is appropriate. Age alone should not be a deterrent to surgery. There are many elderly people in otherwise good health, outside of their spinal stenosis, who benefit greatly from surgical decompression of the lumbar spine (38).

Anterior Thigh Pain

A small percentage of patients have pain that radiates from the back into the anterior thigh or groin (or both). Rest and antiinflammatory medication usually relieve these symptoms. If the discomfort persists after 6 weeks of treatment, an evaluation should be initiated to find any underlying pathology that is contributing to this pain. Several possibilities other than an upper lumbar herniation with radiculopathy should be considered.

The hips should be carefully examined as part of any lumbar examination, and with anterior leg pain, the hips should again be carefully scrutinized. If there is any hint of abnormality on physical examination, an anteroposterior pelvic radiograph should be obtained. An inguinal or femoral hernia can be evaluated with careful physical examination, and referral to a general surgeon for evaluation should be made if this diagnosis is suspected. Kidney stones may also present as anterior thigh pain and can be evaluated by urinalysis, CT scan, or intravenous pyelogram. Peripheral neuropathy in the diabetic patient and meralgia paresthetica are also possible causes of anterior thigh pain or numbness. A glucose tolerance test or an electromyelogram/nerve conduction study should reveal these diagnoses.

Finally, a retroperitoneal tumor can place mechanical pressure on the nerves to the anterior thigh, causing painful symptoms. An MRI of the abdomen or CT scan to evaluate the retroperitoneal space should adequately address this possibility.

If any of these possible causes of anterior thigh pain are found, referral for appropriate care should be made. If no other cause for the back pain with anterior thigh pain can be made, the patient should be treated as a recalcitrant back strain by the protocol already outlined.

Posterior Thigh Pain

This group of patients reports low back pain that radiates into the buttocks and posterior thigh. Like all others entering the algorithm, they should be treated conservatively, and most improve by 6 weeks. Those who do not respond may be given a trial of trigger-point injection. In those who do not improve, it is important to distinguish referred pain from radicular pain.

Referred pain arises from tissues of the same mesodermal origin. The muscles, tendons, and ligaments of the posterior thigh and buttocks have the same embryologic origin as lumbar spine muscles, ligaments, facets, and discs. When the low back tissues are strained and injured, pain may be referred to the thigh or buttock. It cannot be overemphasized that referred pain cannot be cured by surgical decompression, whereas radicular pain is curable.

Radicular pain, as previously mentioned, is caused by compression and inflammation on a nerve root and proceeds along the anatomic dermatome for that root. A herniated disc or stenosis in the midlumbar area (L2-4) can cause radicular pain to the posterior thigh. An MRI scan should reveal nerve root compression if it is present. If it is not, the patient likely has lumbar strain with referred pain and should be treated as such in the algorithm. If compression is present, such as in disc herniation or stenosis, the patient should proceed with epidural or selective nerve root injections as outlined in the sciatica portion of the algorithm. If relief is not obtained, surgical decompression may be considered.

SUMMARY

In most cases, the treatment of low back pain is not a mystery. The algorithm presents a systematic method to guide efficient and effective decision making. It should guide the treating physician toward the appropriate intervention at the appropriate time when pathology is present, while hopefully avoiding unnecessary and costly diagnostic and therapeutic interventions. The algorithm itself is merely a framework into which new information and technology should be integrated as new research and development breach new horizons. In this manner, the algorithm may continue to represent the best and most efficient treatment of those with low back pain.

REFERENCES

1. Cherkin DC, Deyo RA, Loeser JD, et al. An international comparison of back surgery rates. *Spine* 1994;19:1201–1206.
2. Taylor VM, Deyo RA, Cherkin DC, et al. Low back pain hospitalization. *Spine* 1994;19:1207–1213.
3. Porchet F, Vader JP, Larequi-Lauber T, et al. The assessment of appropriate indications for laminectomy. *J Bone Joint Surg* 1999;81B(2): 234–239.
4. Garfin SK, Booth RE, Simeone FA, et al. Results of surgical decompression for lumbar nerve root compression. Presented before the Spine Study Group, March 1986.
5. Spengler DM, Ouellette EA, et al. Elective discectomy for herniation of a lumbar disc. *J Bone Joint Surg* 4990;72A(2):230–237.
6. Weber H. Lumbar disc herniation: a controlled, prospective study with ten years of observation. *Spine* 1984;8:131.
7. Borenstein DG, O'Mara JW Jr, Boden SD, et al. The value of magnetic resonance imaging of the lumbar spine to predict low-back pain in asymptomatic subjects. *J Bone Joint Surg* 2001;83A(9): 1306–1311.
8. Eddy DM. A manual for assessing health care practices and designing practice policies—the explicit approach. *Am Coll Phys* 1991.
9. Furlan AD, Clarke J, Esmail R, et al. A critical review of reviews on the treatment of chronic low back pain. *Spine* 2001;26(7):E155–E162.
10. Andersson GB, Brown MD, Dvorak J, et al. Consensus summary on the diagnosis and treatment of lumbar disc herniation. *Spine* 1996;21(24s):75s–78s.
11. Waddell G, McCulloch JA, Kummel E, et al. Nonorganic physical signs in low-back pain. *Spine* 1980;5(2):117–125.
12. Kostuik JP, Harrington I, Alexander D, et al. Cauda equina syndrome and lumbar disc herniation. *J Bone Joint Surg* 1986;68A: 386–391.
13. Dimaggio A, Mooney V. Conservative care for low back pain; what works? *J Musculoskel Med* 1987;4:27–34.
14. Postacchini F. Results of surgery compared with conservative management for lumbar disc herniations. *Spine* 1996;21(11): 1383–1387.
15. Weber H, Holme I, Amlie A. The natural course of acute sciatica with nerve root symptoms in a double-blind placebo-controlled trial evaluating the effect of piroxicam. *Spine* 1993;18(11):1433–1438.
16. Bush K, Cowan N, Katz DE, et al. The natural history of sciatica associated with disc pathology. *Spine* 1992;17(10):1205–1212.
17. Saal JA. Natural history and nonoperative treatment of lumbar disc herniation. *Spine* 1996;21(24s):2s–9s.
18. Hagen KB, Hilde G, Jamtvedt G, et al. Bed rest for acute low back pain and sciatica. *Spine* 2002;27(16):1736–1741.
19. Malmivaara A, Hakkinen U, et al. The treatment of acute low back pain—bed rest, exercises, or ordinary activity? *N Engl J Med* 1995; 332(6):351–355.
20. Deyo RA, Diehl AK, Rosenthal M. How many days of bed rest for acute low back pain? *N Engl J Med* 1986;315:1065–1070.
21. Basmajian JV. Acute back pain and spasm: a controlled multicenter trial of combined analgesic and antispasm agents. *Spine* 1989;14: 438–439.
22. Nachemson A, Morris JM. *In vivo* measurements of intradiscal pressure: discometry, a method for determination of pressure in the low lumbar disc. *J Bone Joint Surg* 1964;46A:1077.
23. Faas A, Chavannes AW, van Eijk JT, et al. A randomized, placebo-controlled trial of exercise therapy in patients with acute low back pain. *Spine* 1993;18(11):1388–1395.
24. Faas A, van Eijk JT, Chavannes AW, et al. A randomized trial of exercise therapy in patients with acute low back pain. *Spine* 1995;20(8):941–947.
25. Faas A. Exercises: Which ones are worth trying, for which patients, and when? *Spine* 1996;21(24):2874–2878.
26. Taimela S, Diederich C, et al. The role of physical exercise and inactivity in pain recurrence and absenteeism from work after active outpatient rehabilitation for recurrent or chronic low back pain. *Spine* 2000;25(14):1809–1816.
27. Federickson BE, Baker D, McHolick WJ, et al. The natural history of spondylolysis and spondylolisthesis. *J Bone Joint Surg* 1984; 66A:699–707.
28. O'Sullivan PB, Phyty GD, Twomey LT, et al. Evaluation of specific stabilizing exercise in the treatment of chronic low back pain with radiologic diagnosis of spondylolysis or spondylolisthesis. *Spine* 1997;22(24):2959–2967.
29. Hanley EN Jr, Levy JA. Surgical treatment of isthmic lumbosacral spondylolisthesis. *Spine* 1989;14:48–50.
30. Lonn JH, Glomsrod B, Soukup MG, et al. Active back school: pro-

phylactic management for low back pain, a randomized, controlled, 1-year follow-up study. *Spine* 1999;24(9):865–871.

31. Dreyfuss PH, Dreyer SJ, Herring S. Contemporary concepts in spine care; lumbar zygapophysial (facet) joint injections. *Spine* 1995;20(18):2040–2047.
32. Waddell G, Main C, Morris E, et al. Chronic low back pain, psychological distress, and illness behavior. *Spine* 1984;9:209.
33. Koes BW, Scholten RJ, Mens JM, et al. Efficacy of epidural steroid injections for low-back pain and sciatica: a systematic review of randomized clinical trials. *Pain* 1995;63:279–288.
34. Riew KD, Yin Y, Gilula L, et al. The effect of nerve-root injections on the need for operative treatment of lumbar radicular pain, a prospective, randomized, controlled, double-blind study. *J Bone Joint Surg* 2000;82A(11):1589–1593.
35. Karppinen J, Ohinmaa A, et al. Cost effectiveness of periradicular infiltration for sciatica. *Spine* 2001;26(23):2587–2595.
36. Narozny M, Zanetti M, Boos N. Therapeutic efficacy of selective nerve root blocks in the treatment of lumbar radicular leg pain. *Swiss Med Wkly* 2001;131:75–80.
37. Karppinen J, Malmivaara A, Kurunlahti M, et al. Periradicular infiltration for sciatica, a randomized controlled trial. *Spine* 2001;26(9): 1059–1067.
38. Spengler DM. Degenerative stenosis of the lumbar spine. *J Bone Joint Surg* 1987;69A:305–308.

CHAPTER 47

Determining Reasons for Failed Lumbar Spine Surgery

Christopher S. Raffo, Sam W. Wiesel, and William C. Lauerman

The success of lumbar spine surgery is not guaranteed. In fact, although 300,000 new laminectomies are performed yearly in the United States, 45,000 of these patients (15%) remain disabled (1). The patient who has undergone multiple surgeries with persistent or worsening pain and disability presents more frequently now than ever before. This complicated condition is termed *failed back surgery syndrome* (FBSS). As our aged population swells in the upcoming decades, the problem and likewise the cost will also expand. This presents an obvious problem in an era of rigid cost containment. The complexity of a multiply operated patient necessitates a methodical, precise, and cost-efficient evaluation.

It is worth restating the best chance for an excellent outcome from spine surgery is appropriate indications for that surgery. Conversely, surgery with inaccurate or inappropriate indications must be avoided due to its dismal chance for successful outcome (2,3). Precise correlation of symptoms and the physical findings with diagnostic imaging studies is essential, due to the high incidence of clinically false-positive myelograms, discograms, computed tomograms (CT), and magnetic resonance imaging (MRI) studies (4–6). Surgical exploration of the spine is no longer acceptable. The pathology must be well-defined and consistent with data gathered from the examination and advanced imaging. Due to increasing complexity with each revision operation, the first surgical procedure has the greatest chance for success.

The first decision in the evaluation of FBSS is to separate mechanical from nonmechanical pathology. Mechanical pathology includes herniated discs, segmental instability, and spinal stenosis. These conditions often respond favorably to surgical treatment because they directly compress the neural elements. Nonmechanical causes of lumbar spine pain include surgical scar, psychosocial conditions, and general medical problems. Nonmechanical conditions will not improve with surgery and, in fact, will probably further deteriorate. Differentiating between the two is critical in selecting surgical candidates.

The foundation to establishing a good outcome from the treatment of lumbar spine pathology is obtaining an accurate diagnosis. Although this seems intuitive, failure to accomplish this primary goal will lead to treatment failures.

EVALUATION

An organized approach to the evaluation of a multiple-operated low back patient is required both to simplify the evaluation and to prevent missing significant details. The history can be quite detailed and complex. Many patients desire to relate their chronology of back problems, and it is best to allow them the opportunity to do so. After deciphering the complex history, three historical points must be gathered.

The first is to clearly define the number and nature of previous operations on the spine. The number of previous surgeries correlates with the future outcome. The odds of successful results fall dramatically with additional operations. Historically, a second procedure for a given problem had only a 50% success rate, and further procedures often worsened the patient's condition (7–9).

The length of the pain-free interval is the second important historic point that must be obtained. If the patient awoke from the previous operation with the exact pain that brought the patient to surgery, it is likely that the nerve root was not decompressed completely, or the improper nerve root was decompressed. However, if the interval was 6 months or greater, the new pain may result from a recurrent disc herniation at the same or a different level. If the pain-free interval is 1 to 6 months, and the new symptoms gradually progressed, scar tissue is suspected (7,10). Epidural fibrosis and arachnoiditis cause this pain pattern.

The third essential historic point is the patient's pain pattern. If leg pain predominates, a new or recurrent herniated disc or spinal stenosis is likely the diagnosis. Scar tissue may also result in predominantly leg pain. Back pain, however, is suggestive of infection, instability, tumor, or scar tissue, but it may also be idiopathic. When back and leg pain are present in approximately equal intensity, spinal stenosis or scar tissue are suggested.

While gathering historic information, signs of psychosocial problems or psychiatric illnesses should be sought out and probed. Specifically, a history of substance abuse or the presence of known psychiatric diagnoses is of concern. Also, symptoms indicative of depression or anxiety, and the overdramatization of symptoms and physical findings should be noted and weighed during treatment. The presence of unsettled litigation or workers' compensation claims may portend a poor outcome for the treatment of spinal disorders.

After a thorough and detailed history, the physical examination is the next most important aspect of evaluation. Objective neurologic findings and the presence of a tension sign, such as the sitting straight-leg raise, must be sought. A documented and dependable presurgical examination from office notes and medical records is very helpful, as it allows comparison with the current examination. If the neurologic examination is unchanged from before the surgery and no tension sign is present, mechanical compression is unlikely. However, if a new neurologic deficit exists and a tension sign is also present, then radiculopathy is likely. However, as it may also be caused by epidural or perineural fibrosis, the tension sign is not pathognomonic for radiculopathy from a herniated disc or stenosis.

Special attention should be paid to nonorganic physical findings. Red flags include nonanatomic pain distributions or distraction signs. Waddell showed that presence of three or more nonorganic signs predicts a poor outcome from repeat lumbar surgery (8). Formal psychologic testing, such as the Minnesota Multiphasic Personality Inventory, can be useful in detecting nonorganic pain but should not replace the surgeon's attempt to identify well-motivated and adjusted patients (11). These are the patients most likely to benefit from further surgery.

Diagnostic Imaging

The final phase of the diagnostic workup of FBSS is the analysis of imaging studies. The patient should bring all previous studies, especially the original preoperative studies. Plain radiographs, dynamic radiographs, CT, CT-myelograms, and MRIs are all helpful. Do not exclude the possibility that preoperative studies from the previous surgical procedure may indicate that an inappropriate or incorrect procedure was performed. That (potentially) is the reason for failure of that surgery.

The plain radiographs yield valuable information, such as the extent and level of the previous laminectomy and the presence of spondylolisthesis or stenosis. Medially placed or short pedicles, which are readily seen on plain films, may be an indication of stenosis. It should not be assumed that the previous decompression was at the appropriate level. The preoperative studies, the postoperative laminectomy defect, the operative report from the prior surgery, and the patient's neurologic examination all must correlate precisely. Dynamic radiographs, specifically the weightbearing, lateral flexion, and extension films, are useful for assessing iatrogenic instability (12).

Plain CT imaging can show bony stenosis but is rarely used alone in evaluation of FBSS. CT with myelographic enhancement is more sensitive and specific in demonstrating impingement on the thecal sac and the nerve roots, and it also demonstrates arachnoiditis (13). Standard metrizamide myelography without CT is of limited use in the evaluation of FBSS. It identifies compression but cannot distinguish between disc and scar (14).

MRI remains the most useful and most frequently obtained diagnostic imaging modality. Some patients cannot undergo MRI, however, due to the presence of medical implants. For these patients, the other modalities discussed previously are used. MRI clearly differentiates scar from herniated disc material (15). The vascular scar tissue enhances with the intravenous contrast material, gadolinium-labeled pentetic acid. The avascular disc will not enhance.

MRI findings must be reviewed cautiously in the 6 months after surgery. During this time, even asymptomatic patients may have pathologic-appearing changes on MRI that seem to indicate recurrent herniation or scar formation (16,17). This limits the usefulness of this modality in diagnosing recurrent lesions at the operative level during this critical period. Finally, MRI is an excellent screening tool for other pathologic conditions, such as infection or a neoplastic process (16).

Functional tests, such as provocative discography and diagnostic facet injection, are of limited value in this patient population. The predictive value of these expensive, invasive tests has never been proven. Selective nerve root injection is an exception, which can be both diagnostic (by determining the pain contribution of a particular nerve root) and therapeutic. However, selective nerve root injection does not differentiate scar tissue from disc material. The authors also believe electromyography adds little to a thorough physical examination. However, nerve conduction velocity testing can be useful to distinguish peripheral neuropathy from spinal root compression.

DIAGNOSIS

The primary goal in the evaluation of a patient with FBSS is to arrive at the correct diagnosis. Only then can treatment alternative be planned with a reasonable chance for success. The lesions most often responsible for FBSS include persistent or recurrent disc herniation (12 to 16%), lateral (58%) or central (7 to 14%) stenosis, arachnoiditis (6 to 16%), epidural fibrosis (6 to 8%), and instability (less than 5%) (10,18). To standardize and simplify the approach to treatment of this complex problem, an algorithm has been developed. The algorithm assists by organizing the diagnostic criteria, helping to identify the correct diagnostic category, and directing treatment principles. The algorithm is presented in Fig. 1. Also see Table 1.

An important step in the algorithm is identifying nonspinal causes for back pain. Important medical diagnoses to consider are pancreatitis, diabetes mellitus, and abdominal aneurysm. All can mimic FBSS. A general medical evaluation by an internist or equivalent physician should be routinely obtained. In addition, any psychosocial abnormality should be identified, evidenced by

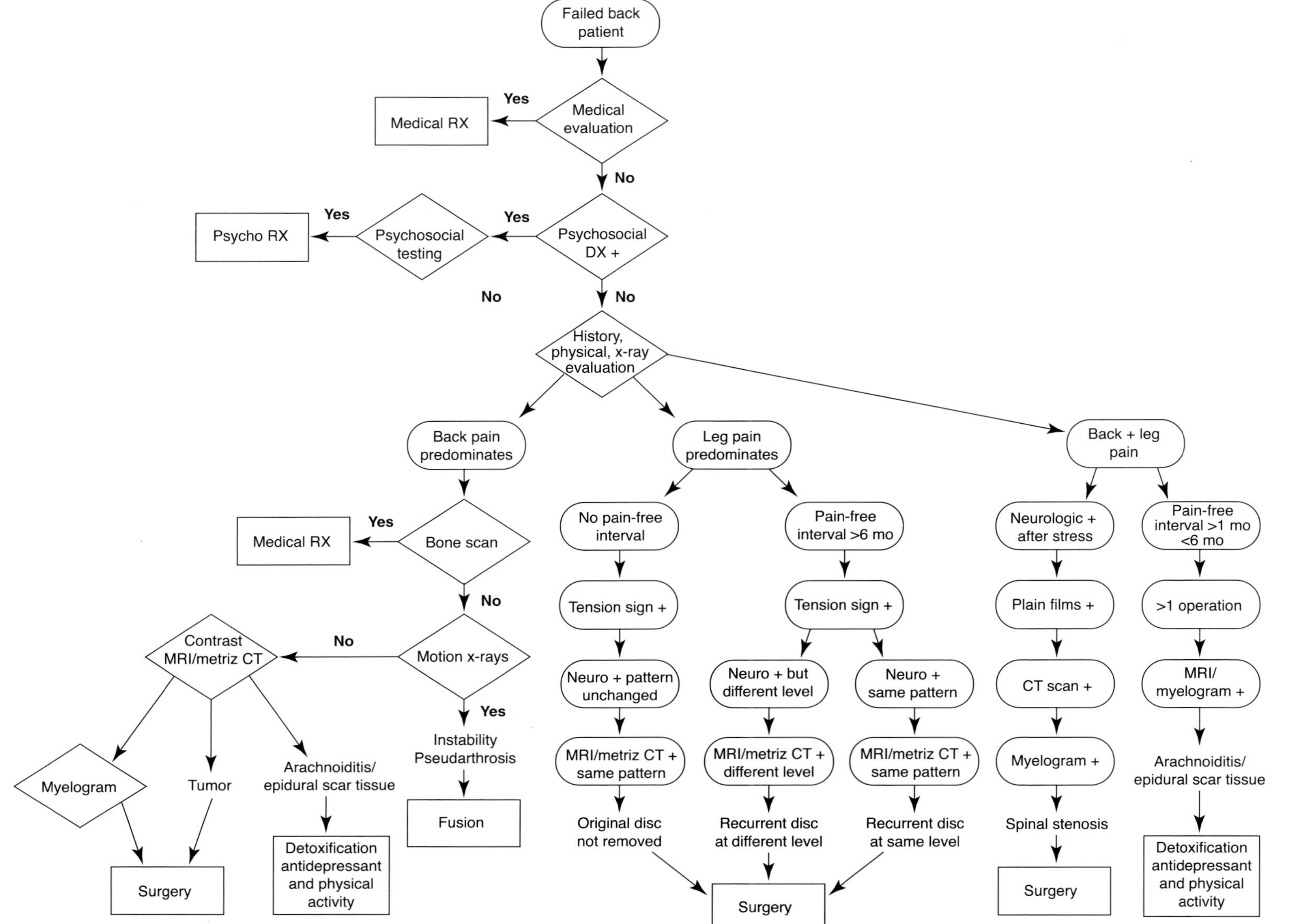

FIG. 1. An algorithm for evaluating failed lumbar spine surgery patients. CT, computed tomography; DX, diagnosis; MRI, magnetic resonance imaging; RX, therapy. (From Boden SD, Wiesel SW, Laws ER Jr, et al. *The aging spine*. Philadelphia: WB Saunders, 1991, with permission.)

TABLE 1. *Differential diagnosis of the multiply operated back*[a]

History and physical radiographs	Original disc not removed	Recurrent disc at same level	Recurrent disc at different level	Spinal instability	Spinal stenosis	Arachnoiditis	Epidural scar tissue
Number of previous operations	—	—	—	—	—	>1	—
Pain-free interval	None	>6 mo	>6 mo	—	—	>1 mo but <6 mo	>1 mo gradual onset
Predominant pain (leg vs. back)	Leg pain	Leg pain	Leg pain	Back pain	Back and leg pain	Back and leg pain	Back and/or leg pain
Tension sign	+	+	+	—	—	May be positive	May be positive
Neurologic examination	+Same pattern	+Same pattern	+Different level	—	+After stress	—	—
Plain x-rays	+If wrong level	—	—	—	+	—	—
Lateral motion x-rays	—	—	—	+	—	—	—
Metrizamide myelogram	+But unchanged	+Same level	+Different level	—	+	+	+
Computed tomography scan	+	+	+	—	+	—	+
Magnetic resonance imaging	+	+	+	—	+	—	+

[a]Table format of algorithm for treatment of failed back surgery syndrome.
From Boden SD, Wiesel SW, Laws ER Jr, et al. *The aging spine*. Philadelphia: WB Saunders, 1991, with permission.

alcoholism, drug dependency, anxiety, or depression. A psychologic or psychiatric evaluation is necessary in these patients. It is worth restating that patients with unresolved litigation or compensation issues do not respond as favorably to further surgery (19).

Of course, patients with psychiatric disorders may also have significant organic pathology. These patients are a particular therapeutic challenge and require careful coordination with the psychiatrist or psychologist. Ideally, addressing the psychosocial issues will reduce the somatic back symptoms and obviate the need for surgery. This is not always the case.

After eliminating those patients with medical or psychiatric diagnoses and those primarily motivated by secondary gain, the goal is to identify which patients have specific mechanical problems that may respond favorably to further surgery from those with symptoms resulting from scar tissue or inflammation.

Mechanical Lesions

Herniated Intervertebral Disc

Three possibilities exist if a herniated disc causes the symptoms associated with FBSS. The original pathologic disc may still be causing symptoms. This occurs when the proper level was insufficiently decompressed, when an incorrect level was decompressed, or when extruded disc material remains in the canal. Typically, leg pain predominates and is identical to the preoperative pain, as the nerve root remains mechanically compressed. The neurologic findings, tension signs, and radiographic pattern will be unchanged from the preoperative findings. The key historic point is the absence of a pain-free interval; the patient awoke in the recovery room with the identical, unrelieved pain. These patients benefit from a proper and complete decompression of the pathologic disc.

A recurrent herniation may also occur at the previous level, despite an adequate decompression at the index procedure. Typically, the patient awoke in the recovery room pain-free and remained so for at least 6 months. The recurrent herniated disc compresses the original nerve root, causing the identical symptoms. If contrast-enhanced CT or gadolinium-enhanced MRI demonstrate herniated disc material, further decompression is warranted. However, it is important to cautiously interpret advanced imaging studies for 6 months after surgery, as previously discussed.

Finally, a herniation may occur at a different level or on the contralateral side at the same level, causing a separate constellation of symptoms. The pain-free interval is typically greater than 6 months, but the process may occur at any time. Leg pain usually predominates, in an anatomic pattern consistent with mechanical compression of a newly affected nerve root. The tension sign should be positive. Again, if contrast-enhanced CT or gadolinium-enhanced MRI demonstrates a disc herniation consistent with the symptoms, the patient should benefit from decompression.

Lumbar Instability

Segmental instability is a poorly understood entity that may be implicated as an etiology in FBSS. *Instability*, defined as the abnormal motion between two vertebral bodies, results from the inability of the spinal motion segments to bear normal physiologic loads. Although deformity and neurologic deficits are potential complications of instability, pain is the most frequent result (20). The cause of instability in the FBSS patient may be related to the underlying degenerative process, spondylolisthesis or iatrogenic. The common iatrogenic causes are excessive surgical facet resection and pseudarthrosis, particularly when the fusion was

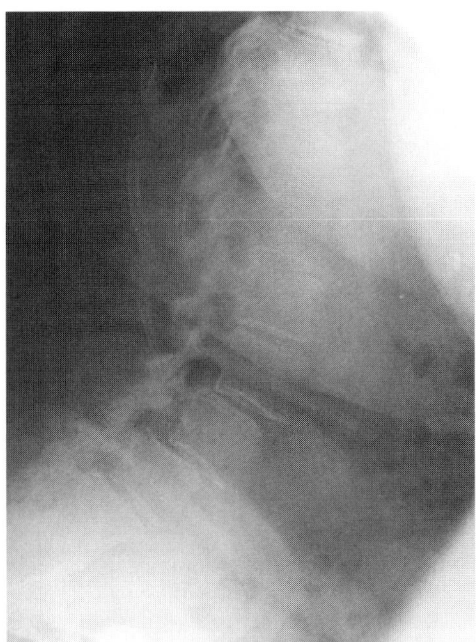
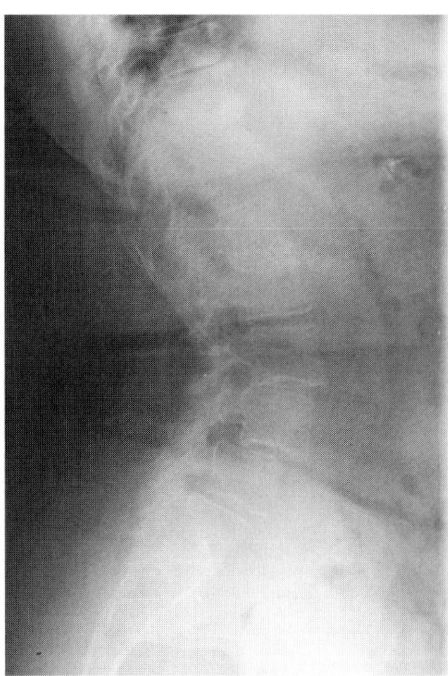

FIG. 2. Flexion and extension lateral radiographs showing instability in a patient who has had multilevel laminectomy.

performed for instability present at the time of the index procedure (e.g., degenerative spondylolisthesis) (21). Less common causes are a frank facet fracture or fracture through the pars.

The pain felt from segmental instability may be episodic. Particular activities, such as rising from a chair or straightening after forward bending, may provoke symptoms. Less commonly, instability can produce a dynamic stenosis, creating leg pain with certain movements. The physical examination is often normal, although a characteristic reversal of normal spinal rhythm may be noted on return from forward bending (22).

Diagnosis usually is based on weight-bearing and lateral flexion and extension radiographs (Fig. 2). Relative sagittal translation of 12% or angulation of 11 degrees is considered diagnostic for instability at L-1 to L-4 or L-5. At L-5 to S-1, however, 25% of translation or 19 degrees of angulation is considered a positive test (12). Progressive scoliosis or listhesis on serial postoperative radiographs is also indicative of instability. Instability has also been identified at previous discectomy levels at long-term follow-up (23). In one study, 30% of patients had excessive motion. The most common pattern was in women with a previous L-4 to L-5 discectomy.

Radiographic evidence of abnormal motion should be interpreted cautiously, because not all patients with this finding are symptomatic. In the absence of another identifiable mechanical cause for pain, patients with both pain and abnormal motion may benefit from fusion of the affected levels (14). Additionally, exploration of a pseudarthrosis may be indicated if abnormal motion can be documented. When abnormal motion is not present, surgery to fuse a pseudarthrosis has a low probability of success (24).

Spinal Stenosis

Lumbar spinal stenosis may produce back and leg pain in any patient, including patients with FBSS. The pain may result from progression of a degenerative spinal disorder, a previous incomplete decompression, or by overgrowth of a fusion mass.

The pain-free interval varies depending on the circumstances. If the previous surgery failed to completely decompress a stenotic canal, there may be no pain-free interval. Alternatively, the patient may be free of symptoms for months to years before the canal becomes sufficiently stenotic to again produce symptoms.

In general, the history and physical examination should be similar to any patient with lumbar spinal stenosis. Back and leg pain are typically present. The leg pain often is exacerbated by walking, although this is not essential to the diagnosis. The neurologic examination is typically normal, unless neurogenic claudication can be produced during an exercise stress test. Tension signs are generally absent (25,26). It is crucial to differentiate true neurogenic claudication from pain produced by vascular insufficiency.

Plain radiographic findings suggestive of stenosis are facet hypertrophy and degeneration, decreased interpedicular distance, decreased sagittal canal diameter, and degenerated and narrow disc spaces. Spondylolisthesis is commonly associated with central and lateral stenosis. Although it occurs most commonly at the L-4 to L-5 level, it can occur at the previous operative level. MRI clearly shows thecal sac narrowing and, with gadolinium enhancement, can help differentiate between compression caused by epidural scar and by hypertrophied soft tissue structures. Postmyelographic CT provides excellent visualization of bony encroachment on the neural elements centrally, as well as in the lateral recesses and foramina. However, CT cannot reliably differentiate scar from hypertrophied soft tissue (27).

If direct evidence of bony encroachment or mechanical pressure from hypertrophied soft tissue can be found on advanced imaging, good results can be expected from further decompression in at least 70% of properly selected patients. However, if gadolinium-enhanced MRI shows substantial scar tissue is present, the likelihood of pain relief is less certain. Perhaps related to this fact, patients who have undergone previous laminectomy and fusion respond less well to repeated surgical decompression (28). This point reiterates that the best chance for a successful outcome occurs at the time of the index procedure.

Nonmechanical Spinal Lesions

The previously discussed entities are all caused by direct compression of the neural elements, causing pain. Scar tissue and discitis are nonmechanical sources of recurrent pain in the failed back surgery patient. Although the pathology and anatomic location of these lesions are distinct, they are commonly discussed in conjunction because neither improves with additional surgery, and the treatment approach is the same. Postoperative scar formation in the spine is divided into two categories. Scar tissue that forms within the dura is referred to as *arachnoiditis*. Scar tissue that forms outside the dura is appropriately termed *epidural fibrosis*. Finally, the explosion of the use of segmental spinal instrumentation in this country in the past decade introduces a new component to the evaluation of nonmechanical back pain after surgery.

Arachnoiditis

Arachnoiditis is strictly defined as inflammation of the pia-arachnoid membrane surrounding the spinal cord or cauda equina (18). The extent of scarring may vary. At its most severe, the subarachnoid space is obliterated, and the flow of cerebrospinal fluid (and contrast agents) is obstructed. Although the precise cause is uncertain, previous lumbar spine surgery, intraoperative dural tears, and the injection of oil-based contrast agents are known precipitating factors (29). Postoperative infection may also play a role in the pathogenesis of arachnoiditis (30,31).

There is no consistent clinical presentation for arachnoiditis. The typical patient has back and leg pain that developed after a brief pain-free interval, classically between 1 and 6 months after the initial surgery. A history of multiple surgeries is common. The physical examination is generally not helpful, with any neurologic deficits attributable to previous surgery or pathology. CT myelography and MRI usually confirm the diagnosis.

At present, there is no effective treatment for arachnoiditis. Surgery has proved ineffective at relieving pain or reducing further scar formation. Several nonoperative therapies may succeed when combined with much-needed encouragement (2,18,31,32). The administration of epidural steroids, transcutaneous electrical nerve stimulation, spinal cord stimulation, operant conditioning, bracing, and patient education have all been tried. None of these therapies cures the condition, but all may relieve the symptoms for varying periods. All narcotics should be eliminated and amitriptyline hydrochloride (Elavil, Astra-Zeneca, Wilmington, DE) begun to help treat the symptoms. Encouraging the patient to remain as active as possible is also important. Treating these patients remains a significant challenge, requiring devotion and patience by both the physician and patient.

Epidural Fibrosis

Formation of scar outside the dura, on the cauda equina or directly on the nerve roots, is relatively common after decompressive spine surgery (33). The epidural scar tissue may act as a constrictive force on the neural elements and cause postoperative pain. However, whereas most postsurgical patients have some extent of epidural scar formation, only an unpredictable few are symptomatic.

Patients with epidural scarring may present with symptoms at any time, from several months to more than 1 year after surgery. The onset is insidious, and patients often report back or leg pain. New neurologic deficits are uncommon, but a tension sign may be present due to constriction and scarring around the nerve root. The condition is best differentiated from a recurrent herniated disc with a gadolinium-enhanced MRI (Fig. 3).

As with arachnoiditis, there is no definitive treatment for epidural scar formation. Therefore, prevention may be the best strategy. Until recently, a free-fat interpositional graft was used after laminectomy to hopefully reduce scar formation (34). However, a study comparing the use of Gelfoam (Upjohn, Kalamazoo, MI), interposed free fat, and placebo showed no statistical difference in preventing or promoting epidural fibrosis (35). Adcon-L, a recently introduced biodegradable gel matrix that was approved by the U.S. Food and Drug Administration for use after single-level laminectomy or laminotomy, reduces epidural scar formation in experimental studies. Although its use is attractive, its clinical efficacy is not entirely proven. Although Adcon-L is available for patients felt to be high risk for scarring, its routine use should be avoided until further studies show a distinct benefit in outcomes (36).

Once epidural fibrosis has formed, surgical treatment is not beneficial. More scar, in fact, forms from repeated surgical exploration. The treatment program described for arachnoiditis should also be used for epidural fibrosis.

Discitis

Discitis is an uncommon but debilitating complication of lumbar spine surgery. It is a localized inflammatory lesion of the intervertebral disc that follows a discectomy. The pathogenesis, although not completely understood, is thought to be direct inoculation of the avascular disc space (37). Severe back pain, usually beginning approximately 1 month after surgery, is the usual presentation. Signs on physical examination that may corroborate the diagnosis are fever, presence of a tension sign, and a superficial abscess.

If discitis is suspected, plain radiographs, blood cultures, an erythrocyte sedimentation rate (ESR), and a C-reactive protein (CRP) should be obtained. CRP is more specific than ESR, especially in the early phases of infection. Also, it normalizes more quickly than the ESR and in other orthopedic infections is commonly used as a marker of response to treatment. The classic plain radiographic findings of disc-space narrowing and end-plate erosion may not be present early in the disease, but a contrast-enhanced MRI should confirm the diagnosis.

The treatment of discitis remains controversial (37). Most commonly, the patient is restricted to short-term bed rest and immobilized with a brace or corset. With symptomatic improvement and normalization of the ESR and CRP, the patient may resume ambulation. Typically, the affected level undergoes autofusion in 6 months to 1 year (38). If pain progresses despite immobilization or constitutional symptoms develop, a needle aspiration is recommended. If an organism is isolated by the aspiration, appropriate intravenous antibiotics are administered, usually for 6 weeks. Often, an organism is not identified and broad-spectrum treatment is required. In an occasional patient, constitutional symptoms persist despite antibiotics, and radiographs show progressive disc space and vertebral destruction. These patients require open débridement and grafting.

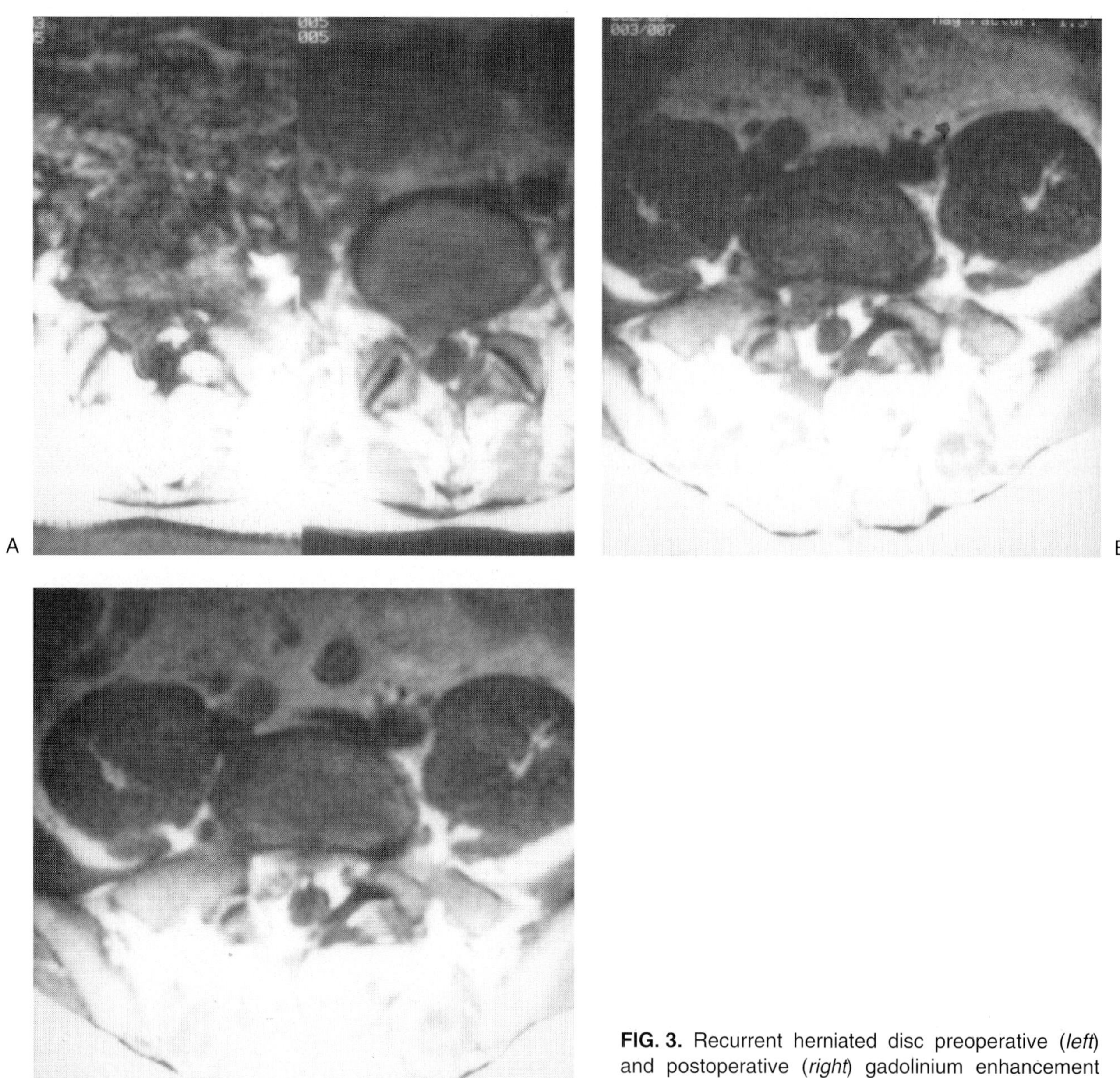

FIG. 3. Recurrent herniated disc preoperative (*left*) and postoperative (*right*) gadolinium enhancement **(A)**, scar-mimicking disc without enhancement **(B)**, and enhancing scar **(C)**.

Instrumentation

The use of instrumentation as an adjunct to lumbar spinal fusion has exploded in the last 10 years, almost exclusively in the form of pedicle-screw–based implants. This complicates the approach to the FBSS patient. It is the authors' anecdotal experience that more patients are undergoing lumbar spine fusion without objective indications, resulting in a high failure rate of clinical success. The presence of the implant itself raises several technical considerations relating to possible revision surgery, including the significance of screw breakage, implant loosening, infection, and aberrant screw placement. Finally, because of adverse publicity surrounding the use of these devices, their presence raises legal implications that at times further cloud a complicated clinical picture.

Pedicle screw instrumentation systems are inert orthopedic implants with an exceedingly low incidence of true allergy. Mechanical failure of the implant does not always represent an indication for removal or revision. The most dramatic mode of failure is breakage of the screw, typically at the shank-thread junction, which has been reported at a rate of 0.5 to 2.5% (39,40). Screw failure was historically quite common, even early in the postoperative period. With advances in material science and manufacturing, implant failure is now far less common. Furthermore, a broken screw often has questionable clinical significance and does not eliminate the possibility of a successful fusion. However, a recent study by Lonstein reported a correlation between screw breakage and pseudarthrosis. In this study, 12 of 19 patients who had a fractured screw had a pseudarthrosis (39). The authors recommended that all symptomatic patients with broken pedicle screws have the implants removed.

Other mechanisms of failure of these systems include screw loosening in the pedicle and vertebral body. This is a more common long-term finding, typically noted as a small zone of radiographic lucency above the screw. Again, no correlation between loosening and symptoms has been reported. Therefore, asymptomatic loosening, in the absence of pseudarthrosis with instability, warrants observation.

Finally, the risk of infection appears to be increased and has been reported as high as 5% (41). Although infection in the perioperative period is more readily diagnosed, late-onset infection has been reported and may represent a source of recurrent back pain after a pain-free interval. The patient with worsening pain several months or even years after an otherwise successful fusion may be manifesting late infection and should be evaluated accordingly. Some abnormality of the complete blood count, ESR, or CRP would raise suspicions of a chronic infection. These laboratory values have been critically evaluated in the total joint arthroplasty literature for their usefulness in identifying chronic, and otherwise undetectable infection, of an indwelling implant (42). A CT scan may reveal a fluid collection around the implant. Aspiration and culture of the wound or the fluid collection may further aid in accurate diagnosis.

SURGICAL TECHNIQUES IN THE MULTIPLY OPERATED SPINE

Surgery on the previously operated lumbar spine can be a considerable technical challenge. The actual technique of a repeat laminectomy is different than the initial procedure. There is increased morbidity, with increased risk of damage to the dura and neural elements. The specific technique for repeated laminectomy and repair of a dural tear are presented.

Repeated Decompression

The goal of decompression in the multiply operated back patient is identical to the goal for any spinal decompression: to safely and completely free the neural elements, without causing excessive hemorrhage. After previous decompression, however, the anatomic relationships are no longer normal, and the presence of scar tissue may complicate exposure and ease of decompression. Thus, several technical aspects of performing a repeated laminectomy are different from those for a primary procedure.

The first difference involves the operative approach. Stripping the paraspinal muscles away with impunity is not possible, because often no lamina or ligamentum flavum is present at the previously operated sites to protect the neural elements. This means the approach must begin at an adjacent anatomic level, which is normal and protected. This allows the surgeon to find the correct depth of the cauda equina (neural elements).

The surgeon may also be tempted, after the depth of the neural elements is determined, to remove the extradural scar tissue directly from the dura. Technically, this is difficult, and there is a great deal of hemorrhage and a high possibility of injury to the dura. Even if the scar tissue is successfully removed, there is no good way to prevent its reformation. Therefore, it is recommended that, in most cases, that extradural scar tissue should be left intact. Only tissue that is covering the area of pathologic change should be removed. Usually, the operative plane can be developed by elevating the scar (and dura) away from the bone at the lateral margin of the old laminectomy.

Finally, the nerve roots must be visualized laterally and any mechanical pressure on them removed. This is accomplished by extension of the laminectomy from the new level down the lateral gutters, leaving the central scar tissue intact. As each nerve root is then identified, any bony encroachment or herniated disc material at that level can be easily removed. It is essential not only to visualize the nerve root to the dorsal root ganglion and to enlarge the foramen, but also to ensure that the root is mobile.

Routine fusion in a multiply operated back patient is not necessary. If there are preoperative signs of instability on the lateral, weight-bearing flexion and extension radiographs, a fusion is indicated. Also, widening the laminectomy so that bilaterally 50% of the facet joints are destroyed at any one level or the pars interarticularis is thinned potentially destabilizes the spine. A bilateral, lateral fusion is recommended in these circumstances. The preoperative patient counseling and the surgical planning should reflect this possibility.

The integrity of a previous fusion mass should be checked during all revision surgeries for the possibility of a pseudarthrosis. A pseudarthrosis can be extremely difficult to detect, even by direct visualization. Unless there are objective signs of instability on flexion-extension radiographs, a nonunited fusion mass can be easily missed. After identifying the fusion mass laterally, an osteotome is used to shave off the outer surface. In a solid fusion, the bone is contiguous throughout. If a defect is identified, the area should be decorticated and new bone graft added. However, even a proven pseudarthrosis may not be responsible for a patient's symptoms. As stated previously, many pseudarthroses are asymptomatic, and caution must be used when deciding to treat an apparently painful pseudarthrosis with revision surgery and fusion.

Repair of Dural Tears

The rate of dural injury or tear is definitely increased in FBSS. The surgeon must be skilled in handling this complication. Although each dural tear is unique, certain basic principles always should be applied.

A dural tear usually occurs as the surgeon is gaining visualization of the spinal canal. After the tear is visualized, the surgeon places a piece of absorbable gelatin sponge (Gelfoam) over the injury site—with a large Cottonoid (Codman, Raynham, MA) covering the entire area—and obtains adequate exposure of the tear. The patient's head should be tilted down to decrease the flow of cerebrospinal fluid in the wound.

After adequate exposure is obtained, the surgeon's attention can be focused on repairing the tear with a watertight closure. If this cannot be accomplished, a cerebrospinal fluid fistula potentially may form, raising the risk of meningitis or the development of a subarachnoid cyst. A subarachnoid cyst can exert mechanical pressure on the neural elements.

The technique used to close the dura depends of the size and location of the tear. For simple lacerations, 4-0 silk sutures on a tapered, one-half circle needle are used. A running locking suture (Fig. 4A) or simple sutures incorporating a free fat graft (Fig. 4B) give a

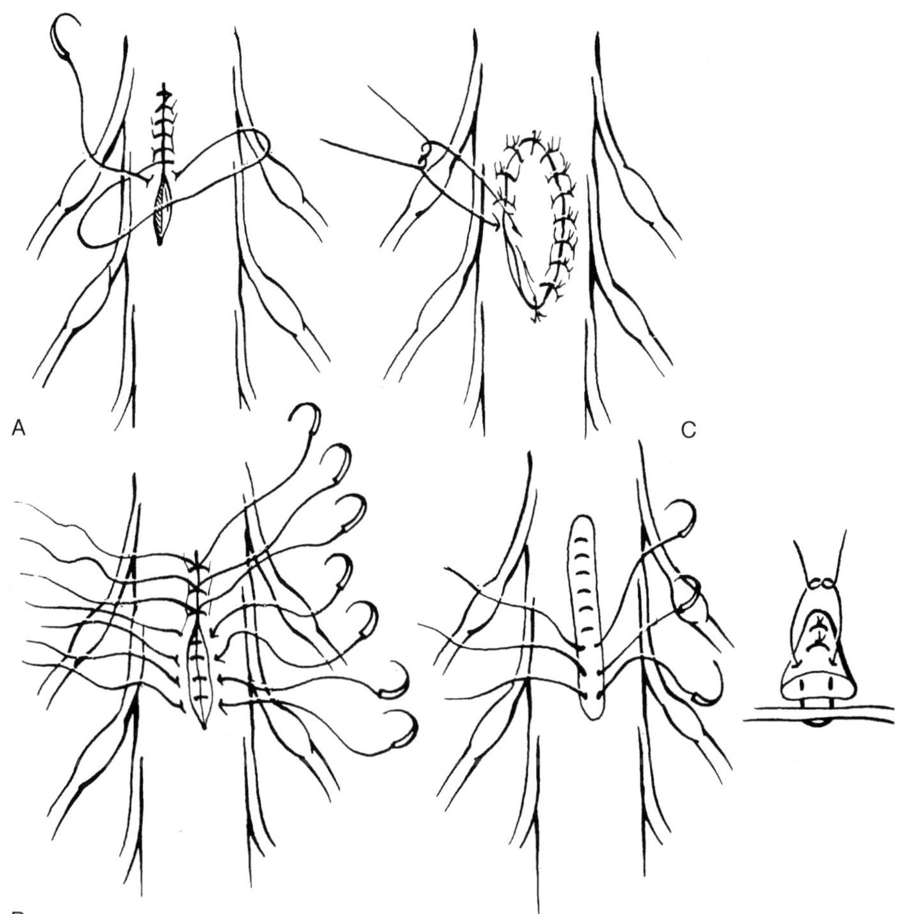

FIG. 4. Technique for dural repair. (From Eismont FJ, Wiesel SW, Rothman RH. Treatment of dural tears associated with spinal surgery. *J Bone Joint Surg* 1981;63A:1132–1137, with permission.)

watertight closure. If a large tear is present, a graft from the lumbar fascia is obtained and sutured in place with interrupted dural silk sutures (Fig. 4C). If the defect is in an inaccessible area, a small tissue plug of muscle or fat is introduced through a second midline durotomy and pulled against a tear from the inside of the dura.

To test the repair, the patient is placed in the reverse Trendelenburg position, and the Valsalva maneuver is performed. This maneuver increases intrathecal pressure and stresses the watertight closure. If no leak is present, the fascia is then closed with a heavy nonabsorbable suture to create another watertight barrier to the egress of cerebrospinal fluid. Drains should not be used, as drains may promote fistula formation. Postoperatively, the patient should be kept flat, on strict bed rest, for at least 3 days. The repair should heal by this time.

Prevention of dural tears is best achieved by excellent visualization and meticulous technique during exposure. Complete hemostasis should always be maintained. If there is any question about the presence of dura in the jaws of a bone-biting instrument, a Cottonoid patty should be placed between the dura and the bony structures to prevent dural injury. This is an easy and safe preventive measure.

CONCLUSION

FBSS will likely continue to rise with the high rate of lumbar spine surgery in our society. Prevention of FBSS is unquestionably more beneficial to the patient, because successful treatment of this condition is limited. Properly selecting candidates for lumbar spine surgery leads to more successful operations; however, many patients with FBSS were inappropriately selected for their original surgery, and further surgery only worsens their conditions. When considering revision surgery in these patients, a clear-cut diagnosis of nerve root compression or instability should be present. Nonoperative measures should be exhausted before operating.

The evaluation of a patient with FBSS is the critical step in the patient's treatment. The cause of the patient's symptoms must be accurately localized and identified, and a thorough investigation of the patient's psychosocial and general medical status is needed. Critical historic points are the number of previous operations, predominance of back or leg pain, and the duration of the pain-free interval. New neurologic deficits and tension signs are sought on physical examination. All imaging studies available should be thoroughly reviewed to corroborate the history and physical examination findings. When all the information is integrated, the physician can usually identify patients with correctable mechanical problems from those with epidural fibrosis, arachnoiditis, and discitis.

Physicians involved in the treatment of FBSS should realize there is little likelihood the patient will return to a pain-free state. Some level of permanent pain or disability generally remains. These patients should be counseled and encouraged to resume as functional a role as possible in society.

REFERENCES

1. Spengler DM, Freeman DW. Patient selection for lumbar discectomy: an objective approach. *Spine* 1979;4:129.
2. Laurie JD. Clinical problem solving: a pain in the back. *N Engl J Med* 2000;343:723–726.
3. Rothman RH, Simeone FA. *The spine*, 2nd ed. Philadelphia: WB Saunders, 1982.
4. Boden SD, Davis DO, Dina TS, et al. Abnormal magnetic-resonance scans of the lumbar spine in asymptomatic subjects. A prospective investigation. *J Bone Joint Surg Am* 1990;72:403–408.
5. Holt EP. The question of lumbar discography. *J Bone Joint Surg Am* 1968;50:720–726.
6. Wiesel SW, Bell GR, Feffer HL, et al. A study of computer assisted tomography. Part I. The incidence of positive CAT scans in an asymptomatic group of patients. *Spine* 1984;9:549–551.
7. Finnegan WJ, Tenline JM, Marvel JP, et al. Results of surgical intervention in the symptomatic multiply operated back patient. *J Bone Joint Surg Am* 1979;61:1077.
8. Waddell G, Kummell EG, Lotto WN, et al. Failed lumbar disc surgery and repeat surgery following industrial injuries. *J Bone Joint Surg Am* 1979;61:201.
9. Loupasis GA, Stanos K. Seven to twenty year outcome of lumbar discectomy. *Spine* 1999;24:2313–2317.
10. Fritsch EW. The failed back surgery syndrome: reasons, intraoperative findings and long-term results. A report of 182 operative treatments. *Spine* 1996;21:626–633.
11. Southwick SM, White AA. Current concepts review: the use of psychological tests in the evaluation of low back pain. *J Bone Joint Surg Am* 1983;65:560–565.
12. Boden SD, Wiesel SW. Lumbosacral motion in normal individuals: have we been measuring instability properly? *Spine* 1990;12:571–576.
13. Teplick JG, Haskin ME. Intravenous contrast-enhanced CT of the postoperative lumbar spine, improved identification of recurrent disc herniation, scar, arachnoiditis, and diskitis. *AJR Am J Roentgenol* 1984;143:845–855.
14. Byrd SE, Cohn ML, Biggens SL, et al. The radiographic evaluation of the symptomatic postoperative lumbar spine patient. *Spine* 1985;10:652–661.
15. Ross JS, Masaryk TJ, Modic MT, et al. Lumbar spine: postoperative assessment with surface-coil MR imaging. *Radiology* 1987;164:851–860.
16. Gundry CR, Fritts HM. Magnetic resonance imaging of the musculoskeletal system: the spine. *Clin Orthop* 1998;346:262–278.
17. Boden SD, Davis DO, Dina TS, et al. Postoperative discitis: distinguishing early MR imaging findings from normal postoperative disk space changes. *Radiology* 1992;184:765–771.
18. Burton CV. Lumbosacral arachnoiditis. *Spine* 1978;3:24–30.
19. Waring EM, Weisz GM, Bailey SI. Predictive factors in the treatment of low back pain by surgical intervention. *Adv Pain Res Ther* 1979;1:939–942.
20. White AA, Panjabi MM, Posner I, et al. Spinal stability: Evaluation and treatment. Presented at AAOS Instructional Course Lectures. St. Louis, MO: Mosby 1981;30:457.
21. Hazlett JW, Kinnard P. Lumbar apophyseal process excision and instability. *Spine* 1982;7:171–174.
22. Paris SV. Physical signs of instability. *Spine* 1985;10:277–279.
23. Frymoyer JW, Hanley EN Jr, Howe J, et al. A comparison of radiographic findings in fusions and non-fusion patients, ten or more years following lumbar disc surgery. *Spine* 1979;4:435–440.
24. Lauerman WC, Bradford DS, Ogilvie JW, et al. Results of lumbar pseudoarthrosis repair. *J Spinal Disord* 1992;5:149–157.
25. Spengler DM. Degenerative stenosis of the lumbar spine. Current concepts review. *J Bone Joint Surg Am* 1987;69:305–308.
26. Hall S, Onofrio BM, et al. Lumbar spinal stenosis: clinical features, diagnostic procedures, and results of treatment in 68 patients. *Ann Intern Med* 1985;103:271–275.
27. Bolender NF, Schonstrom NSR, Spengler DM. Role of computed tomography and myelography in the diagnosis of central spinal stenosis. *J Bone Joint Surg Am* 1985;67:240–246.
28. Nasca RJ. Surgical management of lumbar spinal stenosis. *Spine* 1987;12:809–816.
29. Quiles M, Marchisello PJ, Tsairis P. Lumbar adhesive arachnoiditis: etiologic and pathologic aspects. *Spine* 1978;3:45–50.
30. Epstein BS. *The spine*. Philadelphia: Lea & Febiger, 1962.
31. Coventry MG, Staufer RN. The multiply operated back. In: American Academy of Orthopaedic Surgeons. *Symposium on the spine*. St. Louis: Mosby, 1969;132–142.
32. Mooney V. Innovative approaches to chronic back disability. Instructional course lecture at Dallas. Dallas: American Academy of Orthopaedic Surgeons, January 1974.
33. LaRocca H, Macnab I. The laminectomy membrane: Studies in its evolution, characteristics, effects and prophylaxis in dogs. *J Bone Joint Surg Br* 1974;56:545–550.
34. Lahde S, Puranen J. Disk space hypodensity in CT: the first radiological signs of postoperative discitis. *Eur J Radiol* 1985;5:190–192.
35. Hinton JL Jr, Wreck DJ. Inhibition of epidural scar formation after lumbar laminectomy in the rat. *Spine* 1995;20:564–570.
36. Fischgrund JS. Use of Adcon-L for epidural scar prevention. *J Am Acad Orthop Surg* 2000;8:339–343.
37. Dall BE, Rowe DE, Odette WG, et al. Postoperative discitis: diagnosis and management. *Clin Orthop* 1987;224:138–148.
38. Pilgaard S. Discitis (closed space infection) following removal of lumbar intervertebral disc. *J Bone Joint Surg* 1969;51A:713–716.
39. Lonstein JE, Denis F, Perra JH, et al. Complications associated with pedicle screws. *J Bone Joint Surg* 1999;81A:1519–1528.
40. Steffe AD, Brantigan JW. The variable screw placement spinal fixation system: report of a prospective study of 250 patients enrolled in FDA clinical trials. *Spine* 1993;18:1160–1172.
41. Masferrer R, Gomez CH, Karahalios DG, et al. Efficacy of pedicle screw fixation and the treatment of spinal instability and failed back surgery. A five-year review. *J Neurosurg* 1988;89:371–377.
42. Munjal S, Phillips MJ, Krackow KA. Revision total knee arthroplasty: planning, controversies, and management—infection. *Instr Course Lect* 2001;50:367–377.

CHAPTER 48

Lumbar Spinal Stenosis

A. Pathoanatomy and Pathophysiology

John A. Glaser

PATHOANATOMY

The normal adult lumbar spine is between 11.5 and 30 mm in its anteroposterior diameter and between 17 and 42 mm in width (1–4). Foraminal height is between 20 and 23 mm, and foraminal width is between 8 and 10 mm (1,5,6). The nerve root moves between 2 and 5 mm within the foramen with motion of the lower extremity (7). Reductions in these dimensions can result in spinal stenosis.

Spinal stenosis is generally considered to be of two types, congenital or acquired. Congenital stenosis occurs at a younger age in those patients anatomically predisposed because of a spinal canal of smaller dimensions (8–10). Acquired stenosis is generally seen later in life and is due to encroachment on the neural structures from age-related degenerative changes of the spine or progressing spinal deformities. Compression of the neural elements can occur in one, two, or all three anatomic areas as illustrated in Figure 1. The central area is the portion occupied by the dural sac. The lateral recess extends from the lateral portion of the dural sac to the medial edge of the pedicle. The foraminal region is the area bordered superiorly and inferiorly by the pedicles beneath the facets. The nerve root generally occupies approximately 30% of the foramen (11).

The degenerative process usually starts in the disc (12,13). Declining nutrition within the disc eventually leads to cell death and matrix degradation. This results in annular weakening and bulging or herniation of the disc posteriorly into the spinal canal, osteophyte formation, and degeneration of the facet joints due to transfer of mechanical stresses. With degeneration of the facet joints, further encroachment occurs, particularly of the lateral recess at the level of the pedicle and of the disc (Fig. 2). There is also infolding of the ligamentum flavum leading to compression in the lateral and central regions (14). The size of the foramen is decreased by disc space narrowing and sagittal plane deformity (Figs. 3 and 4) (5,6,15–17).

Attempts have been made to quantify the diagnosis of spinal stenosis, either radiographically or anatomically. Although the variation in the clinical picture makes this difficult, a cross-sectional area of the dural sac of less than 100 mm^2 or a midsagittal diameter of 10 mm or less generally correlates well with clinically symptomatic spinal stenosis (1,10). Similarly, foraminal stenosis, often with nerve root compression, correlates with a posterior disc height less than 4 mm and foraminal height less than 15 mm (5).

PATHOPHYSIOLOGY

It is not known why some individuals with neural compression become symptomatic with anatomic evidence of spinal stenosis and others do not, but this is likely related to the duration, extent, and location of compression. In a cadaver model, increases in intradural pressure are first noted with dural sac constriction to 77 ± 13 mm Hg (18). In patients with spinal stenosis, epidural pressure measurements have shown the pressure to range between 18 ± 6.9 mm Hg in the supine position and 116.5 ± 38.4 mm Hg in the standing extended position. In animal models, Olmarker has shown that constriction of the venules of nerve roots occurs with pressure as low as 10 mm Hg (19,20) accompanied by a 64% reduction in blood flow and 20 to 30% reduction in nutrition. With more severe constriction, Delamarter has shown blockage of axoplasmic flow and wallerian degeneration from the level of constriction in other animal experimental studies (21). Although not

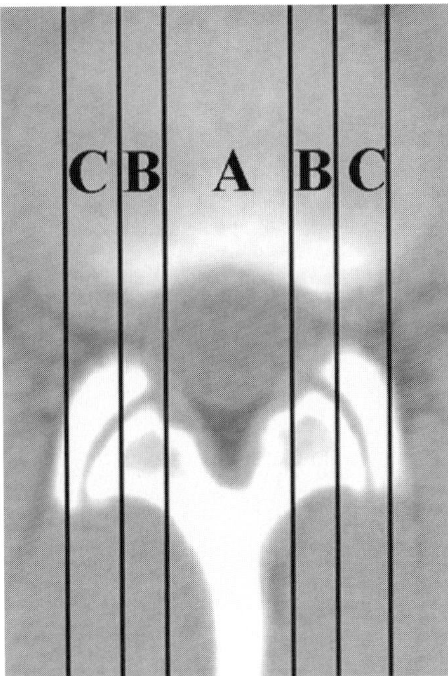

FIG. 1. Axial computed tomography scan showing the central region (*A*), lateral recess (*B*), and foraminal regions (*C*).

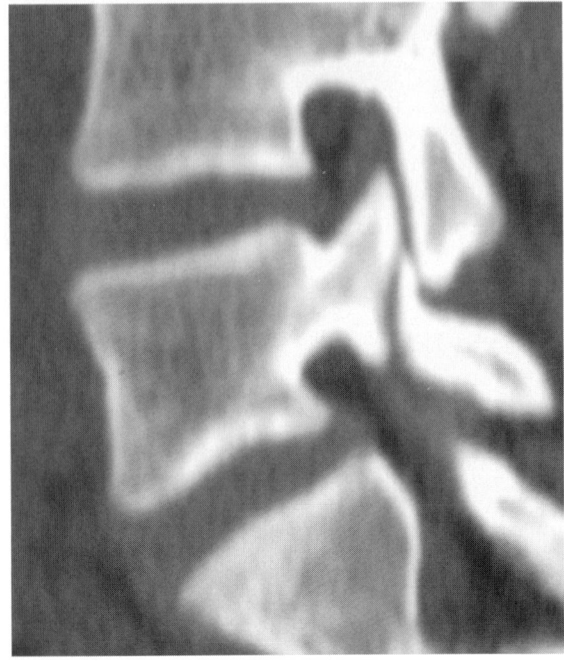

FIG. 3. Normal sagittal computed tomography scan showing foraminal dimensions.

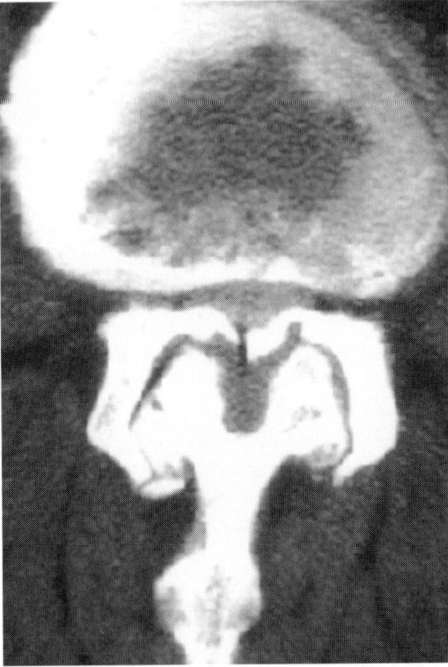

FIG. 2. Axial computed tomography scan showing facet degeneration with hypertrophy and resultant lateral recess stenosis.

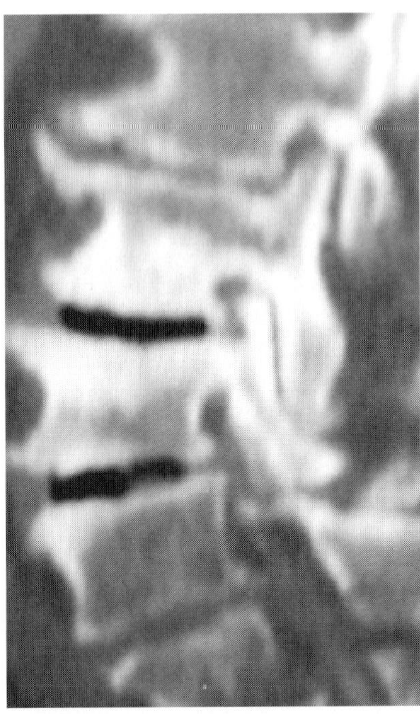

FIG. 4. Sagittal computed tomography scan showing foraminal encroachment due to degenerative changes.

completely comparable to the clinical situation, it has also been shown that acute constriction leads to more edema within the nerve root than does chronic constriction and that constriction at multiple levels slows nutrient transport and electrical conduction more than with single-level constriction (22–25). The latter is consistent with the double-crunch phenomenon seen in humans.

Inflammation clearly plays a role in the pathophysiology as well. Changes in the levels of various neuropeptides, including substance P, vasoactive intestinal polypeptide, calcitonin–gene-related peptide, and brain-derived neurotrophic factor, have all been described in association with nerve root compression (26–28). In addition to this, the activity of the protooncogene c-fos is altered, and there is an increase in bradykinin receptor activity in the injured nerve root (28,29).

REFERENCES

1. Bolender NF, Schonstrom NS, Spengler DM. Role of computed tomography and myelography in the diagnosis of central spinal stenosis. *J Bone Joint Surg Am* 1985;67(2):240–246.
2. Gouzien P, et al. Measurements of the normal lumbar spinal canal by computed tomography. Segmental study of L3-L4 and L4-L5 related to the height of the subject. *Surg Radiol Anat* 1990;12(2):143–148.
3. Postacchini F, Ripani M, Carpano S. Morphometry of the lumbar vertebrae. An anatomic study in two caucasoid ethnic groups. *Clin Orthop* 1983;(172):296–303.
4. Ullrich CG, et al. Quantitative assessment of the lumbar spinal canal by computed tomography. *Radiology* 1980;134(1):137–143.
5. Hasegawa T, et al. Lumbar foraminal stenosis: critical heights of the intervertebral discs and foramina. A cryomicrotome study in cadavera. *J Bone Joint Surg Am* 1995;77(1):32–38.
6. Jenis LG, An HS. Spine update. Lumbar foraminal stenosis. *Spine* 2000;25(3):389–394.
7. Smith SA, et al. Straight leg raising. Anatomical effects on the spinal nerve root without and with fusion. *Spine* 1993;18(8):992–999.
8. Sarpenyer M. Congenital stricture of the spinal canal. *J Bone Joint Surg* 1945;27:70–79.
9. Verbiest H. A radicular syndrome from developmental narrowing of the lumbar vertebral canal. *J Bone Joint Surg* 1954;36B:230–237.
10. Verbiest H. Pathomorphologic aspects of developmental lumbar stenosis. *Orthop Clin North Am* 1975;6(1):177–196.
11. Hasue M, et al. Classification by position of dorsal root ganglia in the lumbosacral region. *Spine* 1989;14(11):1261–1264.
12. Buckwalter JA. Aging and degeneration of the human intervertebral disc. *Spine* 1995;20(11):1307–1314.
13. Butler D, et al. Discs degenerate before facets. *Spine* 1990;15(2): 111–113.
14. Yong-Hing K, Reilly J, Kirkaldy-Willis WH. The ligamentum flavum. *Spine* 1976;1:226–234.
15. Cinotti G, et al. Stenosis of lumbar intervertebral foramen: anatomic study on predisposing factors. *Spine* 2002;27(3):223–229.
16. Crock HV. Normal and pathological anatomy of the lumbar spinal nerve root canals. *J Bone Joint Surg Br* 1981;4:487–490.
17. Garfin SR, et al. Spinal nerve root compression. *Spine* 1995;20(16): 1810–1820.
18. Schonstrom N, Hansson T. Pressure changes following constriction of the cauda equina. An experimental study *in situ*. *Spine* 1988;13(4):385–388.
19. Olmarker K, Rydevik B, Holm S. Edema formation in spinal nerve roots induced by experimental, graded compression. An experimental study on the pig cauda equina with special reference to differences in effects between rapid and slow onset of compression. *Spine* 1989;14(6):569–573.
20. Takahashi K, et al. Epidural pressure measurements. Relationship between epidural pressure and posture in patients with lumbar spinal stenosis. *Spine* 1995;20(6):650–653.
21. Delamarter RB, et al. Experimental lumbar spinal stenosis. Analysis of the cortical evoked potentials, microvasculature, and histopathology. *J Bone Joint Surg Am* 1990;72(1):110–120.
22. Matsui H, et al. Local electrophysiologic stimulation in experimental double level cauda equina compression. *Spine* 1992;17(9):1075–1078.
23. Olmarker K, et al. Effects of experimental graded compression on blood flow in spinal nerve roots. A vital microscopic study on the porcine cauda equina. *J Orthop Res* 1989;7(6):817–823.
24. Olmarker K, Rydevik B. Single- versus double-level nerve root compression. An experimental study on the porcine cauda equina with analyses of nerve impulse conduction properties. *Clin Orthop* 1992;279:35–39.
25. Takahashi K, et al. Double-level cauda equina compression: an experimental study with continuous monitoring of intraneural blood flow in the porcine cauda equina. *J Orthop Res* 1993;11(1):104–109.
26. Cornefjord M, et al. Neuropeptide changes in compressed spinal nerve roots. *Spine* 1995;20(6):670–673.
27. Ha SO, et al. Expression of brain-derived neurotrophic factor in rat dorsal root ganglia, spinal cord and gracile nuclei in experimental models of neuropathic pain. *Neuroscience* 2001;107(2):301–309.
28. Kawakami M, et al. Experimental lumbar radiculopathy. Immunohistochemical and quantitative demonstrations of pain induced by lumbar nerve root irritation of the rat. *Spine* 1994;19(16):1780–1794.
29. Levy D, Zochodne DW. Increased mRNA expression of the B1 and B2 bradykinin receptors and antinociceptive effects of their antagonists in an animal model of neuropathic pain. *Pain* 2000;86(3):265–271.

CHAPTER 48

Lumbar Spinal Stenosis

B. Clinical Presentation and Diagnosis

Alexander J. Ghanayem

One of the earliest records of lumbar decompression for stenosis was in 1893 when W. A. Lane described the removal of dense and thickened lamina (1). After removal, the dura was noted to have been so compressed that it would not expand, and the surrounding bone was removed. Sachs and Fraenkel (in 1900) and Bailey and Casamajor (in 1911) described painful walking conditions relieved by forward flexion (2,3). Van Gelderen proposed hypertrophy of the ligamentum flavum as a potential cause of painful narrowing of the spinal canal (4). In 1954, Verbiest put the clinical, structural, and diagnostic characteristics of spinal stenosis together, clearly defining the clinical characteristics of spinal stenosis (5,6).

CLINICAL PRESENTATION

Epidemiology

In general, spinal stenosis is a disease of the older population. Radiographic spinal stenosis increases with age and can start in the fourth decade. Symptomatic stenosis typically starts to become symptomatic in patients in their mid-fifties and progresses into the sixth and seventh decades of life. The prevalence of symptomatic stenosis is less than in radiographic stenosis (7). Females are affected more than males at a ratio of 3:1 for all types of stenoses, including degenerative spondylolisthesis (8). Patients with congenital narrowing of the spinal canal tend to become symptomatic at an earlier age because there is less "extra" space to accommodate the narrowing associated with degenerative arthritis.

Presentation

The most common clinical symptom of lumbar stenosis is neurogenic claudication. Patients complain of leg pain, usually bilateral, starting in the buttock and radiating into the posterior thigh and, when more severe, the calf. The symptoms can also be described as deep ache, numbness, or rubbery feeling. Patients often note their legs as almost feeling like "they were not their own." Symptoms are relieved by rest—typically sitting or lying down. They observe that if they walk with an assistive device allowing them to flex forward, such as a cane, walker, or shopping cart, their walking tolerance increases. Aerobic exercise tolerance usually is not limited. For example, they can usually ride a stationary bicycle without difficulty (9).

Axial symptoms of back pain are also associated with stenosis. Increasing back pain with walking can be related to the neurologic compression as well as the mechanical pain and fatigue that relates in part to walking in a forward flexed posture. Axial symptoms are also associated with segmental instability that occurs as with degenerative spondylolisthesis.

Bowel and bladder dysfunction is rarely a presenting symptom of spinal stenosis. The sacral roots are located centrally in the cauda equina and are the last to be compressed. Before attributing bowel and bladder dysfunction to stenosis, other causes in this older age group should be explored. In men, prostatic hypertrophy should be considered and a urologic evaluation obtained. In women, pelvic floor muscle incompetence and anatomic changes in the urogenital region should be considered. Referral to a urogynecologist can help to define these issues. In men and women, bowel and bladder dysfunction in the presence of long-tract neurologic signs and symptoms should prompt a search for a cervical or thoracic cord lesion.

Differential Diagnosis

Lumbar spinal stenosis can be mimicked by other musculoskeletal and nonmusculoskeletal conditions. These include myelopathy, osteoarthritis of other joints, vascular disease, and peripheral neuropathy. A careful history and physical examination can usually differentiate between these disease processes. Confirmation with appropriate diagnostic testing can then be directed.

Myelopathy from cord compression is typically involved in the cervical region but can occur in the thoracic region or thoracolumbar junction if the conus medullaris is involved. Gait dysfunction and difficulty walking are usually painless with myelopathy. Upper-extremity and hand dysfunction should also alert the physician to the possibility of a cervical lesion. Bowel and bladder dysfunction is more common with a cervical myelopathy than with lumbar stenosis. Physical findings, such as a broad-based gait, hyperreflexia, long-tract signs (e.g., Hoffman's and Babinski's signs, clonus) and loss of proprioception, are consistent with myelopathy. However, patients may have concomitant cervical stenosis with myelopathy and lumbar stenosis. In these patients, the myelopathy should take precedence in treatment.

Osteoarthritis of other joints can also mimic and coexist with lumbar stenosis. Sacroiliac (SI) joint arthritis can result in standing intolerance as well as walking intolerance, with pain starting in the buttock and referred into the proximal thigh. However, SI joint arthritis also is associated with sitting intolerance, a symptom that typically does not occur with spinal stenosis. A provocative physical test for SI joint dysfunction and anterior-posterior pelvic radiographs can help to clarify this diagnostic possibility. More commonly, lumbar stenosis occurs with hip and knee arthritis. A pain diagram completed by the patient can prompt the physician to consider these sites. Anterior thigh pain is a referral zone from both the hip and knee as well as the upper and middle lumbar regions. Careful observation of a patient's gait reveals hip abductor weakness with a Trendelenburg gait and a decreased stance phase on one limb consistent with hip arthritis. Malalignment at the knee accompanied by lateral thrusting should draw attention to the knee as a source of pain and gait dysfunction. The hips and knees should be examined for loss of range of motion, contracture, pain with motion, and joint line tenderness. Plain radiographs of the hip and knee (standing) can confirm the presence of osteoarthritis in these joints. The order of treatment in patients with both a symptomatic osteoarthritic hip or knee and lumbar stenosis is variable and should be a personal decision between the patient and physician. In general, the author has found that joint replacement done first tends to enhance the overall patient recovery and, in some patients, helps to avoid a lumbar spine procedure because of an enhanced ability to participate in conservative care programs.

TABLE 1. *Characteristics of neurogenic and vascular claudication*

Characteristic	Neurogenic	Vascular
Pattern of symptoms in legs	Proximal to distal	Distal to proximal
Relief of symptoms	Sitting or lying down	Standing
Night pain at bedrest	None	Relieved with standing
Walking on hills	Easier uphill	Easier downhill
Exercise bicycle riding	Comfortable	Painful
Truck posture	Improved symptoms with flexion, worse with extension	No effect
Pulses	Present	Absent
Lower-extremity skin	Normal	Loss of hair, shiny skin, trophic changes in feet and nail beds

Vascular claudication commonly can be confused with neurogenic claudication from lumbar stenosis. History and physical findings can usually differentiate the two and are summarized in Table 1. In general, a patient who complains of leg pain starting distal and moving proximal feels better standing and worse lying down, complains of night or rest pain, has associated diabetes, or has a significant smoking history, probably has vascular disease resulting in claudication. Patients with significant vascular disease often feel better walking downhill, whereas neurogenic patients feel better walking uphill. When walking uphill, patients with spinal stenosis often lean forward, placing the spine in flexion, which tends to relieve stenosis. In contrast, walking downhill requires lumbar extension, which decreases spinal canal area and aggravates stenosis. Physical findings, such as absent pedal pulses and trophic changes in skin and nails of lower extremities and feet, are found in patients with vascular disease. When lumbar spine radiographs are reviewed, the presence of aortoiliac calcifications should prompt a reassessment for vascular disease. On occasion, magnetic resonance imaging (MRI) or computed tomography (CT) scans reveal significant calcifications of the aortoiliac system or (more threateningly) an abdominal aortic aneurysm. It also should be remembered that patients can have both vascular and neurologic claudication (10). Consultation with a vascular surgeon can help to direct the appropriate treatment algorithm.

Peripheral neuropathies can also mimic symptoms of spinal stenosis. Etiologies include diabetic neuropathy, primary peripheral nerve disorders, and neuropathies associated with chemotherapeutic agents. Typically, peripheral neuropathies are distal rather than proximal, are in "stocking-glove" distributions, and are symptomatic with both activity and rest. The history should alert the physician to consider these alternative diagnoses. Patients can have two disease processes with symptomatic lumbar stenosis and a peripheral neuropathy. An electromyogram (EMG) or nerve condition study (NCV) can be useful in differentiating disease process and also can help to identify the particular nerve that should be addressed with spinal decompression (11).

Physical Examination

The clinical diagnosis of symptomatic lumbar stenosis can usually be made from the history. Physical examination can further support the diagnosis or redirect further evaluation for other pathologic conditions. The examination should start with observing how the patient stands up from the chair. Does the patient have to use his or her arms for support because of balance problems (myelopathy) or trunk and lower-extremity weakness? Posture should be observed both initially and after asking the patient to walk. If the patient assumes a forward flexed posture, this finding supports the diagnosis of lumbar stenosis. A limp secondary to hip or knee pathology should be noted as outline above. Palpation of the back is typically benign, with minimal to no pain or muscle spasm. A step-off deformity may be palpable if there is degenerative spondylolisthesis. Coronal imbalance should be noted; this is associated with degenerative scoliosis with stenosis. Lumbar extension is usually poorly tolerated, as this narrows the spinal canal dimensions. Lumbar flexion is well tolerated for the opposite reason—it increases the spinal canal dimensions. Patients may, however, have to use their arms to push off of their thighs to assume a full erect posture. There may or may not be discomfort of palpation in the sciatic notch. The SI joint should be palpated, and the pain response should be noted.

Neurologic examination is frequently normal in patients with spinal stenosis. There may be subtle weakness or sensory deficit in the distribution of the L-5 or S-1 roots. Absent or hypoactive reflexes are relatively nonspecific and are common findings in older patients without symptomatic spinal stenosis. Hyperactive reflexes and the presence of long-tract signs should prompt a search for a compressive lesion affecting the spinal cord. Tension signs, such as the straight-leg raise and femoral nerve stretch test, are typically negative. Finally, the absence of pulses and trophic changes associated with vascular disease should be noted.

Patients and family typically ask whether they become "paralyzed" from lumbar stenosis. They may have seen a friend or other family member with stenosis in a wheelchair. It is important to educate them that most patients will not become "paralyzed." Most are weak from deconditioning as a result of inactivity. Therefore, it is important to convey the idea that the long-term results of ongoing symptomatic disease unresponsive to conservative care is one of disability from loss of strength and endurance, not paralysis. This deconditioning, if progressive, can have other implications from a cardiopulmonary standpoint for patients undergoing surgery, as well as their ability to recover and rehabilitate after surgery. Presurgical cardiac clearance is important in these patients, even without cardiac symptoms.

DIAGNOSIS

In patients with symptomatic lumbar spinal stenosis, further diagnostic testing typically defines the extent of the disease process. The clinical diagnosis can usually be established with a fair degree of confidence after taking a careful history and performing a complete physical examination. At the minimum, standing plain radiographs and some sort of neuroimaging study should be obtained.

Plain Radiographs

Standing plain radiographs are the first line of diagnostic testing. Supine radiographs can miss instability such as occurs with degenerative scoliosis and spondylolisthesis. Routine flexion-extension radiographs are usually not necessary but should be obtained in patients who have had previous low back surgery or clinical suspicion of instability. Plain radiographs can also reveal other pathologic conditions (e.g., osteoporotic compression fractures, absent pedicles, or other destructive lesions associated with metastatic disease) that also affect the elderly population with spinal stenosis.

Magnetic Resonance Imaging

MRI has evolved into the gold standard neuroimaging study for patients with spinal stenosis (Fig. 1). CT-myelography was the neuroimaging study of choice through the 1980s. A transition from CT-myelography to MRI occurred in the 1990s. MRI is noninvasive, safe, and extensile, with the ability to image the entire spinal axis. It can provide data regarding extrinsic neural compression from disc and degenerative changes as well as intradural abnormalities. Other concomitant conditions, such as osteoporotic compression fracture, neoplastic or metastatic disease, and infection, can be evaluated.

Stenosis in the lumbar spine can occur in three locations: the central canal, lateral recess, and foramen. Central stenosis is related to hypertrophy of the ligamentum flavum, as well as buckling and infolding as the intervertebral disc height narrows, thus shortening the distance between its cranial and caudal laminar attachments. The shape of the spinal canal as seen on cross-sectional imaging progresses from the more normal oval appearance to a trefoil shape in affected patients. Disc degeneration with thickening and bulging of the annulus fibrosis can contribute to central stenosis.

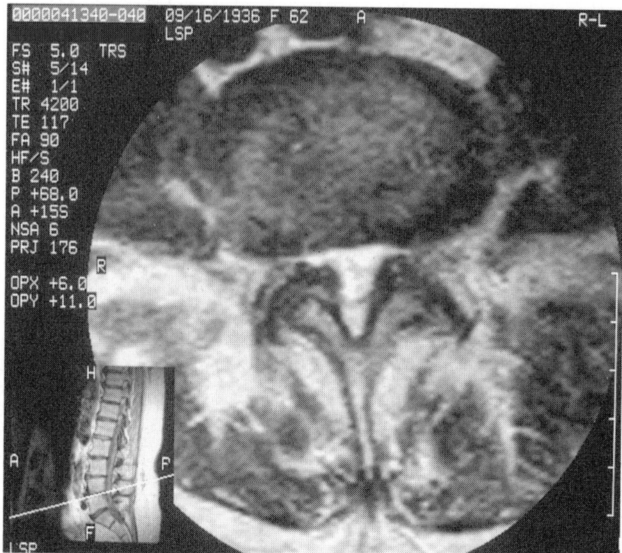

FIG. 1. Typical cross-sectional magnetic resonance image of a patient with symptomatic lumbar spinal stenosis. Note the trefoil shape of the spinal canal and the facet joint hypertrophy.

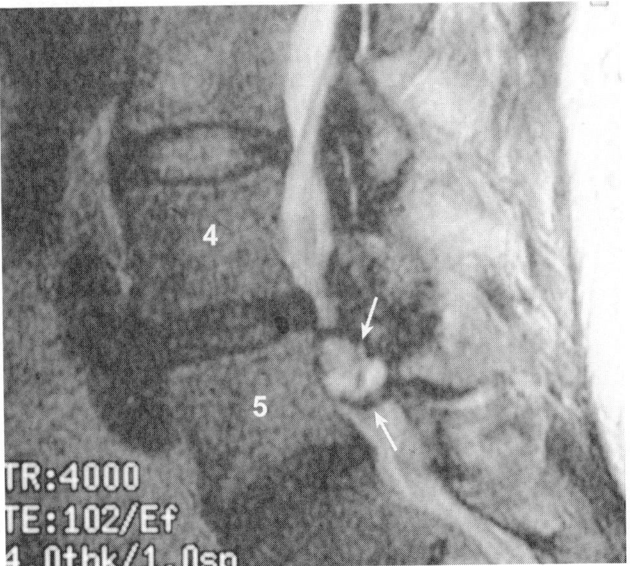

FIG. 2. Sagittal magnetic resonance image of a patient with a large synovial cyst extending from the facet joint into the spinal canal (*arrows*), creating significant spinal stenosis. Also note the subtle degenerative spondylolisthesis between L-4 and L-5.

Lateral recess stenosis is defined anatomically by the portion of the spinal canal lateral to the pedicle extending to the most medial portion of the facet joint. In the lateral recess, stenosis can occur by facet joint or capsule hypertrophy, thickening of the lateral portions of the ligamentum flavum, and posterolateral disc degeneration. Synovial cysts from the facet joint can extend into the lateral recess or central canal (Fig. 2).

The foraminal region is defined by three zones as classified by Lee et al. (12). The entrance zone is the most medial and superior portion of the foramen. It is here that the nerve root shoulder enters the foramen. It can be considered a portion of the lateral recess in that these anatomic areas essentially overlap. The middle zone is caudal to the pedicle and between the pars interarticularis posteriorly and vertebral body anteriorly. The dorsal root ganglion lies in the middle zone. The exit zone sits in front of the lateral portion of the facet joint and behind the posterior far lateral disc.

Care must be taken to review the axial and sagittal MRI sequences to fully assess the entire spinal canal. Central and lateral recess stenosis usually can be appreciated easily on the axial images. The sagittal sequences can help to identify foraminal stenosis, especially the far lateral images (Fig. 3).

Computed Tomography–Myelography

Despite the advances in MRI technology, CT-myelography still has a vital role in the imaging of patients with spinal stenosis. When MRI is contraindicated because of aneurysm clips, metal fragments in the eyes, pacemakers, or bullets near vital structures, CT-myelography becomes the neuroimaging study of choice. Patients with degenerative scoliosis may be difficult to completely and thoroughly assess with MRI alone, and CT-myelography can add important data when planning surgical treatment (Fig. 4). MRI imaging can be degraded with the presence of titanium spinal implants in place and perhaps should not be obtained with stainless steel implants. In patients with previous failed surgery, sometimes one neuroimaging study is not sufficient to fully assess pathology and preoperatively plan the appropriate surgery. MRI and CT-myelography can be complementary studies. Except for assessing bone fusion and implant location in patients with prior surgery, plain CT scanning is of limited value.

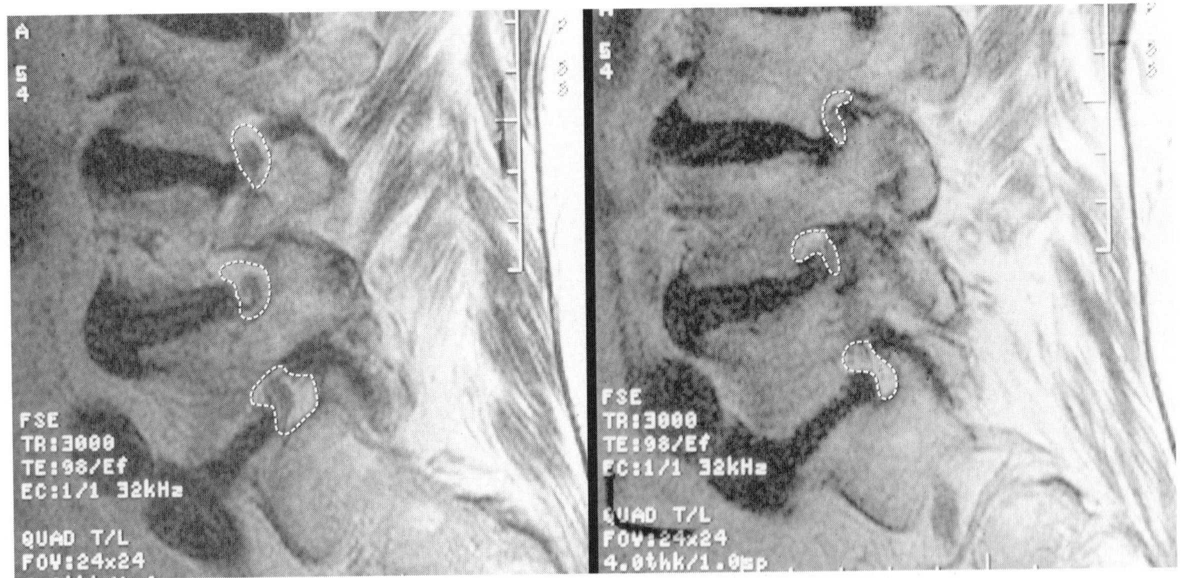

FIG. 3. Far lateral sagittal magnetic resonance images from two different sides of the spinal canal. **A:** The neuroforamina have been highlighted (*dashed lines*). Note the relative area and contrast that to the opposite side in **(B)**. The size of the neuroforamina in **(B)** is much smaller than that in **(A)**.

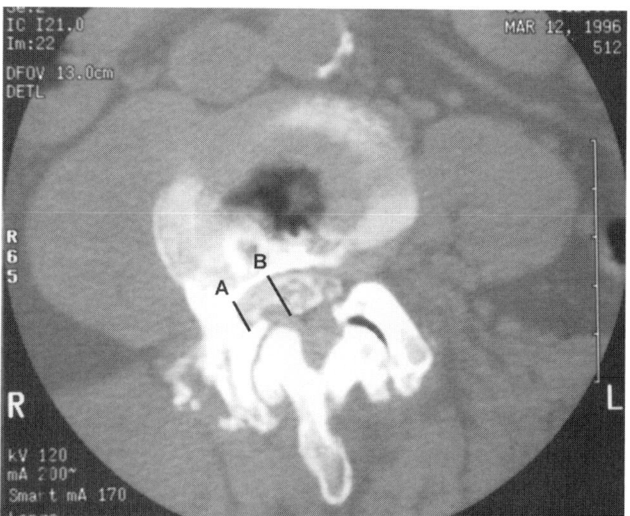

FIG. 4. Cross-sectional computed tomography image postmyelogram in a patient with stenosis and degenerative scoliosis. Note the rotation in the axial plane. The lateral recess, which is stenotic, is lateral to the medial border of the pedicle (*line A*) and bound centrally by the medial extent of the facet joint (*line B*).

Electrodiagnostic Studies

Electrodiagnostic studies are useful adjuvant studies in some patients with spinal stenosis. In the uncomplicated patient with classic symptoms of neurogenic claudication, no comorbid medical problems (e.g., diabetes or peripheral vascular disease), no unexpected physical findings on examination, and straightforward findings of stenosis on neuroimaging studies, there is no added benefit to obtaining electrodiagnostic studies. In patients in whom multiple disease processes might contribute to symptoms (e.g., diabetic neuropathy and stenosis), EMG/NCV can be helpful to delineate the cause of the patient's symptoms (11,13,14). Revision cases and patients with extensive radiographic disease may also benefit from electrophysiologic studies. Typically, EMG reveals bilateral multiradicular findings in patients with stenosis in contrast to the unilateral monoradicular finding in patients with disc herniation (8,14). However, EMG can give false negative results in patients with predominately sensory-claudication–type symptoms, because it only assesses motor nerve fibers, not sensory fibers. The NCV portion of the study can help to differentiate between peripheral neuropathy and radiculopathy (11). Although somatosensory evoked potentials can be positive in patients with lumbar spinal stenosis, their utility is limited in the context of obtaining an adequate history, examination, and appropriate neuroimaging studies.

SUMMARY

Patients with symptomatic spinal stenosis can present with disabling symptoms of leg pain and neurogenic claudication. Many of the patients are otherwise healthy and want to be as active as possible. The care and successful treatment of the patients can be rewarding for patients and their families as their functional capabilities improve. The first step in providing successful care is recognition of the clinical problem followed by accurate exclusion of other disease processes. Testing further confirms the diagnosis or draws attention to other problems that may adversely effect the success of treatment directed at the lumbar stenosis. Although physical findings of lumbar stenosis may be minimal, careful listening and assimilation of the medical data lead the primary or spinal care physician to the proper diagnosis and treatment algorithms as described in the chapters that follow.

REFERENCES

1. Lane WA. Case of spondylolisthesis associated with progressive paraplegia; laminectomy. *Lancet* 1893;1:991.
2. Sachs B, Fraenkel J. Progressive ankylotic rigidity of the spine (spondylose rhizomelique). *J Nerv Ment Dis* 1900;27:1–15.
3. Bailey P, Casamajor L. Osteoarthritis of the spine as a cause of compression of the spinal cord and its roots: with reports of 5 cases. *J Nerv Ment Dis* 1911;38:588–609.
4. Van Gelderen C. Ein orthotisches (lordotisches) Kaudasyndrom. *Acta Psychiatr Neurol* 1948;23:57–68.
5. Verbiest H. A radicular syndrome from developmental narrowing of the lumbar vertebral canal. *J Bone Joint Surg* 1954;36B:230–237.
6. Verbiest H. Further experiences of pathologic influence on a developmental narrowing of the lumbar vertebral canal. *J Bone Joint Surg* 1956;38B:576–583.
7. Boden SD, Davis DO, Dina TS, et al. Abnormal magnetic-resonance scans of the lumbar spine in asymptomatic subjects. *J Bone Joint Surg* 1990;72A(3):403–408.
8. Hall S, Bartleson J, Onfrio B, et al. Lumbar spinal stenosis. Clinical features, diagnostic procedures and results of surgical treatment in 68 patients. *Ann Intern Med* 1985;103:271–275.
9. Dyke P, Doyle J. "Bicycle test" of Van Gelderen in diagnosis of intermittent cauda equina compression. *J Neurosurg* 1977;46:667–670.
10. Dodge L, Bohlman H, Rhodes, R. Concurrent lumbar spinal stenosis and peripheral vascular disease. *Clin Orthop* 1988;230:141–148.
11. Hirsch LF. Diabetic polyradiculopathy simulating lumbar disc disease. *J Neurosurg* 1984;60:183–186.
12. Lee CW, Rauschning W, Glenn W. Lateral lumbar spine canal stenosis. *Spine* 1988;13:313–320.
13. Haldeman S. The electrodiagnostic evaluation of nerve root function. *Spine* 1984;9:42–48.
14. Johnsson KE, Rosen I, Uden A. Neurophysiologic investigation of patients with spinal stenosis. *Spine* 1987;12:483–487.

CHAPTER 48

Lumbar Spinal Stenosis

C. Treatment

Gordon R. Bell

NATURAL HISTORY

A clear understanding of the natural history of any spinal disorder is the basis for determining the efficacy of treatments. Surprisingly, there are no well-designed, long-term, prospective studies describing the true natural history of spinal stenosis, despite the importance of this condition, particularly in an aging society. Several studies describing and comparing different treatments included patients who had no treatment, and symptoms progressed in approximately 20% of them. One study reported a series of 22 patients, only two of whom were not operated on: one patient showed gradual progression of symptoms over a 10-year period, and the other exhibited no progression over 7 years (1). Another study included 13 patients with spinal stenosis, three of whom were treated nonoperatively (2). Only two of these patients were followed, one of whom improved and one who was unchanged.

The largest and best study of the natural course of lumbar spinal stenosis reported on 32 patients with spinal stenosis, followed for an average of 49 months, with a range of 10 to 103 months (3). All patients had been preselected for surgery, but 32 patients did not have it, either because they refused to undergo surgery or the anesthesiologist refused to administer anesthesia. The patients were described as having conservative treatment (i.e., no treatment). Evaluation was by questionnaire, including a visual analog scale (VAS) and by clinical examination. At final follow-up, 41% of patients were improved, 18% were worse, and 41% were unchanged based on the clinical examination. The VAS showed 15% were improved, 15% were worse, and 70% were unchanged. Walking capacity was approximately equally distributed among those improved, made worse, or unchanged (Table 1). When final outcome was compared with anteroposterior (AP) diameter of the dural sac, as measured by water-soluble contrast myelography, patients with a narrower AP diameter had a tendency not to improve. This study concluded that the majority of nonoperated patients with spinal stenosis remained unchanged at 4-year follow-up, and severe deterioration was unlikely. However, this study was a nonrandomized, comparison design.

NONOPERATIVE MANAGEMENT

Conservative treatments of spinal stenosis include nonsteroidal antiinflammatory medications, analgesics, oral and epidural steroids, physical therapy, bracing, and calcitonin (4). Evaluating the efficacy of such treatments, however, is difficult due to a dearth of good, prospective, randomized studies. Indeed, a recent attempt at a metaanalysis of the literature regarding surgery for spinal stenosis failed to identify a single randomized trial comparing surgery with conservative treatment (5). A 1-year prospective study of patients with spinal stenosis treated surgically or nonsurgically in community-based practices in the state of Maine revealed little improvement in symptoms in nonsurgically treated patients over a 1-year period (6). This was an observational cohort study only and, therefore, had several design flaws. These included a short follow-up period (1 year), the nonrandom nature of the study, and the fact that it included only 22% of those who were eligible to be enrolled. In addition, there was no standardization of the type of conservative care rendered. Its conclusions must, therefore, be

TABLE 1. *Outcome of nonoperated patients with spinal stenosis*

	Worse (%)	Unchanged (%)	Improved (%)
Visual analog scale	15	70	15
Clinical exam	18	41	41
Walking capacity	30	33	37

From Johnsson K, Rosen I, Uden A. The natural course of lumbar spinal stenosis. *Clin Orthop Relat R* 1992;279;82–86, with permission.

interpreted with caution. Nevertheless, this study revealed only 28% of the conservatively treated patients reported significant improvement in their predominant symptom at 1 year, compared to 55% of the surgically treated group (Table 2).

Johnsson, Uden, and Rosen compared the outcome of a group of 19 patients treated conservatively with 44 patients treated with surgical decompression (Table 3) (7). The authors found 53% of the nonsurgical patients still had neurogenic claudication at an average follow-up of 31 months. Thirty-two percent of the conservatively treated group reported subjective improvements by VAS, 58% were unchanged, and 10% had deteriorated. In the surgical group, 37% of the patients reported continued neurogenic claudication at an average of 53 months after surgery. Fifty-nine percent of the patients reported improvement, 16% were unchanged, and 25%

TABLE 2. *One-year outcome of surgical and nonsurgical treatment of spinal stenosis*

Outcome variable	Surgical (%)	Nonsurgical (%)
Lower back pain		
Better	77	42
Same	18	38
Worse	5	20
Leg pain		
Better	79	45
Same	15	43
Worse	6	12
Change in predominant symptoms		
Much better	55	28
Same	42	57
Worse	3	15
Patient satisfaction		
Very good	69	36
Satisfied	68	32
Would have surgery again	88	—
Significant improvement in quality of life	81	49

Modified from Atlas S, Deyo R, Keller R, et al. The Maine lumbar spine study, part III. One-year outcomes of surgical and nonsurgical management of lumbar spinal stenosis. *Spine* 1996;21(15):1787–1795.

TABLE 3. *Prospective, randomized study comparing surgical vs. nonsurgical treatment of lumbar spinal stenosis*

	Surgical (%)	Nonsurgical (%)
Stenosis present	37	53
Improved	59	32
Unchanged	16	58
Worse	25	10

From Johnsson K, Uden A, Rosen I. The effect of decompression on the natural course of spinal stenosis. a comparison of surgically treated and untreated patients. *Spine* 1991;16 (6):615–619, with permission.

deteriorated. Results of surgery did not appear to be related to the magnitude of stenosis, as documented by preoperative myelography. Neurophysiologic deterioration showed progression in almost all patients and were therefore not reversed or prevented by the surgery. This study concluded that nonsurgical treatment produced some improvement in approximately one-half of the patients, with only a 10% chance of deterioration during the 2- to 3-year follow-up period. It also suggested the "decision for surgical decompression in spinal stenosis is not a neurological imperative" (7). This study, however, was neither prospective nor randomized, again making comparison between the two groups difficult.

One recent report evaluated the outcome of patients with lumbar spinal stenosis treated with aggressive nonsurgical measures, including therapeutic exercises and epidural steroids (if they were deemed necessary), and suggested that such treatment could be very effective (8). Fifty-two patients were followed for 2 to 8 years, with 33 of the patients (63%) reporting a tolerable pain level controlled with nonnarcotic analgesics and having no major restriction in daily activities. Although 36 patients (69%) reported "no or minimal restriction in walking tolerance," 25 patients (48%) reported "difficulty in standing for long periods." None of the patients experienced any further deterioration in neurologic loss. Four of the 52 patients (8%) required surgery for presumed failure of nonsurgical measures. The exclusion criteria for this study, however, may have produced some element of bias, because patients with preexisting comorbidities, or patients with a "compliance issue that prevented participation in a therapeutic exercise program" were excluded.

SURGICAL TREATMENT

Although surgical treatment of spinal stenosis is generally thought to be the definitive treatment of spinal stenosis, prospective and randomized trials comparing surgery with nonsurgical treatment are uncommon. As noted above, a recent attempted metaanalysis of the literature on surgery for spinal stenosis failed to identify even a single randomized trial comparing surgery with conservative treatment (5). The Maine observational cohort study of patients treated in a community-based practice revealed that, although improvement was reported by only 55% of the surgically treated group, the outcome was nearly twice as good as the 28% improvement reported by conservatively treated patients (Table 2) (6). Because of the study's short follow-up period (1 year), lack of standardization of the conservative care rendered, and inclusion of only 22% of those eligible for enrollment, the results of this study must be interpreted with caution.

Despite its perceived superior outcome compared to either the natural history or conservative treatment, the long-term results of surgery for spinal stenosis have been shown to deteriorate over time (9–11). Katz and associates examined the predictors of outcome after spinal surgery for spinal stenosis (12). Several predictors of poor outcome were identified, including an increased length of follow-up, single-level decompression, and a greater number of comorbidities. Only the comorbidities, however, were found to be statistically significant, after adjusting for multiple comparisons. The most common comorbidities were osteoarthritis (32%), cardiac disease (22%), rheumatoid arthritis (10%), and chronic pulmonary disease (7%). Only 40% of patients with the highest comorbidity score had a good outcome at the time of final follow-up, compared with 75% of patients who had the lowest comorbidity score ($p = .004$). Their data suggested the effect of comorbidities was additive, because no single comorbidity was significantly associated with worse outcome. In a subsequent clinical investigation by the same authors, comorbidity was found to be the second most important determinant of disability in lumbar canal stenosis. The predominant preoperative complaint of low back pain, as opposed to leg pain, was the most important determinant of disability (12).

Because comorbidity is often associated with increasing age of the patient, surgical complication rates generally correlate with age. The relationship between patient age and outcome after lumbar spinal surgery has been investigated (13). As would be expected, hospital morbidity and mortality are greater in older patients. When complications arise, there often is an increasing complexity of diagnosis and greater complexity of surgical treatment. The study by Deyo and associates reported an overall mortality of 0.07% for 18,122 hospitalizations in the state of Washington between 1986 through 1988 in patients undergoing spinal surgery (14). The mortality increased with age, increasing to 0.6% (nine-fold increase) in patients older than 75 years of age. Similar findings were noted for complications, with an overall complication rate of 9.1%, which increased to 17.7% in patients 75 years of age or older.

Associations between outcome and comorbidity, independent of patient age, have also been examined. Outcome measures, such as mortality, perioperative complications, cost, length of stay, and quality of life, have been reported. As would be expected, increase in comorbidity is highly associated with greater in-hospital complications and perioperative mortality (14), independent of age alone. Similar findings were found by Oldridge and associates in an administrative database study of 34,418 patients 65 years of age or older from 1986 Medicare inpatient Health Care Financing Administration claims files (15). There was an age-related increase in mortality only for patients older than 80 years of age. There was, however, a significant increase in in-hospital and 1-year cumulative mortality, again associated with the number of comorbidities.

SURGICAL TECHNIQUES

The ultimate goal of surgery for spinal stenosis is decompression of symptomatic neural compression. The techniques for accomplishing this may be broadly divided into decompressive procedures without concomitant fusion and decompression with fusion. The techniques used to accomplish the goal of decompression vary primarily in the amount of bone and other tissue removed. There is, therefore, a spectrum of surgical techniques ranging from limited procedures, such as single-level unilateral laminotomy for focal neural compression, to more global procedures, such as multilevel bilateral laminectomy with bilateral facetectomies for diffuse stenosis.

The decision to fuse generally depends on the perceived risk of preoperative and intraoperative instability or on the magnitude of back pain complaints present before surgery. The risk of instability is determined by the presence or absence of preexisting instability (e.g., degenerative spondylolisthesis or scoliosis) and by the extent and number of levels of decompression required. Fusion is considered for patients who have significant preexisting back pain, based on the assumption that fusion might ameliorate the back pain. Types of fusion procedures include anterior lumbar interbody fusion, posterior lumbar interbody fusion, transforaminal lumbar interbody fusion, posterior fusion, posterolateral (also known as intertransverse or bilateral lateral) fusion, or combinations of these procedures. Indirect neural decompression may occur after anterior lumbar interbody fusion, posterior lumbar interbody fusion, or transforaminal lumbar interbody fusion, because these procedures usually create an element of disc space distraction, thereby enlarging the central or foraminal canal. Fusion is often augmented by the use of spinal instrumentation, either by anterior fixation devices or by posterior devices, such as those using pedicle screw with plate or rod constructs. Such fixation accomplishes several goals: It provides immediate stability, increases the rate of fusion, and allows correction of spinal deformity. It remains unclear whether increased fusion correlates with better clinical outcome.

Decompressive Procedures without Fusion

Laminectomy

The gold standard surgical procedure for spinal stenosis is surgical decompression. This may involve bilateral laminectomy or hemilaminectomy. Decompression is extended laterally as far as is needed to assure adequate neural decompression. This may involve foraminotomy, partial facetectomy, or even total facetectomy. For bilateral laminectomy, the lamina and ligamentum flavum are removed on both sides of the stenotic level(s) to the level of the lateral recess.

Traditional laminectomy attempts to preserve both facet joints at the operated level if at all possible to minimize the risk of postoperative instability. Because spinal stenosis is a global degenerative process, encompassing multiple levels and involving nerve roots bilaterally, multilevel bilateral laminectomy is commonly required. However, there is some debate as to whether it is more appropriate to decompress only the symptomatic level and side, or whether all stenotic levels should be decompressed. The risk of converting an asymptomatic level exhibiting radiographic neural compression to a potentially symptomatic unstable level by its surgical decompression must be balanced by the risk of symptomatic progression of the degenerative process at a nonoperated stenotic level. This is an important consideration, because long-term deterioration after initially successful surgical decompression is well recognized (10,16,17).

Technique of Laminectomy

The patient is positioned with the abdomen hanging freely to decrease abdominal compression and thereby reduce epidural bleeding. This is usually accomplished by placing the patient in a kneeling position.

Decompression is most safely initiated at the most distal extent of neural compression and proceeds in a caudal-to-cranial manner. This allows the initial part of the procedure to begin at a relatively less-compressed area and avoids beginning the decompression at a stenotic segment. Although the L-5 to S-1 level is rarely compressed centrally due to the capacious nature of the spinal canal at that level, decompression is most safely initiated at that level rather than at L4-5, the most commonly involved level, which is often severely stenotic.

Decompression is performed sequentially, from medial to lateral. The midline decompression is performed initially and is extended throughout the full extent of the anticipated decompression. This is generally performed from the patient's left side for a right-handed surgeon, and from the patient's right side by a left-handed surgeon. The spinous processes of all involved levels are removed with a Horsley rongeur. In areas where severe stenosis is not present, a Leksell rongeur or a relatively large rongeur, such as a 4-mm Kerrison rongeur, may be used to remove or thin the thickened lamina. In stenotic areas, however, the use of such large instruments risks injury to underlying neural structures. Under these circumstances, it is safer to thin the lamina with a high-speed power burr. This allows the surgeon to then use a smaller instrument, such as a 2-mm or 3-mm Kerrison rongeur, to complete the midline decompression.

The key to maintaining proper orientation during the decompression is to identify the level of the pedicle, because the pedicle defines the level of the nerve root as it passes inferior to the pedicle of the same number. If in doubt as to the proper level, localization can be confirmed by an intraoperative x-ray with a bent probe beneath the pedicle within the neural foramen.

Decompression of the lateral recess is performed next. The decompression is extended laterally until the lateral edge of the root is visualized and is determined to be free of compression. Care is taken to preserve the pars interarticularis to minimize risk of producing instability by inadvertent sacrifice of the superior articular facet. Preservation of the facet joint may be accomplished by undercutting the facet joint by the use of either oblique-angled (45-degree) Kerrison rongeurs or osteotomes.

Finally, lateral decompression of the foraminae is performed, if necessary. Once the shoulder of the nerve root is identified and decompressed, it is followed from its origin through the neural foramen. In performing the lateral decompression, it is generally safer to proceed from a cranial-to-caudal direction to minimize risk of injury to the nerve root by inadvertent cutting across the root, which can occur when performing the lateral decompression from a distal-to-proximal direction. Occasionally, the use of an angled Kerrison rongeur can be helpful for foraminal decompression. The adequacy of the foraminal decompression is assessed both visually and by palpation. The use of a bent probe, such as a bent number 4 Penfield elevator, is useful for determining the presence or absence of nerve root compression within the neural foramen. Decompression is generally complete when a bent probe can be gently passed out of the foramen both dorsal and ventral to the nerve root, and the root can be gently retracted approximately 1 cm medially.

After midline and lateral decompression, a check should be made for the presence or absence of a concomitant disc herniation, which could also contribute to neural compression. Unless the disc is contributing to definite and significant neural compression, it is generally best to avoid discectomy in the presence of laminectomy, because resulting instability may occur when both anterior and posterior supporting structures are partially removed. When laminectomy is accompanied by discectomy, strong consideration should be given to performing an arthrodesis at the time of surgery.

TABLE 4. *Patient outcome*[a]

	Preoperative (%)	1 yr (%)	2 yr (%)	5 yr (%)
Improvement in walking capacity	—	63	67	56
Rest pain	59	29	25	53
Overall excellent outcome	—	—	—	52

[a]Includes only 86 patients not undergoing additional surgery within follow-up period.

From Jonsson B, Annertz M, Sjoberg C, et al. A prospective and consecutive study of surgically treated lumbar spinal stenosis. Part II: five-year follow-up by an independent observer. *Spine* 1997;22:2938–2944, with permission.

Results of Surgery

A recent prospective study examined the 5-year outcome of 105 patients undergoing laminectomy without fusion for lumbar stenosis (18). Of the 86 patients available for evaluation at 5 years, 19 (22%) had undergone additional surgery within 5 years. Although 67% of patients reported excellent results related to leg symptoms within the first 2 years of surgery, the results deteriorated over the 5-year follow-up period, and only 48% of all patients reported excellent outcome at 5 years (Tables 4 and 5). Factors associated with good outcome were: a small (≤6 mm) AP central canal diameter and no associated comorbidities and shorter duration (<4 years) of claudication symptoms. The most significant finding of that study was that surgical outcomes were better in patients who had severe canal narrowing than in patients having a lesser degree of constriction. Similar findings, correlating better surgical outcome with increasing size of disc herniation (and hence more neural compression), noted at surgery, have been reported for patients with lumbar disc herniation (19).

In a retrospective review of 88 patients undergoing laminectomy for spinal stenosis, Katz and associates found that the long-term outcome was generally less favorable than had been previously reported (Table 6) (11). Outcome assessment included a questionnaire in which patients rated outcome in terms of pain

TABLE 5. *Long-term (5-year) outcome of all patients*[a]

Excellent (%)	Fair (%)	Same (%)	Worse (%)
48	17	19	16

[a]Includes 19 patients undergoing second surgical decompression within 5 years.

From Jonsson B, Annertz M, Sjoberg C, et al. A prospective and consecutive study of surgically treated lumbar spinal stenosis. Part II: five-year follow-up by an independent observer. *Spine* 1997;22:2938–2944, with permission.

TABLE 6. *Long-term outcome after surgery for spinal stenosis*

	1-yr follow-up (%)	Final follow-up (%)
Poor outcome	11	43
Severe pain	7	30
Reoperation	6	17
Limited function	8	35
Inability to walk 50 ft	8	21

From Katz J, Lipson S, Larson M, et al. The outcome of decompressive laminectomy for degenerative lumbar stenosis. *J Bone Joint Surg* 1991;73-A:809–816, with permission.

and function. The authors reported a surprisingly high failure rate. At 1 year, 11% of patients reported a poor outcome and 6% had a second operation. At final follow-up, 43% reported a poor outcome and 17% had a repeat operation. Risk factors for poor outcome included preoperative comorbidity and limited (single-level) decompression. The authors concluded the long-term outlook for patients undergoing decompressive laminectomy for spinal stenosis is guarded due to progressive deterioration of results over time. Because spinal stenosis is a global condition, often with diffuse degenerative changes occurring at multiple levels, they suggested that consideration be given to more extensive bone removal at the time of initial surgery.

Other reports also suggest poor long-term outcome for patients undergoing surgical decompression for spinal stenosis. A retrospective, nonrandomized, uncontrolled study of 88 patients undergoing decompressive surgery for spinal stenosis with minimum 5-year follow-up reported a high initial success rate after surgery, but by 5 years, the failure rate had reached 27%, with a predicted failure rate of 50% within the anticipated life expectancy of most patients (20). More than one-half (62%) of these failures were due to development of subsequent neurologic symptoms and recurrent stenosis at the same level or at a new level. Because of the high rate of failure from recurrent stenosis, the authors recommended that all impending levels of stenosis be decompressed along with the symptomatic levels.

Hemilaminectomy

Hemilaminectomy is more limited in the amount of bone and ligamentum flavum removed than is traditional laminectomy. It involves unilateral, rather than bilateral, removal of the lamina and ligamentum flavum causing neural decompression. Tissues that are not contributing to neural compression are retained, thereby limiting the risk of developing postoperative instability. With this procedure, the supraspinous and interspinous ligaments and the contralateral hemilamina are preserved. In addition to preserving midline stabilizing structures, hemilaminectomy also avoids exposure of, and therefore potential injury to, the contralateral facet joint. Because the integrity of the unexposed contralateral facet is maintained, more aggressive decompression of a nerve root by partial, or even total, ipsilateral facetectomy can be performed without the need for concomitant prophylactic fusion. As with traditional laminectomy, care is taken to preserve the pars interarticularis laterally to minimize risk of developing postoperative instability from inadvertent sacrifice of the superior articular facet.

Hemilaminectomy is appropriate for patients with unilateral symptoms from unilateral stenosis. It is particularly appropriate for moderate central stenosis. However, foraminal stenosis can be difficult to address from an ipsilateral hemilaminectomy approach because of difficulty in obtaining enough lateral exposure: the presence of an intact spinous process and interspinous-supraspinous ligament complex makes it difficult to angle the Kerrison rongeur laterally enough to decompress the depths of the neural foramen. Under such circumstances, removal of the midline spinous process and interspinous-supraspinous ligament complex may be necessary to allow the proper angulation of the rongeur to perform the foraminal decompression. Alternatively, the use of angled Kerrison rongeurs may facilitate lateral decompression without sacrifice of the spinous process.

Another technical challenge of this procedure is the relative difficulty performing contralateral decompression. Contralateral nerve root decompression may be accomplished by tilting the table away from the operating surgeon. When used in conjunction with the operating microscope, excellent illumination and magnification is obtained, and contralateral decompression can be facilitated without the need for removal of midline bony and ligamentous structures by angling the microscope to visualize the opposite side. The contralateral neural foramen can usually be visualized and decompressed, and its more distal portion can be palpated with a long bent probe, such as a bent number 4 Penfield elevator or a Woodson probe.

Although offering the advantage of preserving normal, noncompressing midline structures and minimizing scar tissue on the opposite side, this technique is more demanding than bilateral laminectomy because decompression is performed through a more limited exposure, and the determination of adequate foraminal patency is more dependent on feel (palpation) than by direct visualization. In addition, there is a greater potential for dural laceration from the Kerrison rongeur when working through a small opening. Should such a dural tear occur, its repair usually necessitates complete (bilateral) laminectomy with adequate exposure of the dural rent.

Other Alternatives to Laminectomy

A potential major problem with laminectomy is long-term deterioration due to recurrence of symptoms from recurrent or new neural compression (10,16,17). Despite this concern, more limited decompressive surgical alternatives to laminectomy and hemilaminectomy have been espoused to further minimize removal of normal, noncompressing structures and thereby minimize risk of postoperative instability. Such procedures include hemilaminotomy, wide fenestration, and laminoplasty.

Hemilaminotomy involves a more limited neural decompression than hemilaminectomy and removes only structures causing neural compression. It is the same procedure used to provide exposure for discectomy, but it involves removal of additional compressing tissue, including removal of adjacent portions of two contiguous hemilaminae and the ligamentum flavum, which is often redundant and buckled. This procedure is more likely to be performed in younger patients with unilateral focal stenosis, in whom extensive laminectomy carries the risk for later development of instability. It may also be considered in older patients

TABLE 7. *Comparison of decompression alone with decompression and fusion in spinal stenosis*

Evaluator	Decompression without fusion	Decompression and fusion (most stenotic segment only)	Decompression and fusion (all decompressed levels)
Patient	13/15 (87%)	12/15 (80%)	10/15 (67%)
Examiner	13/15 (87%)	12/15 (80%)	11/15 (73%)

From Grob D, Humke T, Dvorak J. Degenerative lumbar spinal stenosis: decompression with and without arthrodesis. *J Bone Joint Surg* 1995;77A:1036–1041, with permission.

who do not have extensive global stenosis, where laminectomy would otherwise be the preferred surgery of choice.

In the absence of significant underlying congenital stenosis, neural compression is generally due to primary degeneration and narrowing of the intervertebral disc, with secondary buckling of the ligamentum flavum. Hypertrophy of the facet joints may occur as a consequence of abnormal stresses. Because the superior attachment of the ligamentum flavum is approximately at the midpoint of the deep surface of the superior hemilamina, resection of the distal half of the superior hemilamina is generally required to remove the proximal insertion of the ligamentum. Therefore, hemilaminotomy generally involves removal of the inferior half of the superior hemilamina and the superior portion of the inferior hemilamina, together with the attached ligamentum flavum. Lateral decompression by partial facetectomy is performed, if required, as is done for bilateral laminectomy or hemilaminectomy. Like hemilaminectomy, contralateral decompression with preservation of spinous processes and the midline supraspinous-interspinous ligaments can be performed by tilting the operating table away from the surgeon and by undercutting the midline and contralateral ligamentum flavum with a 45-degree Kerrison rongeur. These minimal decompressive procedures have generally produced acceptable short-term results when compared to decompressive laminectomy (21–23).

Wide fenestration is a procedure described for central stenosis in which only the medial portion of the inferior facets and adjacent ligamentum flavum are removed (24–26). Care is taken to remove only pathologic neural compressing anatomy and to preserve the interspinous-supraspinous ligament complex and spinous processes that act as midline stabilizing structures. This is performed via bilateral laminotomies at each involved segmental level. A 5-year follow-up study of this procedure found that 82% of patients had good or excellent early surgical outcome, but the results deteriorated to only 71% rated as satisfactory by 4 years postoperatively (25). Poor results were thought to be due to instability rather than to symptomatic new bone formation. Although new bone was often formed at the fenestration site, it did not necessarily result in recurrent stenosis and was found to actually provide stability to the operated segments. The long-term problems associated with this procedure are therefore similar to those encountered with laminectomy.

Laminoplasty was originally proposed as an alternative to laminectomy in active manual workers (27,28). This procedure is similar to cervical laminoplasty and involves hinging open the lamina on one side and inserting the excised spinous processes into the open hinge to keep it patent. In a 3-year follow-up study of only ten patients, the mean Japanese Orthopaedic Association evaluation score improved an average of 73%, and the size of the spinal canal increased an average of 119% after surgery.

Decompressive Procedures with Fusion

Fusion is generally considered for spinal stenosis associated with spinal deformity, stenosis requiring multilevel decompression, or stenosis associated with significant back pain. It also is considered when disc excision has been performed, particularly in a younger patient. There is little support in the literature for fusing for focal stenosis with exclusively radicular leg pain and not associated with either degenerative scoliosis or spondylolisthesis. A recent prospective, randomized study of 45 patients undergoing either decompression alone or decompression and fusion for spinal stenosis without associated instability reported no significant differences in outcome between fused and unfused groups (29). Patients in this study were randomized into one of three treatment groups: group I—decompression without arthrodesis; group II—decompression with arthrodesis of only the most stenotic segment; group III—decompression and arthrodesis of all decompressed segments (Table 7). Overall, 78% of patient-reported and 80% of examiner-rated results were rated very good or good. When broken down by type of procedure performed, there were no significant differences in outcome between the three groups with regard to pain relief. Decompression alone produced satisfactory results in 87% of patients. The authors concluded that surgical decompression changed the natural history of spinal stenosis, resulting in generally favorable outcome and improved quality of life in the majority of patients. They further concluded that arthrodesis was not justified in the absence of radiographically proven segmental instability, because there was no statistical difference in outcome between the three treatment groups.

Spinal Stenosis with Degenerative Spondylolisthesis

Degenerative spondylolisthesis was first described in 1930 by Junghanns, who coined the term *pseudospondylolisthesis* to describe the presence of forward slippage of a vertebral body in the presence of an intact neural arch (30). The clinical and pathologic features of this entity were further defined by Macnab, who described the condition as "spondylolisthesis with an intact neural arch" (31). The term *degenerative spondylolisthesis* was originally used by Newman and Stone and is the terminology most commonly used to describe the anterior slippage of one vertebral body on another in the presence of an intact neural arch (32).

Degenerative spondylolisthesis may be asymptomatic, or it may be a source of low back and leg pain. It may cause either radicular or referred leg pain in a characteristic pattern of neurogenic claudication. It is a radiographic diagnosis made on the lateral radiograph. It may have a dynamic component to it such that the slip may reduce in the supine position and may therefore be apparent only on standing or stress radiographs. Such radiographs may include standing lateral views, sitting or standing flexion-extension views, or distraction compression radiography. The distinction between normal and abnormal segmental motion has been described by several authors (33,34).

Both the natural history of degenerative spondylolisthesis and, until recently, its optimal treatment has been incompletely understood. A metaanalysis of the literature on degenerative spondylolisthesis between 1970 and 1993 found that only 25 of the 152 studies reviewed (representing 889 patients) satisfied the inclusion criteria of the investigators (35). Only three of these studies (encompassing 278 patients) described the natural history of degenerative spondylolisthesis (36–38). Overall, 90 of these 278 patients (32%) achieved satisfactory results without specific treatment. The study by Matsunaga et al. represented the best of the three studies and was the only true natural history study (37). In this study, 40 patients who received no treatment were followed from 5 to 14 years, with a mean of 8.25 years. Only 4 of 40 patients (10%) showed clinical deterioration over the course of the study, and all four were in a subgroup of 28 patients who exhibited no slip progression over the follow-up period. Progressive slip was noted in 12 patients (30%), but none of the 12 patients exhibited clinical deterioration. The majority of the patients in this study showed slight improvement in their clinical symptoms over time. In general, no correlation was noted between slip progression and clinical deterioration. The lack of correlation between slip progression and progression of symptoms has also been reported by other authors (39).

One recent report supporting decompression without fusion for degenerative spondylolisthesis reviewed an elderly (average age of 67 years) population of 290 patients, 250 of whom had a one-level slip and 40 of whom had a two-level slip (21). The data from this study were self-reported by the surgeons and was retrospective. The decompressive procedures included laminectomy in 249 patients and fenestration procedures in 41 patients. Fenestration procedures typically involved bilateral laminotomy with partial medial facetectomy and foraminotomy. Only patients with a stable slip (having less than 4 mm of translation and less than 10 to 12 degrees of angulation on dynamic flexion-extension lateral radiographs) were included. At an average follow-up of 10 years (range: 1 to 27 years), 69% of patients reported excellent, 13% good, 12% fair, and 6% poor outcomes. The authors concluded that an 82% excellent/good outcome was very acceptable in this older population, in whom fusion is associated with higher morbidity and mortality. Other studies have confirmed significant morbidity and mortality in elderly patient populations undergoing spinal fusion (13,14,40).

A prospective study that assigned a group of 67 patients with spinal stenosis to either laminectomy or multilevel laminotomy included a small group of patients with degenerative spondylolisthesis (23). Nine of the patients assigned to the laminotomy group crossed over to the laminectomy group, which allowed for some ambiguity in the interpretation of the results. However, no patient undergoing multilevel laminotomies developed instability as a result of the surgery, compared with three patients undergoing laminectomy. The authors concluded that multilevel laminotomies could be recommended for patients with developmental stenosis, mild to moderate degenerative stenosis, or degenerative spondylolisthesis. Total laminectomy was recommended for patients with severe degenerative stenosis or marked degenerative spondylolisthesis.

Another recent study prospectively evaluated 54 consecutive patients who underwent decompression without fusion for spinal stenosis (22). In the small subgroup of 15 patients who had concomitant degenerative spondylolisthesis, 87% (13 of 15 patients) showed no change in the amount of preoperative slip. Overall, 88% of the 54 patients reported good/excellent clinical outcome, and the results were comparable between patients with and without degenerative spondylolisthesis. The study concluded that degenerative spinal stenosis, including patients with degenerative spondylolisthesis, can be decompressed effectively without the need for fusion.

Role of Noninstrumented Fusion for Degenerative Spondylolisthesis

Although the beneficial role of fusion in the surgical treatment of spinal stenosis associated with degenerative spondylolisthesis is less controversial than the role of fusion in the treatment of other degenerative back conditions, incontrovertible evidence supporting its use is sparse. An attempted metaanalysis of literature reported between 1970 and 1993 found only six studies meeting the inclusion criteria that compared results of decompression with fusion and decompression alone for degenerative spondylolisthesis (35). In that review, 79% of patients who had decompression without fusion reported satisfactory outcome, compared to 86% of those who had decompression and a concomitant fusion (Table 8).

Other studies have supported the position that patients undergoing fusion with decompression for degenerative spondylolisthesis do clinically better than those undergoing decompression alone (38,41,42). However, it is difficult to gain a clear understanding of this issue from a review of existing literature, because well-designed studies reporting surgical outcome after surgery for degenerative spondylolisthesis are uncommon. The metaanalysis by Mardjetko and associates found only eleven papers (encompassing 216 patients) reporting outcome measures after decompression without fusion that met their inclusion criteria (Table 9) (35). One of these studies was retrospective and nonrandomized (41), two were prospective and randomized (38,43), and the remaining eight were retrospective, nonrandomized, and uncontrolled. Overall, 69% of patients in this metaanalysis reported satisfactory outcome with decompression alone, with 31% having an unsatisfactory result and 31% having progression of the slip. Although most studies found no correlation between clinical outcome and amount of slip progression, one study suggested that poor outcome was associated with slip progression. That study was a prospective, randomized design that included a subgroup of 11 patients undergoing decompression and noninstrumented fusion for degenerative

TABLE 8. *Results of decompression with noninstrumented fusion: metaanalysis of literature (1970–1993) (six articles)*

Total number of patients	Satisfactory	Unsatisfactory	Fusion
84	59 (79%)[a,b]	16 (21%)[a,b]	62 (86%)

[a]Weighted, pooled proportion.
[b]Data from five of six articles reported.
From Mardjetko SM, Connolly PJ, Shott S. Degenerative lumbar spondylolisthesis. a meta-analysis of literature 1970–1993. *Spine* 1994;19(20S):2556S–2565S, with permission.

TABLE 9. *Results of decompression without fusion: metaanalysis of literature 1970–1993 (11 articles)*

Total number of patients	Satisfactory	Unsatisfactory	Progressive slip
216	140 (69%)[a]	75 (31%)[a]	67 (31%)[b]

[a]Weighted, pooled proportion.
[b]Reported in only 9 of 11 articles.
From Mardjetko SM, Connolly PJ, Shott S. Degenerative lumbar spondylolisthesis. a meta-analysis of literature 1970–1993. *Spine* 1994;19(20S):2556S–2565S, with permission.

spondylolisthesis (43). Of the ten patients available for follow-up, only three (30%) reported improved functional outcome, and seven had an increase in their preoperative spondylolisthesis.

Many studies on the surgical treatment of degenerative spondylolisthesis emphasize the unfavorable outcome after decompression without fusion. One early, small study by two groups of surgeons from two different institutions included two populations of patients with spinal stenosis and degenerative spondylolisthesis: one group underwent decompression alone and the other decompression and fusion (41). In the patient cohort undergoing decompression alone, 5 of 11 (45%) were rated as good (satisfactory) and 6 of 11 (55%) as fair/poor (unsatisfactory). In contrast, five of eight patients (63%) undergoing decompression with *in situ* posterolateral fusion achieved a satisfactory outcome. This study suggested that patients did better when their decompression was accompanied by noninstrumented fusion.

A prospective, randomized study comparing decompression alone to decompression and noninstrumented posterolateral spinal fusion in the treatment of L3-4 and L4-5 degenerative spondylolisthesis with spinal stenosis reported superior results when concomitant fusion was performed with the decompression (39). Satisfactory outcome was more than twice as common in the fused group compared to the unfused group (96% vs. 44%, respectively). Furthermore, the percentage of excellent results was significantly and dramatically greater in the fused group (44% excellent) than in the unfused group (8% excellent; $p = .0001$) (Table 10). This study concluded that the results of surgical decompression with *in situ* arthrodesis were superior to those of decompression alone in the treatment of spinal stenosis associated with L3-4 or L4-5 degenerative spondylolisthesis. Outcome was not influenced by the age or sex of the patient or the preoperative height of the disc space. The authors concluded that the decision for concomitant arthrodesis should be based purely on the presence or absence of a preoperative slip rather than on other preoperative factors such as the age or sex of the patient or the disc height, or on intraoperative factors such as the amount of bone resected during the decompression. Although postoperatively there was a significant ($p = .002$) increased risk for slip progression in nonfused patients compared to those undergoing fusion, 36% of those who did have an arthrodesis were noted to have a pseudarthrosis, but all had an excellent or good result.

TABLE 10. *Prospective, randomized comparison of decompression versus decompression and noninstrumented spinal fusion for degenerative spondylolisthesis*

	Arthrodesis (n = 25)	No arthrodesis (n = 25)
Result		
Excellent	11 (44%)	2 (8%)
Good	13 (52%)	9 (36%)
Fair	1 (4%)	12 (48%)
Poor	0 (0%)	2 (8%)
Mean increase in slip (preoperative to postoperative)	0.5 mm	2.6 mm ($p = .002$)

From Herkowitz HN, Kurz LT. Degenerative lumbar spondylolisthesis with spinal stenosis. A prospective study comparing decompression with decompression and intertransverse process arthrodesis. *J Bone Joint Surg* 1991;73-A:802–808, with permission.

A recent long-term review of 96 patients undergoing decompressive surgery for spinal stenosis followed for at least 5 years included a subset of patients with associated degenerative spondylolisthesis (20). Although this subgroup was not fully analyzed separately, and the study itself was retrospective, nonrandomized, and uncontrolled, some important trends were noted. Twenty-six patients (27%) were considered failures: 16 because of recurrent neural symptoms and 10 because of low back pain. The frequency of degenerative spondylolisthesis was significantly greater in the surgical failures (12 of 26 patients, or 46%) than in the surgical successes (16 of 64, or 25%). The authors concluded that because of the higher incidence of recurrent symptoms in patients with preexisting degenerative spondylolisthesis, all patients with associated slip should be fused.

One well-recognized cause of long-term failure of decompression for spinal stenosis is subsequent bone regrowth causing recurrent neural compression. One recent study reported the relationship between bone regrowth occurring an average of 8.6 years after surgical decompression for spinal stenosis and long-term outcome (17). Sixteen of the 40 patients (40%) in that study had degenerative spondylolisthesis. Ten of the 16 (62%) had a concomitant arthrodesis. Although all 16 patients with degenerative spondylolisthesis showed some bone regrowth, the degree of regrowth was more severe in the six unfused patients than it was in the ten patients who were fused (Table 11). Furthermore, the proportion of satisfactory results was significantly higher in patients who had spinal fusion. Although this study was not randomized and was retrospective, it suggested that arthrodesis stabilizes the spine, resulting in less bone regrowth causing recurrent stenosis and superior long-term results.

Role of Instrumented Fusion

The long-term clinical outcome of surgical decompression with instrumented spinal fusion, particularly when compared to the

TABLE 11. *Relationship between outcome and fusion in patients with degenerative spondylolisthesis*

	Number of patients	Excellent	Good	Fair	Poor
Fusion	10	3	5	2	0
No fusion	6	0	2	1	3

From Postacchini F, Cinotti G. Bone regrowth after surgical decompression for lumbar spinal stenosis. *J Bone Joint Surg* 1992;74-B:862–869, with permission.

outcome of decompression with noninstrumented fusion, is not completely known. Although there is little argument that segmental instrumentation produces a more solid arthrodesis than noninstrumented fusion, conflicting data exist relating the presence of a solid arthrodesis to superior clinical results. The multicenter historical cohort study of spinal fusion using pedicle screw fixation involved a retrospective review of 2,684 patients with degenerative spondylolisthesis (44). Solid radiographic fusion was noted in 89% of patients who had undergone pedicle screw fixation compared to 70% of those treated without instrumentation. It is important to note that the clinical outcomes were also better in the group of patients undergoing instrumented fusion.

A prospective, randomized study followed 124 patients for 1 year after instrumented or noninstrumented fusion for a variety of diagnoses, including degenerative spondylolisthesis (42). Two types of spinal instrumentation were used: a rigid system and a semirigid system. Outcomes were based on radiographic fusion rate. The overall fusion rate was 65% for the noninstrumented group, 77% for the semirigid fixation group, and 95% for the rigid fixation group. A trend for better clinical outcome with increasing rigidity of fixation was also observed. Seventy-one percent of the noninstrumented patients, 89% of the semirigid group, and 95% of the rigid group reported excellent or good results. For the subgroup of patients with degenerative spondylolisthesis, 65% of the noninstrumented patients fused compared with 50% of the semirigid fixation group and 86% of the rigid fixation group.

A retrospective study of 30 patients undergoing decompression and instrumented fusion for degenerative spondylolisthesis reported radiographic outcome as measured by fusion rate and functional outcome as measured by a patient questionnaire and the Short Form 36 survey (45). Fusion rate and a successful outcome as measured by patient satisfaction were 93%. However, 13 patients (43%) had complications, including dural tears (three patients), excessive blood loss (two patients), pseudarthrosis (two patients), pulmonary embolus (one patient), deep infection (one patient), urinary tract infections (three patients), and unstable angina (one patient). The study concluded that patients treated with decompression and fusion for degenerative spondylolisthesis had improved patient-reported functional outcomes.

In contrast, some studies have concluded that the addition of spinal instrumentation to a fusion does not necessarily improve outcome. A recent randomized prospective study of patients undergoing posterolateral lumbar fusion, with and without pedicle screw instrumentation, for a variety of conditions concluded that the addition of instrumentation did not produce an incremental clinical benefit to that obtained from noninstrumented fusion, although there was a slight nonsignificant trend toward a higher fusion rate in the instrumented fusion group (46). Overall, there was no statistical difference in patient-reported outcome between the two groups. There was a slight nonsignificant trend toward increased radiographic fusion rate in the group with instrumentation that did not correlate with an increased patient-reported improvement rate. For the entire group, the results did not indicate a clinical benefit from the addition of instrumentation in elective lumbar fusions. For the subgroup of ten patients who had degenerative spondylolisthesis, five underwent instrumented fusion, and five underwent noninstrumented fusion *in situ*. Four of the five patients with degenerative spondylolisthesis undergoing instrumented fusion achieved excellent/good outcome, compared to two of five of those undergoing noninstrumented fusion. For this small subgroup of patients with degenerative spondylolisthesis, the clinical outcome appeared to be better than that of the overall population studied, although this subgroup was too small to achieve statistical significance.

A prospective, randomized study of 76 patients with spinal stenosis and degenerative spondylolisthesis examined the potential benefit of segmental transpedicular instrumentation (47). Although successful fusion occurred significantly more often in the instrumented group than in the noninstrumented group (82% vs. 45%, respectively), there was not a significant improvement in clinical outcome between the two groups (76% vs. 85% excellent/good outcome, respectively). The authors concluded that the presence of successful fusion did not predict or influence outcome.

From a societal perspective, fusion (particularly instrumented fusion) adds significantly to the incremental costs of treating spinal stenosis with degenerative spondylolisthesis. A recent study looked at the 10-year costs, quality-adjusted life years, and incremental cost-effectiveness ratios (reported as dollars per quality-adjusted year of life gained) for patients undergoing decompressive surgery, with or without spinal fusion, for spinal stenosis with degenerative spondylolisthesis (48). Laminectomy with noninstrumented fusion was found to cost $56,500 per quality-adjusted year of life versus laminectomy without fusion. The cost-effectiveness ratio of instrumented fusion, compared with noninstrumented fusion, was $3,112,800 per quality-adjusted year of life. A cost-effectiveness ratio of $82,400 per quality-adjusted year of life was calculated if the proportion of patients experiencing symptom relief after instrumented fusion was 90% as compared with 80% for patients with noninstrumented fusion. The study concluded that the cost effectiveness of laminectomy with noninstrumented fusion compared favorably with other surgical interventions, although it depended greatly on the true effectiveness of the surgery to alleviate symptoms and also on how patients valued the quality-of-life effect of relieving severe stenosis symptoms. Instrumented fusion was very expensive compared with the modest incremental gain in health outcome. The study further concluded that better data on the effectiveness of such alternative procedures were needed to justify their incremental cost.

An unresolved issue with the use of spinal instrumentation in the elderly patient is its potential biomechanical effect on adjacent, unfused levels. There is evidence that the rigidity afforded by fusion with instrumentation produces significant stresses at the levels above or below the fusion, with the potential for adjacent level failure by vertebral compression fracture or stress fracture. Because of this, it theoretically may be preferable to have a less-rigid noninstrumented fusion or even a stable pseudarthrosis rather than a rigid arthrodesis.

Currently, there does not appear to be a clear consensus as to the optimal way to treat patients with symptomatic degenerative spondylolisthesis. Most studies suggest that patients undergoing surgery do better when the decompression is accompanied by fusion. It is less clear, however, whether the fusion should be augmented with instrumentation. It seems reasonable that if there were clear evidence of instability on flexion-extension radiographs, the immediate stability provided by instrumentation would warrant the additional time, expense, and potential morbidity associated with its use. This would seem to be especially appropriate for young, active patients with good bone stock. On the other hand, the indication for its use in the patient with a collapsed disc space, no motion at the spondylolisthetic level, or osteoporosis is less clear.

CONCLUSION

The optimal surgical treatment of spinal stenosis, particularly when associated with degenerative spondylolisthesis, is still somewhat controversial. Such controversy involves the method and extent of decompression, the role of fusion, and the use of spinal instrumentation. Although spinal stenosis is a global degenerative condition with many segmental levels often showing evidence of radiographic stenosis, decompression of every level showing any degree of radiographic stenosis is clearly not always indicated. Obviously, all symptomatic levels should be decompressed. There is no clear consensus, however, on whether to decompress asymptomatic levels, and this decision depends on many factors. Because restenosis at a previously decompressed level or the development of symptomatic stenosis at a previously asymptomatic and unoperated stenotic level is a common reason for failure of surgery for spinal stenosis, it is generally more prudent to decompress any stenotic level suspected of being potentially symptomatic than not to. When diffuse degenerative changes produce multilevel stenosis, particularly in an elderly patient, decompression by unilateral or bilateral laminotomies, rather than by multiple complete laminectomies, should be considered. Multilevel decompression with bilateral laminectomies carries the risk of development of instability and therefore mandates consideration of fusion to ameliorate this risk. Because fusion is associated with higher morbidity in the elderly population, it is prudent to consider a less expansive surgical decompression that could obviate the need for fusion in these patients. Such an approach reduces the need for concomitant fusion by preserving the uninvolved laminae and ligamentous structures, thereby minimizing the risk of developing late instability.

The decision of whether to fuse a patient with stenosis associated with degenerative spondylolisthesis can be difficult in the elderly patient with multiple comorbidities. Many studies suggest that patients have better clinical outcome when decompression is accompanied by arthrodesis. The issue of whether to augment the fusion with segmental instrumentation is not yet resolved. In a young, healthy patient with spinal stenosis associated with degenerative spondylolisthesis, particularly if associated with well-maintained disc height, it seems reasonable to fuse the listhetic level, usually with segmental fixation, because of the risk of developing subsequent instability. In elderly, debilitated, or low-demand patients, on the other hand, the decision to fuse must be balanced against the increased morbidity associated with arthrodesis. Arthrodesis may not be a therapeutic imperative in the elderly patient with a listhetic level associated with decreased disc height, spur formation, subchondral sclerosis, or ligament ossification, because these degenerative changes may provide stability to the listhetic level and minimize the risk of slip progression. Under such conditions, consideration of unilateral or bilateral laminotomies to preserve uninvolved stabilizing structures seems warranted.

In summary, decompression and fusion with pedicle fixation are reasonable in active, healthy, young patients with spinal stenosis associated with degenerative spondylolisthesis who have relatively few degenerative changes promoting stability at the level of the slip. Elderly and active patients with degenerative changes usually benefit from decompression with noninstrumented fusion. Elderly, low-demand patients with multiple comorbidities who have associated degenerative changes at the listhetic level may often be managed by limited decompression without fusion.

REFERENCES

1. Blau J, Logue V. Intermittent claudication of the cauda equina. An unusual syndrome resulting from central protrusion of a lumbar intervertebral disc. *Lancet* 1961;1:1082–1086.
2. Jones R, Thomson J. The narrow lumbar canal: a clinical and radiological review. *J Bone Joint Surg* 1968;50-B:595–605.
3. Johnsson KE, Rosen I, Uden A. The natural course of spinal stenosis. *Clin Orthop* 1992;279:82–86.
4. Spivak J. Current concepts review. Degenerative lumbar spinal stenosis. *J Bone Joint Surg* 1998;80A(7):1053–1066.
5. Turner J, Ersek M, Herron L, et al. Surgery for Lumbar Spinal Stenosis: attempted meta-analysis of the literature. *Spine* 1992;17:1–8.
6. Atlas S, Deyo R, Keller R, et al. The Maine lumbar spine study, part III. *Spine* 1996;21(15):1787–1795.
7. Johnsson K, Uden A, Rosen I. The effect of decompression on the natural course of spinal stenosis. A comparison of surgically treated and untreated patients. *Spine* 1991;16(6):615–619.
8. Saal JA, Saal JA, Parthasarathy R. The natural history of lumbar spinal stenosis. The results of non-operative treatment. Presented at tenth annual meeting of the North American Spine Society (NASS). Washington, D.C., 1995.
9. Jonsson B, Stromqvist B. Symptoms and signs in degeneration of the lumbar spine. A prospective, consecutive study of 300 operated patients. *J Bone Joint Surg* 1993;75(B):381–385.
10. Katz J, Lipson S, Chang L, et al. Seven- to 10-year outcome of decompressive surgery for degenerative lumbar spinal stenosis. *Spine* 1996;21:92–98.
11. Katz J, Lipson S, Larson M, et al. The outcome of decompressive laminectomy for degenerative lumbar stenosis. *J Bone Joint Surg* 1991;73(A):809–816.
12. Katz J, Lipson S, Brick G, et al. Clinical correlates of patient satisfaction after laminectomy for degenerative lumbar spinal stenosis. *Spine* 1995;20(10):1155–1160.
13. Deyo R, Ciol M, Cherkin D, et al. Lumbar spinal fusion. A cohort study of complications, reoperations, and resource use in the Medicare population. *Spine* 1993;18(11):1463–1470.
14. Deyo R, Cherkin D, Loeser J, et al. Morbidity and mortality in association with operations on the lumbar spine. *J Bone Joint Surg* 1992;74-A:536–543.
15. Oldridge N, Yuan Z, Stoll J, Rimm A. Lumbar spine surgery and mortality among Medicare beneficiaries, 1986. *Am J Public Health* 1994;84(8):1292–1298.
16. Postacchini F, Cinotti G, Gumina S, et al. Long-term results of surgery in lumbar stenosis. 8-year review of 64 patients. *Acta Orthop Scand Suppl* 1993;251:78–80.
17. Postacchini F, Cinotti G. Bone regrowth after surgical decompression for lumbar spinal stenosis. *J Bone Joint Surg* 1992;74-B:862–869.
18. Jönsson B, Annertz M, Sjoberg C, et al. A prospective and consecutive study of surgically treated lumbar spinal stenosis. Part II: five-year follow-up by an independent observer. *Spine* 1997;22(24):2938–2944.
19. Spangfort EV. The lumbar disc herniation: a computer-aided analysis of 2,504 operations. *Acta Orthop Scand Suppl* 1972;142:1–95.
20. Caputy A, Luessenhop A. Long-term evaluation of decompressive surgery for degenerative lumbar stenosis. *J Neurosurg* 1992;77:669–676.
21. Epstein N, Epstein J. Decompression in the surgical management of degenerative spondylolisthesis: advantages of a conservative approach in 290 patients. *J Spin Disord* 1998;11(2):116–122.
22. Kleeman TJ, Hiscoe AC, Berg EE. Patient outcomes after minimally destabilizing lumbar stenosis decompression: the "port-hole" technique. *Spine* 2000;25(7):865–870.
23. Postacchini F, Cinotti G, Perugia D, et al. The surgical treatment of central lumbar stenosis. Multiple laminotomy compared with total laminectomy. *J Bone Joint Surg* 1993;75(B):386–392.

24. Lin PM. Internal decompression for multiple levels of lumbar spinal stenosis: a technical note. *Neurosurgery* 1982;11(4):546–549.
25. Nakai O, Ookawa A, Yamaura I. Long-term roentgenographic and functional changes in patients who were treated with wide fenestration for central lumbar stenosis. *J Bone Joint Surg* 1991;73(A):1184–1191.
26. Young S, Veerapen R, O'Laoire S. Relief of lumbar canal stenosis using multilevel subarticular fenestrations as an alternative to wide laminectomy: preliminary report. *Neurosurgery* 1988;23(5):628–633.
27. Matsui H, Kanamori M, Ishihara H, et al. Expansive lumbar laminoplasty for degenerative spinal stenosis in patients below 70 years of age. *Eur Spine J* 1997;6(3):191–196.
28. Matsui H, Tsuji H, Seido H, et al. Results of expansive laminoplasty for lumbar spinal stenosis in active manual workers. *Spine* 1992;17 [3 Suppl]:S37–S40.
29. Grob D, Humke T, Dvorak J. Degenerative lumbar spinal stenosis decompression with and without arthrodesis. *J Bone Joint Surg* 1995;77-A:1036–1041.
30. Junghanns H. Spondylolisthesen ohne spalt in zwischengelenkstueck. *Archiv fuer Orthopadische Unfallchirurgie* 1930;29:118–127.
31. Macnab I. Spondylolisthesis with an intact neural arch—the so-called psuedo-spondylolisthesis. *J Bone Joint Surg* 1950;32-B:325–333.
32. Newman P, Stone K. The etiology of spondylolisthesis. *J Bone Joint Surg* 1963;45-B:39–59.
33. Boden SD, Wiesel SW. Lumbosacral segmental motion in normal individuals: Have we been measuring instability properly? *Spine* 1990;5:571–576.
34. Hayes MA, Howard TC, Gruel CR, et al. Roentgenographic evaluation of lumbar spine flexion-extension in asymptomatic individuals. *Spine* 1989;14(3):327–331.
35. Mardjetko S, Connolly P, Shott S. Degenerative lumbar spondylolisthesis: a meta-analysis of literature, 1970–1993. *Spine* 1994;19[20 Suppl]:2256S–2265S.
36. Fitzgerald J, Newman P. Degenerative spondylolisthesis. *J Bone Joint Surg* 1976;58-B(2):184–192.
37. Matsunaga S, Sakou T, et al. Natural history of degenerative spondylolisthesis: pathogenesis and natural course of the slippage. *Spine* 1990;15(11):1204–1210.
38. Rosenberg N. Degenerative spondylolisthesis: surgical treatment. *Clin Orthop Rel Res* 1976;117:112–120.
39. Herkowitz H, Kurz L. Degenerative lumbar spondylolisthesis with spinal stenosis: a prospective study comparing decompression with decompression and intertransverse process arthrodesis. *J Bone Joint Surg* 1991;73–A:802–808.
40. Turner JA, Ersek M, Herron L, et al. Patient outcomes after lumbar spinal fusions. *JAMA* 1992;268(7).
41. Feffer H, Weisel S, et al. Degenerative spondylolisthesis: to fuse or not to fuse. *Spine* 1985;10(3):286–289.
42. Zdeblick T. A prospective, randomized study of lumbar fusion: preliminary results. *Spine* 1993;18:983–991.
43. Bridwell K, et al. Role of fusion and instrumentation in the treatment of degenerative spondylolisthesis. *J Spinal Dis* 1993;6(6):461–472.
44. Yuan HA, Garfin SR, Dickman CA, et al. A historical cohort study of pedicle screw fixation in thoracic lumbar, and sacral spinal fusions. *Spine* 1994;19(20S):2279–2296.
45. Nork SE, Serena SH, Workman KL, et al. Patient outcomes after decompression and instrumented posterior spinal fusion for degenerative spondylolisthesis. *Spine* 1999;24(6):561–569.
46. France JC, Yaszemski MJ, Lauerman WC, et al. A randomized prospective study of posterolateral lumbar fusion. outcomes with and without pedicle screw instrumentation. *Spine* 1999;24(6):553–560.
47. Fischgrund J, Mackay M, Herkowitz H, et al. Degenerative lumbar spondylolisthesis with spinal stenosis: a prospective, randomized study comparing decompressive laminectomy and arthrodesis with and without spinal instrumentation. *Spine* 1997;22(24):2807–2812.
48. Kuntz KM, Snider RK, Weinstein JN et al. Cost-effectiveness of fusion with and without instrumentation for patients with degenerative spondylolisthesis and spinal stenosis. *Spine* 2000;25(9):1132–1139.

CHAPTER 49

Segmental Instability: Anatomic, Biomechanical, and Clinical Considerations

William F. Donaldson III, Ezequiel H. Cassinelli, and Eric J. Graham

The human spine has many functions. It must be rigid enough to withstand the large loads the body experiences during strenuous exercise or heavy lifting, while protecting the neural elements. It also has to be flexible enough to allow for sufficient motion to accomplish the multiple activities humans perform. It is extremely difficult to define what constitutes normal spinal motion, other than in generalized, age-adjusted measure of flexor extension, lateral bend, and rotation. The term *spinal instability* attempts to define what motion may be considered pathologic, particularly at individual motion segments. Frymoyer describes degenerative instability as "a loss of spinal motion segment stiffness, such that force application to that motion segment produces greater displacement(s) than would be seen in a normal structure, resulting in a painful condition, the potential for progressive deformity, and which places neurologic structures at risk" (1).

RELEVANT THORACIC AND LUMBAR SPINE ANATOMY

Knowledge of the basic anatomy of the thoracic and lumbar spine is essential to better understand spine biomechanics in "normal" as well as pathologic states. The anatomy of each of these two regions is adapted to best perform their respective unique functions. The rib cage and sternum provide significant additional rigidity and stiffness to the thoracic vertebral column. These anatomic restraints limit the possible range of motion, however, but serve to protect vital internal organs as well as enable upright ambulation. This is in distinct contrast to the lumbar region, which bears significant loads as well as allowing for trunk mobility.

Static Restraints

The major building block is the vertebral body itself. The 12 thoracic and five lumbar vertebra gradually increase in width caudally. The exception to this rule occurs at T1-3, where width is fairly uniform. In the thoracic region, the height of the posterior wall is slightly greater than that of the anterior wall, which results in a physiologic kyphosis ranging from 20 to 50 degrees. In the lumbar region, the anterior wall is slightly greater than the posterior, leading to an overall lordosis ranging from 20 to 70 degrees. The balanced curvilinear shape of the entire spine allows for the transmission of force along the spinal column while maintaining the balance of stiffness and stability at each individual functional unit.

The thoracic spine is unique, as there are costal facets on all 12 thoracic vertebrae. T1-9 possess a dual articulation with adjacent ribs. Every rib articulates with the vertebral body via costotransverse and costocentral joints. Each rib/costovertebral joint level in the thoracic spine responds similarly when subjected to three-point bending stress (2). The presence of an intact rib cage increases stiffness in all planes of motion, which is most pronounced in extension, and increases the stability of the column against compression fourfold. Removal of the sternum significantly decreases this stiffness (3), whereas removal of one or two ribs has no significant effect. The differences in strength of the upper rib cage versus the lower rib cage, therefore, are due to the geometry of the cage rather than differences in the individual ribs. This is evident in the high level of trauma needed to produce fractures of the upper ribs and sternum. The lower thoracic spine represents a transition zone with some characteristics of lumbar vertebral bodies, particularly with respect to facet orientation.

The facet joints in the thoracic spine are coronally aligned, which presents rotational freedom, while relatively limiting flexion/extension. At the thoracolumbar junction, the facet orientation becomes more sagittal, thereby decreasing rotational freedom but increasing flexion/extension mobility. In the lumbar region, the facets become even more sagittally oriented, allowing for greater flexion/extension and decreased axial rotation as one moves caudal. Flexion/extension at the L1-2 level is approximately 12 degrees, and increases gradually to 20 degrees at L-5 to S-1 (4).

An important concept in describing spinal motion is coupling. The individual motion segment can be described as having three axes: cephalocaudad, lateral, and rotational. About each of these axes, rotations and translations can occur in a positive or negative vector. Coupling indicates rotations and translations around one vector. For example, in the thoracic spine, lateral bending is coupled with axial rotation in such a way that the spinous processes point toward the convexity of the curve. This pattern is most evident in the upper thoracic spine. The lumbar spine also exhibits a coupling pattern, but the spinous processes point to the opposite side of the curve (5). Lateral bending is also coupled with flexion/extension (6).

There are seven ligamentous connections between adjacent vertebrae, which are consistently present from C-2 to the sacrum. They function to resist tensile but not compressive forces in a specific plane. Like other ligaments in the body, their load-deformation curves are nonlinear, and offer little resistance to physiologic ranges of motion, but significant resistance to motions beyond that range. Each ligament is oriented parallel to the plane of motion it resists. The anterior vertebral column is supported by the anterior longitudinal ligament (ALL). This ligament travels throughout the spine and increases in tensile strength in a caudal direction (7). The ALL is a significant restraint to hyperextension of the spine. The posterior longitudinal ligament (PLL) extends over the posterior surfaces of the vertebral bodies and has strong attachments to the posterior fibers of the annulus fibrosus. The ALL is twice as strong as the PLL due to the fact that it has double the cross-sectional area. The intertransverse ligaments connect neighboring transverse processes and serve as insertions for some of the deep paraspinal back muscles. The interspinous and supraspinous ligaments run between spinous processes and resist hyperflexion of the spine. The facet capsule itself provides significant stability because it is oriented perpendicular to the plane of the facet. Thus, in the thoracic spine the capsules help resist flexion, whereas in the lumbar spine they are more constrained to rotation. Last, the ligamentum flavum connects adjacent lamina and plays a smaller role in resisting flexion. It is also under tension in its resting state, which might help prevent it from buckling when the spine goes into extension and the flavum shortens.

The intervertebral disc is one of the main stabilizers of the thoracic and lumbar spine. The outer annulus fibrosus (comprised primarily of type I collagen) surrounds the gelatinous, central nucleus pulposus (rich in proteoglycans). The annulus resists tensile stresses and reduces strain caused by compressive, torsional, and transverse loading of the spine (8). The hydrostatic nucleus pulposus serves to limit the deformation of the annulus, as well as providing a "shock-absorbing effect" to dissipate compressive loads. Discs in the thoracic spine are rectangular in shape and have less height than in the lumbar spine. Lumbar intervertebral discs also tend to be wedge shaped, which contributes as well to lumbar lordosis.

Dynamic Restraints

Without all of its muscular attachments, the intact spine is actually a rather unstable structure. These muscles provide postural stability at rest and aid in movement with physiologic activity. The muscles also serve a protective role by helping to stabilize the spine during trauma. Bergmark hypothesized that there were two main muscle systems that play a role in spine stability (9). The first is a "global system," which does not attach directly to the spine but acts to provide general truncal stability. These include the rectus and obliquus abdominis and part of the iliocostalis. The second is a "local system," which does attach directly to the spinal elements and plays a role in segmental stability. These include muscles such as the multifidus, psoas major, quadratus lumborum, the lumbar parts of the iliocostalis and longissimus, and the transversus abdominis.

BIOMECHANICS

To simplify the complex biomechanics of the entire spine, Panjabi introduced the concept of the functional spinal unit (FSU) and multisegmental spinal unit (10). An *FSU* is defined as the smallest segment of the spine that has biomechanical characteristics similar to the spine as a whole and is made up of two adjacent vertebrae, the intervertebral disc, and the spinal ligaments that connect them. The costovertebral articulations are included in the thoracic spine. The use of multiple segments allows for a closer representation of *in vivo* behavior, as many of the structures making up the FSU (i.e., ligaments) are continuous structures.

A load-deformation curve describes the amount of motion (or deformation) a structure demonstrates in response to varying amounts of load. The load-deformation curve of an FSU is similar to those of individual ligaments. At low applied loads, most of the motion of an FSU occurs near its resting position, thus producing very little resistance. This is termed the *neutral zone* (NZ). Increasing loads deflect the FSU even further from its resting position, and this causes the bony and soft-tissue structures to offer increasing resistance to motion (i.e., deformation). This is called the *elastic zone* (EZ). Loads that exceed the FSU's ability to resist deformation result in permanent damage to the FSU. This is called the *plastic zone* (PZ). Panjabi showed that the NZ increased with segmental injury and disc degeneration—that is, greater displacement occurred under the same physiologic loads.

Studies have also shown that motion (and thus decreased resistance to load) of the FSU increases with sequential resection of its components (11). The ability of the FSU to resist displacement is not constant (not linear) and is also dependent on the rate of loading. The changes in dynamic motion (e.g., velocity, acceleration) that occur with progressive FSU destabilization (e.g., sequential discectomy and unilateral facetectomy) have been evaluated (12). The investigators concluded that after destabilization, acceleration parameters were sensitized to motion direction and load condition, suggesting that instability might be related to a change in dynamic motion rather than an abnormality in the overall amount of displacement.

The effect of the muscular stabilizers on spine biomechanics is less understood, as they are difficult to study experimentally. Muscles produce movement; enable the performance of various tasks, such as heavy lifting; and provide dynamic stabilization of the spine. Various studies have suggested there is a neural control system that receives afferent proprioceptive input from the spine and surrounding structures and responds by effects adjustment of paravertebral muscle forces (13,14). Neurons sensitive to mechanical strain have been found in lumbar spine ligaments and facet capsules. Cholewicke and McGill have found that the lumbar spine is more susceptible to instability at low loads with low muscle forces, and that the actions of the local muscle systems served to stabilize the spine under these conditions (15). The multifidus is felt to help maintain lumbar lordosis and stabilize the FSUs within their NZ (16). The deep abdominal muscles provide resistance to lateral bending and rotation via the thoracolumbar fascia.

Abnormal spinal motion is most easily studied in the context of trauma, as it is the condition most easily simulated in an experimental model. The concept of spinal stability with thoracolumbar spine trauma is well described by Dennis' three-column theory (17). The rib cage–sternum complex has been described as the fourth column of support unique to the thoracic spine (18). The validity of the three-column theory is generally accepted. The main disagreement is whether the most important column is the middle or posterior column when stability is compromised after thoracic and lumbar fractures. Denis (17) and Panjabi et al. (19) identified the middle column as the most critical, whereas James and coworkers found that the posterior column integrity was the most crucial (20). Evidence that the majority of the load is borne by the anterior portion of the vertebral body was documented in a study by Edwards et al. (21).

In the thoracic region, the normal thoracic kyphosis makes this region more susceptible to flexion instability. This region of the spine is less mobile and much more difficult to disrupt, as it is further reinforced by the costovertebral articulations. The ribs are believed to impart thoracic stability via two mechanisms (22). The first is the articulation of the rib with the adjacent vertebral bodies. The second is due to the presence of the thoracic cage as a whole, which increases the moment of inertia and thus adds increased resistance. The thoracic spine is much less tolerant of abnormal displacements, however, as it has less free space available for the spinal cord when comparing the cord to canal ratio. The relative contributions of the selective soft-tissue structures and the bony elements have been evaluated in a number of studies. Some investigations have suggested that releasing the anterior elements results in instability when the spine is loaded in extension (22,23). These studies also showed an increase in all motions when the posterior elements were removed.

Oda and associates sacrificed the posterior elements, costovertebral joints, and the rib cage itself in successive testing (24). They concluded that destruction of the posterior elements, as well as bilateral costovertebral articulations, would result in thoracic instability. The importance of the rib cage in lending structural support was confirmed by Andriacchi et al. in another study (3).

Friertag et al. performed a cadaveric study on human torsos with the rib cage–sternum complex intact (25). After selective excision of the spinal elements, they concluded that the disc was the most important stabilizer; however, sacrifice of the costovertebral articulation resulted in an increase in the sagittal and coronal motion of the involved segments. Unilateral facetectomy did not significantly destabilize the thoracic spine. This last finding was corroborated in a biomechanical cadaveric study by Broc et al., who examined the effects of microdiscectomy via unilateral pedicle resection coupled with rib head resection (26).

Oda and associates performed a similar experiment to Friertag et al. (24). After selective anterior destabilization procedures, they concurred that the disc is the primary stabilizer of the thoracic spine. Discectomy alone increased flexion by 193% and axial compression by 111%. Rib head resection resulted in 81% increase in flexion and 72% increase in axial compression. Sacrifice of the lamina and facets compromised less than 30% of the stability of the intact thoracic spine. The rib head was felt to be an important stabilizer in all planes. Another line of inquiry has been the effects of laminectomy on spinal stability.

Many clinical studies have documented iatrogenic kyphosis after laminectomy, particularly in the cervical spine. Yoganandan and peers focused on the effects of laminectomy on the thoracic spine (27). They noted that a two-level laminectomy decreased the strength and stability of the thoracic spine under axial compression, whereas a single-level laminectomy did not significantly destabilize the thoracic column.

The thoracolumbar spine has some unique considerations for traumatic instability (10). This region represents a transition zone between the fixed thoracic region and more mobile lumbar spine. The stability imparted by the rib cage is lost, and the facet orientation becomes more sagittally oriented. This results in a relatively abrupt change in biomechanical properties, which produces a stress concentration in this region. It is not surprising that the thoracolumbar junction is the most common site of failure after the spine trauma.

The lumbar spine is more tolerant of abnormal motion than either the thoracic or thoracolumbar spine due to the absence of the spinal cord and increased room for the nerve roots with a larger canal to dural area ratio. Some studies have shown only a 3% risk of neurologic deficits with fractures or fracture-dislocations of the lumbar vertebrae (28). A large part of the stability of the lumbar spine is imparted by the intervertebral disc (annulus fibrosus in particular), as well as by the ALL. Various studies have shown the facet joints to be critical in providing lumbar spine stability, particularly against axial rotation (29–31). This remittance to axial rotation is due to the orientation of the facet joints as well as the highly developed joint capsule. Abumi et al. showed medial facetectomy did not affect segment stability, whereas complete facetectomy, even if only unilateral, significantly destabilized the lumbar spine (11). Sullivan showed that more than 30 degrees of lumbar spine axial rotation resulted in progressive failure of the neural arch (31). Others have shown the supraspinous ligament to play an important role in lumbar spine stability, whereas the interspinous ligament has little effect (32). The contribution of the muscular attachments was investigated by Panjabi et al., who studied the effects of simulated muscle forces on the lumbar FSUs. He found that muscle forces stabilized intersegmental motion after injury in all planes of motion except for flexion, which increased with muscle force application (33).

Traumatic instability has been easier to study experimentally because acute disruption of bony and/or soft-tissue constraints can be performed in the laboratory setting. The biomechanical changes that occur with degenerative diseases is much harder to analyze. The pathophysiology of degenerative disease is less clear and not uniformly agreed on, although it is likely the result of long-term mechanical overloading.

Kirkaldy-Willis introduced the three-joint complex of the spine (i.e., intervertebral disc and bilateral facet joints) and classified the lumbar spine degeneration into three stages: (a) temporary dysfunction, (b) unstable phase, and (c) stabilization (34). During the stage of temporary dysfunction, facet capsules become slightly lax, the facet articular cartilage becomes fibrillated, and the disc shows early signs of degeneration. During the instability phase, he postulated repetitive minor trauma causes further damage to these structures, which then results in increased and abnormal motion. He opined a clinical entity was identifiable during this stage, and that dynamic instability could be detectable on flexion-extension films. During the stabilization phase, the abnormal mechanical forces produce osteophytes, joint surface irregularities, and facet hypertrophy, resulting in a gradual limitation of motion and stabilization of the deformity.

The biomechanical changes describing degeneration are varied in the literature. Nachemson et al. studied the mechanical behavior in cadaveric FSUs and found no correlation between disc degeneration and range of motion (35). Similar results were reported by others (36,37), but as the biomechanical studies have shown, there are differences between normal and degenerated specimens. An found that motion segments with grade IV degeneration exhibited the greatest range of motion, and this decreased in grade V degenerated segments (38). Mimura et al. found that the NZs were significantly larger with certain motions in degenerated specimens (39). Yang et al. found that the loads produced in the facet joints in the lumbar spine were higher in specimens that had facet arthritis (40).

Clinically, the relationship between abnormal motion and degeneration is also not clear. Fujiwara et al. looked at the relationship between disc degeneration, facet joint arthritis, and instability by using magnetic resonance imaging (MRI) and functional radiography (41). Specifically, they found the magnitude of anterior translation was positively correlated with disc degeneration and facet arthritis, whereas abnormal tilting in flexion and anterior-posterior translation was negatively correlated with facet arthritis only. Others, however, have found no relation between degeneration and instability (42). Murata et al. also compared MRI and functional radiography and were not able to find a significant relationship between degeneration and instability (43).

CLINICAL ASPECTS OF INSTABILITY

There are numerous causes of spinal instability, including trauma, tumors, and infection. A general classification scheme is presented here in Table 1 (44). These causes are addressed in more detail in other sections of this text. Instability due to degeneration of the spine is addressed further in this section, as it is an entity that remains poorly defined and thus is an area of controversy in the literature.

Diagnosing degenerative instability in the clinical setting has proven to be difficult. White and Panjabi have defined *clinical instability* as "the loss of the ability of the spine under physiologic loads to maintain its pattern of displacement so that there is no initial or additional neurologic deficit, no major deformity and no incapacitating pain" (22), but this definition is difficult to apply in the clinical arena. There is no clear consensus on clinical or radiographic diagnostic criteria, and there are few data available on why certain patients with suspected instability develop symptoms while others do not.

Many patients with suspected instability complain of rather nonspecific symptoms, which can be caused by many spinal pathologies. Most complain of low back pain with occasional radiation into the thighs and buttocks. The pain may increase throughout the day and may be relieved with rest or recumbency, and this is described as "mechanical." Paraspinal muscle spasm and tension signs can be present as well. Signs considered to be indicative of instability include a palpable step-off deformity or a lateral deviation between spinous processes, as well as a "catch" felt during flexion-extension range of motion (45). Studies have not, however, been able to establish adequate intra- and interobserver reliability for these clinical observations.

TABLE 1. *Lumbar segmental instabilities*

- Fractures and fracture-dislocations
- Infections involving anterior columns
  - With progressive loss of vertebral body height and deformity despite treatment with antibiotics
  - With progressing neurologic symptoms despite treatment with antibiotics (if accompanied by progressive loss of vertebral body height and deformity)
- Primary and metastatic neoplasms
  - With progressive loss of vertebral body height and deformity
  - With progressing neurologic symptoms not resulting from direct tumor involvement of the spinal cord, cauda equina, or nerve roots (e.g., caused by progressive loss of vertebral body height and deformity)
  - Postsurgical (after resection of neoplasm)
- Spondylolisthesis
  - Isthmic spondylolisthesis
    - L-5 to S-1 progressive deformity in a child, particularly when accompanied by radiographic risk signs (this lesion is rarely unstable in adults)
    - L4-5 deformity (probably unstable in adults)
- Degenerative instabilities
- Scoliosis (any progressive deformity in a child—subclassified by criteria of the Scoliosis Research Society)

Modified from Sullivan JD, Farfan HF. The crumpled neural arch. *Orthop Clin North Am* 1975;6(1):199–214.

Due to the clinical variability with which spinal instability can present, many clinicians rely instead on radiographic parameters to try and define instability. Even these parameters however, are not universally accepted. Historically, studies that attempted to define segmental instability used overall range of motion as their main determinant. Other methods, such as the instability factor (the ratio between translation and rotation) or the centrode of motion, have been used to try to better clarify instability (46,47). The value of these other methods remains to be seen. Traditional radiographic findings indicative of degenerative instability include the vacuum disc sign (Knutsson's phenomenon), as well as traction spurs. These spurs, as described by Macnab, were formed because of the tensile forces placed on the outer fibers of the annulus (48). Abnormal tilting motion with flexion was introduced by Kirkaldy-Willis as a type of instability, though he did not define any specific criteria (34). Other signs of instability are thought to include excessive rotatory motion as well as excessive translation.

Some studies distinguish between instability present on resting films (a so-called static slip) and instability present with range of motion (dynamic slip). A static slip may also coexist with a dynamic slip. Boden and Wiesel recommended that a dynamic slip of greater than 3 mm in flexion/extension be considered suggestive of instability, as only 5% of patients in their study of asymptomatic subjects exhibited that magnitude of displacement (49). Hayes et al., however, found that 20% of asymptomatic volunteers had at least 4 mm of translation (50). White and Panjabi, in their checklist approach to lumbar instability, define sagittal plane displacement or translation of 4.5 mm or 15% of vertebral body anteroposterior diameter as criteria for clinical instability (22).

Criteria for instability also differ with respect to tilting motion observed on flexion-extension films. Boden reported the normal range of motion in the lumbar spine to be 7.7 degrees at L3-4, and 9.4 degrees at L4-5 and L-5 to S-1 (49). Hayes reported mean values of 10 degrees at L3-4, 13 degrees at L4-5, and 14 degrees at L-5 to S-1 (50). Hanley et al. have recommended that angulation greater than 10 degrees be used as a criteria for surgical intervention (51), whereas Soini and Murata define abnormal angular motion as greater than 15 degrees (20 degrees at L-5 to S-1) (42,43). White and Panjabi consider greater than 15 degrees at L1-2, L2-3, and L3-4; greater than 20 degrees at L4-5; and greater than 25 degrees at L-5 to S-1 to be abnormal (22). Sato and Kikuchi helped clarify the natural history of radiographic instability by reporting greater than 10-year follow-up on 50 patients with this diagnosis (52). They found that 20% had their instability resolve. Increased flexion in the sagittal plane alone did not adversely affect the long-term clinical outcome, but increased chronic symptoms were seen when abnormal sagittal flexion occurred in association with increased translation.

Classification of Degenerative Segmental Instabilities

Frymoyer has described a classification system for degenerative segmental instabilities that is an expansion of an earlier classification system (53,54). It is based on radiographic findings, as well as a history of previous spine surgery (Table 2). There is a very important caveat to this clarification: Frymoyer and Boden stated that the patient has a deformity apparent on static radiographs that increases during spinal motion or compressive/tension loads beyond normal measurement errors or that can be documented to increase on serial radiographs in association with progressive symptoms. The underlying concept is that segmental instability is best diagnosed when the deformity progresses over time. Indeed, the classification was based principally on such progressive deformities, rather than abnormal motions and translations identified on a single dynamic flexion-extension radiograph. A primary instability is one that cannot be attributed to any previous interventions (i.e., surgery, chemonucleolysis). Secondary instabilities are those that were created or exacerbated by an intervention.

TABLE 2. *Degenerative segmental instabilities*

Primary instabilities
Axial rotational instability
Translational instability
Retrolisthetic instability
Progressing degenerative scoliosis
Disc disruption syndrome
Secondary instabilities
Post–disc excision—subclassified according to the pattern of instability as described under primary instabilities
Post–decompressive laminectomy
Accentuation of preexistent deformity
New deformity (i.e., no deformity existed at the time of original decompression)—further subclassified as for primary instabilities
Post–spinal fusion
Above or below a spinal fusion, subclassified as for primary instabilities
Pseudarthrosis
Postchemonucleolysis

Type I: Axial Rotational Instability

Axial rotational instability has a rotational malalignment as a major part of the deformity. Because cadaveric studies have shown that degenerative spondylolisthesis can have combinations of rotatory deformity, lateral bend, and translation (55), Frymoyer suggests that this and type II defects might be the same. Clinically, patients complain of recurrent, episodic low back pain provoked by twisting motions. Radiographically, this is manifest by malalignment of the spinous processes as well as pedicle rotation. Myelograms have been reported to show a pedicle-to-pedicle defect (34).

Type II: Translational Instability

Translational instability is synonymous with degenerative spondylolisthesis. Forward displacement of the cephalad vertebrae is the predominant deformity, although some rotational component can exist. Patients may complain of recurrent episodes of back pain along with an extensor lag. Classic radiographic signs described by Knutsson and Macnab, such as traction osteophytes and vacuum discs, are associated with this type of deformity. Women are affected five to six times more often than men, and the instability usually occurs after the age of 40 years. It occurs three times more often in African American women than in white women (56), and usually involves the L4-5 interspace. Facet joint angulation has been implicated as a cause of the deformity. Boden et al. found that patients with degenerative spondylolisthesis had a mean facet orientation of 60 degrees, compared with 41 degrees in asymptomatic volunteers (57).

Type III: Retrolisthetic Instability

Retrolisthetic instability is manifest by posterior displacement of the cephalad vertebra, posterior disc space collapse, and facet subluxation. The symptoms, which may include low back pain and nerve root signs, are most prominent in extension. Radiographically, the retrolisthesis increases with extension as well. Lehmann et al. observed this instability pattern was present in 30% of males with low back pain (58,59).

Type IV: Degenerative Scoliosis

The curve seen in this degenerative scoliosis (60) is usually less than 40 degrees and is associated with central and lateral recess stenosis. The combination of the curve with degenerative disease of the disc and facets reduces canal size, and thus can be associated with central and lateral stenosis. Symptoms usually consist of low back pain with or without neurogenic claudication and/or radiculopathy (61,62). Patients with stenosis due to degenerative scoliosis, however, generally do not get relief from sitting (61).

Type V: Internal Disc Disruption

Various authors have tried to study the relationship between instability and disc disruption but have not found a definitive link. Soini et al. found no association between disc degeneration (as assumed by discography) and abnormal angular movement (42). Murata et al. used MRI to classify disc degeneration and also found no link with abnormal motion using functional radiography (43). Fujiwara et al., however, found disc degeneration to be associated with abnormal anterior translation (41). It is not clear at this time what the relationship is between disc disruption and clinical instability.

Post–Disc Excision

Instability has been seen after discectomy for lumbar disc herniation, but these findings have not always correlated with physical findings. Padua et al. reported on long-term outcome after hemilaminectomy and discectomy for lumbar disc herniation (63), and found that although criteria for radiographic instability were met in 30 out of 50 patients, only nine had any symptoms of low back pain. Tibrewal et al. prospectively correlated lumbar spine motion before and after discectomy for herniation using biplanar radiography and found that discectomy did not produce clinical or radiographic instability (64). Kotilianen, however, reported that 22% of patients who underwent microdiscectomy for a lumbar disc herniation had clinical signs of segmental instability, which correlated with an unsatisfactory long-term outcome (65). It is difficult to establish whether the symptomatology is due to the natural history of degenerative disc disease or is the result of surgery.

Post–Decompressive Laminectomy

Frymoyer subclassifies post–decompressive laminectomy into *de novo* post–laminectomy instability and accentuation of previous instability. Both entities have been described in the literature, but the natural history is unclear. Biomechanically, Abumi et al. have shown that resection of 50% of bilateral facets or complete unilateral facetectomy significantly alters segmental stiffness (11). Boden et al. showed in a cadaver model that although wide laminectomy did not alter segmental motion, resection of the facet capsule and cartilage did have a significant effect (66). New as well as worsening radiographic instability have been seen but are often asymptomatic. There is disagreement in the literature as to the exact clinical relevance of these findings. Some studies have consistently documented progression of deformity after radical facetectomy but without consistent progression of symptoms (67). Fox and colleagues followed 92 patients who underwent decompression without fusion for degenerative lumbar stenosis (68). They found that 31% of patients with normal preoperative alignment showed signs of radiographic instability, compared to 73% of patients who had preoperative subluxation. However, they did not find a consistent correlation between radiographic instability and patient self-reported outcome. Mullin et al., on the other hand, found that postoperative radiographic instability was present in 54% of patients who underwent laminectomy and medial facetectomy for stenosis, and that this was negatively correlated with ambulatory ability (69). Herkowitz and Kurz studied 50 patients with spinal stenosis from degenerative spondylolisthesis who underwent decompression alone versus decompression plus fusion (70). They found that patients who underwent concomitant fusion had significantly less buttock and leg pain (96% vs. 44%), as well as less progression of their spondylolisthesis postoperatively (28% vs. 96%).

Post–Spinal Fusion

As there is normally some degree of spinal motion in the healthy spine, fusion at one or more levels is not physiologic, and thus can alter the mechanics of the rest of the spine. This has been seen clinically, but again, there is little correlation between radiologic instability and clinical symptoms reported by patients. Adjacent segment instability has been studied in *in vitro* as well as *in vivo*. Using a canine model, Nagata et al. found that long fusions caused increased loads at all segments distal to the fusion (71). Chow and colleagues found in an *in vitro* human model that L4-5 and L-4 to S-1 fusions increased motion at segments above and below the fusion, with the longer fusion having a greater increase (72). The *in vivo* studies are mostly retrospective and look for development of degeneration or instability near the site of a previous fusion. Multiple studies have documented degeneration immediately adjacent to as well as a few segments away from a previous fusion (73,74). Frymoyer et al. found in a long-term follow-up that although 20% of patients who underwent an L-4 to sacrum fusion showed radiographic signs of instability, only 4% required an extension of their fusion (75). On the other hand, 20% of the patients who underwent L-5 to sacrum fusion had to have their fusion extended. Aota et al. reported higher rates of radiographic instability above a fusion rather than below it (76). It is not clear if the degeneration and instability seen in these patients is caused by the increased stresses placed on the adjacent segments or rather by a natural progression of their spinal degeneration.

Frymoyer classifies pseudarthrosis after attempted fusion as an instability pattern, but it is debatable whether it is truly an unstable condition. Recognizing the difficulty and variability reported in diagnosing a pseudarthrosis (77), failure of fusion has been reported in up to 36% of patients in various studies (51,75,78). Many of these patients remain asymptomatic, however. Hanley found that success rates after fusion for degenerative spondylolisthesis were high, regardless of whether pseudarthrosis occurred. Some authors suggest that pseudarthrosis may actually lessen the risk of developing adjacent segment degeneration (79) because from a biomechanical standpoint, some motion at the fusion site should theoretically lessen the stresses placed on the adjacent segments.

Definitions of instability and biomechanics as related to the spine are constantly being modified with the addition of new information and research. Instability is a difficult concept to grasp, define, and, particularly, apply clinically. Based on the biomechanical and anatomic studies with destructive testing, a fair understanding of the clinical expression of instability can be gleaned in particularly applicable cases of tumors, fractures, and infections. The concept of degenerative instability remains more elusive.

REFERENCES

1. Frymoyer J. Segmental instability. In: Weinstein JN, Wiesel SW, eds. *The lumbar spine*. Philadelphia: WB Saunders, 1990.
2. Yoganandan N, Pintar F. Biomechanics of human thoracic ribs. *J Biomech Eng* 1998;120(1):100–104.
3. Andriacchi T, et al. A model for studies of mechanical interactions between the human spine and rib cage. *J Biomech* 1974;7:497.
4. White AA III, Panjabi MM. The basic kinematics of the human spine. A review of past and current knowledge. *Spine* 1978;3(1):12–20.
5. Miles M, Sullivan W. Lateral bending at the lumbar and lumbosacral joints. *Anat Rec* 1961;139:387.
6. Pearcy M. Stereoradiography of lumbar spine motion. *Acta Orthop Scand Suppl* 1985;56:212.
7. Nasca RJ, et al. Cyclic axial loading of spinal implants. *Spine* 1985;10(9):792–798.
8. Buckwalter J, Einhorn T, Simon S, eds. *Intervertebral disc structure, composition, and mechanical function, in orthopaedic basic science: biology and biomechanics of the musculoskeletal system*. Chicago: American Association of Orthopedic Surgeons, 2000:582.
9. Bergmark A. Stability of the lumbar spine. A study in mechanical engineering. *Acta Orthop Scand Suppl* 1989;230(60):20–24.
10. Panjabi M, White A, eds. *Physical properties and functional biomechanics of the spine, in clinical biomechanics of the spine*. Philadelphia: JB Lippincott, 1990.
11. Abumi K, et al. Biomechanical evaluation of lumbar spinal stability after graded facetectomies. *Spine* 1990;15(11):1142–1147.
12. Ogon M, et al. A dynamic approach to spinal instability. Part I: Sensitization of intersegmental motion profiles to motion direction and load condition by instability. Part II: Hesitation and giving-way during interspinal motion: a dynamic approach to spinal instability. *Spine* 1997;22(24):2859–2866.
13. Amonoo-Kuofi HS. The density of muscle spindles in the medial, intermediate and lateral columns of human intrinsic postvertebral muscles. *J Anat* 1983;136(Pt 3):509–519.
14. Cavanaugh JM, et al. Sensory innervation of soft tissues of the lumbar spine in the rat. *J Orthop Res* 1989;7(3):378–388.
15. Cholewicke J, McGill S. Mechanical stability of the in vivo lumbar spine: implications for injury and chronic low back pain. *Clin Biomech* 1996;11(1):1–15.
16. Wilke HJ, et al. Stability increase of the lumbar spine with different muscle groups. A biomechanical *in vitro* study [see comments]. *Spine* 1995;19(15):1697–1703.
17. Denis F. The three column spine and its significance in the classification of acute thoracolumbar spinal injuries. *Spine* 1983;8(8):817–831.
18. Berg E. The sternal-rib complex. A possible fourth column in thoracic spine fractures. *Spine* 1993;18(13):1916–1919.
19. Panjabi MM, et al. Validity of the three-column theory of thoracolumbar fractures. A biomechanic investigation. *Spine* 1995;20(10):1122–1127.
20. James KS, et al. Biomechanical evaluation of the stability of thoracolumbar burst fractures. *Spine* 1994;19(15):1731–1740.
21. Edwards CC 2nd, et al. Structural features and thickness of the vertebral cortex in the thoracolumbar spine. *Spine* 2001;26(12):1330–1336.
22. White A, Panjabi M. *Clinical biomechanics of the spine*, 2nd ed. Philadelphia: JB Lippincott, 1990.
23. Hausfeld J. A biomechanical analysis of clinical stability in the thoracic and thoracolumbar spine. New Haven, CT: Yale University School of Medicine, 1977.
24. Oda I, et al. Biomechanical role of the posterior elements, costovertebral joints, and rib cage in the stability of the thoracic spine. *Spine* 1996;21(12):1423–1439.
25. Feiertag MA, et al. The effect of different surgical releases on thoracic spinal motion. A cadaveric study. *Spine* 1995;20(14):1604–1611.
26. Broc GG, et al. Biomechanical effects of transthoracic microdiscectomy: comparative pull-out strength of tapped and untapped pilot holes for bicortical anterior cervical screws. *Spine* 1997;22(6):605–612.
27. Yoganandan N, et al. Biomechanical effects of laminectomy on thoracic spine stability: kinematics of the lumbar spine following pedicle screw plate fixation. *Neurosurgery* 1993;32(4):604–610.
28. Riggins RS, Rucker RB. The risk of neurologic damage with fractures of the vertebrae. *J Nutr* 1977;107(9):1747–1754.
29. Adams MA, Hutton WC, Stott JR. The resistance to flexion of the lumbar intervertebral joint. *Spine* 1980;5(3):245–253.
30. Posner I, et al. A biomechanical analysis of the clinical stability of the lumbar and lumbosacral spine. *Spine* 1982;7(4):374–389.
31. Sullivan JD, Farfan HF. The crumpled neural arch. *Orthop Clin North Am* 1975;6(1):199–214.
32. Myklebust JB, et al. Tensile strength of spinal ligaments: experimental spinal injuries with vertical impact. *Spine* 1988;13(5):526–531.
33. Panjabi M, et al. Spinal stability and intersegmental muscle forces. A biomechanical model. *Spine* 1989;14(2):194–200.
34. Kirkaldy-Willis WH, Farfan HF. Instability of the lumbar spine. *Clin Orthop Rel Res* 1982;165:110–123.
35. Nachemson AL, Schultz AB, Berkson MH. Mechanical properties of human lumbar spine motion segments. Influence of age, sex, disc level, and degeneration. *Spine* 1979;4(1):1–8.
36. Hirsch C, Lewin T. Lumbosacral synovial joints in flexion-extension. *Acta Orthop Scand* 1968;39(3):303–311.
37. Rolander SD. Motion of the lumbar spine with special reference to the stabilizing effect of posterior fusion. An experimental study on autopsy specimens. *Acta Orthop Scand* 1966;[Suppl 90]:1–144.
38. An H, et al. The relationship between disc degeneration and kinematic characteristics of the lumbar motion segment. Atlanta: Orthopaedic Research Society, 1996.
39. Mimura M, et al. Disc degeneration affects the multidirectional flexibility of the lumbar spine. *Spine* 1994;19(12):1371–1380.
40. Yang KH, King AI. Mechanism of facet load transmission as a hypothesis for low-back pain. *Spine* 1984;9(6):557–565.
41. Fujiwara A, et al. The relationship between disc degeneration, facet joint osteoarthritis, and stability of the degenerative lumbar spine. *J Spinal Disord* 2000;13(5):444–450.
42. Soini J, et al. Disc degeneration and angular movement of the lumbar spine: comparative study using plain and flexion-extension radiography and discography. *J Spinal Disord* 1991;4(2):183–187.
43. Murata M, Morio Y, Kuranobu K. Lumbar disc degeneration and segmental instability: a comparison of magnetic resonance images and plain radiographs of patients with low back pain. *Arch Orthop Trauma Surg* 1994;113(6):297–301.
44. Hazlett JW, Kinnard P. Lumbar apophyseal process excision and spinal instability. *Spine* 1982;7(2):171–176.
45. Mirkovic S, Garfin S. Segmental spine instability as related to the degenerative disc. *Semin Spine Surg* 1991;3:119–123.
46. Gertzbein SD, et al. Centrode patterns and segmental instability in degenerative disc disease. *Spine* 1985;10(3):257–261.
47. Weiler PJ, King GJ, Gertzbein SD. Analysis of sagittal plane instability of the lumbar spine *in vivo*: numerical [corrected] analysis of the load capacity of the human spine fitted with L-rod instrumentation. [erratum appears in *Spine* 1991;16(2):175.]. *Spine* 1990;15(12):1300–1306.
48. Macnab I. The traction spur. An indicator of segmental instability. *J Bone Joint Surg* 1971;53(4):663–670.
49. Boden SD, Wiesel SW. Lumbosacral segmental motion in normal individuals. Have we been measuring instability properly? [erratum appears in *Spine* 1991;16(7):855.]. *Spine* 1990;15(6):571–576.
50. Hayes MA, et al. Roentgenographic evaluation of lumbar spine flexion-extension in asymptomatic individuals: clinical and radiological evaluation of lumbosacral motion below fusion levels in idiopathic scoliosis. *Spine* 1989;14(3):327–331.
51. Hanley EN Jr. The indications for lumbar spinal fusion with and without instrumentation. *Spine* 1995;20[24 Suppl]:143S–153S.

52. Sato H, Kikuchi S. The natural history of radiographic instability of the lumbar spine. *Spine* 1993;18:2075–2079.
53. Frymoyer JW. Segmental instability. Rationale for treatment. *Spine* 1985;10(4):325–327.
54. Boden S, Frymoyer J. Segmental instability. In: Frymoyer J, ed. *The adult spine: principles and practice*, 2nd ed. Philadelphia: Lippincott–Raven, 1997.
55. Farfan HF. The pathological anatomy of degenerative spondylolisthesis. A cadaver study. *Spine* 1980;5(5):412–418.
56. Herkowitz HN, et al., Spine update. Degenerative lumbar spondylolisthesis. *Spine* 1995;20(9):1084–1090.
57. Boden SD, et al. Orientation of the lumbar facet joints: association with degenerative disc disease. *J Bone Joint Surg* 1996;78(3):403–411.
58. Lehmann T, Brand R. Instability of the lower lumbar spine. *Orthop Trans* 1983;7:97.
59. Vogt MT, et al. Lumbar olisthesis and lower back symptoms in elderly white women. The Study of Osteoporotic Fractures. *Spine* 1998;23(23):2640–2647.
60. Grubb SA, Lipscomb HJ, Coonrad RW. Degenerative adult onset scoliosis. *Spine* 1988;13(3):241–245.
61. Grubb SA, Lipscomb HJ. Diagnostic findings in painful adult scoliosis. *Spine* 1992;17(5):518–527.
62. Jackson RP, Simmons EH, Stripinis D. Incidence and severity of back pain in adult idiopathic scoliosis. *Spine* 1983;8(7):749–756.
63. Padua R, et al. Ten- to 15-year outcome of surgery for lumbar disc herniation: radiographic instability and clinical findings. *Eur Spine J* 1999;8(1):70–74.
64. Tibrewal SB, et al. A prospective study of lumbar spinal movements before and after discectomy using biplanar radiography. Correlation of clinical and radiographic findings. *Spine* 1985;10(5):455–460.
65. Kotilainen E. Microinvasive lumbar disc surgery. A study on patients treated with microdiscectomy or percutaneous nucleotomy for disc herniation. *Ann Chirurg Gynaecol Suppl* 1994;209:1–50.
66. Boden SD, et al. Increase of motion between lumbar vertebrae after excision of the capsule and cartilage of the facets. A cadaver study. *J Bone Joint Surg* 1994;76(12):1847–1853.
67. Johnsson KE, Willner S, Johnsson K. Postoperative instability after decompression for lumbar spinal stenosis. *Spine* 1986;11(2):107–110.
68. Fox MW, Onofrio B, Hanssen A. Clinical outcomes and radiological instability following decompressive lumbar laminectomy for degenerative spinal stenosis: a comparison of patients undergoing concomitant arthrodesis versus decompression alone. *J Neurosurg* 1996;85(5):793–802.
69. Mullin BB, et al. The effect of postlaminectomy spinal instability on the outcome of lumbar spinal stenosis patients. *J Spinal Disord* 1996;9(2):107–116.
70. Herkowitz HN, Kurz L. Degenerative lumbar spondylolisthesis with spinal stenosis. A prospective study comparing decompression with decompression and intertransverse process arthrodesis. *J Bone Joint Surg [Am]* 1991;73:802–808.
71. Nagata H, et al. The effects of immobilization of long segments of the spine on the adjacent and distal facet force and lumbosacral motion. *Spine* 1993;18(16):2471–2479.
72. Chow DH, et al. Effects of short anterior lumbar interbody fusion on biomechanics of neighboring unfused segments. *Spine* 1996;21(5):549–555.
73. Whitecloud TS III, Davis JM, Olive PM. Operative treatment of the degenerated segment adjacent to a lumbar fusion. [see comments.]. *Spine* 1994;19(5):531–536.
74. Schlegel JD, Smith JA, Schleusener RL. Lumbar motion segment pathology adjacent to thoracolumbar, lumbar, and lumbosacral fusions. *Spine* 1996;21(8):970–981.
75. Frymoyer JW, et al. A comparison of radiographic findings in fusion and nonfusion patients ten or more years following lumbar disc surgery. *Spine* 1979;4(5):435–440.
76. Aota Y, Kumano K, Hirabayashi S. Postfusion instability at the adjacent segments after rigid pedicle screw fixation for degenerative lumbar spinal disorders. *J Spinal Disord* 1995;8(6):464–473.
77. Hamill CL, Simmons ED Jr. Interobserver variability in grading lumbar fusions. *J Spinal Disord* 1997;10(5):387–390.
78. Lehmann TR, et al. Long-term follow-up of lower lumbar fusion patients. *Spine* 1987;12(2):97–104.
79. Rahm MD, Hall BB. Adjacent-segment degeneration after lumbar fusion with instrumentation: a retrospective study. *J Spinal Disord* 1996;9(5):392–400.

CHAPTER 50

Disorders of the Sacrococcygeal Junction

Philip Michael Bernini

The sacrococcygeal junction, although functionally of minor structural importance, can harbor varied and discrete diagnoses that may be hurtful as well as harmful. Moreover, bothersome signs and symptoms may be perceived by the physician and patient alike as arising in the sacrococcygeal area when, in fact, they are referred from other sites. Because the etiology of localized complaints may be ambiguous, treatment is often disappointing and frustrating. These failed therapeutic outcomes relate less to the modality used and more to the difficulty in identifying the discrete or contributory etiologies for the syndromes associated with this anatomic site. Accordingly, successful clinical management of sacrococcygeal junction disorders is linked to a sound diagnosis (Table 1).

EMBRYOLOGY AND CHONDRO-OSSIFICATION

In the third week of gestation, the dorsal layer of the bilaminar embryo invaginates, then proliferates, to form the primitive streak and eventually the tubular notochordal process between the ectoderm and the endoderm. The notochord then induces the overlying ectoderm (neuroectoderm) to thicken. This results in formation of the neural tube, which serves as a nidus for further induction, this time of the third component of the trilaminar embryo, the mesoderm. The mesoderm then differentiates into the intermediate columns, which give rise to the urogenital structures; the lateral mesodermal plates, which enclose the coelomic cavities; and last, the medial paraxial columns, which give rise to the 42-44 somites, the last five and eight of which develop into the sacrum and the coccygeal blastomal vertebra, respectively (Fig. 1). This last development occurs at 5 weeks of intrauterine growth and occurs in a cranial to caudal direction.

The internal specialization of the somites, which has enveloped the notochord, yields a dorsolateral group (i.e., dermomyotome), destined to be the integument and the dorsal musculotendinous tissue, while the ventral medial mass (i.e., sclerotome) migrates in three directions, becoming the skeletal (the osteocartilaginous) components of the spine. A cleft, the fissure of von Ebner, allows for the bisegmental development of each of the sclerotomes so that the caudal aspect of one combines with the cranial aspect of the adjacent level as they surround the notochord (i.e., the eventual nucleus pulposus of the disc) (Fig. 2). This results in the formation of the motion segment consisting of the vertebra and disc, with segmental and bilateral entry and exit of vascular and neurogenic structures. This close proximity of the coalescing components of the pluripotential cells of the trilaminar embryo in the last (caudal) maturing site of the spine is a reason to entertain a broad differential diagnosis while treating patients with sacrococcygeal syndromes.

By the eighth week, the sixth, seventh, and eighth coccygeal segments (i.e., the blastemal vertebrae) involute and the fifth (fourth) coalesce with loss of a recognizable vertebral processes. The residual four (three to five) coccyxes then ossify from one primary center of ossification. Recent magnetic resonance imaging (MRI), computed tomography, and conventional imaging studies have demonstrated these anatomic observations and noted that two other centers of ossification can occur in the first coccygeal segment, contributing to the cornu and transverse processes (1), and fuse anywhere from age 6 years to age 30 years. The five centers of ossification of the sacral vertebra usually fuse by age 25 years, but

TABLE 1. *Sacrococcygeal syndromes: differential diagnosis*

Local
- Gross trauma: fracture/subluxations/dislocations
- Infection
- Neoplasm
- Coccydynia
  - Traumatic (nonfracture/subluxation)
    - Postpartum
  - Idiopathic
- Pseudococcydynia
  - Levator ani syndrome
  - Proctalgia fugax

Referred
- Gastrointestinal
- Genitourinary
- Lumbosacral

Psychogenic: depression and sacrococcygeal pain syndromes

Homo caudatus

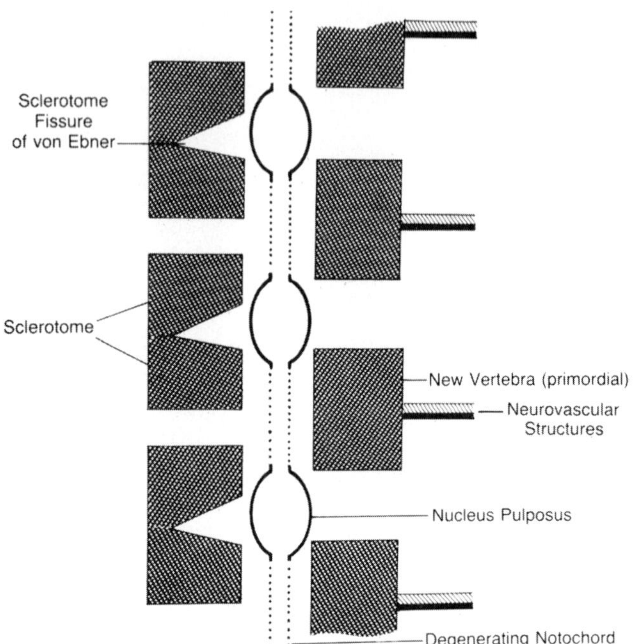

FIG. 2. Anteroposterior view of the lumbosacral spine with sclerotome differentiation occurring on the left about the sclerotome fissure of von Ebner with resegmentation recurring on the right. The bisegmental innervation of each segment of the spine can contribute to difficulties in identifying the specific nidus of irritation locally. (From Wiesel S, Bernini P, Rothman RH. *The aging lumbar spine.* Philadelphia: WB Saunders, 1982:7, with permission.)

the posterior arches of the fourth and fifth sacral vertebra, in general, remain unfused and form the sacral cornua, which defines the entrance to the sacral hiatus. The rudimentary sacral intervertebral disc fuse in a caudad to cephalad direction between ages 18 and 25 years. The notochord and the dorsolateral cells of the somites contribute to the intervertebral disc that may allow motion at the fifth sacral through first coccygeal, and first coccygeal and second coccygeal segments (2,3).

Functional Anatomy

Osteology

The fused concave ventral sacrum articulates with the generally concave ventral coccygeal segments (Fig. 3). The ventral surface of the sacrococcygeal junction and each of the various number of coccygeal segments are smooth without distinguishing characteristics. The word *coccyx* is derived from the Greek word "kokkux" because of its similar shape to the beak of a cuckoo. The sacral hiatus represents the dorsal interface between the sacrum and the coccyx, with the entrance defined by the sacral cornua of the fifth sacral and at times the fourth sacral vertebra, which are the unfused posterior neural arches and entire facet articulations of those vertebra. The inferior aspect of the hiatus is defined by the coccygeal cornua of the first coccygeal segment, which represents the vestigial superior articular process and the posterior neural arch. Small transverse processes are frequently found on C-1, and asymmetric development of these posterior structures is not unusual (1).

The number of mature, full coccygeal bodies varies, but Dieulaffe found four coccygeal segments in 80%, five segments in 17%, and three segments in 4% of 136 anatomic specimens (4). Fifty-four percent of asymptomatic volunteers have motion between the sacrum and C-1; 34% have motion between the sacrum and C-1, and C-1 and C-2; and 5% have three sites of motion (5,6).

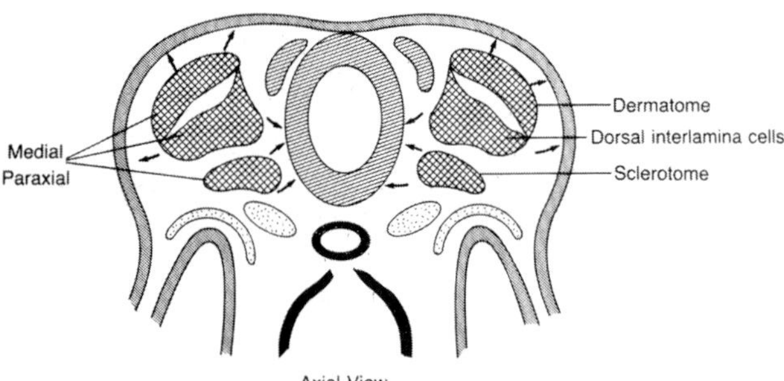

FIG. 1. Axial view trilaminar embryo with subdivision of the primitive mesoderm into the medium paraxial, intermediate, and lateral columns. The proximity of the notochord to mesodermal, ectodermal, and endodermal tissue prompts consideration of a wide differential diagnosis at the sacrococcygeal junction. (From Wiesel S, Bernini P, Rothman RH. *The aging lumbar spine.* Philadelphia: WB Saunders, 1982:6, with permission.)

DYNAMIC AND STATIC STABILIZERS

The sacrococcygeal junction provides stable and mobile moorings for muscles in the pelvic outlet (Fig. 4). Eventually, the distal fibers of the gluteus maximus extend from the lateral aspect of the coccyx to the iliotibial band and the gluteal tuberosity of the femur (i.e., the sickle band), whereas the sphincter ani externa originates on the

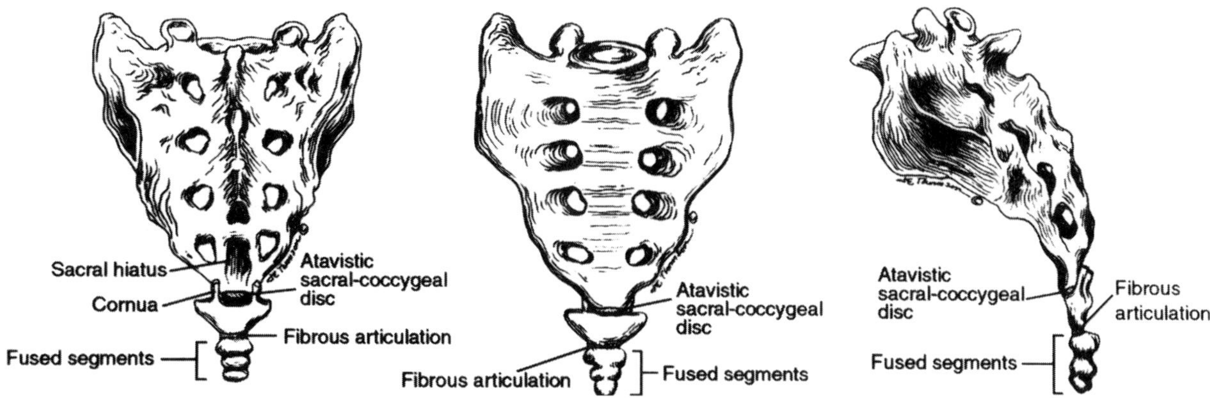

FIG. 3. Dorsal, ventral, and lateral views of the sacrum and sacrococcygeal area.

most distal tip of the coccyx. The coccygeus muscle inserts in the lateral aspect of the lower sacrum and upper coccyx, whereas the iliococcygeus (the posterior fibers of the levator ani) extends from the ischial spine and arcus tendons and inserts on the lateral border of the lower coccyx and the median ano coccygeal raphe (2,5). These muscles may move a mobile coccyx ventral or from side to side, but there is no dynamic extension capability; that is, muscles generating dorsal motion of the coccyx (5).

The static stabilizers include (a) the sacrospinous ligament that runs from the spine of the ischium to a broad attachment on the ventral lateral aspect of the lower sacrum and coccyx; (b) the sacrotuberal ligament, which has its origin on the iliac spine and the dorsolateral aspect of the sacrum and coccyx and converges on the ischial tuberosity; and (c) the long superficial and short, deep portion (i.e., the posterior longitudinal ligament) of the posterior sacral coccygeal ligament (Fig. 5). The dura, which is of mesodermal origin, forms an investment around the filum terminale at the level of the first sacral vertebra and continues caudally as a thin fibrous cord, the coccygeal ligament, to blend in and insert into the periosteum, while also contributing to the posterior longitudinal ligament on the dorsum of the coccyx (7). The sacrum and the first coccygeal segment may articulate by way of a symphysis, an intervertebral disc or a syndesmosis (attached ventrally to periosteum and/or anterior longitudinal ligament), which is a ligamentous attachment, but can also exist as a synovial joint (i.e., diarthrosis) (2,3,8).

Neurovascular Anatomy

The fifth sacral and paired coccygeal nerves are the primary local nerves that supply the posterior perineal musculature and form the coccygeal plexus, which distributes to perineum, perianal, and genital skin (9). Important motor and sensory input to the area includes the first, second, and third sacral roots, forming the sacral plexus from which the pudendal nerve arises, which innervates numerous peroneum structures (e.g., the ischial rectal fossa, dorsal nerves of the penis and the clitoris, the anal canal musculature, the ureteral sphincter, and the anterior perineum musculature), motor branches to the levator ani muscle, and the autonomic pelvic nerves coursing to the inferior hypogastric plexus (9,10). Regarded as "the major neural integration center" (11) within the pelvis, the inferior hypogastric plexi provides an explanation for the ambiguity associated with localizing the peroneal and sacrococcygeal complaints. Sensory nerves, namely the middle and the inferior cluneal nerves from the ventral and dorsal rami from the first, second, and third sacral nerve roots add to the multilevel etiology of afferent nerve supply. According to Wesselmann et al. (11),

> In general, pelvic viscera are innervated by both divisions of the autonomic nervous system, the sympathetic and parasympathetic divisions as well as by the somatic and sensory nervous system. In a broad anatomical view, dual projections from the thoracolumbar and sacral segments of the spinal cord carry out their innervations, converging primarily into discrete peripheral neural plexies before distributing nerve fibers throughout the pelvis. Interactive neural pathways, routing from higher origins in the brain through the spinal cord, add to the complexity of neuronal regulation in the pelvis.

The arterial supply to the sacrococcygeal area is derived from the lateral sacral arteries, from the superior gluteal or the hypogastric and the middle sacral arteries from the aortic bifurcation, which, it is interesting to note, is the caudal artery of tailed quadriceps (8) (Fig. 6). It is important that the termination of the middle sacral and the lateral sacral vessels, coalesce to form Luschka's gland, or the glomus coccygeum, which is a normal arteriovenous anastomosis just anterior to the sacrococcygeal junction, and has branches that have been found intraosseously in the coccyx (8,12).

The venous supply is composed of valveless external and internal plexi, coinciding roughly with the arterial supply.

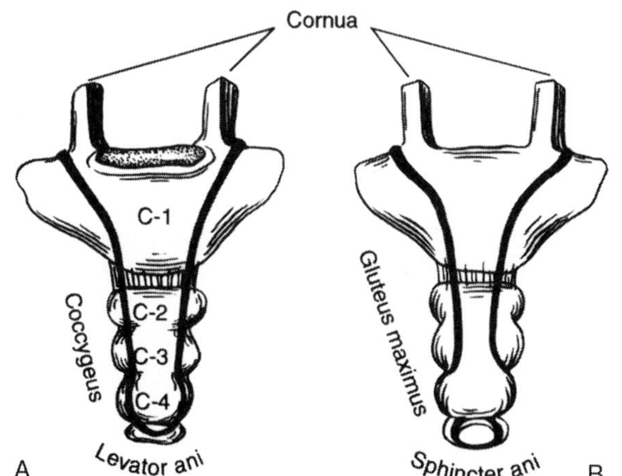

FIG. 4. Ventral **(A)** and dorsal **(B)** surfaces for the dynamic stabilizers at the sacrococcygeal junction.

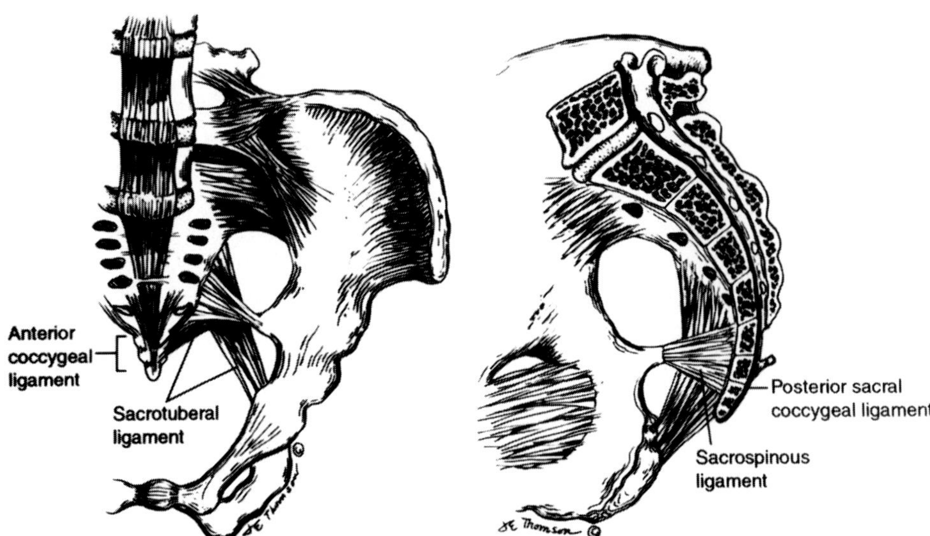

FIG. 5. The ventral and lateral views of the static stabilizers at the sacrococcygeal junction and their relationship to the pelvic ring.

Functional Anatomy

The static (ligamentous) and dynamic (muscle) tissue that finds origin and insertion at the sacrococcygeal junction may provide different loads and vectors of motion, depending on gender, size, and posture. These variables have made the definition of normal motion at the sacrococcygeal junction very difficult, particularly because coccygeal number and the mobility of the individual coccygeal segments on the sacrum, as well as on each other, are defined by varying types and number of articulations.

Anatomic studies have suggested that the typical pelvis bituberous diameter, the anteroposterior diameter, and the greater sciatic notch width, are greater in women than men, making the sacrococcygeal area more prominent and potentially more vulnerable to axial loads in women (13–17).

Roentgenographically, no discrete morphologic or qualitative abnormalities have been defined because the number of segments, mobile or otherwise, and their configuration as they relate to the sacrum, are quite variable. Postacchini and Massobrio attempted to classify the static sacrococcygeal configuration into following four major types (Fig. 7) (6):

Type I: The coccyx is curved slightly forward.
Type II: The curve of the coccyx is more marked with its apex pointing forward.
Type III: The coccyx is sharply angulated forward.
Type IV: The coccyx is subluxated anteriorly.

They also noted, however, that in their 120 patients, nearly 70% had a gentle kyphotic attitude (type I) with the apex of the coccyx pointing downward and slightly caudal on a static, lateral x-ray. An intercoccygeal angle (18), defined as the dorsally measured angle between the first and last segment of the coccyx in 20 normal patients (18 women and 2 men), was calculated again on static lateral x-rays to be 47.9 degrees (range, 25 to 88 degrees) in a sense compatible to the type I and II configuration described by Postacchini and Massobrio (6).

Maigne has contributed significantly to defining normal configuration and mobility by obtaining dynamic roentgenographic measurements in volunteers, recognizing the important role of posture, gender, and body mass index (BMI) on the attitude at the sacrococcygeal junction. In a series of publications, Maigne has attempted to quantify the functional attitude of the sacrococcygeal function as postural changes are made from lateral upright to lateral decubitus and sitting postures (Fig. 8) (3,19–21). He has attempted to describe normal motion with postural changes with

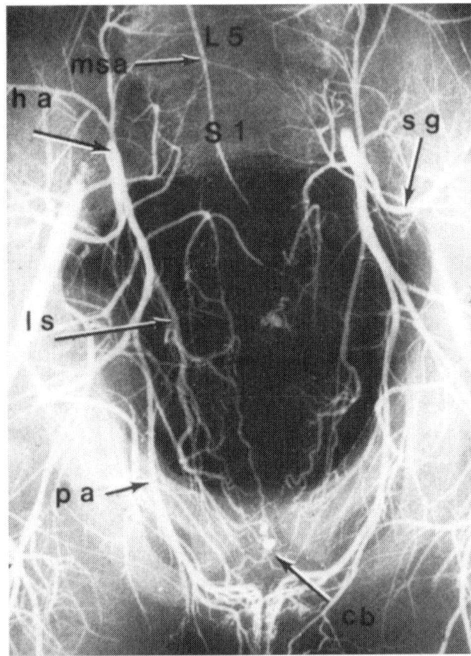

FIG. 6. Just anterior to the coccyx, the small knot of arterial venous anastomoses described as the coccygeal body represents a normal vascular structure in the area of the sacrococcygeal junction. (From Rothman RH, Simeone FA. *The spine,* 2nd ed. Philadelphia: WB Saunders, 1982:4, with permission.)

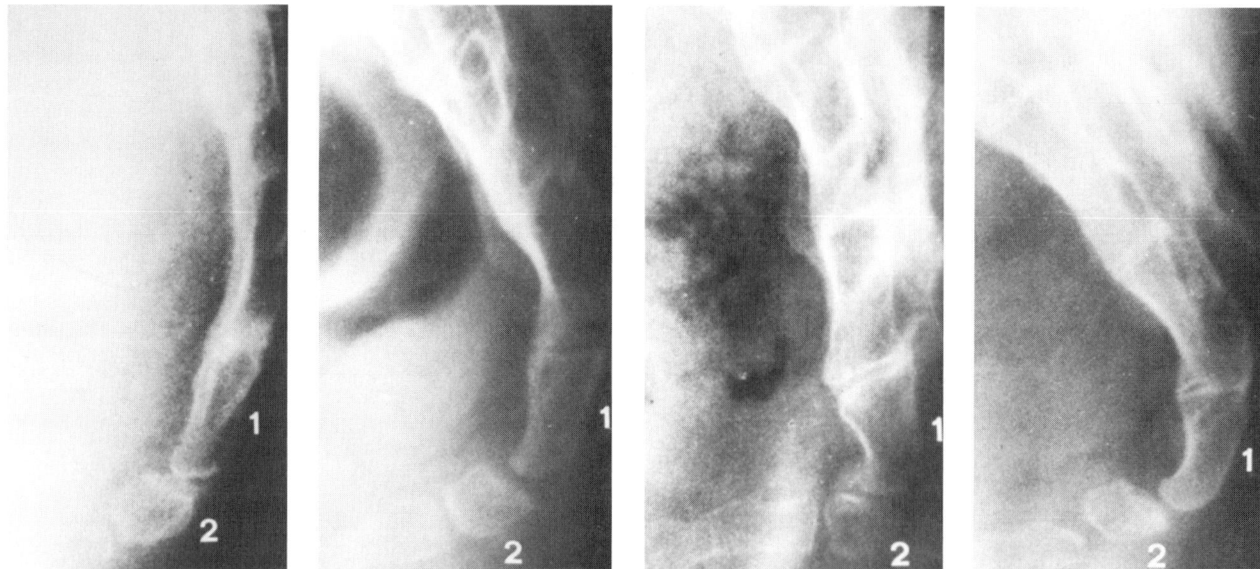

FIG. 7. **A:** Type I configuration consists of three bony segments with a gentle forward flexed attitude. **B:** Type II configuration of the coccyx with a more acute forward-flexed attitude. **C:** Type III configuration with a 90-degree forward flexion of the terminal fused coccygeal segments on C-2. **D:** Type IV configuration of the coccyx with a ventral subluxation of C-2 on C-1. 1, last fused coccygeal segments; 2, mobile coccygeal segment. [From Postacchini F, Massobrio M. Idiopathic coccygodynia. Analysis of fifty-one operative cases and a radiographic study of the normal coccyx. *J Bone Joint Surg* 1983;65A(8):1116–1124, with permission.]

the additional hope of identifying abnormal or excessive motion that may be correlated with patients with bothersome symptoms at the sacrococcygeal junction. The angle of incidence is derived from a sitting film, obtained on a hard stool with the back slightly extended, and is defined as the angle at which the coccyx strikes the seat when sitting down, thus determining the sagittal or anterior-posterior moment of the coccyx (19). The difference in the angular motion of the coccyx on the sacrum is obtained by superimposing the standing and the sitting lateral, with "normal" defined as being less than 20 to 25 degrees but with the direction of movement influenced by the difference in the sagittal pelvic rotation, again determined by superimposing the standing and the sitting lateral films. The smaller the angle of incidence (i.e., the coccyx is more parallel to the seat), the greater the likelihood of forward or a flexed attitude of the coccyx when sitting. With a higher angle of incidence (i.e., the coccyx is oblique or perpendicular to the seat), there is a greater likelihood that the coccyx angles posteriorly, presumably due in part to the increased intrapelvic pressure generated while sitting. With a high sagittal pelvic rotation (i.e., greater than 40 degrees), the angle of incidence is less and therefore mitigates more forward flexion, whereas a low sagittal pelvic rotation allows the angle of incidence to be more and therefore contributes to greater posterior angulation (i.e., extension). It is of interest that in obese patients with a BMI greater than 27.4 in women and 29.4 in men, these high BMIs vary inversely with pelvic rotation and directly with the angle of inclination, thereby contributing to a greater likelihood of extension of the coccyx (20,21). In contrast, a thin individual's greater ability to rotate the pelvis while sitting (i.e., contact made with more lumbar flexion and because less tissue exists between the seat and the buttock) allows the coccyx to assume a more parallel orientation (i.e., lower angle of incidence attitude) and thereby flex and/or sublux forward. Whether the sacrococcygeal junction or the first intercoccygeal joint subluxes anterior or posterior rather than simply flexes and extends are additional variables, not as of yet clearly understood. An immobile coccyx remains another confounding issue and is still within the realm of "normal." These studies provide an admirable preliminary step leading to a better idea of normal variation. Because many of these findings were

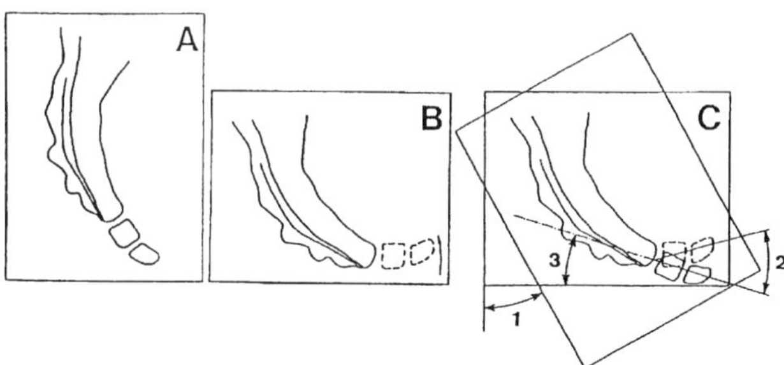

FIG. 8. Functional postural measures of Maigne. **A:** Standing radiograph. **B:** Sitting radiograph showing flexion of the coccyx. **C:** Superimposition of the two radiographs matching the sacrum obtained by pivoting the sitting film through an angle representing sagittal pelvic rotation (angle 1 equals angle of rotation). Coccygeal mobility is indicated by angle 2 (angle of mobility). Angle 3 is the angle at which the coccyx strikes the seat surface (angle of incidence). [From Maigne JY, Doursounian L, Chatellier G. Causes and mechanisms of common coccydynia: role of body mass index and coccygeal trauma. *Spine* 2000:25(23):3072–3079, with permission.]

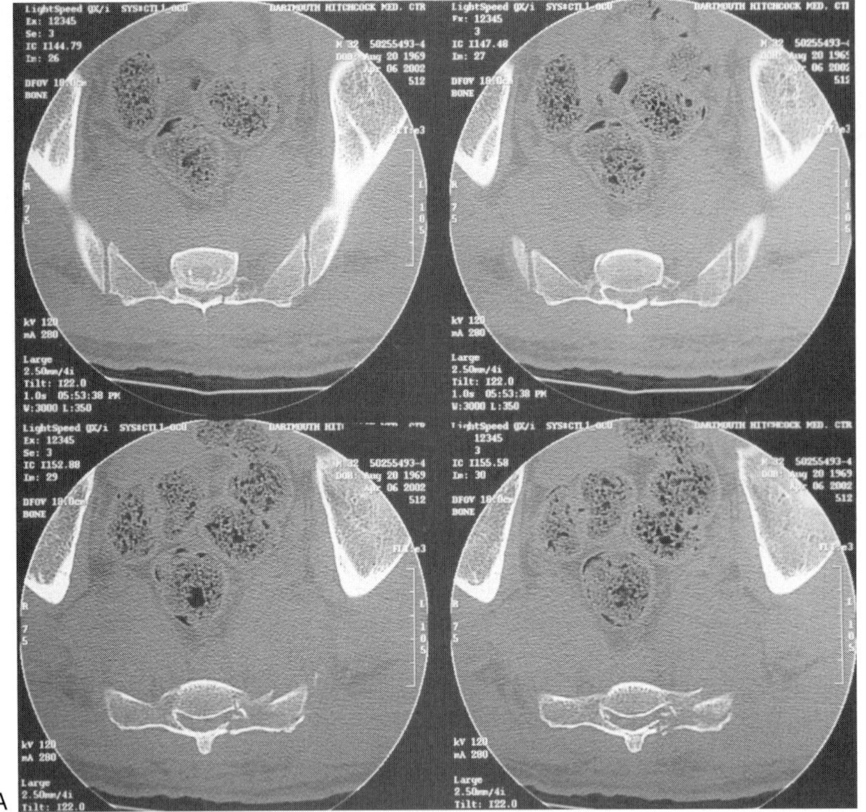

A

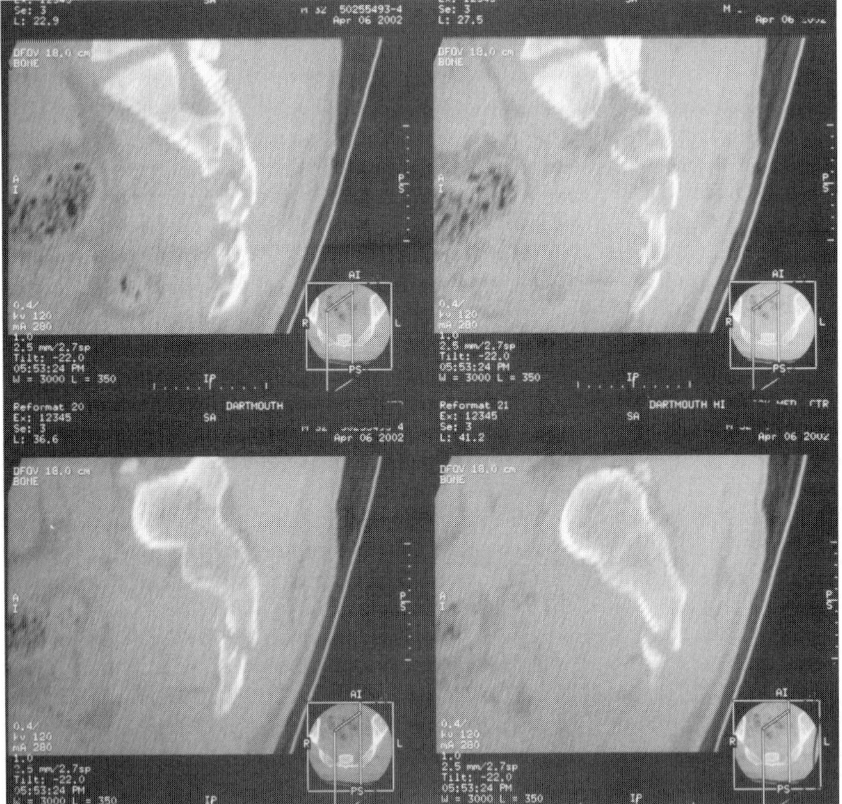

B

FIG. 9. A,B: Axial and sagittal reconstructions of the sacrum showing a comminuted fracture. With the sacrum being rigid and not mobile like the coccyx, the former is far more susceptible to fracture with trauma.

generated comparing symptomatic patients with normal asymptomatic volunteers, further samples are required to assess the significance of these radiographic variables.

DIAGNOSTIC CATEGORIES

The most common syndrome encountered at the sacrococcygeal junction has been called "coccygodynia," a term coined by Simpson in 1861 as a descriptive term defining pain in and around the sacrococcygeal junction, made worse with sitting and various postural changes (22). It is, however, a diagnosis of exclusion and it therefore becomes essential to rule out harmful as well as other hurtful causes of sacrococcygeal discomfort.

History and Physical Examination

The history and the physical examination are crucial in evaluating sacrococcygeal complaints as they are for any other medical problem. The temporal framework within which the symptoms develop; the acute or insidious nature of the symptoms; the aggravating posture; the presence or absence of pain at rest; coincident bowel, bladder, and sexual dysfunction; association with menses; and lower-extremity function both motor and sensory, must be queried. Constitutional signs and symptoms and a thorough review of systems and past medical and surgical history focus one's attention on the likely etiology within the differential diagnosis.

The observations made during the physical examination must include what is seen and palpated at the sacrococcygeal junction. A rectal and, at times, a vaginal digital examination defining the sensitivity and mobility of the coccyx and whether the presenting symptoms are reproductive of or not compatible with the patient's chief complaint is essential. Perianal pinprick sensation, resting and voluntary rectal tone, and a bulbocavernous reflex should all be documented. Abdominal and lower-extremity neuromuscular and vascular examinations are also important parts of this evaluation.

Imaging

At the minimum, plain anteroposterior, lateral films of the lumbosacral spine, the pelvis, and the sacrococcygeal area are required. A 30-degree included anteroposterior radiograph better defines the anatomy of the sacrum and coccyx. More sophisticated imaging, in the form of computerized axial tomography, technetium bone scan, and/or MRI, prompted by the likelihood and concern within the differential diagnosis, particularly if surgical intervention is being contemplated, are then warranted.

DIFFERENTIAL DIAGNOSIS

Gross Trauma (Fracture/Dislocation/Subluxation)

Fractures and dislocations of the coccyx at the sacrococcygeal junction can occur in isolation, although significant falls more often affect the immobile and more vulnerable, lower sacrum (Fig. 9) (23–25). This is particularly true in all patients who have sustained a pelvic ring injury. Kaehr et al.'s classification (26) of sacral fractures (Table 2) does not include specific trauma to the coccyx, but their type I fracture involves avulsion of the sacrotuberous and sacrospinous ligaments, which find origin, in part, on the coccyx (26). Their type II fracture, the transverse sacral injury, can result in

TABLE 2. *Kaehr classification of sacral fractures*

Fracture type	Description	Direction of fracture	Number of cases	Mechanism	Nerve damage (%)	Stability	Treatment
1	Avulsion fractures of SI joint, sacrotuberous sacrospinous ligaments	Ligament avulsions	29	Vertical shear	21	Often highly unstable	Unstable—ORIF SI joint
				Anteroposterior compression			Stable—protected weight bearing
2	Alar fracture (lateral to foramen)	Vertical	41	Lateral compression	12	Impacted—stable	Protected weight-bearing
3	Transforaminal	Vertical	42	Lateral compression	17	Impacted—stable	Protected weight-bearing
				Vertical shear		Displaced—unstable	Closed reduction and percutaneous screws
							Late radiculopathy—posterior decompression
4	Transforaminal with extension into central canal	Vertical	8	Lateral compression	62	Impacted—stable	Protected weight-bearing
				Vertical shear		Displaced—unstable	Closed reduction and percutaneous screws

continued

TABLE 2. *Continued*

Fracture type	Description	Direction of fracture	Number of cases	Mechanism	Nerve damage (%)	Stability	Treatment
5	Transverse (usually at S1-2)	Transverse	2	Axial loading Direct blow	50	Highly unstable	Bed rest Posterior decompression for neurodeficit ? Closed reduction and sacral fixation
6	H-type (bilateral transforaminal with transverse component)	Vertical and transverse	16	Axial loading Direct blow	63	Highly unstable	Bed rest Posterior decompression for neurodeficit

ORIF, open reduction, internal fixation; SI, sacroiliac.
From Kaehr DM, et al. Classification of sacral fractures based on CT imaging. *J Orthop Trauma* 1989;3:163, with permission.

sagittal deformation of the sacrum and alter the location of the sacrococcygeal junction without specific injury to that site.

Meek'ren, in 1862, first reported a dislocation of the coccyx, reduced by manipulation and in 1698, Gahrliep reported a fractured coccyx, although neither case enjoyed the benefit of imaging confirmation (Fig. 10) (27,28). Beach did note an open fracture of the coccyx in 1899, and several other authors (29–35) described trauma in many of their patients, but whether a coccygeal fracture or dislocation was present is uncertain (29). Depalma describes a fracture/dislocation in his fracture atlas, without any references, but recent, isolated case reports do confirm the occurrence of fractures and dislocations, although the incidence is still uncertain (Fig. 11) (36).

End-plate avulsion fractures have also been described (32) and while this phenomenon is an adult injury, a Salter-Harris type I fracture at the sacrococcygeal junction has been described by Gutierrez et al. (37) and is similar to an avulsion of the cartilage end-plate from the subchondral bone, noted by Cameron et al. in 1975 (38). Although plain films of the sacrococcygeal area can confirm these diagnostic categories with subtle end-plate or Salter injuries, MRI may be the best modality to make this specific diagnosis (23).

Symptomatic closed management, with or without manipulative efforts, depending on the extent of the fracture/dislocation deformity, is usually warranted. Care, however, must be demonstrated, particularly with fractures so as to avoid converting these injuries into open contaminated trauma by compromising the integrity of the rectal or vaginal mucosa. Any suggestion of an open injury, such as blood on rectal or vaginal digital examination, would merit emergent general surgical and/or gynecologic consultation.

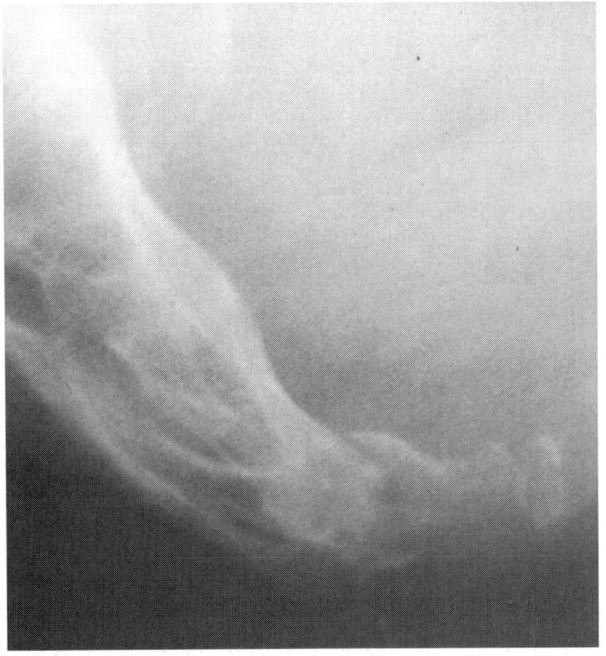
A

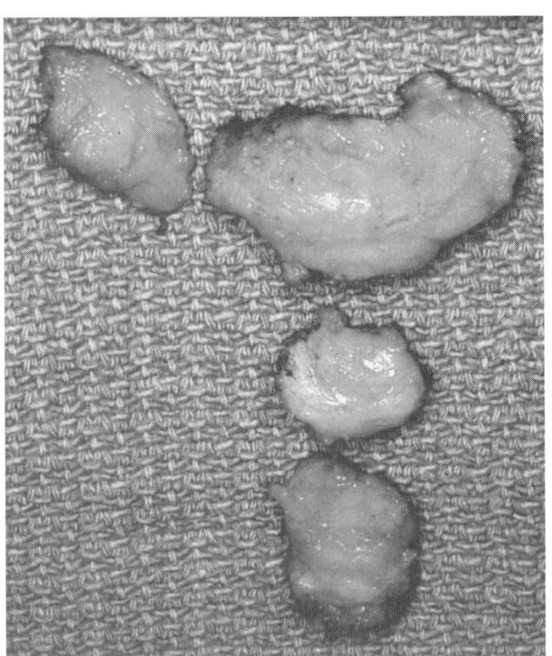
B

FIG. 10. A,B: Fracture of the coccyx seen on lateral radiography with the anatomic specimen retrieved at the time of coccygectomy.

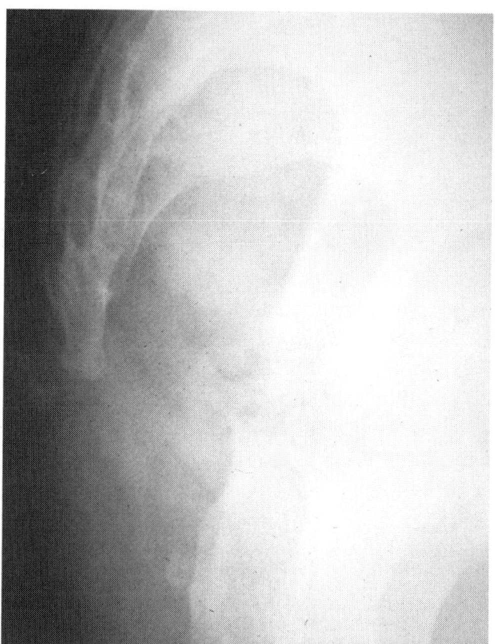

FIG. 11. Posterior dislocation of the coccyx on the sacrum.

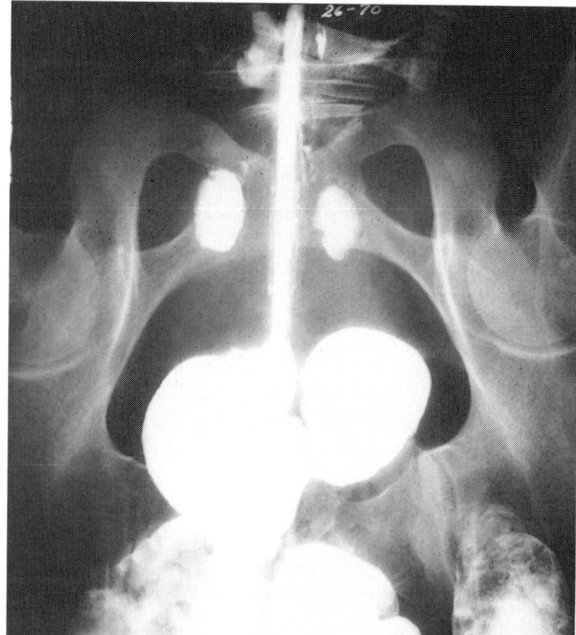

FIG. 12. Barium enema study demonstrating numerous perianal and perirectal abscesses in sacrococcygeal area in a patient with ulcerative colitis.

Open reduction has also been described (35), but this is probably ill advised in light of the results reported with coccygectomy; if symptoms persist, follow nonoperative symptomatic efforts. In any event, no invasive treatment should be afforded without a specific diagnosis.

Infection

Constitutional signs and symptoms, localized pain and swelling, erythema, and perhaps drainage are the hallmarks of soft-tissue or osseous infection at the sacrococcygeal junction. Beyond pilonidal sinuses, perianal fistulas, and abscesses (Fig. 12), infection affecting only the terminal axial skeleton is unusual, with those reports primarily in the old literature (39–43). Appropriate medical and/or surgical management is determined by the presence or absence of an abscess or a sequestered, infected bone. The proximity of the gastrointestinal tract requires imaging to ascertain all of the tissues involved in this suspected infectious process and accordingly a general surgical consultation is warranted.

Neoplasms and Hamartomas

The trilaminar embryo contribution to the sacrococcygeal junction's anatomic components provides a pluripotential etiology to a wide variety of primary neoplastic or hamartomatous lesions. This is particularly true as seen in children with malignant sacrococcygeal teratomas (44,45). A complaint of pain or discomfort at the sacrococcygeal junction, along with gastroenterologic, urogenital, and lower-extremity signs and symptoms, merits the consideration of this diagnostic category while evaluating patients with sacrococcygeal symptoms. Although chordomas, giant cells, carcinoid tumors, lipomas and even avascular necrotic lesions have been described within the coccyx proper (46–50), these are fairly rare occurrences (see Chapter 11). Often, involvement of the lumbosacral spine with symptoms appreciated along the dermatomal course of S-3 to S-5 and the coccygeal nerves due to tumor involvement proximal to the sacrococcygeal junction and perceived at the terminal aspect of the axial skeleton can occur. This can be particularly true with the more commonly encountered axial and retroperineal metastatic lesions.

One lesion not to be confused with a symptomatic tumor is the pericoccygeal and intracoccygeal glomus bodies. These glomi ("balls of yarn" in Latin) are normal arterial venous anastomoses (8), consisting of a vascular channel (the channel of Surquet-Hoyer) that is surrounded by a variant of smooth muscle, and should be considered an incidental finding and not causative of sacrococcygeal symptoms (12,51,52).

Coccydynia

Coccydynia represents a diagnosis of exclusion. This hurtful, not harmful diagnostic category, nevertheless, can be very troublesome and may represent the most common cause of symptoms at the sacrococcygeal junction. When Simpson coined the term "coccygodynia" in 1861, he did not identify an unequivocal pathologic condition but defined a symptom complex of pain in and around the area of the sacrococcygeal joint, made worse with sitting and with various postural changes (22). This ambiguity encourages a classification that may identify separate patient cohorts whose symptoms may be similar but in whom outcomes may differ, suggesting different and varying contributing etiologies.

Traumatic (Nonfracture/Subluxation)

Traumatic coccydynia was first diagnosed in 1588 by Smitz, who observed that his wife's fall had "so injured the coccygeal bone that she cannot sit without pain, nor can she empty her bowel or bladder or cough without much distress" (5). Numerous investigators (30,31,34,53,54) have inculcated trauma as a cause of coccydynia. Although some authors have noted a fracture or dislocation, blunt trauma without deformity can be a causative mechanism, as was first noted by Petit in 1726 (39). This mechanism has been suggested as being responsible for 38 to 65% of cases in a gynecologist's practice (16,17) and has been described in 50 to 89% of cases by several other authors (6,15,20,21,55–57). It has been suggested by several of these authors that these cases of trauma, without obvious fracture or dislocation, were associated with pathologic changes in postmortem evaluations, compatible with degenerative joint disease at the sacrococcygeal junction, end-plate separations, avulsions of the cartilage end-plate, and from bone and cystic inflammatory reactions.

Maigne has suggested using dynamic sitting and standing films and recognizing the importance of BMI, and has gone on to demonstrate that a normally neutrally configured coccyx posteriorly flexes or subluxes, particularly with blunt trauma, which coincidentally increases the intrapelvic pressure, enhancing posterior displacement (3). In female, perhaps more than male, obese patients with high BMI, repetitive trauma with normal sitting may result in the coccyx being posteriorly subluxed or flexed because their pelvic sagittal rotation is usually less and angle of incidence is generally more, enhancing posterior displacement.

Postpartum

Birth trauma to the sacrococcygeal junction is not unexpected (13,16,17,56,58) because the coccyx is the posterior landmark of the anteroposterior diameter of the pelvic obstetrical outlet (2), and in women, its shape makes it more susceptible to injury. Peyton in 1988 found only 6% of 180 patients in a gynecologic practice with postpartum coccydynia who had an obvious history of second-stage labor difficulties. Overall, the reported prevalence of postpartum coccydynia varies from approximately 4 to 15% (16,17,21,44,55,59,60). Only Brunskill in 1987 and Jones in 1997 describe an actual fracture during delivery (61,62).

Idiopathic

Idiopathic coccydynia—that is, pain in the area of the sacrococcygeal junction without any precipitating event—accounts for 20 to 40% of the patients (6,21,22,55,56). Whereas Duncan in 1937 did not identify any roentgenographic abnormality in 262 patients with coccygeal pain compared to asymptomatic patients, Postacchini and Massobrio found that when the coccyx was more anteriorly oriented (types III and IV), patients were more prone to symptoms (6,15). Yamashita likewise found a more anterior (dislocated) orientation in the idiopathic group compared to normals with 4.8% versus 2.6% in men and with 11.1% versus 5.2% in women, respectively (63). Kim in 1999 found a significantly greater intercoccygeal angle in the idiopathic group than that found in normals, but there was no age, gender, or coccygeal number differences (18). Maigne (20,21) has used dynamic (sitting and standing) films and developed the concepts of the pelvic sagittal rotation, the coccygeal angle of incidence, and the direction of coccygeal movement (Fig. 8), and has analyzed the influence of BMI on these roentgenographic measures. His studies suggest varying causes of vulnerability in the idiopathic group, which has led him to develop possible subcategories for patients with coccydynia (3,19–21). Although the blunt or chronically traumatized group, as noted earlier, has less pelvic sagittal rotation and a greater angle of incidence, the idiopathic group may have more pelvic rotation and less angle of incidence, resulting in hypermobility and forward flexion of the coccyx more than 35 degrees, and/or the development of a "spicule of bone" at the mobile (and at times immobile) and susceptible sacrococcygeal or cocccococcygeal junction due to a chronic inflammatory phenomenon or the development of a bursa. An acquired and painful "nodule" over the coccyx, resulting from the chronic trauma of long-distance bicycling, particularly in anteriorly flexed coccyx (64), lends credence to this etiology. In women, two extremes are identified. In one there is a blunt and/or chronically traumatic etiology with no precipitating event, accompanied by a posterior flexed coccyx, particularly in patients with an elevated BMI. At the other extreme there is no precipitating event, there may be coccygeal hypermobility or immobility, an anterior flexed or subluxed coccyx, and a lower BMI.

Pseudococcydynia

Pseudococcydynia, described by Traycoff and others in 1989, represents an important distinction from coccydynia, better defining patients with a variety of sacrococcygeal complaints attributed to a muscular etiology, namely proctalgia fugax and levator ani syndrome (65). Indeed, both have pain in and around the coccyx; that is, "coccygodynia," but the source of pain is most likely muscular and successful treatment may more often be realized with gentle manipulation and relaxation techniques. *Tension myalgia of the pelvic floor*, coined by Sinaki in 1977, is a useful, synonymous term that includes proctalgia fugax and levator ani syndrome as well as piriformis syndrome, obstipation, constipation, and dyspareunia, which are less likely to be confused with coccydynia (66).

Levator Ani Syndrome

Ely in 1910, and later Thiele in 1937, brought attention to the role of muscle spasm and the role for massage in the pelvic floor and described the origins of the spasm in the levator ani and coccygeal muscles and medial fibers of the gluteus medius, producing this pseudococcydynia (59,67). At times, this pain in the coccyx area may be associated with pain in the supragluteal region and thigh due to spasm of the piriformis. The levator ani syndrome, found predominantly in men in a 7:3 ratio, has pain in the coccygeal area but is not classically associated with coccygeal tenderness. The left-side tenderness and spasm on rectal examination is classic (68) and it has been identified on transverse and frontal section MRI involving the puborectal band of the levator ani muscle (69). The etiology of this phenomenon, however, is still uncertain.

Proctalgia Fugax

Proctalgia fugax, due to spasm of the levator ani, rectal wall muscle, and anal sphincter, perhaps associated with contraction of the sigmoid colon, may represent a variant of the levator ani syndrome or a separate muscular cause of pseudococcydynia. Men and women are affected equally (70,71). Episodes of pain that are intense and last for a 15- to 20-minute period can be followed by periods of remission that can last for years (72). Vasospasm of the hemorrhoidal artery with venous engorgement has been demonstrated angiographically (73), but whether this is causal or coincidental is unclear.

Treatment for coccydynia and pseudococcydynia initially merits reassurance for the patient and the use of aggressive, nonoperative intervention, with surgery only warranted after time and continued persistence of symptoms. Furthermore, this guideline would apply only to patients who truly qualify for the diagnosis of coccydynia. Surgery is not indicated for pseudococcydynia patients who do not have associated pain and tenderness with specific coccygeal manipulation.

Conservative measures include protection of the sacrococcygeal area by limited sitting, decompressive orthotics, use of sitz baths, nonsteroidal antiinflammatory medication, mild analgesics, and pelvic relaxation techniques (72,74,75). Pelvic massage has been used with good but varying results, most likely due to specific diagnostic ambiguity, as well as the type of manual techniques used (17,59,76,77). Indeed, joint manipulation, muscle massage, and direct manipulation applied to the coccyx are all manual techniques that may overlap to varying degrees while this modality is afforded. Although the results with manipulation have been reported as successful in 65% of noncontrolled studies, one should anticipate such a result only if the problem is primarily muscular, which probably affects no more than 25% of the patients with coccydynia (76,77). The combination of massage and local infiltration of tissue with steroids and a local anesthetic has been very helpful in 85% of patients (78). Porter, in 1981, found local injections particularly helpful in the majority of patients with idiopathic coccydynia, whereas short-waved diathermy was more helpful in the traumatic cases, although it has also been described as helpful in the nontraumatic cases by Sinaki, in 1977 (66,79). In general, symptomatic treatment with time and patience provides satisfactory results in a majority of patients.

When patients' symptoms persist for an extended period of time, usually in excess of 3 months (6,32), and manipulative and other nonoperative modalities have not been helpful and a diagnosis other than coccydynia has been ruled out, surgery may be warranted. Coccygectomy (total and subtotal) and sacral rhizotomies have been the operative procedures most frequently used.

Pickett in 1758 (5) advised coccygectomy for persistent pain and Blundell, in 1890, recommended this procedure for a variety of causes, with Nott performing the first coccygectomy in the United States in 1844 (41,43). The procedure was not used in earnest until 1923 by Gant, who performed it on numerous patients who probably had a variety of diagnoses (80). Duncan and Key, in 1937, reported, independently, 70 to 80% good or excellent results with this procedure (15,31). Over the years, numerous authors have identified comparable results, with good or excellent results obtained in approximately 80% of patients within 3 to 4 months postoperatively (5,6,18,20,31,32,53,55,56,60,81–84). Whereas most of these results involved total coccygectomy, good results could be obtained with a partial coccygectomy in select patients (6,55,56,78) but may be less reliable (55). Bayne, in 1984, concluded that direct trauma and postpartum patients had a better outcome with coccygectomy—75% had satisfactory results—whereas the insidious or spontaneous onset patients only had a 58% recovery rate, and patients with coccydynia resulting from spinal surgery did not have a satisfactory result at all (56). However, low back pain as a comorbidity with coccydynia has been reported as not to compromise surgical outcomes (6,60).

Coccygectomy

Coccygectomy is best performed with a longitudinal incision centered over the sacrococcygeal joint (6,20,82). Same day or overnight observational status can be anticipated whether surgery is performed with a general or regional anesthetic. A broad-spectrum antibiotic is advised for the surgical procedure. Slight flexion of the waist when the patient is prone, with the buttocks taped apart with skin adhesive to open up the intergluteal region for easier access and exposure, is very helpful. The incision (Fig. 13A,B) is taken down through the soft tissue with a sharp knife and then cautery resection, avoiding trauma to skin; the coccyx is subperiosteally exposed. Once the sacrococcygeal disc space is entered and the cornua and lateral aspect of C-1 are freed from the surrounding tissue, an elevator is placed anterolaterally to the coccyx allowing for tensile traction directed away from the anteriorly located rectum, facilitating the resection with the electrocautery. With gentle traction from proximal to distal and side to side, the entire coccyx can be removed, with the last fibrous attachment released from the most distal coccygeal segment. At times, the prominent sacrum can be beveled down in proximity to the sacral hiatus, where epidural fat can easily be seen. Intraoperative x-rays are usually not required but with anomalies in sacrococcygeal development, x-rays should be used to confirm removal of all mobile segments (Fig. 13C,D).

The wound is copiously irrigated with saline and then closed in layers with absorbable sutures after the buttock tapes are removed from under the drapes by a circulating nurse. The skin is best approximated with subarticular absorbable suture material and the wound dressed with 4 × 4s and elastic tape after the wound is sealed with two separately applied coats of collodium.

Mobilization, protection of the wound with gauze or a feminine napkin, and the avoidance of immersion in water, prolonged sitting, or abrasive clothing is encouraged for a 3- to 4-week period, after which time activity is increased as tolerated. Wound healing delays in excess of 3 weeks can be anticipated in nearly one-half of the patients, but complete healing should take place by 5 to 6 weeks (6,32). Low-grade infection requiring more aggressive wound care and antibiotics coverage is encountered in up to 16% of patients (32,56) but in general, does not compromise the eventual clinical outcome (20).

Sacral Rhizotomies

Rhizotomies of the fourth and fifth sacral roots and the terminal paired coccygeal nerves can result in a sensory denervation of the lower sacrum and coccygeal area and have been recommended with good results in 80% of the patients, as reported by Bohn in 1956 and 1958 (85,86). Because the procedure has the potential for worse pain and neurologic complications (85,87), sacral rhizotomies should be reserved for those patients who have anococcygeal tenderness and pain confined to that area with associated distal cauda equina nerve damage (85,86), particularly when a coccygectomy has failed.

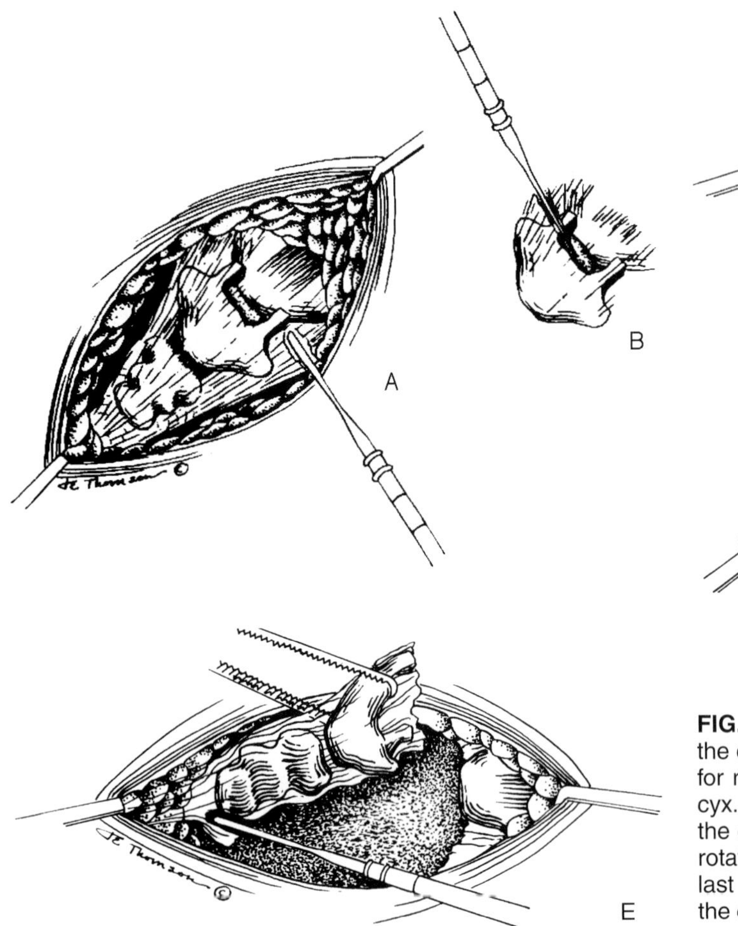

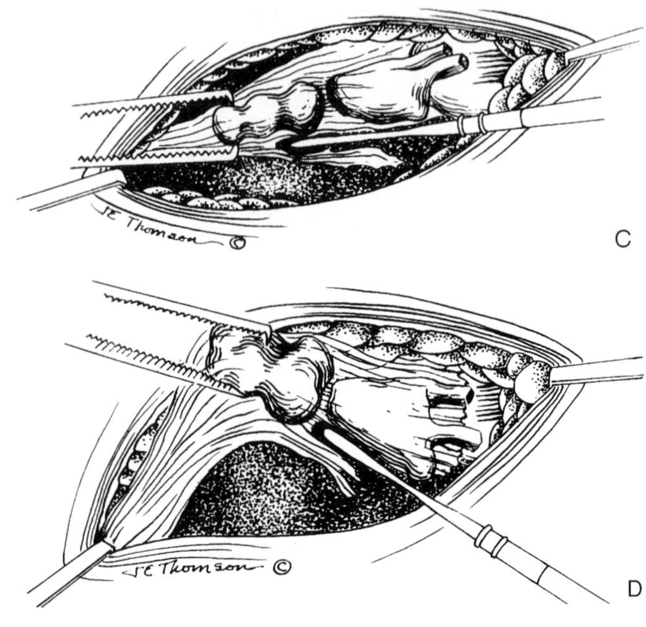

FIG. 13. A,B: Exposure of the sacrococcygeal junction and the excision of the sacrococcygeal disc to mobilize the coccyx for removal. **C:** Releasing the lateral attachments of the coccyx. **D:** Lateral and ventral release of the soft tissue securing the coccyx with tension applied to the tissue as the coccyx is rotated on the sacrum. **E:** The entire coccyx removed with the last ventral attachments released from the terminal aspect of the coccyx.

Referred Pain

As was referenced earlier (72), the gastroenterologic and urogenital organs of the pelvis enjoy autonomic, somatic, and sensory innervation with the inferior hypogastric plexus providing the major neural integration center of those structures. The sensory innervation of the sacral coccygeal area, primarily S-4, S-5, and the coccygeal nerves, transverses the full length of the lumbosacral spine, positioned centrally within the cauda equina, and therefore can be compromised anywhere along its course within the epidural space and its retroperitoneal environment. A thorough history and physical examination with appropriate subspecialty consultation and imaging should identify abnormalities if they exist.

Gastrointestinal and Genitourinary Lesions

In evaluating gastrointestinal complaints, cinedefecograph may provide insight leading to a working diagnosis, such as internal rectoanal intussusception, rectocele, or paraxial puborectalis contraction (68,88). Associated factors coexisting or contributing to perirectal/sacrococcygeal pain (72,89), including constipation, peripelvic, anal, or spinal surgery, anxiety and depression, and irritable bowel syndrome have been described. Although the female genitals receive a different source of innervation than the rectal and anal sphincters (72), the pudendal nerve and the S-4 and S-5 nerve roots are common pathways for the terminal aspects of the gastrointestinal and genitourinary systems, therefore potentially confounding the source of sacrococcygeal pain.

Lumbosacral

Although neurogenic lesions, such as Tarlov's cysts (Fig. 14), arachnoiditis, schwannomas, perineural cysts, benign spinal stenosis, disc herniations and various spondylolisthetic lesions and cauda equina lesions, can anatomically involve the terminal nerve roots, resulting in the perception of pain at the sacrococcygeal junction (49,56–58,75,90,91), the presence of pain and tenderness on palpation of the coccyx with increased pain during active and passive movement of the sacrococcygeal joint would suggest the possibility that local pathology may exist coincidentally and would persist even after the appropriate management of the more proximal lesions. Conversely, proximal problems associated with pelvic or lumbosacral pathology may persist when a tender and reproducible sacrococcygeal lesion is appropriately managed medically and surgically (6,60). As always, a high index of suspicion must guide the diagnostic workup with invasive treatment reserved for those patients with a specific diagnosis.

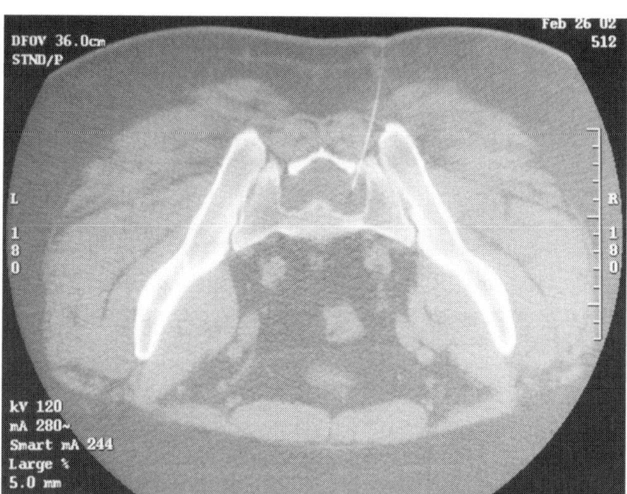

FIG. 14. Computed axial tomography scan directed diagnostic aspiration of a Tarlov's cyst with successful relief of sacrococcygeal pain.

Psychogenic: Depression and Sacrococcygeal Pain Syndromes

Wesselmann and Skevington have observed that like all chronic pain complaints, it is likely that individuals with coccydynia experience higher rates of depression than controls (72,92). A cognizance of that reality should help the clinicians modify their therapeutic suggestions but not deny appropriate care. Bremer's dicta, published in 1896, has not survived the scrutiny of time and the observations of numerous clinicians. Bremer emphasized the hysterical nature of patients with coccydynia when he wrote (93):

> The desperate monotony of an excessively painful and annoying affection engenders a craving for something phenomenal. They look upon their suffering as unique in atrociousness and unexampled in medicine and nothing short of an extraordinary (therapy) will, in their opinion, be of any avail. As a rule, nothing short of an operation will satisfy them and generally they do not meet with any difficulty in finding a surgeon who is willing to operate. To use a knife on such patients is a grave mistake. To cut off a painful coccyx is as irrational as removal of the ovaries in hysterical ovarialgia. The time will come when another generation of medical men will look upon such operations as one of the most remarkable aberrations of the science of medicine. The trouble is in the brain but not at the periphery, neither bone nor skin.

Watson-Jones in 1943 (103), however, more appropriately concluded that "the functional and psychological aspects of coccydynia have been exaggerated," a conclusion reiterated by other authors (6,31) and enduring the passage of time (57).

Maroy, in 1988, reported that highly significant correlation was found between the following parameters: pain evoked on digital rectal examination and depressive status in noncoccydynic patients, coccydynia and evoked pain, and coccygeal and paracoccygeal muscular pain (94). The severity of coccydynia was not correlated with a number of depressive signs, nor was gender, age, or treatment efficacy. He and his co-author actually went on to propose that the mechanism of depressive pain, in this case, a digital rectal examination–evoked pain, may be an "objective" diagnostic sign for identifying "masked" depression, as well as a tool for monitoring needed psychological treatment if depression is present. Caution, not denial of surgical treatment, is warranted in this patient population, but efforts should be made to provide objective evidence of an organic lesion, along with the psychological support of all subspecialty clinicians who would be involved in such complex cases.

Homo Caudatus

If there is a persistence of the nonchondrified lower coccygeal segments (i.e., lower four or five of the original eight coccygeal somites), described as a disturbance in fetal tail regression (95), an ill-defined human tail *homo caudatus* can be manifest (96). Fara and Bar-Maor have provided classification systems to explain clinical cases that are defined by a spectrum of embryologic development that can vary from a soft tissue to a true functional tail (97,98). More than 100 cases have been reported in the literature with no gender preference, but a familial and perhaps racial tendency has indeed been suggested (97,99,100).

Bartel's classification described three separate variations (types I, II, and III) of a "soft tail" presumably arising from the embryologic tail, whereas type IV in his classification defines a bony tail caused by hypertrophy of the usual sacrococcygeal vertebra one to four and his type V, a true animal tail containing additional vertebrae (ossification of the fourth through the eighth coccygeal segments) (5,101,102).

Described associated malformations of the vascular system in the caudal processes may have been a coincidental or a causative mechanism for the persistence of a soft tissue or the chondro-ossification of the original coccygeal somites (95,98). Pain due to the prominence and susceptibility of these "tails" to trauma and/or a cosmetic issue may prompt surgical removal, but the possibility of associated neurovascular, gastrointestinal, and urogenital anomalies should be assessed with CT scan and/or MRI before invasive treatment.

REFERENCES

1. Broome DR, Hayman LA, Herrick RC, et al. Postnatal maturation of the sacrum and coccyx: MR imaging, helical CT and conventional radiography. *AJR Am J Roentgenolol* 1998;170:1061–1066.
2. Gray H. *The anatomical basis of medicine and surgery.* In: Williams PL, ed. *Gray's anatomy*, 38th ed. Edinburgh: Churchill Livingstone, 1995:1282.
3. Maigne J-Y, Guedj S, Straus C. Idiopathic coccygodynia, lateral roentgenograms in the sitting position and coccygeal discography. *Spine* 1994;19(8):930–934.
4. Dieulaffe R. *Le Coccyx; etude osteologique. Arch d'anat, d'histol et d'em bryol.* 1933:1641.
5. Howorth B. The painful coccyx. *Clin Orthop* 1956;14:145–161.
6. Postacchini F, Massobrio M. Idiopathic coccygodynia. Analysis of fifty-one operative cases and a radiographic study of the normal coccyx. *J Bone Joint Surg* 1983;65A(8):1116–1124.
7. Truex RC, Carpenter MB. *Human neuroanatomy*. Baltimore: Williams & Wilkins, 1969.
8. Park WW. Applied anatomy of the spine. In: Rothman RH, Simeone FA, eds. *The spine*, 2nd ed., vol. II. Philadelphia: WB Saunders, 1975.
9. Matzel K, Schmidt R, Tanagho E. Neuroanatomy of the striated muscular anal continence mechanism: implications for the use of neurostimulation. *Colon Rectum* 1990;33:666–673.

10. Dietemann J, Sick H, Wolfram-Gabel R, et al. Anatomy and computed tomography of the normal lumbosacral plexus. *Neuroradiology* 1987;29:58–68.
11. Wesselmann U, Burnet AL, Heinber LJ. The urogenital and rectal pain syndromes. *Pain* 1977;73:269–294.
12. Gatalica Z, Wang L, Lucio ET, et al. Globus coccygeum in surgical pathology specimens. Small troublemaker. *Arch Pathol Lab Med* 1999;123(10):905–908.
13. Frazier L. Coccydynia: a tail of woe. *North Carolina Med J* 1985; 46(4)209–212.
14. Caldwell W, Moloy H. Anatomical variations in the female pelvis and their effect in labor with a suggested classification. *Am J Obstet Gynecol* 1933;26:479–505.
15. Duncan G. Painful coccyx. *Arch Surg* 1937;37:1088–1104.
16. Ryder I, Alexander J. Coccydynia: a woman's tail. *Midwifery* 2000; 16(2)155–160.
17. Peyton FW. Coccygodynia in women. *Indiana Med* 1988;81(8):697–698.
18. Kim NH, Suk KS. Clinical and radiological differences between traumatic and idiopathic coccygodynia. *Yonsei Med J* 1999;40(3):215–220.
19. Maigne J-Y, Tamalet B. Standardized radiologic protocol for the study of common coccygodynia and characteristics of the lesions observed in the sitting position. Clinical elements differentiating luxation, hypermobility and normal mobility. *Spine* 1996;21(22):2588.
20. Maigne J-Y, Doursounian L, Chatellier G. Causes and mechanisms of common coccydynia: role of body mass index and coccygeal trauma. *Spine* 2000;25(23):3072–3079.
21. Maigne J-Y, Lagauche D, Doursounian L. Instability of the coccyx in coccydynia. *J Bone Joint Surg* 2000;82B(7):1038–1041.
22. Simpson JY. Removal of the coccyx in coccygodynia (letter). *Med Times Gaz* 1861;1:317.
23. Raissaki MT, Williamson JB. Fracture dislocation of the sacrococcygeal joint: MRI evaluation. *Pediatr Radiol* 1999;29:642–643.
24. Shore RM, Wilson MA, Rao BK. Sacrococcygeal trauma. *Clin Nuclear Med* 1981;6(3):124–125.
25. O'Keefe RJ, Jones JA, Hurwitz SR. Bilateral sacroiliac joint fracture-dislocation requiring late coccygectomy. A case report. *J Trauma* 1992;33(5):793–794.
26. Kaehr DM, et al. Classification of sacral fractures based on CT imaging. *J Orthop Trauma* 1989;3:163.
27. Meek'ren J. Observationes Medicochirurgicae, ex belgico in latinum, translatae ab Abrahamo Blasio, H & T Boom, Cap. 59 De luxatione ossis caudae, Amsterdam, 273–274, 1682.
28. Gahrliep GC. De luxationis ossis coccygis periculosae, facili, etc. *German Acad Naturae Curiosorum*, Ser 3, A5-6:572, 1697–1698.
29. Beach H. Compound fracture of the coccyx. *Boston Med Surg J* 1899;234.
30. Hamsa W. Coccygodynia: a study of the end result of treatment. *J Iowa State Med Soc* 1937;27:154–156.
31. Key AJ. Operative treatment of coccygodynia. *J Bone Joint Surg* 1937;19(3):759–764.
32. Grosso NP, van Dam BE. Total coccygectomy for the relief of coccygodynia: a retrospective review. *J Spinal Dis* 1995;8(4):328–330.
33. Powers J. Coccygectomy. *South Med J* 1957;50:675–678.
34. Tavel L. Coccygodynia and proctalgia fugax. *J Am Osteopath Assoc* 1976;75:1068–1070.
35. Bergkamp ABM, Verhaar JAN. Dislocation of the coccyx: a case report. *J Bone Joint Surg* 1995;77-B(5)831.
36. Depalma A. *The management of fractures and dislocations, an atlas*, 2nd ed. Philadelphia: WB Saunders, 1970.
37. Gutierrez PR, Martinez JJM, Arenas J. Salter-Harris type I fracture of the sacrococcygeal joint. *Pediatr Radiol* 1998;28:734.
38. Cameron H, Fornaiser V, Schatzker J. Coccyodynia [letter]. *Canadian Med Assoc J* 1975;112, 557–558.
39. Petit JL. *A treatise of the diseases of the bones* (translated from the French). London: T. Woodward, 1726.
40. Bacon HE, Taylor A. Osteomyelitis of the coccyx and sacrum with sinus formation simulating anorectal fistula. *N Engl J Med* 1940; 23:668–671.
41. Blundell J. *Principles and practice of obstetric medicine* (revised by A. Cooper Lee and Nathaniel Rogers), London: J. Butler, 1840.
42. Darrah R. A report of 3 cases of the coccyx. *Boston Med Surg J* 1893;128:36.
43. Nott JC. Facts illustrative of the practical importance of a knowledge of the anatomy and physiology of the nervous system. *New Orleans Med J* 1844;1:57.
44. Raney RB, Chatten J, Littman P, et al. Treatment strategies for infants with malignant sacrococcygeal teratoma. *J Pediatr Surg* 1981;16[4 Suppl 1]:573–577.
45. Capanna R, Briccoli A, Campanacci L, et al. Benign and malignant tumors of the sacrum. In: Frymoyer JW, ed. *The adult spine*, 2nd ed. Philadelphia: Lippincott–Raven, 1987.
46. Lourie J, Young S. Avascular necrosis of the coccyx: a cause of coccydynia? *Br J Clin Pract* 1985;39:247–248.
47. Yamaguchi T, Yamato M, Saotome K. First histologically confirmed case of a classic chordoma arising in a precursor benign notochordal lesion: differential diagnosis of benign and malignant notochordal lesions. *Skeletal Radiol* 2002;31(7):413–418.
48. Genovese AM, Fedele F, Barbera A, et al. Posterior approach in the treatment of sacrococcygeal chordoma: a rare, locally infiltrating, destructive and recurrent tumor. A case report and review of the literature (Italian). *Minerva Chirurg* 2000;55(6):455–458.
49. Dittrich RJ. Coccygodynia as referred pain. *J Bone Joint Surg* 1951;33-A(3):715–718.
50. Samson J, Springfield D, Suit H, et al. Operative treatment of sacrococcygeal chordoma. *J Bone Joint Surg* 1993;75-A(10):1476–1484.
51. Bell RS, Goodman SB, Fornasier VL. Coccygeal glomus tumors: a case of mistaken identity? *J Bone Joint Surg [Am]* 1982;64-A:595–597.
52. Albrecht S, Hicks MJ, Antalffy B. Intracoccygeal and pericoccygeal glomus bodies and their relationship to coccygodynia. *Surgery* 1994;115(1):1–6.
53. Pyper JB. Excision of the coccyx for coccydynia. A study of the results in twenty-eight cases. *J Bone Joint Surg* 1957;39B(4):733–737.
54. Nixon EA. Coccygodynia. *Am J Surg* 1939;44:390–393.
55. Helberg S, Strange-Vognsen H. Coccygodynia treated by resection of the coccyx. *Acta Orthop Scand* 1990;61:463–465.
56. Bayne O, Bateman JE, Cameron HU. The influence of etiology on the results of coccygectomy. *Clin Orthop* 1984;190:266–272.
57. Richards HG. Causes of coccydynia. *J Bone Joint Surg [Br]* 1954;36-B:142.
58. Ziegler DK, Batnitzky S. Coccygodynia caused by perineural cyst. *Neurology* 1984;34:829–830.
59. Thiele GH. Coccygodynia and pain in the superior gluteal region and down the back of the thigh. *JAMA* 1937;109:1271–1274.
60. Wray CC, Easom S, Hoskinson J. Coccydynia: aetiology and treatment. *J Bone Joint Surg* 1991;73-B:335–338.
61. Brunskill P, Swan J. Spontaneous fracture of the coccygeal body during the second stage of labor. *Am J Obstet Gynecol* 1987;7(4):270–271.
62. Jones M, Shoaib A, Bircher M. A case of coccygodynia due to coccygeal fracture secondary to parturition injury. *Injury* 1997;28(8):549–550.
63. Yamashita K. Radiological study of 1500 coccyces. *J Jpn Orthop Assoc* 1988;62(1):22–36.
64. Nakamura A, Inoue Y, Ishihara T, et al. Acquired coccygeal nodule due to repeated stimulation by a bicycle saddle. *J Dermatol* 1995;22:365–369.
65. Traycoff RB, Crayton H, Dodson R. Sacrococcygeal pain syndromes: diagnosis and treatment. *Orthopaedics* 1989;12(10):1373–1377.
66. Sinaki M, Merritt JL, Stillwell G. Tension myalgia of the pelvic floor. *Mayo Clin Proc* 1977;52:717–722.
67. Ely LW. Coccygodynia. *JAMA* 1910;44:968.
68. Ger GC, Wexner SD, Jorge JN, et al. Evaluation and treatment of chronic intractable rectal pain—a frustrating endeavor. *Dis Colon Rectum* 1993;36(2):139–145.
69. Plattner V, Leborgne J, Heloury Y, et al. MRI evaluation of the levator ani muscle: anatomic correlations and practical applications. *Surg Radiol Anat* 1991;13(2)6:129–131.
70. Karra SJD, Angelo G. Proctalgia fugax. *Am J Surg* 1951;82:616–625.
71. Thaysen ET. Proctalgia fugax. *Lancet* 1936;2:243–246.
72. Wesselmann U, Reich SG. The dynias. *Semin Neurol* 1996;16(1):63–74.
73. Pradel E, Hernandez C, Alloy A. Le Syndrome et it de "proctalgia fugax." *Ann Chu* 1967;21:691–699.
74. Johnson PH. Coccygodynia. *J Ark Med Soc* 1981;77:421–424.
75. Stern FH. Idiopathic coccygodynia among the geriatric population. *J Am Geriatr Soc* 1967;15:100–102.

76. Maigne J-Y, Chatellier G. Comparison of three manual coccydynia treatments. A pilot study. *Spine* 2001;26:E479–E484.
77. Segura JW, Ospitz JL, Greene LP. Prostatosis, prostatitis or pelvic floor tension myalgia. *J Urol* 1979;122:168–169.
78. Wray AR, Templeton J. Coccygectomy: a review of thirty-seven cases. *Ulster Med J* 1982;51:121–124.
79. Porter KM, Kahn MA, Piggot H. Coccydynia: a retrospective review. In: Proceedings of the British Orthopaedic Association. *J Bone Joint Surg* 1981;63B(4):635–636.
80. Gant SC. *Diseases of the rectum, anus and colon, including the ileocolic angle, appendix, colon, sigmoid flexure, rectum, anus, buttocks and sacrococcygeal region*. Philadelphia: WB Saunders, 1923.
81. Borgia C. Coccygodynia: its diagnosis and treatment. *Mit Med* 1964;129:335–338.
82. Gardner RC. An improved technique of coccygectomy. *Clin Orthop* 1972;85:143–145.
83. Zayer M. Coccygodynia. *Ulster Med J* 1996;65(1):58–60.
84. Hodge J. Clinical management of coccydynia. *Med Trial Tech* 1979;25(3)277–288.
85. Albrektsson B. Sacral rhizotomy in cases of ano-coccygeal pain. *Acta Orthop Scand* 1981;52(2):187–190.
86. Bohn E, Franksson C, Petersen I. Sacral rhizopathies and sacral root syndromes. *Acta Chir Scand* 1956;Suppl 216.
87. Saris SC, Silver JM, Vieira JFS, et. al. Sacrococcygeal rhizotomy for perineal pain. *Neurosurgery* 1986;19:789–793.
88. Swinton NW. Coccygodynia as a cause of unexplained rectal pain. *Lahey Clin Bull* 1941;2:110–113.
89. Bonica JJ. Pelvic and perineal pain caused by other disorders. In: JJ Bonica, ed. *The management of pain*, 2nd ed. Philadelphia: Lea & Febiger, 1990:1384–1385.
90. Kinnett JG, Root L. An obscure cause of coccygodynia. *J Bone Joint Surg* 1979;61-A(2):299.
91. Dehaine V, Wechsler B, Ziza JM, et al. Coccygodynia disclosing Tarlov's cysts (review) (French). *Revue de Medecine Interne* 1990; 11(4)280–284.
92. Skevington SM. The relationship between pain and depression: a longitudinal study of early synovitis. In: Gebhart GF, Hammond DL, Jensen TS, eds. *Proceedings of the 7th World Congress on Pain. Progress in Pain Research and Management*, vol 2. Seattle: ISAP Press, 1994:201–210.
93. Bremer L. The knife for coccygodynia: a failure. *Medical Record* 1896;154–155.
94. Maroy B. Spontaneous and evoked coccygeal pain in depression. *Dis Col Rectum* 1988;31(30):210–215.
95. Matsuo T, Koga H, Moriyama T, et al. A case of true human tail accompanied with spinal lipoma (Japanese). No Shinkei Geka. *Neurol Surg* 1993;21(10):925.
96. Parsons RW. Human tails. *Plas Reconstruct Surg* 1960;25(6): 618–621.
97. Fára M, Smahil J. Human tail. *Acta ChirurgPlasticae* 1975;15:184–189.
98. Fára M. Coccygeal ("tail") projection with cartilage content. *Acta Chirurg Plasticae* 1977;19(1):50–55.
99. Bar-Maor JA, Kesner KM, Kaftori JK. Human tails. *J Bone Joint Surg* 1980;62-B(4):508–510.
100. Miller C. Tailed humanity. *Med Surg Rep* 1881;45:165–166.
101. Gould GM, Pyle VL. *Anomalies and curiosities of medicine*. Philadelphia: WB Saunders, 1897:277–280.
102. Bartels M, Diegeschwanzten, Menechen. *Arch Antrop* 1883;15:45–131.
103. Watson-Jones R. *Fractures and joint injuries*, 3rd ed., vol. 1, Edinburgh, UK: E & S Livingstone Ltd., 1943.

CHAPTER 51

Bone Grafting and Bone Graft Substitutes in Spinal Surgery: Basic Science and Clinical Applications

Safdar N. Khan and Harvinder S. Sandhu

The step-by-step cellular and molecular events involved in the bone formation cascade during spinal fusion as well as the identification of the various critical growth factors orchestrating this process have been elucidated in some detail in the past few years (1). Based on the pioneering work of Marshall Urist, growth factor technology has been exploited in an attempt to improve rates of spinal fusion, and promising results have been demonstrated in preclinical animal studies and pivotal clinical human studies (2). In this chapter, the authors review the biology of spinal fusion and provide a perspective on the future of spinal fusion, grafting, and bone graft substitutes.

An ideal bone graft or bone graft substitute must consist of the following three essential elements: (a) an osteoconductive matrix, (b) osteoinductive factors, and (c) responsive osteogenic cells. *Osteoconductivity* can be broadly defined as the process of infiltration of capillaries, perivascular tissue, and osteoprogenitor cells within a three-dimensional matrix (3). *Osteoinduction* is the stimulation of undifferentiated cells to produce osteogenic elements (3). This process is mediated primarily by growth factors such as bone morphogenetic proteins (BMPs) that are capable of inducing differentiation of mesenchymal cells into cartilage- and bone-producing cells. *Osteogenetic cells* are mesenchymal-type cells that may be harnessed from host or graft bone marrow (3).

Autogenous cancellous bone graft satisfies all three categories most completely. Hydroxyapatite (HA) and collagen serve as the three-dimensional osteoconductive framework, mesenchymal stromal cells lining the microcavities possess the necessary osteogenic potential, and an endogenous family of growth factors within the bone matrix and adjacent hematoma induce the regenerative and augmentation processes. For these reasons, the autogenous cancellous bone graft is considered the gold standard of bone grafting.

Nearly 250,000 spinal fusions are performed annually in the United States, and almost all require the implantation of a bone graft material (4). Most of these fusions use the transplantation of structured or morselized autogenous corticocancellous bone derived from the iliac crest. Not surprisingly, arthrodesis of the spine has become the most common reason for autogenous bone graft harvest. However, several potential complications involved with autogenous grafting (e.g., donor site morbidity, limited availability for harvest, and increased operative blood loss) have led to the search for viable substitutes that may perform equally well, at best, to autograft in several biologic environments (4,5).

LUMBAR FUSION ANIMAL MODEL: A STUDY IN SPINAL FUSION BIOLOGY

To understand the science behind bone grafting, it is important to review the biology of spinal fusion. Boden et al. have characterized a clinically relevant rabbit model of posterolateral lumbar spinal fusion (6). A sequential histologic analysis of this model revealed a continuum of three bone graft incorporation phases.

Phase I

The first phase, as in fracture healing, is an inflammatory reaction (weeks 1 through 3). An initial hematoma is induced at the fusion site by decortication and disruption of the local blood, followed by an accumulation of inflammatory cells, such as polymorphonuclear leukocytes. The fracture hematoma-clot then turns into a fibrovascular stroma by fibroblast-like mesenchymal cells. The beginning of membranous bone formation is observed at the decorticated surface of the transverse processes, and early evidence of endochondral bone formation is seen between the bone graft fragments.

Phase II

In the middle or reparative phase (weeks 4 and 5), membranous and endochondral bone formation continues at a steady rate. Resorption of necrotic graft tissue and the revascularization of the implanted bone graft progresses. The membranous bone formation is evident at the transverse processes and extends toward the center of the fusion mass, and the endochondral bone formation occurs centrally at the interface between the upper and lower halves of the fusion mass. This central endochondral process is attributed to the tolerance of cartilage to the low oxygen saturation observed centrally or to the motion present between the upper and lower portions of the fusion mass (3).

Phase III

In the late phase (weeks 6 to 10), the early bone fusion mass is remodeled. The fusion mass is initially shown to have a thin cortical rim surrounding a center composed of secondary spongiosa and bone marrow. As the remodeling continues, the cortical rim thickens, and newly formed trabeculae extend toward the center of the fusion (3). This remodeling is deemed a critical element of the biomechanical development of a fusion mass. This sequential histologic analysis of a rabbit lumbar fusion model suggests spinal fusions involving bone grafts are a complex but highly regulated process including necrotic graft resorption, graft revascularization, and membranous bone formation.

AUTOGRAFT

Cancellous autograft has limited use in situations in which structural support is required. However, due to its increased surface area and osteogenic potential in relation to osteogenic cells, this quickly changes secondarily to osseointegration at the host fusion site (7). Cancellous strips, prepared in flat strips approximately 5 mm across, usually tend to incorporate completely. However, cortical bone may lose up to one-third of its biomechanical strength during incorporation and usually takes up to 18 months to remodel and incorporate (8,9). Cortical bone is not preferred, as fewer marrow spaces yield fewer cells with osteogenic potential, and they present less surface area onto which new bone can be laid down. Furthermore, vascular invasion and remodeling is resisted (8).

Essential in the fusion process is the technical preparation of the fusion bed and the handling of the bone graft material. Indeed, volume and density characteristics of autograft bone that lead to predictable fusion are yet to be reported in the literature. Effects of host bone mineral density, wet and dry weight of the implanted autograft, and morselization and mean size of the implanted graft all have potential effects on graft incorporation and fusion, and the implanting surgeon must be aware of each. The fusion bed itself is the primary source of the osteogenic cells. Therefore, proper decortication and preparation of recipient bone, such as maximizing the surface area of exposed cancellous bone while minimizing cellular and mechanical damage, is critical. Overzealous use of the burr may lead to necrotic bone at the fusion bed.

Fusion rates using autograft are generally superior in the posterior cervical and thoracic location compared to the posterior lumbar location. The interbody location is a favorable healing environment throughout the spinal column due to the relatively large surface area of subchondral cancellous bone along the vertebral end-plates combined with the compressive loads present at the fusion site (10–13).

Tricortical iliac crest wedges and bicortical iliac dowels have been used extensively for intervertebral grafting and have been associated with favorable fusion rates but may undergo graft collapse. Weiland and McAfee reported only one pseudarthrosis among 100 consecutive patients undergoing all types of posterior cervical fusions and none in patients requiring subaxial fusion using Bohlman's triple wire technique with autogenous corticocancellous bone blocks (14). Sawin et al. reported a 98.8% fusion rate in 300 patients undergoing posterior cervical fusions with autogenous rib graft compared to 94.2% in patients treated with iliac crest autograft (15). They observed significantly less morbidity associated with the rib graft harvest compared to the iliac crest harvest (3.7% vs. 25.3%). The presence of interbody devices filled with autograft theoretically lessens the likelihood of graft subsidence. These include metallic cages, dowels, and femoral ring allografts (FRAs). More recently, threaded cylindrical metallic cages containing morselized autograft have been implanted in an intervertebral space distracted to the maximal tension of the annulus. Ray, in a prospective series using such devices, observed a 96% fusion rate in 208 patients with 2-year follow-up (16). However, the accuracy of radiographic assessment of fusion through these titanium cages is suspect, as bony consolidation is often obscured by the metallic implants. Longer-term follow-up of patients implanted with threaded cages has been advocated.

Autogenous iliac crest bone graft is still considered the gold standard for most spinal fusion applications. The morbidity associated with autograft procurement continues to be its greatest drawback (17–19).

ALLOGRAFT

Allografts are currently the most common extenders for autogenous bone grafting. They are considered highly osteoconductive, weakly osteoinductive, and not osteogenic, as the cells do not survive implantation. Processing and preservation techniques affect the osteoinductive, osteoconductive, and immunogenic properties of the allografts. After donor screening, allograft bone is harvested under sterile conditions, usually within 24 hours of death, and is processed immediately thereafter. Preservation is accomplished by freezing or freeze-drying (lyophilization), both of which serve to reduce immunogenicity and allow extended storage. If kept at –20°C, the mechanical strength of frozen grafts does not attenuate, and they can be stored for up to 1 year (20–23). Lyophilization and vacuum packing permit room temperature storage and an indefinite shelf life with even less immunogenicity. The mechanical strength of freeze-dried implants, however, can be reduced by 50% compared with frozen grafts. Terminal sterilization using ethylene oxide gas or high-dose gamma irradiation is used, but both methods may further reduce osteoinductivity (24).

Cloward reported that in 46 patients implanted with fresh-frozen allograft for anterior cervical spine surgery, only three grafts resorbed (25). Brown et al. compared the use of frozen allograft to autograft and found that 32 patients treated with frozen allograft for single-level arthrodesis fused equally well as 29 patients implanted with autograft (26). An equal frequency of graft collapse was noted between the autograft group and the allograft group. A higher rate of graft collapse in multilevel fusions implanted with allograft was noted. Zdeblick et al. compared the use of freeze-dried tricortical allograft with autograft for Smith-Robinson–type fusions in 87 consecutive patients and noted an equal fusion rate (95%) 1 year after surgery in patients undergoing single-level fusion (27). Significantly, in patients undergoing two-level fusions, 63% of 16 levels implanted with allograft and 17% of levels implanted with autograft developed nonunions. In this series, 30% of the allograft fusions subsided, compared to 5% of the autograft fusions. Zhang et al. retrospectively reviewed 121 patients undergoing multilevel cervical fusions and reported that 85% of those implanted with autograft fused, compared to only 50% of those implanted with allograft (28). From the clinical data available, it can be surmised that generally poorer results occur in multilevel disease, regardless of the type of graft implanted. These adverse results seem to be a consequence of an increased number of surfaces that require osseous fusion and the increased instability created by multilevel discectomies.

The use of allografts with and without autograft for posterior lumbar fusion in adults has been examined recently. Jorgenson et al. found that patients who were implanted with allograft alone or allograft mixed with autograft had a lower radiographic fusion rate than those implanted with autograft alone (29). Dodd et al. showed that femoral head allograft bone combined with locally decorticated bone can even be considered the graft composite of choice in the adolescent idiopathic scoliotic population (30). They found 100% fusions in 20 patients treated by this method. Although control patients who had been implanted with iliac crest autograft also had no pseudarthroses, 40% complained of persisting pain or paresthesia at the graft site. The rate of spontaneous fusion in the pediatric and adolescent age group in itself remains higher than the older population, and patient age and site of fusion must be taken into consideration before drawing any conclusions about the use of allografts for posterior lumbar fusion. Recently, however, Barnes et al. examined the results of patients undergoing posterior lumbar interbody fusion (PLIF) with allograft cylindrical dowels or wedges (31). Twenty-seven patients underwent PLIF with impacted allograft wedges, and 22 patients underwent PLIF with allograft cylindrical threaded cortical bone dowels (TCBD). The cylindrical TCBD group showed a 13.6% rate of permanent nerve root injury, and the impacted wedge group demonstrated a 0% rate—a statistically significant difference. The fusion rate at a mean of 13.9 months of follow-up was 95.4% in patients in whom the cylindrical TCBD was implanted and 88.9% after a mean of 17.4 months of follow-up in patients in whom impacted wedges were used—an insignificant difference. The authors concluded there was a significant increase in permanent nerve root injury rates with the use of cylindrical TCBD implants as compared with impacted allograft wedges. There was no difference between the two groups in terms of fusion rates, but clinical outcomes with the use of impacted wedges were significantly better.

In the anterior lumbar spine, cortical allografts have successfully been used for structural support and have been combined with autogenous bone graft. Kozak reviewed the results of 45 patients implanted with a ring-shaped femoral allograft filled in the center with morselized iliac crest autograft and found that radiolucencies surrounding the graft persisted for up to 1 year, but established pseudarthroses were rare (32). A recent study by Cohen et al. compared the results of anterior lumbar interbody fusion (ALIF) pseudarthrosis repair with iliac crest autograft or FRAs (33). Two series of patients underwent ALIF with anterior instrumentation to repair pseudarthrosis (group I, 33 patients with tricortical autogenous iliac crest, and group II, 20 patients with FRAs). At minimum 2-year follow-up, there was no difference in fusion rates (group I, 32 of 33 vs. group II, 20 of 20). Patients in group I had radiographic fusion develop more rapidly than patients in group II (12 months vs. 18 months), but a significant proportion of patients in group I (35%) had an average of 2 mm of graft subsidence. Despite excellent fusion rates in both groups, overall functional outcomes were not as good, with only 28% of patients in group I and 36% of patients in group II returning to work. Similarly, Molinari et al. reviewed the long-term outcomes of patients who underwent anterior strut allografting in maintaining long-term sagittal plane correction. Twenty-three consecutive adult patients had a combination of anterior structural fresh-frozen allograft plus posterior autogenous grafting and posterior segmental spinal instrumentation performed. All patients had sagittal plane abnormalities, and all surgeries were performed by the same surgeon. Five-year follow-up was available for 20 of the 23 patients. Of the 67 structural allografts, 66 (98.5%) showed incorporation at final follow-up. None of the 67 structural allografts showed evidence of collapse. In all grafted levels and in any patient, there was no difference in sagittal plane measurements obtained immediately after surgery and those obtained at follow-up examinations 2 years and 5 or more years after surgery. The authors concluded that, at a minimum of 5 years after surgery, there was a high rate of structural allograft incorporation into the adjacent vertebral bodies.

DEMINERALIZED BONE MATRIX

Acid extraction of bone leaves behind growth factors, noncollagenous proteins, and collagen while removing the mineral phase of bone. This demineralized, partially defatted homologous bone matrix is a potent inducer of new bone formation, as it retains the essential growth factors that orchestrate bone formation. Demineralized allograft materials provide a suitable framework for cells to populate and produce new bone and also stimulate the healing response by encouraging mesenchymal cells to differentiate into bone-forming osteoblasts. Hence, at the site of implantation, these factors trigger the endochondral ossification cascade, leading to new bone formation. Processed demineralized bone matrix

(DBM) composites became widely available for clinical use in 1991 and since then have been used widely in all areas of orthopedic bone grafting. The first widely available preparation, known as Grafton Gel (Osteotech Inc., Eatontown, NJ), consists of DBM combined with a glycerol carrier and is easily extricable from a standard syringe onto an operative site. Variations of the Grafton composite, including a putty form and a flex form, are also available, but there are no clinical data available to assess their performance. Various formulations are now being prepared that contain within them demineralized corticocancellous chips, presumably for a greater osteoconduction and osteoinduction. No clinical data have been reported as yet.

Martin et al. used a rabbit model of posterolateral intertransverse process fusion to determine the efficacy of the flex and putty formulations (34). In this study, 108 rabbits underwent bilateral fusions at L5-6, using autograft alone (control), flex alone, putty alone, or flex plus autograft or putty plus autograft. At 6 weeks, the rabbits were sacrificed and outcome was assessed by manual palpation, radiography, and undecalcified histology. The results indicated that the newer forms of DBM were effective as graft extenders and enhancers and appeared to have a greater capacity to form bone than autograft alone in this model. Recently, however, the safety of these materials has been brought under scrutiny. In a preclinical study by Bostrom et al., the relative toxicology of the nonallograft components that make up various commercially available DBM products was examined (35). Six different commercially available bone grafting materials were tested in subcutaneous and intermuscular locations in 30 athymic mice. Of the nine rats implanted with Grafton DBM products, only one rat remained alive after 4 weeks; the other eight rats died 1 to 4 days after implantation. None of the remaining ten animals implanted with the four other grafting materials died. The experiment was then modified and completed with a lower dose of bone graft material. Pathologic analysis indicated that the cause of death was hemorrhagic necrosis of the kidneys, most likely caused by a toxic effect on the glomeruli and tubules. A possible contributing factor might have been the glycerol in the graft material. The authors concluded that although the volume of Grafton product per kilogram of body weight used in the study was approximately eight times the maximum volume used in humans, reporting the data was essential because the product is used substantially in clinical settings.

Sassard et al. retrospectively reviewed patients who had undergone instrumented posterolateral lumbar spine fusion with autogenous bone graft and Grafton gel and compared them with an age-, gender-, and procedure-matched group of patients undergoing instrumented fusions with autograft harvested from the iliac crest (36). Using a bone mineralization rating scale, they did not find any radiographic differences between the groups based on films taken 3, 6, 12, and 24 months after surgery. However, the fusion rates in the autograft with Grafton group and the autograft-only group were only 60% and 56%, respectively, less than has been reported in other studies of instrumented posterior fusion. The choice of instrumentation was significantly related to fusion success and was the most important predictor of 24-month bone mineralization.

CERAMICS

The role of ceramics in reconstructive orthopedics is primarily that of osteoconduction (37–39). The major ceramics that have clinical application are the calcium phosphate biomaterials, either HA, tricalcium phosphate (TCP), or varying combinations of the two. These compounds have been favored because they elicit little or no immunologic reaction in adjacent tissues, are stable in bodily fluids, and are able to withstand sterilization. This biocompatibility is due to the fact that these substitutes are primarily composed of calcium and phosphate, just as host bone is. Systemic toxicity with the use of these substitutes is also minimal (40).

Calcium phosphate, calcium sulfate, and natural coral ceramics have been examined in animal models and in selective clinical studies. Of note are two major preclinical studies conducted by Boden et al. (41–42). In the first study, the efficacy of a coralline HA as a bone graft substitute was investigated in a posterolateral lumbar arthrodesis animal model. Single-level posterolateral lumbar arthrodesis was performed at L5-6 in 48 adult New Zealand white rabbits. Rabbits were assigned to one of three groups based on the graft material they received: 3.0 mL coralline HA plus 1.5 mL bone marrow; 1.5 mL coralline HA plus 1.5 mL autogenous iliac crest bone; or 3.0 mL coralline HA plus 500 μg bovine-derived osteoinductive bone protein extract on each side. Rabbits were killed after 2, 5, or 10 weeks. The coralline HA used with bone marrow produced no solid fusions (0 out of 14). When combined with an equal amount of autogenous iliac crest bone, coralline HA resulted in solid fusion in 50% of the rabbits (7 out of 14). When combined with the osteoinductive growth factor extract, the coralline HA resulted in solid fusion in 100% of the rabbits (11 out of 11). Similarly, the fusion masses in the growth factor group were significantly stronger and stiffer based on tensile testing to failure when normalized to the adjacent unfused level. The authors concluded that coralline HA served as an excellent carrier for the bovine osteoinductive bone protein extract, yielding superior results to those obtained with autograft or bone marrow.

In the second study, a nonhuman primate lumbar intertransverse process arthrodesis model was used to evaluate recombinant human BMP-2 (rhBMP-2) in an HA-TCP carrier as a complete bone graft substitute. Twenty-one adult rhesus monkeys underwent a laminectomy at L4-5 followed by bilateral intertransverse process arthrodesis via the same midline incision ($n = 16$) or a minimally invasive video-assisted posterolateral approach ($n = 5$). Bone graft implants on each side consisted of 5 cm^3 of autogenous iliac crest bone or 60:40 HA-TCP blocks (1.2 cm × 0.5 cm × 3.7 cm) loaded with a solution containing 0, 6, 9, or 12 mg of rhBMP-2 per side. Twenty-four weeks after surgery, fusion was not achieved in any of the monkeys treated with autogenous iliac crest bone graft. Both of the monkeys treated with the HA-TCP blocks with 0 mg rhBMP-2 achieved fusion. All 15 monkeys treated with the HA-TCP blocks and either of the three doses of rhBMP-2 achieved solid fusion. The results in animals fused via the minimally invasive video-assisted technique were the same as in those fused with the open technique. There was a dose-dependent increase in the amount and quality of bone throughout the ceramic carrier when rhBMP-2 was added based on qualitative histologic assessment. Based on the results of this study, HA-TCP proved to be a suitable carrier for rhBMP-2 in the posterolateral spine fusion model in rhesus monkeys. The results of this study thus formed the basis for using biphasic calcium phosphate with rhBMP-2 in a pilot human clinical trial (Bone Morphogenetic Proteins).

Passuti et al. reported a study of 12 adolescent patients with severe scoliosis who underwent internal fixation and fusion in which they used blocks of HA-TCP (3:2) with or without autogenous cancellous bone graft for facet joint fusion. Biopsies of the fusion mass were taken in two patients, and all patients underwent clinical and radiologic assessment after an average follow-up of 15 months (43). All patients were deemed radiographically and clinically fused, and histologic analysis of the two specimens indicated *de novo* bone ingrowth into the macropores of the ceramic.

Ransford et al. reported a prospective, randomized study of 341 patients undergoing correction of idiopathic scoliosis and posterior spinal fusion (44). The patients were randomly implanted with autograft (iliac crest or rib) or synthetic porous ceramic blocks. Curve correction and maintenance were similar in both groups 18 months after surgery. Pain and function were also comparable between the groups.

Delecrin et al. reported the results of 58 patients who were enrolled in a prospective randomized study to assess the clinical and radiographic performance of synthetic porous ceramic as a bone graft substitute for scoliosis surgery (45). Posterior spinal fusion was performed using local bone graft combined with autograft in 30 patients and combined with porous biphasic calcium phosphate ceramic blocks comprised of HA and TCP in another 28 patients. Mean follow-up time was 48 months. Patients in the ceramic plus local bone graft group had a lower average blood loss than the control group, and they were also free from local complications at the graft donor site as seen in the control group. Radiographic incorporation and maintenance of correction of deformity was equivalent and satisfactory in both groups.

McConnell et al. recently reported the results of a prospective randomized trial with clinical and radiographic outcome review of patients receiving HA or tricortical iliac crest graft for cervical interbody fusion (46). In this study, 29 patients undergoing anterior cervical fusion and plating were randomized to receive coralline HA (ProOsteon 200) or iliac crest bone graft. There was no significant difference in clinical outcome or fusion rates between the two groups. Significantly, graft fragmentation occurred in 89% of the HA grafts and 11% of the autografts. Significant graft settling occurred in 50% of the HA grafts as compared with 11% of the autografts. One patient in the ProOsteon 200 group required revision surgery for graft failure. Based on the results of this study, ProOsteon 200 did not seem to possess adequate structural integrity to resist axial loading or maintain segmental lordosis during cervical interbody fusion. Thalgott et al. conducted a retrospective review of 20 patients undergoing circumferential lumbar fusion with coralline HA blocks anteriorly and autograft with transpedicular or translaminar facet screw fixation posteriorly (47). At a minimum of 3-year follow-up, radiographic data yielded a solid arthrodesis rate of 93.8% by level (30 of 32 disc spaces) and 90% by patient (18 of 20). Clinical follow-up generated a mean pain reduction of 61.8%, with clinical success demonstrated in 80% (16 of 20) of all patients who reported good or excellent pain relief. A testament to the fact that spinal fusion biology is clearly dependent on fusion environment and biomechanical stability, the authors concluded that coralline HA is a good alternative to autograft and allograft as part of a circumferential fusion, albeit with rigid posterior fixation. They did not recommend coralline HA for stand-alone ALIF.

BONE MORPHOGENETIC PROTEINS

Marshall Urist identified a collection of low-molecular-weight glycoproteins within the demineralized bone and later identified them as BMPs (48). It was not until 1988, however, using molecular cloning, that Wozney identified the specific molecules, of which all but one belong to the transforming growth factor–beta superfamily of proteins (49). Currently, rhBMP-2 carried on a type I collagen sponge is available to be used with a tapered and threaded intervertebral fusion cage (LT cage, Medtronic Sofamor Danek, Minneapolis, MN) for the clinical treatment of degenerative lumbar disc disease. RhBMP-7, also known as osteogenic protein-1, is available for humanitarian use for the treatment of recalcitrant tibial nonunions.

A large number of preclinical studies for efficacy and feasibility purposes were performed to establish the efficacy of BMP in animal models of spinal fusion (50). This section, however, is devoted entirely to the clinical relevance of these growth factors, which include rhBMP-2 and rhBMP-7.

Laursen et al. reported a pilot study performed in five patients with unstable thoracolumbar spine fractures treated with transpedicular rhBMP-7 transplantation, short-segment instrumentation, and posterolateral fusion (51). Follow-up time was 12 to 18 months, and patients were evaluated clinically by plain radiographs and serial computed tomography scans. In all five patients, there was a loss of correction of anterior and middle column height and sagittal balance at last follow-up. The authors were forced to discontinue the study in the face of these results and concluded that rhBMP-7 was not capable of inducing an early sufficient structural bone support in the spine. Similarly, Jeppsson et al. used rhBMP-7 on a bovine collagen type I carrier for cervical spine fusion in four patients with atlantoaxial instability due to rheumatoid arthritis (52). No autograft or DBM was used as a carrier for the rhBMP-7. Conventional radiography was used postoperatively at 2, 6, and 10 months to assess fusion. Their results were again unsatisfactory. In three patients, no new bone was detectable, whereas only one patient had evidence of atlantoaxial arthrodesis at 6 months. Perhaps the most promising study regarding rhBMP-7 and spinal arthrodesis was performed in a preliminary trial using the growth factor as an adjunct to iliac crest autograft in lumbar fusion by Patel et al. (53). Sixteen patients with the diagnosis of spinal stenosis and single-level degenerative spondylolisthesis in the lower lumbar spine (L-3 to S-1) were enrolled in a multicenter trial after U.S. Food and Drug Administration and institutional review board approval. The patients were randomized to an rhBMP-7 group (12 patients) or a control group (4 patients). The control group received iliac crest autograft alone, whereas the experimental group received iliac crest autograft plus 3.5 mg of rhBMP-7 in a putty carrier per side. Clinical outcomes were measured using the Oswestry score and radiographically by two independent, blinded radiologists. At 6 months, 9 of 12 (75%) patients receiving autograft with rhBMP-7 were deemed radiologically fused versus 2 of 4 (50%) patients in the control group. Clinical success was defined as a minimum 20% improvement in the Oswestry score. With that criterion, at 6 months, 10 of 12 (83%) of rhBMP-7 plus autograft implanted patients were deemed clinical successes, compared to two of four (50%) of the control group. This pilot study demonstrated the effectiveness of rhBMP-7 when used in concert with autograft in human posterolateral lumbar fusion.

Johnsson et al. conducted a randomized trial of noninstrumented posterolateral fusion using rhBMP-7 or autogenous bone graft for grade I and grade II L-5 to S-1 spondylolytic spondylolisthesis (54). The patients were brace immobilized for 5 months after surgery. The stability of posterior spinal fusion was evaluated with 0.8-mm metallic markers positioned in L-5 and the sacrum to allow for radiostereometric analysis. One year after surgery, radiostereometric analysis was performed by evaluating the positional change from supine posture to standing and sitting. Although radiographic fusions were not seen in all patients, there were no significant differences in residual motion at the L-5 to S-1 segment between the two cohorts.

Recently, a U.S. Food and Drug Administration–approved investigational device–exempted multicenter pilot study was performed to report the early results of the first human trial attempting to use rhBMP-2 in lumbothoracic-interbody fusion cages (55). Fourteen patients with single-level lumbar degenerative disc disease refractory to nonoperative therapy were entered into the prospective randomized trial. The control group received autogenous bone graft inside tapered titanium fusion cages, whereas the investigational group received rhBMP-2 delivered in a collagen sponge inside the fusion cages. Patients were followed at regular intervals with radiographs, sagittally reformatted computerized tomography scans, and Short Form (SF)-36 and Oswestry outcome questionnaires. At 3-month follow-up, 91% (10 of 11) were judged to be fused. At 6 months, 1 year, and 2 years, 100% (11 of 11) patients were noted to have solid fusion. Of the three control patients, two had solid union, and one had an apparent nonunion at 1 year. After 3 months, the Oswestry scores of the rhBMP-2 group improved sooner than the control group, with both groups demonstrating similar improvement at 6 months. This study clearly showed evidence of osteoinduction by a recombinant growth factor in humans.

The results of this study led to the further examination of rhBMP-2 in a larger pivotal clinical trial. In this trial, 143 patients were implanted with the LT cage filled with rhBMP-2, and 136 patients were implanted with the LT cage filled with autograft (56). This trial used an open retroperitoneal approach to the spinal column and was designed as a prospective multicenter randomized trial. The operative time and blood loss were significantly less in the rhBMP-2–treated cohort. Thirty-two percent of control patients experienced some degree of donor site pain even 2 years after surgery. There were no significant differences in Oswestry scores between the rhBMP-2–treated cohort and the autograft-treated cohort. Similarly, SF-36 outcome scores and back pain scores were not different between these groups. Two years after surgery, 100% of rhBMP-2–treated patients achieved radiographic fusion, and 95.6% of autograft-treated patients also fused. Serology testing indicated that the incidence of a positive antibody response to rhBMP-2 was 0.7% in the rhBMP-2–implanted group and 0.8% in the autograft-implanted group. A positive antibody titer to type I collagen was noted in 13.1% of rhBMP-2 patients and 12.9% of autograft patients. There was no association between the presence of antibodies to collagen and the presence of adverse sequelae or clinical outcome.

RhBMP-2 has also been examined in lumbar posterolateral transverse process fusion (57). In this case, the molecule was combined with a granular biphasic calcium phosphate carrier consisting of 60% HA and 40% TCP to provide a more structured scaffolding for this environment. In an investigational device–exempted study, 25 patients undergoing posterior lumbar arthrodesis were randomized (1:2:2 ratio) to an arthrodesis technique: autograft with Texas Scottish Rite Hospital (TSRH) pedicle screw instrumentation (n = 5), rhBMP-2 and TSRH (n = 11), and rhBMP-2 only without internal fixation (n = 9). On each side, 20 mg of rhBMP-2 was delivered on the biphasic calcium phosphate carrier (10 cm per side). All 25 patients were available for follow-up evaluation. The radiographic fusion rate, determined by plain radiography and computed tomography scan, was 40% (two out of five) in the autograft/TSRH group and 100% (20 out of 20) with rhBMP-2 group with or without TSRH internal fixation. A significant improvement in Oswestry score was seen after 6 weeks in the rhBMP-2–only group and after 3 months in the rhBMP-2/TSRH group, but not until 6 months in the autograft/TSRH group. At the final follow-up assessment, Oswestry improvement was greatest in the rhBMP-2–only group. The SF-36 showed similar changes. This pilot study was the first with at least 1 year of follow-up evaluation to demonstrate successful posterolateral spine fusion using a BMP-based bone graft substitute. Consistently, rhBMP-2 was able to induce bone in the posterolateral lumbar spine when delivered at a dose of 20 mg per side with or without the use of internal fixation.

Kleeman et al. compared laparoscopic ALIF using rhBMP-2 in titanium tapered cages to autogenous bone in TCBD (58). In a prospective clinical study, a total of 47 patients were studied, 22 of whom underwent a laparoscopic ALIF with an rhBMP-2–soaked collagen sponge within a tapered titanium cage. Twenty-three patients underwent a laparoscopic ALIF with TCBD packed with autograft. Results indicated that the group undergoing laparoscopic ALIF with rhBMP-2 resulted in shorter operative times and length of hospital stay compared to fusion with TCBD. Both groups reported improvement of back pain, leg pain, and overall satisfaction, although the rhBMP-2 group improved to a higher level based on full restoration of function, which was statistically significant.

FUTURE DIRECTIONS

In the last 15 years, our understanding of bone graft biology has continually evolved. The description of the cellular and molecular processes involved in the bone induction cascade during spinal fusion and the identification and characterization of various growth factors have set the stage for a new outlook in bone grafting for spinal surgery. Recently, significant interest has arisen in gene therapy principles for the induction of spinal fusion in laboratory animals and has met with admirable success (59). These principles are based on two fundamental strategies: the introduction of the complementary DNA of a single BMP by a viral vector at the fusion site or the delivery of an intracellular transcription factor that upregulates the expression of multiple BMPs and other growth factors. As is true for the recombinant growth factors, important issues regarding dosing, vector, carrier, and cost will eventually factor into the clinical applicability of gene therapy for spinal fusion.

REFERENCES

1. Morone MA, Boden SD, Hair G, et al. The Marshall R. Urist Young Investigator Award. Gene expression during autograft lumbar spine fusion and the effect of bone morphogenetic protein 2. *Clin Orthop* 1998;(351):252–265.
2. Sandhu HS, Boden SD. Biologic enhancement of spinal fusion. *Ortho Clin North Am* 1998;29(4):621–631.
3. Burchardt H. The biology of bone graft repair. *Clin Orthop* 1983; 174:28–42.

4. Banwart JC, Asher MA, Hassanein RS. Iliac crest bone graft harvest donor site morbidity. A statistical evaluation. *Spine* 1994;20:1055–1060.
5. Fernyhough JC, Schimandle JJ, Weigel MC, et al. Chronic donor site pain complicating bone graft harvesting from the posterior iliac crest for spinal fusion. *Spine* 1992;17:1474–1480.
6. Boden SD, Schimandle JH, Hutton WC. An experimental lumbar intertransverse process spinal fusion model. Radiographic, histologic, and biomechanical healing characteristics. *Spine* 1995;20(4):412–420.
7. Beresford JN. Osteogenic stem cells and the stromal system of bone and marrow. *Clin Orthop* 1989;240:270.
8. Burwell RG. The function of bone marrow in the incorporation of a bone graft. *Clin Orthop* 1985;200:125–141.
9. Burwell RG. The Burwell theory on the importance of bone marrow in bone grafting. In: Urist MR, O'Connor BT, Burwell RG, eds. *Bone grafts, derivatives, and substitutes*. Boston: Butterworth-Heinemann, 1994:103–155.
10. An HS, Simpson JM, Glover JM, et al. Comparison between allograft plus demineralized bone matrix versus autograft in anterior cervical fusion. A prospective multicenter study. *Spine* 1995;20:2211–2216.
11. Brodsky AE, Khalil MA, Sassard WR, et al. Repair of symptomatic pseudarthrosis of anterior cervical fusion. Posterior vs anterior repair. *Spine* 1992;17:1137–1143.
12. Butterman GR, Glazer PA, Hu SS, et al. Revision of failed lumbar fusions: a comparison of anterior autograft and allograft. *Spine* 1997;22:2748–2755.
13. Connolly PJ, Esses SI, Kostuik JP. Anterior cervical fusion: outcome analysis of patients fused with and without anterior cervical plates. *J Spinal Disord* 1996;9:202–206.
14. Weiland DJ, McAfee PC. Posterior cervical fusion with triple-wire strut graft technique: one hundred consecutive patients. *J Spinal Disord* 1991;4:15–21.
15. Sawin PD, Traynelis VC, Menezes AH. A comparative analysis of fusion rates and donor-site morbidity for autogeneic rib and iliac crest bone grafts in posterior cervical fusions. *J Neurosurg* 1998;88(2):255–265.
16. Ray CD. Threaded titanium cages for lumbar interbody fusions. *Spine* 1997;22(6):667–679.
17. Cockin J. Autologous bone grafting complications at the donor site. *J Bone Joint Surg Br* 1971;53:153.
18. Cowley SP, Anderson LD. Hernias through donor sites for iliac bone grafts. *J Bone Joint Surg Am* 1983;65:1023–1025.
19. Silber JS, Anderson DG, Daffner SD, et al. Donor site morbidity after anterior iliac crest bone harvest for single-level anterior cervical discectomy and fusion. *Spine* 2003;28(2):134–139.
20. Bugbee WD, Convery FR. Osteochondral allograft transplantation. *Clin Sports Med* 1999;18:67–75.
21. Burwell RG, Friedlaender GE, Mankin HJ. Current perspectives and future directions: The 1983 Invitational Conference on Osteochondral Allografts. *Clin Orthop* 1985;200:141–157.
22. Kumta SM, Leung PC, Griffith JF, et al. A technique for enhancing union of allograft to host bone. *J Bone Joint Surg* 1998;80B:994–998.
23. Hanley EN, Harvell JC Jr, Shapiro DE, et al. Use of allograft bone in cervical spine surgery. *Semin Spine Surg* 1989;1:262.
24. Malanin TI. Acquisition and banking of bone allografts. In: Habal MB, Reddi AH, eds. *Bone grafts and bone substitutes*. Philadelphia: WB Saunders, 1992.
25. Cloward R. The anterior approach for removal of ruptured cervical discs. *J Neurosurg* 1958;15:602.
26. Brown MD, Malinin TI, Davis PB. A roentgenographic evaluation of frozen allografts versus autografts in anterior cervical spine fusions. *Clin Orthop* 1976;119:231.
27. Zdeblick TA, Ducker TB. The use of freeze-dried allograft bone for anterior cervical fusions. *Spine* 1991;16:726–729.
28. Zhang ZH, Yin H, Yang K, et al. Anterior intervertebral disc excision and bone grafting in cervical spondylitic myelopathy. *Spine* 1983;8:16.
29. Jorgenson SS, Lowe TG, France J, et al. A prospective analysis of autograft versus allograft in posterolateral lumbar fusion in the same patient: a minimum of 1-year follow-up in 144 patients. *Spine* 1994;19:2048.
30. Dodd CA, Ferguson CM, Freedman L. Allograft versus autograft bone in scoliosis surgery *J Bone Joint Surg* 1988;70(B):431–434.
31. Barnes B, Rodts GE Jr, Haid RW Jr, et al. Allograft implants for posterior lumbar interbody fusion: results comparing cylindrical dowels and impacted wedges. *Neurosurgery* 2002;51(5):1191–1198.
32. Kozak JA, Heilman AE, O'Brien JP. Anterior lumbar fusion options: technique and graft materials. *Clin Orthop* 1994;300:45.
33. Cohen DB, Chotivichit A, Fujita T, et al. Pseudarthrosis repair. Autogenous iliac crest versus femoral ring allograft. *Clin Orthop* 2000;(371):46–55.
34. Martin GJ Jr, Boden SD, Titus L, et al. New formulations of demineralized bone matrix as a more effective graft alternative in experimental posterolateral lumbar spine arthrodesis. *Spine* 1999;24(7):637–645.
35. Bostrom MP, Yang X, Kennan M, et al. An unexpected outcome during testing of commercially available demineralized bone graft materials: how safe are the nonallograft components? *Spine* 2001;26(13):1425–1428.
36. Sassard WR, Eidman DK, Gray PM, et al. Augmenting local bone with Grafton demineralized bone matrix for posterolateral lumbar spine fusion: avoiding second site autologous bone harvest. *Orthopedics* 2000;23(10):1059–1064.
37. Muschler GF, Lane JM, Dawson EG. The biology of spinal fusion. In: Cotler JM, Cotler HB, eds. *Spinal fusion, science and technique*. New York: Springer-Verlag, 1990.
38. Muschler GF, Lane JM. Orthopaedic surgery. In: Habal MB, Reddi AH, eds. *Bone grafts and bone substitutes*. Philadelphia: WB Saunders, 1992.
39. Muschler GF, Negami S, Hyodo A, et al. Evaluation of collagen ceramic composite graft materials in a spinal fusion model. *Clin Orthop* 1996;328:250.
40. Flatley TJ, Lynch KL, Benson MD. Tissue response to implants of calcium phosphate ceramic in rabbit spine. *Clin Orthop* 1983;179:246.
41. Boden SD, Martin GJ Jr, Morone M, et al. The use of coralline hydroxyapatite with bone marrow, autogenous bone graft, or osteoinductive bone protein extract for posterolateral lumbar spine fusion. *Spine* 1999;24(4):320–327.
42. Boden SD, Martin GJ Jr, Morone MA, et al. Posterolateral lumbar intertransverse process spine arthrodesis with recombinant human bone morphogenetic protein 2/hydroxyapatite-tricalcium phosphate after laminectomy in the nonhuman primate. *Spine* 1999;24(12):1179–1185.
43. Passuti N, Daculsi G, Rogez JM, et al. Macroporous calcium phosphate ceramic performance in human spine fusion. *Clin Orthop* 1989;248:169–176.
44. Ransford AO, Morley T, Edgar MA, et al. Synthetic porous ceramic compared with autograft in scoliosis surgery. A prospective, randomized study of 341 patients. *J Bone Joint Surg Br* 1998;80(1):13–18.
45. Delecrin J, Takahashi S, Gouin F, et al. A synthetic porous ceramic as a bone graft substitute in the surgical management of scoliosis: a prospective, randomized study. *Spine* 2000;25(5):563–569.
46. McConnell JR, Freeman BJ, Debnath UK, et al. A prospective randomized comparison of coralline hydroxyapatite with autograft in cervical interbody fusion. *Spine* 2003;28(4):317–323.
47. Thalgott JS, Klezl Z, Timlin M, et al. Anterior lumbar interbody fusion with processed sea coral (coralline hydroxyapatite) as part of a circumferential fusion. *Spine* 2002;27(24):E518–E525.
48 Urist MR. Bone formation by autoinduction. *Science* 1965;150:893–899.
49. Wozney JM, Rosen V, Celeste AJ, et al. Novel regulators of bone formation: molecular clones and activities. *Science* 1998;242(4885):1528–1534.
50. Sandhu HS, Khan SN. Animal models for preclinical assessment of bone morphogenetic proteins in the spine. *Spine* 2002;27[16 Suppl 1]:S32–38.
51. Laursen M, Hoy K, Hansen ES, et al. Recombinant bone morphogenetic protein-7 as an intracorporal bone growth stimulator in unstable thoracolumbar burst fractures in humans: preliminary results. *Eur Spine J* 1999;8(6):485–490.
52. Jeppsson C, Saveland H, Rydholm U, et al. OP-1 for cervical spine fusion: bridging bone in only 1 of 4 rheumatoid patients but pred-

nisolone did not inhibit bone induction in rats. *Acta Orthop Scand* 1999;70(6):559–563.

53. Patel TS, Vaccarro AR, Truumees E, et al. *A safety and efficacy of osteogenic protein-1 (OP-1) as an adjunct to posterolateral lumbar fusion.* Presented at the Sixteenth Annual Meeting of the North American Spine Society. New Orleans, 2001.
54. Johnsson R, Stromqvist B, Aspenberg P. Randomized radiostereometric study comparing osteogenic protein-1 (BMP-7) and autograft bone in human noninstrumented posterolateral lumbar fusion: 2002 Volvo Award in clinical studies. *Spine* 2002;27(23): 2654–2661.
55. Boden SD, Zdeblick TA, Sandhu HS, et al. The use of rhBMP-2 in interbody fusion cages. Definitive evidence of osteoinduction in humans: a preliminary report. *Spine* 2000;25(3):376–381.
56. Burkus JK, Gornet MF, Dickman CA, et al. Anterior lumbar interbody fusion using rhBMP-2 with tapered interbody cages. *J Spinal Disord Tech* 2002;15(5):337–349.
57. Boden SD, Kang J, Sandhu H, et al. Use of recombinant human bone morphogenetic protein-2 to achieve posterolateral lumbar spine fusion in humans: a prospective, randomized clinical pilot trial: 2002 Volvo Award in clinical studies. *Spine* 2002;27(23): 2662–2673.
58. Kleeman TJ, Ahn UM, Talbot-Kleeman A. Laparoscopic anterior lumbar interbody fusion with rhBMP-2: a prospective study of clinical and radiographic outcomes. *Spine* 2001;26(24):2751–2756.
59. Boden SD, Titus L, Hair G, et al. Lumbar spine fusion by local gene therapy with cDNA encoding a novel osteoinductive protein (LMP-1) *Spine* 1998;23(23):2486–2492.

Operative Techniques

Editor: William C. Lauerman

CHAPTER 52

Surgical Approaches to the Thoracic and Thoracolumbar Spine

Daniel D. Lee, Mesfin A. Lemma, and John P. Kostuik

ANATOMY OF THE THORACIC SPINE

The bony anatomy of the thoracic spine differs from that of the lumbar spine in a number of respects. The thoracic vertebrae are smaller; their facets are more frontally oriented in the anteroposterior view, and only begin to resemble the lumbar spine at the thoracolumbar junction; the spinous process is longer and more distally angled; the transverse processes are shorter and are oriented posterolaterally; the pedicles are smaller in diameter and length; the bodies are heart shaped with a circular vertebral canal; the ribs articulate with the vertebral body; and there is an overall physiologic kyphosis (Fig. 1). The thoracic canal surrounded by bony elements is smaller, containing less free space than the cervical and lumbar region.

There is inherent stability of the thoracic spine provided by the ribs. Each vertebra has a superior and inferior costal articulation bilaterally. The thoracic spine is mechanically stiffer and less mobile. Considerable force is required, especially in the upper thoracic spine, to disrupt the contiguous bony anatomy and result in paraplegia.

The blood supply to the spinal cord in the thoracic spine is variable and tenuous (Fig. 2). Cross-clamping of the aorta and bilateral ligation of thoracic segmentals may lead to paraplegia. The artery of Adamkiewicz (80% from T-10 from the left but origin may vary from T-5 to L-5) supplies the thoracic cord.

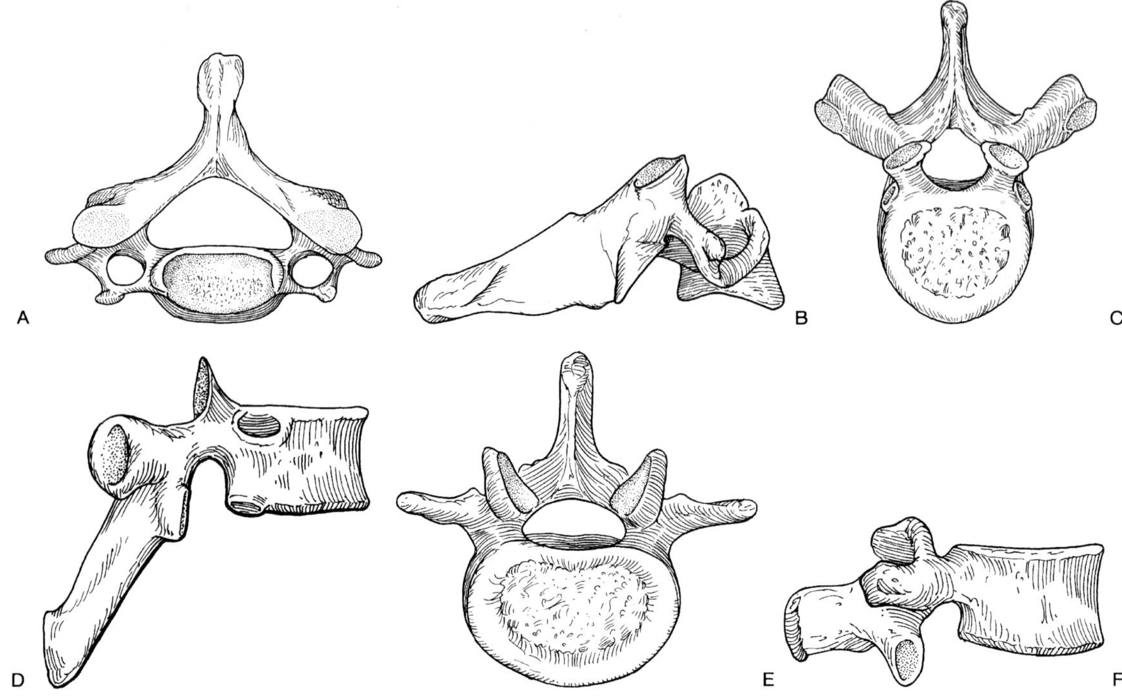

FIG. 1. A–F: Comparative sectional and sagittal bone anatomy of the cervical, thoracic, and lumbar spine.

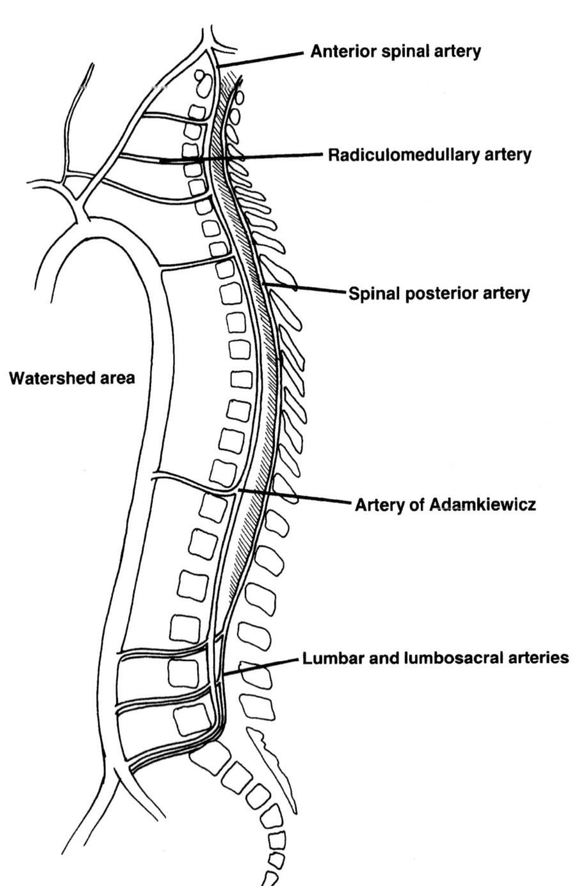

FIG. 2. Blood supply to the thoracic spine.

INDICATIONS FOR SURGERY

As a general rule, the surgical approach is guided by the site of pathology, as well as dependent on the pathology. Anterior or anterolateral approaches and sometimes even a posterolateral costotransversectomy are reserved for anterior pathology, whereas posterior approaches are readily used for posterior pathology. On occasion, especially for primary tumors of the anterior and posterior columns, both approaches may be necessary. This may also be true in some cases of metastatic disease to the spine.

The following indications are listed, in order of frequency:

- Posterior approaches
  - Trauma
  - Scoliosis
  - Kyphosis—developmental or congenital
  - Posttraumatic kyphosis
  - Tumor stabilization
  - Segmental instability (degenerative)
- Anterior approaches
  - Trauma
  - Infection
  - Tumor
    - Metastatic
    - Primary
  - Deformity
    - Scoliosis
    - Kyphosis
  - Spinal cord decompression
  - Thoracic and thoracolumbar disc herniation
  - Segmental instability (degenerative)

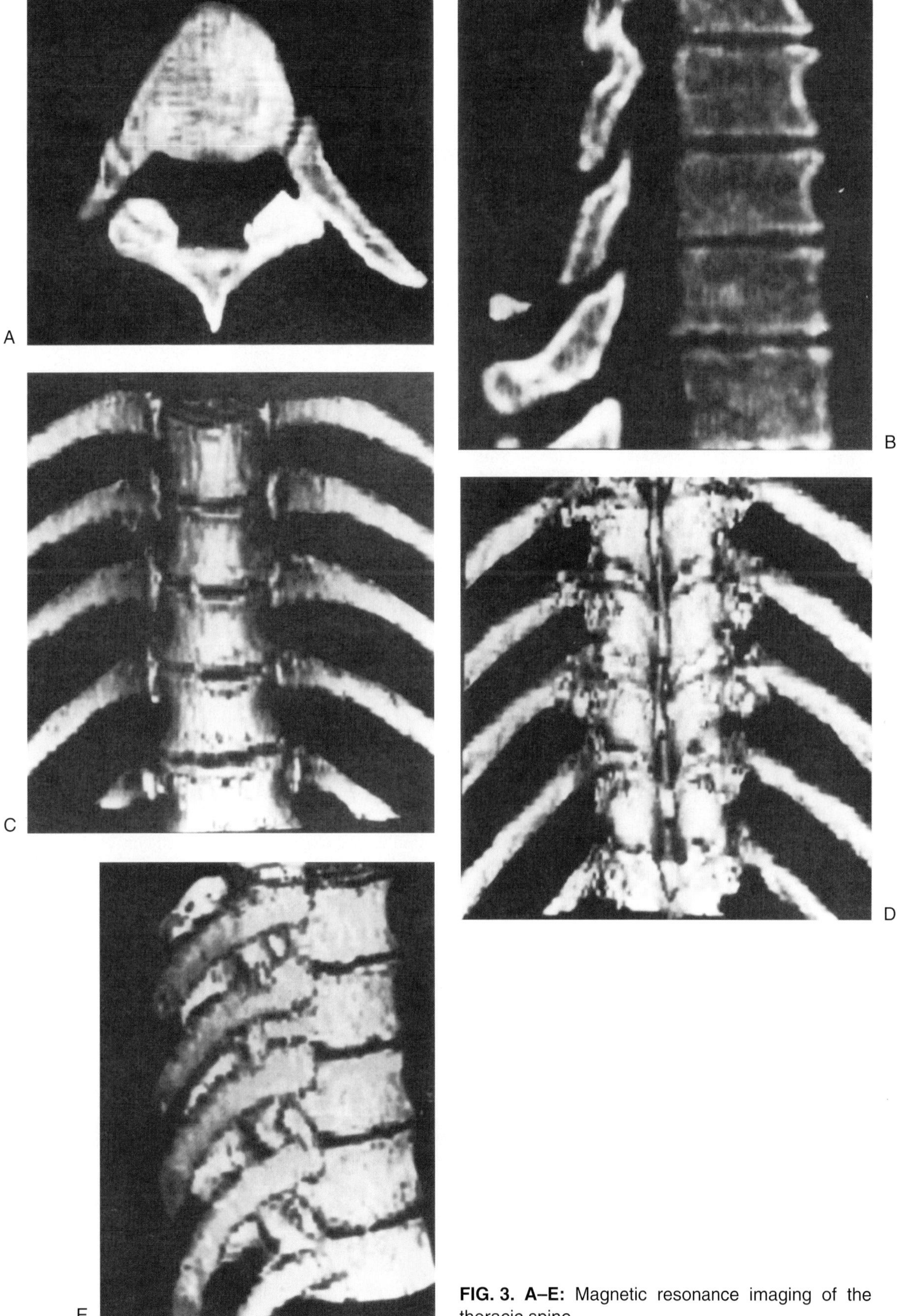

FIG. 3. A–E: Magnetic resonance imaging of the thoracic spine.

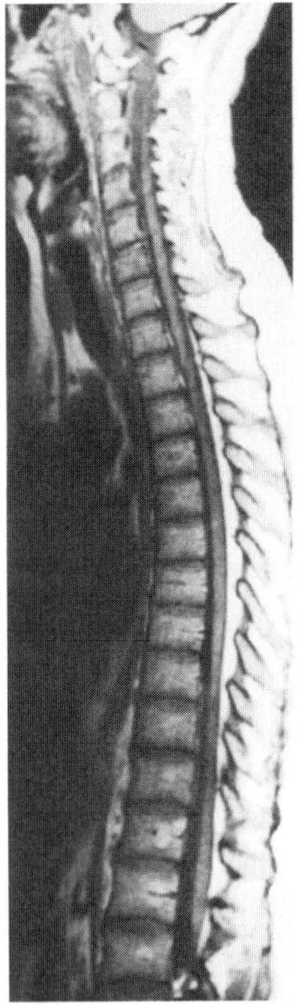
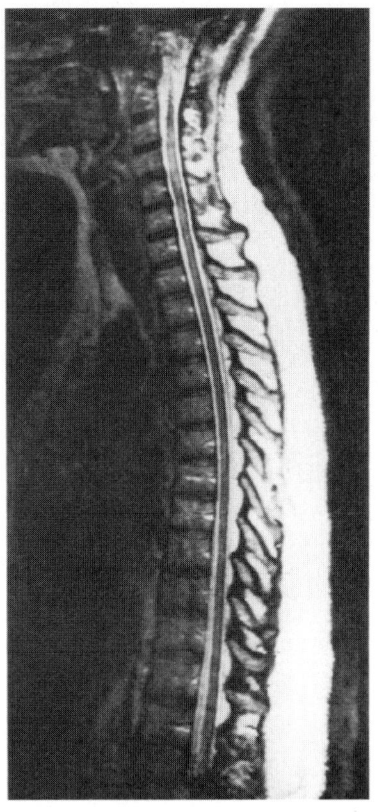
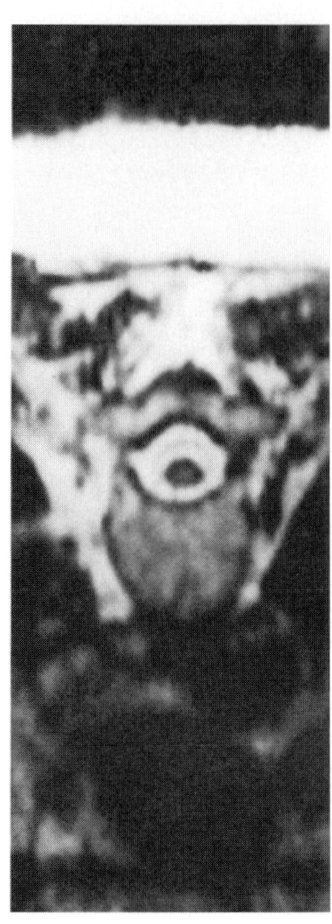

A–C

FIG. 4. A–C: Computed tomographic images of the thoracic spine.

Preoperative Planning

A thorough history is the basis for deciding the surgical approach. This should include a history of the pain, neurologic symptoms, functional disturbances, medical and surgical history, and disability, including socioeconomic issues. The physical examination contributes further and should include an analysis of deformity and gait, palpation for local tenderness, range of motion of spine and joints, pulses, signs of impaired nerve root conduction (i.e., reflexes, sensory and motor examination), upper-motor neuron signs, and abdominal and rectal examination as well.

Radiologic Imaging

Plain radiographs of the involved areas are paramount. They provide not only insight into pathology, but are also important for preoperative planning of the degree of resection, the length of the construct, and the insertion of implants, particularly pedicle screws.

Magnetic resonance imaging (MRI) is the image of choice for most procedures to assess the pathology and the soft tissues, such as ligaments and spinal cord. In the region of the spinal cord, MRI is preferred over computed tomography (CT)–myelography for assessment of cord compression. In contrast, CT-myelography and MRI may be of comparable value in the cauda equina. In cases with implants, CT-myelography is invaluable (Figs. 3 and 4).

For assessment of bony elements, CT is preferred. In addition to axial sequences, sagittal reconstruction cuts should be obtained, and occasionally, three-dimensional CT imaging may be of value (Fig. 4). Quite frequently, in cases of metastatic disease, MRI and CT scanning are complementary, as the former allows a good view of the soft tissues and the latter of the bony structures, and they aid significantly in preoperative planning of the extent of the resection necessary.

SURGICAL APPROACHES

The choice of approach is dictated by the site of primary pathology. Anterior approaches through the thorax, abdomen, or flank are best used for pathology involving the vertebral bodies, whereas pathology involving the posterior elements is best approached posteriorly through a vertical midline approach. Posterolateral structures may be approached through a midline posterior approach or a posterolateral muscle-splitting approach. Approaches should be planned so that they can be extended if necessary at the time of surgery. The general methods available are as follows:

- Anterior upper thoracic spine
  - Sternocleidomastoid
  - Transthoracic
  - Transpleural axillary thoracotomy
  - Anterior sternocleidomastoid with medial resection of clavicle and proximal sternotomy
  - Anterior sternotomy
  - Anterior transthoracic: The transthoracic approach may be transpleural or retropleural. Both allow good access to the vertebral body, including the pedicle nearest to the operator, but access is poor to the opposite vertebral pedicle (Fig. 5).
- Anterior thoracoabdominal
  - Transpleural retroperitoneal
  - Retropleural retroperitoneal
  - Posterior: This approach is used to access the vertebral arch and is most appropriate for laminectomies and posterior or pos-

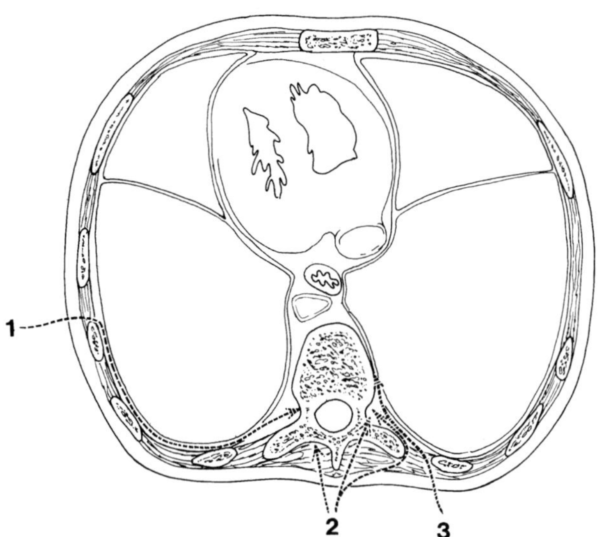

FIG. 5. Possible approaches to the thoracic spine. 1: Transthoracic. 2: Posterior or extended posterior. 3: Posterolateral (costotransversectomy).

terolateral fusions. However, it may be possible to visualize the lateral or even the anterior part of the spine in scoliotic deformities, depending on the degree of rotation in the thoracic spine (Fig. 6).

Posterolateral: These include costotransversectomy or an extensile posterior approach, which can be made bilaterally or unilaterally.

Transpedicular (eggshell)

Laminoplasty

Thoracoscopy

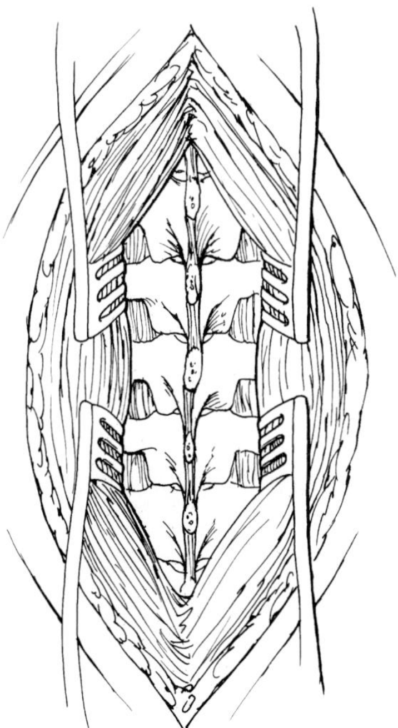

FIG. 6. Exposure is extended laterally to include the transverse processes.

If the pathology involves the cervical as well as the thoracic spine, four basic strategies are available: (a) posterior approaches, (b) approaches anterior to the sternocleidomastoid, (c) cervicosternotomy, and (d) transpleural axillary thoracotomy, or some combination thereof.

Approaches to the thoracolumbar spine include posterior and anterolateral approaches. The posterior approaches are simple and well known and are usually indicated for procedures such as laminectomies and posterior or posterolateral fusions. Anterolateral approaches may be retroperitoneal, transpleural retroperitoneal, or transpleural transdiaphragmatic retroperitoneal. The last approach is the most extensive.

Thoracolumbar approaches may, of course, be extended to involve the entire lumbar spine, Indeed, the entire thoracolumbar spine can be accessed through a thoracoabdominal approach. In addition to the cervicothoracic, thoracic, thoracolumbar, and lumbar approaches, approaches may be performed in combination, such as combined posterior and anterior or anterolateral approach. These procedures are usually reserved for patients requiring an osteotomy, or for primary malignant tumors.

Posterior Approaches to the Cervicothoracic, Thoracic, and Thoracolumbar Spine

The indications for posterior approaches are laminectomy and fusions, with or without instrumentation. These incisions are straightforward, because of the superficial presentation of the spinous processes. The patient is placed in the prone position, usually on a Jackson table or Relton-Hall four-poster frame, which allows the abdomen and thorax to be free from pressure and venous reflux. The anterosuperior aspect of the iliac crest is carefully protected, because the lateral femoral cutaneous nerve of the thigh is vulnerable and meralgia paresthetica may be a problem postoperatively. This complication is usually transitory, however. The positioning of the head is determined by the anesthetist, but a neutral position with the eyes well protected is recommended.

Before the injection of hypotensive medications, the skin is scored with a scalpel. Then the skin and the underlying musculature is infiltrated with a weak solution of 1 cc of 1/1,000 adrenaline and 500 cc of normal saline. If the patient is younger than 50 years, hypotensive anesthesia, which maintains the upper systolic blood pressure between 80 to 90 mm Hg, is used as another means to control bleeding, provided there are no medical contraindications (e.g., a history of hypertension or stroke). The fascia typically is incised in line with the skin incision, and the spinous processes and laminae are exposed by subperiosteal dissection. In cases of scoliosis, a plumb line is dropped from the spinous process of C-7 to the gluteal cleft and a straight incision is made over the operative segments. Some undermining at the junction of the fascia and subcutaneous tissues is necessary in cases in scoliosis to identify the tips of the spinous processes.

In children, the cartilaginous spinous process apophyses are split in the midline with a sharp knife together with the interspinal ligaments. A Cobb elevator then can be used to strip the apophyses with the adherent periosteum. In adults, cautery is used to strip the fascia.

In contrast to the lumbar spine, the laminae of the thoracic spine run obliquely. When using the periosteal elevator to remove soft tissues, this anatomic perspective must be kept in mind to decrease bleeding (Fig. 6). Care must be taken to cau-

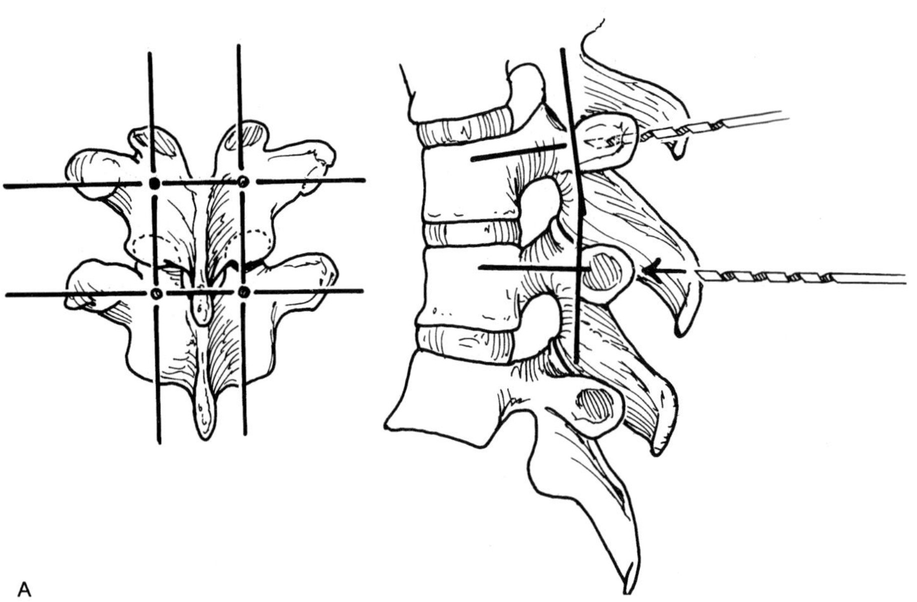

FIG. 7. Localization of the pedicular holes in the thoracic spine **A:** Posterior view. **B:** Lateral view.

terize the small artery that appears between the transverse processes as the soft tissues are dissected from the structures.

Instrumentation is common in the posterior thoracic spine. Anatomic variations of the thoracic pedicles are minor when compared to the lumbar spine. The ideal entry point is located on two bisecting lines in the upper corner of the outer inferior quadrant. A horizontal line from the midpoint of the transverse process is intersected by a vertical line that passes through the midportion of the facet joint. A drill or awl may be inserted.

The drill or awl must be angled no more than 5 degrees medially, whereas angulation in the sagittal plane depends on an analysis of the lateral radiograph. Also, the pedicle is closer to the superior aspect of the vertebral body in the thoracic spine than it is in the thoracolumbar spine. It is useful to obtain a lateral radiograph on the operating table as the sagittal angle may change when the patient is positioned supine.

In terms of the morphometry of the pedicles in the thoracic spine, various studies have shown that pedicle diameter uniformly diminished between T1-6. In fact, at T-6, 75% are too small to accept a 5.5-mm screw. However, screws up to 115% of pedicle diameter may be inserted without causing decrease in screw holding power because of plasticity of the pedicular cortex.

According to the literature, several methods may be used to assess the placement of thoracic pedicle screws. The use of blunt-tip probes, biplanar fluoroscopy, intraoperative CT, and intraoperative electromyographic (EMG) stimulation can effectively aid in their appropriate placement. Suk et al. reviewed 4,604 thoracic pedicle screws placed with the help of a blunt-tip probe and determined that there was a high margin of safety and excellent correction of deformity. In this study, 1.5% of screws were malpositioned mostly in the inferior direction and only one case of transient paresthesias was reported.

Extended Posterior Approach (*En Bloc* Spondylectomy)

The extended posterior approach is used primarily for tumors. It gives access to the entire spine including the contents of the spinal canal, allows the combined exposure of the posterior and anterior structures of the spine, and may be unilateral or bilateral. Total vertebrectomies can be performed in the thoracic spine with one

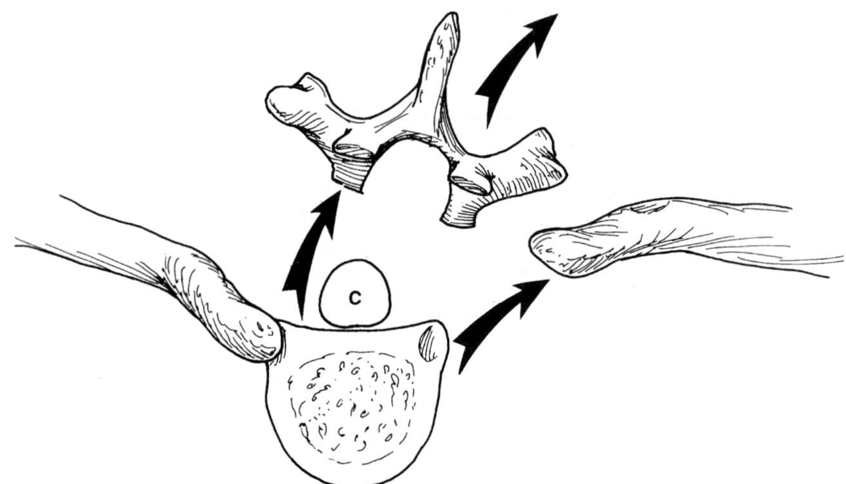

FIG. 8. Bilateral laminectomy and resection of transverse processes, pedicles, and one rib. C, spinal cord.

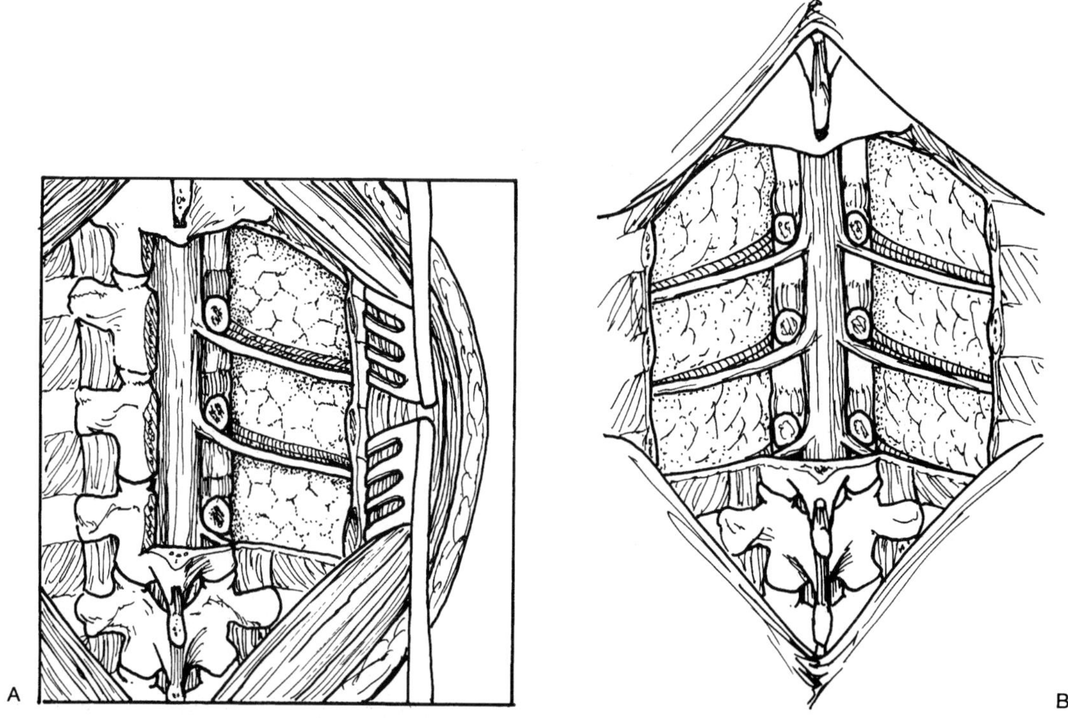

FIG. 9. A: Resection of three ribs allows the posterior mediastinum to be approached. **B:** Completion of laminectomy, bilateral costotransversectomy, and pedicular resection.

procedure. Because the approach is so extensive, there is a high risk of neurologic damage from direct damage to neurostructures or interruption of the blood supply in the watershed area of the thoracic spine (Fig. 2).

The patient is placed in the prone position (Fig. 7). A midline posterior incision is used to permit complete visualization of the posterior vertebral arch and the posterior aspect of the ribs for at least 5 cm. The incision must be three to four levels proximal and distal to the area of resection in order to allow sufficient retraction. In some cases, exposure is facilitated by dividing the paravertebral muscles transversely (Fig. 5).

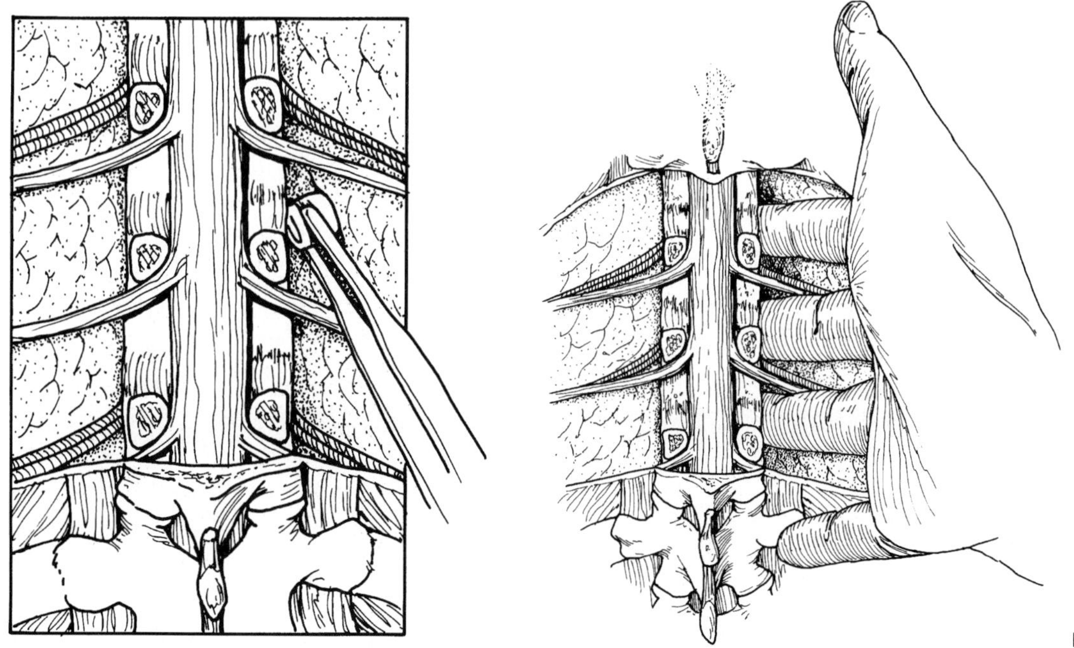

FIG. 10. A: The posterior mediastinum is separated from the vertebrae with swab mounted on a forceps, and then with fingers. **B:** Anterior pleural dissection on either side of the vertebral bodies is carried out using fingers.

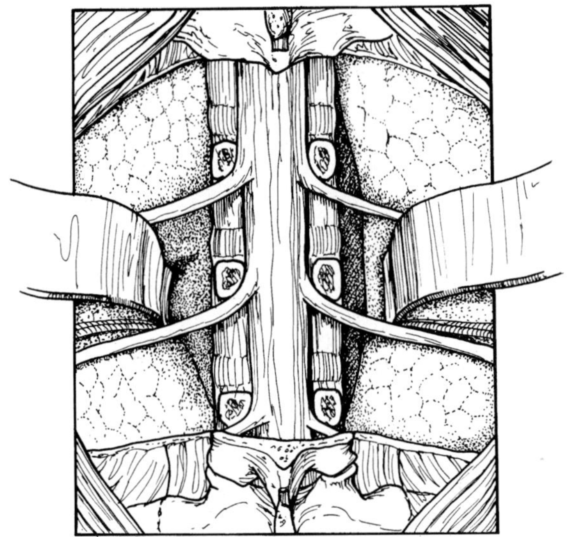

FIG. 11. The pleura and lungs are retracted anteriorly with malleable retractors.

A complete laminectomy of the desired number of segments is performed (Figs. 8 and 9), thus permitting the spinal canal and its contents to be visualized. The ribs are divided 3 cm lateral to the costotransverse joints. The neurovascular pedicles are preferentially not ligated. Usually, a minimum of three levels is necessary. The posterior mediastinum can then be entered. Ideally, resection of the ribs is done extrapleurally, but in most adults the pleura is very thin and tenuous. It is common for an intrapleural approach to result in a pneumothorax, necessitating insertion of a chest tube at the completion of the procedure.

The articular processes and the pedicles are resected. The posterior mediastinal structures are swept away from the vertebral body, preferably by hand with use of swabs (Fig. 10). Mobilizing the vascular structures requires that the segmental vessels be ligated. A malleable retractor is inserted to protect and displace the anterior structures (Fig. 11). The vertebral bodies are excised, generally through the disc spaces above and below the pathology. There is usually less blood loss with this procedure, but the length of the resection is greater. Alternatively, vertebral bodies may be sectioned with a modified Gigli saw, starting anteriorly and extending through vertebral bodies from anterior to posterior, through the anterior two-thirds of the vertebral body. The osteotomy is then completed in the remaining posterior one-third of the vertebral body from either side with a thin osteotome. The posterior longitudinal ligament is then easily cut with a knife (Figs. 12 and 13).

Before the anterior resection, the posterior part of the spine should be stabilized. Otherwise, the spine is temporarily completely destabilized and at even greater risk of neurologic compromise (Fig. 14). After resection of the vertebral bodies, posterior stabilization and grafting can be added. The extended posterior approach is often long, laborious, and tedious, and it must be done with great care (Fig. 15).

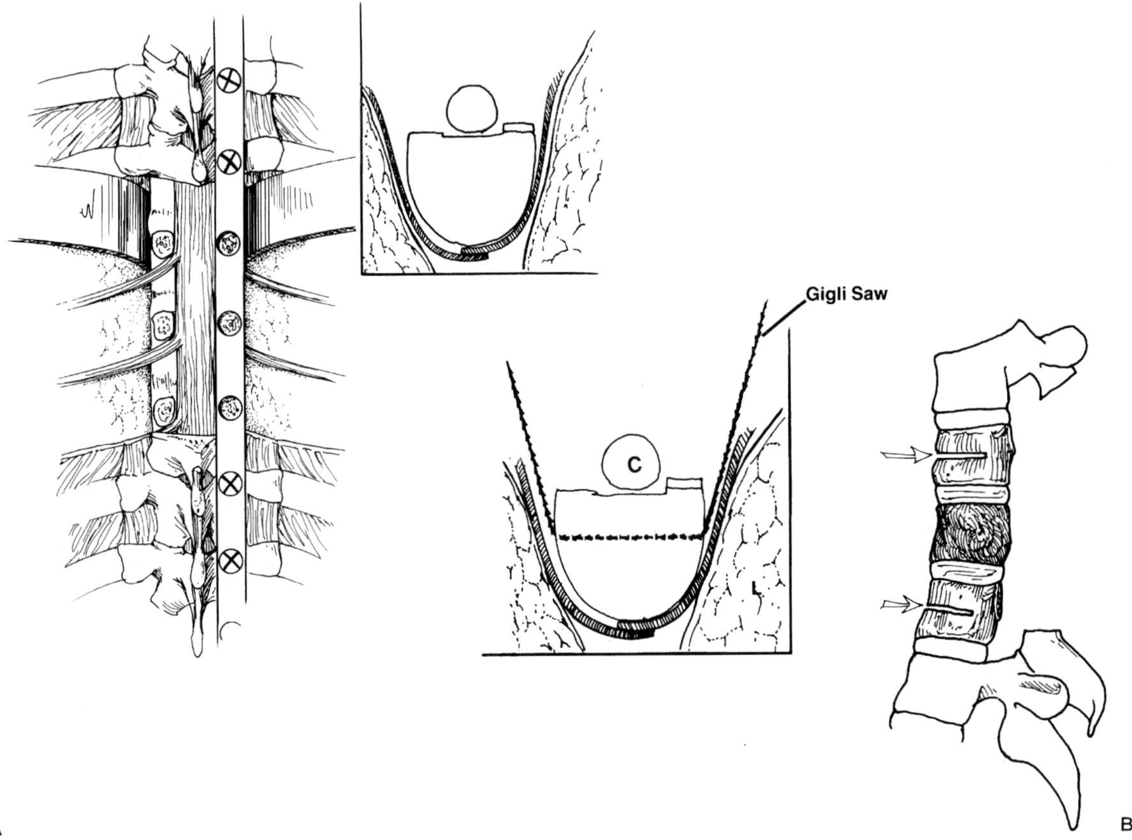

FIG. 12. A: Malleable retractors to protect posterior mediastinum. **B:** Partial anterior vertebral body section with Gigli saw. C, cord; L, lung.

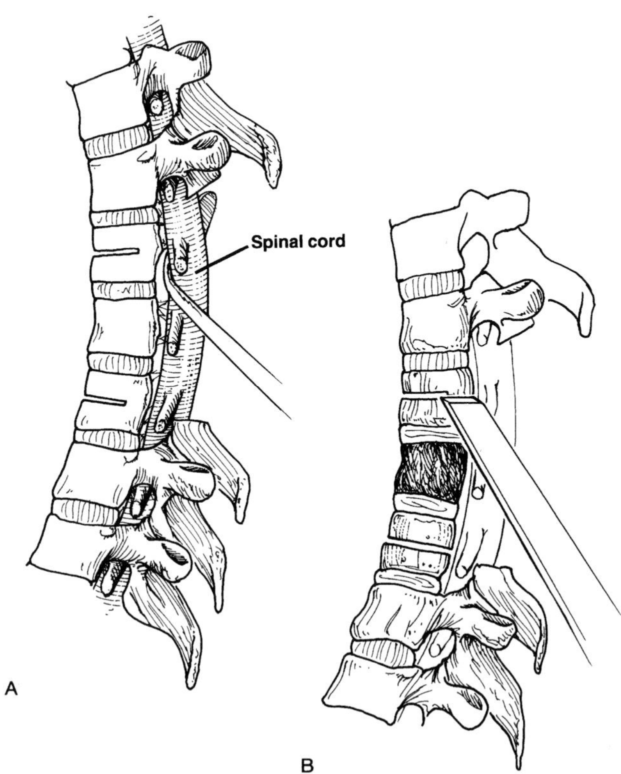

FIG. 13. A: The dura is dissected from the posterior vertebral body. **B:** Transverse posterior vertebral body wall osteotomy using fine osteotomes is done to join the Gigli saw vertebral section.

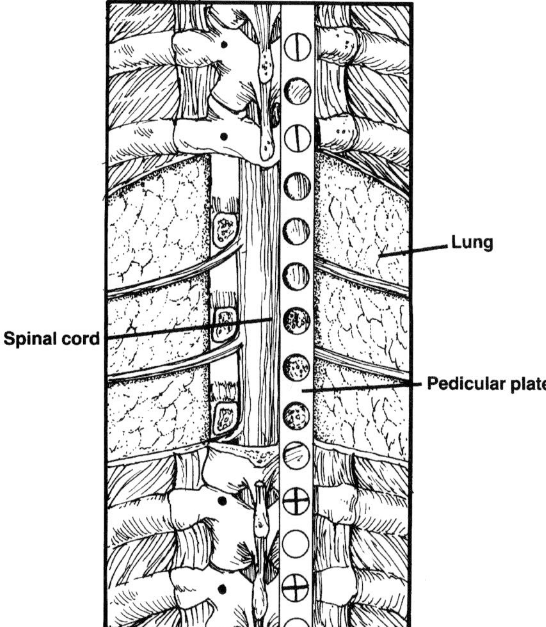

FIG. 14. Provisional pedicular plate stabilization.

Transpedicular Approaches

Transpedicular approaches (i.e., the eggshell procedure) have been popularized for the treatment of kyphotic deformities, particularly of a congenital type. Another indication is biopsy through the pedicle to prevent spread of tumor cells in case of potential malignancy (Figs. 16–18). As well, it is recommended for the use in cases of ill senior patients who require an anterior decompression, for example for treatment of an osteoporotic fracture in an otherwise somewhat debilitated person who might not tolerate a transthoracic or retropleural approach. The transpedicular approach allows anterior decompression access and posterior stabilization through a single posterior approach. It is prudent to use intraoperative evoked potentials, as this technique is used to address both sides of the neural tube.

The posterior spine is exposed. The spinous process is removed, and the laminae are thinned down or may be removed. The cortical bone over the pedicle is removed, and the pedicle hole is enlarged using progressively larger curettes. This allows access to the vertebral body (Fig. 18A–C). Angled curettes are then used to remove the cancellous bone of the vertebral body to the limits of the anterior and posterior cortex of the vertebral body, to gain greater access to the vertebral body; the lateral wall of the pedicle is fractured and retracted laterally. A curette may then be directed in a more lateral to medial direction. This allows removal of the bone directly anterior to the spinal canal (Fig. 18D). The pedicle on the contralateral side is similarly approached. The contents of the spinal canal are still protected by the laminae, the medial walls of the pedicle, and the posterior wall of the vertebral body. If there is anterior impingement of the dural sac by retropulsed bone, an elevator placed between the dura and the fragment allows the retropulsed bone to be forced anteriorly into the vertebral body. After this, internal fixation and transpedicular bone grafting, if desired, can be used. After removal of the posterior aspect of the vertebral body, the spine is malleable and correction of the deformity may be carried out (Fig. 18E–G).

If a kyphectomy is to be performed instead, the entire posterior arch pedicle and posterior wall of the vertebral segment must be removed. The retropulsed fragments are removed as well. Increased mobility may be obtained by disc removal. Greater correction may also be achieved by fracturing the lateral vertebral body walls of the involved segment. This can be accomplished by the use of an osteotome to cut the side of the cortical shell. With this degree of mobility, severe fixed-flexion deformities of the spine can be corrected. During the process of correction of the kyphotic deformities, it is necessary to ensure that no bony impingement occurs on the neural elements by the posterior laminae; such impingement requires removal. Also, in revision cases with epidural scarring, it is important to thin out the excessive scar to prevent buckling of the dura. Finally, a radiograph to assess the amount of sagittal correction is important as well.

The "eggshell" technique encompasses procedures ranging from simple transpedicular decompression and posterior fusion to more complex procedures, including transpedicular vertebrectomy and strut grafting or pedicle subtraction osteotomy. The morbidity of the procedure has been reported most recently in the range of 17%. This series included primary and revision deformity, and tumor and infection cases. Historically, pulmonary complication rates ranged from 10 to 17%, neurocomplication rates from 0 to 5%, and pseudarthrosis rates from 5 to 41%. On average, in cases of kyphotic deformity, a closing-wedge osteotomy through the pedicle with removal of 2 to 3 cm of posterior elements, the correction is approximately 25 degrees per level.

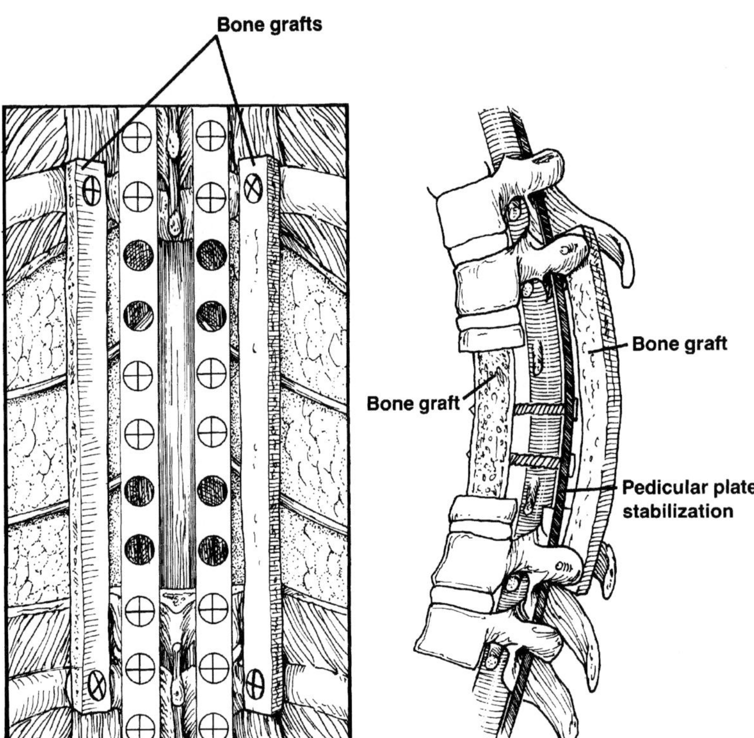

FIG. 15. Posterior stabilization, anterior reconstruction, and lateral grafts.

Posterolateral Approaches

Costotransversectomy

The costotransversectomy provides access to the lateral aspect of the vertebral bodies and to the posterior elements.

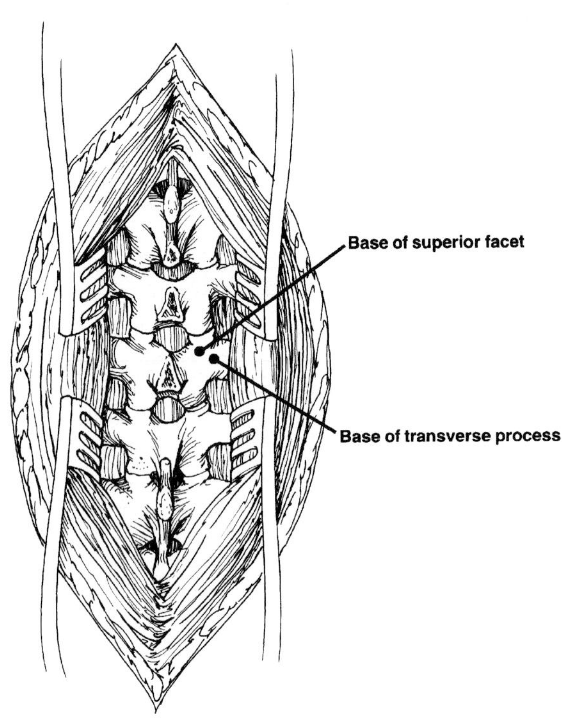

FIG. 16. Point of entry into the pedicle at the lumbar level.

This approach was originally developed for the drainage of tuberculosis abscesses, its major advantage being to avoid contamination of the thoracic cavity and associated morbidity of a thoracotomy. It offers limited access to the anterior vertebral elements when compared to a formal thoracotomy, however.

If the approach is extended, the anterior part of the vertebral bodies can also be accessed. It is particularly valuable in the upper thoracic spine, where access to the bodies may be difficult

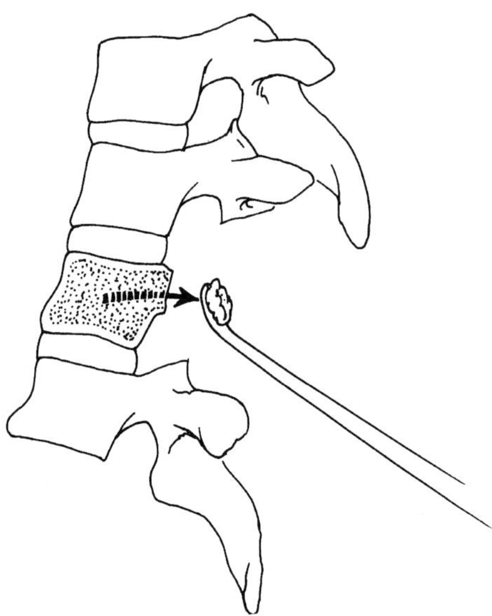

FIG. 17. Biopsy using a straight curette and then a curved curette. This vertebral body may be evacuated, producing an "eggshell" as described by Heinig.

by a more conventional anterior approach. Usually the approach is extrapleural, but it need not be.

The patient is in the lateral position, with an axillary roll padding the contralateral side to avoid compression of the neurovascular structures. The rib to be excised is determined by the pathology. Proximal to T-7, the incision is made posteriorly in a straight line, midway between the vertebral border of the scapula and spinous processes. This selection of incision depends to some degree on the extent of exposure to the posterior elements required. As an alternative, the skin incision may be made in a line directly over the spinous processes. When this incision is done, the paravertebral muscles must be divided horizontally. In the upper thoracic spine, tumor resections may require mobilization of the entire scapula. This maneuver allows a complete approach to the cervicothoracic spine.

Between T-7 and T-10, the longitudinal part of the incision usually lies at the lateral quarter of the vertebral muscles. The distal limb of the incision is slightly oblique and follows the rib to be approached (Fig. 19).

During mobilization of the scapula for upper thoracic spine lesions, the trapezius and rhomboid muscles are divided. The lateral border to the trapezius and medial border of the latissimus dorsi and serratus are also cut. The paravertebral muscles are lifted and retracted to expose the costotransverse joint and transverse processes; alternatively, these muscles may be divided. The approach may be extrapleural, dividing the periosteum of the rib longitudinally, or an intrapleural violation may occur. The rib is cut at a distance of approximately 8 cm from the costotransverse joint to permit easy access. The ligaments of the costotransverse joint are released, consisting of a superior costotransverse ligament, medial capsular ligament, lateral costotransverse ligament,

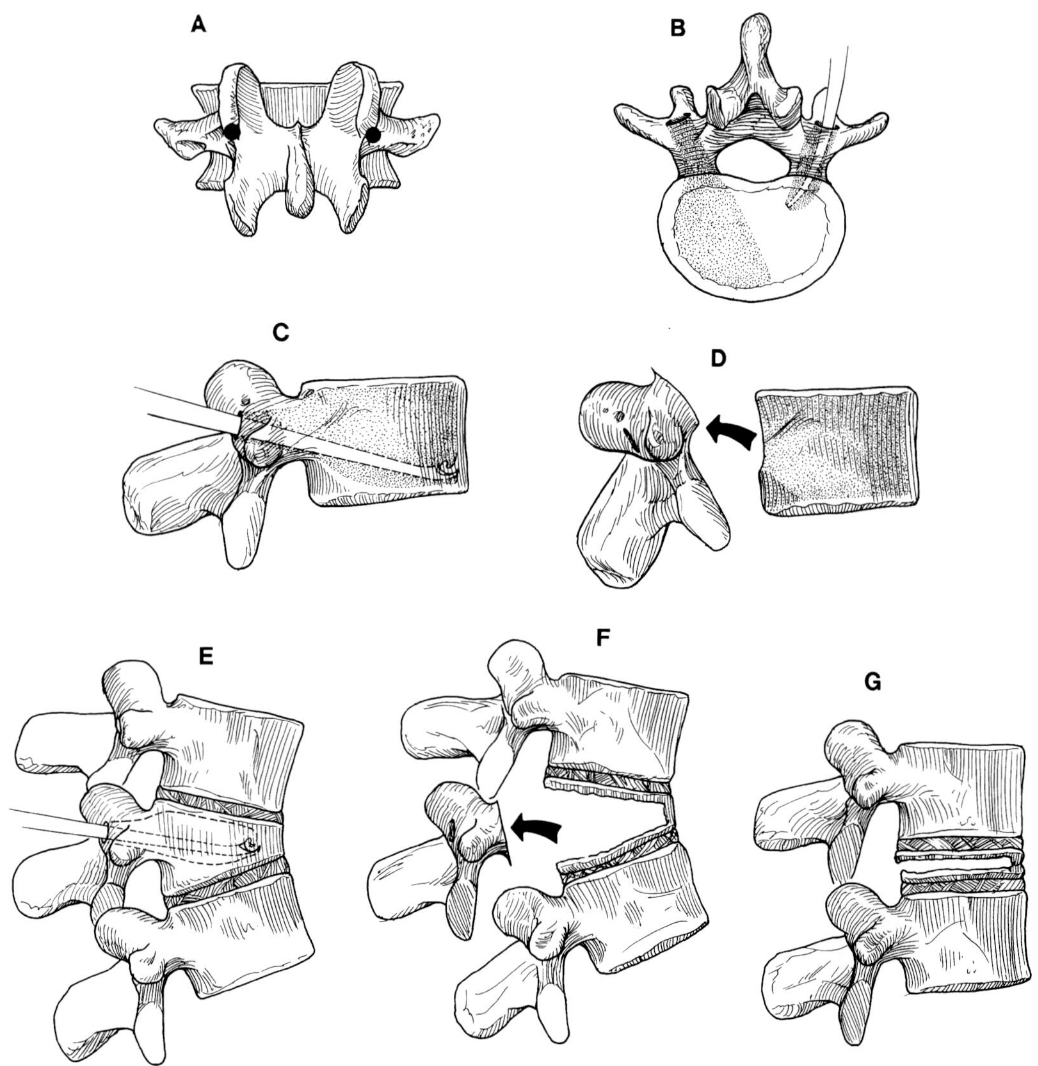

FIG. 18. Heinig's eggshell procedure. **A:** Locate the pedicle. **B:** Remove cortical bone directly over the pedicle. Place a probe within the medullary canal of the pedicle. **C:** Use curettes and rongeurs to remove bone. **D:** Remove the posterior elements, pedicles, and the posterior wall of the vertebral body. **E–G:** For correction of deformity: remove cancellous bone **(E)**; remove posterior elements, pedicles, and posterior wall of the body **(F)**; and close the osteotomy **(G)**.

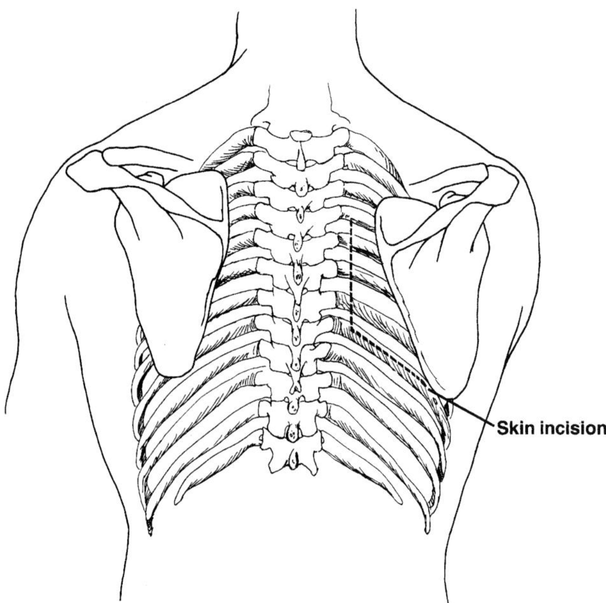

FIG. 19. Position of the patient and skin incision.

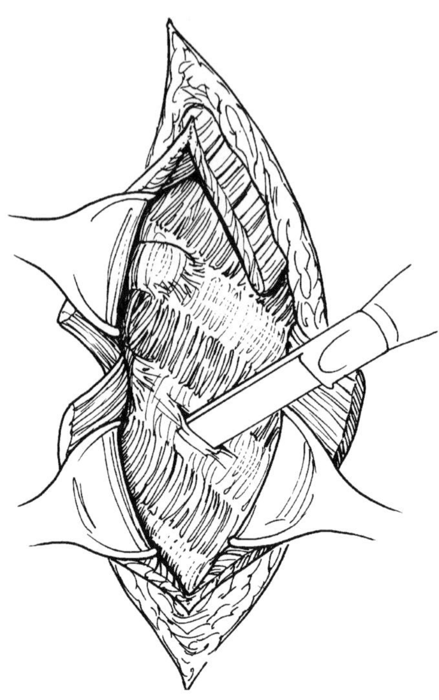

FIG. 21. The paravertebral muscles are retracted, and the ribs are stripped of their periosteum.

and anterior costotransverse ligament. The pleura is usually protected anteriorly, before cutting the rib. The anterior ligaments are cut, and the rib is removed. Alternatively, the rib may be released at its neck rather than through its ligamentous attachments (Figs. 20–24), followed by removal of the stump of the main rib. The approach may be enlarged by removing the adjacent ribs. Intercostal vascular pedicles may be ligated, if necessary. Access to the intervertebral foramina is facilitated by removal of the transverse process. The pleura and lung should be protected by use of malleable retractors (Fig. 25B,C). The posterior mediastinum is opened and lateral surface of the vertebral bodies is exposed. The approach on the vertebral bodies may be extended above and below. A one- or two-rib costotransversectomy permits two and sometimes three vertebrae to be accessed. Greater exposure may be obtained by resection of more of the chest wall, particularly for the resection of larger tumors.

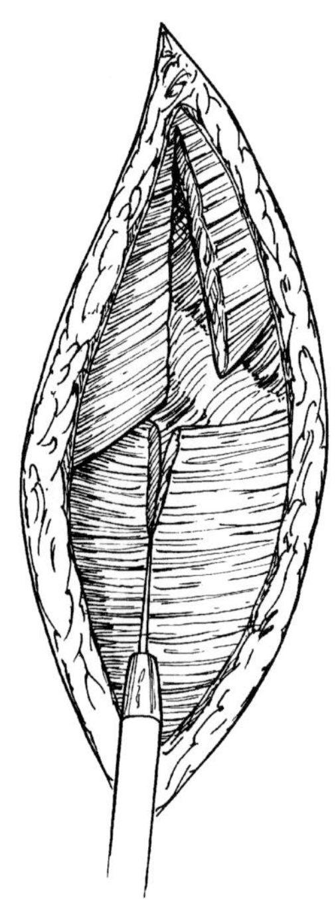

FIG. 20. Division of the muscles of the chest wall with cutting diathermy.

It is important to recognize that if a pleural tear occurs, it should be repaired if possible and a chest tube placed. Also, injury to the vascular pedicle and dura may occur, especially in the small and confined working space. Dural tears should be repaired to prevent fistula formation. Finally, potential iatrogenic thoracic instability may occur with resection of more than three ribs. Assessment intraoperatively with attempted manipulation of the vertebral column should be done with appropriate fixation if necessary.

Transcostovertebral Approach

The transcostovertebral approach is much like the costotransversectomy technique, but limited in scope, indication, and dissection. It has been mainly used for excision of herniated thoracic discs. A midline incision is used to gain access of the costovertebral junction. A posterolateral corridor is used, and the costovertebral joint and lateral edge of the vertebral end-plates are drilled to expose the lateral annulus. The ribs are preserved. The visualization is limited, but adequate for disc excision at any thoracic disc level. It offers the potential advantages of shorter operating time, less blood loss, less dissection, less pain, and shorter hospital stays.

Laminoplasty

Although laminoplasty has been well described for use in the cervical spine, it has also been used in the thoracic and lumbar

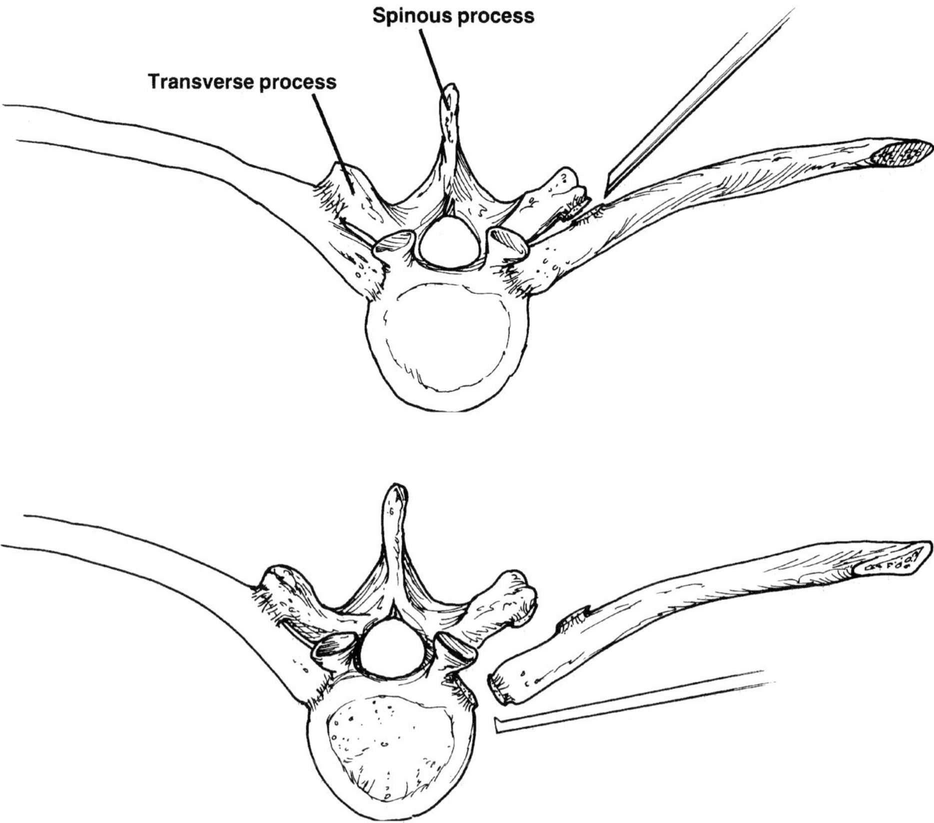

FIG. 22. Division of the posterior costotransverse ligaments is made under direct vision.

FIG. 23. The anterior costotransverse ligament is shown divided.

spine. The open-book technique of Hirabayashi has been used in the thoracic spine and has particular value in achondroplastic dwarfs (Fig. 26). In addition, Tsuzuki has described laminopediculoplasty as a method of reconstructing the posterior elements of the thoracic spine.

A wide posterior approach is used. A circumferential decompression of the thoracic cord may be achieved through a single posterior approach. The posterior elements, including the laminae, facet joints, and medial two-thirds of the pedicle, are removed (Figs. 27 and 28). The lateral one-third of the pedicle is preserved for reconstruction. To gain access to the anterior central one-third of the vertebral body immediately beneath, the vertebral body is deepened with use of an air drill. The base of the remaining bony masses is removed, leaving untouched the part of the bone in contact with the anterior dura. After this, the remaining portion of bone may be gently freed or resected. If the dural tube is ossified, it is opened and expanded with a fascial patch. Tsuzuki reconstructs the posterior elements using a thin cortical cancellous graft taken from the other aspect of the iliac crest and bent into a semicircle (Figs. 29 and 30). Posterior instrumentation may be used to supplement stabilization above or below the level of decompression. Tsuzuki has advocated this technique in cases of thoracic myelopathy. Other techniques of laminoplasty include the lobster-shell technique (Fig. 31) and pars interarticularis osteotomy (transversoarthropediculectomy) (Figs. 32 and 33).

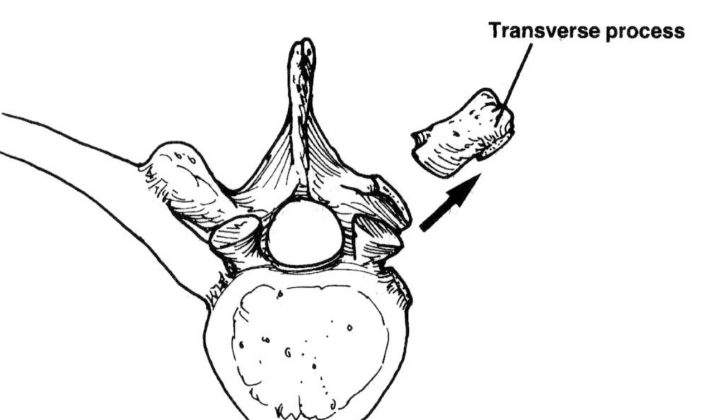

FIG. 24. The transverse process is usually divided.

Lateral Extracavitary Approach (Transversoarthropediculectomy)

The lateral extracavitary approach is similar to the costotransversectomy but enlarges the scope of the exposure. It entails resection of a longer segment of rib, dissection of the intercostal neurovascular bundle, and pleural retraction to provide a far-lateral exposure of the entire spinal canal. Again, it allows exposure of the lateral aspect of the thoracolumbar vertebrae without entering the thoracic cavities from a posterior incision. Better visualization of the anterior dural surface is gained, as well as greater access to disc and vertebral body. Posterior instrumentation, vertebrectomy, and anterior bone grafting can be done through this approach. Exposure at the proximal or distal ends can be more difficult. Although technically demanding, it creates a line of sight tangential to the dorsal musculature. The most common complications for this approach are pneumonia

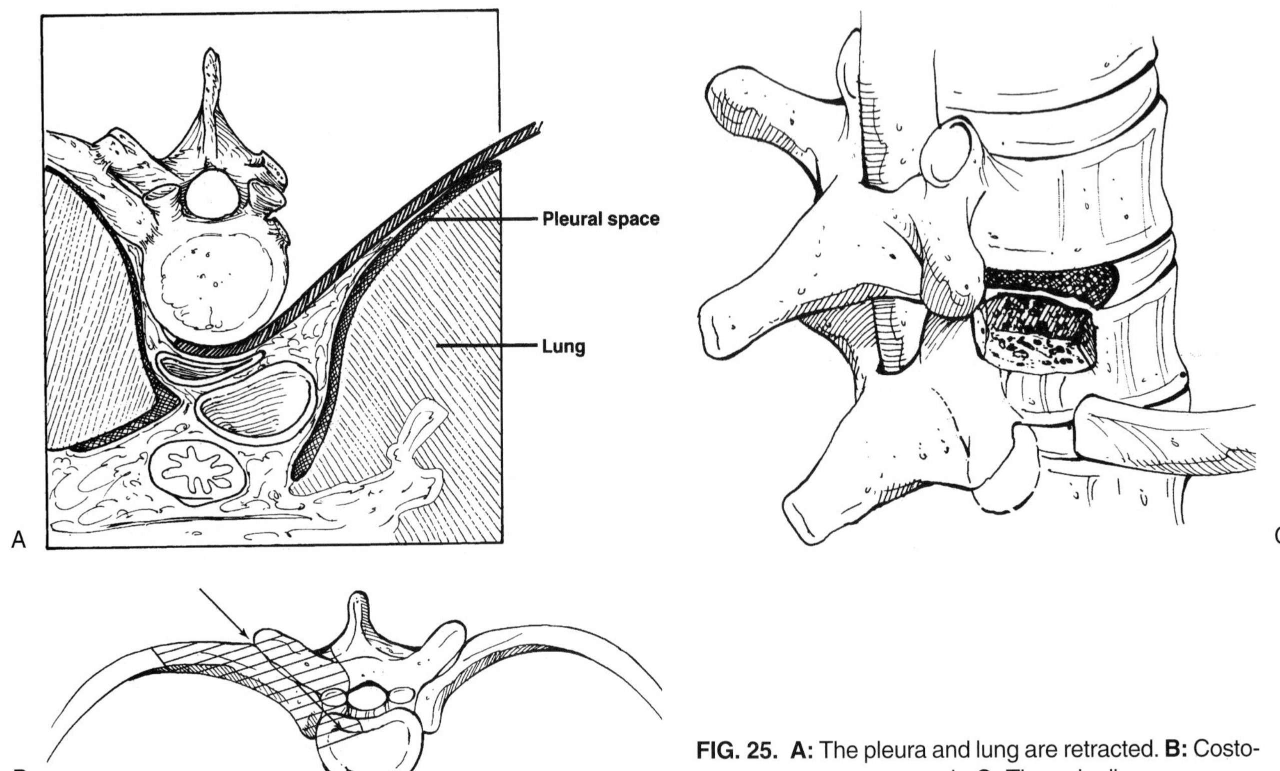

FIG. 25. A: The pleura and lung are retracted. **B:** Costotransversectomy approach. **C:** Thoracic disc exposure.

or atelectasis (4%), wound infections (3%), pleural tear (3%), and thoracic radiculopathy in the sacrificed nerve root (3%).

Anterior Approaches to the Thoracic and Thoracolumbar Spine via the Sternomastoid

The first thoracic vertebra and the T1-2 disc can be reached through a standard anterior approach to the cervical spine. Resection of the body of T-2 or correction of deformity to the T1-2 level is, however, difficult (Fig. 34). The T1-2 levels can also be reached through an upper-thoracic thoracotomy, particularly through the third rib. In the anterior sternomastoid approach, hyperextension of the neck, if not contraindicated, aids in the exposure. Intraoperative radiographic confirmation is difficult to obtain, and it may be necessary to apply traction to the shoulders to obtain satisfactory views. The approach is through a vertical incision anterior to the medial border of the sternomastoid muscle that, if possible, is made from the left side to prevent damage to recurrent laryngeal nerves. The omohyoid and inferior thyroid vascular pedicle are divided. Exposure may be difficult and significant retraction necessary. The caudal extent of exposure is limited to T-3 by the great vessels of the mediastinum, whereas the angle of the approach to the cervicothoracic junction is dictated by the manubrium.

Danger to the great vessels, particularly the innominate artery and especially vein, must be considered.

Cervical Sternotomy

The lower cervical and upper three thoracic vertebral levels may be accessed through a cervical sternotomy. Again, it is preferable to use the left side to avoid damage to the recurrent laryngeal nerves. The head is, therefore, rotated right.

A vertical incision is made (Fig. 35) anterior to the sternomastoid, then distally toward the jugular notch and the xiphisternum. The brachiocephalic vein at the upper border of the manubrium sterni is ligated. The innominate veins can be well visualized. The sternum is divided by an oscillating saw, usually proximal to distal, along its entire length. The sternum is retracted after coating the bone edges with wax to decrease bleeding. The pericardium and costomediastinal pleural recesses are separated. The esophagus and trachea are retracted anteriorly to the right, and the common carotid artery posteriorly to the left. The best exposure may be obtained by ligation of the left brachiocephalic vein. Care must be taken to avoid vascular damage (Fig. 36). Mobilization of the esophagus and trachea with displacement to the right allows exposure of the thoracic spine to the third thoracic level.

Partial division of the sternum can achieve the same exposure. In this case, the sternum is longitudinally osteotomized to the third or fourth intercostal level, where it is divided transversely. This approach is rarely used, but may assist in tumor excision at the cervicothoracic junction or correction of the deformity at this level. Again, the danger lies in damage to the vascular structures, particularly the innominate vein (Fig. 37).

A disadvantage of both of these techniques is that sternotomy carries a relatively high risk of infection or dehiscence.

An anterior approach to the upper thoracic spine in which the medial portion of one clavicle and part of the manubrium sterni are excised has also been described. A left-sided approach is preferred to decrease risk of damage to the recurrent laryngeal nerves.

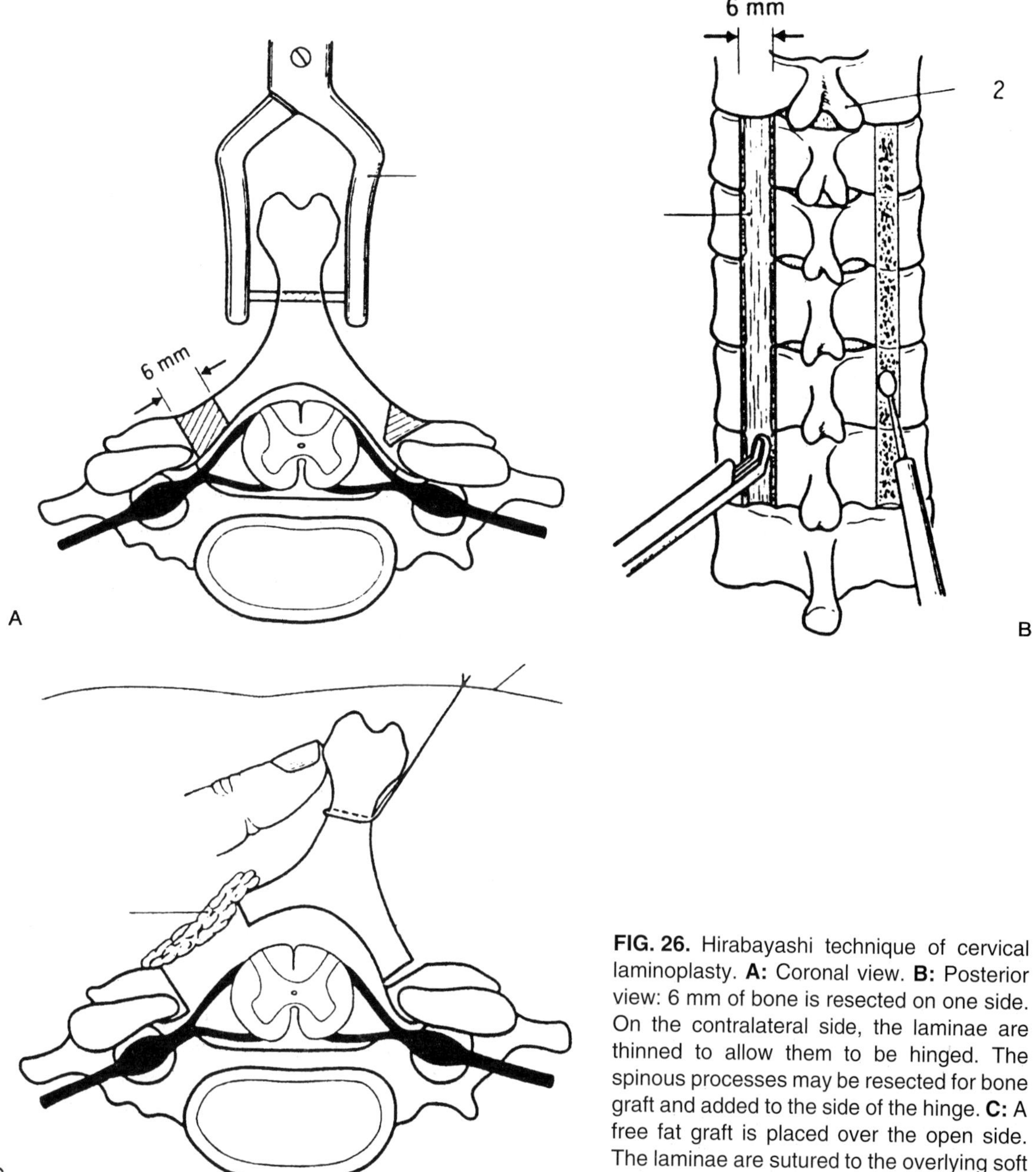

FIG. 26. Hirabayashi technique of cervical laminoplasty. **A:** Coronal view. **B:** Posterior view: 6 mm of bone is resected on one side. On the contralateral side, the laminae are thinned to allow them to be hinged. The spinous processes may be resected for bone graft and added to the side of the hinge. **C:** A free fat graft is placed over the open side. The laminae are sutured to the overlying soft tissue.

Transpleural Axillary Thoracotomy

The transpleural axillary thoracotomy approach has been used for resection of cervical ribs in thoracic outlet syndrome. It may be used for unusual conditions affecting the cervicothoracic or upper thoracic spine. The exposure is difficult, however, because of the depth of the wound.

When this approach is used, the patient is positioned in the left lateral decubitus position, in which the aorta and thoracic duct are more prominent. The shoulder is in full abduction and is positioned in external rotation with the patient's hand behind the neck, opening the axilla. The upper extremity on the side to be operated must be prepared out and mobile. The incision is carried from behind, downward and forward along the intercostal space, usually the third space. The incision averages approximately 15 cm in length and lies between the latissimus dorsi posteriorly and the pectoralis major anteriorly. It may be extended into the submammary crease. In retracting the latissimus dorsi, care must be taken to avoid injury to the long thoracic nerve of Bell and the nerves of the latissimus dorsi. For greater exposure, the inferior portion of the pectoralis major may be released (Fig. 38). The chest may be opened along the upper border of the fourth rib. If the pleura is opened and the chest entered, the apex of the lung is retracted distally to reveal the costovertebral region. The mediastinal pleura is then divided, and the intercostal vessel and esophagus are retracted anteriorly. Closure is achieved by approximation of the ribs.

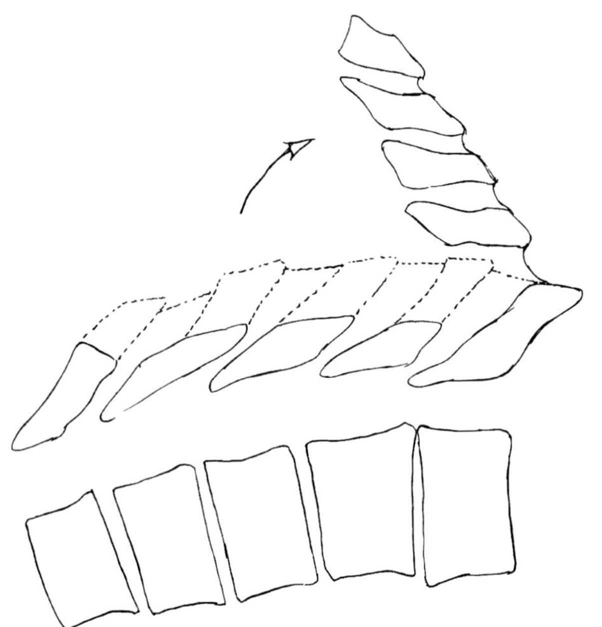

FIG. 27. The spinous process ligament complex is preserved before the laminectomy.

Transthoracic Approaches

The thoracic spine from T2-12 may be exposed through a transthoracic approach (Fig. 39). These approaches may be used for biopsies, anterior spinal cord decompression and instrumentation, spinal osteotomy, correction of kyphosis, correction of scoliosis, vertebral body resection and reconstruction for tumor or infection, and anterior interbody fusion. For the uninitiated, these approaches may be done with assistance of an experienced cardiovascular or thoracic surgeon.

Many surgeons prefer a retropleural rather than a transpleural approach, but the authors have found that in adults the pleura frequently becomes torn in the former method. Also, the authors do not feel that a transpleural approach is generally more traumatic or requires more postoperative care.

Transpleural Approach

The authors' preference is to approach the patient from the left side. Release of segmental vessels at the midpoint of the vertebral body allows the great vessels (i.e., aorta, inferior vena cava, azygos system) to fall away from the spine. The aorta protects the more fragile venous structures. Some surgeons prefer to approach

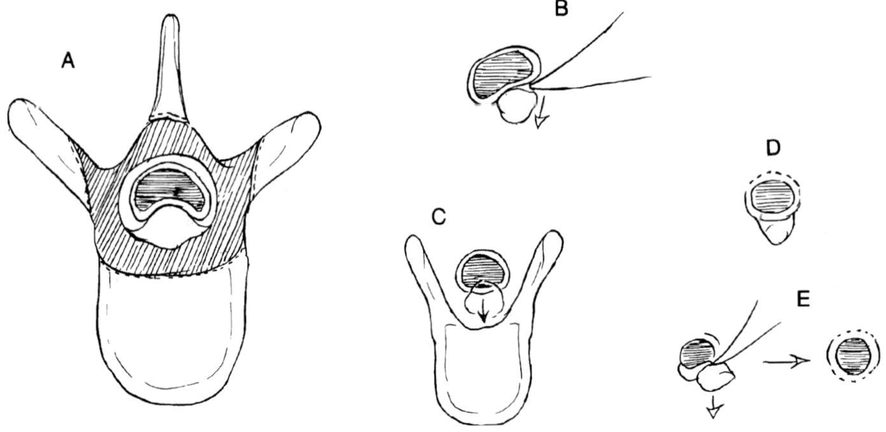

FIG. 28. Anterior decompression of the thoracic cord through the wide posterior approach. **A:** Area of bone resected. **B:** Bony remnant separated from the anterior dura. **C:** Where bony remnant cannot be separated from the dura, both are allowed to fall forward into prepared cavity. **D:** Expansion of involved dura with a patch. **E:** Resection of involved dura and posterior longitudinal ligament.

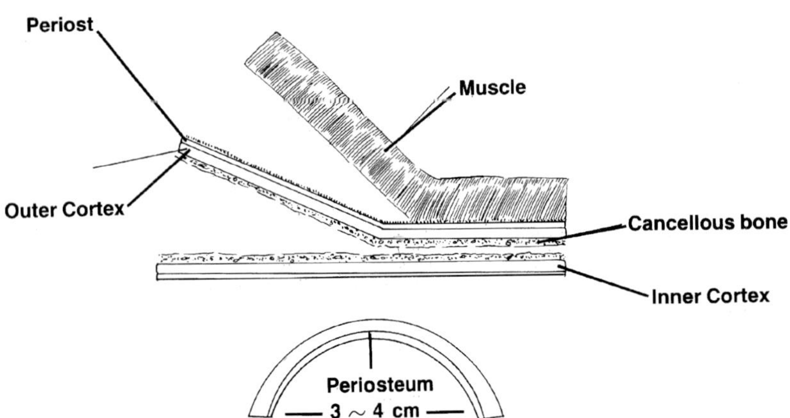

FIG. 29. Obtaining the osteoperiosteal graft. A thin corticocancellous graft with the periosteum (Periost) intact is taken from the outer corticocancellous portion of the iliac wing.

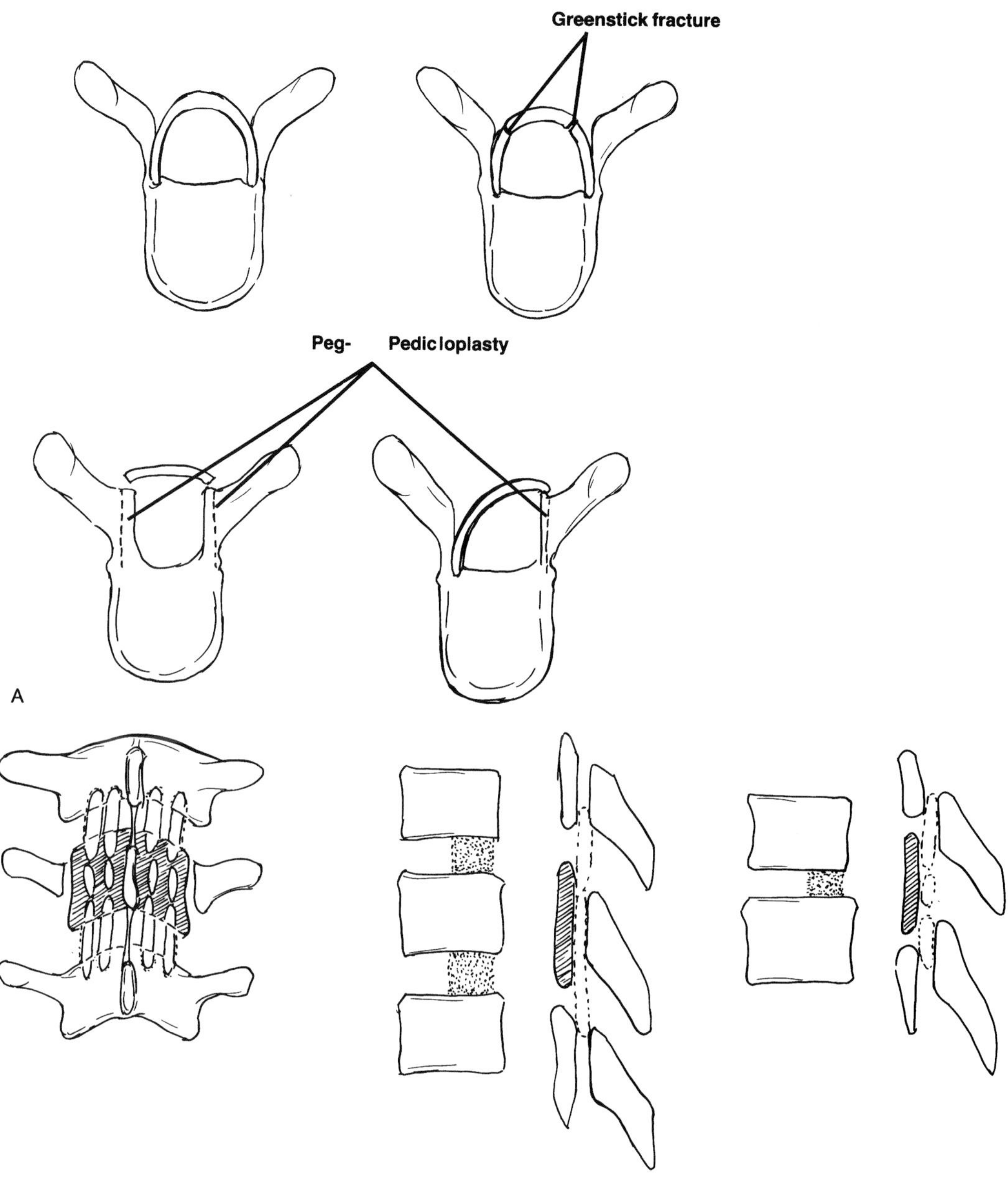

FIG. 30. Reconstruction of the posterior elements of the spine. **A:** Patterns of laminopediculoplasty. **B:** Sites for grafting. The spinous process ligament complex is replaced on a new lamina.

the thoracic and lumbar spine from the right side unless the pathology dictates otherwise, especially when internal fixation devices are to be used (Figs. 38 and 39). They feel that the proximity of the internal fixation devices to the arterial structures may result in traumatic aneurysms. Indeed, the Dunn device on the left side did cause aneurysms from the left side, but none in the inventor's hands. In the senior author's experience of more than 2,000 cases of anterior instrumentation of the spine, this complication has not been encountered from an internal fixation device inserted from the left side. Release of two segmental vessels proximal and, if possible, distal to the site of the insertion of the implants allows the great vessels to fall away to the opposite side. However, care must be taken not to place the internal fixation devices directly anterior. An anterolateral position is preferred. Venules and arterioles may be cauterized and intermediate vessels clipped, whereas larger vessels are preferably tied off, because the release of a clip may result in significant blood loss.

The patient is placed on his or her side tilting at a 60-degree angle toward the horizontal, ideally over a break in the table to improve exposure or correct deformity. An axillary roll is used on the down side. The upper extremity on the side of the surgical approach usually rests over the other arm, with a pillow between them (Fig. 39). Selective bronchial intubation may permit collapse of the lung on the ipsilateral side, creating more space within the field (Fig. 40).

The level of the incision depends on the vertebra to be reached. Ideally, the incision should be two ribs above the vertebral lesion, but this depends to some degree on the obliquity of the ribs. The incision usually runs from the lateral border of the vertebral muscles as far anterior as necessary. The muscles are divided with cautery. The rib is removed and saved for bone

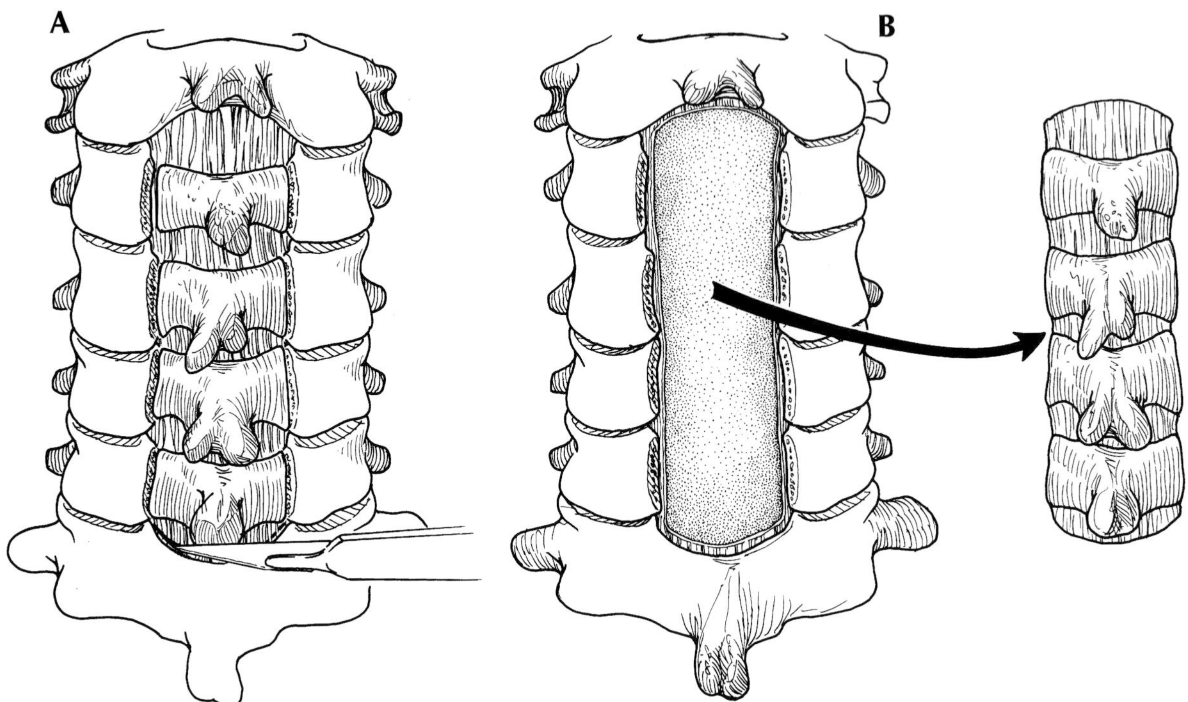

FIG. 31. Lobster-shell technique. **A:** Division of the ligamentum flavum distally. **B:** Removal of posterior arches in one piece.

grafting (Fig. 41). Thoracotomy may be done without rib resection, but excision of the rib gives better exposure. The latissimus dorsi and the lateral part of the trapezius muscle or the rhomboids in the upper approach may be divided, but it is rarely necessary to cut the rhomboids.

The entire thoracic spine from T-1 to the diaphragm can be exposed through the fifth rib, if necessary, in some patients. This is relatively easily achieved in short patients. In taller patients, two incisions are required—one through the fourth rib and one through the eleventh rib. With the lung selectively deflated, exposure of the spine is easy. If the lung remains inflated, it may have to be retracted out of the field.

The mediastinal pleura is excised, exposing the intercostal vessels, which are usually easily visualized, depending on the amount of fat present (Fig. 42). The intercostal vessels should be ligated or clipped in the midpoint of the spine (Fig. 43). Large veins are preferably ligated, or else locking clips may be applied. The vertebral bodies are exposed subperiosteally or extraperiosteally. The periosteum becomes adherent to the annulus of the disc at each level and results in more difficult exposure. Subperiosteal dissection results in greater and earlier blood loss, but it may be preferable at the time of closure (Figs. 44 and 45). The neurovascular intercostal bundle is vulnerable and is often coagulated.

At the time of closure, the mediastinal pleura is usually left open, as it is thin and difficult to approximate (Fig. 46). A large chest tube is necessary to evacuate the postoperative accumulations of fluid. It is not necessary to have an airtight pleural closure in the transpleural approach, as the muscles become rapidly repleuralized.

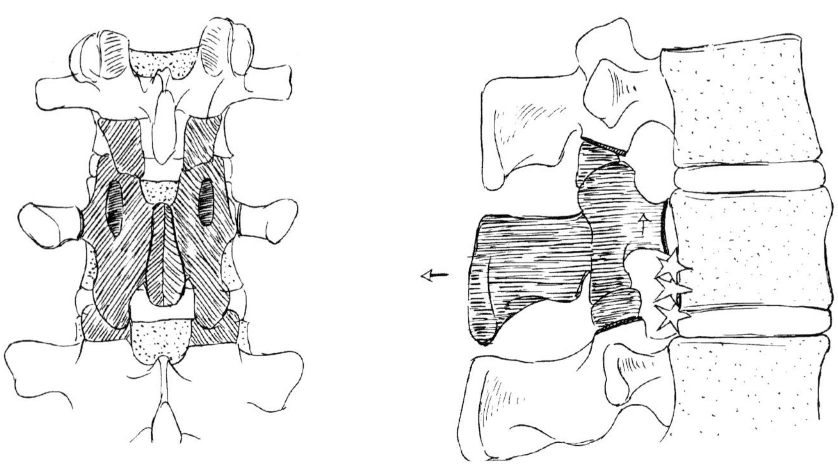

FIG. 32. Hemitransversoarthropediculotomy osteotomies for foraminal disc herniation.

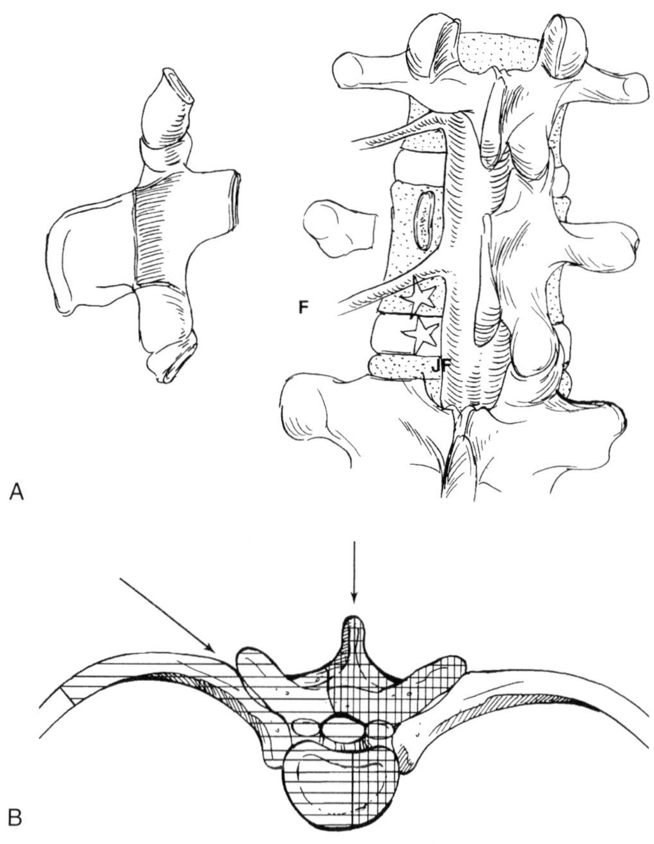

C

FIG. 33. **A:** Monobloc removed. Foraminal (*F*) and juxtaforaminal (*JF*) neurogenic structures. **B:** Lateral extracavitary approach. **C:** Line-of-sight view of lateral dural sac and nerve roots and lateral vertebrae.

Retropleural Approach

The retropleural approach is similar to the transpleural approach and is generally performed one rib proximal to the involved vertebra. The rib is exposed subperiosteally and resected. The parietal pleura is then separated from the rib and muscle layers with fingers or swabs (Figs. 47 and 48). This is best started posteriorly at the posterior mediastinum. Resection of the head and neck of the rib helps at this point. At the lateral part of the thoracic wall, the pleura is more adherent. If the pleura is torn a transpleural approach may be made, or the pleura can be closed and an extrapleural dissection continued. It is not necessary to open the parietal pleura as the vertebral bodies are approached.

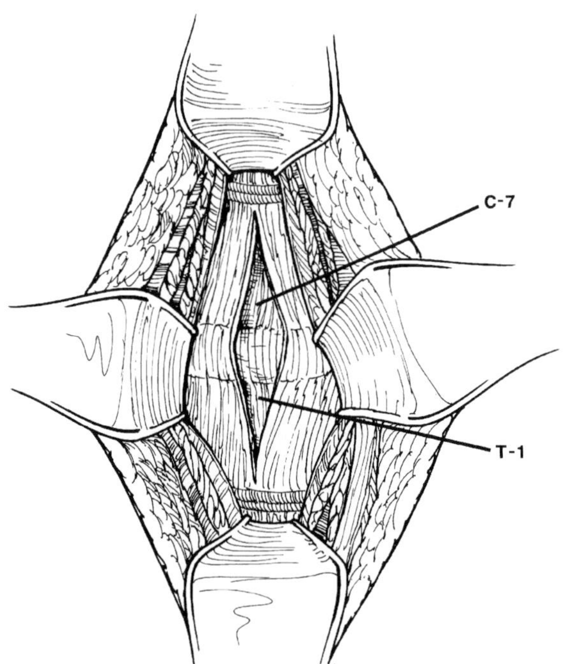

FIG. 34. Cervicothoracic lordosis limits access distal to T-1. Exposure of T-1 is relatively easy, although the wound is deep.

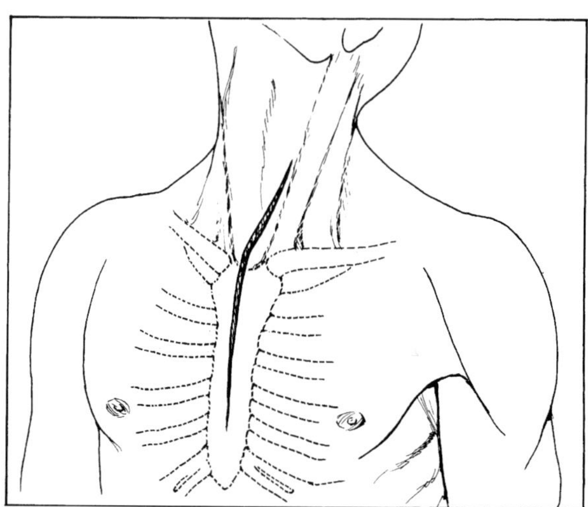

FIG. 35. Cervical sternotomy. The approach is anterior to the sternomastoid and is extended distally by a vertical midline sternal incision.

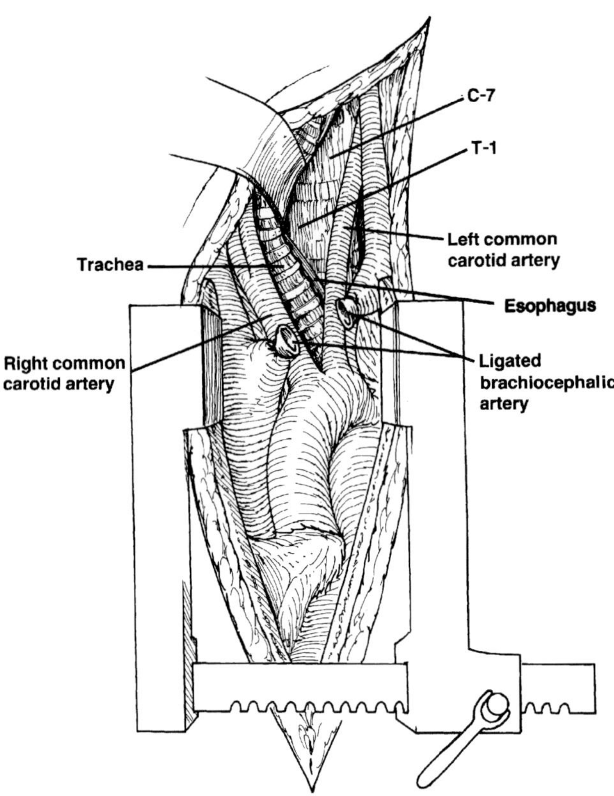

FIG. 36. The left common carotid lies laterally. The trachea and esophagus are identified with the finger and are retracted medially and anteriorly to expose the spine. The arch of the aorta and the left brachiocephalic (innominate) vein are in the lower part of the wound. Ligation of the brachiocephalic vein increases exposure but is not essential. A thorough knowledge of the vasculature is important.

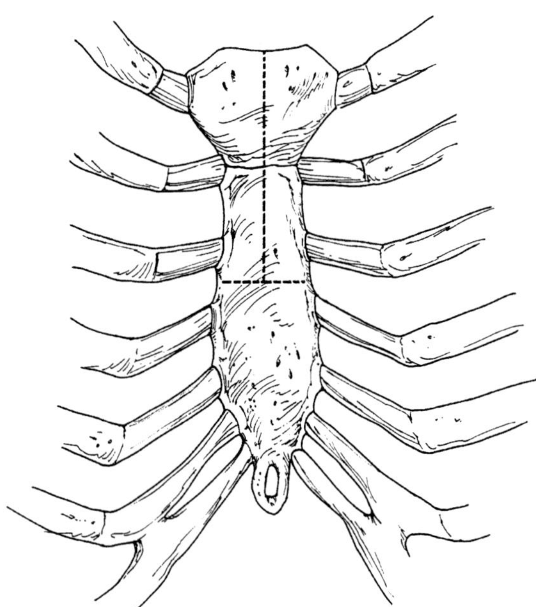

FIG. 37. A variation of vertical division of the sternum is possible. The sternal division stops at the level of the third or fourth intercostal space, where the sternum is divided transversely.

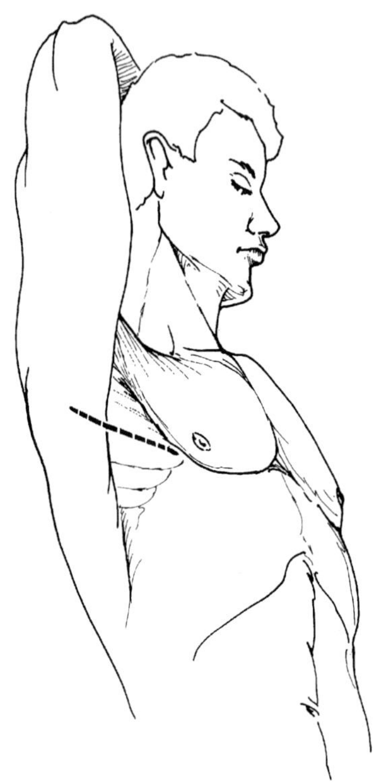

FIG. 38. Transpleural axillary thoracotomy. An approach from the right is preferable. The shoulder is in full abduction, with patient's hand behind the head and neck. The incision is oblique from behind, downward, and forward along the third intercostal space for a length of 15 cm.

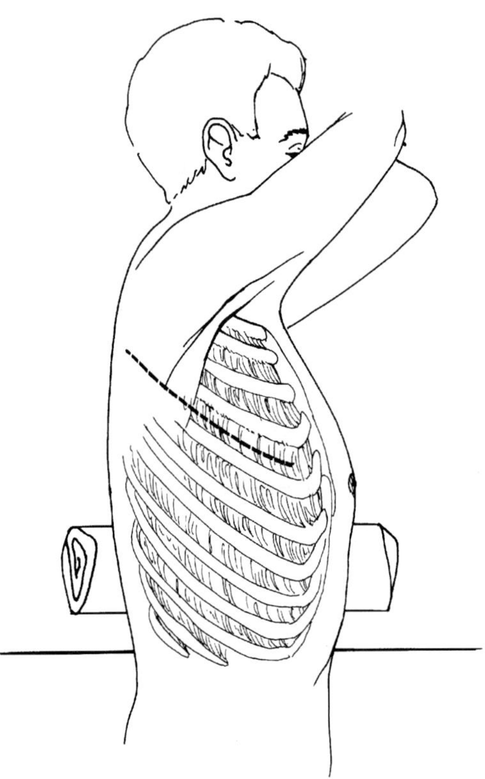

FIG. 39. Rib incision is usually two levels proximal to the vertebral body to be approached.

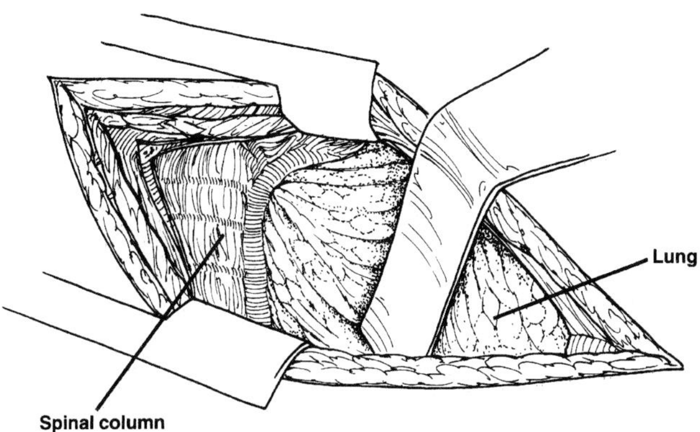

FIG. 40. The retracted lung allows visualization of the spine. It is helpful if the anesthesiologist collapses the ipsilateral lung.

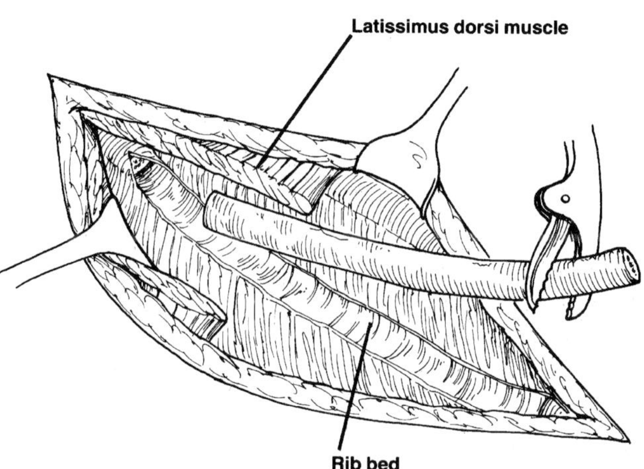

FIG. 41. Resection of the rib is helpful in adults with a rigid thorax.

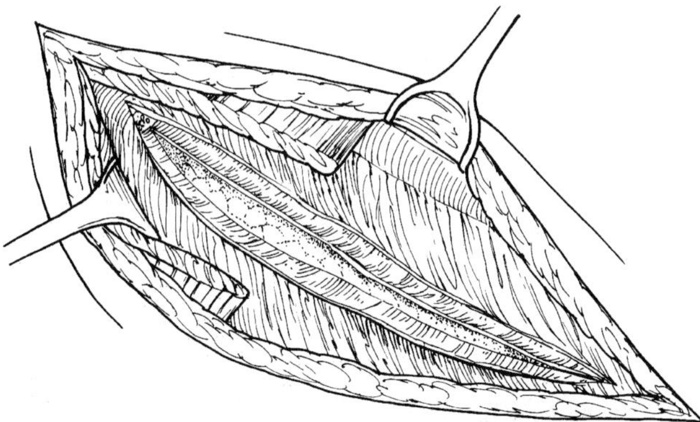

FIG. 42. The pleura is opened in the bed of the rib.

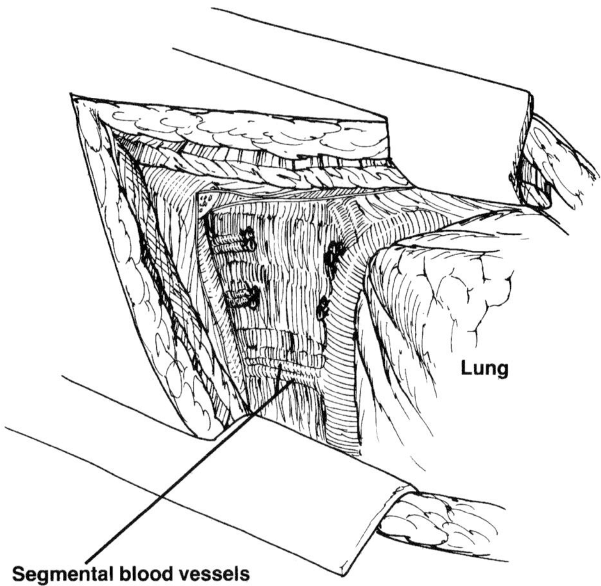

FIG. 43. The segmental vessels are ligated in the midline. The pleural foramina must be avoided to not interfere with the blood supply to the spinal cord.

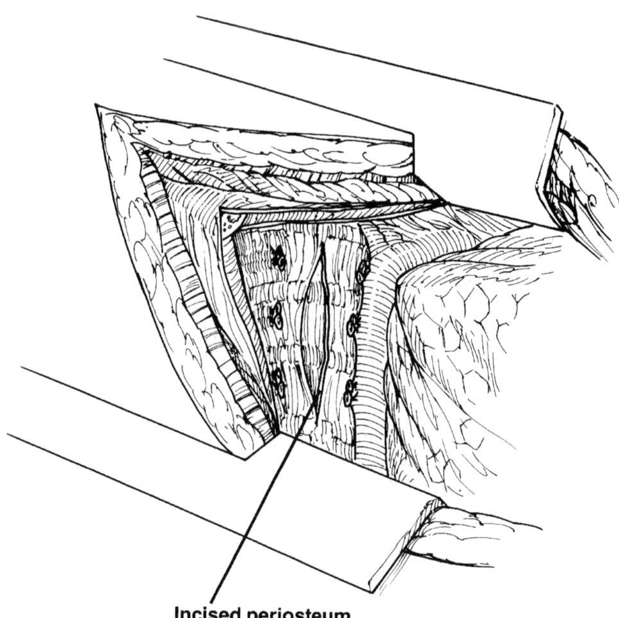

FIG. 44. The periosteum may be incised with cutting diathermy after ligation of the vascular pedicles (subperiosteal dissection).

The intercostal vessels in the plane of the dissection can be ligated easily. An intercostal nerve often serves as a guide to the intravertebral foramina. However, care must be taken to avoid coagulation of these vessels near any of the foramina so as not to damage the blood supply to the spinal cord, particularly in the watershed area.

When more limited access to the spine is desired, for example to a thoracic disc, the rib excised is dictated by the pathology. The rib that lies directly horizontal to the vertebral level at the midaxillary line of the anteroposterior chest x-ray is usually chosen. The rib removed must be proximal to the lesion and provide adequate exposure while working down on the lesion. For example, the eighth rib is resected for a T7-8 disc. In the thoracic spine, the disc is the most prominent anterior structure. It is soft and white, relatively avascular, and provides a safe area

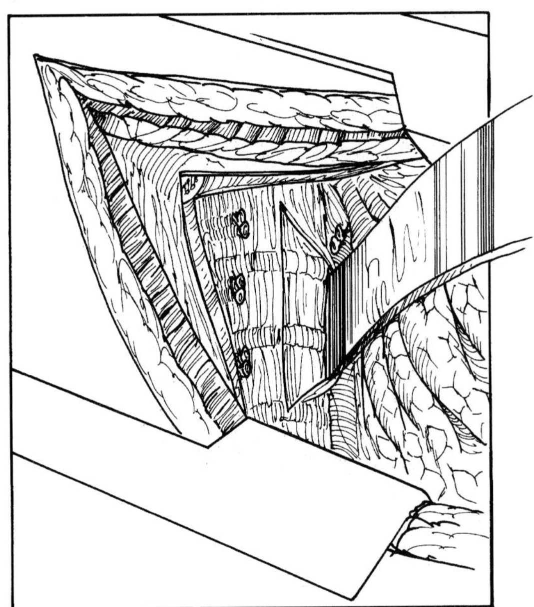

FIG. 45. A malleable retractor is placed on the opposite side of the vertebral body to protect structures on that side from damage.

for dissection. The intercostal vessels cross the midportion of each vertebral body and are easily delineated. If the segmental vessels are cut in the midline over the vertebral body, damage to the spinal cord blood supply is not a problem. Coagulation in the intervertebral foramina must be avoided. The thoracic duct usually passes from right to left in the T4-5 area. The sympathetic chain should be preserved, but interruption is not of major consequence except in the upper thoracic spine, where disruption may result in Horner's syndrome. Resection of the rib may be necessary to gain access to the posterior disc in the spinal canal in decompressive procedures. For greater exposure of a verte-

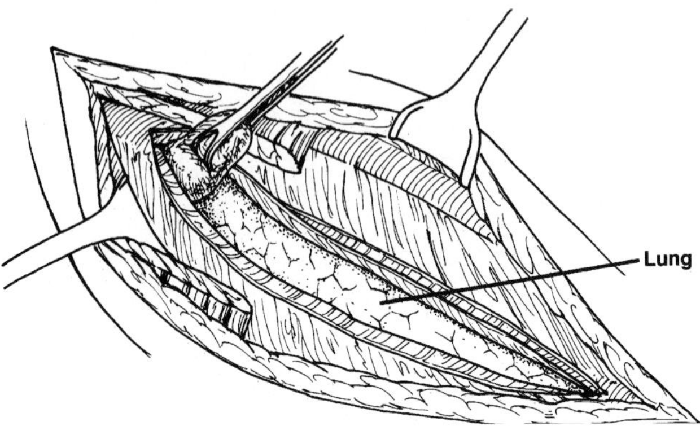

FIG. 47. Separation of the parietal pleura begins in the posterior mediastinum.

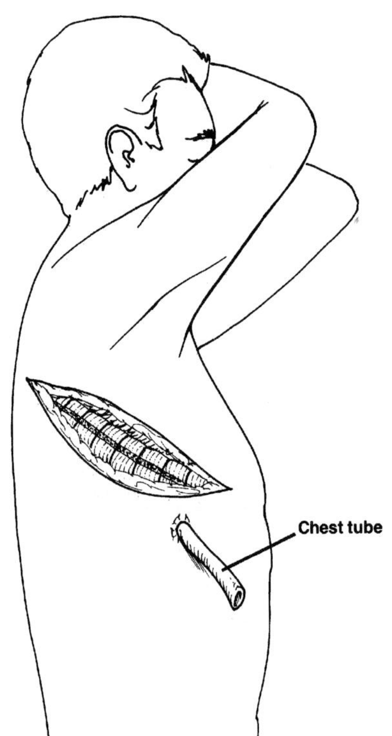

FIG. 46. Closure is obtained by bringing the adjacent ribs together with sutures. Drainage of the thoracic cavity is essential. The chest tube emerges in line with the midaxillary line.

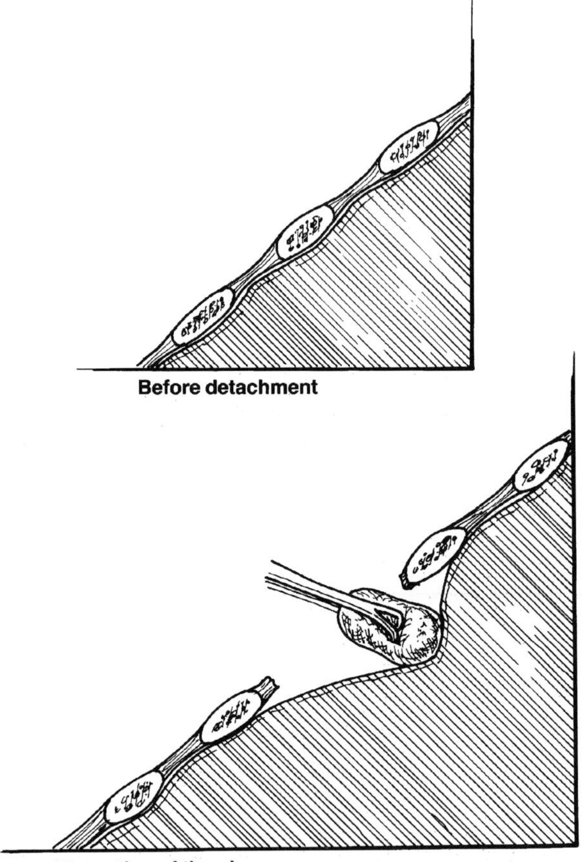

FIG. 48. The pleura is gradually pushed away.

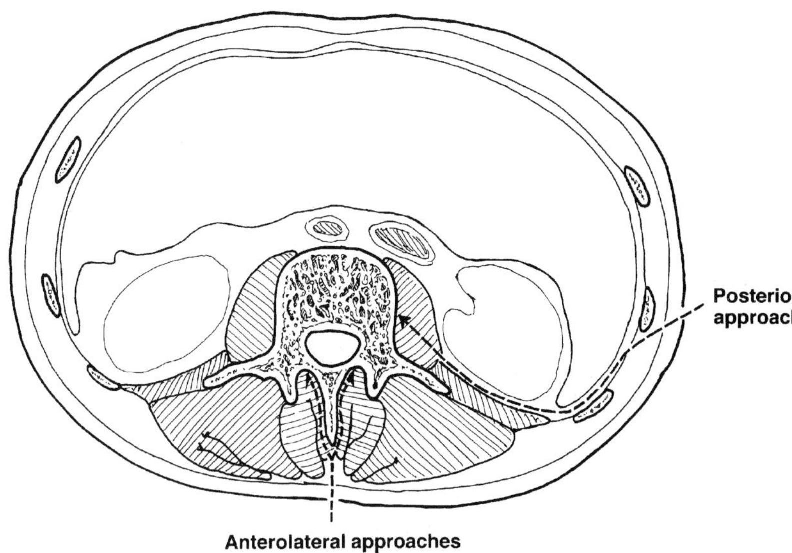

FIG. 49. Anterolateral approaches to the thoracolumbar spine, whether retropleural and retroperitoneal, or transpleural, transdiaphragmatic, and retroperitoneal, give access to the vertebral bodies. An anterolateral approach gives exposure to T-11, T-12, and L-1 and is not extensive. The classic posterior approach gives access to all vertebrae from T-4 distally.

bral body, the discs above and below are resected, allowing for identification of the posterior vertebral body wall and the canal.

Anterolateral Approaches to the Thoracolumbar Spine

Two main types of anterolateral approaches are available, and the choice depends on the required exposure (Fig. 49). A retropleural retroperitoneal approach gives limited access to only the lower thoracic spine from T-10 distally, and exposure to the sacrum may be difficult. Generally, a transpleural retroperitoneal approach allows full access at all levels. In this approach, incising and detaching the diaphragm from the chest wall is preferable. Some surgeons prefer a transpleural retroperitoneal approach, in which the diaphragm is incised but not detached. However, the authors use the more extensive transpleural diaphragmatic retroperitoneal approach in almost all patients.

For all of these approaches—retropleural retroperitoneal, transpleural retroperitoneal, and the extended anterior transpleural transdiaphragmatic retroperitoneal—the patient is usually positioned on the lateral side, with an axillary roll under the contralateral axilla. The patient is rolled slightly posterior at approximately 60 to 70 degrees. If radiographs are to be taken, an adjustable radiolucent table is necessary. As an alternative position, the patient may be placed directly lateral. This is necessary if the spine is also to be approached posteriorly, or if a corrective procedure, such as an osteotomy, is planned.

Retropleural Retroperitoneal Approach

The incision in the retropleural retroperitoneal approach is centered over the eleventh rib (Fig. 50). The twelfth rib may be resected or osteotomized. The incision extends from the lateral border of the paravertebral muscles, but generally it aims anterior to the anterosuperior iliac spine, depending on the exposure required to the lumbar level. Musculature is cut with cutting diathermy to decrease bleeding and improve hemostasis. The thoracic portion of the procedure is done first. The rib is located, and the periosteum stripped. Care must be taken to remain outside of the pleura, which in older adults is difficult. If the pleura is torn, it may be sewn or left open with subsequent insertion of a chest tube for drainage. The retroperitoneal space is entered by following the eleventh rib tip, which is usually detached and then

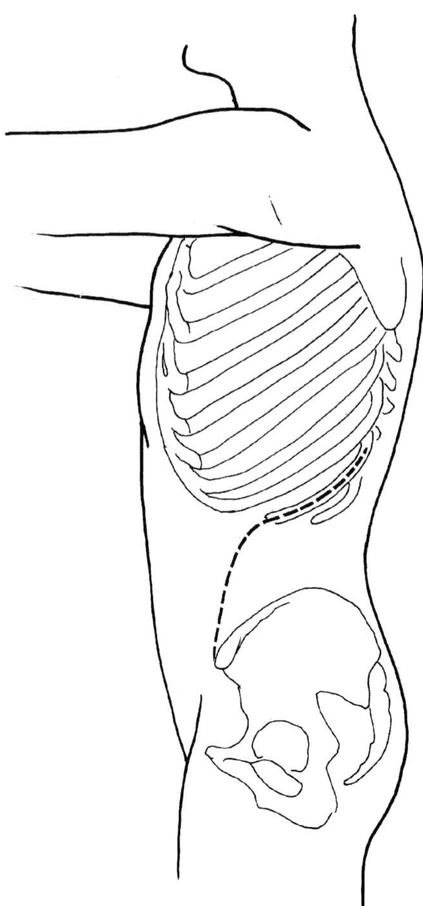

FIG. 50. Lateral position and skin incision.

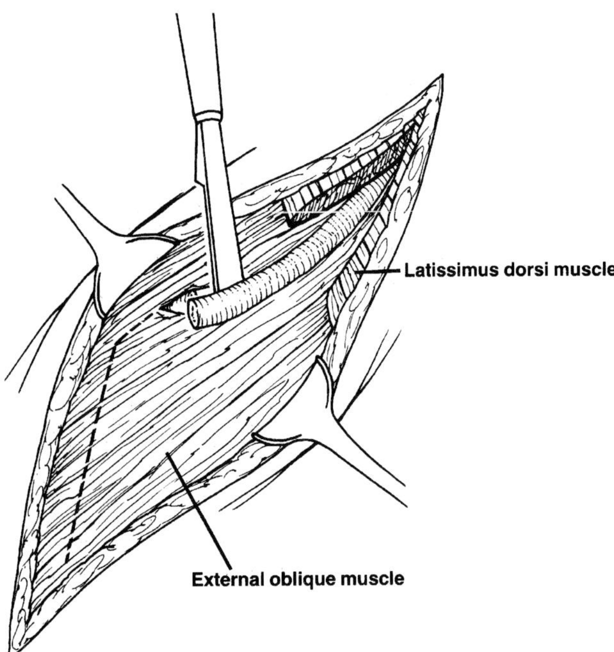

FIG. 51. Incision of the muscles, resection of the eleventh rib, and opening of the retroperitoneal space at the tip of the rib. If a more proximal rib is chosen, the distal ribs may have to be osteotomized in a transpleural, transdiaphragmatic, and retroperitoneal approach.

split (Fig. 51). The diaphragm usually attaches to this cartilaginous tip. After osteotomy of the rib posteriorly, the approach passes anteriorly, dividing the musculature after stripping the periosteum from the ribs under the surface (Fig. 52).

Mobilization of the parietal pleura is preferably done with blunt dissection using fingers, or a sponge on a forceps. This

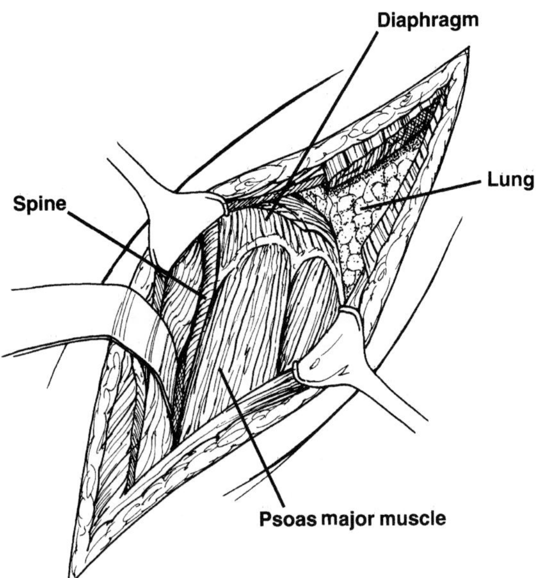

FIG. 52. Anatomic cross-section after removal of the peritoneum to show the relationship between the lungs, diaphragm, crura, arcuate ligaments, and spine.

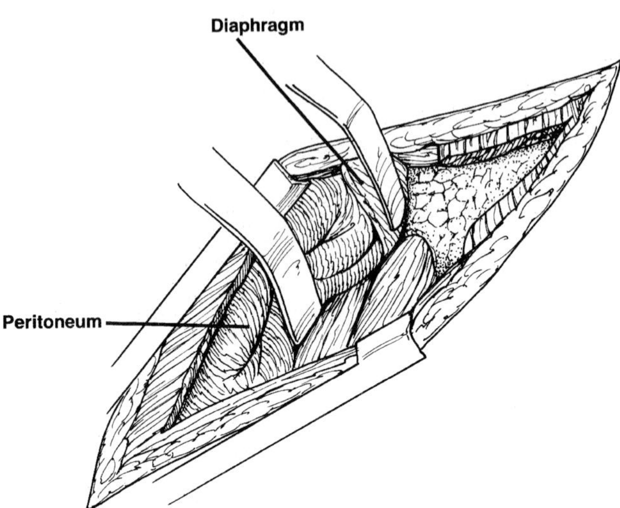

FIG. 53. Gradual mobilization of the peritoneal sac. The pleura above, the diaphragm in the middle, and the peritoneum below are mobilized simultaneously *en bloc.*

begins anteriorly and progresses posteriorly. The pleura, diaphragm, and the peritoneum are mobilized (Fig. 53). After release of the diaphragm from the eleventh rib, mobilization continues posteriorly and through the twelfth rib and lateral arcuate ligament (Fig. 54). The medial attachment of the lateral arcuate ligament and the lateral attachment of the medial arcuate ligament are divided close to the tip of the transverse process of L-1. Sufficient tissue must be left to reapproximate the diaphragm (Fig. 54).

The crus of the diaphragm is divided approximately 2 cm away from the vertebral body. Blood vessels in the midline may be ligated or clipped, but care must be taken to avoid coagulation near the foramina to prevent any damage to blood supply to the spinal cord. After division of the arcuate ligament, chest retractors are inserted. The viscera and diaphragm are retracted (Figs. 55 and 56). The parietal pleura is detached as far as T-10. The pleura may be more adherent to the vertebral bodies in the

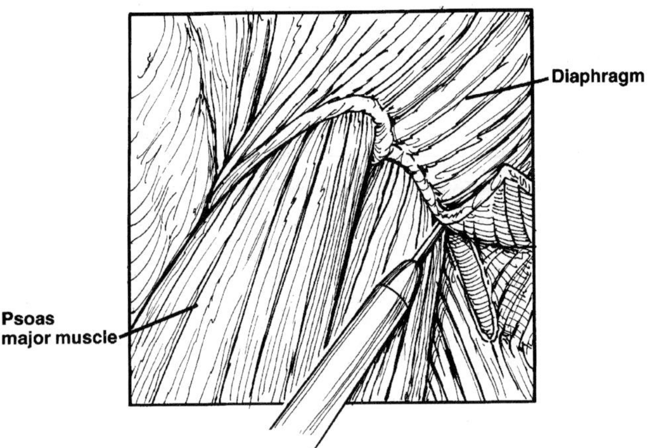

FIG. 54. The release of the peripheral attachment of the diaphragm is achieved by manual traction and cutting diathermy.

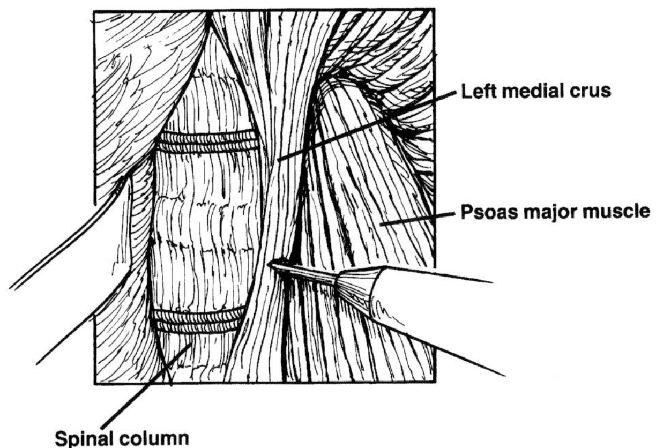

FIG. 55. Division of the fleshy body of the crus to permit its later reattachment. It should be tagged for reattachment.

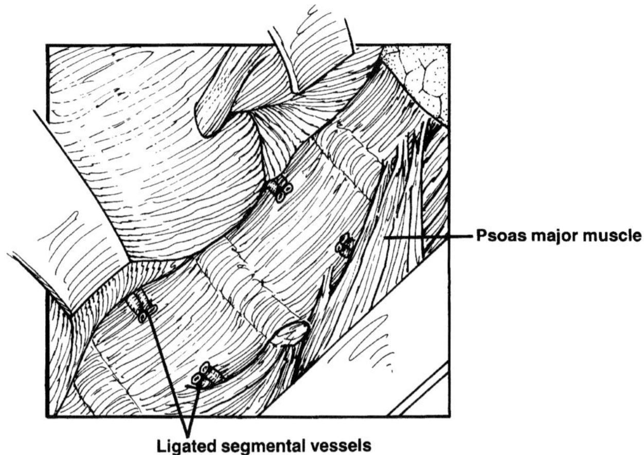

FIG. 57. Ligation of the segmental vessels.

area of the posterior mediastinum. The intercostals and lumbar vessels are ligated in the midline of spine or as close to the aorta as possible (Fig. 57). This maneuver allows the great vessels (i.e., aorta, inferior vena cava) to be displaced. With dissection, the pleura can be detached from the mediastinum to T-10 (Fig. 58). It is preferable to mobilize the psoas to allow full exposure to the lumbar motion segments required. The psoas may be detached as far lateral as the pedicle. Care must be taken to avoid coagulation in the area of the intravertebral foramina.

Some authors prefer to incise the periosteum with cutting diathermy (Fig. 59), and subsequently to expose the vertebral body with a periosteal elevator (Fig. 60), but this method often results in excessive bleeding from the body.

A dissector must be inserted in the vertebral foramen at the base of the pedicle if one wishes to gain access to the posterior vertebral wall. It is preferable to identify the root in the area of each foramen first. A preferable and safer alternative is to approach the posterior wall of the vertebral body by excising the intervertebral disc. Dissection then may proceed proximally or distally. In the area of the thoracolumbar spine, the posterior longitudinal ligament is very thin and usually incised. Indeed, in burst fractures, it may be torn.

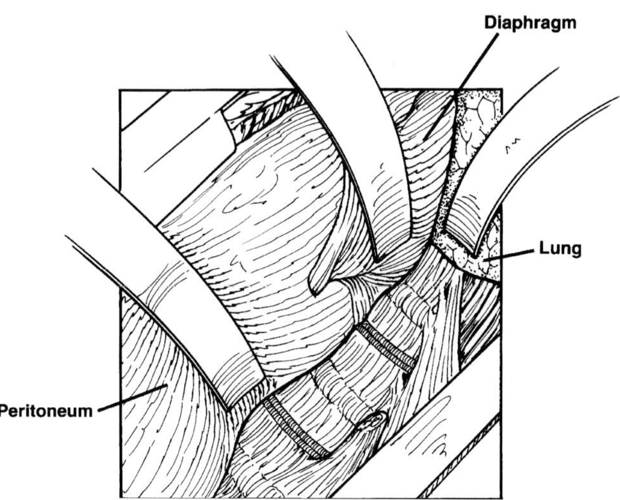

FIG. 56. The two viscera sacs and the diaphragm are retracted anteriorly to the spine and held by malleable retractors.

The diaphragm at the closure is reattached by repairing the crus to the medial and lateral arcuate ligaments. The abdominal and chest walls are then closed in layers. Those who prefer the retropleural retroperitoneal approach feel that postoperative care is easier. The authors have not found this to necessarily be the case in their experience, however.

Transpleural Retroperitoneal Approach

In the transpleural retroperitoneal approach, considerable exposure is achieved by selective intubation and collapse of the ipsilateral lung. This is not necessary, however, especially if exposure is at the lower part of the thoracic spine. Again, exposure through the left side is preferable. The preferable rib to excise is two levels proximal to the most proximal level of path-

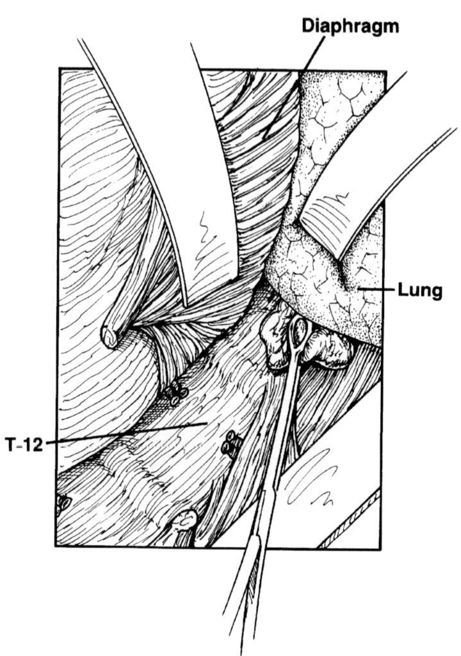

FIG. 58. Detachment of the mediastinal pleura can be extended proximally.

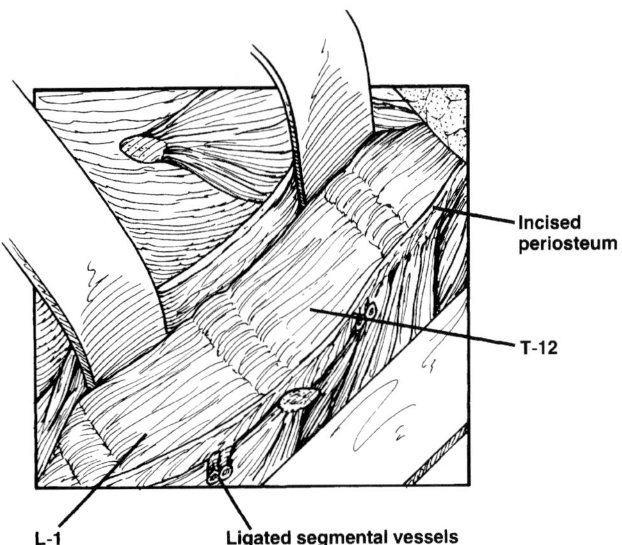

FIG. 59. After incision and elevation of the periosteum in a subperiosteal approach, malleable retractors are placed on the side opposite the vertebral bodies, protecting the viscera and great vessels.

ology. The incision begins posteriorly from the lateral border of the paravertebral muscles and continues for the length of the rib (Fig. 61). If there is a need to be proximal to the tenth or eleventh rib, the incision is carried anteriorly toward the costal margin, and then the distal rib is osteotomized (Fig. 62). The intercostal vessels require ligation in this more proximal approach to mobilize the chest wall. If the approach is through the tenth or eleventh rib, the incision is carried to the midaxillary line by turning the incision distal toward the anterosuperior iliac crest and the lateral margin of the rectus abdominis.

In this approach, the rib is removed and used as graft, although occasionally the incision through the intercostal muscle may be carried out on the superior border of the rib. The rib is removed extraperiosteally, and the pleura is opened. After careful division of the abdominal muscles, the peritoneum is swept from under the transversalis muscle. The eleventh costal cartilage is divided at the junction of the retroperitoneal space and thoracotomy. After this, the peritoneum and its contents are swept off the abdominal wall laterally and from the undersurface of the diaphragm. The diaphragm is then cut approximately 1 cm from the costal margin using cutting diathermy (Fig. 63). The vertebral bodies are approached as for the extrapleural extraperitoneal approach. Closure for the transpleural retroperitoneal transdiaphragmatic approach is performed in a standard manner with repair to the diaphragm. The retroperitoneal space is drained, as is the chest.

Anterior Corpectomy—Surgical Technique

The most common reason to perform a corpectomy is for trauma secondary to a burst injury. The next most common reason is for metastatic disease of the spine. The techniques have some similarities in these two conditions.

When the area of pathology has been reached, it is important that the great vessels be mobilized. This is done by ligating segmental vessels, preferably two levels proximal and two levels distal to the site of pathology. This allows ease of retraction of the great vessels and a safe approach to the contralateral side. The great vessels should be protected by a malleable retractor.

To minimize blood loss, discs at the level above and the level distal to the corpectomy should first be removed. The most proximal and distal end-plates on the normal vertebral bodies should be left intact at this point.

In case of a burst injury (Fig. 64), the part of the body most opposite the side of the approach may be preserved, and typi-

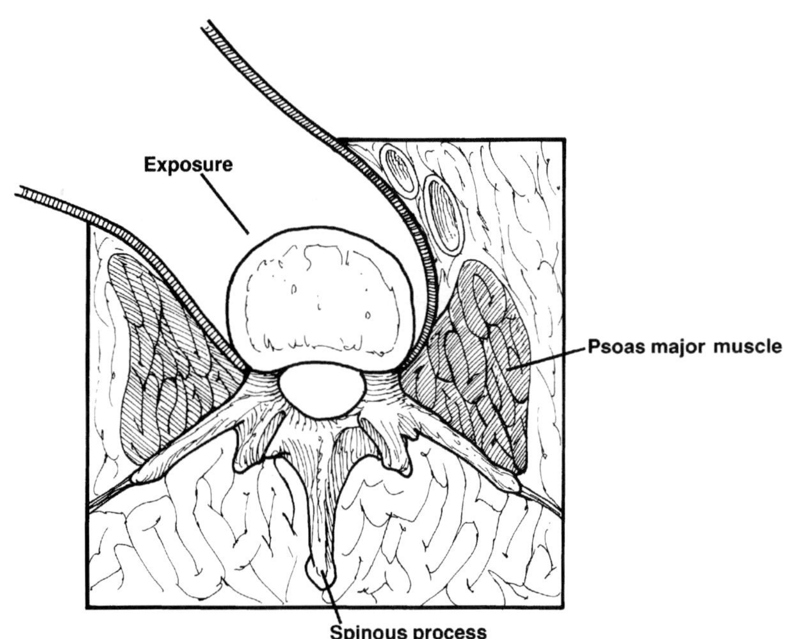

FIG. 60. A malleable retractor retracts and protects the opposite psoas and great vessels. The ipsilateral psoas is dissected off the vertebral body.

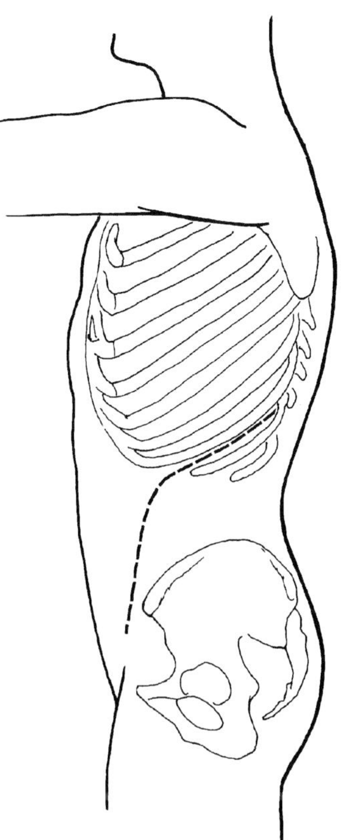

FIG. 61. Oblique incision of the intercostal space. It curves down onto the abdomen at the lateral border of the rectus abdominis to the level of the anterior superior iliac spine. The incision should be placed at least two levels proximal to the most proximal vertebral body chosen in the reconstructive process.

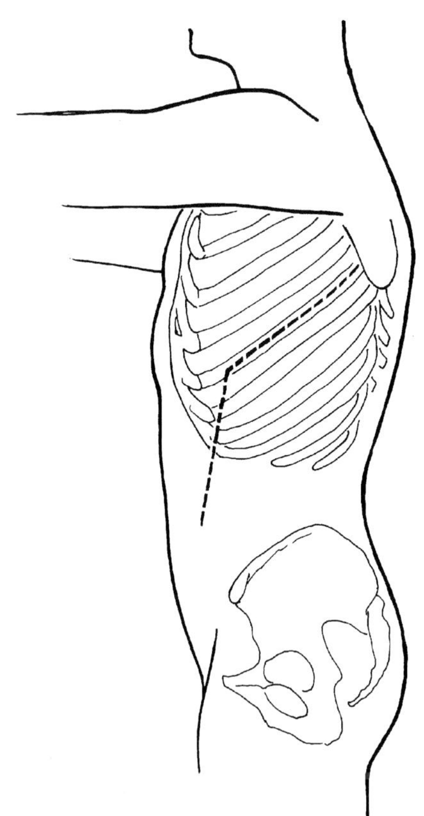

FIG. 62. Position of the patient and skin incision centered on the seventh rib, giving access to T-7 and T-8. Distal ribs are osteotomized.

cally approximately one-fourth of the body can be osteotomized and left attached to the soft tissues. After this, the majority of the body is removed with aid of sharp chisels, taking progressively thinner slices. As one approaches the posterior aspect of the body, these can be approximately 1 mm thickness. Use of rongeurs or high-speed burrs may also be helpful. Once the epidural space is entered, antral punches of various angles aid in increasing exposure of the underlying dura.

In case of a fracture, fragments may remain attached to the disc, and sharp dissection of the disc with a scalpel can help to remove these fragments. Also, the use of a small, sharp chisel on the superoinferior end-plate of the uninvolved vertebral bodies can help detach fragments. Undermining on the upper side can be carried out with antral punches. On the contralateral side, it is the authors' technique to remove a piece of bone, leaving 2 to 3 mm intact against the dural sac. After the trough has been established to the depth of 3 to 4 mm, the ridge closest to the dural sac may be removed, completing decompression. After this, the end-plates of the intact superior and inferior vertebral bodies may be removed. Bleeding is controlled by bipolar cautery; if there is significant bleeding, it may be necessary to arrest the procedure for a short period of time, compressing the dural veins with large pieces of thrombin-soaked Gelfoam with overlying gauze.

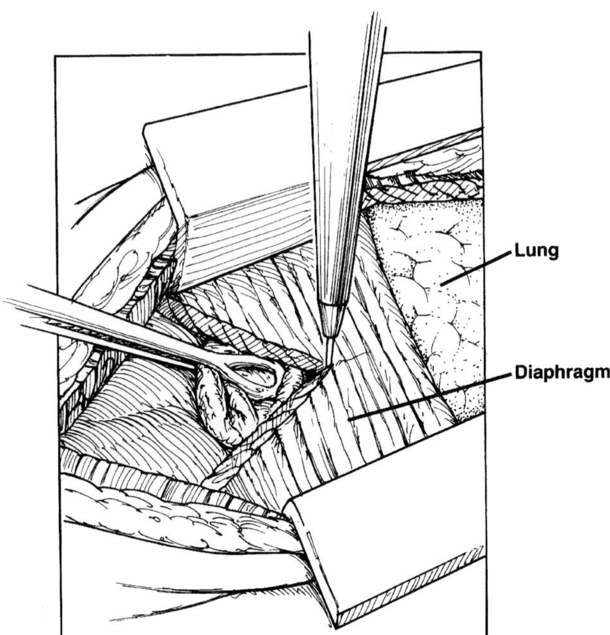

FIG. 63. Division of the periphery of the diaphragm under direct vision after retroperitoneal and transpleural exposure.

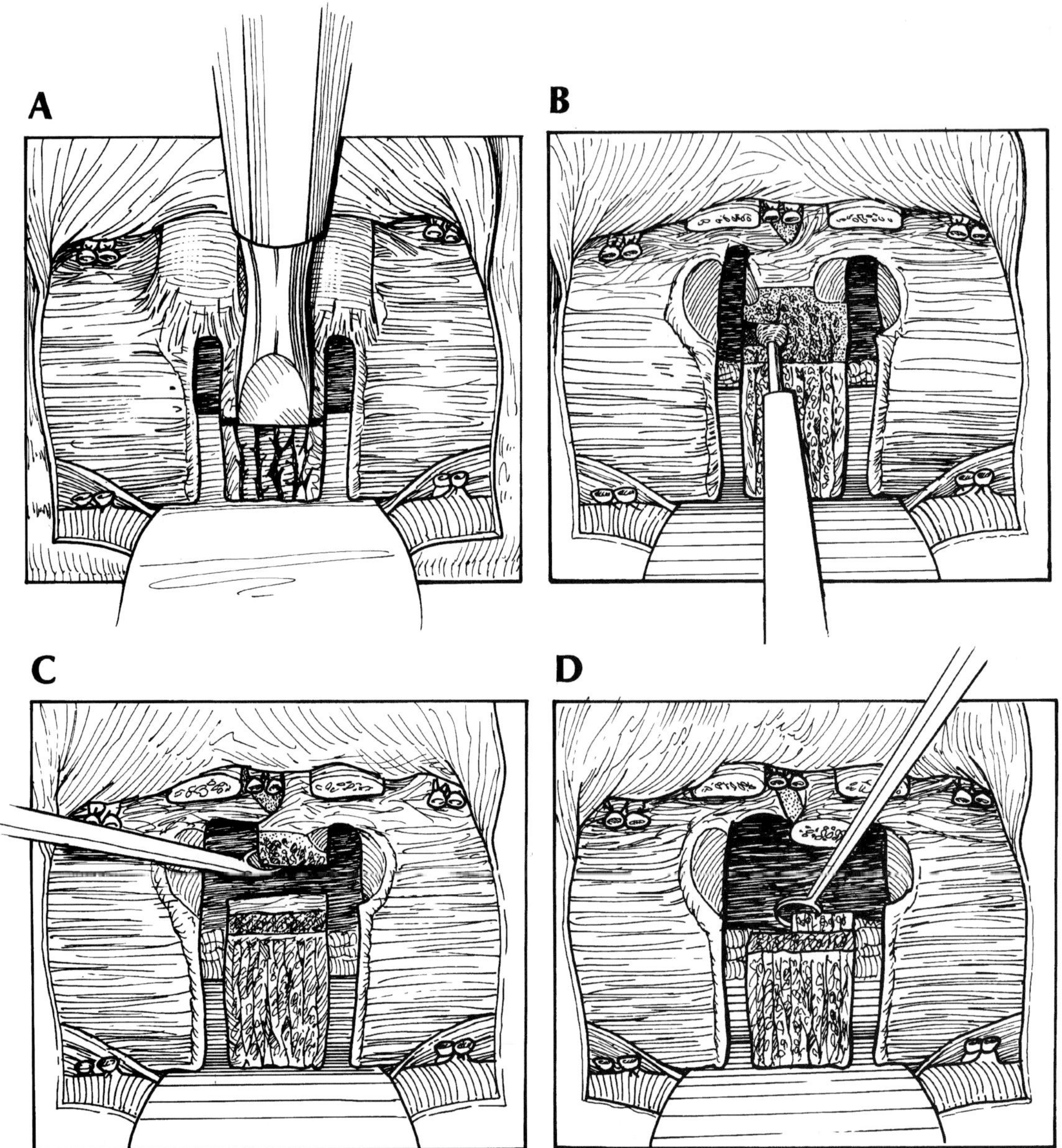

FIG. 64. A: Corpectomy. After exposure, the anterior one-fourth of the body is osteotomized with a chisel and levered forward; it is usually left as a graft. **B,C:** The dura is decompressed using a burr or rongeurs. **D:** Bone from the contralateral side can be removed with a curette.

In the case of tumor, segmental vessels should be similarly ligated. In most cases of tumor that are suspected of being vascular, especially those secondary to renal cell carcinoma, preoperative embolization significantly decreases blood flow and may safely be carried out up to 24 hours before surgery.

These procedures for metastatic disease are not curative. Tumor spill is not important. After isolating the disc space above and below, rongeurs and curettes are usually the instruments most valuable in achieving the corpectomy. This one approach is a dural sac, and smaller curettes may be used. An alternative is to use a Cavitron. The remaining tumor attached to the dural sac should be removed by finding a plane between the dura and the tumor by sharp dissection using a scalpel or by use of a small elevator.

Video-Assisted Thoracoscopic Surgery

The benefits of thoracoscopic surgery are still debated; it potentially could reduce operative times, blood loss, hospital length of stay, and recuperative periods without performing a thoracotomy and its associated potential risks. It has been most useful in patients with spinal deformity, but it has been used in a wide variety of pathologies from thoracic burst fractures and sympathectomies to epidural abscesses and tumor treatment.

General anesthesia is administered with double-lumen intubation, allowing the ipsilateral lung to collapse. The patient is then placed in the direct lateral decubitus position. An axillary roll is placed under the recumbent arm. Usually the portals are placed on the right side, where the hemiazygous vein exists.

Two television monitors are used, one in direct visual line across from the surgical team and a second "slave" monitor in direct visualization for the second assistant.

The C-arm is used to mark levels and portal sites. Portal site placement is key for the procedure. The portals are placed to enable the surgeon to reach the superior and inferior levels of the spine to be released or instrumented. The spine surgeon positions himself at the patient's back, as it orients the surgeon in the same direction as the endoscopic view.

After lung deflation, the initial portal is usually placed in the sixth or seventh interspace, in line with the spine, positioned according to the amount of spinal rotation. Inserting the first portal at this level avoids injury to the diaphragm. The endoscope is inserted into the chest, and additional portals are placed under direct observation. Portal incisions are usually placed directly over the ribs, two interspaces apart. Three or four incisions are used. The portals are 10.5 to 11.0 mm in size.

The pleura is incised longitudinally and dissected along the entire spine. Next, the electrocautery is used to incise the disc annulus. The disc is removed using various commercially available endoscopic instruments. After the disc has been removed and the end-plate completely removed, the disc space is directly inspected with the endoscope to ensure homogeneous bleeding surface.

Using the endoscopic rib cutter, two incisions are made on the superior aspect of the rib. An osteotome is used to cut through the rib along the longitudinal axis. The segmental vessels are grasped at the mid–vertebral body level and cauterized with the electrocautery. A corpectomy can be done or implants are placed with the appropriately designed instruments.

Patients may complain of postoperative dysesthesia over the anterior chest wall, but it is usually transient. Also, mucous plugs in the ventilated lung can be a problem. The major risks of thoracic surgery still exist, and one must be prepared to convert to open procedure if necessary.

INTRAOPERATIVE COMPLICATIONS

Intraoperative complications depend on the pathology and the site of surgery.

Skin

If there has been a previous incision, the old skin scar should be excised. To control hemorrhage, the authors use a diluted solution of 1/500,000 epinephrine (1/1,000 adrenaline in 500 cc of saline) is used. This is injected intraarticularly, subcutaneously, and in the muscle planes. This technique appears to decrease considerably soft-tissue bleeding for up to 2 hours during surgery. Meticulous coagulation of bleeding points should be achieved as the layers are dissected. Skin edges should be sutured so that edges are everted. Staples are excellent for wound closure and decrease the risk of postoperative wound healing difficulties. If there is considerable subcutaneous fat, the compartment should be drained as well. The risk of infection is also minimized by use of pulsatile irrigation, used periodically during the procedure to wash out the wound. All necrotic tissues should be débrided before closure.

Hemorrhage

The degree of blood loss depends on the extent and the time of surgery. Most cases requiring spinal cord decompression should have a cell saver available. If suction of blood greater than 2,000 cc through the cell saver occurs, then the patient should receive fresh-frozen plasma as well as platelets to prevent coagulopathy, which can be frequent under such circumstances. Most blood loss is secondary to oozing from tissues. This may be minimized in bony tissues by the use of bone wax, which, however, may interfere with subsequent arthrodesis and, therefore, should be used judiciously. In anterior decompressions, during corpectomy, the use of large pledges of Gelfoam gently compressed with patties of gauze can aid in controlling bleeding. Epidural bleeding, should it be encountered, can also be controlled by the use of Gelfoam or bipolar coagulation, or both. Epidural bleeding may be extensive in cases requiring anterior decompression, such as in acute burst injuries and in certain tumor types, such as renal cell carcinoma. Such tumors are best dealt with by preoperative angiographies and embolization of feeding vessels. This may also be true for primary tumors, particularly those that are malignant.

The greatest blood loss, however, may be encountered through inadvertent division of large vessels, particularly large veins, which are more difficult to repair than large arteries. When the lesions are in the distal spine, there may be large blood loss from the iliolumbar veins; similarly, it may be encountered from the azygos veins in a thoracotomy. For this reason, the authors prefer to use the left-sided approach when possible, because the aorta protects venous structures. A knowledge of anatomy and the judicious tying off of large veins is important for exposure. The cell saver is a useful adjunct and can decrease transfusion requirements.

Dural Tears

A dural tear during a posterior approach is usually relatively easy to repair using Prolene on a very small noncutting needle. It may be necessary to remove further bone to gain easy access. Anterior dural tears are much more difficult to repair, and it may not be possible to remove more bone to gain access. These tears may be controlled by applying Gelfoam and allowing time for the dural tear to close spontaneously. The addition of free soft-muscle tissue to the site of a dural tear may also help to control bleeding. Large dural tears may require repair with free dural grafts, fascial grafts, or synthetics such as Duragen sutured or glued in place. Also, fibrin glue has proven to be effective as an additional level of barrier and protection of a dural repair.

Neurologic Injury

Major neurologic injury is rare in spinal surgery regardless of pathology, and occurs in approximately 1% of patients. Patients with pre-existing neurologic problems are probably best given a dose of dexamethasone preoperatively, which is then tapered off over a period of 4 to 5 days.

The use of somatosensory evoked and/or motor evoked potentials has greatly aided the operating surgeon in assessing neurologic difficulties. However, there may be a latency period of up to 20 minutes after injury before they can be recorded, particularly for the somatosensory evoked potentials. These potentials may be obtained through cortical evoked or spinal evoked means.

In the lower lumbar spine, the risk of neurologic injury during the application of pedicle fixation may be minimized through the use of direct pedicle hole stimulation and EMG peripheral recordings. During the procedure, after development of the pedicle hole and before insertion of the pedicle screw, the hole may be stimulated for an EMG response. After insertion of the screw, restimulation is important as well. If there is any positive response at a low threshold, then a new hole should be developed.

Infection Control

Antibiotics are administered prophylactically at the commencement of the operation and maintained for a minimum of 24 hours. In patients who are at high risk or debilitated, they may be continued for a longer period of time. The authors like to redose antibiotics for every 1,000 cc of blood loss. Also, the authors minimize the amount of preoperative dry shaving as it can increase infection rates.

POSTOPERATIVE MANAGEMENT

Management of the patient after spinal surgery of the thoracic, thoracolumbar, or lumbar spine depends very much on the pathology, the level of surgery, and the general condition of the patient.

For transpleural approaches, an evacuation of the pleural cavity by chest suction of 20 cm of water is necessary. On the average, tubes are removed approximately 48 hours postoperatively, but they may be left in significantly longer depending on drainage. Once drainage has decreased to less than 50 cc a day, they may be safely removed. A chest x-ray must be taken to ensure the patient does not have pneumothorax.

It is the authors' current practice to drain all cavities in retroperitoneal approaches, as well as posterior approaches with the use of suction drainage for approximately 48 hours.

Pain Management

Thoracotomy incisions are best managed by the injection of bupivacaine on the intercostal nerves at the site of incision. This decreases pain resulting from respiratory movements, and it decreases possible morbidity related to atelectasis and other respiratory problems. Above T-11, the intercostal nerve at that level of the incision is best excised to diminish postoperative incisional pain and postthoracotomy syndrome. Epidural morphine is also of value in controlling pain.

The mainstay of postoperative pain management is patient-controlled analgesia, and this is maintained until bowel sounds return, at which time early administration of mild narcotics such as acetaminophen with 30 mg codeine is administered.

Antiembolism Measures

Pulsatile stockings may be used intraoperatively and maintained postoperatively with TED hose. In addition, most patients undergoing extensive surgery are anticoagulated. The anticoagulation regimen the authors use currently entails low-molecular-weight heparin that starts on the first postoperative day. Anticoagulation is maintained until the patient is discharged. In patients who have a previous history of thrombophlebitis or thromboembolism, anticoagulation is maintained for a period of approximately 3 months.

Nutrition

In the immediate postoperative period, fluid is administered, usually in the form of a 2/3 to 1/3 solution. In patients who are undergoing multiple-stage surgery, parenteral peripheral nutrition is administered. In patients who are debilitated, total parenteral nutrition may be administered.

Respiratory Toilet

Patients who have undergone a prolonged procedure require considerable fluid replacement. As a result, there may be some degree of fluid overload and there exists a risk of pulmonary edema or respiratory distress syndrome. Vigorous chest physiotherapy is mandated. This includes sitting the patient up early, using spirometry, breathing exercises, chest manipulation, good fluid control, and adequate moisture.

It may be necessary to administer a diuretic. Respiratory assistance through continued intubation may be necessary, depending on the patient's age, the level of surgery, and the degree of pulmonary retraction required during surgery for thoracic procedures. The authors prefer to have a double-lumen tube for high thoracic problems when the procedure was transpleural. This allows decompression of the lung on the affected side without retraction, and it is less traumatizing. It is important that the lung be fully reinflated before the chest cavity is closed. Monitoring with periodic x-rays and blood gas measurements may be necessary.

Positioning in Bed

During the first 12 hours after posterior approaches, the patients are allowed to lie on their wounds to compress the wound and decrease the possibility of hematoma development. After this, the patients are rolled and are kept off their backs, positioned with pillows to prevent accumulation of perspiration and other fluids that may macerate a posterior wound. Dressings are changed at 48 hours and daily thereafter. Sutures are taken out at a minimum of 10 days after surgery. The wounds are kept dry during this time.

Ambulation

Patients are usually mobilized by postoperative day 1. If there is any neurologic deficit, they are log-rolled every 2 hours to prevent skin breakdown and mobilized to a chair and ambulation when possible. Those who may have a residual neurologic deficit that precludes standing are helped into a chair for continued respiratory toilet. Patients with neurologic deficit commence muscular rehabilitation 48 hours after surgery in their hospital bed, through a combination of passive and active exercises designed in conjunction with physiotherapy. Resistive exercises with springs and weights are usually used. Orthoses may be used to prevent the development of contractures in patients with neurologic deficits (e.g., drop foot).

Radiologic Control

X-rays should be taken immediately postoperatively to assess position of internal fixation implants. They should be done again before the patient is discharged. Films should allow assessment of coronal and sagittal balance as well as the implants on a single cassette.

Wound Infection

Wound infection after anterior surgery is extremely rare and in the authors' experience has been approximately 1:500. The risk for posterior surgery is greater and ranges from 2 to 4%. When an infection is suspected, an aspiration should be performed and cultures taken. If a wound infection fails to respond to local dressings and systemic antibiotics after 4 to 5 days, the wound should be opened and débrided and a decision made as to whether to leave the wound open or to close it, primarily over suction drainage. Suction drainage may be used to instill regional antibiotics and provide constant irrigation as well.

If internal implants have been used for fixation and if they are not loose, then they should be left in place. If they are loose, they should be removed and an alternate form of fixation should be used, externally (e.g., braces, casts, complete bed rest) or internally from the side of the spine opposite the site of infection.

If neither the local opening and packing of the wound nor the use of irrigation is effective in controlling infection, consideration should be given to the use of implantable antibiotic polymethylmethacrylate beads. If the implants are loose, then they should be removed and the back should be stabilized with reimplanted internal devices or external fixation regardless of the antibiotic treatment. If the wound is left open, delayed closure may be obtained by wet to dry dressings. Also, vacuum-assisted wound closure therapy has been a useful addition in improving outcomes in difficult cases, especially those patients who have diabetes or are immunocompromised. If the tissues are too rigid, then a rotation flap may be necessary.

Finally, it is important to note the nutritional status of the patient. Nutritional supplement between meals is important. It is important to track the albumin and total lymphocyte count to asses the patient's status, especially if the operation is staged.

REFERENCES

1. Bradford DS, Lonstein JE, Ogilvie JW, et al. *Moe's textbook of scoliosis and other spinal deformities*, 2nd ed. Philadelphia: WB Saunders, 1987:135–189.
2. Canale ST. *Campbell's operative orthopaedics*, 9th ed. St. Louis: Mosby, 1998:2691–2695.
3. Dwyer AF, Newton NC, Sherwood AA. An anterior approach to scoliosis. *Clin Orthop* 1969;62:192–202.
4. Freebody D, Bedall R, Taylor RD. Anterior trauma transperitoneal lumbar fusion. *J Bone Joint Surg (Br)* 1971;53(4):617–627.
5. Hall JE. The anterior approach to spinal deformities. *Orthop Clin North Am* 1972;3(1):81–98.
6. Harmon PH. Anterior extraperitoneal lumbar disk excision and vertebral body fusion. *Clin Orthop* 1963;16:169–198.
7. Hodgson AR, et al. Anterior spinal fusion: the operative approach and pathological findings in 412 patients with Pott's disease of the spine. *Br J Surg* 1960;58:172.
8. Hodgson AR, Yau AC. Anterior approach to the spinal column. In: Appley G, ed. *Recent advances in orthopaedics*. Baltimore: Williams & Wilkins, 1964:289–326.
9. Hoppenfeld S, deBoer P. *Surgical exposures in orthopaedics*, 2nd ed. Philadelphia: JB Lippincott Co, 1994:216–279.
10. Laurin CA, Riley LH, Roy-Camille R. *Atlas of orthopaedic surgery: general principles and spine*. Vol. 1. Paris: Masson, 1989.
11. Moskovich R, Benson D, Zhang ZH, et al. Extracoelomic approach to the spine. *J Bone Joint Surg (Br)* 1993;75(6):886–893.
12. Riseborough EJ. The anterior approach to the spine for the correction of deformity of the axial skeleton. *Clin Orthop* 1973;93:207–214.
13. Watkings RG. *Surgical approaches to the spine*. New York: Springer-Verlag, 1983.
14. Suk SI, Kim WJ, Lee SM, et al. Thoracic pedicle screw fixation in spinal deformities. *Spine* 2001;18:2049–2057.
15. Cinotti G, Gumina S, Ripani M, et al. Pedicle instrumentation in the thoracic spine. *Spine* 1999;24(2)114–119.
16. McLain RF, Ferrara L, Kabins M. Pedicle morphometry in the upper thoracic spine. *Spine* 2002;27(22):2467–2471.
17. Shi YB, Martin WH, Pearson JM, et al. Electrical stimulation for intraoperative thoracic pedicle screw placement. *Spine* 2003;28(6):595–601.
18. Ridenour TR, Haddad SF, Hitchon PW, et al. Herniated thoracic disks: treatment and outcome. *J Spinal Disord* 1993;6(3):218–224.
19. Dinh DH, Tompkins J, Clark SB. Transcostovertebral approach for thoracic disc herniations. *J Neurosurg* 2001;94(1):38–44.
20. Vaccaro AR, Albert T. *Spine surgery*. New York: Thieme, 2003:78–80.

CHAPTER 53

Positioning and Approaches to the Thoracolumbar Spine

A. Traditional Approaches

Robert F. McLain

Any portion of the thoracolumbar, lumbar, or lumbosacral spine can be completely exposed through a properly chosen surgical approach. By understanding the three-dimensional anatomy of the lumbar spine and establishing a well-considered surgical plan, the spine surgeon can choose an approach or combination of approaches that will provide direct access to the critical lesion and permit extensile exposure. Although the vast majority of surgical procedures can be carried out through a posterior approach, there are a wide variety of surgical problems that call for an anterior or combined approach, and the surgeon with a diverse practice should be well prepared to apply any of these approaches (1,2). Depending on the situation, the surgeon may be required to enlarge an exposure, extend it cranially or caudally through important structures, or complete an anterior procedure by adding a posterior approach. Preoperative planning is crucial if such contingencies are to be appreciated ahead of time.

The choice of exposure dictates, to a great extent, the specific complications for which the surgeon must prepare: Preoperative testing of pulmonary function is more often necessary for patients in whom the diaphragm may be taken down, and wound complications may be anticipated when a posterior approach is carried through irradiated skin. When possible, the surgeon should choose the approach that exposes the individual patient to the least risk, avoiding old scars, damaged tissue, or potential systemic complications. Most often, however, the approach used is dictated by the location of the spinal lesion itself. Anterior lesions are usually best addressed through an anterolateral approach, and posterior lesions and compressive radiculopathies are best approached through a posterior or posterolateral exposure. The treatment of complex lumbar disorders—tumors, infections, complex reconstructions, or severe trauma—often requires a combined approach using both anterior and posterior exposures.

Even as surgical procedures become more complex and technically challenging, surgical exposures are being progressively reduced and minimized. Although laparoscopic and endoscopic techniques have greatly altered the approach to certain kinds of spinal disorders, minimally open procedures have produced similar improvements by modifying more traditional surgical exposures. Minimally invasive approaches promise (and have delivered) reduced blood loss, reduced morbidity, and more rapid functional recovery. The small skin incisions should not disguise the fact that these patients have still had major surgery and need to be cared for and observed as carefully as any of the more traditionally treated patients.

The principles for success remain the same for each of the standard approaches discussed below: careful assessment of the patient, fundamental knowledge of the three-dimensional anatomy of the spine, anticipation of complicating factors and hazards, careful preoperative preparation and positioning, and skillful technique in executing the surgical approach. A skillful exposure that is well positioned greatly enhances the rest of the surgical procedure.

PREOPERATIVE PLANNING

Once an appropriate surgical plan has been made, the surgeon must address a number of issues to ensure that the preferred approach can be safely and successfully carried out. In assessing patients preoperatively, consider their capacity to tolerate the given approach, their likelihood of developing serious complications, and their medical and surgical history. Although an anterior exposure may be the best or even the only reasonable approach to a given lumbar lesion, previous infection, local irradiation, or surgery through the same region considerably increases the likelihood of complications and may make surgical treatment unwise. Even when the anterior approach is absolutely necessary, previous surgery, irradiation, infection, or tumor mass may make the standard, left-sided approach impossible, leaving the more difficult right-sided approach as the best option.

Preoperative studies, such as magnetic resonance imaging, along with a careful history and physical examination, should alert the surgeon to these factors, allowing the team to establish an alternate plan or even choose another treatment modality; it should rarely happen that an approach is abandoned because of inability to complete the exposure. In cases of tumor or infection, however, this possibility may exist, and the surgeon must recognize and warn the patient that some procedures may not be carried to conclusion without exposing the patient to an excessive risk of catastrophe, and that the surgeon may then have to retreat rather than gamble with the patient's life.

After selecting the best approach and establishing the patient's capacity to tolerate both the surgery and the recovery, plans must be made to carry out the operation successfully. Have the right instruments and appliances available to carry out the principle operation. It is a good idea to have the tools needed for the most likely back-up plan, as well as those needed to deal quickly and effectively with the most likely complications. If the surgeon carrying out the approach is not very experienced in dealing with certain types of problems (e.g., vascular injuries, dural tears), a more experienced surgeon should at least be available and in all likelihood should assist or perform the exposure. Having the support of an experienced surgical team is equally important; for this reason, complex surgical procedures that can tax the surgeon in the best of circumstances should not be carried out in the evenings or on weekends unless the nurses, circulators, and anesthesia staff that usually participate in these cases can also be assembled. Even then, it is often prudent to postpone these kinds of cases until a more routine starting time is available.

Finally, preparation and positioning of the patient plays a role in the success of any procedure and of any given exposure. Spinal cord monitoring and cell-saver equipment routinely should be arranged in advance, and the need for routine x-ray or fluoroscopic imaging should be communicated to the appropriate staff. Arrange the appropriate operating table and positioning frame in advance, and familiarize the operating room staff with their uses. Posterior approaches may be carried out with the patient positioned on any of a number of prone frames, ranging from the Wilson frame or Pheasant frame (used with a standard operating room table) to the radiolucent Jackson turning frame; the situation frequently dictates a preference for one type or the other. Patients with lumbar fractures requiring posterior stabilization need to be positioned so that the normal lumbar lordosis is reestablished before instrumentation is carried out and may be as well positioned on a standard operating table using transverse bolsters as on a more elaborate frame. Patients undergoing lumbar decompression may be better treated in the knee-chest position, using an Andrews frame or table. In this position, the abdomen hangs free, reducing intraabdominal pressure and central venous pressure, and the lumbar spine is flexed, spreading the spinous processes and opening the interlaminar space for easier decompression. If instrumentation and fusion are planned after decompression, a table should be chosen that allows the surgeon to shift from knee-chest to the prone position to allow instrumentation in normal lordotic alignment. Finally, any frame used during pedicle screw placement should allow fluoroscopic visualization, and any table used must allow access of the fluoroscope.

POSTERIOR AND POSTEROLATERAL APPROACHES

The vast majority of thoracolumbar, lumbar, and lumbosacral procedures are carried out through one of these two approaches, with some minor variation. The incision and dissection in this region seem quite straightforward and simple, yet the ease with which subsequent procedures are carried out, the success of the procedures attempted, and the likelihood of postoperative scarring and disability are all dependent on the quality of the exposure. Inadequate or poorly placed incisions invite excessive retraction on skin and muscle, leading to wound complications, scarring, and infection. Overzealous incisions result in unnecessary tissue damage and increase the risk of infection. Poorly placed incisions make subsequent decompression or screw placement unnecessarily difficult or dangerous. Finally, inadequate exposure resulting from undue haste or poor technique is often a contributor to pseudarthrosis and surgical failure.

Percutaneous Biopsy and Discectomy Techniques

The simplest surgical procedures carried out in the lumbar spine are aspirations, injections, and biopsies performed by percuta-

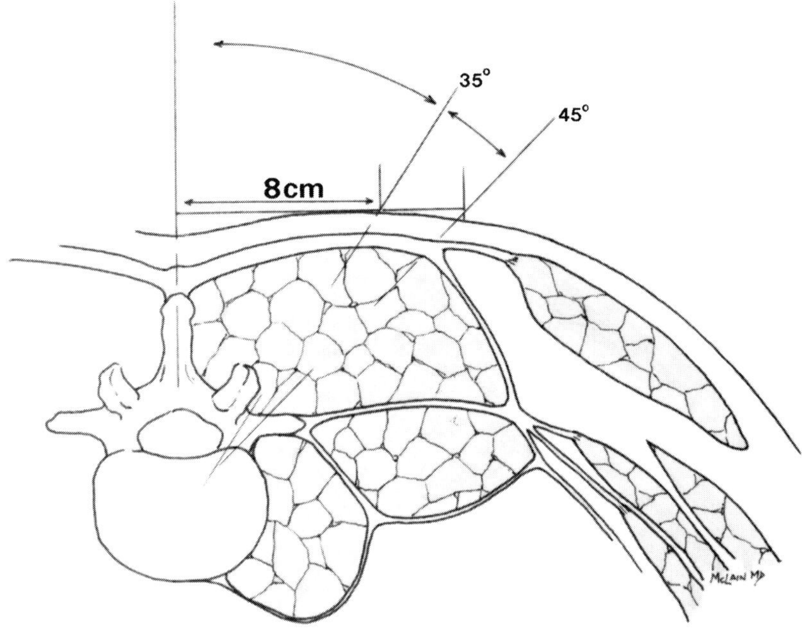

FIG. 1. Surgical approach to the intervertebral disc or vertebral body for discography, biopsy, chymopapain injection, or percutaneous nucleotomy.

neous technique. The vertebral bodies and intervertebral discs L-1 to L-5 to S-1 can be accessed by fine or Craig needle with little risk to the patient and limited need for anesthesia (3). Aspirations for discitis or osteomyelitis, soft- and hard-tissue biopsies for tumor or infection, as well as needle placement for discography, chymopapain injection, or percutaneous nucleotomy can be carried out in the prone or decubitus position using fluoroscopic control for guidance. In the upper lumbar spine, the entry point for needle placement is 8 cm lateral to the posterior midline, whereas at the lower lumbar levels, the starting point drifts 2 to 4 cm more laterally (Fig. 1). In either case, the patient is positioned on a radiolucent operating table, and, after properly preparing the skin and draping the operative field, the needle or guide-pin is positioned over the correct level under fluoroscopic guidance. Using the C-arm to check both anterior-posterior and lateral views, the needle is advanced at a 45-degree angle to the annulus or biopsy site (4).

If a percutaneous nucleotomy or Craig needle biopsy is intended, make a small skin incision with an 11 blade to allow passage of the trocar. Otherwise, advance the trocar or needle directly to the intended disc or vertebral level. At the upper lumbar level, the angle of inclination from the entry site should be between 35 degrees and 45 degrees and parallel to the end-plate; at L-4, the appropriate angle is approximately 45 degrees (5). The most difficult region to access is the L-5 to S-1 disc space. A parasagittal approach to this structure is possible, but it is difficult to accomplish. Discography at L-5 to S-1 is often performed via a transthecal posterior puncture; this is not an appropriate avenue for chymopapain injection or aspiration of a suspected infection.

Midline Posterior Approach

The midline posterior approach is the most common surgical approach in thoracolumbar and lumbar surgery. Place the patient in the prone position on the appropriate surgical frame. If lumbar decompression is planned, place the patient in the knee-chest position, with the abdomen hanging free and the lumbar spine flexed. If fusion is anticipated, the patient may be placed on a four-poster frame or across transverse bolsters, with the knees and hips flexed to release the hamstrings and permit normal lumbar lordosis. If pedicle screw instrumentation is planned, use a radiolucent table with transverse bolsters or a radiolucent frame designed for pedicle screw placement. Once positioned, prep the back widely, from the top of the buttocks to the midthoracic region, including one or both iliac crests, and drape the patient for surgery.

Depending on the size of the incision, take a localizing x-ray before or just after the exposure is begun. For discectomy procedures, place a spinal needle at the appropriate level, based on the best estimate from surface anatomy. After verifying the correct starting point radiographically, incise directly to the underlying spinous process and mark the spine with a single suture. For multilevel reconstructions, the surgeon may easily estimate the midpoint of the surgical field and adjust the dissection one or two levels cranial or caudal, depending on intraoperative localizing film. As the intercrestal line generally falls over the L4-5 interspace, the surgeon should be able to estimate the underlying spinal anatomy to within a single interspace cranial or caudal in any but the most obese patients. In these patients, a more extensive incision is usually necessary in any event.

Incise the skin in the midline. Minimize cutaneous hemorrhage by scoring the skin prior to incision and infiltrating the subcutaneous tissues and paraspinous muscles with a 1:500,000 solution of epinephrine in saline. Divide the subcutaneous tissues sharply or with cautery and place shallow self-retaining retractors to encourage hemostasis before deep dissection. In routine dissections, the cautery dissection is carried directly to the supraspinous ligament and spinous processes through the lumbodorsal fascia. At this point, the spine may be stripped bilaterally, or if a unilateral laminotomy or hemilaminectomy is planned, the paraspinous muscles can be taken down on one side while leaving the other side intact. The lumbodorsal fascia is

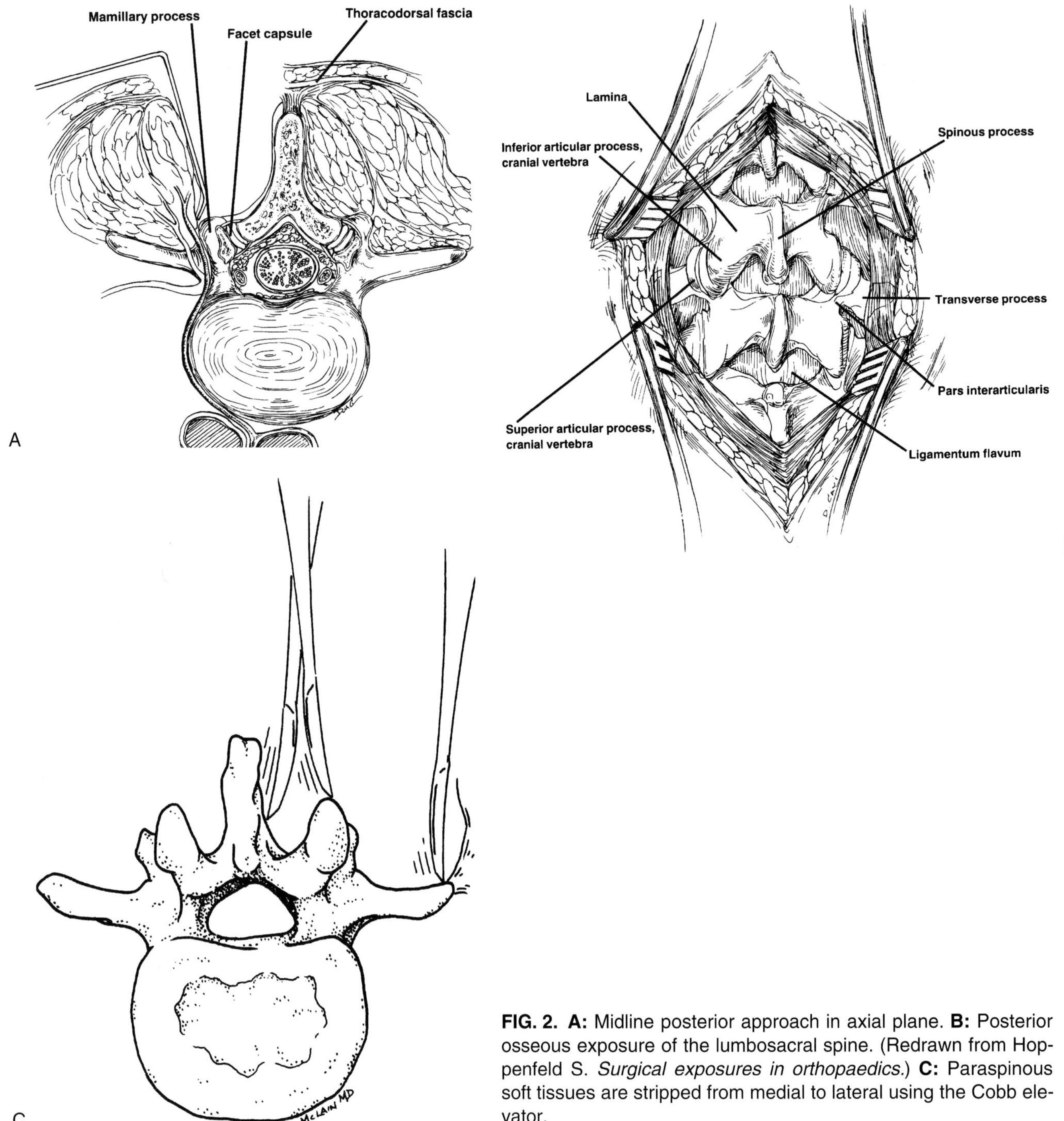

FIG. 2. A: Midline posterior approach in axial plane. **B:** Posterior osseous exposure of the lumbosacral spine. (Redrawn from Hoppenfeld S. *Surgical exposures in orthopaedics.*) **C:** Paraspinous soft tissues are stripped from medial to lateral using the Cobb elevator.

divided just off the centerline, and a Cobb elevator is placed at the superior margin of the spinous process. Subperiosteal dissection proceeds from dorsal to volar along the flank of the spinous process, working from caudal to cranial along the spine. In the case of fracture, approach the zone of injury with care, completing the dissection down to normal tissues proximally and distally before approaching the actual fracture site. This is done to protect neural tissues that may have been extruded posteriorly through a laminar fracture or flexion-distraction injury. By keeping the surgical dissection subperiosteal, muscular damage and hemorrhage are minimized. After stripping the paraspinous muscles down to the level of the lamina, the Cobb elevator is turned over, and the facets and transverse processes are exposed (Fig. 2A). Care is taken not to damage facet capsules at levels that will not be fused.

Exposure of the facets and transverse processes is key to reliable fusion surgery and should be done in a meticulous, routine fashion. After placing the deep self-retaining retractors (cerebellar or large Gelpi retractors), the assistant should retract the paraspinous musculature to expose the insertion of the multifi-

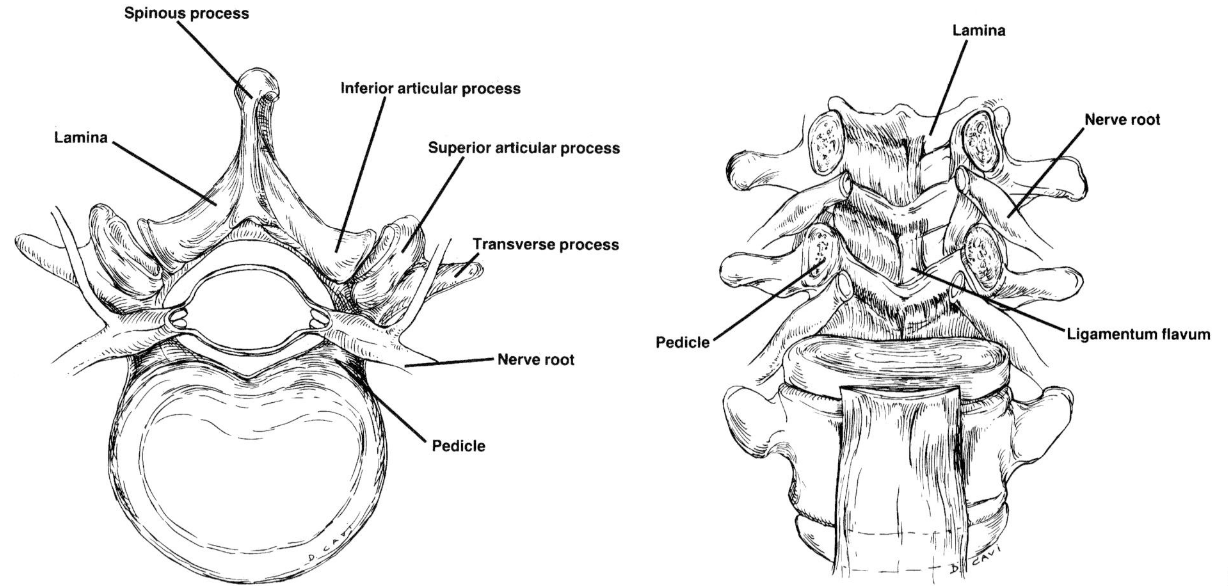

FIG. 3. A: Transverse (axial) plane section of a lumbar segment emphasizing orientation of spinous process bulbous tip, facet articular processes, pedicle, and neuromotor elements. **B:** View from the inside of the canal looking posteriorly demonstrates the anatomy of the ligamentum flavum. The ligamentum flavum originates approximately midway under the cephalad lamina and inserts onto the cephalad edge of the caudal lamina below. The ligamentum flavum is thinnest in the midline, providing the easiest point of entry into the spinal canal. (Redrawn from Watkins RG. Anterior retroperitoneal flank approach to L5-S1. In: *Surgical approaches to the spine*. New York: Springer-Verlag, 1983.)

dus onto the facets. This musculotendinous insertion and the accompanying intermuscular septum form a wall along the lateral side of the facets that must be divided longitudinally to allow access to the lateral gutters and the transverse processes (Fig. 2B). If spinal fusion is intended, the facet capsule should be removed at each level to be fused with a rongeur or chisel, and the muscular insertions along the lateral margin of the facet should be released with the cautery. Cobb dissection is then directed down over the lateral margin of the superior facet onto the transverse process (Fig. 2C). Reversing the Cobb again, the multifidus and intertransverse muscles can be swept from the surface of the process in one or two passes. Bleeding vessels encountered over the lateral margin of the facet and along the superior and inferior margins of the transverse process at its base can be controlled with bipolar cautery (6) (Fig. 3A). If fusion is not intended, this dissection is unnecessary, and the facet capsules should be left alone.

Access to the spinal canal is gained by removing the ligamentum flavum, with or without some portion of the vertebral lamina. If a wide exposure is desired, the interspinous ligament may be taken down with a large rongeur, exposing the whole width of the ligamentum (7). The yellow hue and vertical striations of the ligamentum make this tissue easy to recognize in primary procedures, but in revision surgery, scar and adhesions force a more painstaking and meticulous approach (Fig. 3B). The bulk of the ligamentum may be taken down in the midline using the rongeur, and as the structure is thinned, smaller bites are taken until epidural fat becomes visible through the median raphe. At this point, the Kerrison rongeur is introduced through the midline rift, and the ligamentum is resected back to the facet on either side. After protecting the dura and epidural veins with a small cottonoid, laminotomy or laminectomy may be carried out as desired (Fig. 4).

Posterolateral Approach

The posterolateral approach to the lumbar spine allows direct access to the facets and transverse processes without stripping

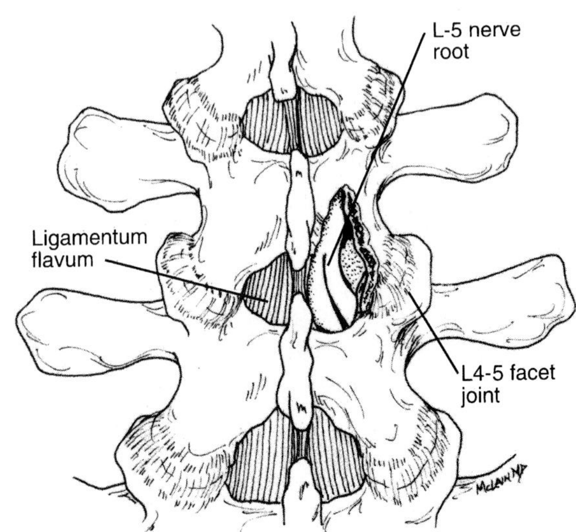

FIG. 4. A laminotomy at L4-5 with medial facetectomy is used to expose the compressed L-5 nerve root, the cauda equina, and the herniated fragment of nucleus pulposus.

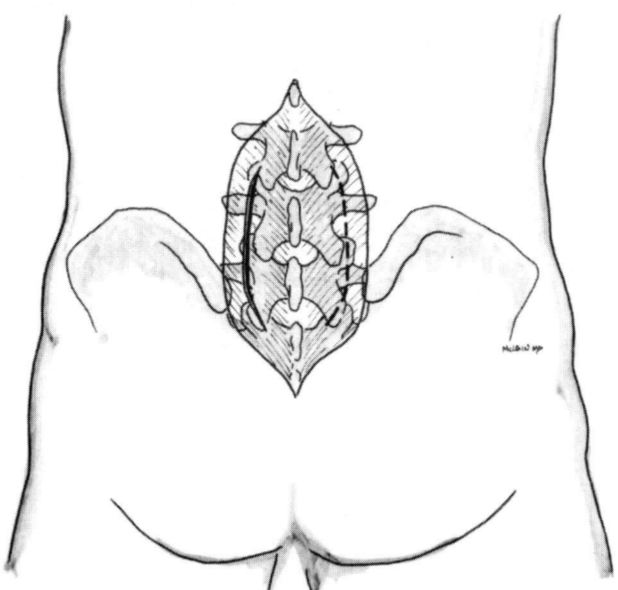

FIG. 5. The paraspinous approach to the lumbar spine can be carried out through either a single midline skin incision or paired paraspinous skin incisions. The muscle-splitting incision is carried out through a paraspinous fascial incision in either case.

the paraspinous musculature from the spinous processes. Taking advantage of the fascial plane between the multifidus and the erector spinae muscles, this approach provides excellent exposure for lower lumbar fusion and pedicle screw instrumentation procedures. By exposing the lateral aspect of the facet and transverse process, this approach also provides access to the spinal nerve root as it exits the lateral boundary of the intervertebral foramen, permitting decompression of far lateral disc herniations or lateral margin osteophytes. Access is also available to the lateral aspect of the pedicle and vertebral body (8).

This approach has been popularized by Wiltse and colleagues (9,10); it requires less retraction of the medial paraspinous musculature and may reduce operative blood loss by taking advantage of the anatomic plane between the multifidus and the longissimus. The approach also encourages a more lateral starting point for lower lumbar pedicle screws, minimizing damage to adjacent facets and assuring a lateral to medial orientation. Stripping of the facet capsule and lamina can still be carried out from this approach, and medial foraminotomies, medial facetectomies and foraminotomies, or complete foraminal decompression can be carried out through this approach. The primary advantage of the approach, however, remains the excellent access to the transverse processes and facets, and its classic application is in the instrumentation and *in situ* fusion of lumbosacral spondylolisthesis.

Start this exposure by incising the skin in the midline, as in the standard posterior approach, or bilaterally, two to three finger breadths off the midline (Fig. 5). The midline incision is carried through the skin and subcutaneous tissue to the lumbodorsal fascia, after which skin flaps are elevated laterally to expose the fascia over the lower lumbar facets, approximately 5 cm to either side of the midline. Bilateral paraspinous incisions are then made through the fascia, creating a gentle medial curve at the cranial and caudal extremes of the incision. The fascial incision will lie over the muscular interval between the multifidus and longissimus, which is bluntly developed to expose the facet joints and transverse processes below (Fig. 6). Alternatively, a paraspinous skin incision can be used directly over the sacrospinalis muscle group without creating the skin flap. Once the facet joint has been identified, a deep Williams or Gelpi retractor may be placed and the Cobb elevator used to strip the soft tissues from the transverse process laterally and from the facet and lamina medially. A bipolar cautery is used to obtain hemostasis around the transverse process and facet by identifying and coagulating the communicating and intraarticular branches of the segmental artery (Fig. 7).

After stripping the remaining soft tissues from the inferior and lateral margins of the superior facet, the junction of the pars, facet, and transverse process is easily identified and prepared for pedicle screw insertion. The articular surfaces of the facet joint are also accessible for débridement and decortication. If the spinal nerve root requires decompression, the dissection is carried down to the extraforaminal region by carefully incising and removing the intertransverse ligament (Fig. 8). The nerve root lies just below this layer, in line with the fibers of the ligament. Care must be taken to distinguish the fibrous bands of the intertransverse ligament from the nerve root itself during dissection to avoid injury to the nerve. The nerve root is then mobilized to allow examination of the lateral aspect of the intervertebral disc. A protruding disc may be excised directly, and any posterolateral osteophytes may be removed to decompress the nerve. A ball-tipped probe is then passed retrograde through the foramen to insure an adequate decompression. If exposure of the lateral pedicle or vertebral body is required (e.g., for biopsy or drainage of a vertebral body lesion), the transverse process may be osteotomized at its base and retracted laterally along with the posterior attachment of the psoas muscle. The nerve roots exiting above and below the pedicle will be exposed and must be protected, but a limited, direct portal may be gained into the posterolateral aspect of the vertebral body at the base of the pedicle.

Microdiscectomy Approach

The operating microscope provides two advantages in lumbar disc surgery. First, magnification permits more meticulous and precise handling of neural tissues, scar, and disc fragments. Second, the orientation of the magnifying lens allows the surgeon a view from directly above the incision, rather than angled from one side. The end result is that a complete disc excision can be completed through a small incision with minimal soft tissue stripping and almost no disruption of the paraspinous muscular attachments. Placement of the skin incision is critical in microdiscectomy, and localizing x-rays should be taken with a spinal needle before the incision is made.

After carefully confirming the level, make a 2- to 3-cm midline incision centered over the disc space (not over the spinous process). Carry cautery dissection down to the lumbodorsal fascia and use the Cobb elevator to develop the plane over the fascia. Divide the fascia just lateral to its insertion into the supraspinous ligament, on the side of the herniation, along the length of the spinous process and subjacent interspinous liga-

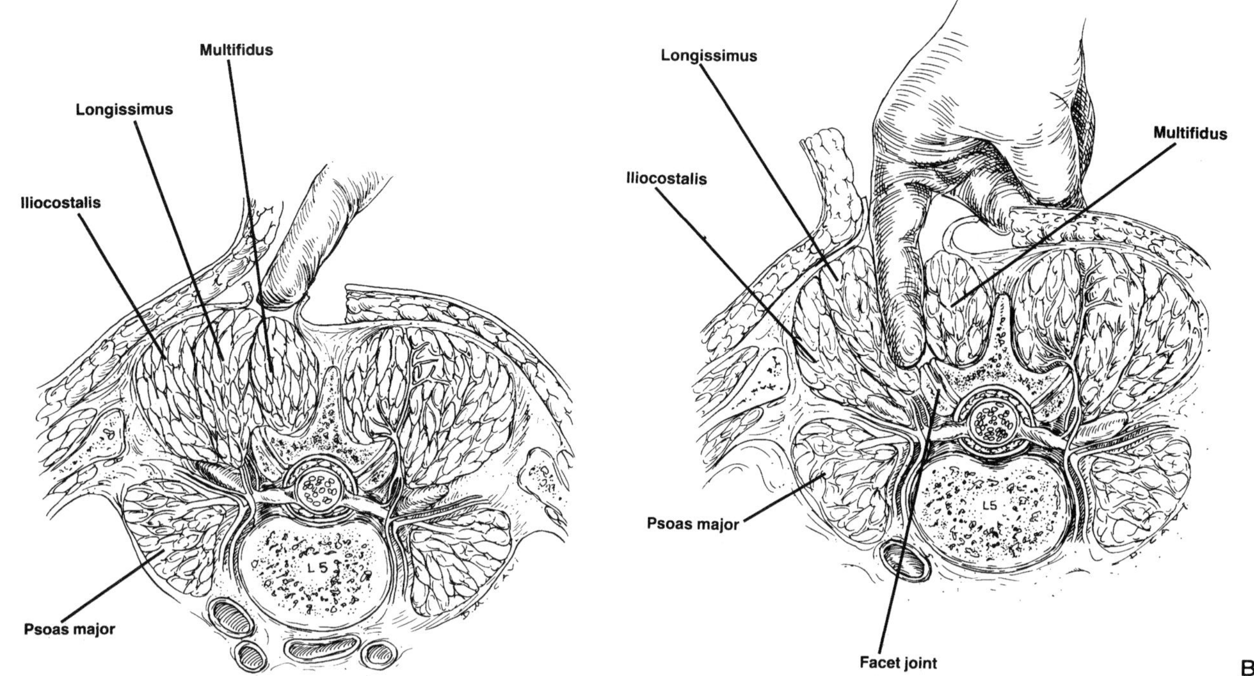

FIG. 6. A: Paraspinal approach through midline incision and muscle-splitting exposure to facets and transverse processes. An interval is developed between the multifidus and longissimus muscle groups. **B:** Further digital dissection places the surgeon's finger easily onto the facet joint. Multifidus, longissimus, and iliocostalis muscles are often collectively termed the *sacrospinalis group.* (Redrawn from Wiltse LL, Spencer CW. New uses and refinements of the paraspinal approach to the lumbar spine. *Spine* 1988;13:696–706.)

ment. Use the Cobb elevator to gently strip the periosteum and paraspinous muscle over that process. With the Cobb holding the elevated tissues laterally, place a deep retractor, such as a Williams retractor, to maintain the exposure. A smaller Cobb, along with gauze sponges and peanuts, can sweep away the remaining soft tissue overlying the ligamentum flavum, and a small, curved curette can be used to develop the margin between the ligamentum and the lamina. After using Kerrison rongeurs to remove the margin of the lamina, carefully release and remove the flavum to reveal the nerve root underneath. Use a high-speed burr to thin down the inferior margin of the supradjacent lamina and remove the remnant with a fine Kerrison to reveal the most cranial edge of the ligamentum flavum. This margin can then be lifted up, and after packing a small cottonoid underneath, the flavum may be dissected back to the facet capsule and removed, revealing the nerve root and underlying disc. A cottonoid paddy placed between the lamina and the epidural fat helps to reduce bleeding and protect the neural elements. Bone wax applied with the tip of a Freer or number 4 Penfield limits bleeding from the laminar rim. This hemilaminotomy technique provides excellent visualization of the lateral border of the nerve root without affecting the facet joint or segmental stability (11,12).

Pedicle Screw Placement

Proper placement of lumbar pedicle screws limits complications and maximizes biomechanical stability. Studies have determined the size of the pedicle isthmus, the angular orientation of the pedicle relative to the vertebral body, and the optimum entry point for pedicle screw insertion (13–16) and have determined the accuracy with which screws may be placed (17).

The starting point for pedicle screw placement is caudal to the superior facet, just lateral to a line drawn vertically through the base of the facet, and on a line drawn horizontally along the axis of the transverse process. This point is located more medially in upper lumbar segments and progressively more laterally as one proceeds caudally (Fig. 9). Likewise, the angle of inclination from lateral to medial of the pedicle increases from 7 to 14 degrees at the L1-2 level and from 25 to 35 degrees at the L-5 level (16). Degenerative spondylosis, individual variations in anatomy, and previous surgical assaults may distort the landmarks used to locate the pedicle entry point. Fluoroscopic confirmation is often essential to avoid inadvertently placing the screw outside the pedicle. Not only do such breaches of the pedicle cortex increase the risk of neurologic injury, but they significantly reduce pullout strength and initial stiffness of the construct.

After broaching the cortex at the junction of the pars, superior facet, and transverse process, a number 4 Penfield or gear shift pedicle finder is passed with little force down the axis of the pedicle. Lateral muscular dissection is necessary to obtain the proper lateral to medial orientation in the lower lumbar segments. Once the gear shift is removed, a tap may be passed, again under fluoroscopic control. After this is removed, a small nerve hook or ball probe is used to check the threads down the inner margin of the pedicle. This determines whether the inner cortex has been breached and whether a screw can be safely passed. If all is well, the screw may then be placed.

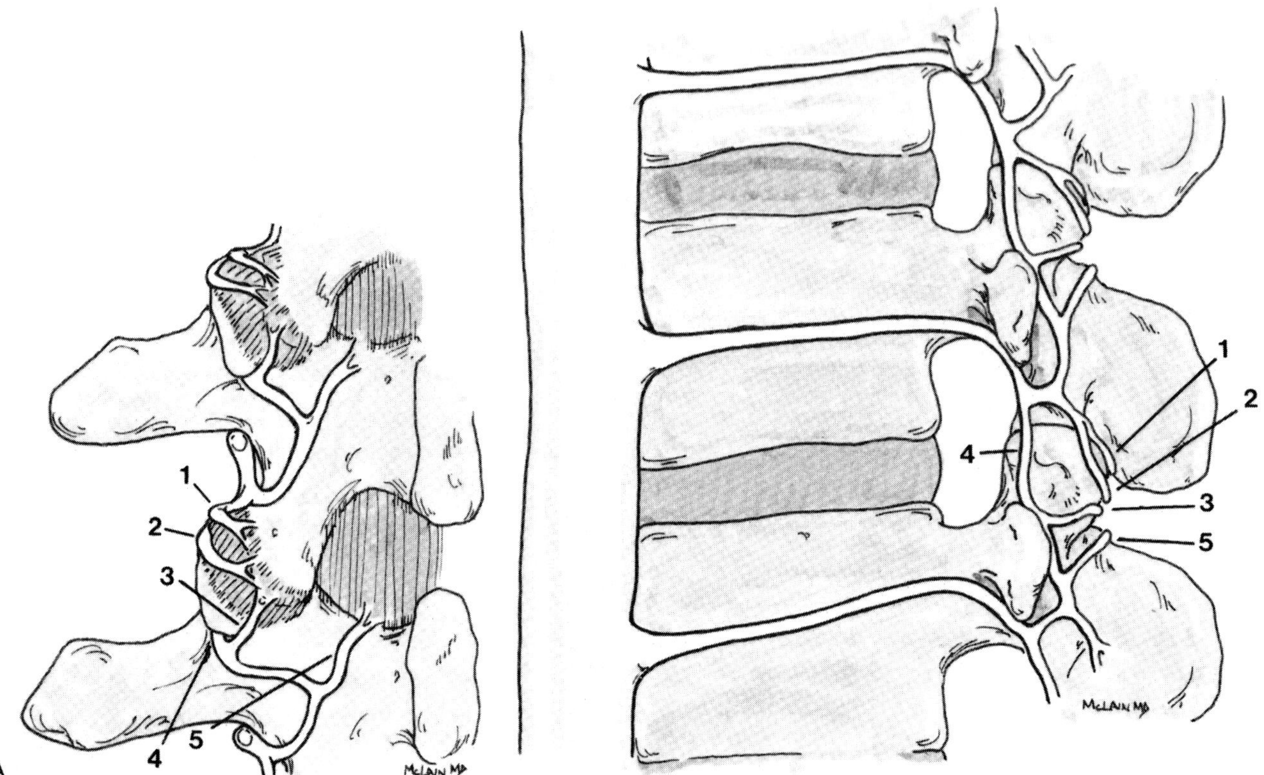

FIG. 7. A: The muscular branches of the lumbar segment vessels: posteroanterior view. Each segmental vessel provides five major branches to the posterior elements. Interarticular artery, found immediately lateral to the pars interarticularis (*1*). Two superior articular arteries lie immediately lateral to the tip of the superior articular facet (*2,3*). The communicating artery is a large vessel that lies immediately lateral to the facet joint, crossing the dorsal surface of the transverse process at its base (*4*). The inferior articular artery lies at the inferior margin of the facet joint in the angle formed by the transverse process and the superior articular facet (*5*). **B:** The muscular branches of the lumbar segmental vessels: lateral view.

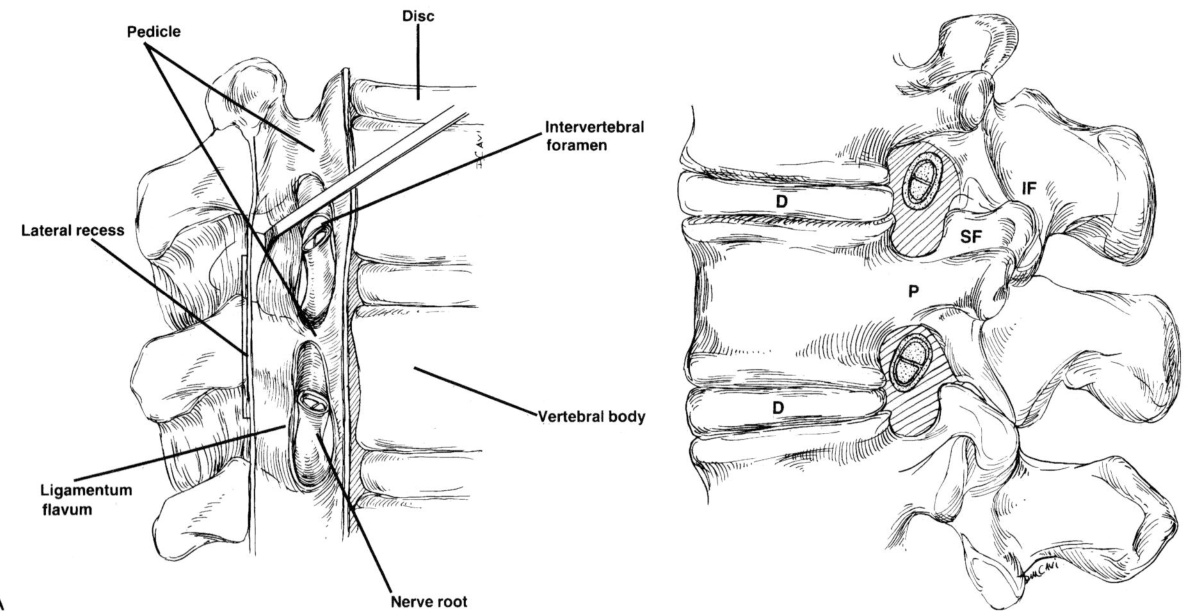

FIG. 8. A: The boundaries of the neural foramina as viewed from inside the spinal canal, looking out. (Redrawn from Watkins RG. Anterior retroperitoneal flank approach to L-5 to S-1. In: *Surgical approaches to the spine*. New York: Springer-Verlag, 1983.) **B:** The neural foramen and its boundaries viewed laterally. D, disc; IF, inferior facet; P, pedicle; SF, superior facet.

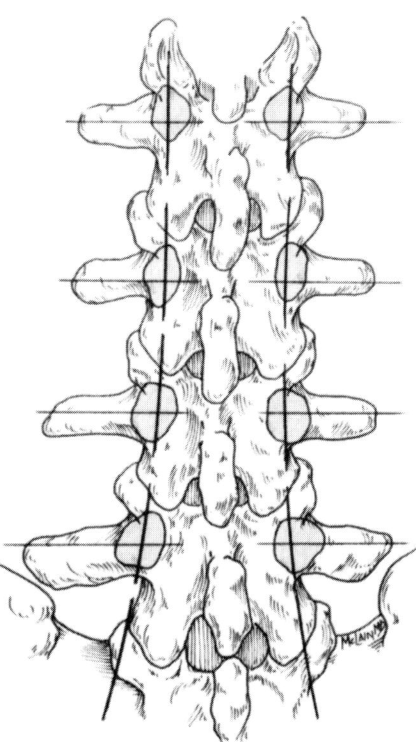

FIG. 9. Entry points to the lumbar pedicles based on intact posterior anatomy. As instrumentation proceeds caudally, the entry point shifts further from the midline.

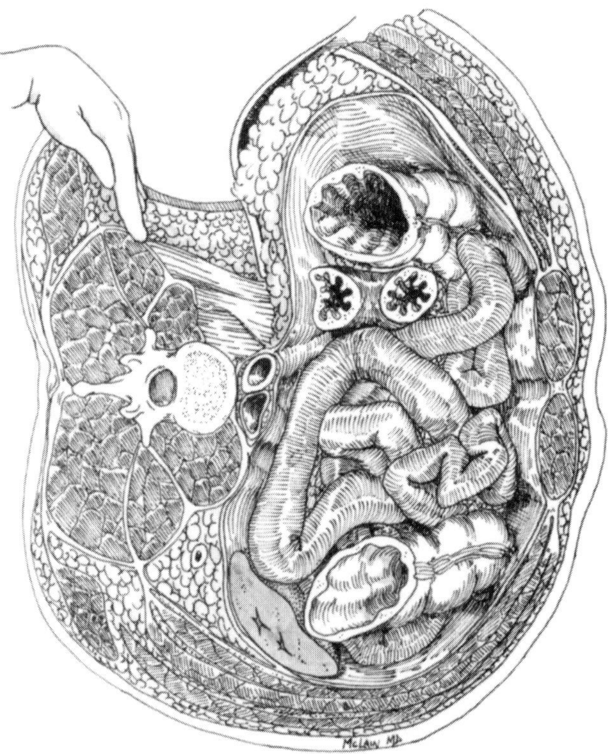

FIG. 10. The natural plane between the peritoneal contents and posterior muscular wall of the trunk allows a relatively bloodless approach to the anterior vertebral body, the lumbar sympathetic plexus, and the great vessels. A Deaver retractor is used to retract the kidney, ureter, and retroperitoneal fat anteriorly away from the vertebral column.

Anterior Approaches

Certain pathologic processes affecting the lumbar spine may only be reached through a direct anterior approach. Osteomyelitis, vertebral abscess, or tumor of the vertebral body, fractures causing neural compression or focal kyphosis, and rigid scoliotic curves may require an anterior approach to the spine as either the primary or part of a combined procedure. In cases of lumbosacral pseudarthrosis or lumbar osteotomy, the anterior procedure may improve chances of a successful fusion or surgical correction. The type of anterior approach chosen is determined by the level of the pathologic process, but most lumbar lesions can be adequately and safely exposed through a standard retroperitoneal approach. This approach may be combined with a transthoracic (thoracoabdominal) approach to expose those vertebral segments obscured by the crus of the diaphragm (see Chapter 60). This exposure may be extended caudally by ligating the iliolumbar vein to allow access to the L-5 to S-1 interspace.

Anterolateral Retroperitoneal Approach to T-12 to L-5

The entire lumbar spine can be accessed through the anterolateral retroperitoneal approach (18). Cranially, the vertebral body of T-12 can be reached by dissecting part of the left diaphragmatic crus away from the anterior lumbar ligament, and caudally, the L-5 to S-1 disc space can be reached by ligating the iliolumbar vein and artery and mobilizing the common iliac vessels. However, the standard retroperitoneal approach provides the best exposure for the L1-5 vertebral bodies and their intercalary discs.

The anterolateral approach takes advantage of the natural plane formed between the visceral peritoneum and the posterior muscular wall of the abdomen and is a modification of a classic surgical approach used for lumbar sympathectomy (19,20) (Fig. 10). By elevating the psoas muscle on the near side and releasing and retracting the great vessels toward the far side, the surgeon gains access to the full circumference of the vertebral body and disc. In primary approaches carried out by skillful hands, the exposure can be accomplished with minimal blood loss, as little muscular dissection or stripping is needed until the psoas is elevated. Approaches through irradiated tissues, infection, tumor, or scar can, on the other hand, be quite challenging, and additional experience is needed to carry these off with an acceptable risk of complications.

In most cases, the surgeon should approach the lumbar spine from the left. This approach exposes the aorta, a tougher, more easily repaired structure, and limits the risk of direct vena caval injury or accidental avulsion of one of the fragile segmental veins from its base. Retraction of the liver may easily result in injury when the upper lumbar segments must be exposed from the right side. Although the spleen may be injured during an exposure from the left (21), this occurs less commonly and is more easily prevented through routine care. Furthermore, in the event of injury, the spleen may be removed to control hemorrhage.

To perform a standard retroperitoneal approach, place the patient in the right decubitus position with the arms protected in

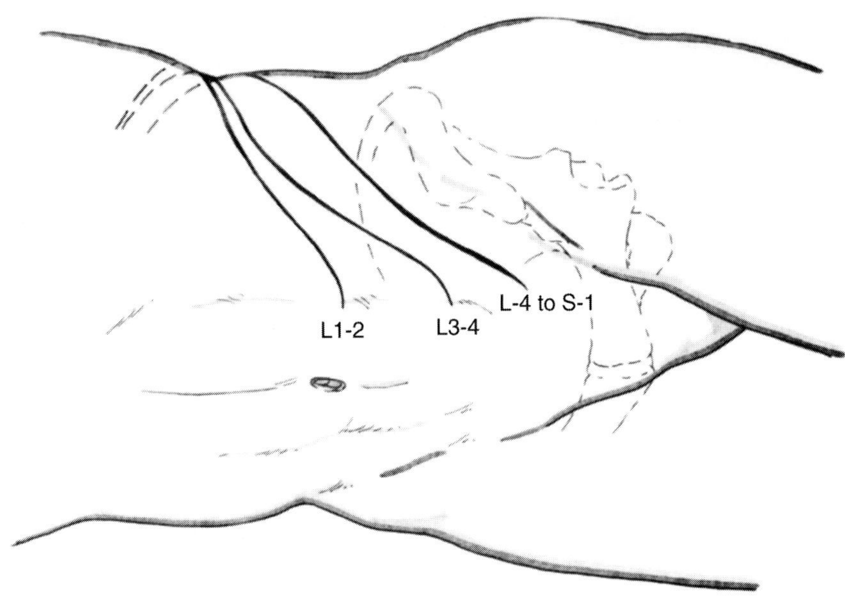

FIG. 11. Patient in right lateral decubitus position. Level of skin incision is determined by the level of the spinal segment to be approached. Incisions for L-5 to S-1 approaches cross just above the iliac crest. Incisions for L2-3 approaches pass just below the twelfth rib.

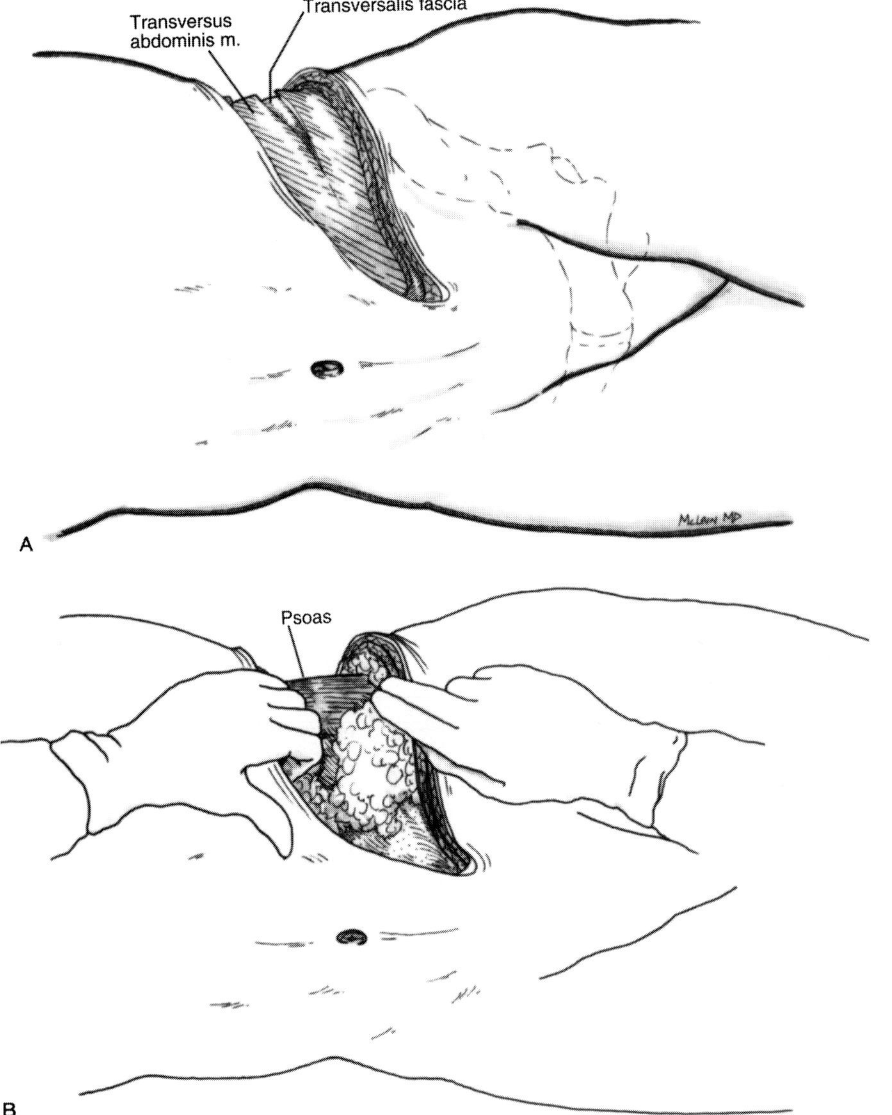

FIG. 12. A: Anterior retroperitoneal approach. Subcutaneous fat and the abdominal muscular layers are divided in line with the skin incision. The transversalis fascia is exposed by dividing the transverses abdominis muscle. **B:** The interval between the peritoneum and the transversalis is developed by carefully dividing the fascia and entering the retroperitoneal cavity. (*continued*)

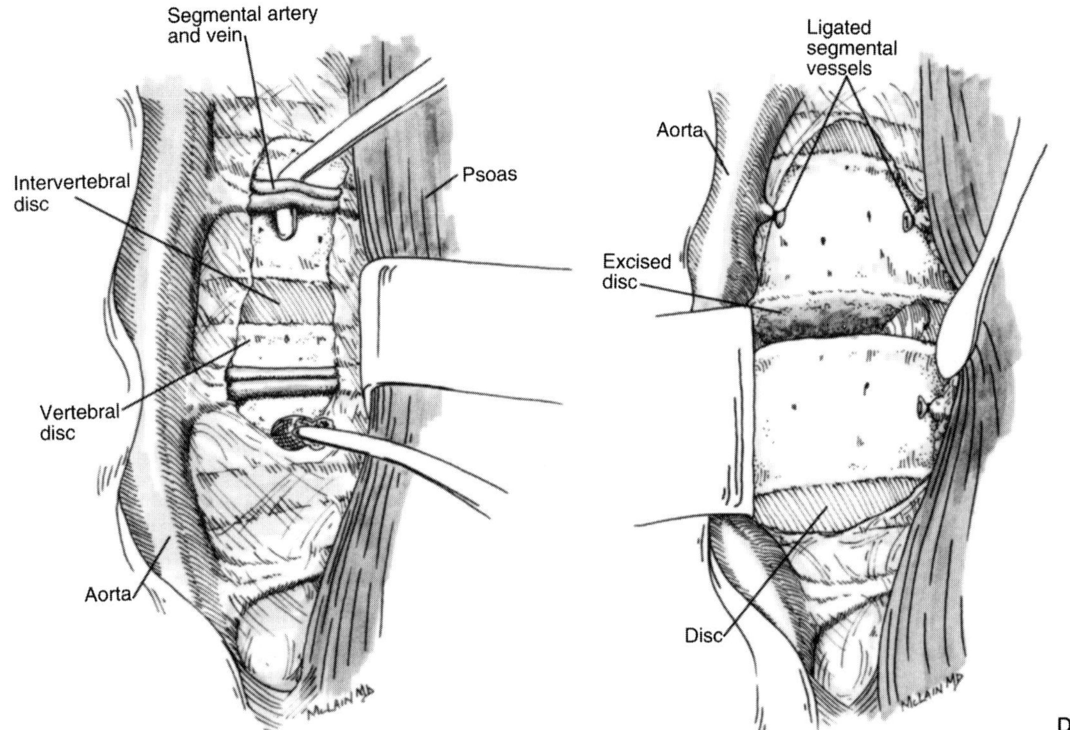

FIG. 12. *Continued.* **C:** The peritoneal contents and retroperitoneal fat are swept forward to expose the psoas muscle dorsally and the aorta ventrally. The segmental vessels are seen crossing the vertebral body midway between the intervertebral discs. **D:** The segmental vessels are ligated and divided, allowing access to the intervertebral disc and the lateral and anterior aspects of the vertebral body. By elevating the anterior longitudinal ligament and surrounding soft tissues, the full circumference of the vertebral body can be exposed. Discectomy is carried out with rongeurs and curettes.

a biplane splint and an axillary roll positioned under the chest wall. Elevate the kidney rest and flex the table to open the left flank. Place pillows between the knees to prevent pressure points, and flex the left hip across the right in a slight figure-of-four position to relax the iliopsoas muscle. The patient is then rolled back 5 to 10 degrees from the true lateral position and the bean bag is deflated to hold this position.

The level of incision is determined by the level of the lumbar lesion and the extent of the exposure required (Fig. 11). After sharply incising the skin, the electrocautery is used to divide the abdominal wall musculature one layer at a time. The external oblique and internal oblique muscles and their fascia are divided in turn, and the transversus abdominis is identified and divided if present (Fig. 12A). The transversalis fascia is then carefully opened in the posterior aspect of the wound to avoid inadvertently entering the peritoneum. Pick-ups are used to lift the fascia up and away from the underlying peritoneum, and the cautery is used to gently nick the surface. Once an entrance is made through the fascia, a digit may be introduced to separate the two layers and expedite division of the transversalis (Fig. 12B). The peritoneum is thickest posterior-laterally and thins toward the midline, where it joins the transversalis fascia beneath the rectus sheath. Rents in the visceral peritoneum should be closed primarily when identified before proceeding with the exposure.

After completing the abdominal wall incision, a large self-retaining retractor is inserted anteriorly. The retroperitoneal fat, containing the ureter and kidney, is gently elevated away from the posterior abdominal wall (Fig. 10) and packed off with moist laparotomy sponges. A C-shaped malleable retractor may be contoured to hold the abdominal contents out of the way. The psoas muscle covers the lateral and anterior aspects of the lumbar spine, with the aorta and segmental vessels apparent anteriorly (Fig. 12C). Digital palpation in the midline reveals the raised, soft intervertebral discs, and placement of a spinal needle in the appropriate interspace permits radiographic confirmation of the correct surgical level. Elevate the psoas muscle laterally to expose the vertebral bodies and intervertebral discs, but note that (a) the retropsoas space between the quadratus lumborum and psoas muscles is a blind pouch that may be entered inadvertently, (b) the genitofemoral nerve is exposed to injury as it exits the iliopsoas muscle belly at the L-3 level, and (c) the segmental vessels are easily traumatized during dissection and may be disrupted by excessive tension during elevation of the psoas or by incidental contact by any of a number of dissecting instruments. For this reason, the segmental vessels over the area of dissection should be isolated by blunt dissection, ligated, and divided. The Adamkiewicz's artery is typically located in the lower thoracic spine, but particularly large vessels may be spared if neural blood supply is a concern. A small vascular clip may be applied temporarily to assess whether occlusion of the vessel affects neural function (22). Any unusually large artery may be so tested, and care may be taken to protect it if somatosensory evoked potential changes are seen following transient occlusion.

After ligating and dividing the segmental vessels, the periosteum overlying the vertebral bodies is elevated and the remaining soft tissues stripped away to expose the vertebral body and annulus fibrosis, and the psoas is elevated and retracted with the Cobb elevator to expose the entire anterior and lateral surface of the lumbar spine (Fig. 12D). A malleable retractor may be placed anteriorly between the vertebral body and the great vessels to provide additional protection. The anterior longitudinal ligament may then be elevated from the midportion of the vertebral body and dissected free of the discs to provide a soft-tissue cuff to protect the vessels anteriorly, or it may be resected with the outer annulus during the disc excision, according to the surgeon's preference. If retained, this cuff provides an anchor for the psoas muscle during closure, loosely sealing the operative site and preventing extrusion of bone graft material into the retroperitoneum.

Exposure of the lower lumbar spine can be obtained through this exposure, but extra care must be taken to mobilize the common iliac vessels and protect them during surgery. The skin incision is carried more anteriorly and inferiorly, with the anterior limit running distally along the border of the rectus. The external oblique is divided in line with its fibers at this point, whereas the internal oblique and transversus are divided as before. After exposing the lower lumbar spine, the L-4 segmental vessels are isolated and divided, and the ascending iliolumbar vein is likewise identified, ligated, and divided to allow mobilization of the common iliac vessels. The common iliac vessels can also be mobilized laterally to allow access to the L-5 to S-1 disc anteriorly, but this requires ligation of the middle sacral vessels and puts the hypogastric plexus at risk. Large, smooth Steinmann pins, shod with rubber catheters, may be impacted into the sacral and lumbar vertebral bodies to maintain retraction of the vessels, but great care must be taken in placing and removing the pins to avoid perforating or scoring the vessel wall (23,24). Because of the difficulty exposing the L-5 to S-1 interspace from the lateral approach, an anterior transperitoneal or retroperitoneal approach is generally preferred.

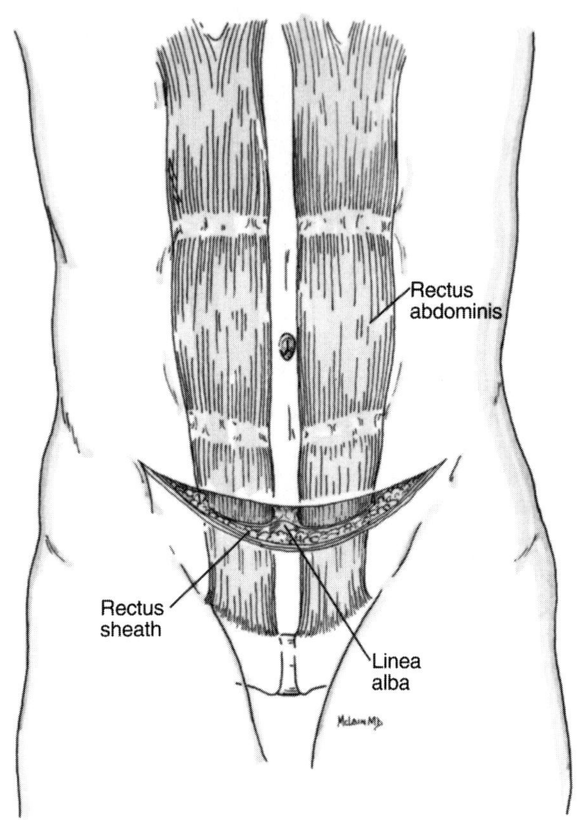

FIG. 13. The Pfannenstiel's incision can be combined with a longitudinal incision splitting the linea alba, a longitudinal paramedian incision through the rectus sheath, or with a transverse incision dividing the rectus musculature in line with the skin incision.

ANTERIOR EXTRACAVITARY APPROACH TO T-10 TO L-5

Anterior Transperitoneal Approach to L-5 to S-1

This approach accesses the lumbosacral junction anteriorly and can be made through either a longitudinal paramedian incision or through a transverse Pfannenstiel's incision. The first provides exposure through the linea alba or rectus sheath, whereas the second is more cosmetic but provides a more limited exposure unless the rectus muscles are transected. The lumbosacral junction is approached directly from anterior, allowing careful blunt dissection and mobilization of the hypogastric plexus and complete access to the width of the L-5 to S-1 disc between the common iliac vessels.

The patient is positioned supine on a standard operating table, and the entire lower abdomen is prepped and draped from the xiphoid to the pubis. The table should be slightly hyperextended. If the Pfannenstiel's incision is used, it should be placed approximately 8 cm above the pubis and gently curved from side to side (Fig. 13). The upper margin is raised as a full thickness flap, exposing the rectus sheath and linea alba. The peritoneum may then be entered one of three ways:

1. The linea alba may be divided in the midline, taking care to identify and protect the bladder in the inferior portion of the wound; the peritoneum is then incised at its attachment to the transversalis fascia, and the omentum and abdominal contents are mobilized proximally and packed off from the incision to expose the posterior peritoneum.
2. The rectus fascia may be incised longitudinally over its lateral margin and the rectus muscle mobilized medially to expose the posterior rectus fascia; this is opened longitudinally in line with the anterior fascial incision, exposing the peritoneum beneath. At this point, the surgeon may proceed transperitoneally (23,25) or retroperitoneally (26).
3. The rectus musculature may be divided transversely, in line with the skin incision; exposure of the lumbosacral junction can be made either transperitoneally or retroperitoneally from this point as well.

If the paramedian skin incision is used, the skin is divided from just above the umbilicus to the upper edge of the pubis (Fig. 14). The subcutaneous fat is divided to expose the rectus sheath and linea alba, and the peritoneum is then entered through the linea or through the rectus fascia, as described above.

After exposing the posterior peritoneum, the sacral promontory and L-5 to S-1 intervertebral disc can be identified by palpation. The posterior peritoneum should be carefully divided to expose the disc space and retroperitoneal vessels (Fig. 15A). The aorta bifur-

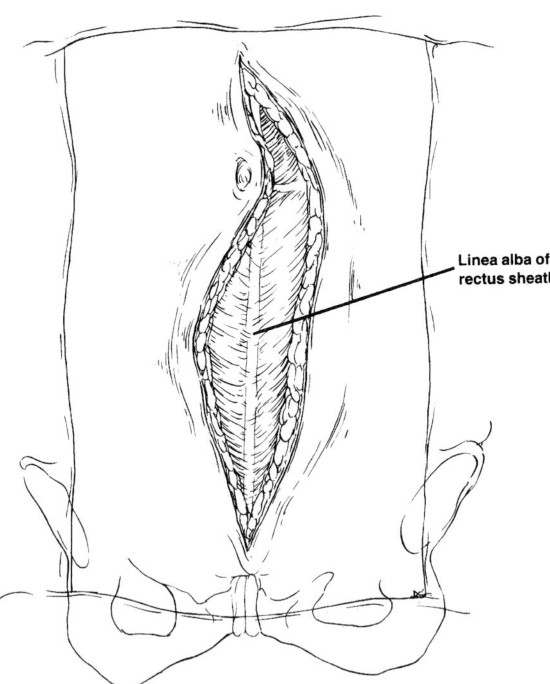

FIG. 14. Longitudinal midline incision with identification of the rectus sheath. (Redrawn from Hoppenfeld S. *Surgical exposures in orthopaedics.*)

cates over the anterior surface of the iliac artery, and the left and right common iliac arteries and veins pass to either side of L-5, giving the middle sacral vessels over the L-5 to S-1 disc space. The hypogastric plexus, the sympathetic contribution to the urogenital system, passes caudally around and over the surface of the aorta, following one or the other branch of the bifurcation to the presacral retroperitoneal space. The mass of the plexus typically courses over the left iliac vessels and the surface of the sacral promontory to reach the anterior surface of the sacrum (Fig. 15B). To expose the intervertebral disc without damaging the plexus, the posterior peritoneum should be opened carefully on the right-hand side of the bifurcation, and sharp and blunt dissection should be used to extend the peritoneal incision longitudinally along the right common iliac vessels (27). The peritoneal incision should be carried distally to the bifurcation of the internal and external iliac vessels, and the right ureter should be identified and protected. After bluntly dissecting down to the anterior vertebral cortex and disc on the right side of the interspace, the presacral tissues may be elevated from the periosteum and swept from the front of the sacrum as a block. Care must be taken to avoid dissecting directly through the plexus, cutting transversely across it, or using cautery during the dissection. If cautery is used, the bipolar coagulator is safer than the unipolar cutting cautery unit. Damage to the hypogastric plexus may result in retrograde ejaculation in male patients, and care must be taken to avoid transverse incisions or cautery among these tissues (28). The middle sacral artery and vein may be ligated.

Anterior Extracavitary Approach to T-10 to L-5

An extracavitary approach can also be used to provide thoracoabdominal exposure in those cases where the thoracolumbar spine is involved in the spinal pathology. The thoracic cavity is opened through the tenth rib bed, and the incision crosses the costochondral junction before turning obliquely across the abdominal wall toward the lateral border of the rectus sheath. The subcutaneous tissues are divided by cautery down to the rib. The erector spinae muscles are elevated and retracted medially but do not need to be divided. The periosteum of the rib is elevated, and the full length of the rib is exposed. After stripping the inner periosteum with a Doyen elevator, the rib is cut posteriorly and disarticulated from the chondral junction anteriorly. The rib bed is then carefully incised to expose the parietal pleura.

After incising the periosteum, a blunt dissector is introduced to gently separate the periosteum from the loosely adherent parietal pleura. Once an initial separation is created, the dissection is continued using a stick sponge or digital dissection to separate the layers cranially and caudally.

The periosteal incision is then extended as the dissection is carried anteriorly to the costochondral junction, and posteriorly to the rib head and the anterior vertebral column. Moist sponges are packed over the exposed surface of the parietal pleura, and the pleura, visceral pleura, and underlying lung are generally retracted to the midline with fans or a malleable retractor. The rib is then disarticulated from the costochondral junction, and the costal cartilage is split longitudinally to enter the abdominal cavity. The external oblique muscle is split along the line of its fibers, then the internal oblique muscle is divided with electrocautery. The transverse abdominis fascia is entered near the rectus sheath, where it is thinnest. After developing the interval between the fascia and the peritoneum, dissect bluntly along the abdominal wall while splitting the fascia with electrocautery. If there is scarring in the retroperitoneum, the surgeon must take particular care to identify the ureter before introducing electrocautery. Usually, the ureter follows the parietal peritoneum and is easily dissected out of the plane. Identify and stay anterior to the psoas muscle.

By dissecting proximally and distally through the retroperitoneal and the extrapleural space, the attachment of the diaphragm is identified along the insertion into the chest wall. The diaphragm is then bluntly detached from the chest wall and dissection carried posteriorly to the crus. Wet sponges are then used to retract the lung, diaphragm, and peritoneal contents anteriorly away from the spine, allowing exposure from the midlumbar to the midthoracic spine through a single incision.

On completion of the spinal procedure, the pleural and peritoneal tissues are allowed to fall back into their normal position. The diaphragm is not directly reattached to the chest wall but is allowed to reapproximate to the wall through the adhesion of peritoneal and pleural tissues. A large intercostal chest tube is placed in the extrapleural space, and the costal cartilages are reapproximated to initiate the closure of the abdominal incision. The rapid readhesion of the parietal pleura to the entire chest and abdominal wall provides fixation of the diaphragm and early restoration of normal diaphragmatic and pulmonary function.

Anterior Retroperitoneal Approach to L-5 to S-1

The surgeon may use the anterior paramedian incision to accomplish a retroperitoneal exposure. Once the anterior abdominal incision is made, the peritoneum is swept to the right side, and the retroperitoneal fat and renal fascia are bluntly dis-

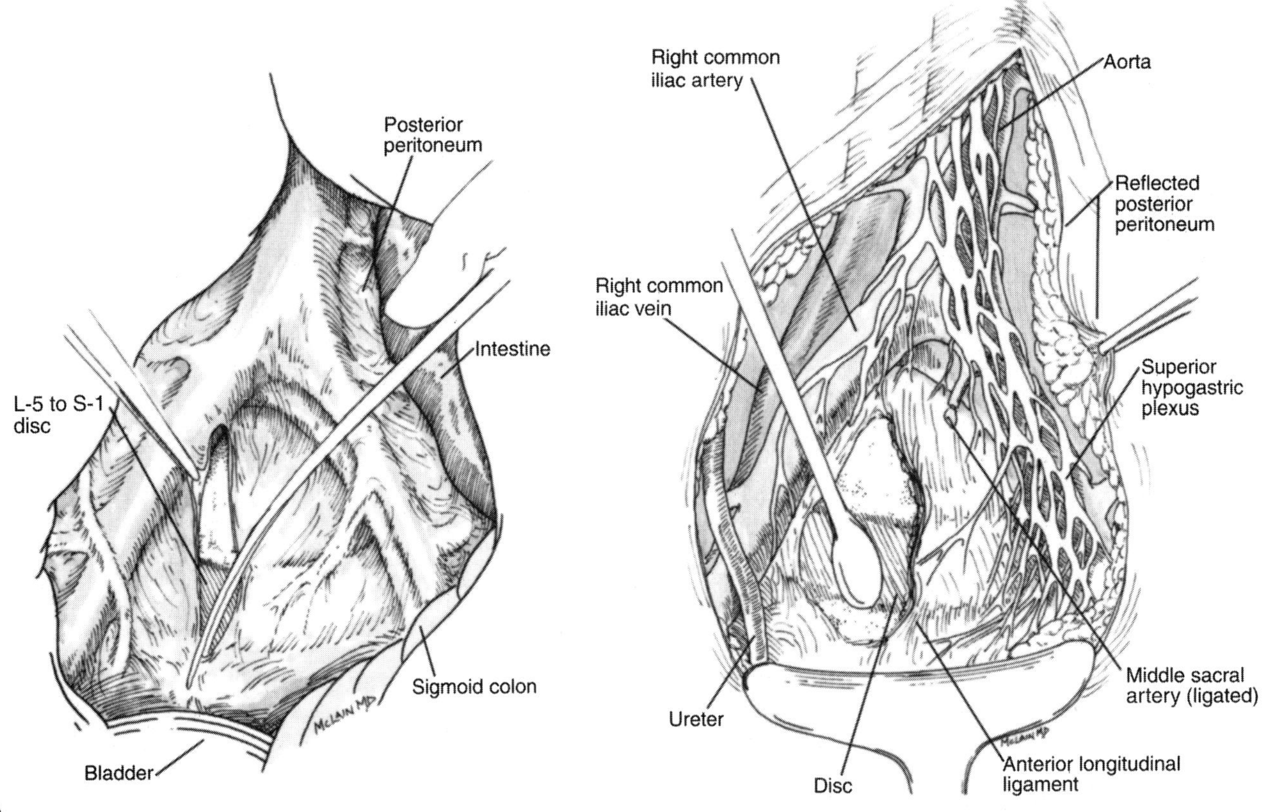

FIG. 15. **A:** Transperitoneal approach. After packing the bowel out of the field, the posterior peritoneum is carefully incised to expose the lumbosacral interspace nestled in the bifurcation of the iliac arteries and veins. Care is taken to avoid damaging the hypogastric plexus. **B:** The hypogastric plexus typically follows the left branch of the iliac artery before passing caudally over the L-5 to S-1 interspace onto the presacral periosteum.

sected away from the posterior abdominal wall until the psoas is exposed. From this point, the dissection of the anterior lumbar spine proceeds as previously described. The right-sided anterior retroperitoneal approach is a very useful variation of the standard approach to the lumbosacral spine. The right-sided approach takes advantage of the bifurcation of the vena cava at L-4 and avoids the sigmoid colon, allowing a wide exposure to the lumbosacral interspace (Fig. 16). The likelihood of ileus is greatly reduced by the retroperitoneal approach, and access to the anterior L-5 to S-1 intervertebral space is not limited. The approach begins lateral to the right rectus muscle at the level of the umbilicus and extends distally to just above the iliac crest, where it curves medially along the margin of the crest. The external and internal oblique muscles are divided in the line of the incision, and the transversus and transversalis fascia are divided carefully to avoid entering the peritoneal cavity. An abdominal retractor is placed to maintain exposure, and the peritoneum is gently mobilized away from the posterior abdominal wall and packed off to the upper-left quadrant. The sigmoid colon does not need to be mobilized from this approach and does not interfere with the exposure. The bifurcation of the aorta and vena cava is visualized, and the common iliacs and right ureter are identified by blunt dissection and careful spreading of tissues (Fig. 17). The iliolumbar vein does not come into play through this exposure, but the middle sacral artery and vein must be identified and ligated; these are often densely adherent to the anterior sacral periosteum and may be controlled with vascular clips.

The right-sided approach offers two other advantages. First, the orientation of the common iliac arteries and veins at the bifurcation puts the left iliac vein medial to the artery and the right vein lateral to the artery. The right vein is, therefore, relatively less susceptible to injury during exposure, making approach from that side more logical. Second, the majority of sympathetic fibers from the superior hypogastric plexus follow the left iliac branch as they cross the bifurcation. By carefully mobilizing the prevertebral soft tissues from the right side of the lumbosacral disc toward the left, the surgeon is least likely to disrupt sympathetic function, again making an approach from the right more comfortable (23,29).

Combining Surgical Approaches

Indications for combined anterior and posterior surgical approaches are varied: resection of a low-grade chondrosarcoma may require a wide resection anteriorly and posteriorly to ensure removal of all neoplastic tissue; a patient with vertebral osteomyelitis may need a formal débridement anteriorly, followed by a posterior stabilization to insure spinal stability; and

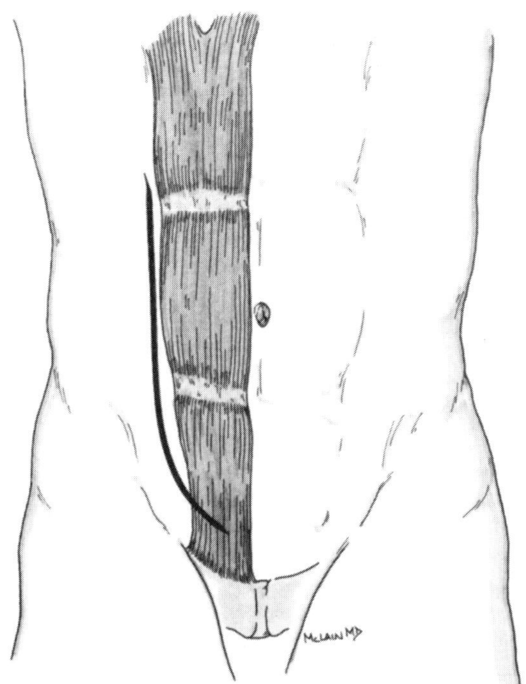

FIG. 16. Incision for right-sided retroperitoneal approach parallels the lateral margin of the rectus before curving medially just above the iliac crest.

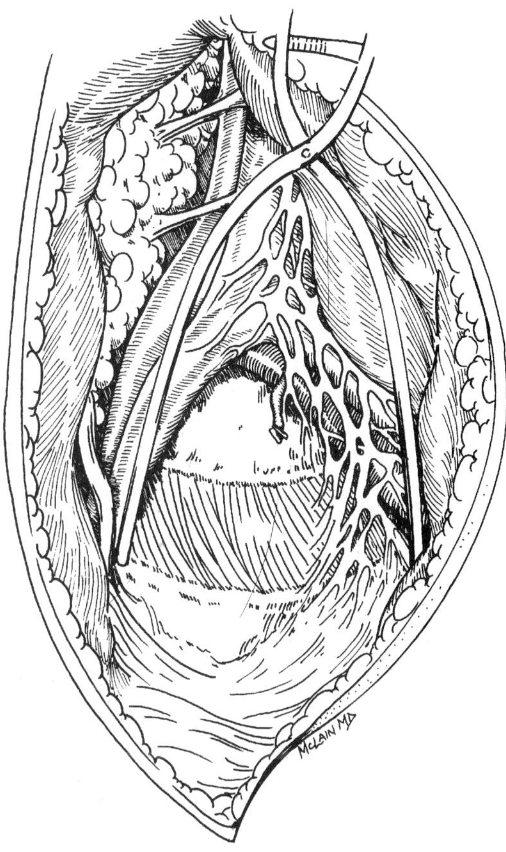

FIG. 17. Right-sided anterior approach allows exposure of the L-5 to S-1 interspace without interference from the sigmoid colon, away from the hypogastric plexus, and from the side exposes the iliac vein to the least risk of trauma.

a patient with a lumbosacral pseudarthrosis may benefit from a combination of an anterior interbody fusion and posterior instrumentation to assure a solid arthrodesis. Depending on the situation, a combined surgical approach can be performed simultaneously, as a single-stage procedure (two operations under a single anesthetic) or as a two-stage procedure with a delay between operations.

Simultaneous Approaches

The need for a combined, simultaneous approach is limited, as most situations permit the surgeon to complete one approach before repositioning the patient, closing the wound, and beginning the second. In some tumor resections, however, and in occasional fracture reconstructions, the surgeon gains a significant benefit by performing both exposures simultaneously. This requires that the patient be positioned in the lateral decubitus position, and that the posterior procedure be performed in this position. The anterior approach is typically begun first, and any decompression or bony work necessary should be completed before beginning the posterior procedure. If a tumor resection is planned, the anterior approach should be carried as far as mobilizing the great vessels and excising the adjacent discs, but the tumor tissue should be left intact to prevent hemorrhage or spillage of tumor cells. The posterior exposure is then begun through a standard midline incision, using a clean instrument setup in cases of tumor or infection.

Tactile feedback available from the simultaneous approaches helps to confirm the appropriate levels. Posterior decompression and resection of the pedicles can be carried out to release the vertebral body posteriorly, allowing an *en bloc* resection anteriorly without risk of tumor seeding from hematoma and without having to reposition the patient while the spine is destabilized. Strut graft reconstruction and posterior instrumentation can then be carried out simultaneously, the anterior wound being closed while the posterior instrumentation is placed. Similarly, highly unstable fractures may be addressed in this manner, carrying out an anterior decompression and strut grafting along with a posterior instrumentation without turning the patient and risking graft displacement. In these cases, the operating table may be flexed to start the anterior approach but must be returned to neutral before the posterior instrumentation is begun.

Single-Stage Procedures

Most combined procedures can be carried out as separate procedures performed under a single anesthetic. These single-stage procedures include anterior-posterior fusions for pseudarthrosis, decompressions and fusions for burst fractures, débridement and stabilization procedures for osteomyelitis, and osteotomies and high-grade spondylolistheses for some complex deformities. In any case, the surgeon has the option of postponing the second procedure if surgical conditions dictate the need or proceeding under the same anesthetic to complete both anterior and posterior procedures.

Most often, the anterior procedure is carried out first. Anterior decompression, vertebral débridement, or tumor resection is carried out through a standard retroperitoneal approach. Bone grafting or strut graft reconstruction is carried out as indicated. If frank pus is encountered, strut graft reconstruction and posterior instrumentation may be delayed until a course of antibiotics can be started and the graft bed adequately prepared. Otherwise, an appropriate strut graft may be prepared and keyed into the resection site to provide provisional stability during closure and turning. The anterior wound is then closed in layers, and the patient is turned gently onto transverse bolsters or a turning frame for posterior exposure, instrumentation, and fusion.

In other situations, it may prove more feasible to perform the posterior stabilization initially. Here, the posterior midline approach may be used to expose the lumbar spine for instrumentation and fusion before turning the patient onto the side for an anterior interbody fusion. In either case, care should be taken to harvest as much bone as is necessary for both procedures when the graft is taken for the first. This minimizes the need to perform two iliac crest harvests through separate incisions.

Two-Stage Combined Procedures

There is a number of reasons to delay the second portion of a combined procedure until another day. Excessive blood loss, patient instability, and surgeon fatigue may make an otherwise manageable second procedure unwise; active infection may provide a clear contraindication to instrumentation and reconstruction as a single-stage procedure. In these situations, the second procedure may be delayed for a period and completed under a separate anesthetic as a two-stage combined procedure.

In patients undergoing anterior reconstruction as the initial portion of a two-stage operation, the postoperative management is dictated by the stability of the spine at the end of the reconstruction. A well-fashioned graft, keyed in to good-quality vertebral bone, may provide adequate stability to get the patient up and ambulating before posterior fixation is attempted. Complete débridement of a pyogenic infection, however, may leave an extensive anterior defect and may not be immediately reconstructible. In this case, the patient may need to be kept at complete bed rest until a second-stage procedure can be performed. The interval between surgeries is generally 7 to 10 days, allowing the patient to recover pulmonary and gastrointestinal function before undergoing another anesthetic. This is also time enough for the patient to recover from fluid shifts incurred during the first procedure and for the hemoglobin levels to stabilize.

Nutritional problems may require a longer delay between operations, particularly in elderly patients and those with neuromuscular disorders. In some cases, it may be helpful to begin nutritional augmentation before the first procedure and continue parenteral nutritional supplements until the second procedure has been completed. In cases of infection, timing of the second procedure must take into account the organism involved, the extent of the infection, and the patient's response to antibiotics. If the second procedure requires reopening the initial incision, this may be done with little difficulty 7 to 10 days after the first procedure, but longer delays will land the surgeon in the midst of a dense vascular scar, making dissection and identification of planes difficult.

COMPLICATIONS

Anterior Approaches

Complications vary depending on the surgical approach chosen. Anterior procedures have the potential for excellent exposure with little blood loss when performed skillfully in uncomplicated patients. The risks of catastrophic complications go up dramatically in patients with previous surgery or prior irradiation or infection or those undergoing radical resections or reconstructions. Adhesions and scars obscure the planes and margins leading to the great vessels and may invest the vessel walls. Tumor tissue may also invest the vessels themselves, making dissection around the aorta and vena cava most challenging. Vessels made friable by irradiation or infection are more easily damaged, and minor missteps during dissection may result in severe hemorrhage and vascular injuries that may be very difficult to control and repair. Avulsion of segmental vessels at their base requires a careful closure of the vessel wall, which is sometimes very difficult in the vena cava. Vena caval perforations or lacerations are similarly difficult to control. Badly diseased aortic tissues may also prove unusually friable, and laceration of the aortic wall may necessitate excision and graft interposition before perfusion can be restored to the lower extremities. Obviously, life-threatening hemorrhage may accompany any of these injuries.

Injury to abdominal viscera can occur through excessive retraction on the liver or spleen or direct penetration by a surgical instrument. The spleen may occasionally be damaged during a left-sided exposure, whereas the liver is at somewhat more risk when the right-sided exposure is used (21). The surgeon must check and recheck the position of the retractors during anterior surgery and be sure that the assisting surgeon knows what lies behind the retractor.

The cauda equina, individual nerve roots, and the sympathetic plexus are at risk from the anterior approach. Injuries to cauda equina and spinal nerves may occur during exposure and bony decompression, and injuries to the sympathetic plexus may occur during exposure of the lower lumbar spine and lumbosacral junction. Great care must be taken in positioning and exposing the spine of any patient with marked compromise of the canal and an impending cauda equina lesion. Inadvertent pressure over the fracture site at the thoracolumbar junction may force fracture fragments back into the canal and injure the conus medullaris or elements of the cauda equina. Placement of fine instruments inside the canal during decompression of tumor or fracture may injure already compromised nerves. Somatosensory evoked potential monitoring should be carried out before and after positioning the patient and throughout the decompression.

Sympathetic injury occurs in a small number of patients during exposure of the lower lumbar spine (30). Damage to the superior hypogastric plexus may interrupt normal sympathetic control of urogenital function, resulting in retrograde ejaculation and sterility in some men (28). Sympathetic injury is unlikely to result in impotence in young, healthy men, but may result in erectile impotence in older patients and those with peripheral vascular disease (31,32). Because women lack a genital sphincter, the effects of sympathectomy are less obvious, and rarely result in significant dysfunction. Nonetheless, care should be taken to protect the hypogastric plexus in any patient undergoing an anterior procedure at the lumbosacral junction.

Knowledge of the course of the superior hypogastric plexus and careful handling of the prevertebral tissues can minimize the risk of complications.

One very rare complication of anterior surgery in the thoracolumbar region is anterior spinal artery ischemia. Ischemic cord injury occurs with some regularity in aortic trauma or aortic aneurysm repair, procedures requiring prolonged cross-clamping at levels above the renal arteries (33) and is a rare complication of anterior scoliosis surgery or osteotomy (33–35). Although cord injury due to unilateral, segmental vessel ligation seldom (if ever) occurs when only one or two levels are addressed, Apel et al. have described a method of evaluating segmental contribution intraoperatively by monitoring somatosensory evoked potential changes while temporarily occluding unusually prominent segmental arteries with a small vascular clip (22). This technique may be particularly useful in the thoracolumbar region and in patients requiring multilevel procedures.

Posterior Approaches

Errors in identifying or selecting levels for fusion and instrumentation can easily occur in posterior surgery. Anatomic markers are inexact and vary from patient to patient. Exposure of the incorrect spinal level can lead to excision of the incorrect intervertebral disc, resulting in a complete failure to treat the existing pathology and in an iatrogenic injury to normal segments of the lumbar spine. Localizing radiographs can eliminate these types of mistakes but are not always simple to interpret; the surgeon must recall that the intervertebral disc at the L4-5 level lies directly volar to the L4-5 interlaminar space, but that the disc at the L1-2 level sits more cranially, under the lamina of L-1. Failure to confirm surgical levels early in the procedure can also lead to inadvertent injury of facet joints at levels that will not be fused. The surgeon may be forced to extend fusion or instrumentation to an unintended level because of iatrogenic injury to facets or disc. Any of these complications can lead to a compromised surgical result or complete treatment failure.

Vascular injuries are far less common from the posterior approach, although careless discectomy technique can result in penetration of the aorta, iliac arteries and veins, or vena cava, which is an often fatal vascular injury (36,37). Less commonly, renal, urethral, and bowel perforation may occur. Persistent hemorrhage from muscle and exposed bone can result in unacceptably large blood losses during extensive posterior surgeries. Careful attention to dissection technique can prevent this complication. Intraoperative blood loss can be minimized by meticulous subperiosteal dissection, electrocautery during muscular division, and cautery control of segmental vessels around facets and transverse processes. Patients with bleeding diathesis, neuromuscular scoliosis, or recent use of antiinflammatory prostaglandin inhibitors may prove difficult to manage even when good technique is used; cell-saver blood collection systems are invaluable in these cases, but management of any underlying bleeding problem should be addressed as well. The surgeon should also keep an eye on coagulation parameters during prolonged and combined procedures. Patients undergoing multiple unit transfusions of cell-saver blood, volume expansion with crystalloid and colloid solutions, and extensive surgical insult to the musculoskeletal system frequently manifest a prolonged bleeding time and elevated coagulation times by the end of a combined procedure. If oozing seems to be increasing toward the end of such a procedure, a prothrombin time and partial thromboplastin time should be sent and fresh-frozen plasma ordered as necessary.

Neurologic injuries occurring during posterior spine surgery range from transient irritations, such as paresthesias or mild paresis of a nerve root, to out-and-out catastrophes of irreversible paraplegia, cauda equine injuries, or intractable pain. Knowledge of the anatomy of the spinal canal is crucial in avoiding neurologic complications, as is patience and adherence to technique when performing disc excisions, decompressing neural elements, and placing instrumentation. Proper exposure and hemostasis are necessary before the canal is entered. Spinal cord monitoring should be used routinely, and changes in signal magnitude or latency related to pedicle screw placement, reduction of deformity, or manipulation of the cauda equina must be appreciated and distinguished from changes related to body temperature or blood pressure.

REFERENCES

1. Cauthen JC. *Lumbar spine surgery*. Baltimore: Williams and Wilkins, 1988.
2. White AH, Rothman RH, Day CD. *Lumbar spine surgery: techniques and complications*. St. Louis: Mosby, 1987.
3. Craig FS. Vertebral body biopsy. *J Bone Joint Surg* 1956;38:93–102.
4. Hoppenfield S. Percutaneous removal of herniated lumbar discs. *Clin Orthop* 1989;238:92–97.
5. Kambin P, Schaffer JL. Percutaneous lumbar discectomy. *Clin Orthop* 1989;238:24–34.
6. Macnab I, Dall D. The blood supply to the lumbar spine and its application to the technique of intertransverse lumbar fusion. *J Bone Joint Surg* 1971;53:628–638.
7. Gill GG, Manning JG, White HL. Surgical treatment of spondylolisthesis without fusion. Excision of the loose lamina with decompression of the nerve roots. *J Bone Joint Surg* 1955;37:493–494.
8. Watkins MB. Posterolateral fusion of the lumbar and lumbosacral spine. *J Bone Joint Surg* 1953;35:1014–1018.
9. Wiltse LL, Bateman JG, Hutchinson RH, et al. Paraspinal sacrospinalis-splitting approach to the lumbar spine. *J Bone Joint Surg* 1968;50:919–926.
10. Wiltse LL, Spencer CW. New uses and refinements of the paraspinal approach to the lumbar spine. *Spine* 1988;13:696–706.
11. Hudgins WR. The role of microdiscectomy. *Orthop Clin North Am* 1983;14:589–603.
12. Wisneski RJ, Rothman RH. Microdiscectomy techniques. *Sem Spine Surg* 1989;1:54–59.
13. Berry JL, Moran JM, Berg WS, et al. A morphometric study of human lumbar and selected thoracic vertebrae. *Spine* 1987;12:362–367.
14. Krag MH, Weaver DL, Beynnon BD, et al. Morphometry of the thoracic and lumbar spine related to transpedicular screw placement for surgical spinal fixation. *Spine* 1988;13:27–32.
15. Panjabi MM, Takata K, Goel V, et al. Thoracic human vertebrae: quantitative three-dimensional anatomy. *Spine* 1991;16:888–901.
16. Zindrick MR, Wiltse LL, Doomik A, et al. Analysis of the morphometeric characteristics of the thoracic and lumbar pedicles. *Spine* 1987;12:160–166.
17. Weinstein IN, Spratt KF, Spengler D, et al. Spinal pedicle fixation: reliability and validity of roentgenogram-based assessment and surgical factors on successful screw placement. *Spine* 1988;13:1012–1018.
18. Burrington JD, Brown C, Wayne ER, et al. Anterior approach to the thoracolumbar spine—technical considerations. *Arch Surg* 1976;111:456–463.
19. Lilly GD, Smith DW, Biggane CF. An evaluation of "high" lumbar sympathectomy in arteriosclerotic circulatory insufficiency of the lower extremities. *Surgery* 1954;35:1–8.
20. Pearl FL. Muscle splitting extraperitoneal lumbar ganglionectomy. *Surg Gynecol Obstet* 1937;65:107–112.

21. Hodge WA, DeWald RL. Splenic injury complicating the anterior thoracoabdominal approach for scoliosis. A report of two cases. *J Bone Joint Surg* 1983;65:396–397.
22. Apel DM, Marrero G, King J, et al. Avoiding paraplegia during anterior spinal surgery: the role of somatosensory evoked potential monitoring with temporary occlusion of segmental spinal arteries. *Spine* 1991;16:S365–S370.
23. Freebody D, Bendall R, Taylor RD. Anterior transperitoneal lumbar fusion. *J Bone Joint Surg* 1971;53:617–627.
24. Watkins RG. Anterior retroperitoneal flank approach to L5-S1. In: *Surgical approaches to the spine*. New York: Springer-Verlag, 1983.
25. Lane JD, Moore ES Jr. Transperitoneal approach to the intervertebral disc in the lumbar area. *Ann Surg* 1948;127:537–551.
26. Southwick WO, Robinson RA. Surgical approaches to the vertebral bodies in the cervical and lumbar regions. *J Bone Joint Surg* 1957;39:631–635.
27. Duncan HJM, Jonck LM. The presacral plexus in anterior fusion of the lumbar spine. *Suid-Afrikaanse Tydskrif Vir Chirurgie* 1965;3:93–96.
28. Johnson RM, McGuire EJ. Urogenital complications of anterior approaches to the lumbar spine. *Clin Orthop* 1981;154:114–118.
29. LaBate JS. The surgical anatomy of the superior hypogastric plexus "Presacral nerve." *Surg Gynecol Obstet* 1938;67:199.
30. Flynn JC, Price CT. Sexual complications of anterior fusion of the lumbar spine. *Spine* 1984;9:489–492.
31. Appell RA, Shield DE, McGuire EJ. Thoridiazine induced priapism. *Br J Urol* 1977;49:160–166.
32. Whitelaw GP, Smithwick RH. Some secondary effects of sympathectomy with particular reference to disturbance of sexual function. *N Engl J Med* 1951;245:121.
33. Kiem HA, Sadek KR. Spinal angiography in scoliosis patients. *J Bone Joint Surg* 1971;53:904–912.
34. Dommisse GF, Enslin TE. Hodgson's circumferential osteotomy in the correction of spinal deformity. *J Bone Joint Surg* 1970;52:778.
35. Dommisse GF. The blood supply of the spinal cord. A critical vascular zone in spinal surgery. *J Bone Joint Surg* 1974;56:225–235.
36. DeSaussure RL. Vascular injury coincident to disc surgery. *J Neurosurg* 1959;16:222–229.
37. Freeman DG. Major vascular complications of lumbar disc surgery. *West J Surg Gynecol Obstet* 1961;69:175–177.

CHAPTER 53

Positioning and Approaches to the Thoracolumbar Spine

B. Endoscopic and Minimally Invasive Approaches

Isador H. Lieberman, Robert F. McLain, Eeric Truumees, and Gregory T. Brebach

INTRODUCTION AND HISTORY

Endoscopic and minimally invasive approaches include rapidly evolving sets of techniques that offer equivalent surgical outcomes with the potential for lower surgical morbidity. The philosophy behind spinal endoscopy and minimally invasive surgery is to apply a therapeutic intervention to the targeted pathology while minimizing damage to surrounding nonpathologic tissues (1–3). These techniques include percutaneous, endoscopically, and fluoroscopically guided treatment.

Endoscopy uses a fiberoptic camera and light source for visualization and magnification through small percutaneous portals. Jacobaeus first applied endoscopic principles in clinical treatment in 1910 as a tool for diagnosing and treating tuberculosis (4). Orthopedic applications of endoscopic principles began with the advent and acceptance of knee arthroscopy. In 1991, Lewis popularized video-assisted thoracic surgery (VATS) for pulmonary diseases. Over a short time, endoscopic techniques have become standard for many abdominal and knee procedures, such as cholecystectomy and meniscectomy (5). Endoscopic spinal surgery was first performed in the lumbar region, and experience with lumbar surgery still outweighs that with thoracic endoscopy (6). The first description of VATS for thoracic spinal diseases was published by Mack and others in 1993 (7).

Regan et al. successfully used endoscopic technique to perform interbody grafting and, more recently, instrumentation, in diverse thoracic spinal pathology, including deformity and degenerative disease (8–10). Rosenthal et al. reported the use of VATS for ventral decompression and stabilization in patients with metastatic tumors of the thoracic spine (11). The initial results using VATS and minimally invasive surgery are encouraging. Although these techniques are characterized by less pain and shorter hospital stays, techniques and instruments continue to evolve rapidly (2,6,12). Endoscopic assistance may also have advantages during posterior approaches to the thoracic spine (13,14).

TABLE 1. *Advantages and disadvantages of thoracic endoscopic spine surgery*

Advantages
Improved visualization
Decreased postoperative incisional pain
Cosmetically acceptable scars
Opportunity to perform simultaneous anterior-posterior procedures
Reduced blood loss
Reduced infection risk
Decreased compromise of respiratory mechanics and rib splinting
Decreased postoperative shoulder girdle dysfunction
Reduced intensive care and hospital stay
Disadvantages
Surgical novelty (learning curve)
Monocular visualization (triangulation, depth perception)
Loss of tactile feedback (increased working distance)
Need for second surgeon
Technical limitations in treating intraoperative complications
Anesthetic demands of double lumen intubation and single-lung ventilation
Currently limited ability to perform endoscopic reconstruction
Currently limited ability to perform dural repair
Specialized, costly, and often single-use instruments

PRINCIPLES OF SPINAL ENDOSCOPY

Vertebral tissues are located centrally within the body. Open surgical approaches require significant soft-tissue dissection, increasing surgical risk, recovery time, and long-term functional consequences. Minimally invasive approaches attempt to perform the same operation while decreasing the size of the incision and damage to otherwise normal surrounding tissues. This, in turn, should decrease morbidity, pain, and hospitalization while leaving a more aesthetically acceptable scar.

Anterior Approaches

Although no direct, randomized trial has compared endoscopic techniques with traditional, open approaches, there are many theoretical and apparent advantages (Table 1) (1,3,5,6,8,9,12,15–25). First, a quality endoscopic system affords the surgeon improved visualization through direct illumination and up to 15 times magnification. By manipulating portal placement, scope angle, and camera trajectory, the surgeon can see directly into areas that cannot be viewed from an open approach.

Second, VATS requires less muscle dissection and no rib spreading and, therefore, decreases incisional pain. Similarly, decreased soft-tissue injury results in more cosmetically acceptable scars, lower risk of postoperative infection, and decreased compromise of respiratory and shoulder mechanics. In the prone position, anterior and posterior procedures may be undertaken simultaneously. Taken together, these advantages may reduce intensive care and hospital stays.

On the other hand, VATS has some disadvantages over open surgery as well (1,3,5,6,8,9,12,15–25). First, these procedures require substantially different technical skill sets compared to traditional, open approaches. There is a significant learning curve requiring that a considerable amount of time be spent with animal, cadaveric, and proctored cases before proceeding with independent VATS spine surgery. Endoscopy changes the surgeon's binocular vision to monocular video-assisted vision and compounds this loss of depth perception with a loss of tactile feedback through the long instruments needed to pass through endoscopic portals. Visualization and manipulation of delicate structures also requires triangulation from widely separated starting points on the chest wall. Ultimately, the surgical procedures are the same as with the traditional open approaches, but the methods are different enough to challenge even the most experienced spinal surgeon.

Although the pulmonary insult may be decreased with endoscopic approaches to the thoracic spine, double lumen intubation and single-lung ventilation are still required. Long periods of single-lung ventilation are physiologically demanding to the patient and technically demanding to the anesthesiologist and may not be tolerated in compromised patients.

Posterior and Combined Approaches

Combined approaches are being increasingly described in the literature. These approaches include simultaneous anterior and posterior surgery for tumors and deformity (23,26). Combined approaches may also refer to combining endoscopic and open techniques in mini-open or endoscopically assisted spine procedures to exploit the advantages of both techniques (21,22). The dissection and retraction of the paraspinal muscles may lead to dead space formation and extensor muscle disruption. Such disruption has been referred to as *fusion disease* (27) and may be associated with early fatigability and other long-term symptoms. Endoscopic techniques, used in combination with minimally invasive posterior approaches, may allow for less disruption of the posterior musculature and a smaller laminotomy.

Relative Indications

In considering the role of endoscopic and minimally invasive surgery as part of a continuum of spine care, it is useful to remember that the most minimally invasive modality is nonoperative care. Nonoperative management should remain the first consideration for most degenerative conditions, especially those involving axial pain in the absence of neurologic dysfunction. Surgical indications must not be liberalized simply because the procedure can be completed through a smaller incision.

VIDEO-ASSISTED THORACOSCOPIC SPINE SURGERY

The majority of endoscopic thoracic spine surgery is directed anteriorly. A traditional thoracotomy requires a large incision, division of the shoulder girdle musculature, rib resection, and forcible rib retraction. This approach can result in desiccation of the exposed lungs and vessels, measurable reduction in pulmonary and shoulder girdle function, postthoracotomy intercostal pain syndrome, and an unsightly scar (2,23). On the other hand, thoracoscopic approaches visualize the anterior spinal elements from the T1-2 to L1-2 disc spaces from the side of approach to the midline (12). VATS affords easier exposure of the extremes of the thoracic spine than open thoracotomy (28). For example, a T-12 corpectomy can be performed without diaphragmatic take-down, and T-3 can be accessed without mobilizing the scapula, as would be required with an open technique.

Indications and Contraindications

Currently, VATS may be used for a number of pathologies, including infections, selected tumors, trauma, corpectomy/decompression, and stabilization and correction of deformity.

Contraindications to thoracoscopic spinal surgery include the inability to tolerate single-lung ventilation, for example, a patient with severe or acute respiratory insufficiency (8). However, patients with chronic obstructive pulmonary disease or interstitial fibrosis and marginal pulmonary function may benefit from the improved postoperative pulmonary mechanics associated with VATS. Similarly, in patients with significant restrictive lung disease from deformity, such as children with neuromuscular scoliosis, a thoracoscopic approach may be better tolerated than thoracotomy.

Other contraindications stem from difficulty visualizing and manipulating instruments through a scarred chest cavity. VATS should not be offered to patients with pleural symphysis, failed prior open anterior surgery, or bullous lung pathology. Relative contraindications include empyema, previous thoracotomy, or previous tube thoracostomy.

Relevant Anatomy for Video-Assisted Thoracic Surgery

The rib cage and chest wall form a rigid open space in which endoscopic surgery may be performed. Unlike the abdomen, carbon dioxide insufflation is not required to maintain a working space. Through most of the thoracic spine, the rib number corresponds to the lower vertebral body at the disc space (e.g., the sixth rib comes off the T5-6 disc space). Because the rib comes directly off the disc space from demifacets just above and below the disc, rib resection is required to adequately access the posterolateral corner of the disc. In the lower thoracic region, T-11 and T-12, the rib head may be well caudal to the disc space, permitting unobstructed access.

The segmental vessels lie at the waist of each vertebral body. Various spinal procedures require sacrifice of these vessels. Discectomy and anterior release procedures, on the other hand, may be done with or without vessel ligation. Some authors argue that these vessels should be preserved, noting that, although slightly more disc area can be excised with ligation of the vessels, sparing the segmental vessels may provide blood supply that aids in fusion. Other authors contend that sacrificing the segmental vessels provides better visualization through improved pleural reflection that allows for a more complete discectomy (24,25,29). In a report of 1,197 procedures in which more than 6,000 vessels were sacrificed, there were no adverse neurologic consequences (30). The surgeon should consider sparing the segmental vessels in patients with a high risk for cord perfusion–related neurologic injury, such as revision surgery, severe kyphosis, and congenital anomalies (31).

Other important structures include the superior intercostal veins and the sympathetic chain. The veins empty into the azygos circulation at or near the T3-4 interspace (1). Branches from the sympathetic chain run over the rib heads, just below the parietal pleura (32). Over the fifth to the tenth ribs, these coalesce as the greater splanchnic nerve, which then courses into the abdomen.

Regional differences in thoracoscopic anatomy dictate different exposure techniques. In the upper thoracic region, unless there are apical adhesions, the collapsed lung readily falls away from the spine, allowing excellent visualization (33). In the midthorax, there is unrestricted space for placement of camera and retractor portals, but the lung tends to intrude into the operative field. A fan retractor or strategically placed sponges are typically needed to keep the collapsed lung out of the operative field. A second retracting port may be needed to retract a bullous or stiff lung (33). In the lower thoracic region, it may be necessary to retract the diaphragm, but lung retraction is not usually a problem.

Anesthesia for Video-Assisted Thoracic Surgery

Safe implementation of thoracoscopic spine surgery begins with anesthesia. Selective double lumen endotracheal intubation allows full collapse of the lung on the operative side. The anesthesiologist may need to periodically assess tube position and should be comfortable using a bronchoscope to confirm airway position intraoperatively (34). In patients who weigh less than 45 kg, even the smallest double lumen endotracheal tube may not fit, and bronchial blockers may be required (3,24). Blockers are technically more difficult to use and have a higher rate of incomplete lung deflation, which may seriously impair visualization (3). Prone positioning may reduce the need for double lumen intubation in deformity cases (35). Hypotensive anesthesia should be avoided in myelopathic patients or in those undergoing segmental artery sacrifice (9).

For patients with no cardiorespiratory disease, tidal volumes of 10 to 15 mL/kg and 100% oxygen content are appropriate (6,34). The respiratory rate is adjusted to titrate the end-tidal partial pressure to between 35 and 40 mm Hg. If oxygen saturation decreases during the procedure, endotracheal tube position should be reassessed.

Patient and Operating Room Positioning

The use of a radiolucent operating frame is ideal for lateral decubitus or prone positioning during endoscopic spinal exposures. The lateral decubitus position, identical to open thoracotomy, is most typical for VATS spine surgery. The patient should be well padded and an axillary roll positioned under the chest wall.

The patient should be secured in place with belts or tape so that the table may be tilted into the Trendelenburg position or to the right or left as necessary to improve intraoperative visualization. Ensure that the patient stays in a strict lateral position during the initial approach to the spine so as to maintain surgeon orientation. In some approaches, particularly in the lower thoracic spine, it may be useful to "break" the table to improve access to the lateral body wall. In patients with significant cord compression, this may increase the risk of iatrogenic neurologic complications (36).

Prone positioning may be used during a simultaneous anterior-posterior approach (23,35). Simultaneous surgical exposures

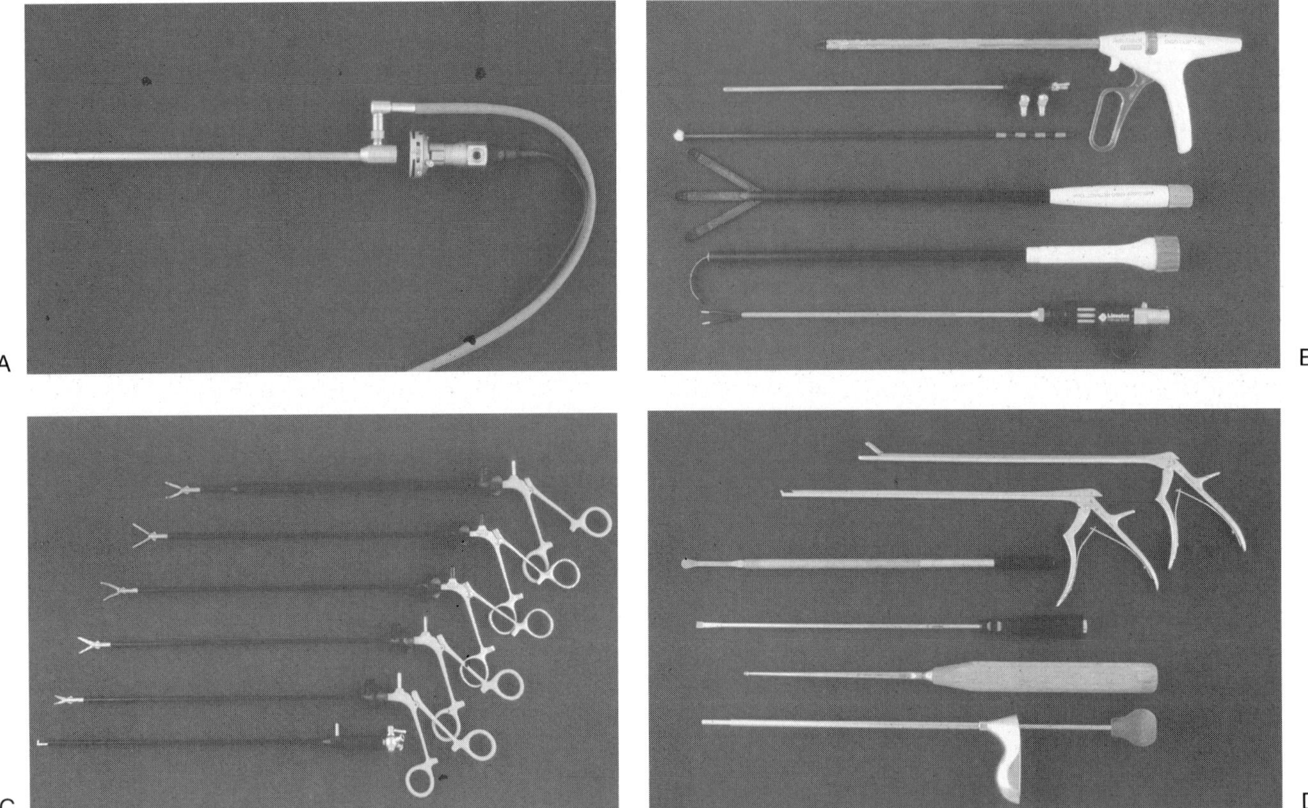

FIG. 1. Spinal thoracoscopy benefits from an ever-increasing array of available instruments. Important among these are the endoscope itself **(A)**, standard endoscopic instruments **(B)** (including a fan retractor and autosuture device), endoscopic dissecting tools **(C)**, and typical spine instruments modified for thoracoscopic use with long hands and uniform diameter shafts **(D)**.

eliminate the need to stage the procedures, along with the added time and costs for repositioning, redraping, and a new operating room set-up. The prone position is particularly advantageous in cases of marked instability or kyphosis. The prone position allows a gravity reduction of hyperkyphosis after osteotomy (35) and has the additional advantage of allowing the lungs to fall away from the spine, decreasing the need for retraction.

The endoscopic surgeon and spine surgeon typically work on the same side of the patient (facing the patient in lateral decubitus position). Instruments for an open thoracotomy should be readily available for emergency use. In the prone position, open access can be achieved with an extended costotransversectomy approach. As the lung has already been mobilized, it is easy to enter the chest. Once access to the thorax is accomplished, the surgeon is readily able to access bleeding and identify and control major vascular structures (23).

Instruments are introduced into the chest through trocars (Fig. 1). Hard trocars may protect the thoracoscope against the rigid fulcrum of the ribcage (1), but soft trocars may be less traumatic to the intercostal nerves.

Initial Surgical Approach

The thoracic spine may be approached from either side depending on the eccentricity of the pathology (Fig. 2). With a left-sided approach, the thick resilient aorta is less prone to injury than the more fragile and tortuous veins of the azygous system. Some authors prefer a right-sided approach when the pathology is not lateralized, because there is greater spinal surface area lateral to the azygos vein than there is lateral to the aorta (12). Below T-9, a left-sided approach avoids the more cranial reflection of the hemidiaphragm on the right.

The main viewing portal is placed in the anterior axillary line at the sixth or seventh intercostal space, giving a broad view of the entire hemithorax. The trocar is inserted after blunt dissection with a Kelly forceps, just over the top of the rib, to avoid damage to the neurovascular bundle or deep structures. This first portal is the only one to be inserted blindly. A digital exploration is undertaken to exclude adhesions and avoid parenchymal lacerations of the lung. Once the chest cavity is open to the atmosphere, the lung falls away from the thoracic wall, allowing insertion of the thoracoscope. The surgeon can then perform an exploratory thoracoscopy and release minor pleural adhesions.

The camera and instruments should work in the same 180-degree arc to avoid creating a mirror image. The camera will have to be removed for cleaning at various intervals. It should be reinserted carefully, as the lung may partially reinflate, and injury to the lung parenchyma is possible (36).

Only one object at a time should be manipulated during endoscopic surgery. The camera may zoom in to the operative site, but as each new instrument is introduced, the camera should pan out to follow the instrument into the operative field. Similarly, retractors and other instruments should be positioned or removed only

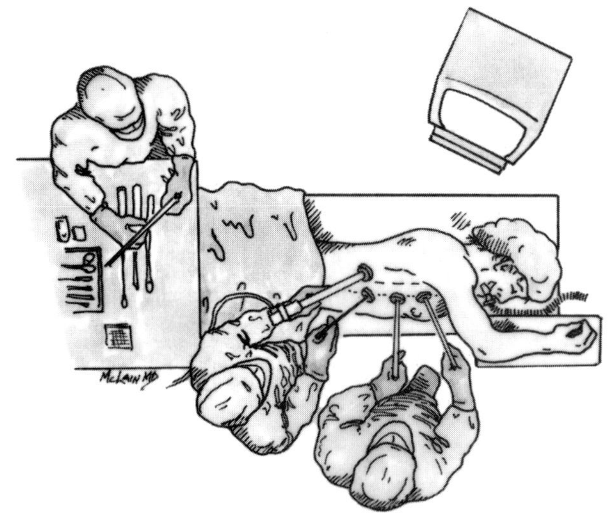
A

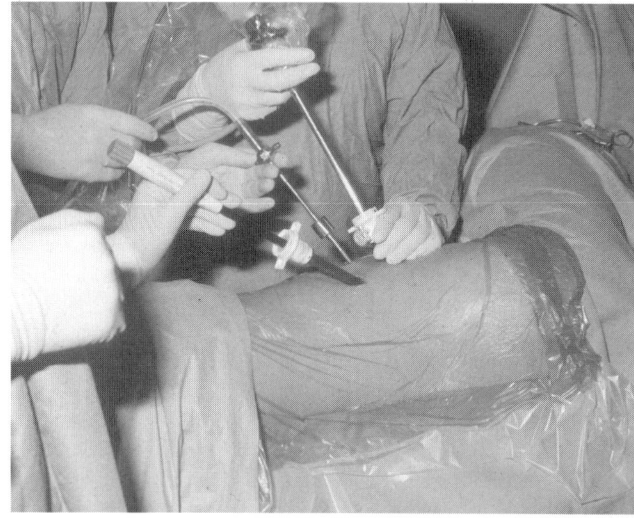
B

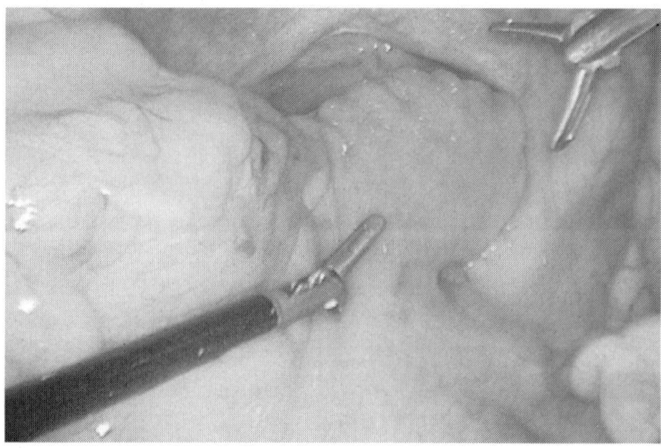
C

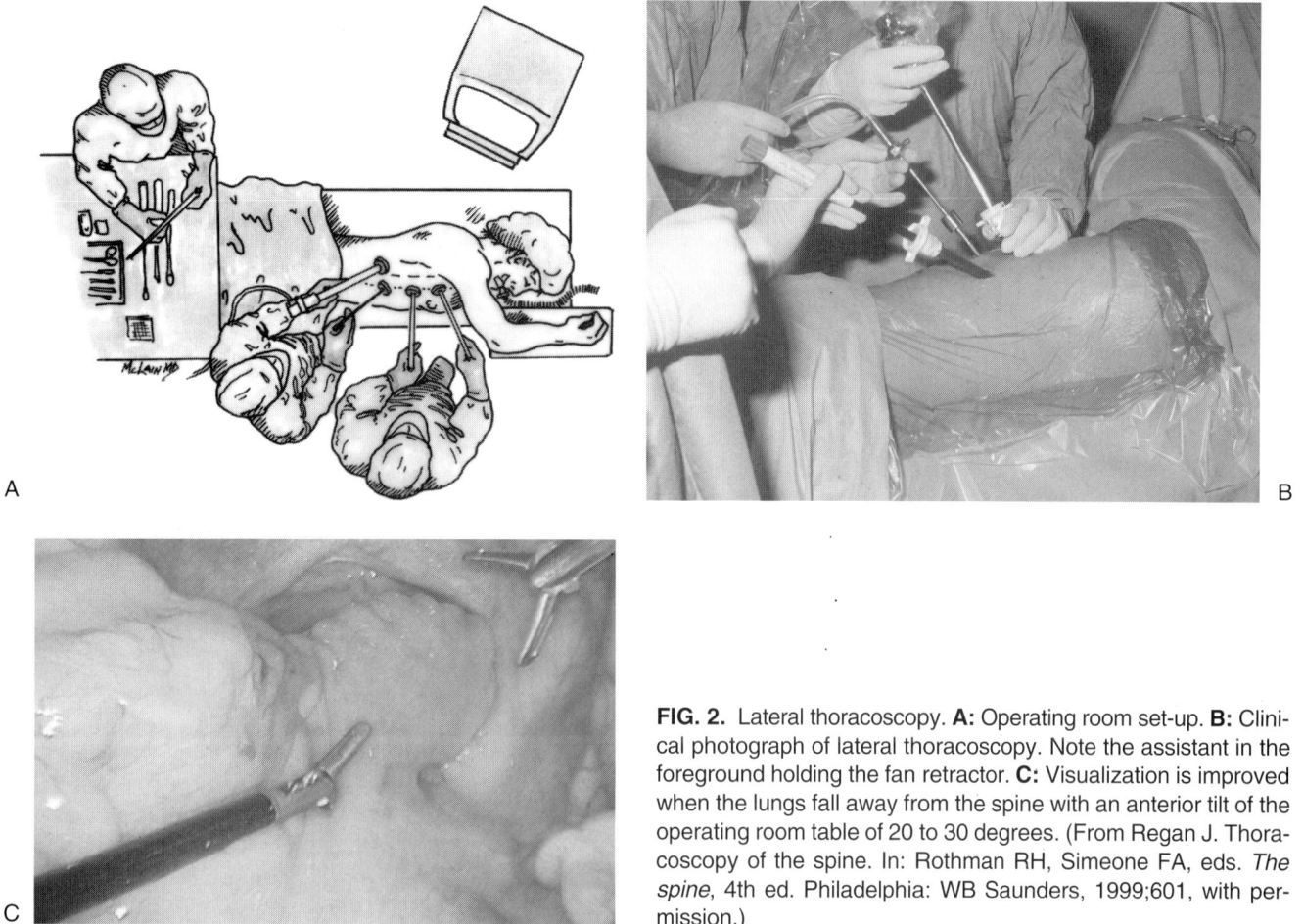

FIG. 2. Lateral thoracoscopy. **A:** Operating room set-up. **B:** Clinical photograph of lateral thoracoscopy. Note the assistant in the foreground holding the fan retractor. **C:** Visualization is improved when the lungs fall away from the spine with an anterior tilt of the operating room table of 20 to 30 degrees. (From Regan J. Thoracoscopy of the spine. In: Rothman RH, Simeone FA, eds. *The spine*, 4th ed. Philadelphia: WB Saunders, 1999;601, with permission.)

under direct visualization. Fan retractors should be removed in the fully closed position only. Avoid levering instruments on the rib cage, as this may injure the intercostal nerve.

Deep Approach

Once in the chest, the surgical levels are identified. Study preoperative radiographs for variant anatomy, such as accessory ribs, then find the surgical level by counting down from the first rib. Mark the disc space and confirm the level radiographically. A Steinmann pin passed directly through the chest wall into the pathologic level confirms localization and also demonstrates the optimal location for the working portal. Anteroposterior radiographs are typically more helpful than lateral (32). In some centers, marking beads are placed at each spinal level, and radiographs or fluoroscopy are obtained before entering the operating suite. The appropriate level bead is maintained on the patient for intraoperative confirmation.

Additional instruments need to be inserted into the chest through two or three additional working portals. During the procedure, the instruments and scope are interchanged between these portals to facilitate work at different levels. Portals are typically created under direct video visualization with the lung protected. Either the chest is percussed and the percussions visualized from within, or 18-gauge spinal needles can be placed through the interspace to verify the level and trajectory. Organize the remaining portals to center the instruments at the level of pathology. Space portals far enough apart that instruments do not "fence" with each other. The final viewing portal should be far enough away from the lesion to allow a panoramic view and to allow room to manipulate instruments (3).

When the correct level has been identified and the appropriate portals have been placed, incise the parietal pleura over the rib head using monopolar cautery. Alternatively, the harmonic scalpel can dissect with less smoke and char (17,37). Avoid monopolar cautery at the inferior margin of the rib head where the intercostal nerve may be injured (36). The degree of pleural dissection depends on the extent of the intended surgery but may include longitudinal approaches parallel to the spine or transverse approaches parallel to each disc space. If the segmental vessels are to be preserved, smaller pleural incisions are created parallel to the disc space. Bluntly dissect the incised parietal pleura proximally, distally, and anteriorly to expose as much of the vertebral margins as is necessary.

At each step, maintain meticulous hemostasis. Control bleeding with monopolar or bipolar electrocautery, harmonic scalpel, argon beam coagulation, or hemostatic packing. Uncontrolled bleeding may necessitate conversion to an open procedure.

At the conclusion of the procedure, irrigate out any disc or bony debris. Most clinicians do not attempt to close the parietal pleura. Some recommend an intercostal bupivacaine block to decrease postoperative pain (38).

To drain the chest cavity and maintain lung expansion, a 20-French, 24-French, or 28-French chest tube (depending on the patient's size) should be inserted through the inferior-most portal and advanced cranially along the vertebral column. Rosenthal uses two chest tubes, one apical tube for air and a second, basilar tube for effusions (11). Depending on the nature of the procedure, the tube can be maintained at water seal or at 20 cm of water suction, and can typically be removed 1 to 2 days postoperatively.

In the postoperative period, most patients are extubated immediately. A chest radiograph is obtained in the recovery room to verify full inflation of the lungs (6). In some conditions, a brief period of intensive care unit (ICU) monitoring is recommended. Aggressive respiratory care is required to prevent down-lung atelectasis and pneumonia. This may include bronchodilators, deep suctioning, and deep coughing.

General Results and Complications

Despite physiologic stressors, VATS has proven a reasonable alternative to open thoracotomy from the anesthesia perspective due to the clinical benefits of accelerated return to activity and decreased ICU and hospital stays. Clinical outcomes have, however, paralleled more traditional approaches.

The complications associated with thoracoscopically assisted spine surgery are essentially the same as with an open approach and are categorized as incomplete operation, neurologic injury, lung injury, and vascular injury (11,19,36).

As in any spinal cord–level procedure, dural laceration, cord injury, or ischemia are possible. Most common, however, is intercostal neuralgia, identified in up to 21% of patients and most often transient (36). Transection of the sympathetic chain causes little or no morbidity, but the surgeon should inform the patient and family of possible temperature and skin color changes below the level of surgery.

Long periods of lung deflation increase pulmonary complications. To reduce the risk of prolonged atelectasis, the deflated lung should be reinflated for 5 to 10 minutes for each hour of operating time (6). Trocars or instruments may directly injure the lungs. Larger air leaks should be repaired with an endoscopic suture ligature. Other common postoperative lung problems include pleural effusions and diaphragmatic injury, and more unusual pulmonary complications may stem from anesthesia or single-lung ventilation mishaps. Pneumomediastinum, pneumoperitoneum, and subcutaneous emphysema have occurred after intubation with a double lumen tube.

Serious vascular injuries can occur. Either penetrating trocars or surgical instruments may injure the heart, great vessels, azygos vein, esophagus, or segmental arteries. Injury to the thoracic duct producing lymphatic leakage should be occluded using an endoscopic clip applier.

Huang and coworkers reported a total of 30 complications occurring in 22 of 90 consecutive patients (24.4%) treated thoracoscopically for a variety of pathologies. Two of these complications were fatal, including one case of massive blood loss and another of pneumonia. Four patients had to be converted to an open procedure.

Applications

Video-Assisted Thoracic Surgery in Deformity

Endoscopic surgery, alone or with other procedures, may serve to arrest curve progression, maximize and maintain curve correction, improve fusion rates, and decompress and protect the neural elements (Table 2) (39). In scoliosis, the anterior longitudinal ligament and concave-side costotransverse ligaments form a structural tether that restricts curve correction (39). Anterior release of these tethers allows correction of coronal and sagittal plane deformities.

The surgeon should consider anterior release in large scoliotic curves greater than 75 degrees and in rigid curves with less than 50% correction on bending films. Anterior epiphysiodesis is typically indicated to prevent the crankshaft phenomena in skeletally immature children with curves greater than 50 degrees or in those with progressive congenital deformities (40). Patients with kyphotic deformities greater than 70 degrees or curves that require rebalancing into the stable zone in the coronal or sagittal plane are also candidates for anterior release. Interbody fusion further minimizes pseudarthrosis risk.

Spinal endoscopy should be given particular consideration in the patient with preexisting pulmonary compromise due to the spinal deformity or associated neurologic syndromes (i.e., polio). Finally, endoscopic techniques should be considered in any situation where the cosmetic result is of particular concern to the patient.

Relative contraindications to the use of endoscopy in spinal deformity include a narrow anterior posterior chest diameter, significant vertebral rotation at the apex, or thoracic scoliosis curves greater than 75 degrees, which may preclude safe visualization and instrumentation of the spine. When the chest anteroposterior diameter is too restricted, there is no room for retraction of even the fully deflated lung, and visualization of the surgical site may prove impossible. In curves greater than 75

TABLE 2. *Indications and contraindications to thoracoscopic surgery in spinal deformity*

Indications: Thoracoscopy is an alternative to thoracotomy in patients with the following:
- Curves >60 degrees with <50% correction on bending
- Curves >75 degrees
- Curves requiring rebalancing into the stable zone in either the coronal or sagittal planes
- Crankshaft prevention in skeletally immature patients with curves >50 degrees
- Kyphotic deformities >70 degrees
- Progressive congenital deformities requiring epiphysiodesis
- Patients at high risk of pseudarthrosis from posterior fusion alone
- Patients with compromised pulmonary mechanics

Contraindications
- See text
- Deformity-specific relative contraindications
  - Narrow anterior-posterior chest diameter or other anatomic variants that limit working space in the chest
  - Significant vertebral rotation at the apex

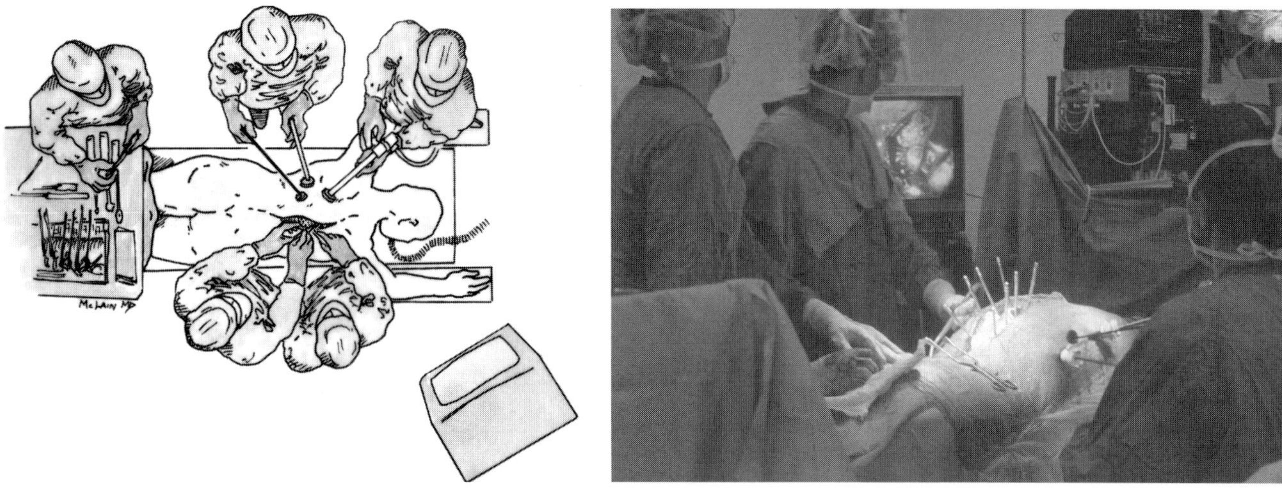

A B

FIG. 3. Prone thoracoscopy. **A:** Operating room set-up for prone thoracoscopy. **B:** Clinical photograph of a simultaneous anterior thoracoscopic release with posterior fusion.

degrees, the chest cavity on the concave side and the rib interspaces are too small to accommodate the 10-mm endoscopic portals and instruments. With spinal rotation, the mediastinal organs begin to obstruct exposure. In certain cases, these problems may be overcome by adding more working portals. For the novice spinal endoscopist, however, formal open thoracotomy may be more prudent.

During deformity correction, the spine may be exposed on either the convexity or concavity, depending on clinical circumstances or the surgeon's preference. Because the structural tether is on the concavity, anterior releases through that side were recommended by Stagnara (23). This approach requires working deep in the concave portion of the deformity between the narrowed rib spaces. Here, the segmental vessels are clumped together and are more likely to be injured, and the mediastinal structures must be meticulously dissected and mobilized. On the other hand, working in the concavity allows access to more disc spaces with fewer portals and a direct approach to the structural tether in the posterolateral corner of the disc space.

Working from the convexity may require more portals to gain parallel access to each disc space. If thoracoplasty is planned, a convex side approach is required. For kyphosis correction, the spine can be approached from either side at the surgeon's discretion.

The lateral decubitus position, mimicking open thoracotomy, is typically selected for spinal deformity procedures (1–3,8,17). Some investigators report simultaneous prone anterior thoracoscopic release with posterior instrumentation (Fig. 3) (23,35).

In gaining access to the spine, the first portal is created opposite the apex of deformity at the middle axillary line. The lung is retracted, and the sympathetic chain is bluntly dissected out of the operative field. Incise the anterior longitudinal ligament and annulus. In scoliosis, the aorta may need to be mobilized with blunt dissection, as it frequently lays in the acute angle between the rib head and lateral vertebral body. Once mobilized, place a small sponge or peanut retractor in the interval between the vertebral body and the aorta to protect the great vessels during the preparation of the disc space.

Once access to the disc space is achieved, the nucleus pulposus is evacuated with rongeurs and curettes down to bleeding subchondral bone end-plates (Fig. 4). This evacuation is extended to but not beyond the posterior longitudinal ligament. For the scoliosis cases approached from the concavity, release the posterolateral corner, costotransverse ligaments, and rib heads on the concave side under direct view to optimize correction. Leave the convex lateral annulus intact as a tether and pivot point to prevent overdistraction during the posterior correction. If working from the convexity, the concave posterolateral corner must be released to achieve a complete correction. For kyphosis releases, incise the entire anterior longitudinal ligament and annulus. During simultaneous front-back cases, lever the disc spaces open with transpedicular instrumentation in place posteriorly to improve visualization of the posterior longitudinal ligament.

Once all levels are released, insert a periosteal elevator and rotate slightly to ensure that proper release has been achieved (1). Then, graft the disc spaces with morcellized cancellous iliac crest graft delivered by a funnel. Alternatively, use allograft or autologous rib grafts from an internal thoracoplasty. A structural tricortical crest graft or femoral allograft ring may prevent postoperative loss of correction.

Internal thoracoplasty can be performed just after anterior endoscopic release or as an independent procedure as described by Mehlman, Crawford, and Wolf (41). Preoperatively, ribs to be resected are identified radiographically and by physical examination. From the lateral decubitus position, thoracoplasty is performed on the convex side. Drape the patient's arm free to allow intraoperative scapular motion. Tilt the operating room table 15 degrees toward the prone position to help with lung retraction.

Plan rib resections as an ellipse to ensure the chest contours are smooth. Work from a cephalad to caudal direction to preserve maximum visibility as the deformity corrects. Expose the ribs to be resected linearly using a harmonic scalpel or monopolar cautery. Then, subperiosteally strip the segment of rib to be removed with an endoscopic curved elevator. Pay careful attention to the inferior margins of each rib to avoid the intercostal vessels. Insert a high-speed burr through the portal-most perpendicular to rib in question and create medial and lateral osteotomies. Use a metal sucker tip

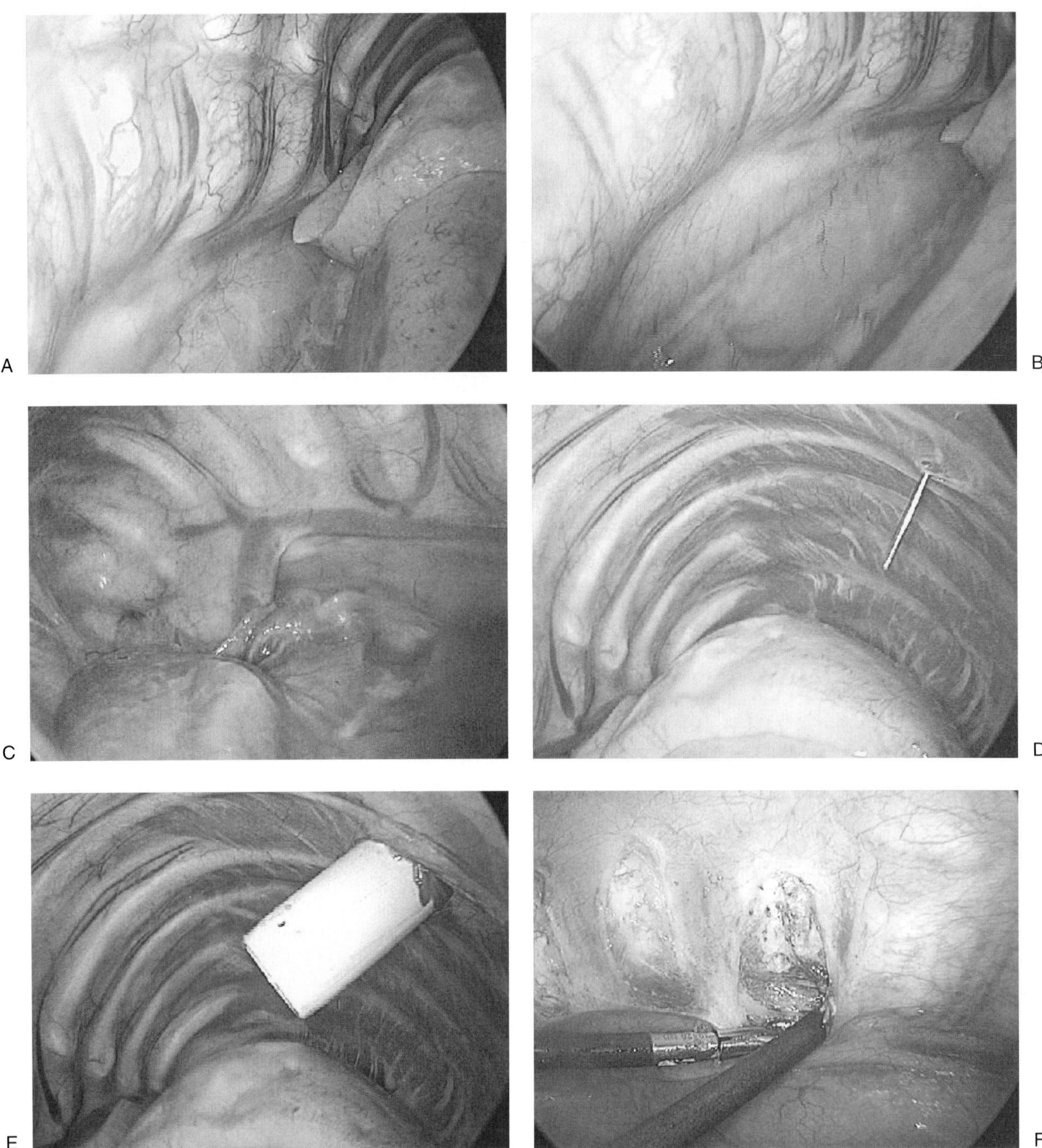

FIG. 4. Multiple releases for scoliosis. **A:** Typical thoracoscopic anatomy. **B:** Further thoracoscopic exploration of the chest. Note the azygos vein and superior vena cava. **C:** Here, in the upper thoracic spine, the superior intercostal vein can be seen feeding into the azygos system. **D:** Further portal placement can be planned with a needle to ensure appropriate alignment. **E:** The portal itself is inserted. **F:** An endoscopic dissector is used to take down a portion of the parietal pleura. This view shows three disc levels exposed without sacrifice of the segmental vessels. (*continued*)

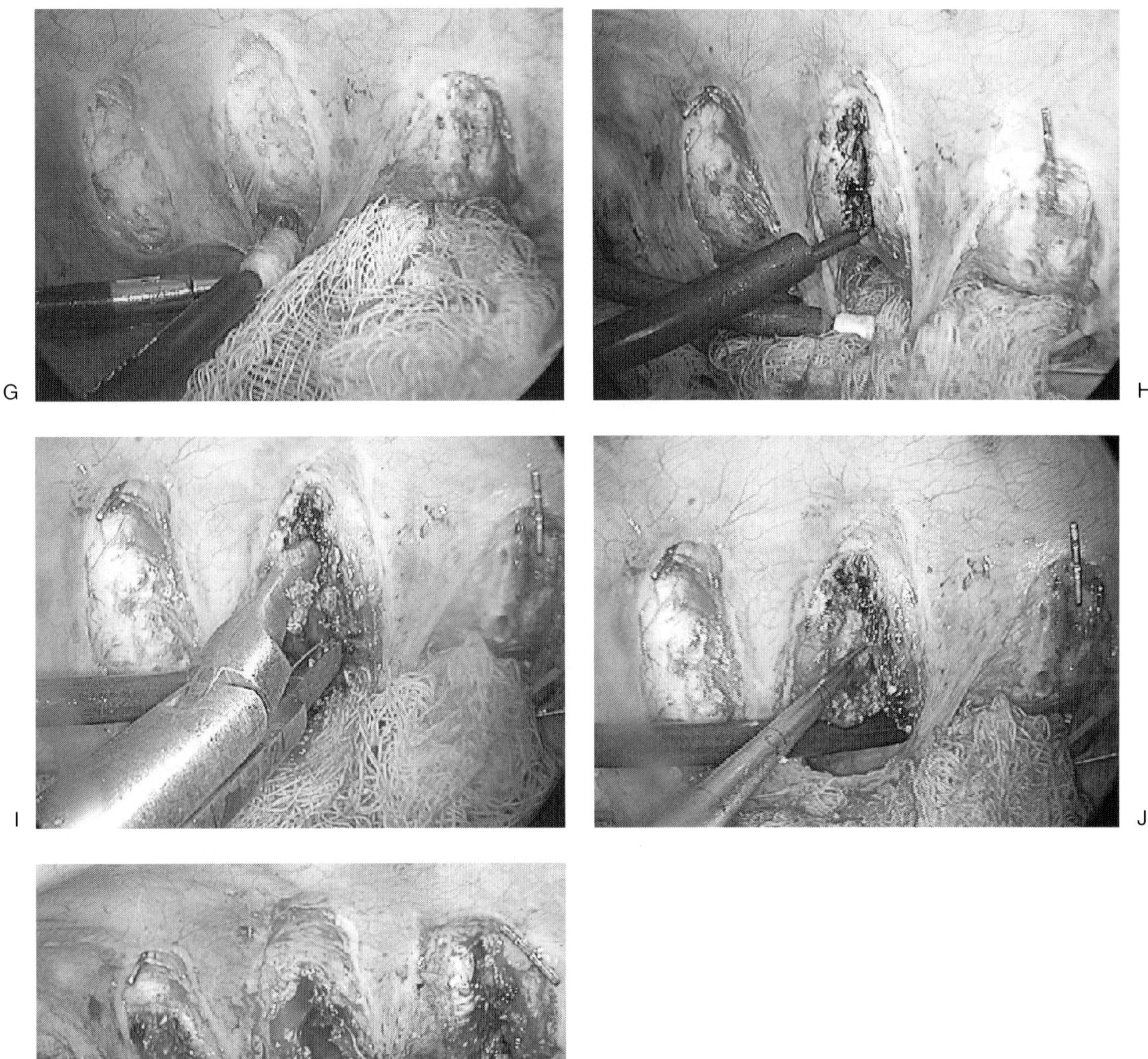

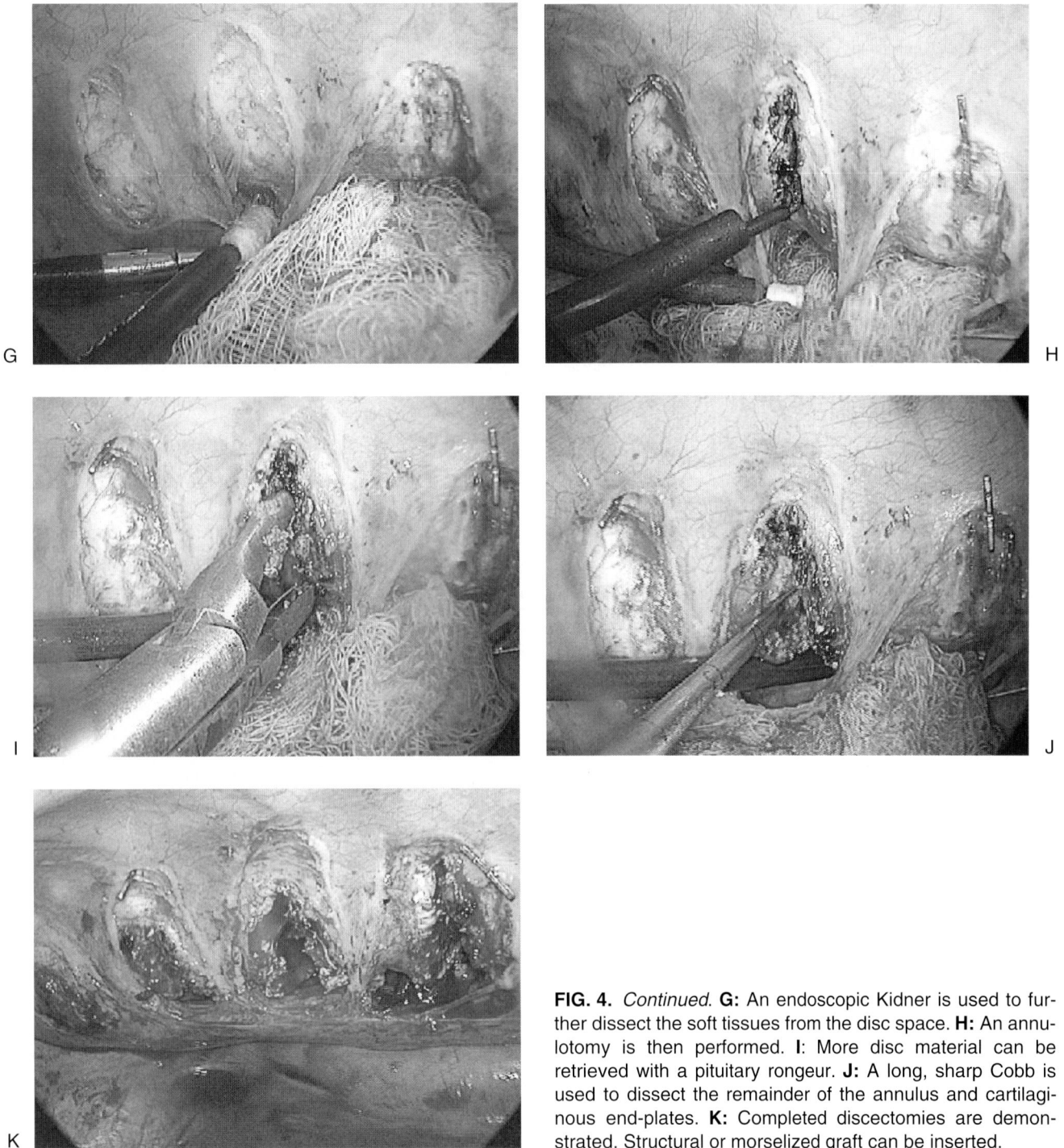

FIG. 4. *Continued.* **G:** An endoscopic Kidner is used to further dissect the soft tissues from the disc space. **H:** An annulotomy is then performed. **I**: More disc material can be retrieved with a pituitary rongeur. **J:** A long, sharp Cobb is used to dissect the remainder of the annulus and cartilaginous end-plates. **K:** Completed discectomies are demonstrated. Structural or morselized graft can be inserted.

both as a retractor and to protect the vessels below. After ribs are cut with the burr, dissect the segment free with a long handled periosteal elevator and deliver it out of the chest cavity with long-handled forceps. Occasionally, ribs are cut but subsequently left in place to ensure adequate thoracic cage stability (41).

The average correction achieved with thoracoscopic techniques appears to be at least equivalent to that obtained with traditional approaches (Figs. 5 and 6) (23,24). Yet Arlet found that thoracoscopic procedures cost 28% more than thoracotomy, and that, 7 years after the first report, the literature still contained only 151 patients. There were no long-term follow-up or significant outcomes data regarding spinal balance, fusion rate, rib hump correction, cosmesis, pain, or patient satisfaction. From that respect, the data do not yet support widespread implementation, and the individual surgeon must consider whether they do enough of the appropriate cases to make learning the technique worthwhile.

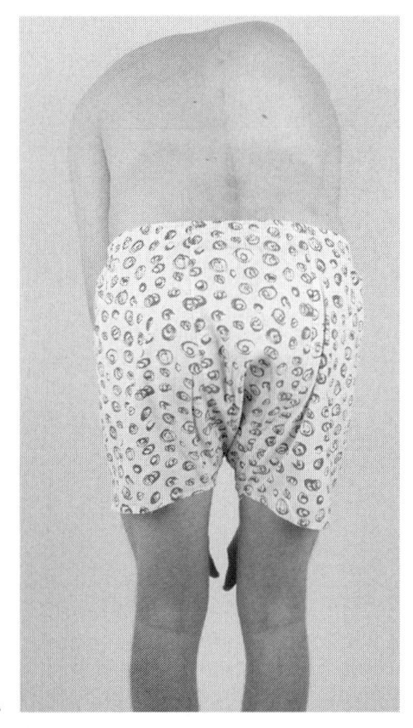

A

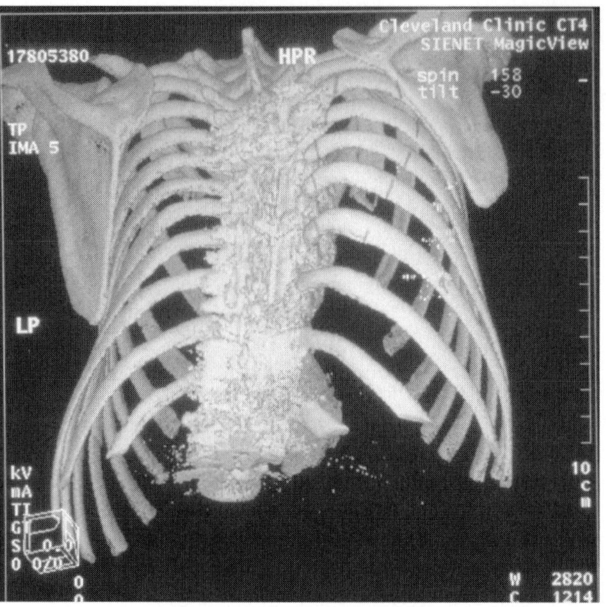

B

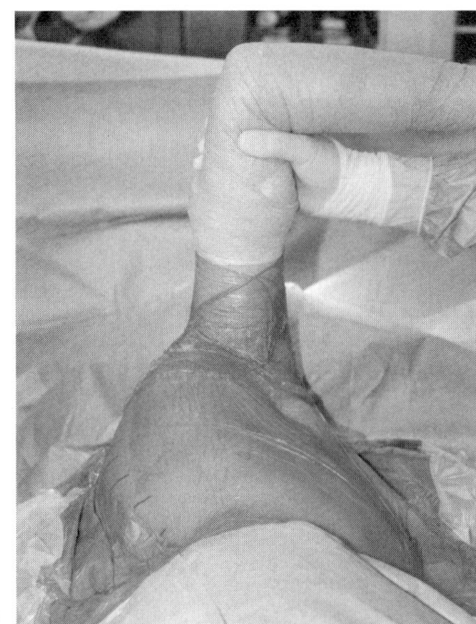

C

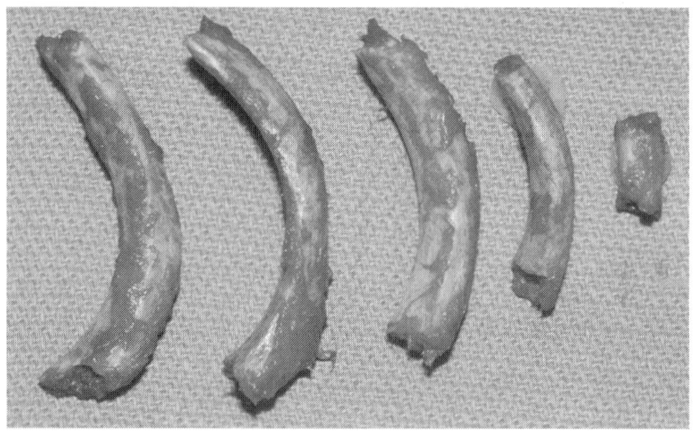

D

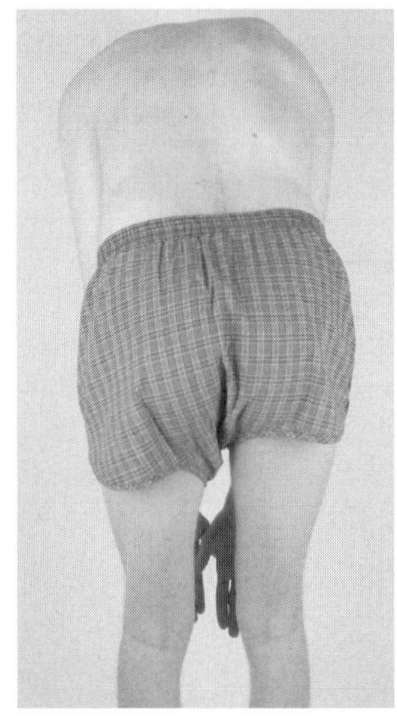

E

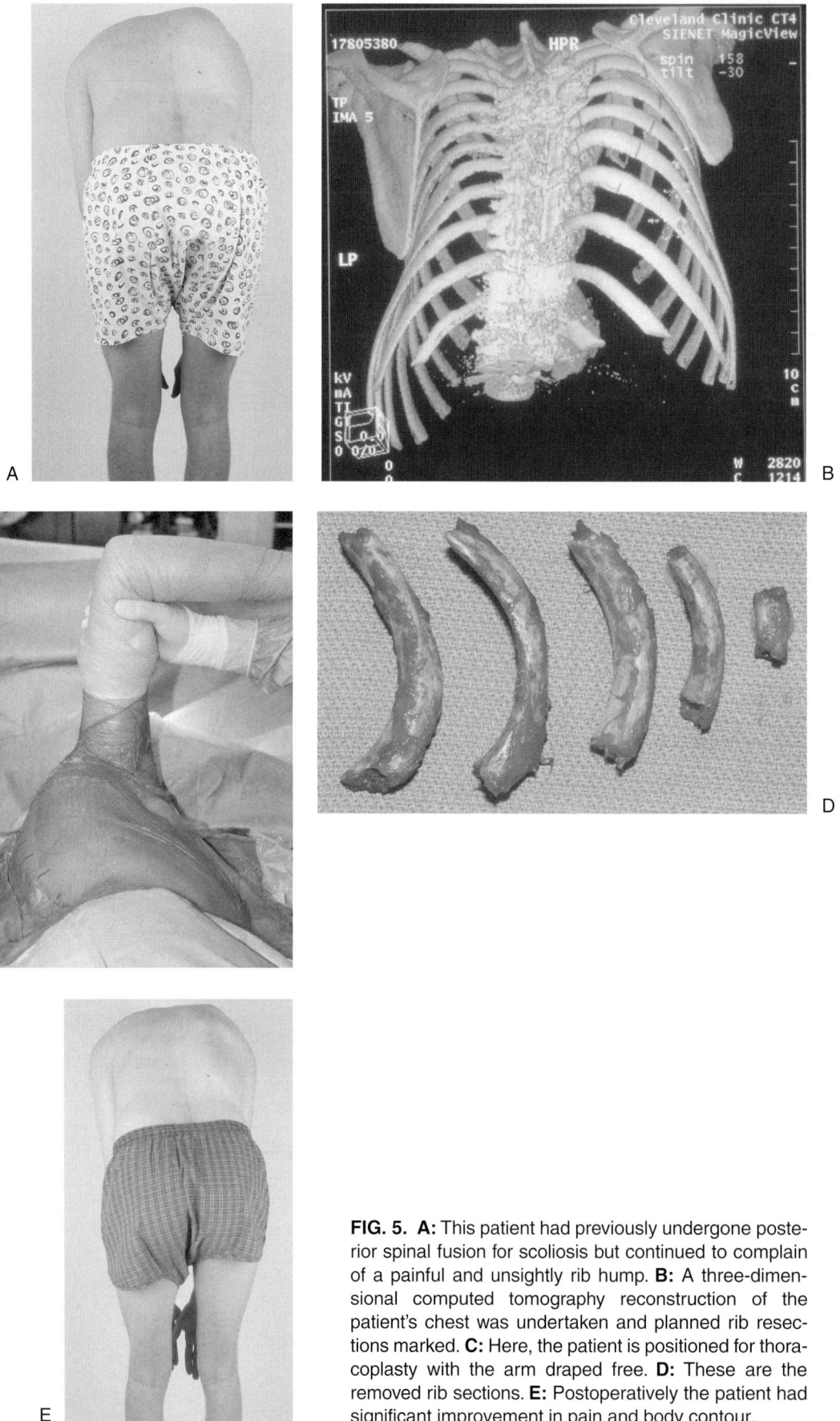

FIG. 5. A: This patient had previously undergone posterior spinal fusion for scoliosis but continued to complain of a painful and unsightly rib hump. **B:** A three-dimensional computed tomography reconstruction of the patient's chest was undertaken and planned rib resections marked. **C:** Here, the patient is positioned for thoracoplasty with the arm draped free. **D:** These are the removed rib sections. **E:** Postoperatively the patient had significant improvement in pain and body contour.

Video-Assisted Thoracic Surgery for Thoracic Spine Degenerative Disease

The use of VATS for treatment of herniated thoracic disc and disc degeneration is becoming increasingly common (2,3, 42,43). Although costotransversectomy and lateral extracavitary approaches have the advantages of being able to decompress and stabilize the spine through a single incision in one stage, they are limited by their time-consuming and technically demanding nature (44). In one report, traditional anterior approaches were found to have a complication rate ranging from 14 to 31%, although dorsal approach–related complications ranged from 17 to 51% (44).

When considering a patient for endoscopic thoracic discectomy, it should be remembered that true radicular or myelopathic symptoms from thoracic disc herniations are rare. More commonly, the patient presents with diffuse midthoracic back pain and multiple degenerative segments with or without herniations. These patients are not ideal candidates for discectomy of any form, either open or endoscopic.

Symptomatic thoracic herniations amenable to endoscopic decompression are typically approached from the side of the herniation. If there has been previous surgery, a contralateral approach may be used. The first trocar is inserted at sixth or seventh interspace, as described previously. Then insert two to three additional portals under direct vision, with one to two portals inserted at the anterior axillary line and one at the posterior axillary line. Use a 30-degree angled rigid scope to see into the disc space and around the bony edges. Identify the appropriate level and resect the proximal 2 cm of rib head, if above T-11. Cut the foraminal ligaments from the superior edge of the pedicle. Resection of the superior part of the pedicle exposes the dura. Some surgeons excise the entire pedicle, particularly for larger and more central herniations (43).

Next, with the spinal cord continuously visualized to prevent inadvertent entry into the canal, create a cavity in the disc space and vertebral bodies anteriorly. Increase the size of this space for larger or more central herniations. A corpectomy may be required for larger or ossified herniations.

Find the disc herniation by tracing the superior edge of the pedicle to the vertebral body and disc space. Fine instruments can then be used to pull the disc herniation into the created cavity. Once the decompression has been completed, document its medial-lateral and cranial-caudal extent by placing a Penfield across the intervertebral space and using fluoroscopy or a radiograph.

Rosenthal and Dickman reported outcomes of 55 consecutive patients undergoing video-assisted thoracoscopic discectomy (43). In patient cohort, 65% presented with myelopathic signs and symptoms due to spinal cord compression, and the remainder had severe thoracic radiculopathy. After surgery, 60% of the myelopathic patients recovered neurologically, whereas 79% of the radiculopathic patients recovered completely, and 21% improved. They compared their thoracoscopic patients with patients treated by costotransversectomy or thoracotomy and found that thoracoscopy was associated with 1 hour less operating room time and one-half the blood loss.

Subsequently, Anand and Regan reported a mean operative time of 173 minutes and average blood loss of 259 mL after 117 thoracoscopic discectomy procedures in 100 consecutive patients (38). The authors concluded that VATS was a safe and efficacious method for the treatment of thoracic disc herniations.

Video-Assisted Thoracic Surgery in the Treatment of Spine Tumors

The traditional approach to cord compression from spinal tumors was posterior or posterolateral. However, as most compression is

A–C

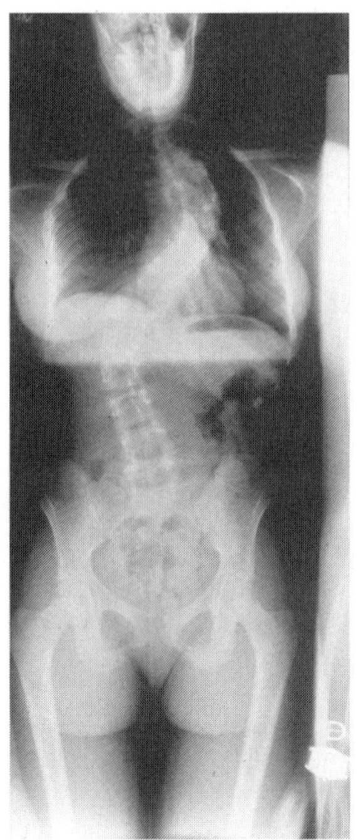

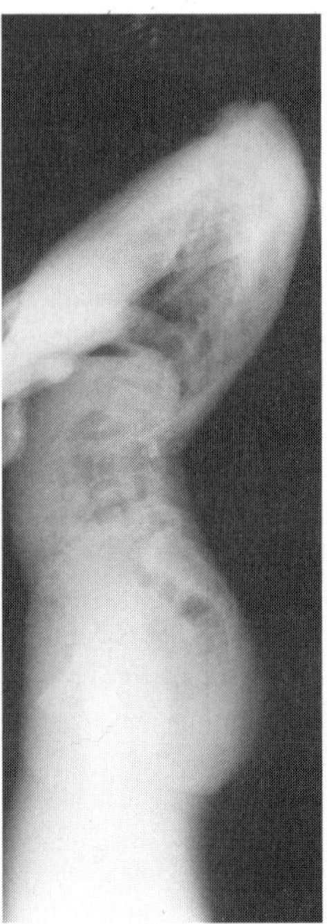

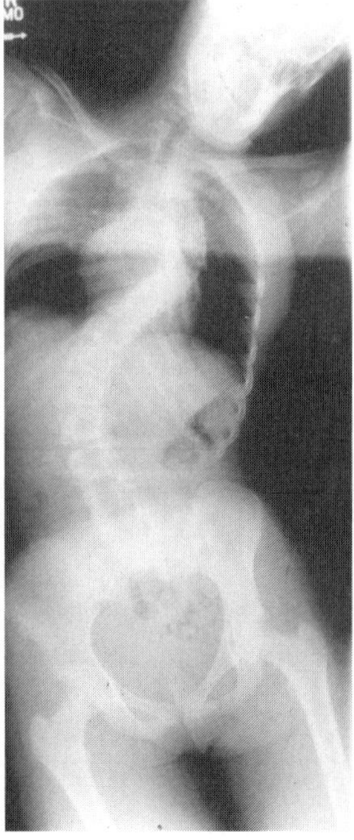

FIG. 6. This patient presented with a progressive, rigid thoracic scoliosis. Anterior-posterior, lateral, and side-bending films are shown **(A–C)**.*(continued)*

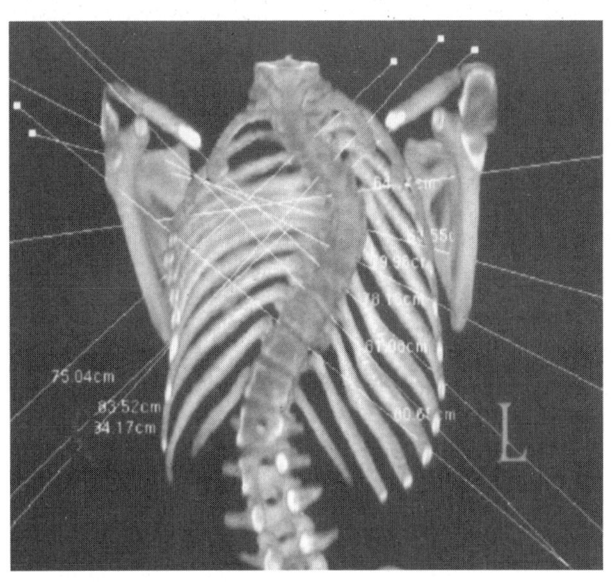

D

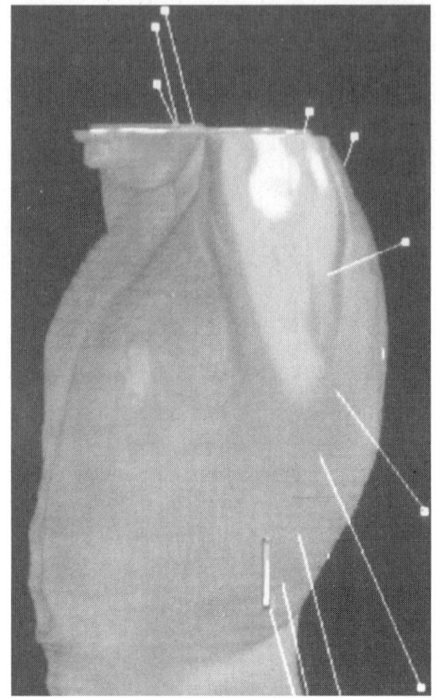

E

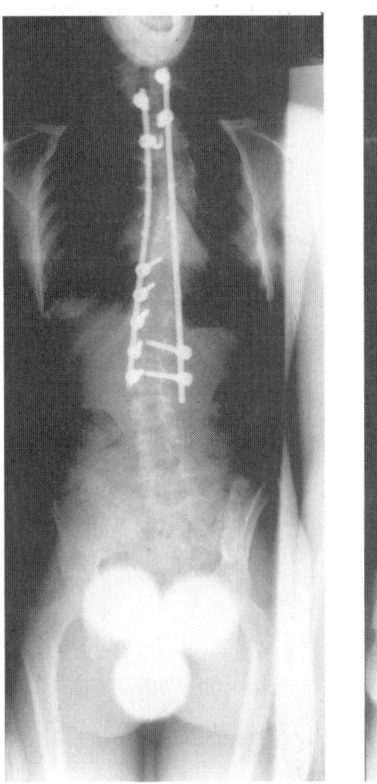

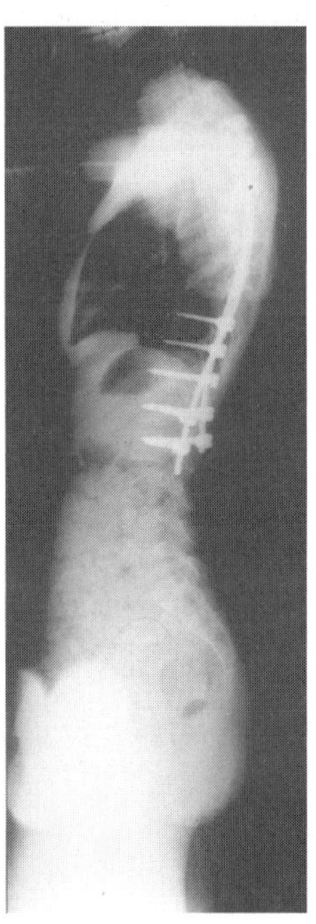

F,G

FIG. 6. *Continued.* Three-dimensional computed tomography reconstructions are useful for surgical planning and portal preparation **(D,E)**. A simultaneous anterior release and posterior instrumented fusion were undertaken. Postoperative films are shown **(F,G)**.

caused by ventral lesions, it is not surprising that results after posterior decompression have been poor. Recently, more aggressive and potentially more morbid thoracotomy approaches have been espoused for successful cord decompression.

The need to limit the invasiveness of an operative approach for neurologic decompression or spinal stabilization is even more acute in patients with spinal malignancy. VATS techniques can be used solely in intralesional or piecemeal tumor resections (45), but solitary tumor *en bloc* resections always require some form of open approach.

The technique of decompression in patients with spinal tumors is similar to that in degenerative disease. Embolization is critical for most rapidly growing neoplasms, especially renal cell cancer. When removing fragments of tumor material, it may be appropriate to drop the material into a tumor bag before bringing it through the body wall. This limits exposure of the thoracic cavity to neoplastic cells. Reconstruction techniques in malignancy may be liberalized, depending on the anticipated life span of the patient. To avoid the morbidity of graft harvest and to achieve early stability, Rosenthal described reconstruction by injection of semiliquid methylmethacrylate (46). The polymethylmethacrylate is injected through a tube into the cavity and allowed to polymerize *in situ*. For patients with a longer anticipated survival, a fusion should be performed. Anterior instrumentation options are improving. In Rosenthal's series, special equipment was used to dilate the skin incision to allow insertion of a ventral plate. Special instruments are used to handle the plates and screws in the chest cavity.

Citow et al. described a single-stage, combined laminectomy and thoracoscopic resection of a 4-cm by 5-cm by 5-cm mass filling 60% of the spinal canal at the T-3 level (16). The lesion was first detached from the spinal cord by a laminectomy with medial facetectomy. Then, a three-portal thoracoscopic approach was undertaken in which the parietal pleura was incised and the tumor bluntly dissected and removed through an expanded anterior portal in a specimen bag. The authors noted that potential limitation to this approach was possible communication between the subarachnoid space with the low-pressure pleural cavity, which would increase the risk of cerebrospinal fluid fistula. They recommended an endoscopic suture of the parietal pleura. Further, because of the potential for malignant lesions to encase or invade the mediastinal structures, they suggested distinguishing between benign and malignant lesions before proceeding with the endoscopic approach.

Van Dijk, Cuesta, and Wuisman described another combined technique for solitary spine tumor resection wherein thoracoscopically assisted ventral releases were followed by a dorsal *en bloc* spondylectomy and reconstruction (47). This approach allowed thoracoscopic access and release of the involved spinal segments to achieve surgical and histopathologic wide margins while avoiding the disadvantages inherent to thoracotomy.

Video-Assisted Thoracic Surgery in the Treatment of Thoracic Spine Trauma

Thoracoscopic approaches to trauma offer similar benefits as to those in other patient groups. Thoracoscopic techniques may be particularly helpful in elderly patients who may not tolerate a thoracotomy and diaphragmatic release. Similarly, protection of shoulder mechanics may be helpful in paraplegic patients by allowing earlier rehabilitation and independent transfers.

Vertebral corpectomy or osteotomy for spinal fracture may be performed in the lateral or prone positions, depending on the subsequent procedures anticipated. During prone procedures, posterior instrumentation can be manipulated to increase intervertebral exposure, as described for kyphosis correction in deformity patients.

The initial trocar is inserted as described previously, and the chest is explored. The injured level is easily identified in acute fractures by the subpleural hematoma covering it. After identification of the level, a second trocar is inserted ventrally to allow lung retraction toward the mediastinum.

Because a significant portion of thoracic trauma occurs at the thoracolumbar junction, the extended manipulating channel method described by Huang et al. may be useful (48). For these injuries, an approach from the left is recommended because the aorta lies just left of the midline, and there is more space available next to the vertebral surface. After the initial portal has been made at the seventh intercostal space, an extended portal 5 to 6 cm in length is placed at the injured level or slightly behind the posterior axillary line at the T9-10 interspace. A length of underlying rib is removed, and a small, self-retaining rib spreader is then placed, allowing introduction of larger instruments and direct palpation of the spine. Gently push the diaphragm down with a sponge forceps introduced through the manipulating channel. The approach-side pedicles are key landmarks and are removed at the vertebrectomy level and the next caudal level (6). With the dura exposed, discectomy of the superior and inferior disc space are undertaken using curettes and pituitary rongeurs.

A defect is created in the anterior portion of the vertebral body with a high-speed burr or rongeur. This allows compressive fragments, such as the posterior vertebral cortex, to be pulled away from the dura. Complete decompressive corpectomy requires direct palpation of the contralateral pedicle.

Reconstruction after trauma includes morselized or structural anterior grafting followed by anterior or posterior instrumented stabilization. Morselized bone placed into partial corpectomy defects is typically stabilized posteriorly with short segment transpedicular instrumentation (21). Alternatively, a corpectomy reconstruction can be completed by negotiating allograft struts or mesh cages into the anterior defect after inserting them into the chest through one of the portals. Then, either anterior or posterior instrumentation is used to stabilize the construct with respect to extension, rotation, and side flexion.

Dickman et al. reported on six patients undergoing thoracoscopic vertebrectomy for fracture (19). They found that the operative time and blood loss were similar to that of a comparable open-thoracotomy group. Narcotic use, ICU stay, and hospital length of stay were all dramatically reduced in the thoracoscopic group.

Video-Assisted Thoracic Surgery in the Treatment of Spine Infection

Treatment of spinal infection begins by identifying the offending organism through blood culture or biopsy. When clear identification of the organism is not provided by fluoroscopically or computed tomography–guided biopsy, surgical biopsy is needed. Endoscopic techniques offer an ideal, less invasive means to obtain an adequate tissue sample.

After the organism has been identified, surgery is indicated in any patient with neurologic deficits, failure to improve with medical management, or continued vertebral collapse. When cord compression occurs, the pathology is most often anterior, and wide approaches such as thoracotomy or costotransversectomy traditionally have been indicated. VATS can be used in patients with spinal infections to accomplish biopsy, débridement, cord decompression, and reconstruction.

Typically, a four-portal technique is used, starting with an initial viewing portal at the T-7 level. There may be a higher rate of pleurodesis secondary to inflammation, requiring either meticulous thoracoscopic release of adhesions or a conversion to an open procedure. Because of adhesions, the risk of postoperative air leak is higher as well.

Frequently, a paraspinal subpleural mass is identified. The pleura is incised parallel to the spine with careful control of the segmental vessels at the midbody level. The extraspinal necrotic material is débrided, and the disc levels above and below the infected segment are identified. Discectomies are performed, and the end-plates are prepared for subsequent fusion. This process affords the surgeon excellent orientation to the spinal anatomy. The pedicles of the affected vertebral bodies are removed. Then, the corpectomies themselves are undertaken from disc space to disc space, progressing in a cranial to caudal direction. As with trauma, begin by creating a hollow in the vertebral body anteriorly. Then, posterior cortex and compressive material can be delivered anteriorly with a curette or small Kerrison rongeur. The magnification and lighting afforded by the endoscope allows the decompressed dura to be inspected at close range to ensure adequate decompression (22).

LUMBAR APPROACHES

Background

Anterior lumbar spinal surgery is currently being performed to treat symptomatic degenerative disc disease, spondylolisthesis, augmentation of posterior spinal fusions, reconstructions for tumor or trauma, and as a salvage procedure for failed posterior approaches. Anterior surgery has allowed the surgeon access to the spine without disrupting intact posterior elements. Reports describing anterior lumbar interbody fusion (ALIF) in the early 1960s stimulated interest in further approaches that minimize soft-tissue trauma while affording the surgeon comparable results to the more accepted posterior approaches. Several approaches have been popularized, including the retroperitoneal muscle-splitting and the transperitoneal routes. The expertise gained in minimally invasive laparoscopic techniques in gynecologic, general, and urologic surgery has now been applied to spinal surgery to take advantage of the potential benefits of a minimally invasive approach.

Laparoscopy was first applied to treating spinal pathology in 1991. Obenchain reported the use of laparoscopy to approach the spine for discectomies (49). By the mid-1990s, several other authors described using minimally invasive techniques to aid ALIF surgery in animal models (50,51). Prospective studies comparing different approaches in lumbar fusion surgery began appearing soon after. Laparoscopic ALIF surgery is now more common in many centers but has not reached the popularity that laparoscopy has achieved in other surgical disciplines. The use of this technology has afforded spinal surgeons with valuable experience in understanding important issues in lumbar spine exposures.

As with any spinal surgical procedure, patient selection is the single most important outcome issue. As knowledge and technology of laparoscopic surgery evolves, the surgeon must adhere to strict indications and exhaust conservative modalities before offering patients a new seductive and potentially wrong option. Patients with mechanical back pain who have failed physical therapy and pharmacologic interventions may benefit from surgery. Back pain secondary to grade I or II spondylolisthesis, degenerative disc disease, postlaminectomy instability, and failed posterior surgery may be helped by fusion surgery. Once the patient has been offered surgery, the most appropriate procedure and surgical approach must be determined on an individual basis. Consultation with a laparoscopist is warranted if the spinal surgeon determines the pathology is better approached anteriorly and if the patient is interested in minimally invasive techniques.

Laparoscopic spine surgery demands a highly specialized team of professionals. The spine surgeon must accept the responsibility and challenge of this new procedure in the face of proven posterior approaches. The spine surgeon must trust the ability of the laparoscopist to determine the feasibility of a minimally invasive approach. The laparoscopist must be skilled technically and have an understanding of the spine surgeon's goals before surgery. During the preoperative workup, magnetic resonance or computed tomography imaging may help to visualize not only the pathology but also the aorta, vena cava, and iliac vessels. Anatomic variations may dictate the feasibility of the approach and also the portal of entry to the disc. This is especially true in cases of L4-5 disc surgery. To undertake a laparoscopic approach, the operating suite must be conducive to a large surgical procedure with specialized equipment, and the surgical technicians must be familiar with both general and spinal surgical instruments and implants. Finally, laparoscopic approaches should not be performed without immediate access to conversion instruments and surgeons capable of dealing with the potential complications.

Technique

Any successful surgery begins with preoperative planning. The spinal surgeon, laparoscopist, patient, and ancillary staff must be cocoordinated and agreeable in terms of goals and expectations of surgery.

The surgical setting is important. Laparoscopic surgery should only be performed in a setting with facilities to deal with potential major complications. The trend toward outpatient or short-stay surgery centers is appealing; however, most of these centers do not have the staff to deal with potential complications on a round-the-clock basis.

Preoperative bowel preparation is at the surgeon's discretion. Occasionally after preparation, the bowel fills with fluid that can be even more bothersome when trying to mobilize the bowel (Fig. 7). Preoperative prophylactic antibiotics are also at the surgeon's discretion.

The patient is positioned supine on a radiolucent table in a steep Trendelenburg position with the pressure points padded. General anesthesia is always used. The radiolucent table is necessary for image intensification during implant insertion. Trendelenburg positioning assists with bowel retraction out of the pelvis. The patient's arms are folded over a chest pillow and secured with tape or are secured at the patient's side. The patient is prepped from the nipples down to the inguinal folds. The iliac crests should be accessible bilaterally for bone graft (Fig. 8).

To gain access, the peritoneum is first insufflated to 15 mm Hg via trocar after direct cutdown or using a Verres needle in the infraumbilical midline. The insufflation site is used for a 10-mm camera portal. In the right lower quadrant, two working portals are inserted under direct vision, one being 10 mm to allow for larger instruments (i.e., the vascular clip applier), the other 5 mm. A 5-mm, left lower quadrant portal is used for retraction purposes. The video monitor is placed to the left of the patient's feet. The general surgeon stands to the right of the patient and works through the two right lower quadrant portals. The assistant stands to the left of the patient and operates the camera and retracts from the infraumbilical and left lower quadrant portals, respectively. The spinal surgeon stands to the right of the patient and operates through a fifth portal placed infraumbilical after the annulus of the targeted level is exposed and verified by image intensifier.

To expose the L-5 to S-1 disc level for interbody fusion, the small bowel is first swept out of the pelvis. The assistant then lifts and retracts the sigmoid colon to the patient's left to tent the mesentery. The parietal peritoneum is then incised with short controlled bursts of cautery over the disc annulus. Monopolar cautery is preferred to prevent any arcing to adjacent tissues and to minimize the risk of retrograde ejaculation in male patients. The harmonic scalpel may also be used. The incision is longitu-

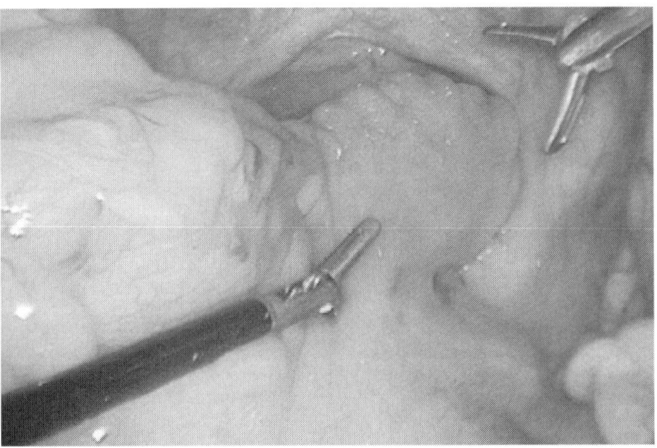

FIG. 7. Intraoperative video image of bowel mobilization to the L-5 to S-1 level.

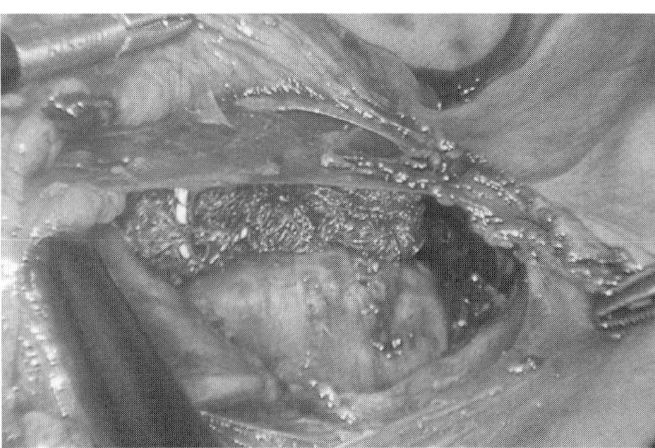

FIG. 9. Intraoperative video image of L-5 to S-1 annulus exposed, left iliac vein retracted to expose annulus.

dinal and deepened using blunt dissection with dental pledgets to move the tissue laterally. This method preserves the autonomic plexus that runs on both sides. The median sacral vessels are carefully mobilized, ligated, and divided. The left common iliac vein usually overlies the lateral third of the annulus and can be mobilized with blunt dental pledget dissection (Fig. 9). The right iliac vein is rarely in the way. The ureters are more lateral at this level and are not exposed. The vascular anatomy allows exposure to the L-5 to S-1 disc without significant manipulation of the nearby vascular structures. The abdominal aorta usually bifurcates at the level of the L4-5 disc or L-5 vertebral body. The common iliac arteries usually bifurcate lateral to the L-5 to S-1 disc.

Once the L-5 to S-1 annulus has been exposed, the annulus is excised, and the disc space is prepared for the surgeon's choice of interbody implant. As a general principle, one should aim to minimize any vessel mobilization, and thus work sequentially,

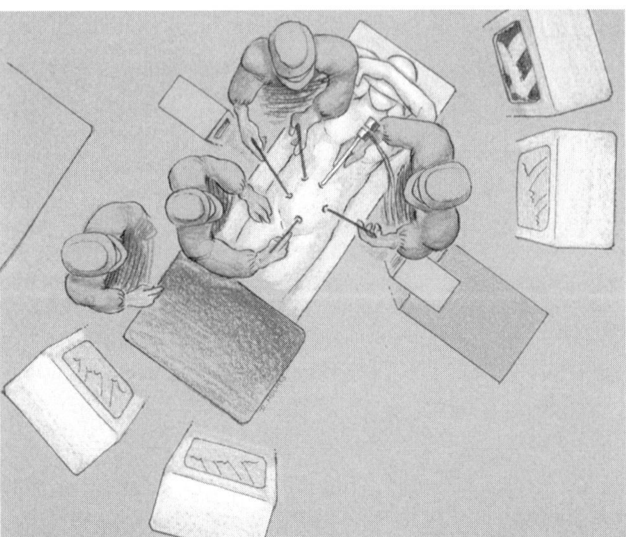

FIG. 8. Surgical setup for standard thoracoscopy and two-team combined thoracic approach.

finishing the surgery on one side while protecting the vessels and not returning to that side again.

Exposures to levels above L-5 to S-1 are technically more demanding due to the need to identify and divide the iliolumbar vein and the need to dissect and retract the aorta and inferior vena cava. The positioning, setup and portal sites are similar to that previously discussed. For more proximal levels, the camera portal may be positioned supraumbilically 1 to 2 cm cephalad to the umbilicus.

The initial dissection is similar to the L-5 to S-1 level. A longitudinal incision is made through the parietal peritoneum overlying the L4-5 level just left of the aorta. Blunt dissection is taken caudal along the aorta and left common iliac artery. To mobilize the aorta, common iliac artery, and inferior vena cava, the iliolumbar vein and one or two lumbar segmental vessels must be mobilized and divided. These vessels are usually substantial and should be ligated with a generous cuff of tissue and divided between vascular clips. The vasculature usually allows for insertion of the interbody implants with the aorta retracted to the right. Occasionally, the anatomy dictates that the interbody devices be implanted between the aorta retracted to the left and the inferior vena cava retracted to the right. The surgeon must be cognizant of the left ureter, which can come into view with dissection and retraction of the great vessels to the left. If multiple levels are being instrumented, multiple portals may be used for insertion of the working sheath. A more lateral exposure of the upper lumbar levels is also possible by mobilizing the sigmoid colon to the right and dissecting in the interval between the psoas and the vertebral bodies. Mobilizing the psoas laterally and posteriorly allows exposure to the lateral aspect of the annulus while minimizing the need to mobilize the great vessels.

The variations in vascular anatomy dictate the route of implant insertion into the L4-5 disc space. Regan et al. described their experience in 58 patients. In 30 patients, the disc was accessed above the bifurcation, with mobilization of the great vessels to the same side (52). In 18 patients, the disc space was below the bifurcation, making access similar to the L-5 to S-1 level. In the remaining ten patients, the disc was accessed between the aorta and inferior vena cava.

An alternate transperitoneal psoas splitting route to the L4-5 level was described by Brody et al. (53). This approach allowed for

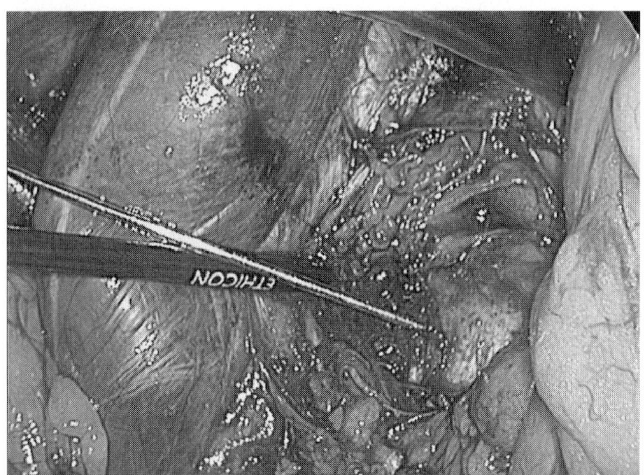

FIG. 10. Intraoperative video image of lateral L4-5 annulus exposure.

standard laparoscopic exposure of L-5 to S-1 and lateral exposure of L4-5 thus obviating the need to dissect and mobilize the inferior vena cava, aorta, and left common iliac vein (Fig. 10). Access to the L4-5 annulus is achieved through a portal inserted directly over the iliac tubercle. Through the transperitoneal approach, a peritoneal window is opened over the psoas muscle, and the psoas is then split in line with its fibers. Alternatively, the psoas, if not too bulky, can be raised off the annulus in the interval between it and the aorta. Once the annulus is exposed, the remaining procedure is performed as would be done with any lateral interbody fusion.

Most surgeons with experience in laparoscopic spinal surgery would agree accessing the L4-5 level is technically more demanding than L-5 to S-1. Once the L4-5 annulus has been exposed, extension to more cephalad levels is fairly simple and easy. Isolation, mobilization, and retraction of the significant abdominal vascular structures may increase morbidity and the need to convert to an open procedure.

Postoperatively, the patient should be monitored for the return of bowel function. A liquid diet can be started on the night of the operation and advanced as tolerated. This is usually done as a 1- to 2-day acute care hospital stay. The return of bowel function can be assessed by diminished or lack of abdominal distention, absence of nausea and vomiting, and the presence of flatus or bowel movements. Deep venous thrombosis prophylaxis should be considered while the patient is in the hospital. Preoperative fitting of a lumbosacral corset or off-the-shelf orthosis can facilitate quicker mobilization. Orthoses and abdominal binders are for patient comfort only and should not be needed to provide stability to the fusion construct. Neurologic checks of the lower extremities are imperative. The first postoperative check should be at baseline or improved from the preoperative status. A change in neurologic function postoperatively should alert the surgeon to the possibly of a hematoma or malpositioned fusion construct. The patient's activity should be limited to activities of daily living while avoiding bending, lifting, and twisting maneuvers until there is radiographic evidence of fusion.

Results

Results of prospective analyses are still needed to determine the practicality of laparoscopic lumbar spine surgery. Most studies were initiated in the mid-1990s and are descriptions of prospective cohorts.

Zucherman et al. was first to report on 17 consecutive patients undergoing laparoscopic fusion with threaded cylindrical cages (54). Fourteen patients had single-level fusions, 12 at L-5 to S-1, two at L4-5. Three patients had two-level fusions at L4-5 and L-5 to S-1. Two patients had to be converted to an open procedure because of intraoperative bleeding. Neither of these required transfusion. Four patients developed a postoperative ileus. One patient required a posterior decompression for a displaced endplate fracture behind the fusion cage. Average follow-up was 8 months. Fifteen patients were pleased with their surgical result, whereas two continued to have disabling back pain.

Mathews et al. commented on the short-term results of six patients. Five patients underwent successful laparoscopic ALIF surgery (55). The sixth was converted to a retroperitoneal approach secondary to an iliac vein injury and excessive bleeding. Average follow-up was 6 months. All patients were determined to be clinically fused by absence of motion with flexion and extension views of L-5 to S-1.

Olsen et al. attempted laparoscopic ALIF in 75 patients (56). Seventy-three were completed successfully. In two patients, the attempt had to be aborted for extensive pelvic adhesions and dense presacral scarring. Two patients had bladder lacerations repaired endoscopically. One patient reported retrograde ejaculation, and one patient required reoperation for a posteriorly placed cage. Average hospital stay was 36 hours. Only 23 patients (30%) were followed for 2 years. Eighteen considered their symptoms significantly improved, five moderately improved. Mean preoperative pain scores were 8.7 compared to 2.3 postoperatively.

Mahvi and Zdeblick operated on 20 consecutive patients and concluded that laparoscopic ALIF is safe, and the early results were encouraging (57). Nineteen patients had single-level L-5 to S-1fusion, whereas one had a two-level L4-5, L-5 to S-1 fusion. Three patients had complications: two bleeding and one neurologic. Two procedures were converted to open secondary to vein injuries. Neither of these required transfusions. A third patient required a posterior decompression for a posterior disc herniation. These complications occurred in the first four patients in the study. The authors concluded the complications were related to the laparoscopic technique of exposing the space and the interbody devices.

Regan, Yuan, and McAfee published a prospective multicenter study comparing open and laparoscopic lumbar fusion in 1999 (58). Two hundred forty consecutive patients undergoing laparoscopic lumbar fusion were compared to 591 patients undergoing open anterior fusion with the same threaded cylindrical interbody device. Twenty-five patients (10%) had to be converted to an open procedure: Six were secondary to bleeding complications; five were due to anatomic variations precluding adequate exposure; eight were attributed to dense scar or adhesions; and only six were attributed to technical reasons. The laparoscopic group had an increased operative time compared to the open group. Hospital stay and blood loss were both reduced in the laparoscopic group. Operative complications were comparable in both groups. The device-related reoperation rate was higher in the laparoscopic group. The need for another operation was most consistently attributed to intraoperative disc herniation. The authors concluded once the learning curve was overcome, laparoscopy was as effective and safe as more traditional open approaches.

Zdeblick, in a second paper, reported on 25 L4-5 fusions performed after his initial learning curve (59). He matched the laparoscopic group with 25 mini-open approaches. He reported more complications in the laparoscopic group and concluded there was no significant advantage to a laparoscopic approach when addressing the L4-5 disc.

Lieberman et al. reported on 47 consecutive laparoscopic patients undergoing one-level, two-level, and three-level fusions (60). Three patients were converted to an open procedure: one secondary to bleeding from the presacral veins that made visualization unacceptable; a second was due to difficult mobilization of the great vessels; whereas the third conversion was in a patient who could not tolerate abdominal insufflation. Two patients needed repeat endoscopy for malpositioned cages. One patient required a laparotomy for a small bowel obstruction. Lieberman concluded transperitoneal laparoscopic exposure can be performed with low risk for single-level and multiple-level anterior lumbar fusions.

In a more recent and ongoing evaluation, the authors matched nine patients undergoing laparoscopic two-level ALIF using threaded cylinders with nine patients undergoing mini-open two-level ALIF using femoral ring allografts augmented with posterior translaminar screw fixation. In the laparoscopic group, one patient sustained an iliac vein tear that required conversion to an open procedure. This patient had an 8,000-cc blood loss, spent 3 days in the surgical ICU, and had a 7-day hospital stay. There were no complications in the mini-open group, although the operative time was on average twice that of the laparoscopic group.

Issues

As with any new procedure, there are risks associated with laparoscopic spinal surgery. Most of these risks involve injury to vascular structures, often causing the surgeon to convert to an open procedure. From published reports, most of these injuries are venous and occasionally can be controlled with laparoscopic vascular instruments. A vascular injury can necessitate blood transfusions, lengthen hospital stay, increase morbidity, and impair functional outcome. Presently, the reported risk of this complication seems low enough to go forward with developing technical skills and instrumentation.

A second issue relates to the risk of retrograde ejaculation. This clinical situation is usually caused by transurethral prostatectomy, diabetic neuropathy, and retroperitoneal lymph node dissection. It is a sympathetic nervous system–mediated lesion through injury to the superior hypogastric plexus. The sympathetic trunks lie anterior to the lumbar segmental vessels and give off a fine reticular network of branches that lie anterior to the parietal peritoneum. The mechanism of injury is proposed to be excessive manipulation or damage of the fine reticular branches when the parietal peritoneum is incised, dissected, and retracted laterally.

The diagnosis of retrograde ejaculation is usually made by a urologist or fertility specialist when sperm is detected in post-ejaculatory urine in clinically infertile males. With open ALIF procedures, the risk is anywhere from 0 to 22%. Some clinicians feel the risk is proportional to the amount of dissection needed. Multiple-level procedures are theoretically at a higher complication risk than single-level procedures. In the 1980s, the complication was believed to be exaggerated, but now many surgeons feel the complication is underreported. Most surgeons would agree the issue must be addressed preoperatively with informed consent, and caution must be taken with all men when an anterior approach is considered.

The future of laparoscopic spinal surgery is promising, however. The technology is evolving rapidly. The advances in interbody device technology, be it fusion or disc replacement, may give surgeons more confidence in pursuing laparoscopic approaches.

POSTERIOR SPINAL ENDOSCOPY

Direct posterior approaches to neurocompressive thoracic pathology have largely been abandoned because laminectomy alone does not adequately decompress a ventral mass and may actually worsen instability and neurologic injury in the presence of kyphotic deformity. Attempts to indirectly decompress central pathologies have been unsuccessful or, worse, have resulted in neurologic decline (61,62). On the other hand, traditional costotransversectomy and lateral extracavitary approaches are associated with large incisions, increased postoperative morbidity, wound healing problems, difficulty with visualization, and less success in decompression and removal of compressive bone or tumor tissue (1,6). Using video-assisted techniques, modified transpedicular approaches use an extrapleural dissection and a 70-degree endoscope to complete the corpectomy with better visualization of the anterior dura, obviating the need for a formal anterior approach. This technique allows the surgeon to operate without collapsing the lung and avoids the postoperative chest tube drainage required of either thoracoscopy or thoracotomy.

This approach is particularly useful in patients with radioresistant metastases of the upper thoracic spine where thoracotomy is difficult and highly morbid (7,13). Contraindications to the currently available techniques include the following: failed previous open surgery, primary vertebral malignancies, and large lesions. Posterior transpedicular instrumentation is another area in which endoscopic assistance may allow for smaller incisions and decreased muscle injury. These resection techniques are intralesional and are therefore not indicated in patients with primary neoplasms (7).

Osman and Marsolais described a posterior endoscopic approach to the thoracic disc space in a cadaver (63). The authors found that above T-10, the rib neck was an ideal guide to the disc space and prevented lateral excursion into the lung. They concluded that this approach would be technically feasible for soft lateral discs.

Jho described a minimally invasive posterior approach to thoracic disc herniations, using a 2-cm transverse paramedian incision at the pedicle level of the involved vertebra (64). Patients are positioned 60 degrees forward inclined to keep the lesion side facing upward. The paraspinal muscles are dissected from the spinous process, lamina, and transverse processes using a periosteal elevator. A tubular retractor is passed into the wound over the facet and lamina. The medial portion of the facet, the lateral portion of the lamina, and the rostral one-third of the pedicle are removed with a high-speed burr to gain access to the disc space and to expose the very lateral margin of the spinal cord dura. A 2-mm burr removes the bone spurs rostral and caudal to the herniated disc and creates a cavity into which more material from the decompression is moved. When an appropriate 1.5-cm cavity has been created, a 4-mm diameter rigid endoscope with a 70-degree lens is mounted to a custom-made endoscope holder. Surgical decompression of the ventral cord can then be performed using 90-degree curved surgical instruments (Fig. 11). For example, a down-biting curette can be used to push more osteophyte away from the cord and into the created cavity. Material can be removed from the cavity with a curved pituitary.

McLain's technique for decompression of thoracic metastases is similar, but it is undertaken through a longitudinal incision (7,13). The initial approach is similar to that of costotransversectomy wherein the proximal rib is removed with the entire pedicle. Here, too, a cavity is created anteriorly and anterior

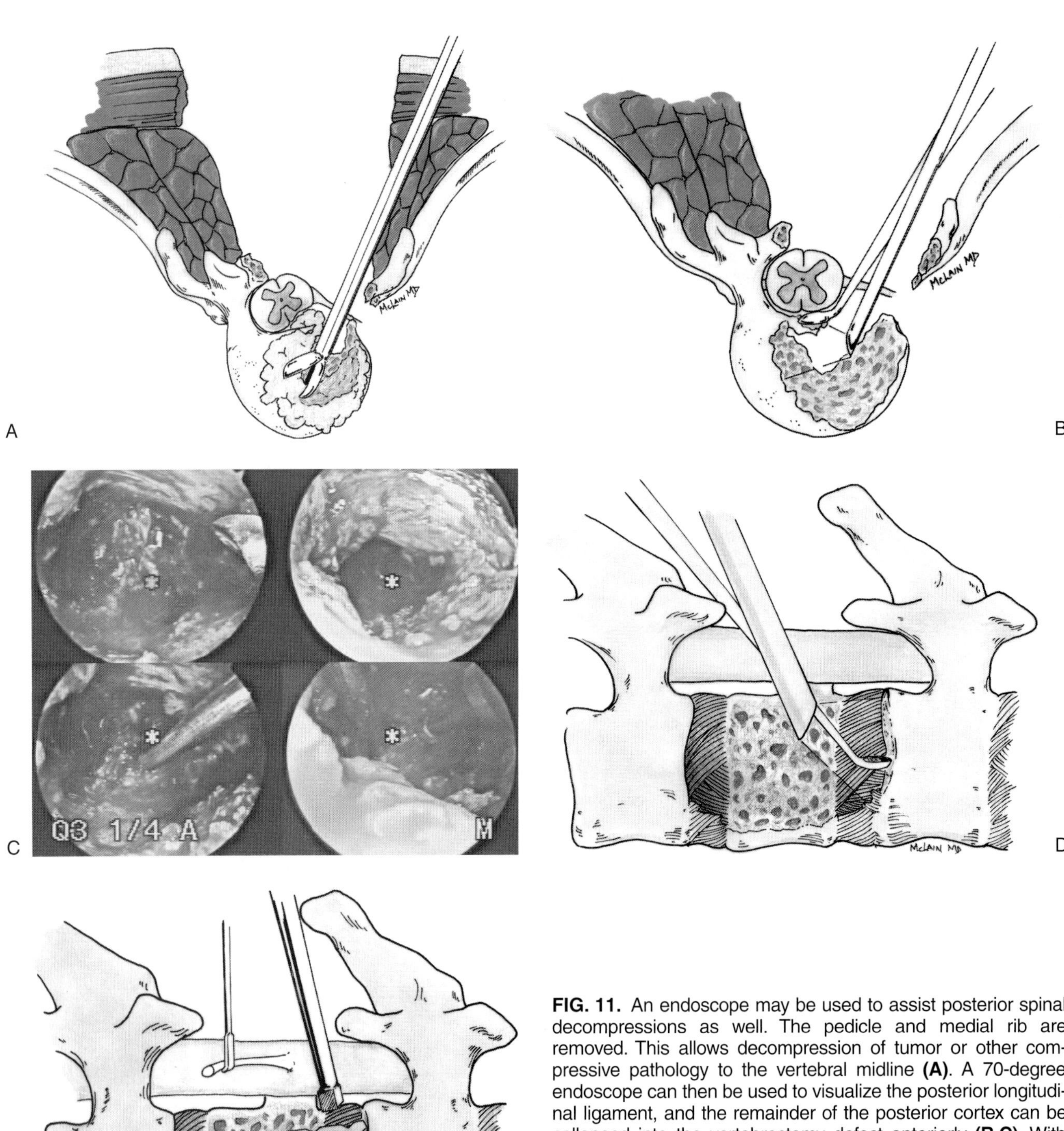

FIG. 11. An endoscope may be used to assist posterior spinal decompressions as well. The pedicle and medial rib are removed. This allows decompression of tumor or other compressive pathology to the vertebral midline **(A)**. A 70-degree endoscope can then be used to visualize the posterior longitudinal ligament, and the remainder of the posterior cortex can be collapsed into the vertebrectomy defect anteriorly **(B,C)**. With the decompression completed, the vertebrectomy can be further prepared by removing the adjacent discs and end-plate cartilage with a curette or rongeur **(D)**. Finally, the defect is reconstructed using a strut graft or cage **(E)**. [From McLain RF. Endoscopically assisted decompression for metastatic thoracic neoplasms. *Spine* 1998;23(10):1130–1135, with permission.]

compressive pathology is collapsed into this cavity using Epstein curettes. After complete decompression, a corpectomy defect is created, and the space can be reconstructed using titanium mesh cages followed by posterior, segmental instrumentation (Fig. 7).

CONCLUSION AND FUTURE DIRECTIONS

Endoscopic and minimally invasive spine surgery refer to changes in approach, not in the operation itself. Therefore, the indications for operative intervention are not relaxed merely because these procedures may be performed through smaller incisions. As in any spine surgery, careful patient selection is the critical factor predicting successful outcomes.

Endoscopic thoracic spinal surgery confers many proven and potential advantages to both the surgeon and patient, including improved surgical visualization through magnification and lighting, decreased perioperative morbidity, and shorter hospital stays. But these advantages must be counterbalanced with disadvantages of these approaches, including lack of familiarity, decreased three-dimensional perspective, and a loss of tactile sense. The early surgical experience may be associated with higher complication rates and longer operating times. Ultimately, a less efficacious technique should not be used merely because it is endoscopic.

As endoscopic techniques are also personnel and equipment intensive, involvement of operating room and hospital-wide administrative personnel may smooth the adjustment. A laparoscopic surgeon may be needed for a given endoscopic procedure but might not be required in an open procedure. Specialized and often single-use instruments are required. These additional operating room costs may be recouped with earlier patient discharge. However, the potential benefits of a minimal approach will not be realized by every surgeon.

REFERENCES

1. Crawford AH, Wall EJ, Wolf R. Video-assisted thoracoscopy. *Orthop Clin North Am* 1999;30(3):367–385.
2. Mack MJ, Regan JJ, Bobechko WP, et al. Application of thoracoscopy for diseases of the spine. *Ann Thorac Surg* 1993;56:736–738.
3. Regan JJ. Percutaneous endoscopic thoracic discectomy. *Neurosurg Clin North Am* 1996;1(7):87–98.
4. Kuklo TR, Lenke LG. Thoracoscopic spine surgery: current indications and techniques. *Orthop Nurs* 2000;19(6):15–22.
5. Regan JJ, Yuan H, McCullen G. Minimally invasive approaches to the spine. AAOS *Instr Course Lec* 127–141.
6. Dickman CA, Detweiler PW, Porter RW. Endoscopic spine surgery. *Clin Neurosurg* 2000;46:526–553.
7. McLain RF. Endoscopically assisted decompression for metastatic thoracic neoplasms. *Spine* 1998;15;23(10):1130–1135.
8. Regan JJ, Guyer RD. Endoscopic techniques in spinal surgery. *Clin Orthop* 1997;225:122–139.
9. Regan JJ, Ben-Yishay A, Mack MJ. Video-assisted thoracoscopic excision of herniated thoracic disc. Description of technique and preliminary experience in the first 29 cases. *J Spinal Disord* 1998;11(3):183–191.
10. Regan JJ, Mack MJ. Endoscopic thoracic fusion cage. In: Regan JJ, McAfee PJ, Mack MJ, eds. *Atlas of endoscopic spine surgery*. St. Louis: Quality Medical Publishing, 1995.
11. Rosenthal D, Marquardt G, Lorenz R, et al. Anterior decompression and stabilization using a microsurgical endoscopic technique for metastatic tumors of the thoracic spine. *J Neurosurg* 1996;84:565B–572B.
12. Dickman CA, Karahalios DG. Thoracoscopic spine surgery. *Clin Neurosurg* 1996;43:393–422.
13. McLain RF. Spinal cord decompression. An endoscopically assisted approach for metastatic tumors. *Spinal Cord* 2001;29:482–487.
14. Magerl FP. Stabilization of the lower thoracic and lumbar spine with external skeletal fixation. *Clin Orthop* 1984;189:125B–141B.
15. Birnbaum K, Pieper S, Prescher A, et al. Thoracoscopically assisted ligamentous release of the thoracic spine: a cadaver study. *Surg Radiol Anat* 2000;22(3-4):143–150.
16. Citow JS, MacDonald RL, Ferguson MK. Combined laminectomy and thoracoscopic resection of a dumbbell neurofibroma. Technical case report. *Neurosurgery* 1999;45(5):1263–1266.
17. Crawford AH, Wolf RK, Wall EJ. Pediatric spinal deformity. In: Regan JJ, McAfee PJ, Mack MJ, eds. *Atlas of endoscopic spine surgery*. St. Louis: Quality Medical Publishing, 1995.
18. Cunningham BW, Kotani Y, McNulty PS, et al. Video-assisted thoracoscopic surgery versus open thoracotomy for anterior thoracic spinal fusion. A comparative radiographic, biomechanical, and histologic analysis in a sheep model. *Spine* 1998;23(12):1333–1340.
19. Dickman CA, Rosenthal D, Karahalios DG, et al Thoracic vertebrectomy and reconstruction using a microsurgical thorascopic approach. *Neurosurgery* 1996;38:279.
20. Dickman CA, Mican CA. Multilevel anterior thoracic discectomies and anterior interbody fusion using a microsurgical thoracoscopic approach. Case report. *J Neurosurgery* 1996;84:104–109.
21. Hertlein H, Hertl WH, Dienemann H, et al. Thoracoscopic repair of thoracic spine trauma. *Eur Spine J* 1995;4:302–307.
22. Huang TJ, Hsu RW, Chen SH, et al. Video-assisted thoracoscopic surgery in managing tuberculous spondylitis. *Clin Orthop* 2000;379:143–153.
23. Lieberman IH, Salo PT, Orr RD, et al. Prone position endoscopic transthoracic release with simultaneous posterior instrumentation for spinal deformity: a description of the technique. *Spine* 2000;25(17):2251–2257.
24. Newton PO, Shea KG, Granlund KF. Defining the pediatric spinal thoracoscopy learning curve: sixty-five consecutive cases. *Spine* 2000;25(8):1028–1035.
25. Newton PO, Wenger DR, Mubarak JS, et al. Anterior release and fusion in pediatric spinal deformity. A comparison of early outcome and cost of thoracoscopic and open thoracotomy approaches. *Spine* 1997;12(22):1398–1406.
26. Heltzer JM, Krasna MJ, Aldrich F, et al. Thoracoscopic excision of a posterior mediastinal dumbbell tumor using a combined approach. *Ann Thorac Surg* 1995;60:431–433.
27. Zdeblick TA. A prospective, randomized study of lumbar fusion—preliminary results. *Spine* 1993;18(8):983–991.
28. Parker LM, McAfee PC, Fedder IL, et al. Minimally invasive surgical techniques to treat spine infections. *Orth Clin North Am* 1996;27(1):183–199.
29. Arlet V. Anterior thoracoscopic spine release in deformity surgery. A meta-analysis and review. *Eur Spine J* 2000;9[Supp 1]:S17–S22.
30. Winter RB, Lonstein JE, Denis F, et al. Paraplegia resulting from vessel ligation. *Spine* 1996;21(10):1232–1233.
31. Sucato DJ, Welch RD, Pierce B, et al. Thoracoscopic discectomy and fusion in an animal model: safe and effective when segmental blood vessels are spared. *Spine* 2002;15-27(8):880–886.
32. Vissochi M, Masferrer, Sonntag VKH, et al. Thoracoscopic approaches to the thoracic spine. *Acta Neurochir (Wien)* 1998;140:737–744.
33. Ikard RW, McCord DH. Thoracoscopic exposure of intervertebral discs. *Ann Thorac Surg* 1996;61:1267–1268.
34. Lischke V, Westphal K, Behne M, et al. Thoracoscopic microsurgical technique for vertebral surgery. Anesthetic considerations. *Acta Anaesthesiol Scand* 1998;42:1999–1204.
35. King AG, Mills TE, Loe WA, et al. Video-assisted thoracoscopic surgery in the prone position. *Spine* 2000;25(18):2403–2406.
36. McAfee PC, Regan JJ, Zdeblick T, et al. The incidence of complications in endoscopic anterior thoracolumbar spinal reconstructive surgery. A prospective multicenter study comprising the first 100 consecutive cases. *Spine* 1995;14:1624–1632.
37. Picetti G III, Blackman RG, O'Neal K, et al. Anterior endoscopic correction and fusion of scoliosis. *Orthopedics* 1998;21(12):1285–1287.
38. Anand N, Regan JJ. Video-assisted thoracoscopic surgery for thoracic disc disease: classification and outcome study of 100 consecu-

tive cases with a 2-year minimum follow-up period. *Spine* 2002;15-27(8):871–879.

39. Johnson JR, Holt RT. Combined use of anterior and posterior surgery for adult scoliosis. *Orthop Clin North Am* 1988;19:361–370.
40. Gonzalez-Barrios I, Fuentes Caparrios S, Avila Jurado MM. Anterior thoracoscopic epiphysiodesis in the treatment of crankshaft phenomenon. *Eur Spine J* 1995;4:343–346.
41. Mehlman CT, Crawford AH, Wolf RK. Video-assisted thoracoscopic surgery (VATS), endoscopic thoracoplasty technique. *Spine* 1997;22(18):2178–2182.
42. Regan JJ, Mack MJ, Picetti GD, et al. A comparison of video-assisted thoracoscopy surgery (VATS) with open thoracotomy in the thoracic spinal surgery. *Today Therap Trend* 1994;11:203–218.
43. Rosenthal D, Dickman CA. Thoracoscopic microsurgical excision of herniated thoracic discs. *J Neurosurg* 1998;89(2):224–235.
44. Resnick DK, Benzel EC. Lateral extracavitary approach for thoracic and thoracolumbar spine trauma. Operative complications. *Neurosurgery* 1998;43:796–803.
45. McLain RF, Lieberman IH. Controversy: endoscopic approaches to metastatic thoracic disease. *Spine* 2000;15-25(14):1857–1858.
46. Rosenthal D. Endoscopic internal fixation of the thoracic spine. In: Regan JJ, McAfee PJ, Mack MJ, eds. *Atlas of endoscopic spine surgery*. St. Louis: Quality Medical Publishing, 1995;333.
47. van Dijk M, Cuesta MA, Wuisman PI. Thoracoscopically assisted total *en bloc* spondylectomy: two case reports. *Surg Endosc* 2000;14(9):849–852.
48. Huang TJ, Scu RWW, Hsu KY, et al. Video-assisted thoracoscopic treatment of spinal lesions in the thoracolumbar junction. *Surg Endosc* 1997;11:1189–1193.
49. Obenchain TG. Laparoscopic lumbar discectomy: case report. *J Laparoendosc Surg* 1991;1:145–149.
50. Southerland SR, Remedios AM, McKerrell JG, et al. Laparoscopic approaches to the lumbar vertebrae: an anatomic study using a porcine model. *Spine* 1995;20:1620–1623.
51. Hildebrandt U, Pistorius G, Olinger A, et al. First experience with laparoscopic spine fusion in an experimental model in the pig. *Surg Endosc* 1996;10:143–146.
52. Regan JJ, Aronoff RJ, Ohnmeiss DD, et al. Laparoscopic approach to L4-L5 for interbody fusion using BAK cages: experience in the first 58 cases. *Spine* 1999;24:2171–2174.
53. Brody F, Rosen M, Tarnoff M, et al. Laparoscopic lateral L4/L5 disc exposure. *Surg Endosc* 2002;16;650–653.
54. Zucherman JF, Zdeblick TA, Bailey SA, et al. Instrumented laparoscopic spinal fusion, preliminary results. *Spine* 1995;20:2029–2034.
55. Mathews JJ, Evans MT, Molligan HJ, et al. Laparoscopic discectomy with anterior lumbar interbody fusion. *Spine* 1995;20:1797–1802.
56. Olsen D, McCord D, Law M. Laparoscopic discectomy with anterior lumbar interbody fusion of L-5 to S-1. *Surg Endosc* 1996;10:1158–1163.
57. Mahvi D, Zdeblick TA. A prospective study of laparoscopic spinal fusion. *Ann Surg* 1996;224:85–90.
58. Regan JJ, Yuan H, McAfee PC. Laparoscopic fusion of the lumbar spine: minimally invasive spine surgery. *Spine* 1999;24:402–411.
59. Zdeblick TA, David SM. A prospective comparison of surgical approach for anterior L4-L5 fusion. *Spine* 2000;25:2682–2687.
60. Lieberman IH, Willsher PC, Litwin DE, et al. Transperitoneal laparoscopic exposure for lumbar interbody fusion. *Spine* 2000;25:509–514.
61. Larson SJ, Holst RA, Hemmy DC, et al. Lateral extracavitary approach to traumatic lesions of the thoracic and lumbar spine. *J Neurosurg* 1976;45:628–637.
62. Hulme A. The surgical approach to thoracic intervertebral disc protrusions. *J Neuro Neurosurg Psychiatr* 1960;23:133–137.
63. Osman SG, Marsolais EB. Posterolateral arthroscopic discectomies of the thoracic and lumbar spine. *Clin Orthop* 1994;304:122–129.
64. Jho HD. Endoscopic transpedicular thoracic discectomy. *J Neurosurg* 1999;91:151–156.

CHAPTER 54

Microdiscectomy and Microsurgical Spinal Laminotomies*

David A. Wong

Advances in diagnostic and surgical technology continue to change the face of spinal surgery. Microscopic, minimally invasive spine surgery rides firmly on the crest of this new wave of technology. However, the most critical factor in achieving satisfactory patient outcomes is not the use of the newest technology or the smallest incision. Rather, skilled clinical judgment in patient evaluation, physical examination, and correlation of imaging studies guide the spinal microsurgeon to appropriate patient selection. Identification of the ideal clinical situation allows optimal use of the microscope as a precision instrument. This technology helps the surgeon attain the best outcomes while reducing patient morbidity through a minimally invasive approach.

Given competent surgical expertise, there is little apparent difference in long-term patient outcomes between a microsurgical discectomy and a standard laminectomy/discectomy with magnifying loupes (1–7). The advocates of microsurgical discectomy believe that once the learning curve has been traveled, the microscope not only offers advantages over loupes, it forces one to think at a much higher level of clarity in the analysis of the pathology of nerve root encroachment. The surgical correction of canal pathology becomes self-evident as a result of more exacting analysis. Equally important, the patient attains these clinical outcomes with less morbidity and an earlier hospital discharge compared to standard or limited discectomy (4,6,8).

* Readers who have enjoyed prior editions of this textbook will note that this chapter was previously coauthored by my partner, John A. McCulloch, along with R. B. Delamarter. Tragically, John McCulloch died in March 2002 from injuries sustained in a skiing accident. John's contributions to the field of spinal microsurgery were substantial and vital to the advancement of minimally invasive lumbar surgery. Key concepts such as the "three-story" anatomic analysis to locate critical pathology in the spinal canal are McCulloch themes. It is a sad but essential duty to present John's concepts to a new generation of microsurgeons.

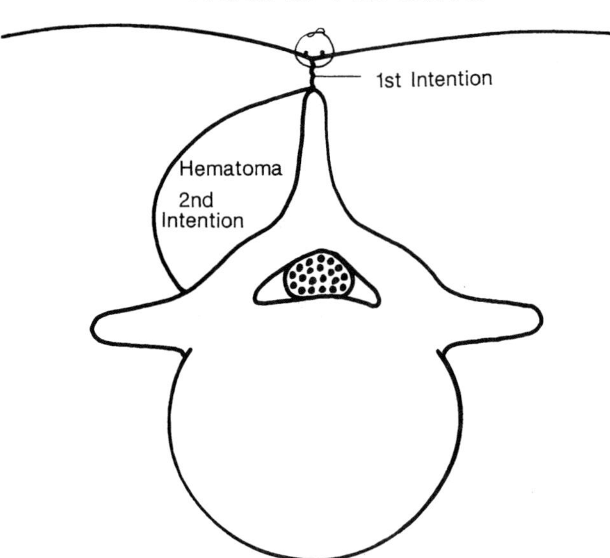

FIG. 1. Skin is expected to heal by primary intention, but if dead space is left behind by a longer paraspinal incision, it fills with hematoma and heals by secondary intention (scar). Dead space is reduced when the smallest possible invasion (i.e., microsurgery) is used.

BIOLOGIC BASIS FOR LEAST INVASIVE SPINAL SURGERY

The model for wound healing represents the foundation for minimally invasive surgical techniques. Older dogma would suggest that the length of the incision is not important, as "wounds heal side to side, not end to end." However, this principle ignores the concept of wound hematoma and its relation to the magnitude of peridural scar (Fig. 1) (9). La Rocca and Macnab studied the laminectomy membrane and observed: "The fibrous response was always more marked when a wide operative exposure was employed" (10).

It also follows that the less muscle dissection that occurs, the less potential dead space exists for hematoma. When a limited wound incision is made, there is a reduced requirement for healing by secondary intention and in the final analysis, less scar (Fig. 2).

The hematoma is such an organized mass of cells, and the events involved in its physiology occur in such a specific, ordered sequence that the healing wound can be considered a "temporary organ unto itself" (9). Figure 3 demonstrates the advancing front of wound healing that encircles the dead space hematoma filling a paraspinal incision. This process of wound healing is affected by local factors, such as the amount of tissue damage inflicted at the time of the incision, the number of sutures inserted, and the presence or absence of other necrotic debris (e.g., cauterized tissue). Infection further exacerbates the associated inflammatory reaction. In the end, the healed wound is represented by superficial, deep, and perineural scars.

An additional disadvantage of a long incision is the muscle denervation. This problem was illustrated by Macnab et al., whose clinical study of 113 patients documented denervation of the paravertebral muscles on electromyelogram in 96% (11). Denervation was shown to persist for many years after surgery with minimal reinnervation potential.

A further advantage of microsurgery is the capability to accomplish a disc excision with limited reflection of the ligamentum flavum and laminal excision (12). Epidural scar can thus be limited, and mobility of the root maintained.

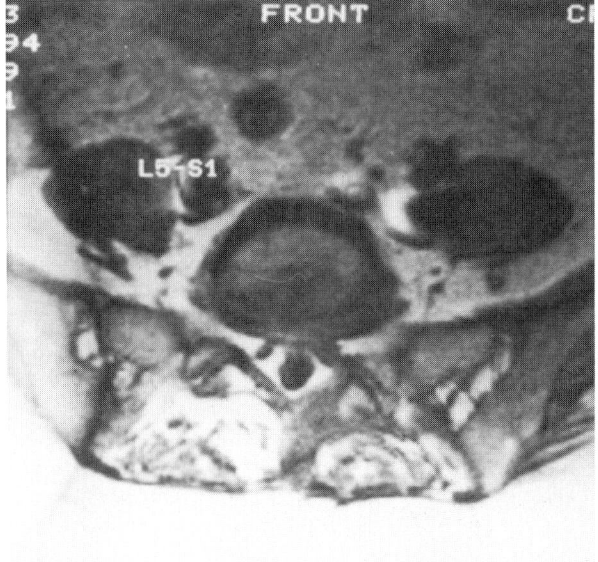

A

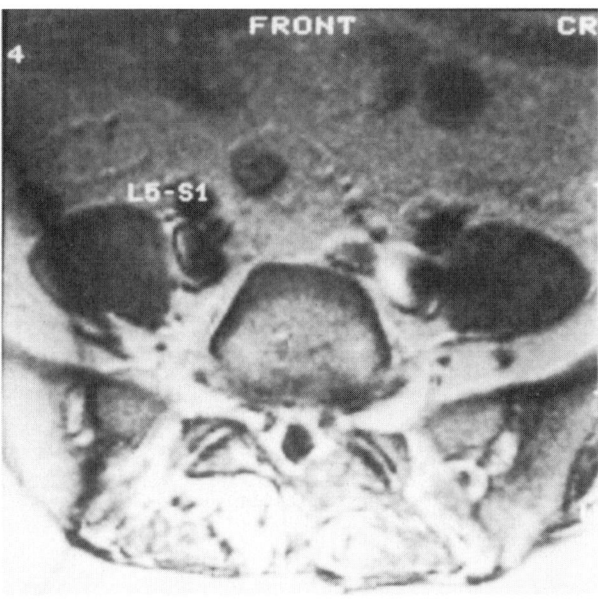

B

FIG. 2. A postoperative microdiscectomy on magnetic resonance imaging (MRI). Note the laminectomy membrane **(A)** and very little scar around the dura and root (left L-5 to S-1), which is covered by a residual ligamentum flavum flap. The postgadolinium MRI **(B)** reveals very little scar tissue deep to the ligamentum flavum flap.

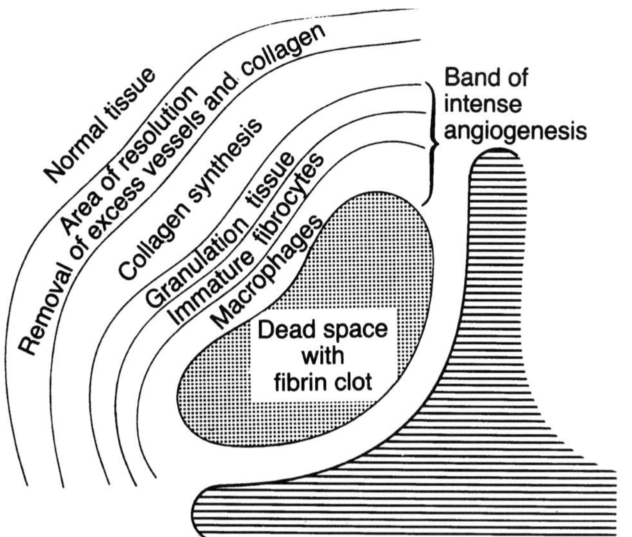

FIG. 3. The module of wound healing—a complicated, multifaceted "organ unto itself." The advancing front heals as scar tissue and retracts.

Finally, one of the major benefits of microsurgery for lumbar disc disease is early mobilization. Kahanovitz et al. compared a cohort of patients who had standard laminectomy to a group of patients with microsurgical exposure (13). Outcomes were identical between the two groups except for postoperative morbidity and length of stay in hospital. The patients undergoing a microsurgical approach had a much shorter hospital stay. A patient who can get out of bed the same day as having a microsurgical procedure and be home as an outpatient on the day after surgery has an advantage over the patient who has a more painful wound and requires longer bed rest and hospitalization (14,15). The potential benefits of early mobilization include a reduced risk of pulmonary and vascular complications (e.g., atelectasis and thrombophlebitis). In the present era of limited health care resources, shorter hospital stays allow more effective use of financial assets.

Early mobilization affects the basic physiology of wound healing. Peacock outlined the three basic molecular steps in local wound healing in 1967: intracellular synthesis of tropocollagen molecules, extracellular assembly of fibrils and fibers, and formation of ground substance (9). An important fundamental property of the healing wound is its tensile strength, which is directly related to collagen formation and orientation. Salter and coworkers studied wounds healed with continuous passive motion versus immobilization (16). The continuous passive motion wounds healed better qualitatively and quantitatively. The investigators postulated that the tension of continuous passive motion enhanced the formation and alignment of collagen.

Halstead predicted the progression to a minimally invasive approach in 1913. He stated, "I believe that the tendency will always be in the direction of exercising greater care and refinement in operating, and that the surgeon will develop increasingly a respect for tissues; a sense which recoils from inflicting, unnecessarily, insult to structures concerned in the process of repair." This historic observation accurately reflects modern-day microsurgical practice.

DISADVANTAGES OF THE MICROSCOPE

Before using a microscope for lumbar disc surgery, it is best to understand its disadvantages and limitations. Every new technique or technology has a learning curve and new and different challenges. The most striking problem of the microscope is its limited field of vision, with an associated loss of orientation to peripheral structures. Within the 5-cm diameter field of vision of the microscope, there is enhanced visualization of tissues. Outside that field, nothing is visible. Thus, as the surgical procedure crosses the edge of the microscopic field, the microscope must be adjusted so that the center of the operation remains within that field. This is known as "maintaining the field of vision" and is the single biggest hurdle in adapting to the microscope. The circumferentially 360-degree–mobile microscope head and base greatly facilitate the necessary maneuvers (Fig. 4). When the field of vision is adjusted, adjacent soft tissues may restrict the surgeon's view. The offending tissue needs to be excised to maintain optimum clarity. Remember, "Overhang is the enemy!" (Fig. 5).

The second difficulty in adapting to the microscope is the recognition of tissues under higher magnification. For example, empty severed epidural veins, strands of ligamentum flavum, and annulus or herniated disc tissue may at one time or another bear a startling resemblance to "strands of nerve rootlets." However, actual rootlets visualized from a damaged root sleeve have a stark whiteness and a central vein that quickly distinguish them from the dull and yellowish tinge of other tissues. Such instances of mistaken identity actually may make

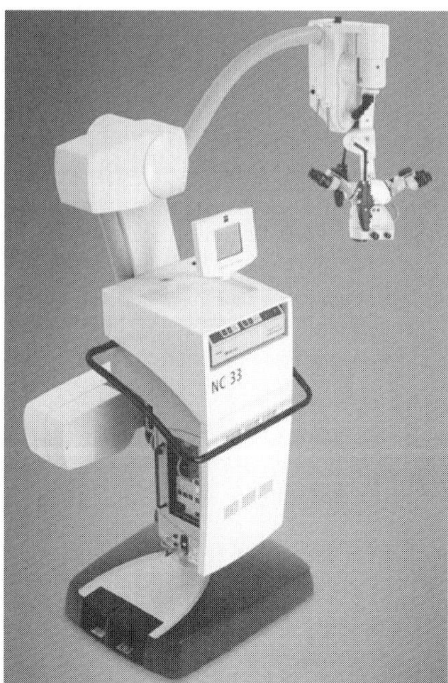

FIG. 4. The latest fully mobile computerized operating microscope stand from Carl Zeiss (NC-33). (Courtesy of Carl Zeiss, Inc., Thornwood, NY.)

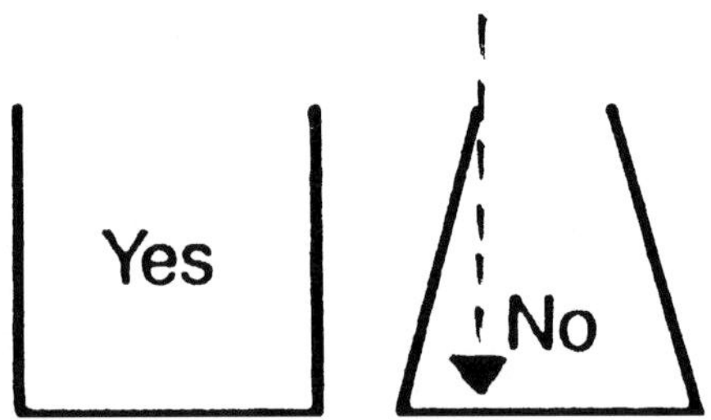

FIG. 5. "Overhang is the enemy!" To maintain the field of vision, maintain a wound as in **Yes**, and do not operate in a wound with overhang of soft tissue, bone, or anything as in **No**. "Overhang" in this wound interferes with the line of vision (*arrow*).

the surgeon more cautious and reduce the rate of dural tears and root damage.

Bleeding

Even a small amount of bleeding into a limited operative field interferes with visualization. The difference between 25 cc and 100 cc of blood loss under the microscope can be significant. Preoperative efforts to reduce bleeding include cessation of all antiinflammatory medications, blood thinners, and herbal supplements. Postoperative interventions include patient positioning on the operating frame with the belly free and intraoperative control of hemorrhage from cancellous bone and epidural veins. Generally, bone wax for cancellous bleeding and Gelfoam with thrombin for epidural hemostasis are effective and minimize the requirement for electrocautery.

Infection

Wilson and associates reported an increased rate of postmicrosurgery disc space infections, which they thought was due to the presence of the microscope head directly over the wound (17,18). Although the microscope is covered with a sterile drape, the unsterilized eyepieces are exposed. The outside of the plastic drape can be contaminated during the draping and repositioning process. The limited operating space between the lens and the wound introduces another element for a potential break in surgical technique that can result in wound contamination. More recent reviews indicate no difference in infection rate between microsurgical and routine lumbar decompressive techniques (19).

COMPLICATIONS INHERENT IN MICROSURGERY

Complications are a risk in all spinal decompressions. Two are particularly likely with microscopic techniques, as explained in this section.

Exploration of the Wrong Level

Because the size of a wound is limited, the sacral ala is not available for assisting in the identification of levels. Only the interlaminar window to be opened and the adjacent edges of the lamina are exposed; thus, it is very important to identify the correct level. A reliable fluoroscopic method of marking the level of intervention is outlined in Figure 6.

Alternatively, the spinous processes and the interspinous intervals can be palpated, and a mini-incision can be made based on the usual location of the intercrestal line at L4-5. A marker positioned on an exposed spinous process gives a reliable bony marker. Because up to 10% of patients have congenital lumbosacral anomalies, preoperative plain x-rays can assist in avoiding misidentification. If on entering the interlaminar space the expected pathology (e.g., a large extruded fragment) is not encountered, the exposure is likely at the wrong level and an intraoperative x-ray is imperative. Radiographic control should be used to ensure that the correct interspace is being approached. If there is any doubt, a radiograph should be taken before the annulotomy is performed. Initial exposure of the wrong level is such a common occurrence that one must constantly check the level. Particularly during the early exposure phase of a microsurgical procedure, repeat confirmation should be performed against the marks initially made to locate anatomic structures. When using the fluoroscopic marking method, a reliable check is to mark the inferior edge of the disc space to be exposed, and also to have the marking needle inferior to the spinous process. The medial hook of the retractor can then be placed on this line (Fig. 7). From the hook, follow the inferior edge of the spinous process to the inferior edge of the lamina and the correct interlaminar level. This is easy to do for a microdiscectomy at L4-5 and L-5 to S-1, but it is more difficult to achieve in degenerative disc disease, high lumbar levels, and patients in hyperlordosis on kneeling frames. If using the mini-incision and marking a spinous process as the bony reference point, a rongeur or Bovie is used to create a mark for future reference. Also, a mark is placed on the skin opposite the position as an additional reference point. A copy of the fluoroscopic localization picture or the lateral x-ray film should be easily visible so that the anatomic landmarks at the surgery site can be easily and repetitively reoriented to the

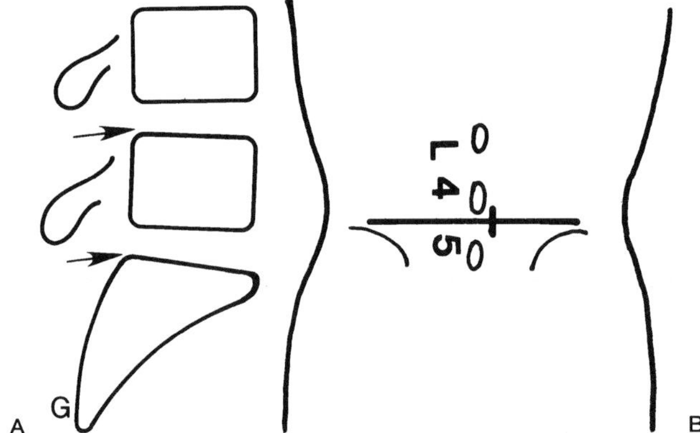

FIG. 6. A: After a preliminary preparation, use a marking needle and an image intensifier control to mark a line **(B)** that is at the inferior edge of the disc space and the inferior tip of the spinous process. This is very difficult in a lordotic back, in degenerative disc disease, and in the higher lumbar levels. Put all three together, and you have an impossible task: Be prepared for a wrong-level exposure.

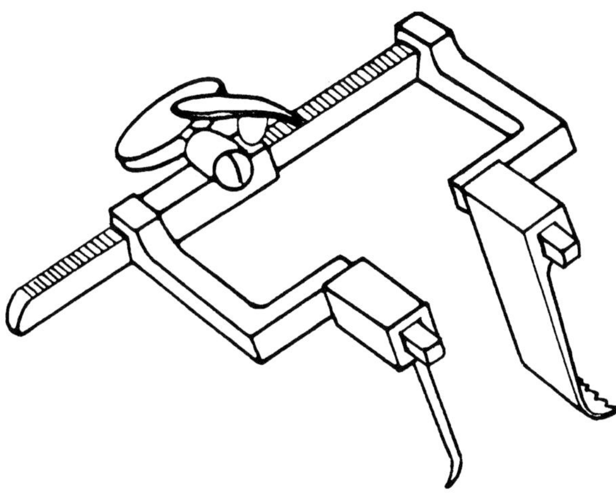

FIG. 7. The frame retractor assembled with the lateral muscle blade and medial hook that fits in the interspinous ligament interval. Make sure the hook is on the skin-marking line.

imaging studies. Some surgeons inject a small amount of dye through the localization needle as a further guide to the desired interlaminar space.

Missed Pathology

Missed pathology is a major and valid criticism of microsurgery. To avoid this pitfall, two principles are important:

1. The preoperative imaging studies, particularly magnetic resonance imaging (MRI), must be studied in detail. Establish a three-dimensional picture of the pathology and its relation to principal anatomic landmarks of the appropriate surgical window. Construct a surgical plan based on the type and location of root encroachment before the limited skin incision is made (Fig. 8).

2. The key principle of any decompression procedure, including microdiscectomy and lumbar microlaminectomy, is to free the nerve root. The root must be free and mobile at the completion of the procedure. Various probes are useful adjuncts to confirm that complete decompression has been accomplished (Fig. 9).

Other Complications

Battered Nerve Root

Gentle handling of neural structures is a basic tenet of surgery involving the spine. With a limited exposure, a deep wound, and the close proximity of the dural sac and roots, excessive force involving retractors, probes, and elevators is a constant concern. Vigilance is particularly necessary when using a Cobb elevator to expose a spinal bifida occulta at the L-5 to S-1 interlaminar space. Careful evaluation of preoperative plain radiographs alerts the surgeon to this potential danger.

Particular attention should also be paid to the nerve root retractor, which acts as a long lever. Thus, small "toeing in" motions of the hands result in exaggerated motions of the retractor shoe against the root. Frequent checks of the retractor position are necessary to avoid excess force and manipulation of the root, which can result in epidural scarring and new neurologic dysfunction.

Dural Tears and Root Damage

Early in a surgeon's microsurgical career, the small opening and deep wound are often very constraining. In this environment, it is easy to tear the dura and damage rootlets. Instrumentation sets have been specifically designed for spinal microsurgery and can reduce these risks. It is recommended that these be used. Should an inadvertent durotomy occur, treatment is based on the potential for dural tamponade. If the dural rent is anterior, where self-

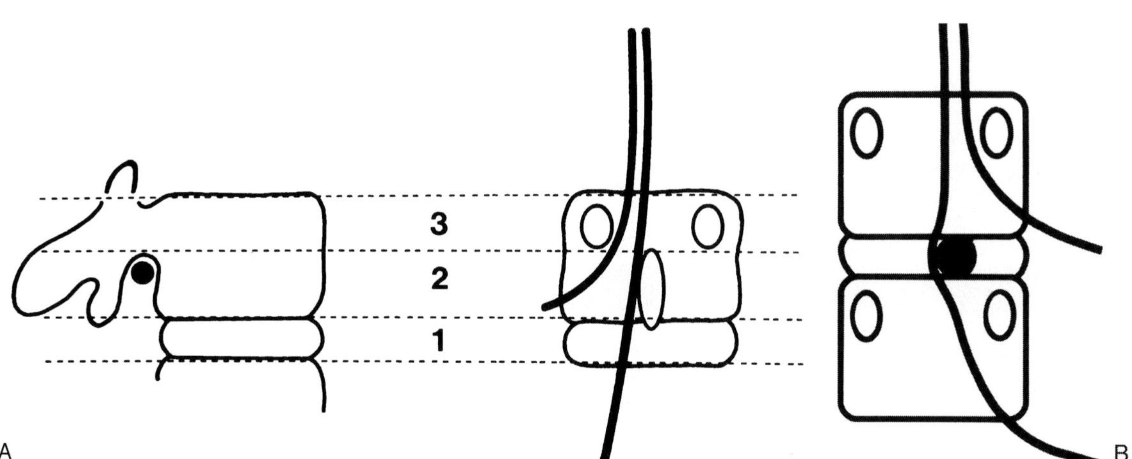

FIG. 8. A: Read the interface between the disc–vertebral column and the common dural sac as if each segment is a three-story house. **B:** A schematic of a first-story disc herniation. (*continued*)

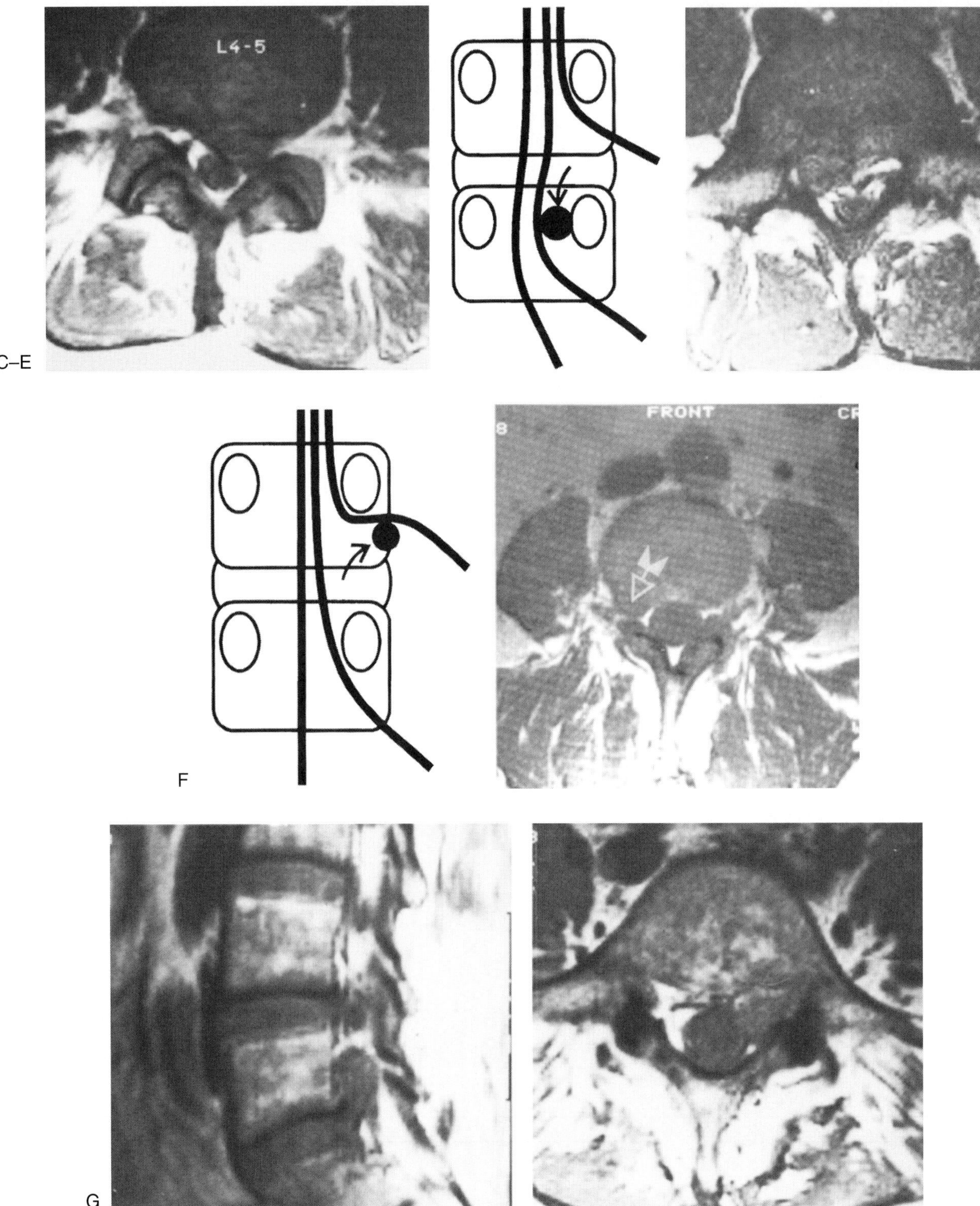

FIG. 8. *Continued.* **C:** A T1-axial magnetic resonance image (MRI) of a first-story disc herniation. **D:** A schematic of a ruptured disc that has left the first story of one anatomic segment and migrated into the third story of the anatomic segment below. **E:** An MRI of a third-story disc herniation. **F:** A rare second-story disc herniation on schematic. **G:** Sagittal and axial MRI slices showing a disc herniation rupturing not only into the second story, but also as high as the third story.

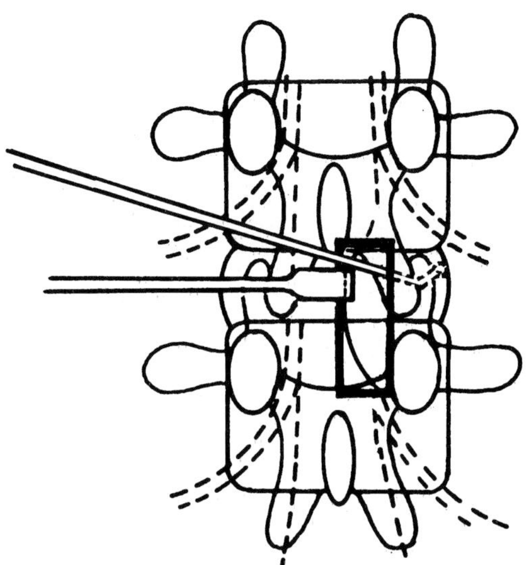

FIG. 9. A probe out into the foramen of the exiting root.

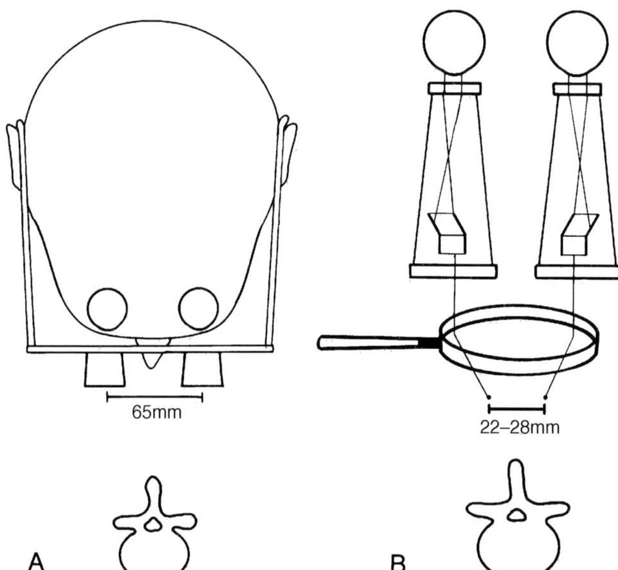

FIG. 10. Stereopsis (three-dimensional) visualization requires at least 65 mm for interpupillary distance with loupes **(A)**. Through the optics of the microscope, this distance is compressed to 22 to 28 mm **(B)**, meaning a much smaller incision is needed to maintain three-dimensional vision in the depth of the wound.

tamponade can be expected, Gelfoam is packed around the defect and a formal repair is unnecessary. Dorsal tears are unlikely to tamponade and must be repaired with a watertight closure, which may be enhanced with the addition of fibrin glue (20). Bed rest for 24 to 48 hours is usually required. However, a recent study shows that ambulation is appropriate for patients with small durotomies sutured and sealed with fibrin glue. Seventy-five percent of patients did not develop a spinal headache (21). Incidental durotomy does not appear to have a long-term detrimental effect on clinical outcome (22).

ADVANTAGES OF USING THE MICROSCOPE

The microscope offers considerable advantages to the spine patient and the surgeon. The obvious advantage is to the patient who has a small wound and corresponding limited morbidity. Many microsurgical procedures are being performed as outpatient surgeries (14,15).

TABLE 1. *The advantages of the microscope over loupes*

Factor	Loupes	Microscope
Magnification	Limited	Relatively unlimited
Illumination	Not parallel to line of vision (paraxial)	Parallel to line of vision (coaxial)
Three-dimensional vision	Limited with less than 65-mm skin incision	Maintained with 25-cm skin incision
Patient size	The larger the patient, the bigger the wound	Neutralized (every patient is made the same size by the optics)
Teaching	Assistants excluded	Assistants included
Surgeon's neck	Flexed	Spared

For many reasons (Table 1), the operating microscope is superior to loupes. The most important reason is maintenance of stereopsis (three-dimensional viewing) in the depths of the wound. For surface surgery, the loupes are fine. For surgery deep in the lumbar spine, three-dimensional vision can be maintained with loupes only if the wound is long enough to accommodate the surgeon's fixed interpupillary distance, which is approximately 65 mm (Fig. 10). Maintenance of three-dimensional vision is impossible with the surgical combination of loupes and a small incision. Every surgeon wants better visualization, so spinal surgeons who wish to see the greatest possible depth in a small wound and maintain three-dimensional vision have adopted the microscope. Additional reasons for using a microscope for spine surgery include the following:

1. A parallel rather than an offset light source (Fig. 11).

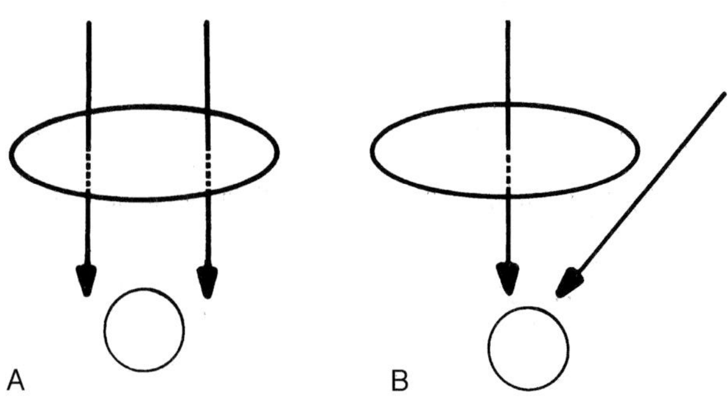

FIG. 11. Coaxial **(A)** versus paraxial **(B)** illumination. With paraxial illumination (loupes and headlight) **(B)**, a wider incision is needed to get the light into the depth of the wound.

2. The ability to go to a very high magnification for fine work (up to 10×).
3. The fact that residents, fellows, and the operating room staff can see what you are doing and participate in a positive learning environment.
4. The microscope is fixed in focus, allowing the surgeon to move around the room without having to refocus on the surgical field.
5. More important for those older surgeons with cervical degenerative disease, it offers relief from the flexed neck position necessary when using loupes.

PRINCIPLES OF THE MICROSCOPE

Before embarking on microsurgery, the surgeon needs to select the microscope that works best and understand the function if its components.

Microscope Head and Optics

The operating microscope is a combination of binocular field glasses and a magnifying glass (Fig. 12). Interposed between the binoculars and the magnifying glass is a magnifying chamber that allows for increasing or decreasing the side of the image (Fig. 13). A series of lenses and prisms then allow for the transformation of an image to the retina. Optical deficiencies, such as reflection and glare, are factored out of the system to improve image quality. The contemporary microscope has a very complicated design that is impossible to explain in this brief chapter. There are excellent technical books that explain the microscope in more detail (23). This section serves as a very basic summary of the microscope assembly important for lumbar disc surgery.

Objective Lens (Magnifying Glass)

The *objective lens* is the large lens on the bottom of the microscope head, closest to the surgical field. Lenses with focal lengths ranging from 150 to 400 mm are available in 25-mm increments. The focal length of an objective lens is a close approximation of the distance between the lens and the point of anatomy that is in focus (Fig. 14).

For spine surgery, a 300-, 350-, or 400-mm lens usually is used. The surgeon must try the various lenses to choose the most comfortable position relative to standing at the microscope and operating on the patient. Also, there must be a comfortable distance between the bottom of the microscope and the depth of the wound so that instruments can be manipulated. The author's preference is for a 350-mm lens.

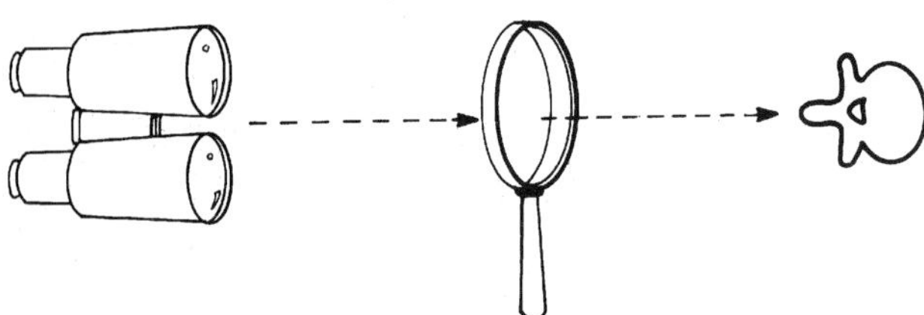

FIG. 12. The microscope, simply stated, is a pair of binoculars looking through a magnifying glass.

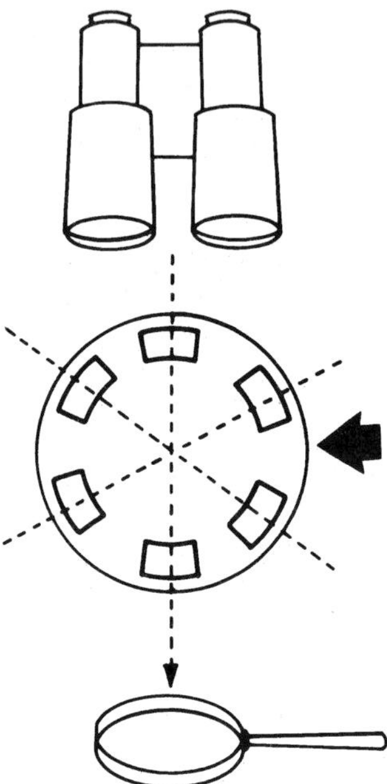

FIG. 13. A magnifying chamber (*thick arrow*) allows for greater or lesser magnification during the procedure, as called for by the surgeon.

Binocular Assembly

The *binocular assembly* consists of two components: the binocular tube and the eyepieces. The image formed by the objective lens is in turn magnified by the binocular assembly. The function

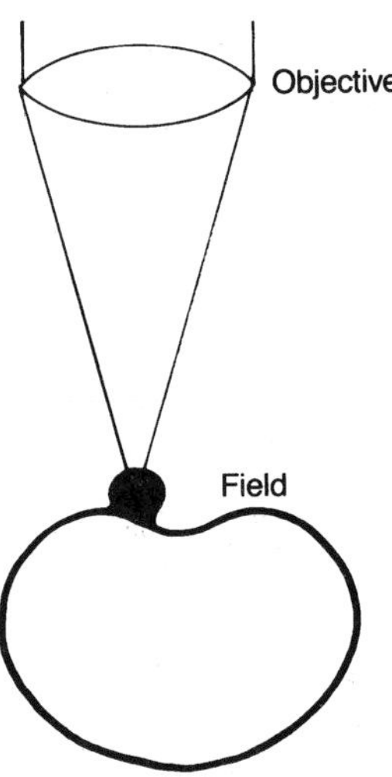

FIG. 14. The focal length of the objective lens determines the distance between the bottom of the microscope and the field in focus.

of the binocular tubes is to take the image of the object, which is translated in infinity, and converge it to something that can be viewed by the human eye. With the addition of eyepieces, the optical system in the binocular assembly becomes convergent.

Binocular tubes can be straight or inclined. The most popular model today is the tiltable binocular tube, which allows for individual adjustment of the angle of the binocular tube. This is most helpful when the surgeon and assistant are of different heights.

Eyepieces

The *eyepieces* add another component to the magnification potential of the microscope. The convergent system in the binocular tube produces an intermediate-sized image, which is magnified by the eyepieces for viewing by the human eye. Eyepieces for the Zeiss microscope are 10×, 12.5×, 16×, and 20×. For the Wild microscope, the eyepieces are 10×, 15×, and 20×. The eyepieces on each of these microscopes are adjustable, with eight diopters to correct for visual acuity problems so the surgeon can operate without glasses. It is possible to wear eyeglasses when using the binocular-tube-eyepieces assembly by folding back the rubber cups on the eyepieces. The use of eyeglasses is recommended when correction for astigmatism is necessary.

Interpupillary Distance

Interpupillary distance varies between surgeons. The eyepieces must be adjusted for interpupillary distance so that the two images are fused and stereoscopic or three-dimensional appreciation of the image occurs. An average interpupillary distance is approximately 65 mm.

Magnification Chamber

The final piece of the microscope that determines the size of the image is the magnification chamber, as depicted in Figure 13. It is a Galilean telescope system that allows for alteration in the magnification setup between the binocular assembly and the objective lens. The actual magnification factor achieved with the chamber can be 0.4×, 0.6×, 1.0×, 1.6×, or 2.5×. The magnification chamber can be a turret-drum setup that clicks in at the previously listed magnifications, or a zoom-magnifying chamber. The zoom system is a mechanized chamber controlled by a foot pedal or dial on the microscope that gives a continuous magnification range from 0.5× to 2.5× using a single optical system.

Controls

Newer microscopes have a computerized program allowing individualized preferences for multiple surgeons to be entered in the memory. This allows rapid and accurate setup of the microscope at the start of a procedure. The computer also facilitates balancing the microscope. Modern hand controls have integrated toggles for zoom and focus, as well as buttons for light intensity. The headpiece also locks.

Illumination Systems

The major advantage of the illuminating system of the microscope is the coaxial paths of the surgical observation and the illumination beams (Fig. 11).

The ideal illumination system provides sufficient brightness for the anatomy to be seen clearly. As magnification increases, the amount of illumination generally decreases. The reduction in brightness is not enough, however, to interfere with surgery. Most microscopes allow adjustment of brightness from the hand control and computer screen. A constant problem with all microscope lighting sources is the generation of heat. The least amount of heat generation is the most desirable.

The choices for illuminating the microscope are as follows:

1. Incandescent (tungsten coil) light: This is the oldest and least expensive source of light in the operating microscope. A 6-volt, 30-watt and a 6-volt, 50-watt bulb have been used. The higher wattage is used when photographic equipment is attached to the microscope. In early microscopes, the bulb was close to the microscope head and the heat generated was significant.
2. Halogen (tungsten coil) bulb: The halogen bulb is the most popular choice for illumination today. It is a more sensitive light than the incandescent bulb, with a greater blue spectrum. This causes the surgical site to appear whiter and brighter. The standard halogen bulb used is 12 volts, 100 watts. This produces light with a brightness of 160,000 lux, or 14,860 foot-candles.
3. The metal vapor lamp: This system forms the basis of the Superlux40 by Zeiss (Carl Zeiss Inc., Thornwood, NY). More than 40,000 foot-candles of power can be produced.

Light Transfer Systems

Light may be transferred through the microscope in two ways. If an incandescent bulb is used close to the microscopic head, then its light source is transferred through the objective with a series of prisms and filters (Fig. 15).

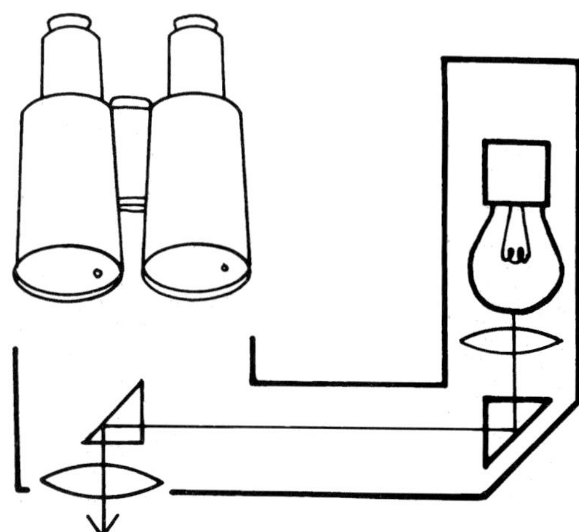

FIG. 15. A light source close to the microscope has to be reflected into the wound via prisms.

A more efficient method is fiberoptics (Fig. 4), which allows for placement of the light source at a distance from the microscope head. Heat is easier to control, and changing bulbs is facilitated if one burns out during the procedure. The fiberoptic system is more expensive, however, and breakage of individual glass cables can result in reduced light over time.

MICROSURGERY IN HERNIATED NUCLEUS PULPOSUS

Indications

The natural history of lumbar disc disease and herniated disc (herniated nucleus pulposus) remains somewhat controversial. Studies by Weber (24) and Hakelius (25) (Table 2) suggest that sciatica as a result of herniated nucleus pulposus is a self-limiting condition, which resolves over time regardless of surgical or conservative treatment. Concerns have been raised, however, about the statistical methodology used in the Weber study, in particular where patients "crossed over" from one randomized treatment group into the other. Specifically, Weber counted patients as having a successful outcome from conservative treatment even if surgery ultimately was required. When these "crossover" patients are counted as "failures" of conservative treatment, Bell reports that the outcomes with surgery were superior to conservative treatment at 5- and 10-year follow-up (26). These studies are all in agreement that surgery has a higher rate of initial success.

In this light, the indications for microsurgical discectomy and standard discectomy are identical. They are generally felt to include the following (27):

1. Bladder and bowel involvement. This is the least frequent but most definite indication for surgery. The problem is usually part of a more generalized cauda equina syndrome secondary to an acute, massive, sequestered central disc herniation. Although uncommon, cauda equina syndrome requires urgent surgical decompression. Large disc herniations can be removed through a microsurgical wound.
2. Progressive neurologic deficit. If, in spite of conservative treatment, increasing motor and/or sensory loss is documented on repeated physical examination, discectomy is indicated.
3. Significant neurologic deficit with persistent limitation of straight-leg raising. This is a relative indication supported by the work of Weber (24) and Hakelius (25). The duration of treatment is controversial. The study by Hakelius indicated that a delay of up to 12 weeks had no adverse effects on neurologic recovery. Others do not agree and recommend earlier intervention.
4. Failure of conservative treatment. This is the most common reason for surgical intervention (28). Typical nonsurgical treatment is discussed elsewhere.
5. Recurrent episodes of sciatic syndrome. Repeated episodes of sciatic syndrome are an indication for surgical intervention as outlined in Table 3.

TABLE 2. *Weber's results (1983)*

	Nonsurgical results	Surgical results
1 yr	60% better	92% better
4 yrs	No statistical difference between the two groups	No statistical difference between the two groups
10 yrs	No difference between 4-yr and 10-yr follow-up	No difference between 4-yr and 10-yr follow-up

TABLE 3. *Recurrent sciatica: indications for surgery*[a]

First episode	90% of patients will get better and stay better
Second episode	90% of patients will get better, but 50% of the patients will have a recurrence of symptoms—consider surgery
Third episode	90% of the patients will get better but almost all will have recurrent episodes of sciatica—propose surgery

[a]This condition is to be distinguished from recurrent herniated nucleus pulposus.

Technique

The frame and position most universally used are shown in Figure 16. The patient is stable in the kneeling position, and there is no hyperflexion at the hips and knees. The abdomen is free, thereby relieving pressure on the abdominal venous system and, in turn, decreasing venous backflow through Batson's plexus into the spinal canal. Some surgeons use a four-poster frame. Patient positioning is easier than for the knee-chest frame. A lordotic spine is maintained. If foraminotomy is required, a decompression in the lordotic position may be more reliable.

It is easy to obtain good-quality intraoperative level lateral x-ray using a grid on these surgical frames. An anteroposterior x-ray is rarely necessary but can be obtained using the four-poster frame and not the knee-chest position. The anteroposterior x-ray

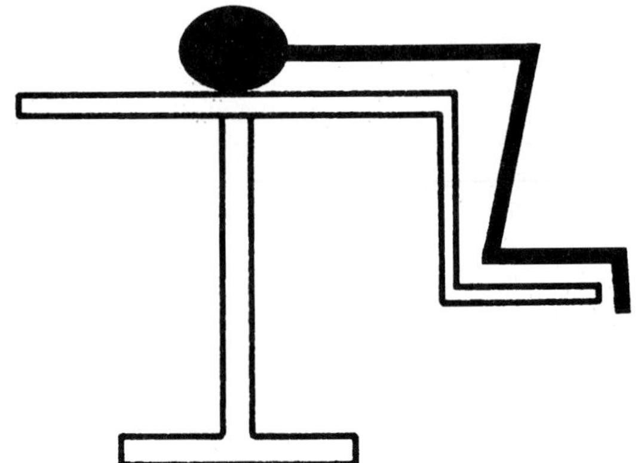

FIG. 16. The kneeling position, taking pressure off of the abdomen and allowing blood to flow from the epidural veins, through Batson's plexus, into the vena cava.

is usually less detailed, as a grid cannot be positioned between the posts. General anesthesia is preferable because of airway and sedation control. More important, it provides the opportunity for hypotensive anesthesia.

Identification of Level and Side

As previously discussed, identification of level and side is a critical factor in lumbar microsurgery. The North Americal Spine Society Task Force on Patient Safety has developed the "Sign, Mark, and X-Ray" (SMaX) program to reinforce a systems approach to this essential step. The SMaX strategy includes a preoperative checklist correlating the medical record, consent form, imaging studies, verbal verification with the patient, and an indelible ink mark of the appropriate side (29). An intraoperative imaging confirmation of the levels completes the SMaX approach. As a further check, the canal pathology should correlate with the findings on preoperative imaging. If necessary, obtain additional films with a marker in the canal or disc space before opening the annulus.

Skin Incision and Exposure of the Interlaminar Space

The skin incision is made one-half to three-fourths of an inch on either side of the primary marking line. The incision is located beside the spinous processes, rather than in the midline. Blunt dissection is used to expose the lumbodorsal fascia. The fascia is opened in a curvilinear fashion (Fig. 17). The skin opening and fascial incision are designed to do the least amount of damage to the supraspinous/interspinous ligament complex. The subperiosteal muscle dissection and elevation are confined to the interlaminar level being exposed. Once the level is exposed, the frame retractor is positioned. The curvilinear fascial incision tilts the frame hook away from the midline. This helps remove the edges of the frame from the line of vision of the microscope. Additional adjustment of the frame can be obtained by attaching a ball and chain weight to the appropriate side. It is at this juncture that the microscope is positioned for the interlaminar exposure and the microdiscectomy/microdecompression.

Entry into the Spinal Canal

It is at the point of entry to the spinal canal that the advantages of the microscope can be best appreciated. With the magnification and illumination inherent in the microscope, a ligamentum flavum–sparing technique can be used. Preserving the ligamentum flavum and epidural fat in microdiscectomy is thought to minimize postoperative epidural fibrosis.

The ligamentum flavum–sparing approach retains the ligamentum flavum as a medially based flap. To release the superior border of the ligamentum flavum flap, a burr or small Kerrison rongeur can be used to remove a few millimeters of bone from the cephalad lamina and 2 to 3 mm of the medial aspect of the inferior facet (Fig. 18). The lateral attachment of the ligamentum flavum is then released from the medial edge of the superior facet using a small cup curette (Fig. 19). Finally, the inferior border is released from the edge of the lamina below with a small curette. It is easiest to release the ligamentum in this order,

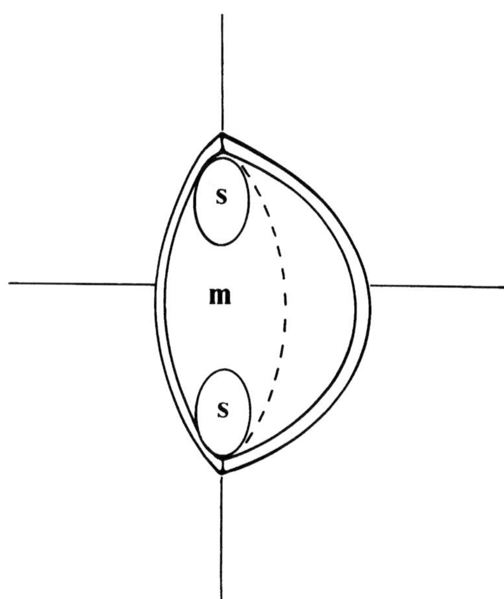

FIG. 17. The curvilinear incision through lumbodorsal fascia and erector spinae fascia that spares the supraspinous/interspinous ligament complex. s, spinous process; m, midline supraspinous ligament area.

as tension on the ligamentum can be maintained if the proximal attachment to the undersurface of the lamina is freed first.

After development of the medially based ligamentum flavum flap, the medial side of the superior facet may need to be resected with a small Kerrison rongeur (Fig. 20). This resection decompresses lateral recess stenosis to the level of the pedicle and up into the foramen. The lateral disc space and the nerve root adjacent to the pedicle can be identified. The nerve root and dura are mobilized with a ball-tip right-angle probe. At this point, the nerve root retractor is placed in the lateral disc space. The ligamentum flavum flap, epidural fat, and nerve root are retracted across the herniated disc toward the midline. This maneuver allows excellent exposure of the disc herniation. A bipolar cautery is used to coagulate epidural veins, which cannot be mobilized off the area of herniation. Cautery is used sparingly to avoid stimulation of epidural fibrosis. The herniation is opened with a small blade or an elevator. The herniated disc material is removed with pituitaries (Fig. 20). The deeper opening through the annulus itself is generally easy to identify. The annular defect is used as a portal via which a limited discectomy of loose disc material can be performed. The disc space is irrigated with antibiotic solution to dislodge and flush out any missed loose fragments. A 14-gauge plastic Angiocath, short intravenous extension tubing, and 20-cc syringe are assembled as the irrigation instrument. The surgeon should watch the anular defect while the solution is injected under pressure. Continue irrigation until no further fragments are flushed. Good return flow of fluid should be observed. If not, a defect in the anterior annulus is suspected, and vital signs must be monitored closely to ensure that there is no ongoing blood loss from possibly injured vascular structures anterior to the disc.

The spinal canal is then checked for any residual disc fragments. A ball-tip or flat Woodson probe is used to palpate under-

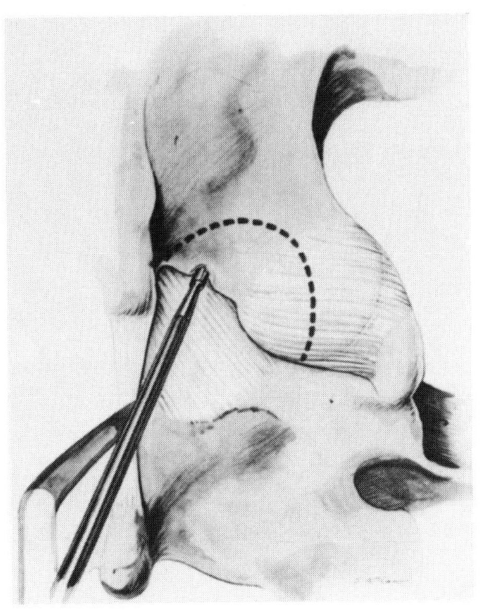

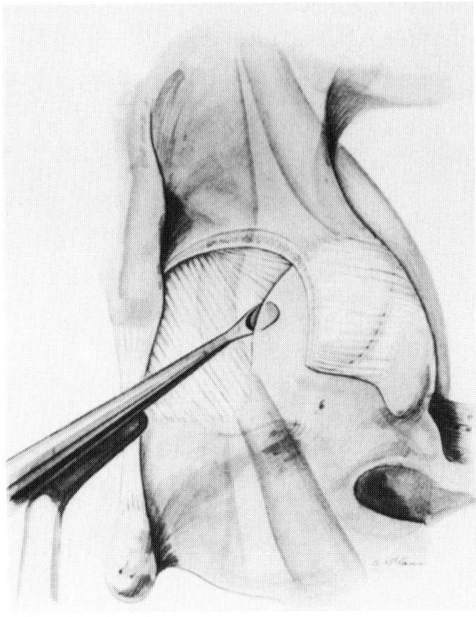

A,B

FIG. 18. A: After exposure of the intralaminar space through a 2- to 3-cm incision, several millimeters of the cephalad lamina and 2 to 3 mm of the medial edge of the inferior facet are removed with the Midas Rex AM-8 burr. This bone can be safely removed, as the undersurface is protected by the ligamentum flavum. **B:** This illustration shows the small forward-angled curette freeing the ligamentum flavum from its attachments to the medial edge of the superior facet. The ligamentum flavum can be freed from the undersurface of the upper and lower laminae, if necessary.

neath the nerve root and across the vertebral body toward the midline. Also, pass the probe laterally out the foramen at the operated segment and distally along the exposed nerve root, around the pedicle and out the foramen of the segment below. The dura and nerve root are given a final inspection to ensure that no areas of incidental durotomy exist. A fat graft from the patient's subcutaneous tissue or the peri-facet fat pad is placed over the laminotomy. Closure is begun with the dorsal lumbar fascia using 0 or #1 Vicryl sutures, followed by the subcutaneous layer with 2-0 Vicryl and the skin with a 3-0 Dexon subcuticular suture. Using this ligamentum flavum–sparing approach, blood loss should be no more than 10 to 20 cc. After closure, the skin is injected with 0.2%

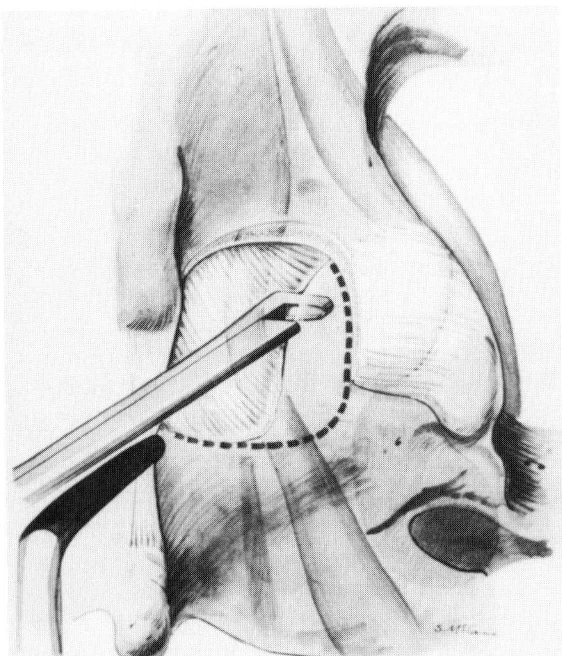

FIG. 19. The 2- and 3-mm Kerrison rongeurs are used to remove the lateral recess (subarticular) stenosis (i.e., the medial edge of the superior facet) back to the pedicle of the lower vertebra and cephalad to the tip of the superior facet. This bony resection removes the lateral recess (subarticular) stenosis and allows exposure of the lateral disc space.

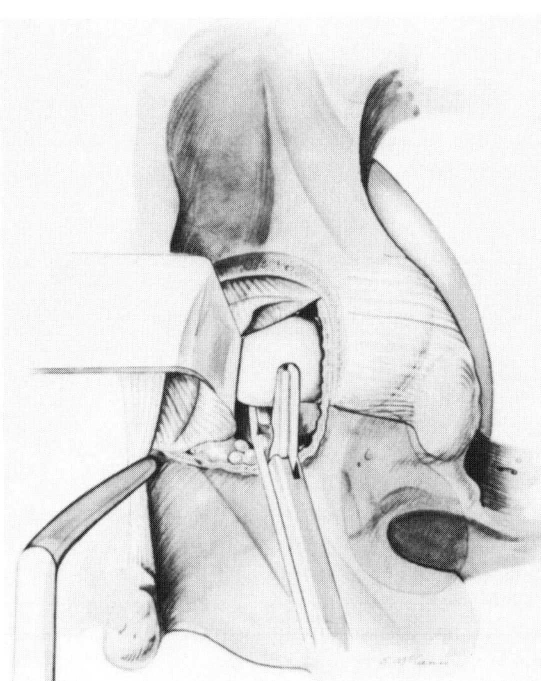

FIG. 20. A nerve root retractor is used to retract the ligamentum flavum, nerve root sleeve, and epidural fat toward midline over the herniated disc. The bipolar cautery can be used to cauterize the epidural plexus over the disc herniation, and, after exposure of the disc herniation, the disc is incised with a blade, and pituitary rongeurs are used to remove the herniated nucleus pulposus. After removal of loose nucleus pulposus, the disc is irrigated with a long angiocatheter, and the nerve root retractor is released, allowing the ligamentum flavum and nerve root sleeve to return to their normal anatomic position.

ropivacaine as a local anesthetic because it provides a sensory block but does not affect motor control. Any postoperative motor changes can thus be reliably ascribed to a true radicular problem and not an effect of the local anesthetic. Toradol (ketorolac tromethamine), 30 to 60 mg, is given 20 minutes before closure of the skin, and 30 mg is given intramuscularly or intravenously every 6 hours for the first postoperative day. Single-level microdiscectomy patients are generally sent home in less than 24 hours, and many times may be sent home the same afternoon as surgery.

Lateral Edge of the Nerve Root

The classic teaching is that once inside the spinal canal, it is essential to identify the lateral border of the nerve root before using any degree of force in manipulating the nerve root and before entering the disc space. The ligamentum-sparing approach described in the previous section does not allow for a clear view of the lateral edge of the nerve root and is not generally recommended. It is safer to remove part of the lateral ligamentum, clearly define the lateral border of the nerve root, and then retract the toe root medially. Only then is it possible to become more aggressive with the Kerrison rongeurs to achieve the cephalad or caudad laminar excision necessary to deal with the pathology.

If the lateral edge of the nerve root cannot be found, the following are important considerations: (a) an axillary disc may be displacing the root laterally; (b) there may be osteophytic lipping of the medial edge of the superior facet, which is obstructing the view and requires removal; (c) adhesions are present; or (d) there is an anomalous root.

Should identification of the lateral edge of the nerve root prove difficult, or if there are concerns that there may be an anomalous root even further lateral to the root in the field of vision, it is important to remember the basic rule that nerve roots are intimately related to pedicles (Fig. 21). If a nerve root cannot be found, a pedicle is identified and the root is immediately beside it. Once the nerve root is identified, probe the medial bony wall of the pedicle just lateral to the root, as proof that no other nerve tissue is lateral. Before retracting the nerve root, the lateral border must be clearly defined. There should be no adhesions tethering it. It is often best for the surgeon to hold the root retractor. However, improved optics on the assistant's side allow the assistant to hold the retractor and the neural structures within the field of view, thus reducing the risk of excess manipulation.

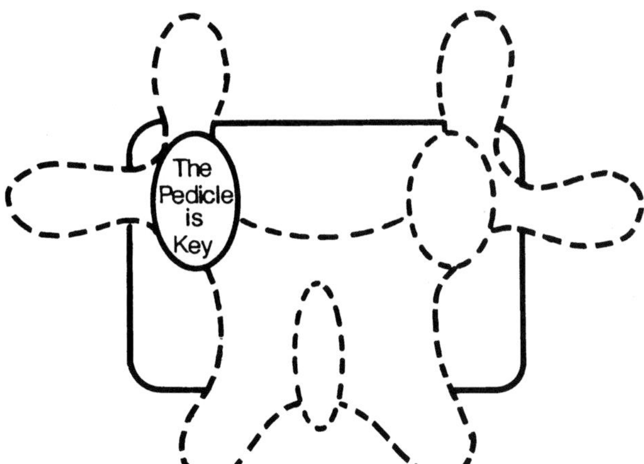

FIG. 21. To find your way in the spinal canal, locate the medial border of the pedicle. Immediately medial is the nerve root. At the superior edge of the pedicle is the disc space.

Stretched Root over Annulus

The root is at greatest risk when there is a moderate- or large-sized disc herniation. The traversing nerve root may be stretched, thinned, adherent, and virtually invisible over the apex of a large herniation that is displacing it. If particular care is not taken to identify the nerve root before incision, it can be inadvertently cut as part of the annulotomy. To facilitate the identification of the root when a large herniation is present, the laminotomy may have to be larger than average so that the proximal and distal extent of the herniation can be assessed. A larger laminotomy allows the root to be reliably found as it hugs the inferior surface of the pedicle. The root can be freed from any adhesions to the adjacent tissues and disc with a blunt nerve hook of the small ball-tip probe. The tip of the instrument is left under the corner of the root/dura and the lateral edge of the root and dura dissected free with a gentle sweeping motion.

Approach to Canal Pathology

The object of the surgical procedure is to leave a freely mobile nerve root. This requires removal of the obvious portion of ruptured disc, and it also includes a diligent search of the canal, along with probing of the foramen, for residual discal or bony pathology.

Removing Intradiscal Tissue

How much disc to remove from within the discal cavity is an unresolved issue. Removal of as much disc as possible implies curettage of the interspace, including the end-plates. Critics of this approach point out the following:

1. It is not possible to remove all intradiscal material in this manner, no matter how diligently the surgeon works.
2. This aggressive approach increases the risk of damage to visceral structures anterior to the disc space.
3. The risk of chronic back pain produced by conditions such as sterile discitis and instability is increased.

Although there are some articles in the literature to suggest that this extensive intradiscal débridement decreases the recurrent herniated nucleus pulposus rate, there are other articles refuting that position. The most compelling is Spengler's, which suggests that clinical limited disc excision is all that is necessary (30).

The advantages of limited disc removal are as follows:

1. Less trauma to end-plates and less dissection
2. Less nerve root manipulation
3. A lower prevalence of infection
4. Reduced risk of damage to structures anterior to the disc space (vessel perforation)

5. Less disc space settling postoperatively, which theoretically reduces the incidence of back pain.

UNIQUE DISC HERNIATION SITUATIONS

Several types of disc herniations are particularly suited to a microsurgical approach, as described in the following sections.

Foraminal Disc Herniation

Foraminal disc herniations constitute approximately 3 to 10% of all disc herniations (31,32). They migrate superiorly and laterally to lie in what Macnab termed the "hidden zone" (Fig. 22). There, they irritate and compress the exiting nerve root (Fig. 22). An attempt to remove this disc herniation through the standard interlaminar window may result in loss of a facet joint, potentially destabilizing the level (1).

Clinical Presentation

Most foraminal disc herniations occur at the L4-5 and L3-4 levels, affecting the L-4 and L-3 roots, respectively. They tend to occur in older patients (average age, 50 years) who have a wide, rather than degenerative and narrowed disc space. The onset of symptoms is usually sudden and the usual presentation is severe anterior thigh pain, interfering with all functions except sitting. Sleep patterns are often grossly interrupted because patients cannot lie on their back or in the prone position with the thigh extended. Neurologic examination, especially the sensory examination, usually gives a clue as to which root is involved, as will an absent knee jerk or weak quadriceps. The very positive femoral stretch test, together with a negative straight-leg raising test, alert the examiner to the possibility of a higher lumbar disc lesion.

Often, these disc ruptures do not respond to conservative care, or else the pain is so severe that the patient is not prepared to accept a prolonged conservative treatment program.

Operative Technique

The lateral zone can be divided into three regions (Fig. 23). A foraminal disc herniation can lie within the foramen or in an extraforaminal position. The key to understanding the boundaries of the foramen is depicted in Figure 24. The best way to obtain a full view of the pathology without sacrificing the facet joint is through an intertransverse window. A lateral disc herniation is best approached through Wiltse's muscle-splitting paraspinal approach (33) (Fig. 25).

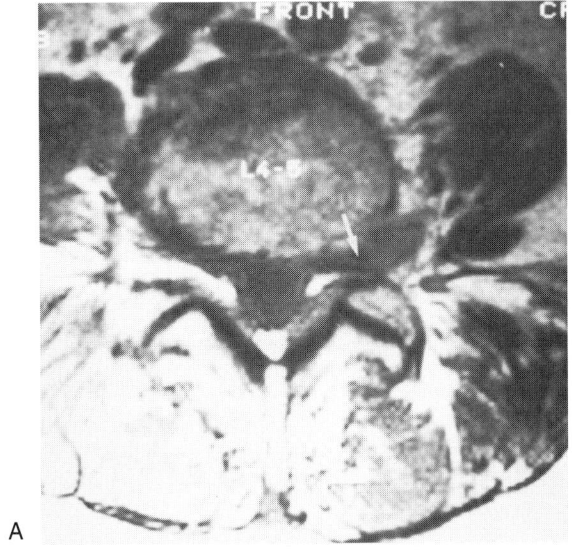

A

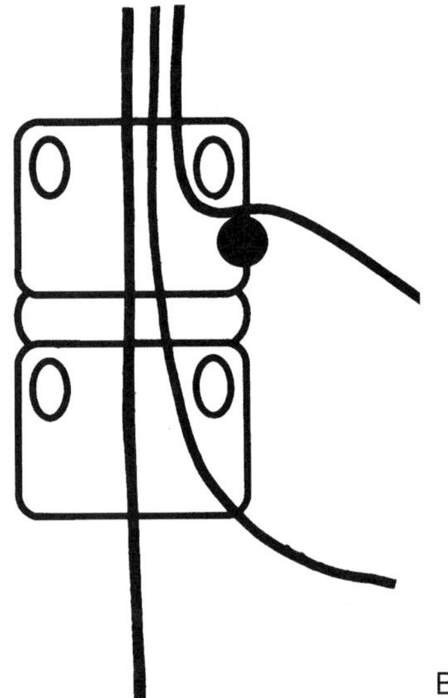
B

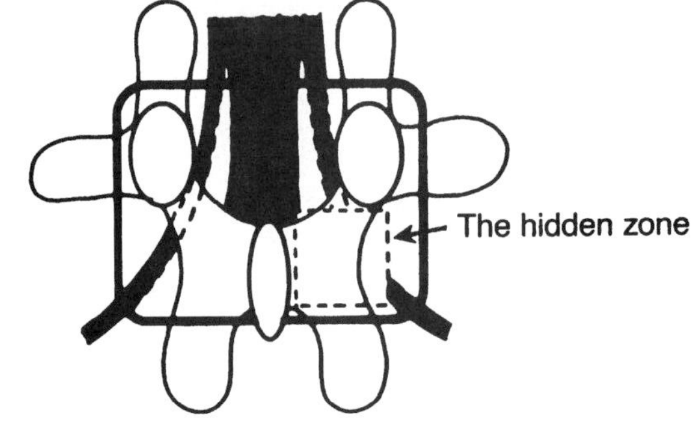

C

FIG. 22. A,B: A foraminal herniated nucleus pulposus, L-4 (*arrow*). **C:** The disc herniation lies in Macnab's hidden zone. But why is that zone "hidden"?

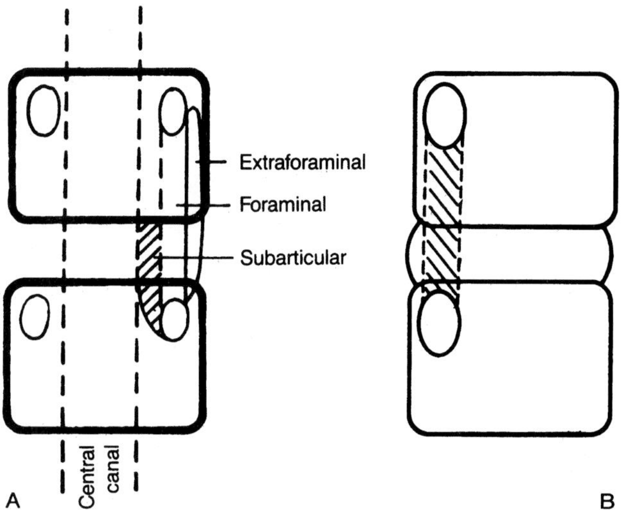

FIG. 23. A: The three regions of the lateral zone: (a) the subarticular, (b) the foraminal, and (c) the extraforaminal. **B:** The boundaries of the foraminal zone (pedicle-to-pedicle and pedicle-to-pedicle).

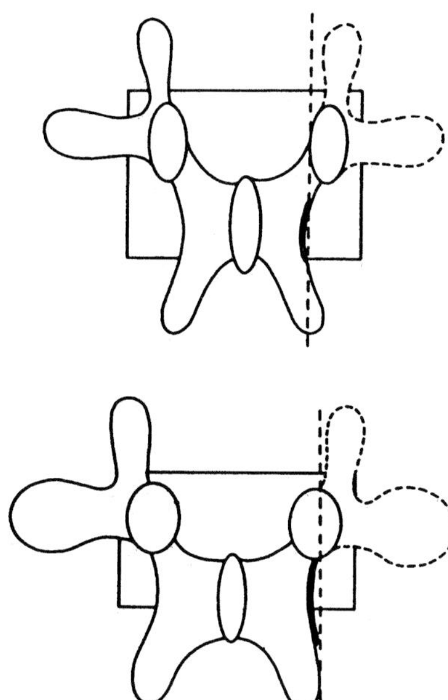

FIG. 24. The key to understanding the boundaries of the foramen, noting that the lateral border of the pars is on the same sagittal plane as the medial border of the pedicle. Another way of understanding this concept is to note that there is no bony roof to the foramen; the posterior boundary is the intertransverse ligament. This applies to all lumbar levels except L-5, shown at the bottom.

Axillary Disc Herniations

There are two mechanisms by which an axillary disc herniation occurs (Fig. 26):

1. A disc fragment can migrate downward and laterally into the axilla (Fig. 27). This usually occurs at the L-5 to S-1 level and most commonly forces the first sacral root tightly into the subarticular recess underneath (i.e., anterior to) the medial edge of the superior facet of S-1. A surgeon unaware of this anatomy can damage the S-1 root with the Kerrison rongeur while attempting to decompress the lateral recess by trimming the facet spurs. There are occasions on which the root cannot be mobilized because of the axillary location of the disc rupture. In these situations, the disc fragment has to be removed carefully from the axilla of the root. The root is then mobilized to complete the discectomy.
2. A disc fragment can migrate upward into the axilla of the nerve root, exiting above (Fig. 27). This also is most common at the L-5 to S-1 level, but the disc herniation migrates cephalad into the axilla of the fifth lumbar root. The fragment usually is anterior to the root and forces it up against the fifth lumbar lamina. The surgeon must take care not to damage the fifth root with the Kerrison rongeur or drill when doing a partial hemilaminectomy of L-5.

Multiple Root Involvement

There are a number of special situations in which the microscope may be useful.

First, after a routine or microdiscectomy, recurrent herniations are reported in 2 to 5% of patients (34). The microscope is especially valuable for dealing with this problem because neurologic tissues and scars are more easily discerned with the aid of higher magnification.

Second, in cauda equina syndrome, traditional lore teaches the following:

1. Any patient with perineal symptoms, bladder or bowel upset, and leg pain has a cauda equina syndrome. Diagnosis and surgery should be performed immediately.
2. Surgery often requires a wide decompression and bilateral approach to the disc fragment.

The first statement is probably true but not necessarily the second. There is no disc herniation too big to be removed through a microsurgical approach. A microdiscectomy in these situations usually can be accomplished through a wide laminotomy from the most symptomatic side or the side to which the disc rupture appears to be eccentric on investigation. The plane between the severely compressed cauda equina and the disc rupture is more easily dissected under the microscope, and further excessive compression of the cauda equina during disc excision is more readily observed (and prevented) under high magnification. If the disc herniation cannot be easily excised unilaterally, a bilateral exposure is indicated. Of nine emergency microdiscectomies performed by the author, cauda equina syndromes all have been managed by a unilateral exposure with no complications.

Results

There are many articles in the literature supporting or negating the value of using the microscope for lumbar disc surgery. The thrust of the articles can be summarized as follows:

1. Terminology such as *microdiscectomy* and *microlumbar discectomy* is irrelevant. What is relevant is a fully decompressed

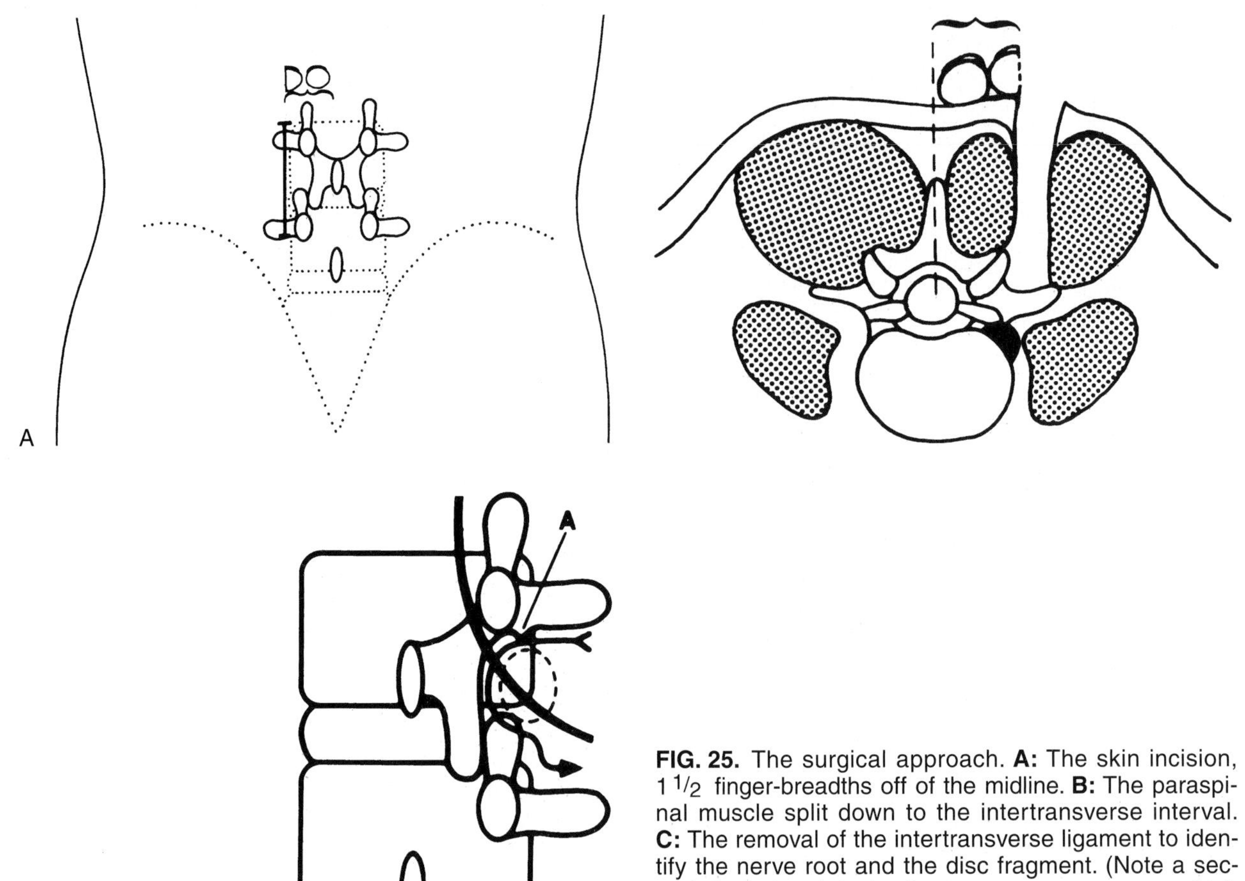

FIG. 25. The surgical approach. A: The skin incision, 1 1/2 finger-breadths off of the midline. B: The paraspinal muscle split down to the intertransverse interval. C: The removal of the intertransverse ligament to identify the nerve root and the disc fragment. (Note a second A that points to the accessory process, which marks the lateral border of the pedicle.)

nerve, removed of all its bony and soft tissue encroachment. Equally irrelevant is the length of the skin incision, the method of entry into the disc space (35), and the amount of lamina removed, providing that instability is not produced. Critics of microdiscectomy suggest that it is an acceptable technique as long as it is the standard operation assisted with the microscope and not a "minuscule operation" that misses pathology.

2. There is no objective evidence from controlled randomized studies that microdiscectomy delivers better overall results than standard discectomy (1,4,6,13). There are many

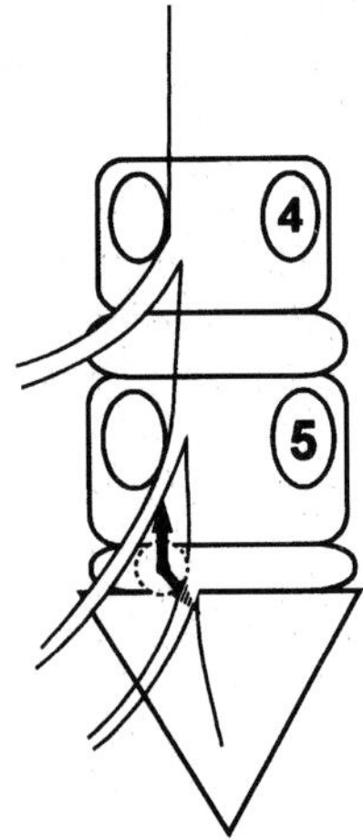

FIG. 26. A schematic of the two migratory patterns of disc ruptures that result in dangerous axillary locations.

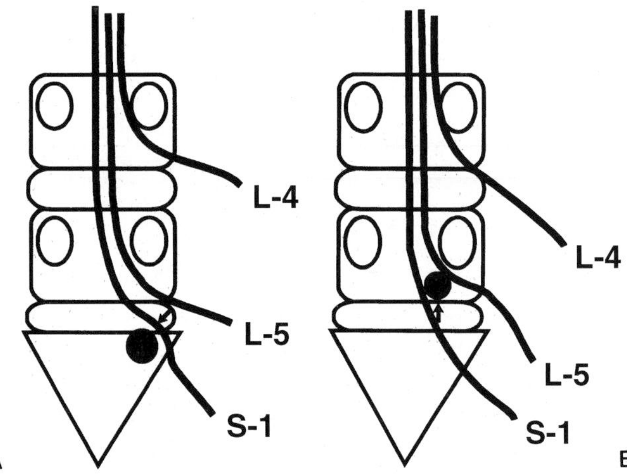

FIG. 27. A: Downward migration into the axilla of the first sacral root. B: Upward migration into the axilla of the fifth lumbar root.

articles claiming that microdiscectomy results in superior outcomes (36–44), but these claims are not scientifically based on controlled, randomized, prospective studies. On the other hand, there is enough evidence to support the idea that the microsurgical discectomy delivers a result as good as a standard discectomy. It is also evident that varying assessment criteria make comparison of one study to others extremely difficult (45).

3. There seems to be widespread agreement that the smaller wound of microsurgical intervention for a disc rupture causes less morbidity than a larger incision. Although the annual incidence of surgeries is increasing (46,47), the length of hospital stay is decreasing. The length of stay is consistently shorter for a microdiscectomy than for the standard procedure (4,6,48–51,52). Furthermore, microsurgical patients require less postoperative medication and recover faster, returning to work sooner. A smaller wound (i.e., smaller muscle dissection and less laminar removal) is the likely reason for these benefits. Some believe that microdiscectomy may turn out to be faster and cheaper than conventional discectomy (4).

4. For years, Williams (50,51,53) dominated the field of "microlumbar discectomy," because he was the first to describe the approach in the North American literature. John McCulloch and many other spine surgeons visited him to learn the technique and were impressed with his surgical skills. In turn, they accepted his minimalist approach to disc excision, following his teaching that only the herniated fragment of disc be removed. Numerous authors had the same experience as Williams, with a high recurrence rate (9%) (5,49). This led them to abandon his "fragmentectomy" approach. There are many reasons why Williams and others have had a high recurrence rate. The evidence today supports the hypothesis that the rate of recurrence directly relates to the type of disc pathology.

5. Today's visible choices for procedures within the disc space are two: a limited intradiscal procedure (i.e., removing loose fragments with rongeurs and lavaging the disc space), or a more aggressive attempt at discectomy with curettage. There is no definitive scientific support in the literature for one choice over the other, and randomized, controlled studies are needed. In nonrandomized standard discectomy studies, the evidence supports the limited approach (30).

6. The recurrence rate after microdiscectomy averages 5% ± 2% (2,4,54,55) and is no different from that of standard lumbar discectomy (52,56). Most recurrences are same level, same side (2,4,55,57–59), with the majority occurring within the first year (58). Within the first month, recurrent symptoms necessitating repeat surgery can result from (a) missed fragments, (b) continuing bony encroachment, (c) an unrecognized second disc, or (d) a massive recurrent disc at the same level, same side (57).

7. There is a learning curve involved in completing nerve root decompression in a limited microsurgical field, as evidenced by the decreases in infection rate (1 to 7%) (17,58, 60,61) and dural tear rate (1.0 to 6.7%) (2,4,8,54,58) that occur with experience. Dural tears are signaled by the appearance of cerebrospinal fluid, and part of the reason for the reported higher incidence of dural tears is that cerebrospinal fluid is more obvious under the microscope. Support for this position comes from the higher rate of root damage (a more significant dural tear) and pseudomeningocele (a missed dural tear) with standard discectomy (5). The author thinks it is reasonable to conclude that the higher incidence of dural tear results from the introduction of a new technique, rather than the new technique itself.

8. The incidence of multilevel intervention is less in almost all microsurgical series compared to standard discectomy. There are many reasons for this, the most important of which is the merging of better surgical techniques with better preoperative investigation (e.g., MRI). This fact, however, still supports the idea that if you are going to limit your incision, you should know in advance what you are going to do when you arrive at the scene of the pathology.

9. Abramovitz and Neff, in a multicenter, prospective trial, proved again what cannot be repeated often enough—if you select patients with dominant radicular pain (compared to back pain), with neurologic changes and significant straight-leg raising changes, and with a study confirming a disc rupture, you can anticipate a high level of success for discectomy, with or without the microscope (1). The rate of successful outcome drops precipitously when these inclusion criteria for surgery are not met. Their study also showed that loss of a facet joint often leads to a poorer outcome.

10. The use of epidural steroids, instilled at the completion of surgery, does not improve the results (62). With the theoretical considerations that steroids may delay wound healing, increase infection, and exacerbate dural tears, it seems reasonable not to use epidural steroids intraoperatively.

11. Persistent back pain occurs in up to 25% of patients undergoing microdiscectomy (55,63). This has led to the opinion that it is important to save the supraspinous/interspinous ligament complex, remove as little lamina as possible, save the ligamentum flavum as a flap, and do a limited discectomy. Again, there is no proof that these steps, facilitated by the microscope, reduce the risk of long-term back pain.

12. There is little discussion in the literature of wrong-level exposure, which is a major problem in all of spine surgery, and more so in microsurgery.

13. Reoperation is probably safer and easier with a microsurgical assist because scar, dura, adhesions, nerve roots, and disc fragments are more readily seen (55). This allows for more aggressive sharp dissection around nerve roots. Results of repeat surgery, regardless of the use of the microscope, are not as good as primary surgery because of scar tissue and the higher incidence of bilateral exposures and multilevel interventions.

Summary

The modern operating microscope enhances the spinal surgeon's ability to effectively correct spinal canal pathology. However, spinal microsurgery is most valuable as a comprehensive surgical discipline. Exacting technical requirements inherent in microsurgery compel the surgeon to enhance his or her clinical skills. A limited, minimally invasive exposure of precisely localized pathology is required. Preoperatively, skillful evaluation of the patient history and physical examination are required to identify clinical syndromes. Ultimately, the clinical situation needs to be correlated with the analysis of pathology from sophisticated imaging studies. Only then can the operating microscope function to optimally assist the surgeon and the patient to obtain the best clinical outcome.

MICROSURGICAL SPINAL LAMINOTOMIES

The merging of the technology of MRI with the magnification and illumination characteristics of the microscope has dramatically changed the surgical treatment of spinal canal stenosis (SCS) (53). The use of the microscope to limit the surgical exposure in SCS has been made possible by the ability of MRI and CT-myelogram to pinpoint the soft tissue and bony stenotic lesion. The surgical procedure that has evolved has been variously named the *intersegmental resculpturing* or *laminoplasty procedure*, or, simply, a *laminotomy* (64). The advantage of considering this limited surgical approach lies in the fact that it is possible to save all the important soft tissue and bony stabilizing structures, and at the same time remove the pathology stenosing the cauda equina.

Classification

Before describing the technical approach, this section outlines the limited types of spinal stenotic lesions that are amenable to a microsurgical operation. Acquired stenosis is described as a lesion developing in mobile spine segments as part of the aging process. Abnormal motion, usually secondary to disc degeneration, results in osteophyte formation, ligamentum infolding or hypertrophy, facet hypertrophy, and/or annular bulging. In turn, these changes encroach on neural structures and reduce the space available to the cauda equina and nerve roots.

The classic symptom of spinal stenosis is limitation of walking distance because of claudicatory leg pain, and feelings of heaviness, fatigue, numbness, or unsteadiness. The common denominator is that all these symptoms limit the walking distance and cause the patient to limp or be lame, hence the term *claudication*. The symptom complex associated with spinal stenosis has become known as *neurogenic claudication*. It forms the foundation of the definition of SCS, which is claudicant limitation of leg function in the presence of a stenotic spinal canal lesion on x-ray, and in the absence of vascular impairment in the lower extremities.

The standard classification of SCS has been outlined elsewhere (65). This etiologic classification and the term *spinal stenosis* are used by most authors to describe canal and "lateral recess" stenosis. This arbitrary division of spinal stenosis into lateral zone stenosis and SCS helps in understanding the two conditions, but at best it is an artificial separation that often has no value when a patient presents with stenosis involving both anatomic regions (Fig. 28).

Purely congenital spinal stenosis is uncommon. It is a disease affecting multiple spinal segments (Fig. 29) and cannot be dealt with by a limited laminotomy procedure.

The three most common forms of spinal stenosis, two of which lend themselves to one procedure, are acquired degenerative conditions. The most common form is SCS resulting from a degenerative spondylolisthesis (Fig. 28) (66,67). Because of the forward and/or lateral translation (slip) of one vertebral segment on the caudal level, a vertebral segmental instability is implied, for which many surgeons would propose a combined decompression and stabilization procedure.

The next two conditions are approachable through limited surgical intervention with the microscope: SCS resulting from degenerative changes in the soft tissue and joints of the lumbar spine without a degenerative spondylolisthesis (Fig. 30) (68), and lateral zone stenosis resulting from degenerative changes in the subarticular, foraminal, and extraforaminal regions of the lateral zone (69).

Pathoanatomy of Spinal Canal Stenosis

The surgical anatomy of the structural lesion in SCS is the key to understanding the limited surgical procedure to relieve

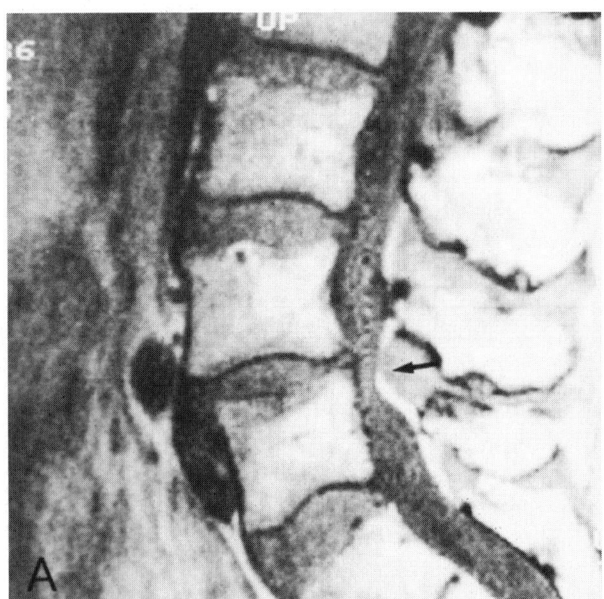

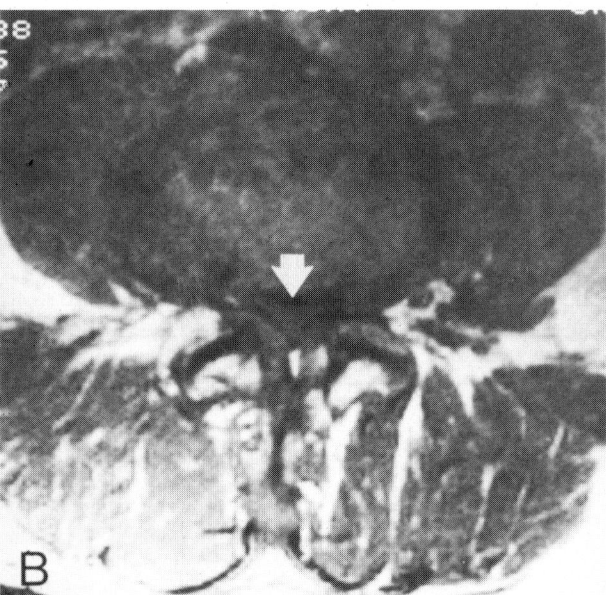

FIG. 28. The classic spinal stenosis, on sagittal **(A)** and axial **(B)** magnetic resonance imaging, showing a degenerative spondylolisthesis at L4-5, canal stenosis (*arrow*), and subarticular stenosis laterally.

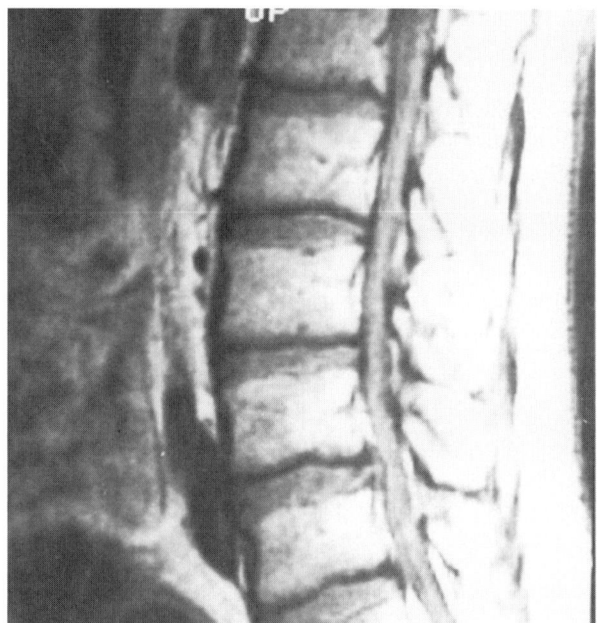
A

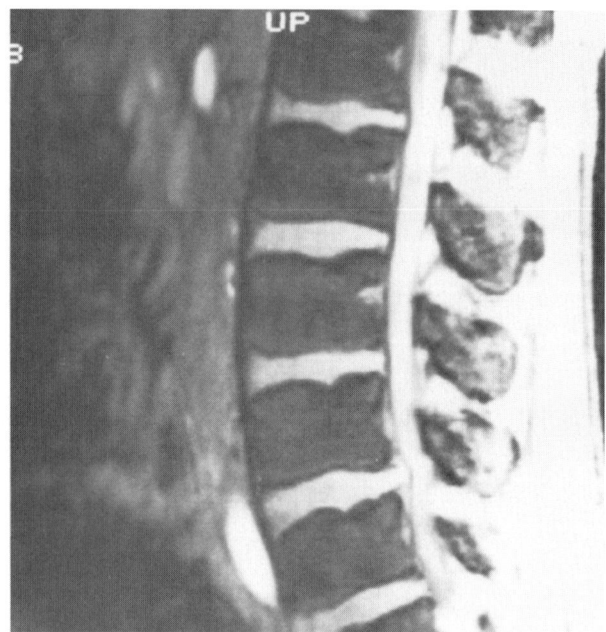

B

FIG. 29. Congenital spinal canal stenosis. The entire canal, all three stories (see Fig. 8) of each segment, and multiple segments are narrowed in this sagittal magnetic resonance image. A small disc protrusion is present at L4-5, which tipped this patient into symptoms.

the cauda equina stenosis (70). Each vertebral segment can be divided into three layers (Fig. 8), corresponding to three stories in a house. Reviewing Figure 28, one can see that the stenotic lesion is largely confined to the first story of the anatomic segment, with some extension into the third story of the anatomic segment below and some extension above into the second story of the same anatomic segment. Figures 29, 31, and 32 show a predominant "first-story" lesion resulting from degenerative changes in the facet joints, disc space, and ligamentum flavum. These degenerative changes are in the form of hypertrophy and unfolding of the ligamentum flavum, annular bulging of the degenerating and collapsing disc, and osteophyte formation at the edges of the vertebral bodies or lips of the facet joints (71). Of the three, infolding of the ligamentum flavum is the major lesion. Note again that the major location of stenosis in Figures 28, 30, 31, and 32 occurs predominantly in the first story of each segment, extending somewhat down into the third story of the segment below, and even less so up into the second story of the same segment. Between the midpoints of the pedicles and at the junction of the third and second stories, there is virtually no stenosis (Figs. 28, 30, 31).

Linking a series of fragments together and being aware that canal stenosis is always most prominent in the first story, one can appreciate that the constriction of canal stenosis occurs between the takeoffs of nerve roots. Thus, canal stenosis at the disc space level of L4-5 (i.e., the first story of L-4) is a constricting ring between the takeoff of the fourth root above and fifth lumbar root below (Fig. 32). Because the ligamentum flavum is such an important contributor to stenosis, some details of its anatomy and degeneration are important to understanding the operative approach.

Ligamentum Flavum

The *ligamentum flava* are paired structures that connect adjacent lamina. The elastin/collagen content of the ligamentum

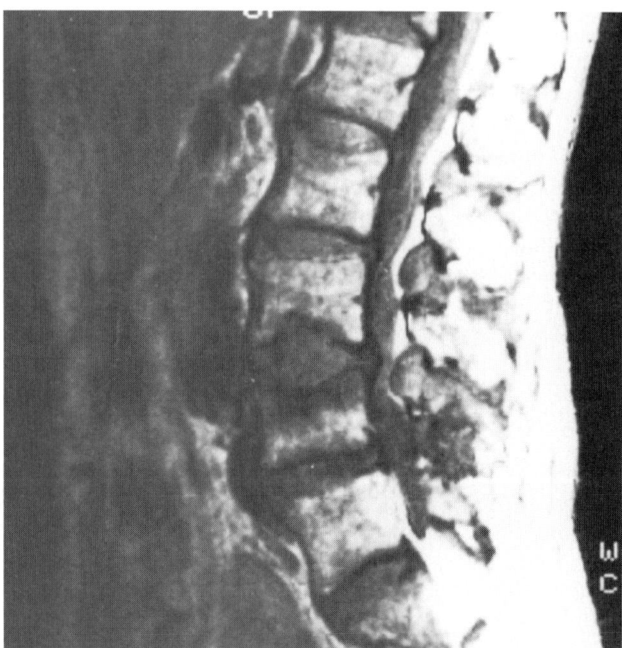

FIG. 30. Sagittal T1-weighted magnetic resonance image showing spinal canal syndrome in multiple segments without a degenerative spondylolisthesis (slip). There is a very early slip, L-4 on L-5, but the stenotic levels are at L2-3 and L3-4.

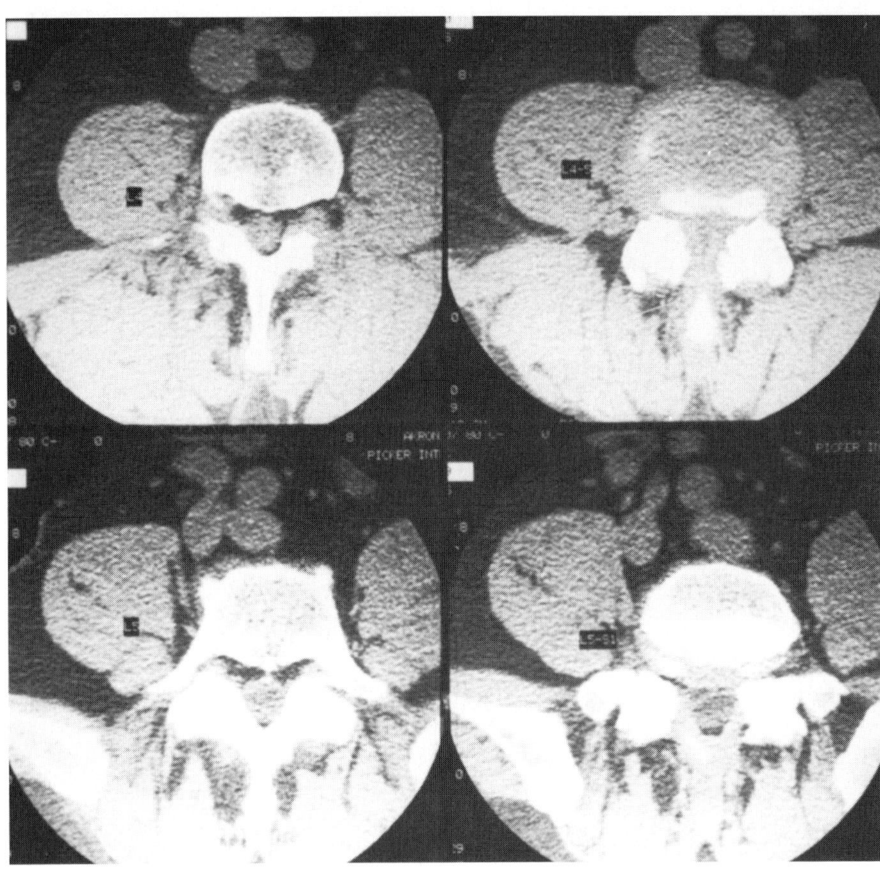

FIG. 31. Axial computed tomographic scans showing stenosis of cauda equina (*top right*). Above and below this "napkin ring" is a patent canal.

flavum and its attachment to the laminae make it a unique structure.

Elastin/Collagen Content

The elastin content of the ligamentum flavum is approximately 80%, versus a collagen content of 20%. This high elastic content gives the ligament a yellow appearance, hence the name "yellow ligament." It is probably a passive structure, acting much like a rubber band when lumbar vertebrae flex and extend. During flexion, the ligamentum flavum stretches but does not inhibit that motion. On return to neutral and extension, it returns to its resting, but still taut, position without buckling. With aging, the ligamentum flavum loses its elastic properties, becomes more collagenous in nature, and as a result can permanently buckle or fold into the spinal canal as seen in Figures 28 and 30.

Attachment of Ligamentum Flavum

The paired ligamentum flava are separated by a midline cleft. Laterally, they extend to the anterior aspect of the facet joint, blending with the anterior capsule of the facet joint. The important attachments are to the cephalad and caudal laminae. Note that the insertion of the proximal edge of the ligamentum is into the anterior surface of the midportion of the cephalad lamina. Its distal edge inserts along the superior border of the caudad lamina (Fig. 33). Total unilateral excision of the ligamentum flavum requires removal of the inferior one-half of the cephalad lamina, the superior edge of the caudal lamina, and the medial margin of the facet joint (Fig. 34). In completing this limited excision, the stenosis of the canal can be allevi-

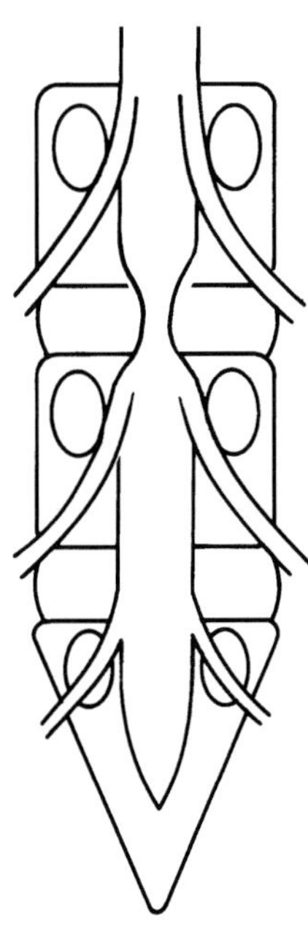

FIG. 32. The napkin ring stenotic lesion in the first story of L-4, stenosing the canal between the L-4 and L-5 roots.

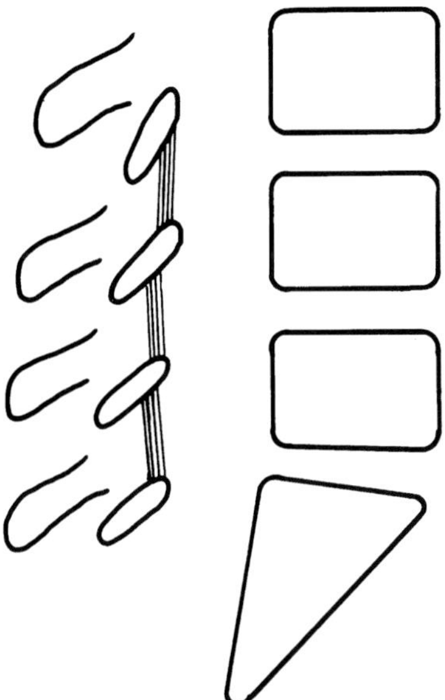

FIG. 33. A lateral schematic showing the attachment of the ligamentum flavum to the anterior aspect of the cephalad lamina and to the posterior edge of the caudal lamina.

ated. Furthermore, this limited interlaminar approach is facilitated by the microscope.

Segments Involved in Spinal Canal Stenosis

Most often, SCS is a multisegmental disease or presents at a "slip" or "listhetic" level, which precludes a microsurgical approach. Less than one-third of SCS patients have unisegmental involvement at a nonslip level and are possible candidates for a microsurgical approach. Although it is theoretically possible to use this microsurgical approach at two stenotic levels, its use in multisegmental decompressions is tedious and inadvisable. Multilevel cases are probably best handled with loupes. The single, most frequently affected level is L4-5, and the least affected level is L-5 to S-1.

Establishing a diagnosis of SCS can be difficult. Because of the older age group affected, it is important to rule out other conditions, such as infection, tumors, and other nonmechanical causes of back pain. Many of these patients may also have vascular disease, and it is necessary to establish that aortoiliac or femoral artery insufficiency is not the dominant cause for their symptoms. Neurologic symptoms require consideration of all possible causes, including generalized neurologic disorders unrelated to the spine, or a myelopathy from cervical spine spondylosis.

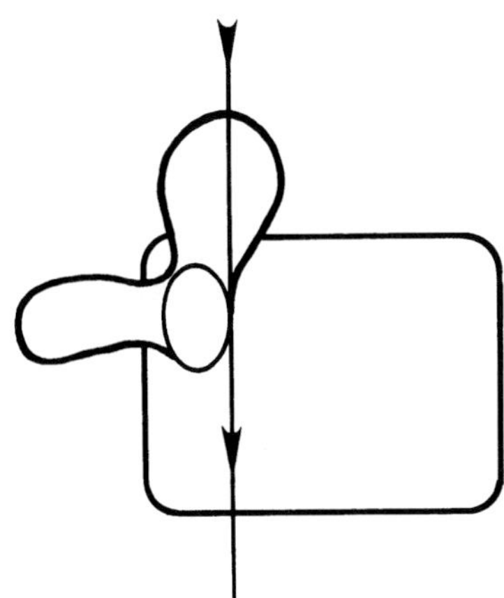

FIG. 34. The medial edge of the superior facet is removed laterally as far as the medial edge of the pedicle.

Radiologic Investigation

Plain x-ray films of most patients are routinely ordered but yield little information about a patient with SCS. Their greatest use is to rule out other conditions, such as tumors or infection. Spinal deformities, such as scoliosis and degenerative spondylolistheses, are also obvious on plain x-ray films.

Many investigators have attempted to define SCS by using plain x-ray measurements of the spinal canal (72). This has routinely failed. Until recently, myelography was the gold standard for the investigation of a patient with SCS, most often in conjunction with CT. More recently, MRI has had a major influence on the diagnosis of SCS and is used as the only preoperative investigative imaging procedure (other than plain x-rays) by many surgeons. The exception to this statement is the patient with degenerative scoliosis and spinal stenosis who still needs a CT-myelogram. These imaging modalities are all preoperative tools that simply document a structural lesion that must be correlated with the clinical presentation. The contraindications for microsurgical intervention are now almost nonexistent in SCS.

MICROSURGICAL LAMINOPLASTY FOR SPINAL CANAL STENOSIS

The principles that must be adhered to when considering a limited microsurgical procedure for SCS are the following:

1. The disease must be confined to one, or at the most, two segments.
2. If the decompression is going to be confined to the central canal, the surgeon must not leave behind encroachment in the lateral zone that may be causing symptoms.
3. Through a limited microsurgical approach, the soft tissue and bony encroachment of the cauda equina can be visualized and removed.
4. The limited surgical approach must spare the other important soft tissue and bony supporting structures of the segment (i.e., the supraspinous/interspinous ligament complex), the facet joints (except for their medial edges), and the annulus/posterior longitudinal ligament complex, in an attempt to maintain as much stability as possible.

Although the primary goal is to relieve the patient's leg symptoms that limit walking ability, one must not lose sight of the mechanical back pain that is present. It is important to explain to patients before surgical intervention that although significant relief of leg pain most often occurs, it may not be complete, and some back pain almost certainly remains. It is unusual, however,

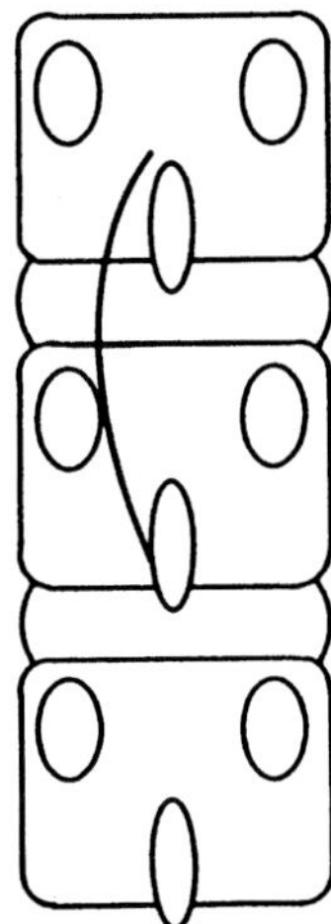

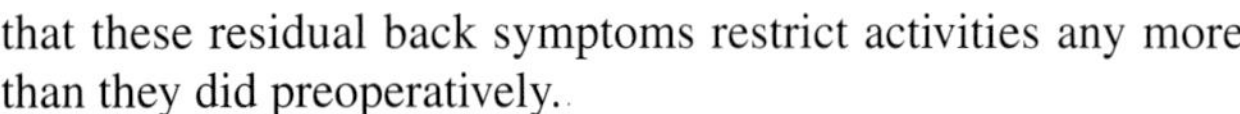

FIG. 35. A unilateral incision is made in the lumbodorsal fascia to save the supraspinous/interspinous ligament complex during decompression of each side.

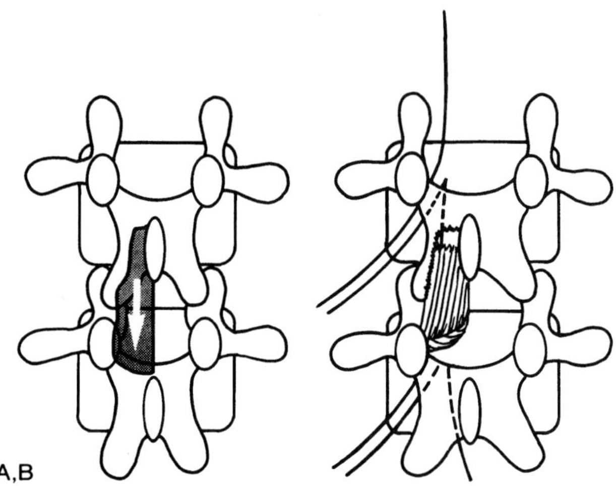

FIG. 37. Working in a proximal-to-distal direction, the inferior one-half of the cephalad lamina is removed **(A)**, and the interspace is decompressed **(B)**.

that these residual back symptoms restrict activities any more than they did preoperatively.

Operative Procedure

It is usual that a patient with unilateral leg pain due to SCS shows radiologic evidence of bilateral disease. Given the limited mortality associated with the procedure, however, it is the author's practice in these circumstances to perform a bilateral decompression. For example, in a decompression at L4-5, the following steps are taken to complete a bilateral interlaminar decompression or laminoplasty from one side.

The procedure is generally done with the patient in the kneeling position, starting with image intensifier localization of the segment to be decompressed. The bilateral decompression should be done from the more symptomatic side. Assuming the more symptomatic side is the left, the skin and fascial incisions for L4-5 are shown in Figure 35. Subperiosteal muscle dissection is carried out such that the entire lamina of L-4 and the upper one-half of the lamina of L-5, as well as the interlaminar space of L4-5 are visible (Fig. 36).

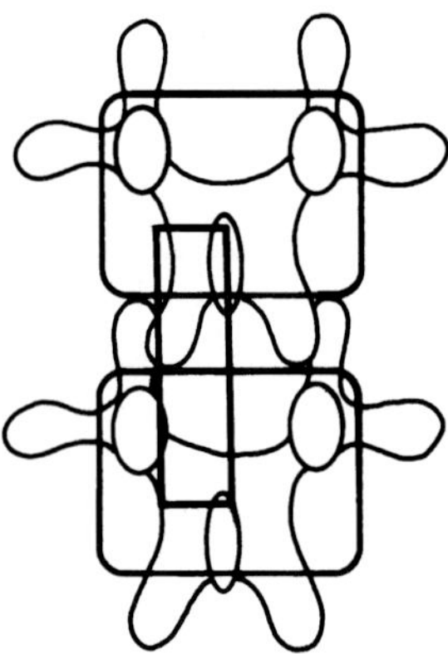

FIG. 36. The extent of the exposure reveals all of the lamina above and the upper one-half of the lamina below the interspace to be decompressed.

Because of the interlaminar narrowing and shingling of SCS, it is rarely possible to directly cross the ligamentum flavum to gain entry into the epidural space. In this situation, one of two approaches is used: removal of the inferior one-half of the cephalad lamina up to the origin of the ligamentum flavum, followed by the removal of the ligamentum flavum in a proximal-to-distal direction (Fig. 37), or identification of the distal attachment of the ligamentum flavum from the caudal lamina and then peeling it off of the superior edge of the caudal lamina, followed by the removal of the ligamentum flavum in a distal-to-proximal direction.

Regardless of the method used, the entire ligamentum flavum must be removed, as well as the medial edges of the inferior facet of L-4 and the superior facet of L-5. The medial edge of the superior facet is removed laterally as far as the medial edge of the pedicle (Fig. 34). This results in a complete decompression of the first story, the adjacent portions of the second story above, and the third story below. Removal of the medial edge of the superior facet also decompresses the subarticular zone, but the foraminal and extraforaminal zones are not decompressed with this approach. When the decompression is finished, the supraspinous/interspinous ligament complex is intact, the facet joints are intact, and the disc space is undisturbed. There are rare occasions on which a ruptured lumbar disc is associated with SCS and requires removal. The routine opening of the disc space at the time of an SCS decompression is to be discouraged, however, as this may result in progressive instability.

Once the unilateral laminoplasty has been completed, the decompression of the opposite side is started. The most anterior fibers of the interspinous ligament are removed. The bony masses that form the confluences of the spinous processes and the two laminae are then removed. Finally, the bulk of the opposite ligamentum flavum is removed, a procedure best accomplished by tilting the operating table away

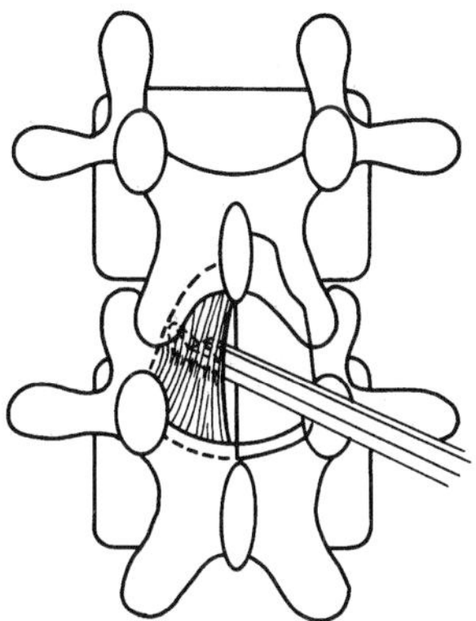

FIG. 38. Operating from one side and retracting the dura to the operating side, the opposite ligamentum flavum can be decompressed. This is facilitated by angling the microscope across to the opposite side.

from the surgeon and angling the microscope across the spinal canal (Figs. 38 and 39). During this portion of the laminoplasty, it is essential to retract the cauda equina. Eventually, the laminar attachments of the ligamentum flavum and the lamina itself are excised to complete the interlaminar decompression. The opposite-side laminoplasty is not considered complete until the roots above and below the constrictive lesion are seen along with the far edge of the dural sheath and its adjacent disc space.

If a second-level laminoplasty is necessary, a similar procedure is carried out, as described previously. The usual situation is for an L3-4 decompression to accompany an L4-5 interlaminar decompression. A two-level, bilateral laminoplasty can be accomplished through a unilateral approach, using a 2- to 3-inch incision, sacrificing only ligamentum flavum, lamina, and the medial edges of the facet joints causing the stenosis, while saving the supraspinous/interspinous ligament complexes, preserving the integrity of the facet joints, and not violating the disc. The resulting postoperative stability allows for early postoperative ambulation and, most often, a hospital discharge within 2 to 3 days.

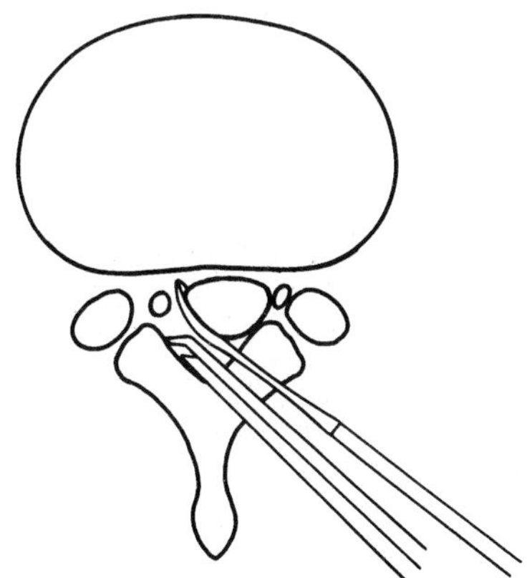

FIG. 39. Retracting the dura to the operating side.

Results

Before mid-1988, the author was not using the microsurgical laminoplasty for SCS. A review of 72 standard, nonmicrosurgical SCS surgeries (minimum, 1-year follow-up; maximum, 4-year follow-up) revealed that 21 were decompressions alone, and 51 were decompressions and fusions. Of the 21 nonsurgical decompressions, there were four failures involving continuing leg symptoms thought to be due to inadequate decompression. Ten decompressions were single level and eleven were multilevel, with L4-5 the most common level decompressed and L-5 to S-1 the least common. No significant complications occurred.

With the increased use of MRI, especially sagittal sections, it became evident that the main lesion in acquired SCS occurs in the first story of the anatomic segment (Figs. 28 and 30). This led to the introduction of the microsurgical decompression of the offending level of the anatomic segment through a bilateral midline exposure in 1988 (73). By early 1989, it became evident that when completing the second decompression on one side, the prior contralateral decompression could be seen through the ipsilateral operating side. Personal communication with Young led to the next step in evolution: the bilateral interlaminar decompression laminoplasty through a unilateral interlaminar portal (Figs. 38 and 39) (74). Since 1989, this technique has been used with no complications except for one postoperative phlebitis, and has yielded good initial results. Acceptable scientific follow-up is not yet available.

The concept of a limited laminotomy for the treatment of SCS has been published by Aryanpur and Ducker (64) and Cherkin et al. (46), describing a 90% successful outcome in 32 patients with "focal lateral recess stenosis." Although this is not midline SCS, as reported in this chapter, the concept of limited surgical intervention for one variety of spinal stenosis has proven useful in their hands with no complications reported.

Complications

The specific perils of operating with the microscope have been covered in the preceding portion of this chapter on microsurgery for lumbar disc disease. The added complications in bilateral laminotomies through a unilateral portal include inadequate decompression of the opposite side and dural tears from inadequate retraction with the use of Kerrison rongeurs on the opposite side.

CONCLUSION

SCS is a relentlessly progressive narrowing of the lumbar spinal canal that insidiously decreases the space available for the cauda equina. The resulting symptoms are quite disabling, yet patients present little clinical evidence of nerve root involvement. The diagnosis is often elusive until the patient undergoes myelographic and/or CT investigation. MRI is playing an increasing role in the diagnosis of SCS.

For patients with unisegmental disease or two-level involvement without a slip level, a laminoplasty or resculpturing procedure represents a very limited surgical option that in its early development offers good results (6,40,45). It is the author's opinion that this approach is facilitated by the microscope, so much that a bilateral laminoplasty can be completed through a unilateral interlaminar window.

ACKNOWLEDGMENT

Many thanks to Paul Young, neurosurgeon, St. Louis University, St. Louis, Missouri, for demonstrating the bilateral decompression of SCS through the unilateral interlaminal portal.

REFERENCES

1. Abramovitz JN, Neff SR. Lumbar disc surgery: results of the prospective lumbar discectomy study of the Joint Section on Disorders of the Spine and Peripheral Nerves of the American Association of Neurological Surgeons and the Congress of Neurological Surgeons. *Neurosurgery* 1991;29:301–308.
2. Barrios C, Ahmed M, Arrotequi J, et al. Microsurgical versus standard removal of the herniated lumbar disc. *Acta Orthop Scand* 1990;61:399–403.
3. Findlay A, Hall B, Musa B, et al. A ten year follow-up of lumbar microdiscectomy. *Spine* 1998;23:1168–1171.
4. Silvers HR. Microsurgical versus standard lumbar discectomy. *Neurosurgery* 1988;22:837–841.
5. Striffeler H, Gröger U, Reulen HJ. "Standard" microsurgical lumbar discectomy vs "conservative" microsurgical discectomy. *Acta Neurochir (Wien)* 1991;112:62–64.
6. Tullberg T, Isacson J, Weidenhielm L. Does microscopic removal of lumbar disc herniation lead to better results than standard procedure? *Spine* 1993;18:24–27.
7. Wenger M, Mariani L, Kalbarczyk A, et al. Long term outcome of 104 patients after lumbar sequestrectomy according to Williams. *Neurosurgery* 2001;49:329–335.
8. Caspar W, Campbell B, Barbier DD, et al. The Caspar microsurgical discectomy and comparison with a conventional standard lumbar disc procedure. *Neurosurgery* 1991;28:78–87.
9. Peacock EE Jr. Dynamic aspects of collagen biology, I: synthesis and assembly. *J Surg Res* 1967;7:433–445.
10. La Rocca H, Macnab I. The laminectomy membrane. *J Bone Joint Surg Br* 1974;56:545–550.
11. Macnab I, Cuthbert H, Godfrey C. The incidence of denervation of the sacrospinales muscles following spinal surgery. *Spine* 1977;2:294–298.
12. Song J, Park Y. Ligament-sparing lumbar microdiscectomy: technical note. *Surg Neurol* 2000;53(6):592–596.
13. Kahanovitz N, Viola K, McCulloch J. Limited surgical discectomy and microdiscectomy: a clinical comparison. *Spine* 1989;14:79–81.
14. Bookwalter JW, Buxch MD, Nicely D. Ambulatory surgery is safe and effective in radicular disc disease. *Spine* 1994;19:526–530.
15. Zahrawi F. Microlumbar discectomy. Is it safe as an outpatient procedure? *Spine* 1994;9:1070–1074.
16. Van Royen BJ, O'Driscoll SW, Dhert WJ, et al. A comparison of the effects of immobilization and continuous passive motion on surgical wound healing in mature rabbits. *Plast Reconstr Surg* 1986;8:360–368.
17. Wilson DH, Harbaugh R. Microsurgical and standard removal of the protruded lumbar disc: a comparative study. *Neurosurgery* 1981;8:422–427.
18. Wilson DH, Kenning J. Microsurgical lumbar discectomy: preliminary report of 83 consecutive cases. *Neurosurgery* 1979;4:137–140.
19. Snook D, Kruse J, McCulloch JA. Operative demographics for 500 consecutive lumbar microsurgeries (single surgeon). *Submitted for publication.*
20. Sawamura Y, Asaoka K, Terasaka S, et al. Evaluation of application techniques of fibrin sealant to prevent cerebrospinal fluid leakage: a new device for the application of aerosolized fibrin glue. *Neurosurgery* 1999;44:332–337.
21. Hodges S, Humphreys S, Craig MD, et al. Management of incidental durotomy without mandatory bed rest: a retrospective review of 20 cases. *Spine* 1999;24:2062–2066.
22. Jones AM, Stambough JL, Balderston RA, et al. Long term results of lumbar spine surgery complicated by unintended incidental durotomy. *Spine* 1989;14:443.
23. Lang WH, Muchel F. *Zeiss microscopes for microsurgery*. Berlin: Springer-Verlag, 1981.
24. Weber H. Lumbar disc herniation: a controlled, prospective study with 10 years of observation. *Spine* 1983;8:131–140.
25. Hakelius A. Prognosis in sciatica: a clinical follow-up of surgical and non-surgical treatment. *Acta Orthop Scand* 1970;129[Suppl]:1–76.
26. Bell GR. Conservative vs. surgical management of lumbar disc herniation: Is outcome following conservative treatment equal to surgical management? In: Bell GR, ed. *Contemporary issues in spine surgery*. Rosemont, IL: AAOS,1999:3–7.
27. Wong D, Mayer T, Watters W, et al. *NASS Phase III Clinical Guidelines: herniated disc.* La Grange, IL: North American Spine Society, 2000.
28. Bell GR, Rothman RH. The conservative treatment of sciatica. *Spine* 1984;9:54–56.
29. Wong D, Mayer T, Watters W, et al. *Sign mark and x-Ray (SMaX): a NASS patient safety program*. LaGrange, IL: North American Spine Society, 2001.
30. Spengler DM. Lumbar discectomy. Results with limited disc excision and selective foraminotomy. *Spine* 1982;7:604–607.
31. Abdullah AF, Wolber PG, Warfield JR, et al. Surgical management of extreme lateral lumbar disc herniations: review of 138 cases. *Neurosurg* 1988;22:648–653.
32. Postacchini F, Montanaro A. Extreme lateral herniations of lumbar disks. *Clin Orthop* 1979;138:222–227.
33. Zindrick MR, Wiltse LL, Rauschning W. Disc herniations lateral to the intervertebral foramen. In: White AH, Rothman RH, Ray DV, eds. *Lumbar spine surgery*. St. Louis: Mosby, 1987:195–207.
34. Pappas CTE, Harrington T, Sonntag VKH. Outcome analysis in 654 surgically treated lumbar disc herniations. *Neurosurgery* 1992;30:862–866.
35. Sachdev VP. Microsurgical lumbar discectomy: a personal series of 300 patients with at least 1 year of follow-up. *Microsurg* 1986;7:55–62.
36. Abernathey CD, Yasargil MG. Results of microsurgery. In: Williams RW, McCulloch JA, Young PH, eds. *Microsurgery of the lumbar spine*. Rockville, MD: Aspen, 990:223–226.
37. Caspar W. A new surgical procedure for lumbar disc herniation causing less tissue damage through a microsurgical approach. *Adv Neurosurg* 1977;4:74–80.
38. Caspar W. Results of microsurgery. In: Williams RW, McCulloch JA, Young PH, eds. *Microsurgery of the lumbar spine*. Rockville, MD: Aspen, 1990:227–231.
39. Goald HJ. Microlumbar discectomy: follow-up of 477 patients. *J Microsurg* 1980;2:95–100.
40. Goald HJ. A new microsurgical reoperation for failed lumbar disc surgery. *J Microsurg* 1986;7:63–66.
41. Nygaard OP, Kloster R, Solberg T. Duration of leg pain as a predictor of outcome after surgery for lumbar disc herniation: a prospective cohort study with 1-year follow up. *J Neurosurg* 2000;92[2 Suppl]:131–134.
42. Papavero L, Caspar W. The lumbar microdiscectomy. *Acta Orthop Scand* 1993;251[Suppl]:34–37.
43. Yasargil MG. Microsurgical operation of herniated lumbar disc. *Adv Neurosurg,* 1977;4:81.
44. Schmid UD. Microsurgery of lumbar disc prolapse. Superior results of microsurgery as compared to standard and percutaneous procedures (review of literature). *Nervenarzt* 2000;71:265–274.
45. Prolo DJ, Oklund SA, Butcher M. Toward uniformity in evaluating results of lumbar spine operations. *Spine* 1986;11:601–606.
46. Cherkin D, Deyo R, Loeser J, et al. An international comparison of back surgery rates. *Spine* 1994;19:1201–1206.
47. Davis H. Increasing rates of cervical and lumbar spine surgery in the United States 1979–1990. *Spine* 1994;19:1117–1124.
48. Andrews DW, Lavyne MH. Retrospective analysis of microsurgical and standard lumbar discectomy. *Spine* 1990;15:329–335.
49. Rogers LA. Experience with limited versus extensive disc removal in patients undergoing microsurgical operations for ruptured lumbar discs. *Neurosurgery* 1988;22:82–85.

50. Williams RW. Microlumbar discectomy: a 12-year statistical review. *Spine* 1986;11:851–852.
51. Williams RW. Results of microsurgery. In: Williams RW, McCulloch JA, Young PH, eds. *Microsurgery of the lumbar spine.* Rockville, MD: Aspen, 1990:211–214.
52. Spangfort EV. The lumbar disc herniation: a computer-aided analysis of 2,504 operations. *Acta Orthop Scand* 1972;142:[Suppl]1–95.
53. Williams RW. Microlumbar discectomy: a conservative surgical approach to the virgin herniated lumbar disc. *Spine* 1978;3:175–182.
54. Leung PC. Complications in the first 40 cases of microdiscectomy. *J Spinal Disord* 1988;1:306–310.
55. Schutz H, Watson CPN. Microsurgical discectomy: a prospective study of 200 patients. *Can J Neurolog Sci* 1987;14:81–83.
56. Weir BK, Jacobs GA. Reoperation rate following lumbar discectomy. An analysis of 662 lumbar discectomies. *Spine* 1980;5:366–370.
57. Ebeling U, Kalbarcyk H, Reulen HJ. Microsurgical reoperation following lumbar disc surgery. *J Neurosurg* 1989;70:397–404.
58. Ebeling U, Reichenberg W, Reulen HJ. Results of microsurgical lumbar discectomy. *Acta Neurochir (Wien)* 1986;81:45–52.
59. Hirabayashi S, Kumano K, Ogowa Y, et al. Microdiscectomy and second operation for lumbar disc herniation. *Spine* 1993;18:2206–2211.
60. Dauch WA. Infection of the intervertebral space following conventional and microsurgical operation on the herniated lumbar intervertebral disc. *Acta Neurochir (Wien)* 1986;82:43–49.
61. Ferrer E, Garcia-Bach M, Lopez L, et al. Lumbar microdiscectomy: analysis of 100 consecutive cases. Its pitfalls and final results. *Acta Neurochir Suppl* 1988;43:39–43.
62. Lavyne MH, Bilsky MH. Epidural steroids, postoperative morbidity, and recovery in patients undergoing lumbar discectomy. *J Neurosurg* 1992;77:90–95.
63. Thomas AMC, Afshar F. The microsurgical treatment of lumbar disc protrusions. *J Bone Joint Surg* 1987;69B:696–698.
64. Aryanpur J, Ducker T. Multilevel lumbar laminotomies: an alternative to laminectomy in the treatment of lumbar stenosis. *Neurosurgery* 1990;26:429–433.
65. Arnoldi CC, Brodsky AE, Cauchoix J, et al. Lumbar spinal stenosis and nerve root entrapment syndromes: definition and classification. *Clin Orthop* 1976;115:4–5.
66. Macnab I. Spondylolisthesis with an intact neural arch—the so-called pseudospondylolisthesis. *J Bone Joint Surg* 1950;32:325–333.
67. Epstein NE, Epstein JA, Carras R, et al. Degenerative spondylolisthesis with an intact neural arch: a review of 60 cases with an analysis of clinical findings and the development of surgical management. *Neurosurgery* 1983;13:555–561.
68. Johnsson K. *Lumbar spinal stenosis: a clinical, radiological and neuro-physiological investigation.* Special publication of Dept. of Orthopaedics, Malmö General Hospital, Lund University, Malmö, Sweden, 1987
69. Epstein JA, Epstein BS, Lavine LS. Nerve root compression associated with narrowing of the lumbar spinal canal. *J Neurol Neurosurg Psychiatry* 1962;25:165–176.
70. Schonstrom HSR, Bolender NF, Spengler DM. The pathomorphology of spinal stenosis as seen on CT scans of the lumbar spines. *Spine* 1985;10:806–811.
71. Verbiest H. Pathomorphologic aspects of developmental lumbar stenosis. *Orthop Clin North Am* 1975;6:177–196.
72. Hamanishi C, Matukura N, Fujita M, et al. Cross-sectional area of the stenotic lumbar dural tube measured from the transverse views of magnetic resonance imaging. *J Spinal Disord* 1994;7:388–393.
73. McCulloch JA. Microsurgery for spinal canal stenosis: the resculpturing or laminoplasty procedure. In: Williams RW, Young PH, McCulloch JA, eds. *Microsurgery of the lumbar spine*. Rockville, MD: Aspen, 1990:199–210.
74. Young PH. Results of microsurgery. In: Williams RW, McCulloch JA, Young PH, eds. *Microsurgery of the lumbar spine*. Rockville, MD: Aspen, 1990:215–222.

CHAPTER 55

Decompression for Lumbar Spinal Stenosis

Hyun W. Bae, David M. Fribourg, and Rick B. Delamarter

Decompression for lumbar spinal canal stenosis (SCS) is becoming the most commonly performed spinal operation (1). With an increasing population of active older adults, the frequency of this procedure is certain to grow even further. Improvements in technology and surgical technique allow the surgeon to pinpoint the specific location of the pathology and relieve neural encroachment in many cases with minimal disruption of the surrounding tissues (2–4).

ETIOLOGY OF LUMBAR SPINAL STENOSIS

SCS may be congenital or acquired. Purely congenital spinal stenosis is uncommon, and it is a disease affecting multiple spinal segments (Fig. 1), with most of the compression occurring at the disc level (5,6).

In most cases, SCS is acquired as the spine ages (Fig. 2). The degenerative changes of disc desiccation with annular bulging, osteophyte formation, ligamentum infolding or hypertrophy, and/or facet hypertrophy all contribute to reduce the space available to the cauda equina and cause the classic symptoms of neurogenic claudication. Facet joint osteophytes contribute to narrowing of the neural foramina and encroachment on the nerve roots (6–8). Less commonly, facet joint cysts can cause similar neural encroachment (Fig. 3).

Another common form of SCS results from degenerative spondylolisthesis (Fig. 4). Vertebral segmental instability leads to forward translation of one vertebral segment on the caudal level. Here, the pathologic compression is circumferential, secondary to the anterior displacement of the lamina combined with the posterior displacement of the disc and body below (9,10).

PATHOANATOMY OF SPINAL CANAL STENOSIS

An understanding of the surgical anatomy of SCS is essential in limited and open decompression. The use of magnetic resonance imaging (MRI) and computed tomography (CT) with three-dimensional reconstruction can now pinpoint the offending lesion or lesions and differentiate whether they are from bone or soft tissue. This information can be transformed into a three-dimensional model of pathology and provide a surgical roadmap. John McCollugh (3) provided a superb organization of this anatomy in his description of the three-story house (Fig. 5). The first floor is the disc level, which contains most of the offending pathology involved in SCS. This level includes the bulging and herniated disc, hypertrophied and infolding ligamentum flavum, and hypertrophied facets. The second, or foraminal level includes the space between the inferior end-plate and the inferior border of the pedicle. Foraminal stenosis often occurs at this level from intrusion of the tip of the superior facet, frequently secondary to a collapsed or degenerative disc (Fig. 6). The third, or pedicular level includes the regions between the superior end-plate and inferior border of the pedicle. Lateral or subarticular recess stenosis is usually seen from the superior edge of the pedicle to the superior end-plate, caused by the hypertrophied superior facet.

In most cases of lumbar spinal stenosis, the stenotic lesion is largely confined to the first story of the anatomic house, with

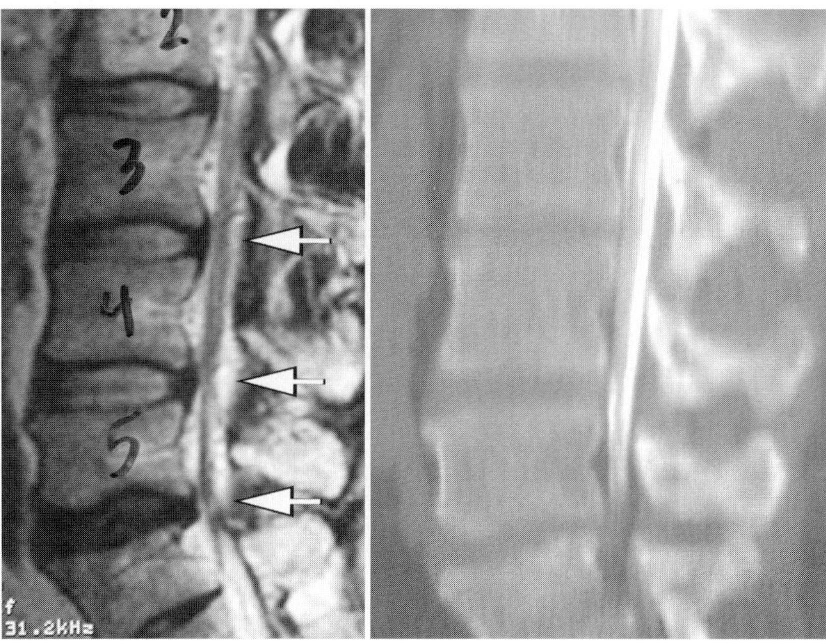

A,B

FIG. 1. Congenital spinal canal stenosis. The entire canal is narrowed in this patient, whose sagittal magnetic resonance image **(A)** and computed tomography–myelogram **(B)** are shown here. Even the small disc bulges seen here at L3-4, L4-5, and L-5 to S-1 are enough to cause symptoms in this young patient.

some extension into the second level above and the third level of the segment below. The example (Fig. 7) shows a typical patient with predominant stenosis at the first story. The pathology at this level is a result of hypertrophy and buckling of the ligamentum flavum, annular bulging of the degenerative and collapsing disc, and osteophyte formation at the edges of the vertebral bodies and facet joints. The major culprit of the three pathoanatomic changes in canal stenosis is the infolding ligamentum. Anatomically, the first-level constriction correlates with the area between the takeoff of the nerve roots. Between the midpoints of the pedicles and at the junction of the second and third level there is virtually no stenosis.

Stenosis can be further classified by its location in the coronal plane (Fig. 8). *Central*, *lateral recess*, *subarticular recess*, *foraminal*, and *extraforaminal* are all terms used by authors to describe stenosis in the coronal plane. These distinctions are easily confused because they tend to overlap one another. In general, cen-

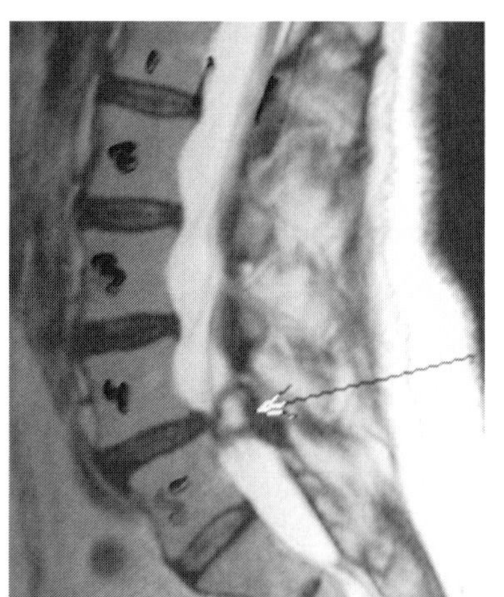
A

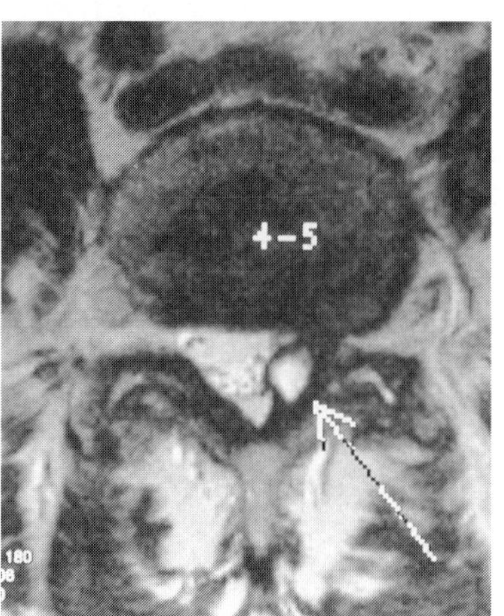

B

FIG. 3. This 75-year-old patient had a large left-sided facet cyst at L4-5 (*arrows*), with severe left leg pain. After laminectomy and microscopic excision of the facet cyst, she resumed her regular daily activities without pain.

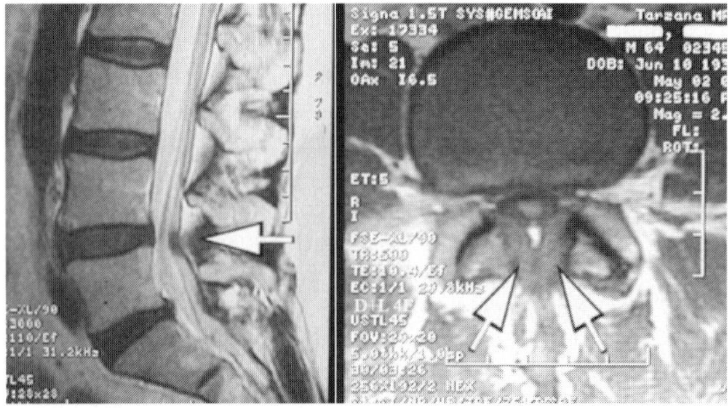

FIG. 2. These sagittal and axial magnetic resonance imaging scans show spinal canal stenosis at L4-5 without degenerative spondylolisthesis. On the axial cut, note the thickened ligamentum flavum (*arrows*).

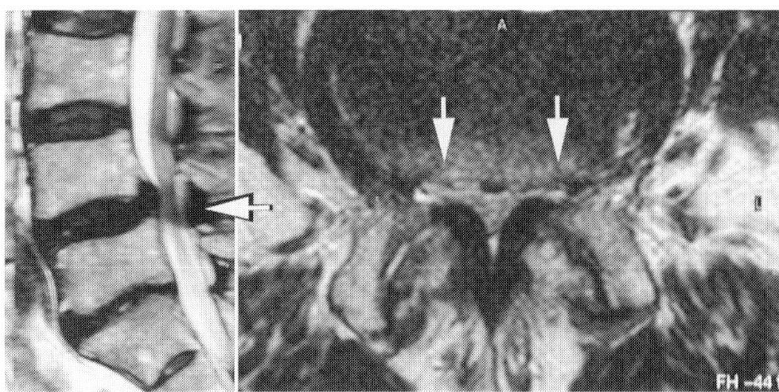

FIG. 4. These magnetic resonance imaging scans show classic spinal stenosis with degenerative spondylolisthesis at L4-5, and subarticular stenosis laterally.

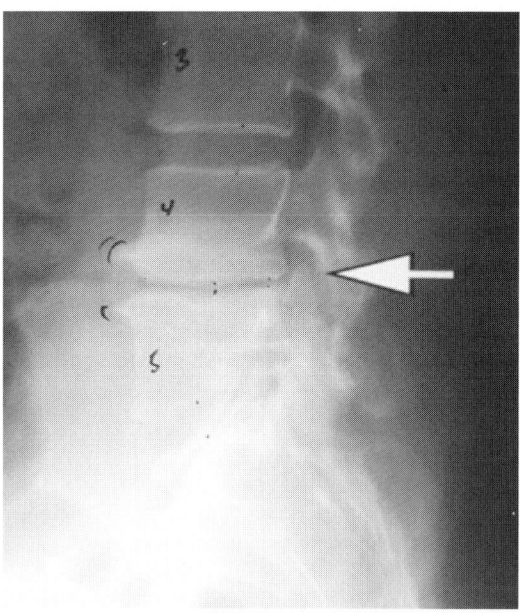

FIG. 6. This radiograph clearly shows the tip of the superior facet of L-5 protruding into the neuroforamen, where it impinges on the exiting L-4 nerve root.

tral stenosis is caused by the ligamentum hypertrophy directly under the lamina posteriorly, and the bulging disc anteriorly. Subarticular recess stenosis is caused by facet hypertrophy, specifically entrapment of the shoulder of the inferior nerve root between the medial edge of the superior facet and the canal floor or bulging disc (10a). The lateral border of the subarticular recess is the medial pedicle wall. Its medial border is more difficult to distinguish and often overlaps with central ligamentous pathology. The medial border begins at the most medial edge of the facet articulation. Lateral recess stenosis is synonymous with subarticular recess stenosis (11–13). Further laterally, foraminal stenosis occurs between the medial and lateral border of the pedicle, where the exiting nerve root may be compressed by ventral cephalad overhang of the superior facet and the bulging disc below (Fig. 9) (13a,13b). The extraforaminal zone is located lateral to the lateral edge of the pedicle, where lateral disc herniation may cause impingement of the existing nerve root (14). These anatomic distinctions are useful in verifying that all potential pathology has

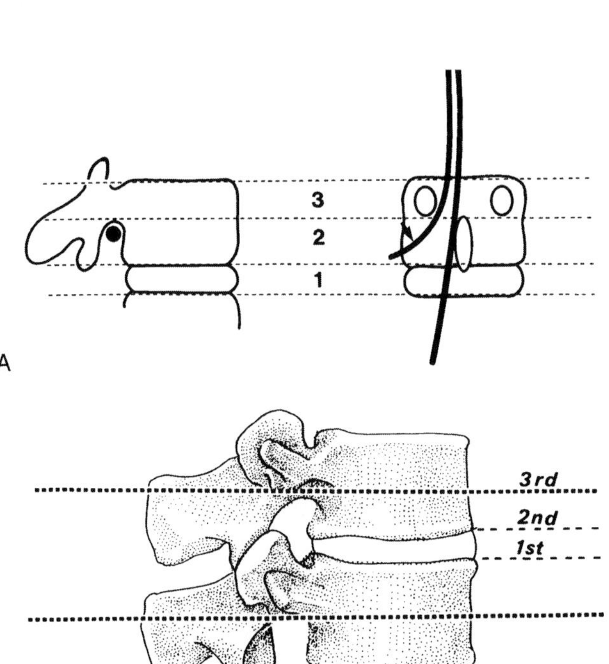

FIG. 5. A: The three stories of each anatomic segment: 1, disc level; 2, foraminal level; 3, pedicle level. Two nerve roots are shown with the arrow pointing to the exiting nerve root of the anatomic segment. **B:** Anatomic lateral view showing three stories. (From McCulloch JA, Young PH, eds. *Essentials of spinal microsurgery.* New York: Lippincott Williams & Wilkins, 1998.)

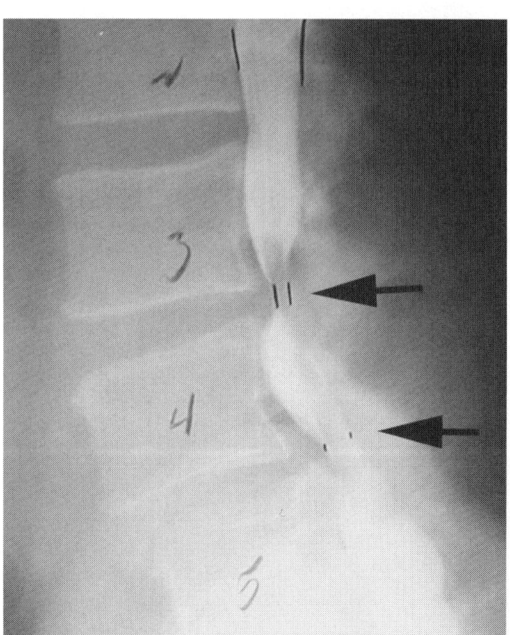

FIG. 7. The myelogram of this patient reveals the typical pattern of stenosis, worst at the first anatomic story of L3-4 and L4-5. Degenerative spondylolisthesis also contributes to the stenosis at L4-5.

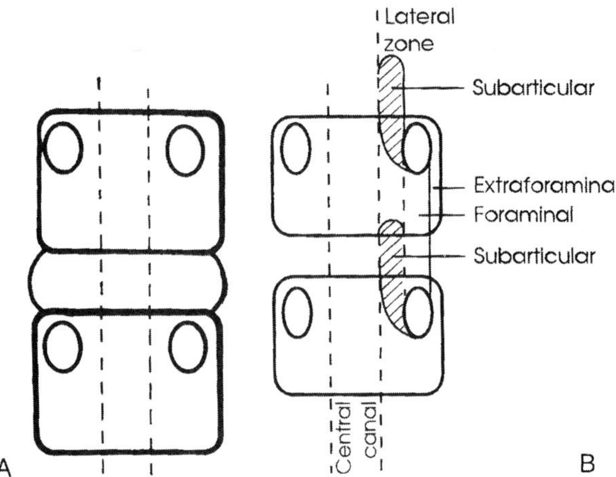

FIG. 8. **A:** The central canal lies between the dotted lines; the lateral zone, outside those lines. **B:** The lateral zone is subdivided into subarticular, foraminal, and extraforaminal zones. (From McCulloch JA, Young PH, eds. *Essentials of spinal microsurgery.* New York: Lippincott Williams & Wilkins, 1998.)

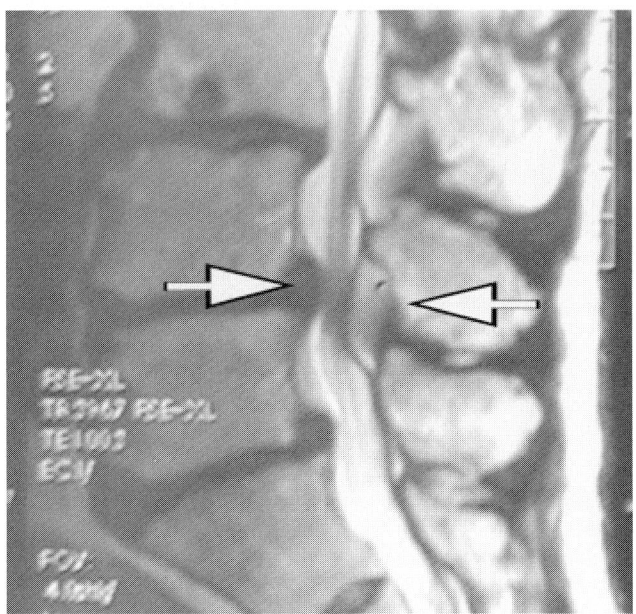

FIG. 10. This patient has multilevel degenerative disease, stenosis, low-grade degenerative spondylolisthesis of L-5 on S-1, and retrolisthesis of L-3 on L-4. This sagittal magnetic resonance image clearly shows the cauda equina pinched between the bulging disc ventrally and the buckling ligamentum flavum dorsally (*arrows*).

been identified and decompressed (14a,14b). Practically, most patients with lumbar spinal stenosis have involvement in several of these coronal plane zones.

LIGAMENTUM FLAVUM

Because the ligamentum flavum is a main contributor to SCS, its specific pathoanatomy is important in understanding the operative approach (15). The ligamenta flava are paired structures separated by a midline cleft. They extend laterally to the anterior portion of the facet joint and blend with facet capsule. Proximally, the ligament extends to the midportion of the cephalad

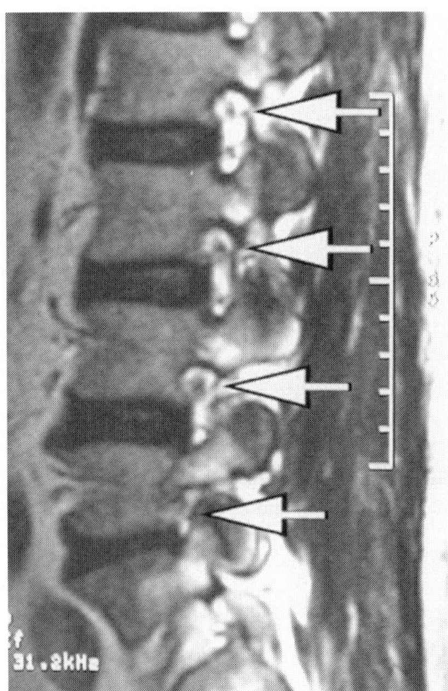

FIG. 9. This sagittal magnetic resonance image (MRI) depicts foraminal stenosis at L-5 to S-1. On this fast spin-echo MRI, there is a bright fat signal that surrounds the normal exiting roots (*upper arrows*). The L-5 to S-1 nerve root exhibits very little fat signal around it, confirming its compression (*lower arrow*).

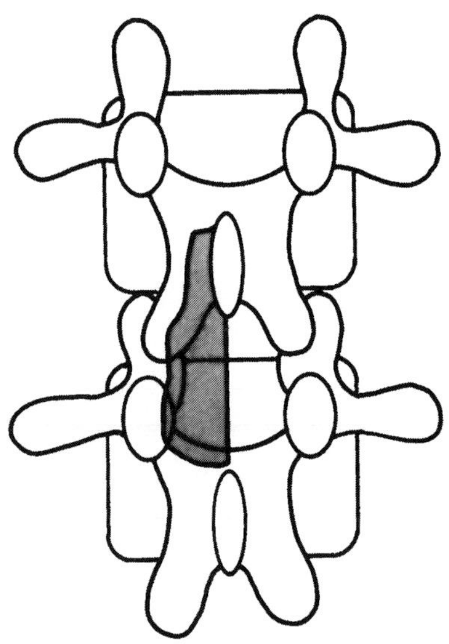

FIG. 11. The ligamentum flavum is shown underlying the lamina in this drawing. It extends superiorly to the halfway point of the lamina above. With central and lateral recess stenosis, the ligamentum must be completely removed to decompress the spinal canal.

lamina ventrally, while distally it inserts to the superior edge of the caudad lamina. With aging, as their composition changes to contain less elastin and as disc collapse decreases the vertical space available, the ligamentum buckles and folds into the spinal canal (Fig. 10). Excision of the ligamentum flavum includes its bony attachments, and requires removal of the inferior one-half of the cephalad lamina, the superior edge of the caudal lamina, and the medial margin of the facet joint (Fig. 11). In many cases, this complete excision of the ligamentum flavum and its bony attachments is all that is required to relieve central canal stenosis.

MICROSURGICAL TECHNIQUES IN LUMBAR DECOMPRESSION

When there is competent surgical expertise, there is little apparent difference in the long-term outcome between microsurgical technique and the standard approach to decompression for lumbar spinal stenosis (14,16,17). The advantage of a microscope is that complete decompression can be accomplished through a smaller incision with less resection of muscle, ligament, and bone. Even in cases in which a wide laminectomy is required to address the pathology, the illumination and magnification provided by the microscope can be helpful in completing the procedure. There are disadvantages of the microsurgical technique, which are most evident as the learning curve is being traveled. There are also significant advantages for the patient and the spinal surgeon, however, which have led to increasing acceptance of microsurgery (18).

The microscope is superior to loupes for many reasons, one of the most important of which is stereopsis in the depths of a spinal wound. Its optics allow for three-dimensional vision through a 22- to 28-mm incision, whereas stereopsis for the surgeon with loupes requires an incision the length of his interpupillary distance, typically 65 mm (Fig. 12). Other advantages include a parallel light source (Fig. 13), high magnification for fine work, and the fact that residents and everyone else in the operating room can see what is happening and stay involved in the operation. For surgeons with cervical degenerative disease, the microscope offers a comfortable position of the neck that loupes cannot provide.

When learning to use the microscope, the surgeon must avoid operating in a wound with overhang of tissues, which could obscure the line of vision (Fig. 14). The microscope may be translated or angulated to maintain the field on the area of interest. During the learning process, the superior visibility of the microscope can occasionally be cause for alarm, causing empty severed epidural veins and residual deep strands of ligamentum flavum to appear alarmingly like strands of nerve rootlets. With experience, one learns to distinguish the stark whiteness of the root from the dull yellowish tinge of the other structures.

The other advantages of the microscope are to the patient. The incision is not only more cosmetic, but there is less iatrogenic damage to supporting muscle, ligament, and bony structures. This leads to less pain and, in some studies, a shorter hospital stay (19). Retraction of the multifidus muscle beyond the midpoint of the facet joint tethers the medial branch of the dorsal ramus and risks denervation of that segment, but with a more focused exposure, segmental denervation can be avoided (20). When compared to a wide laminectomy, the microscopic laminotomy allows preservation of the interspinous and supraspinous ligaments. With a unilateral approach, their attachment to the lumbodorsal fascia is preserved as well. This ligamentous complex helps stabilize the spine in flexion, and may be even more important in cases in which there is degenerative disc disease and facet joint laxity often associated with lumbar spinal stenosis. With the improved lighting and magnification afforded by the microscope, it may be possible to preserve more of the pars interarticularis than a standard laminectomy-medial facetectomy. By preserving the interspinous/supraspinous ligamentous complex and more of the pars interarticularis, the risk of iatrogenic instability is minimized.

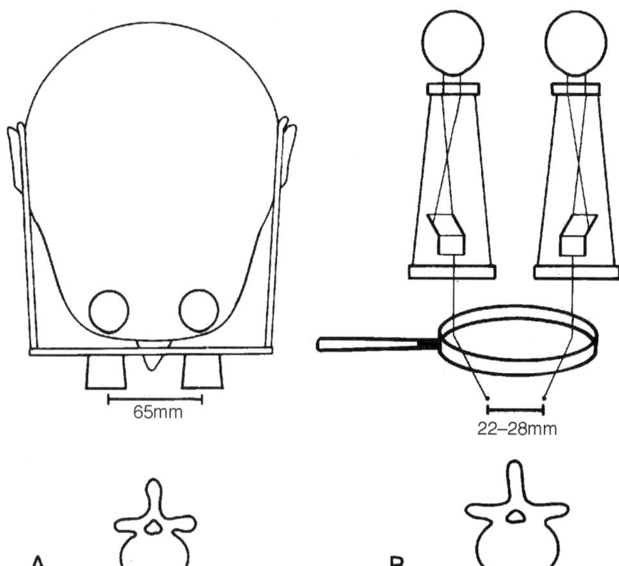

FIG. 12. Stereopsis (three-dimensional) visualization requires at least 65 mm for interpupillary distance with loupes **(A)**. Through the optics of the microscope, this distance is compressed to 22 to 28 mm **(B)**, meaning a much smaller incision is needed to maintain stereopsis in the depth of the wound. (From Delamarter RB, McCulloch JA. Microdiscectomy and microsurgical spinal laminotomies. In: Frymoyer JW, ed. *The adult spine*, 2nd ed. Philadelphia: Lippincott–Raven, 1997:1961–1988.)

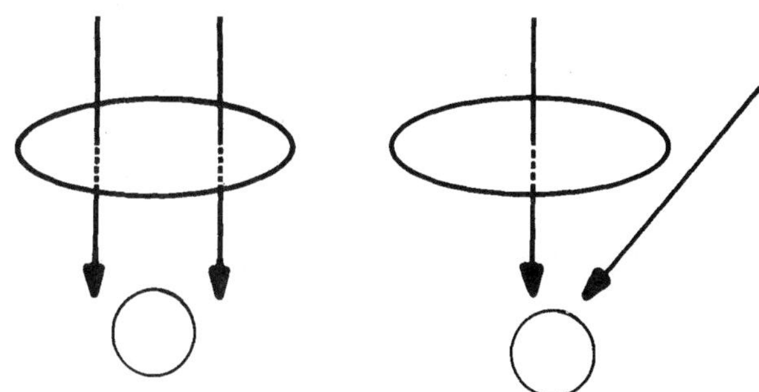

FIG. 13. Coaxial versus paraxial illumination. With loupes and a headlight, a wider incision is needed to get the light into the depth of the wound. (From Delamarter RB, McCulloch JA. Microdiscectomy and microsurgical spinal laminotomies. In: Frymoyer JW, ed. *The adult spine: principles and practice*, 2nd ed. Philadelphia: Lippincott–Raven, 1997:1961–1988.)

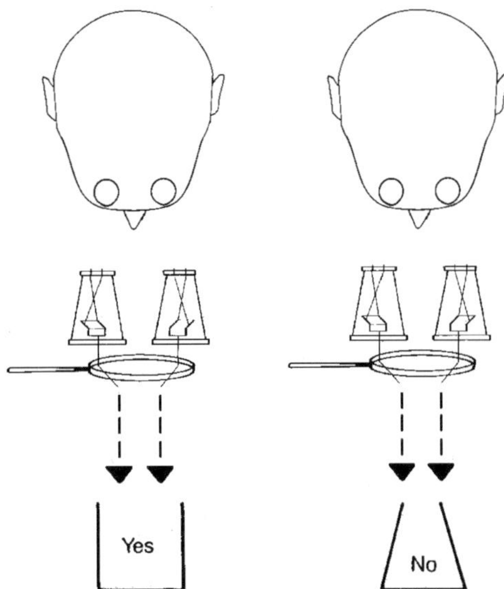

FIG. 14. Overhang is the enemy. To maintain the field of vision, maintain a wound as in **Yes**, and do not operate in a wound with overhang of soft tissues or bone as in **No**. Overhang in this wound interferes with the line of vision (*arrows*).

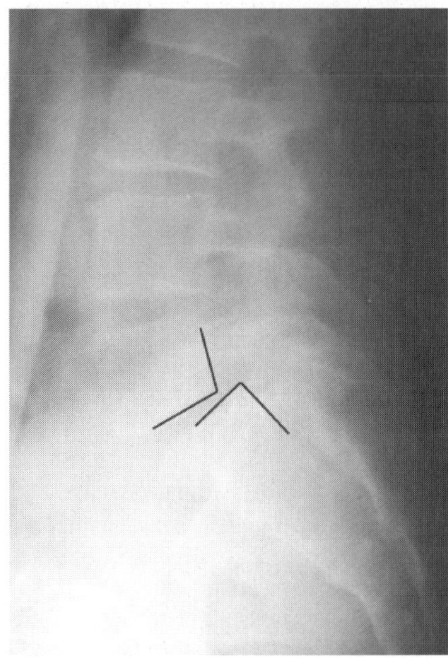

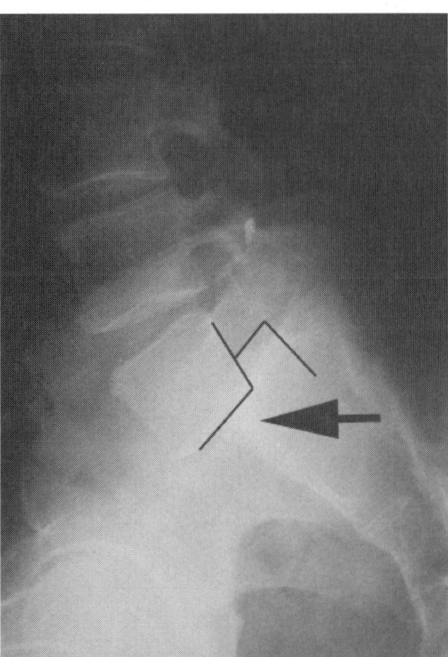

FIG. 15. Preoperatively, this patient had spinal stenosis with a grade I degenerative spondylolisthesis at L-5 to S-1. Three months after decompression at L-5 to S-1, the patient returned with worsening back pain from an iatrogenic pars fracture and grade 2-3 slip.

PLANNING THE PROCEDURE

Preoperative radiographic studies include plain radiographs, flexion-extension lateral views, and at a minimum MRI or myelographically enhanced CT, or both. Flexion-extension radiographs are scrutinized for signs of instability (Fig. 15), which may necessitate a fusion. MRI and/or the post-myelogram CT are used to identify the location and type of pathology. All anatomic zones, central, subarticular, foraminal, and extraforaminal are systematically evaluated for stenosis. At this point, a decision is made on how much bone needs to be removed to complete the decompression. In general, the authors prefer the least invasive technique that allows adequate decompression of all neural encroachment.

In patients with one- or two-level stenosis without instability, the authors favor the microsurgical laminoplasty. In this technique, a unilateral hemilaminotomy is performed through which an ipsilateral and contralateral decompression is completed. This allows the most decompression with minimal tissue violation. Another option is bilateral hemilaminotomies, also known as a *fenestration procedure*. This technique requires more soft-tissue dissection, but is preferred when the unilateral approach is made technically difficult by dense midline adhesions (i.e., from previous surgery), significant lumbar lordosis, or a large body habitus. In those patients with congenital stenosis or more severe multilevel stenosis, a standard laminectomy is preferred. These patients have more global confluent pathology and need a more comprehensive decompression. Patients with degenerative scoliosis or spondylolisthesis generally have more severe stenosis secondary to the abnormal translation of one vertebra on another. These patients may require not only a wide laminectomy, but also some type of stabilization. It has been demonstrated convincingly that patients with degenerative spondylolisthesis have an improved outcome from a concomitant spinal fusion procedure (10,21–24). Those with hypermobility, degenerative scoliosis, or severe axial back pain also need to be critically evaluated for a spinal fusion.

The orientation of the facet joints also plays a critical role in how much bone can be sacrificed and still maintain stability. In facet joints that are oriented sagittally, more care has to be taken in decompressing the lateral recess. In these cases, a more oblique angle of decompression is used to preserve the facet joint while undercutting to decompress the lateral recess (Fig.

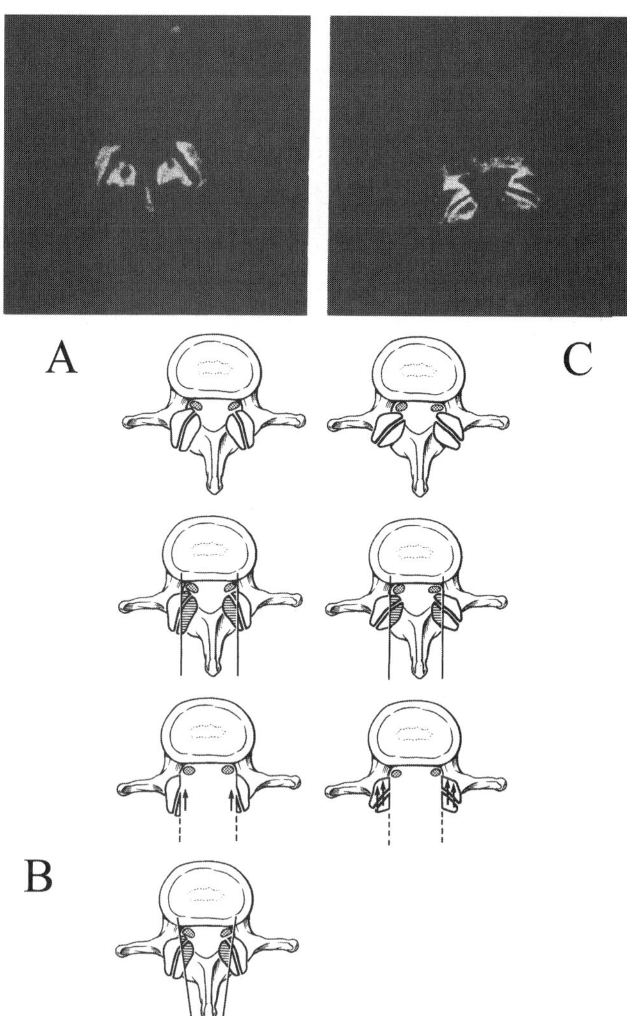

FIG. 16. When the facets are sagittally oriented, a direct approach would significantly destabilize the motion segment **(A)**, and a more oblique approach must be used **(B)**. A more direct route can be used in coronally oriented facets, because they have more inherent stability **(C)**. (From Frymoyer JW, ed. *The adult spine*, 2nd ed. Philadelphia: Lippincott–Raven, 1997:1906.)

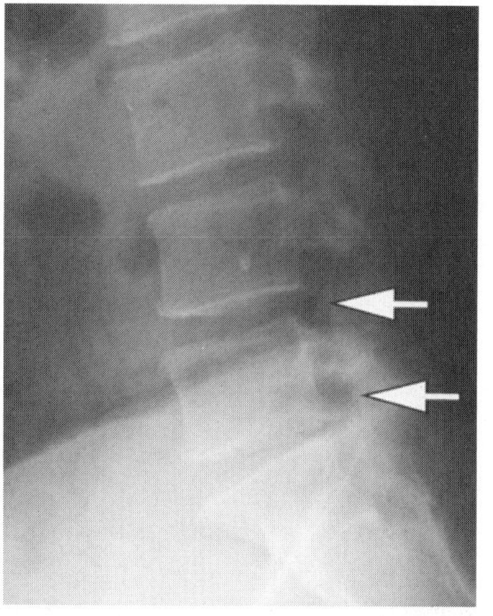

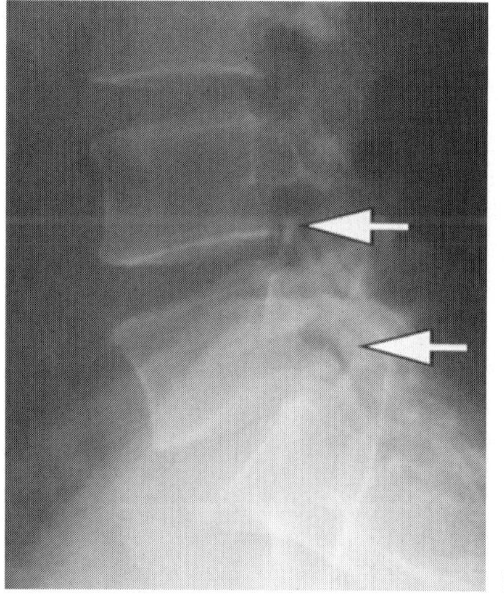

FIG. 17. In this patient with stenosis at L4-5 and L-5 to S-1, notice the change in size of the neuroforamina in flexion (A) compared to extension (B). When the decompression is performed in flexion, one must allow for the natural settling that occurs when the patient stands upright with the spine extended.

16A,B). Facet joints that are oriented coronally have more inherent stability and more direct route can be used to decompress the lateral recess (Fig. 16C).

PATIENT POSITIONING

Unless a fusion is anticipated, the patient is positioned with the lumbar spine in mild flexion. The authors use an Andrews table with the patient in knee-chest position, or a standard radiolucent table with a Wilson frame, which may be cranked up to flex the lumbar spine. This position widens the interlaminar spaces, making it easier to enter the epidural space and perform the decompression. The neuroforamina are also widened in this position, so one must be careful that the decompression is extensive enough to allow for the natural diminishment of this space that occurs when the patient is upright with the lumbar spine extended (Fig. 17). If the patient is to undergo a lumbar fusion after the decompression, the lumbar spine should be taken out of flexion before the spine is fused to avoid iatrogenic flatback deformity.

In addition to flexing the lumbar spine, the frame selected for patient positioning should allow the abdomen to hang free. This decompresses the epidural venous plexus of the lumbar spine by drainage through Batson's venous plexus into the vena cava and helps minimize blood loss during the procedure.

The bony prominences of the elbows, anterior iliac crest, and knees should be padded. The authors place an extra folded towel under the anterior shoulder and axilla to decrease extension-external rotation of the shoulder and thus decrease tension on the brachial plexus. The elbows should not be flexed greater than 90

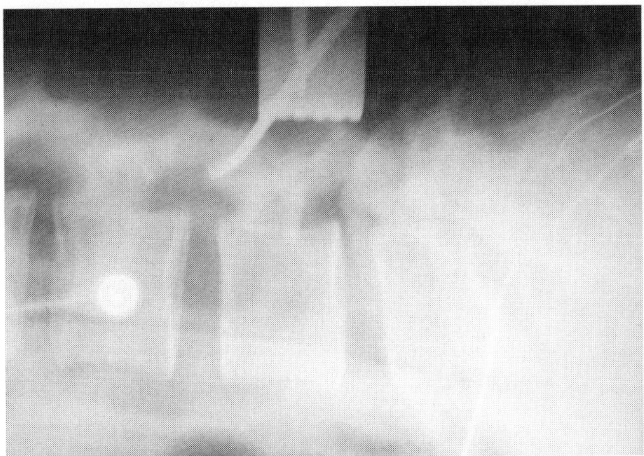

FIG. 18. Here, the tip of the curette is in the interlaminar space. It is imperative to confirm the level before beginning the decompression.

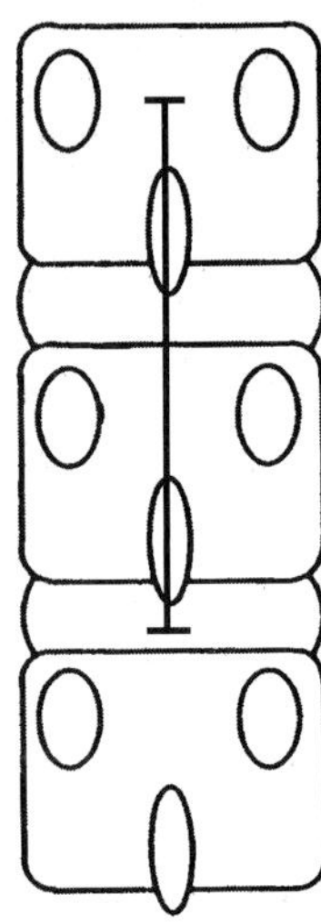

FIG. 19. The skin and fascial incision for the bilateral hemilaminotomy.

degrees, as this may cause undue tension on the ulnar nerve. A foam headrest is used to avoid pressure on the eyes and chin.

All patients are given a prophylactic dose of intravenous antibiotics before the skin incision is made.

LOCALIZING THE LEVEL

Intraoperative radiographic confirmation of the correct level is imperative. In the standard open decompression, two Kocher clamps are placed on adjacent spinous processes to confirm the level. By comparing the distance between the clamps on the radiograph and in the patient, the magnification factor of the radiograph can be determined.

When performing the microscopic decompression techniques, percutaneous needle localization is performed before a skin incision is made. A single needle is placed 1.5 cm lateral to the midline, aiming for the facet joint. At the L4-5 level, for example, a needle placed along the inferior margin of the L-4 spinous process, 1.5 cm lateral to the midline, should arrive at the L4-5 facet joint. By placing the needle on the facet joint, one avoids inadvertent penetration of the dura or the retroperitoneum. Localization of the level before the incision is made allows for the smallest possible incision. The level is routinely confirmed a second time intraoperatively with a forward-angled curette placed under the most cephalad lamina (Fig. 18). The extra time expended in carefully localizing the level intraoperatively can avoid all of the issues inherent in a wrong-level surgery.

SURGICAL TECHNIQUE

Hemilaminotomy

The hemilaminotomy is the cornerstone of microsurgical decompression. Perfecting this technique is important, because laminectomies and laminoplasties are extensions of this procedure. With the use of the microscope, the hemilaminotomy is the first stage of the microsurgical laminoplasty that allows a thorough bilateral decompression. For surgeons who prefer not to use the microscope, a bilateral hemilaminotomy or fenestration procedure may be performed, which still allows preservation of the inter-/supraspinous ligamentous complex, although its attachment to the lumbodorsal fascia is divided.

Typically, even the patient with unilateral leg pain from SCS shows radiologic evidence of bilateral disease. Given the limited morbidity of the procedure, many surgeons perform a bilateral decompression. For a standard bilateral hemilaminotomy, the incision is made in the midline (Fig. 19). Subperiosteal muscle dissection is carried out to reveal the entire lamina of L-4 and the upper one-half of the lamina of L-5.

The central canal is decompressed first. Because of the interlaminar narrowing and shingling of SCS, it is rarely possible to directly cross the ligamentum flavum to gain entry to the epidural space. A portion of the cephalad and caudad lamina, as well as the medial facet, must be removed. The extent of this dissection is determined by the precise anatomy of the ligamentum flavum as described previously. The authors use the high-speed drill to thin out the inferior one-third to one-half of the cephalad lamina and the medial 2 mm of the inferior facet (Fig. 20). By removing bone only in this location, the epidural space is always protected by ligamentum flavum. Bone can now be safely removed to the depth of the ligamentum. In addition to visual cues, the surgeon learns to recognize the difference in feedback of the drill as it enters a bone and the ligamentum, signaling that the appropriate depth has been reached. To complete the laminotomy, the decompression must travel beyond the safe zone where the ligamentum is protective. In this area, the drill is used only to thin the bone, and the Kerrison rongeur is used to complete the laminotomy.

The ligamentum flavum can now easily be freed from the bone by using a forward-angled curette to elevate the ligamentum from the cephalad lamina, the medial edge of the superior facet, and then the caudad lamina (Fig. 21). This facilitates the removal of ligamentum that is essential for the decompression. The authors finish the decompression by using a Kerrison rongeur to complete the laminotomy to the desired extent. At least 6 to 7 mm of pars

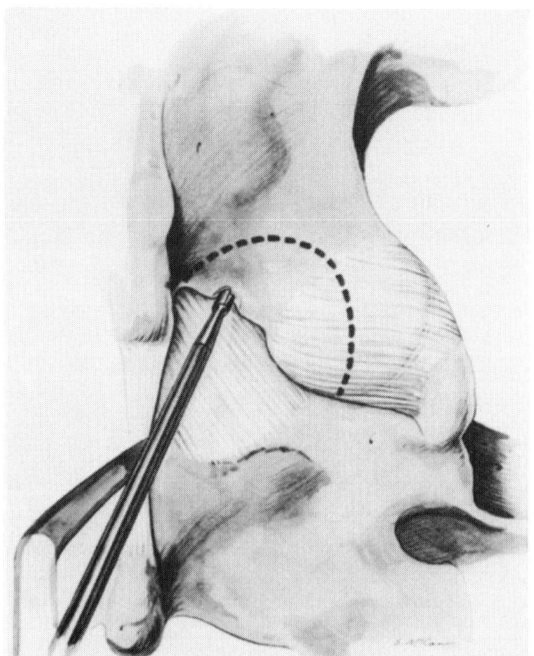

FIG. 20. The dissection for the hemilaminotomy is complete. The high-speed electric burr may now be used to thin the inferior one-half of the lamina and medial 1 to 2 mm of the inferior facet. (From Delamarter RB, McCulloch JA. Microdiscectomy and microsurgical spinal laminotomies. In: Frymoyer JW, ed. *The adult spine*, 2nd ed. Philadelphia: Lippincott–Raven, 1997:1961–1988.)

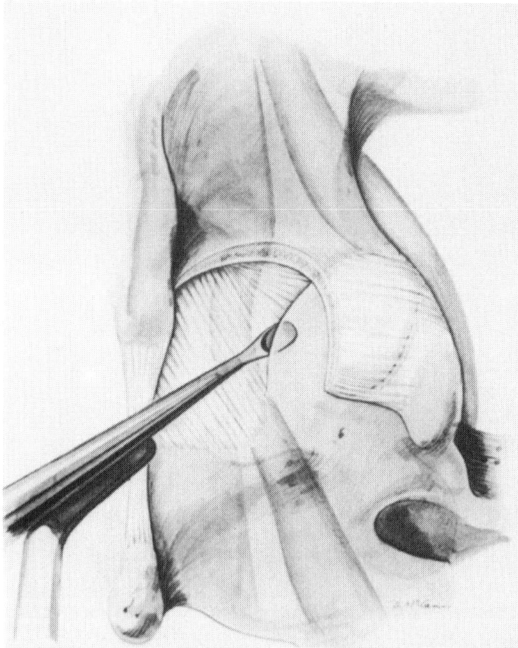

FIG. 21. The ligamentum is elevated and removed from the medial border of the superior facet and the upper and lower lamina. (From Delamarter RB, McCulloch JA. Microdiscectomy and microsurgical spinal laminotomies. In: Frymoyer JW, ed. *The adult spine*, 2nd ed. Philadelphia: Lippincott–Raven, 1997:1961–1988.)

interarticularis must be preserved to prevent a later iatrogenic fracture. This completes the central decompression.

The lateral zone and subarticular recess are addressed next. The Kerrison rongeur is used to undercut the medial edge of the superior facet as far as the medial edge of the pedicle (Fig. 22). This is usually approximately one-third of the facet joint. No more than 50% of the facet joint should ever be sacrificed. Medial facetectomy of the inferior facet is relatively safe. In contrast, the superior facet lies immediately adjacent to the nerve roots and must be approached more cautiously. This can be accomplished by following the superior border of the caudad lamina laterally to the medial wall of the pedicle. Locating the pedicle is the key to performing a safe decompression. The traversing nerve root can routinely be identified just medial to the medial border of the pedicle. This nerve root is freed with the Kerrison by removing overhanging bone on the medial and inferior border of the pedicle, keeping the Kerrison above the root. The subarticular recess above the pedicle is decompressed next, by working the Kerrison around the medial superior edge of the pedicle. This interval is often quite collapsed secondary to the bulging disc and osteophytes below. In severe cases, the collapsed superior facet can be mistaken for the pedicle itself, although the true pedicle lies just more laterally and inferiorly. In these cases, a 2- or 3-mm Kerrison is used to start the decompression, until a larger Kerrison can be fit into this space (Fig. 23). Ultimately, this frees the edge of the traversing root sleeve and allows retraction of the dural sac and visualization

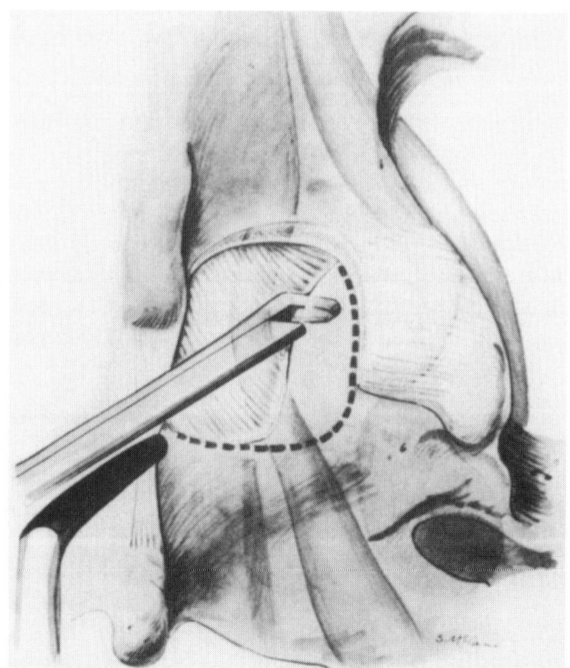

FIG. 22. Lateral recess stenosis is eliminated by removing the medial border of the superior facet. (From Delamarter RB, McCulloch JA. Microdiscectomy and microsurgical spinal laminotomies. In: Frymoyer JW, ed. *The adult spine*, 2nd ed. Philadelphia: Lippincott–Raven, 1997: 1961–1988.)

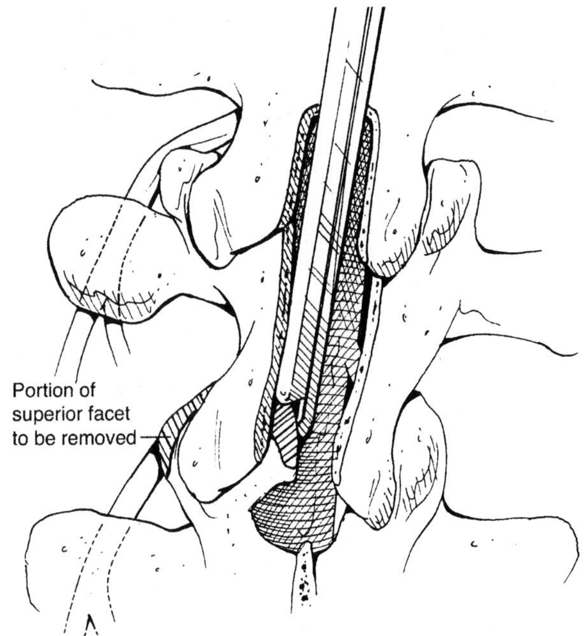

FIG. 23. The superior facet is resected to free the lateral recess of bony impingement.

of the disc space below. This completes the decompression of the first anatomic floor described by McCollugh.

The decompression is completed by working down again along the medial inferior edge of the pedicle, following the root into the foramen, and underbiting the remaining facet. As one undercuts further laterally, the Kerrison must be angled as much as possible out into the foramen, parallel to the exiting nerve root (Fig. 24). Finally, a probe is used to verify that the foramen is clear of any encroachment.

The completed hemilaminotomy leaves the supraspinous/interspinous ligament complex, the facet joints, and the disc space all intact. Rarely, a ruptured lumbar disc is associated with SCS and requires removal, but the routine opening of the disc space is discouraged as this may result in progressive instability. If bilateral pathology is present, the surgeon may choose to repeat the hemilaminotomy on the contralateral side, or continue with a microsurgical laminoplasty.

Microsurgical Laminoplasty

The hemilaminotomy window is now used to approach the contralateral side. The most anterior fibers of the interspinous ligament are removed. The bony mass forming the confluence of the spinous processes and the two laminae is then removed (Fig. 25). Next, the microscope is angled radically across the spinal canal to view the contralateral side. If necessary, the operating table is tilted away from the surgeon to aid in this view. A blunt dissector is then used to separate the dura from the overlying ligamentum flavum. Epidural bleeding is controlled with bipolar electrocautery, Gelfoam and thrombin, and Flo-Seal if need be. During this portion of the laminoplasty, it is essential to retract and protect the cauda equina. The surgeon gradually works laterally, excising contralateral ligamentum to visualize the contralateral laminae. Eventually, the laminar attachments of the ligamentum and lamina themselves are excised to complete the interlaminar decompression.

At this point, it is helpful to identify the cephalad and caudad pedicles on the contralateral side, which allow identification of the facet joint dorsally, the disc space ventrally, and the foramen between the pedicles. If the pedicles cannot be identified, one must continue to undercut further lamina. Once the pedicles are identified, the traversing nerve root may be gently retracted to allow undercutting of the superior facet and decompress the lateral recess.

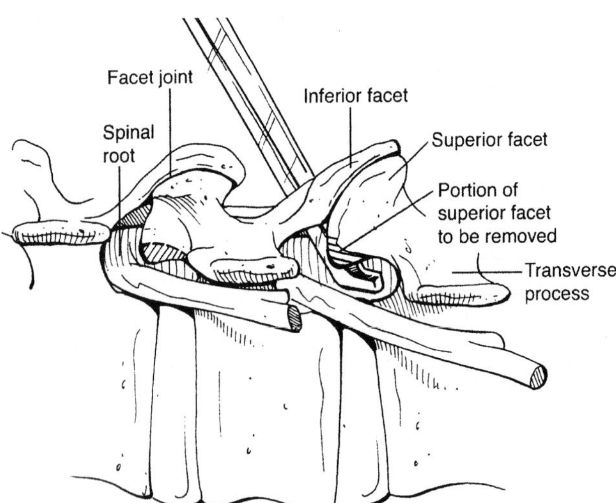

FIG. 24. The foraminal decompression is completed by angling the Kerrison rongeur far out into the foramen. This lateral cartoon view shows the position of the rongeur in a safe position above the exiting nerve root.

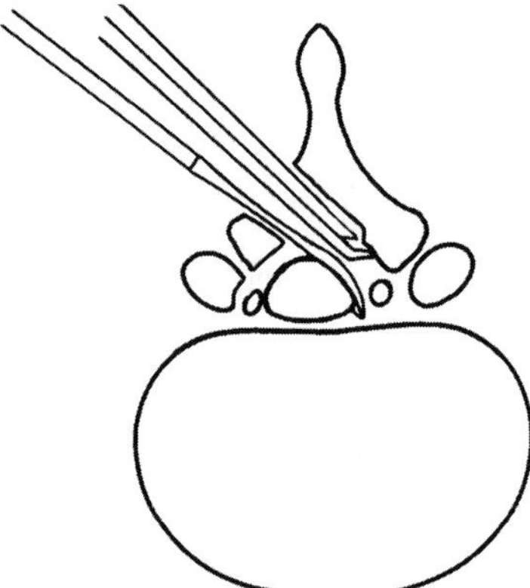

FIG. 25. Microsurgical laminoplasty: After completing the ipsilateral decompression, the dura is retracted to allow access to the contralateral side. The contralateral lamina is thinned with a high-speed burr and further resected with a Kerrison rongeur. (From Delamarter RB, McCulloch JA. Microdiscectomy and microsurgical spinal laminotomies. In: Frymoyer JW, ed. *The adult spine*, 2nd ed. Philadelphia: Lippincott–Raven, 1997:1961–1988.)

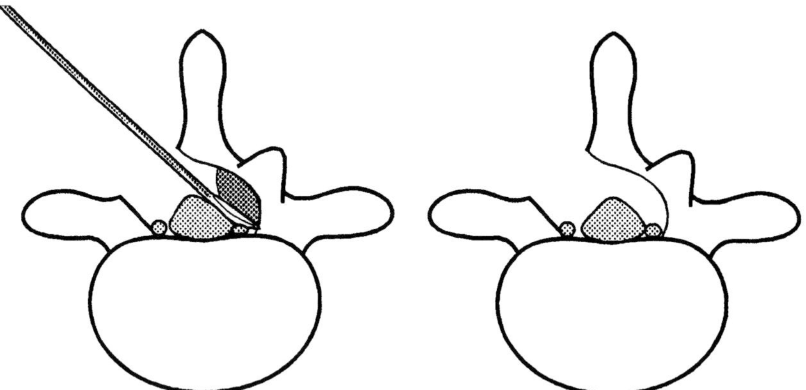

FIG. 26. Microsurgical laminoplasty: Decompression of the contralateral side is complete when all the ligamentum and hypertrophic facet have been resected, from the pedicle above to the pedicle below. (From McCulloch JA, Young PH, eds. *Essentials of spinal microsurgery.* New York: Lippincott Williams & Wilkins, 1998.)

Further medial attachments of the ligamentum flavum must often be removed to complete this decompression. It is helpful to have a variety of Kerrison rongeurs available to reach the contralateral side. The contralateral laminoplasty is considered complete when the exiting and traversing nerve roots are seen and palpated to be free of any encroachment (Fig. 26). If excessive bleeding or adhesions prevents a full decompression, the laminoplasty may be aborted and converted to a bilateral hemilaminotomy.

Laminectomy

After the skin incision, electrocautery is used to divide the subcutaneous tissue down to the deep lumbar fascia. Once the midline has been identified, the lumbodorsal fascia is incised and the paraspinal muscles dissected away from the spinous process and lamina using electrocautery or a Cobb elevator, or both. Care is taken not to expose all of the facet and facet capsule. The width of the dissection is to the lateral edge of the pars interarticularis, which is an essential landmark and should be clearly visible.

Only when the identification of levels is certain can the procedure continue. Meticulous exposure of the lamina and pars must be performed before starting the decompression (Fig. 27). A rongeur may then be used to remove the spinous processes along with the attached ligaments and residual soft tissue. If local bone is to be harvested for a fusion, it is preferable to remove the soft tissue attachments from the intact spine first, rather than from morselized pieces on the back table later. A portion of the most cephalad and caudad spinous process is preserved whenever possible to maintain the ligamentous attachments to the adjacent level. By maintaining the stability of the adjacent levels, the risk of a transitional syndrome may be decreased.

At this point, the decompression begins in earnest by using the high-speed drill to dissolve away the medial edge of the inferior facet and distal lamina, using the ligamentum as a protective buffer. The authors use the Stryker TPS electric drill with a "neuro" drill tip, designed to be aggressive with bone and gentle on soft tissues. Stabilizing the surgeon's hand firmly against the patient sets the depth of the drill and provides a second check to inadvertent drilling. Staying in the "safe zone" directly above the ligamentum greatly decreases the risk of dural tear (Fig. 28). Using the drill, bone is removed from the inferior one-half of the cephalad lamina and the medial aspect of the inferior facet. Careful exposure of the lateral border of the pars prevents an overzealous resection of this stabilizing structure. Although there are good data on how much of the facet can be removed without causing instability (25), it is not clear how much of the pars can be removed without risking a later fracture or instability. In general, the authors leave at least 6 mm of intact pars from its lateral border. The procedure is then repeated on the contralateral side, resecting approximately 2 to 3 mm of the medial border of the inferior facet and the inferior one-half of the cephalad lamina. At this point, a #2 Karlin forward-angled curette is used to free the underlying ligamentum as well as any adhe-

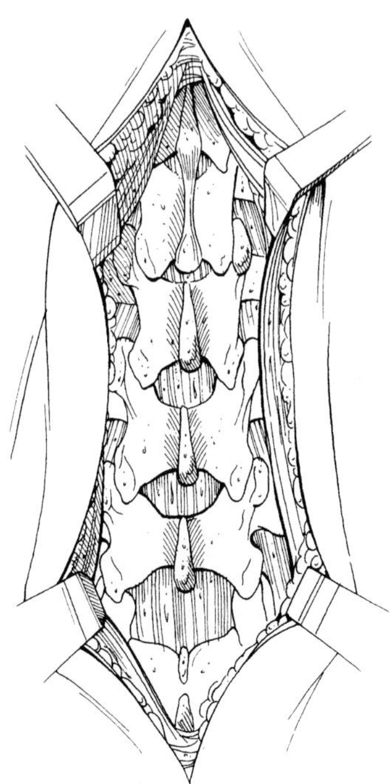

FIG. 27. The bony landmarks of the lamina and pars interarticularis must be clearly identified before the decompression is started.

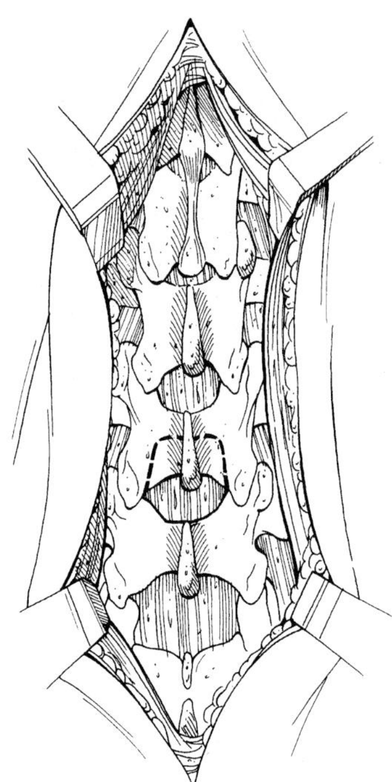

FIG. 28. The ligamentum defines a "safe zone" for the high-speed drill.

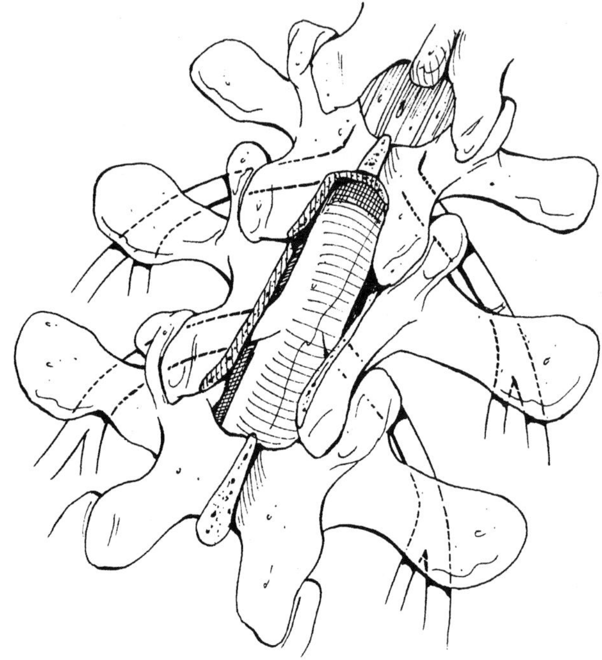

FIG. 29. At the completion of drilling, only the cephalad edge of the lamina remains.

sions from the remaining cephalad lamina and from the medial border of the superior facet. A Kerrison rongeur is then used to remove remaining cephalad lamina and ligamentum to complete the laminectomy. Because the ligamentum attaches directly to the superior edge of the caudad lamina, a curette or a Kerrison is used to remove the distal portion of that structure. The Kerrison is also used to complete the decompression of the cephalad edge of the inferior lamina (Fig. 29). Decompression of the lateral zone and foramen are addressed sequentially exactly as for the hemilaminotomy (see previous). Again, a complete decompression extends from pedicle above to pedicle below. A probe is used to ensure the adequacy of the decompression.

Special Considerations

The techniques described previously generally function well even for complex lumbar decompression. However, certain unusual situations do require modification of these techniques. These include synovial cysts, severe foraminal stenosis, and severe SCS with atrophic or absent dura.

In the case of a synovial cyst, the ligamentum and lamina are decompressed as for the hemilaminotomy. An attempt is made to identify the stalk of the cyst. In many cases, the cyst origin appears to come from the ligamentum itself rather than the facet joint as one might expect. The cyst is gently teased away from the dura and typically can be removed in its entirety without causing a durotomy.

As described previously, foraminal stenosis is typically caused by collapse of disc height causing impingement of the superior facet into the foramen. Once the hemilaminotomy has been completed and the nerve root takeoff is visualized, the foraminal decompression can be completed safely by keeping the back of the Kerrison rongeur to the nerve root. Again, at least 50% of the facet joint must be preserved to prevent instability, so the Kerrison is angled radically into the foramen to undercut the impinging superior facet while maintaining integrity of the joint. If the probe reveals persistent encroachment in the lateral foramen, special curved "foraminal" Kerrison rongeurs may be helpful to complete the decompression. If resection of the facet joints totals more than 100% (i.e., 50% of each facet, or 30% of one facet and 70% of the contralateral side), careful consideration must be given toward fusion of the involved segment. If the patient can tolerate the additional blood loss and operative time required for a fusion, it is most prudent to do so.

In the most severe cases of spinal stenosis, the dura may become atrophic or even absent. This occurs most commonly with severe congenital stenosis, such as that seen in achondroplastic dwarves (Fig. 30). In these cases, neurologic monitoring may be helpful to provide early warning of excessive canal intrusion. Rather than placing even the smallest Kerrison rongeur into the spinal canal, these cases may require careful burring to leave just a thin shell of lamina over the dura. A dental pick or nerve root hook can then be used to gently peel the thin bony shell off the dura. In these cases, incidental durotomies are common and should be repaired. If the dura is found to be absent, it may be reconstructed using bovine pericardium or a fascial graft. This repair is supplemented with fibrin glue, and a subarachnoid drain for larger defects. The deep muscle and the deep fascia are closed in separate layers to ensure a watertight closure, and patients are kept on bedrest for 3 to 5 days depending on the size of the defect.

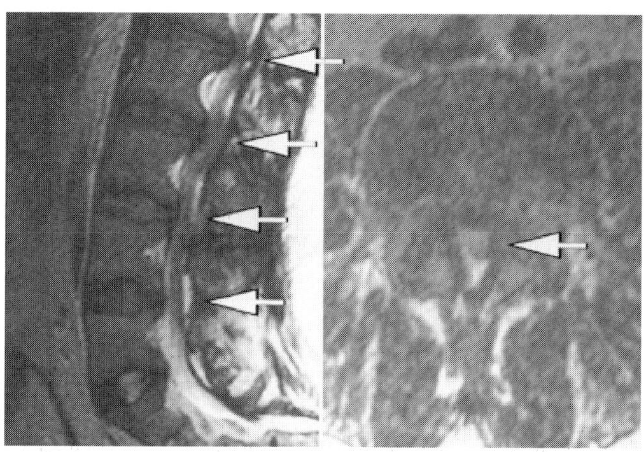

FIG. 30. This 27-year-old patient with achondroplasia experienced severe bilateral leg pain and weakness. The sagittal image shows severe spinal stenosis at L1-2, L2-3, L3-4, and L4-5 (*arrows*). The axial image reveals severe lateral recess stenosis (*arrow*). After a multilevel lumbar laminectomy, he experienced full relief of his symptoms.

Results

The first decompressive laminectomy for spinal stenosis was performed by Lane in 1893 (26). Verbiest first clearly identified the signs and symptoms of neurogenic claudication and the anatomic pathology of spinal stenosis in his classic paper published in 1949 (27,28). Since that time, the standard laminectomy has been shown to be safe and effective, and forms the benchmark to which other decompressive procedures must be compared (28–37).

A retrospective review of laminectomies in 77 patients by Jolles showed 79% good or excellent outcome scores at mean long-term follow-up of 6.5 years (38). Twelve patients with preoperative instability had a concomitant fusion. Of 65 patients without a concomitant fusion, seven (9%) developed some radiographic instability after the laminectomy, but this was not correlated with clinical symptoms.

Amundsen compared conservative and surgical management of lumbar spinal stenosis in 100 patients followed prospectively for 10 years. The 19 patients with the most severe symptoms had decompressive surgery, with 84% good results at 4 years and 71% still reporting good results at 10 years. The 50 patients with milder symptoms at presentation had conservative treatment with 74% good results at 10 years. The third group of 31 patients had intermediate symptoms initially and was randomized to surgery versus conservative care. Those randomized to surgery had 91% good results at 10 years, whereas of those initially randomized to conservative care, 71% had good results with some crossing over to surgery. The main conclusion of the authors was that surgery appears to be good treatment for approximately four-fifths of severely afflicted patients (39).

Lin first described multiple laminotomy for lumbar stenosis in 1982 (40). Postacchini later compared multiple laminotomy to total laminectomy in a series of 67 patients (41). The patients were assigned alternately to one of two groups: 26 patients had multiple laminotomies and 32 had laminectomy. An additional nine patients were selected for multiple laminotomy but were converted to laminectomy by the surgeon primarily for inadequate decompression with multiple laminotomies, although one had a large dural tear requiring laminectomy for visualization and repair. Bilateral laminotomy at two or three levels required a significantly longer operating time than laminectomy at the same number of levels. The clinical results at average follow-up of 3.7 years was similar, with 78 to 81% reporting good or excellent results in the three groups.

Although this study was not randomized or blinded, the authors reported a highly significant difference in the mean subjective improvement in back pain. The multiple laminotomy group had a mean score of 50% better than the laminectomy group. The authors postulated that the higher levels of back pain in the laminectomy group might be due to increased vertebral instability. Three laminectomy patients experienced marked postoperative vertebral instability, whereas none of the multiple laminotomy patients developed this problem. The authors did note, however, that motion segments that were stable preoperatively were not destabilized by the laminectomy.

Microdecompression for lumbar stenosis was originally described by Young in 1988 (4) and subsequently modified by McCulloch in 1991 (42) to include unilateral multifidus retraction, ipsilateral laminotomy, and contralateral microdecompression leaving the spinous processes and midline ligaments intact. Weiner reported on 30 patients treated with this technique at 9-month follow-up (17). They used the neurogenic claudication outcome score to assess functional outcome. The average score improved from 32 to 67. Twenty-six of thirty patients (87%) were satisfied with their outcome. There were no intraoperative complications. Postoperatively, four patients had wound drainage successfully managed with dressing changes and oral antibiotics.

Complications

The overall morbidity and mortality after lumbar spine surgery is determined by patient risk factors and the type of procedure. A review of 18,122 procedures on the lumbar spine included 2,899 patients who had laminectomy alone, without discectomy or arthrodesis (43). The mean age of the laminectomy patients was 63 years; 13.9% had complications during the hospital stay. The relative risk for complications in the laminectomy group was 1.6 when compared to the simple discectomy patients using logistic regression models. For comparison, the relative risk for laminectomy plus arthrodesis was 2.6. The relative risk imparted by age was 1.3 for each 10-year increment. The overall mortality in this study was 0.07%.

Complications specific to lumbar decompressive surgery may be considered in two groups: intraoperative and postoperative.

Intraoperative

In general, the most common intraoperative complication of the lumbar decompressive procedures is incidental durotomy. A dorsal tear in a laminotomy defect does not tamponade itself and generally requires a watertight repair. The dura is closed with a 6-0 suture. The repair is tested by asking the anesthesiologist to provide a Valsalva maneuver to 40 mm Hg. In contrast, an anterior dural rent typically tamponades itself and rarely requires repair. In both cases, the patients are put on bed rest with the head of the bed flat for 24 to 72 hours. Long-term sequelae from these injuries are rare (44,45).

Nerve roots may be temporarily irritated or permanently damaged by intraoperative manipulation. With good technique and knowledge of the anatomy, this complication can be minimized. If the dura must be retracted for any length of time, it is beneficial to allow intermittent periods of relaxation of the retractors. The high-speed drill must be handled with caution. By stabilizing the hand on the patient, any inadvertent plunging can be avoided. The Kerrison rongeur should always be used parallel to the nerve root. Care and attention to these details should keep the rate of permanent injury to a minimum.

Bleeding is typically not severe enough to lead to hemodynamic instability, but it may interfere with visualization and completion of the surgery. Steps to decrease bleeding include stopping antiinflammatory and antithrombotic medication well in advance of the surgery date, assuring proper positioning with the abdomen free of pressure, and controlling intraoperative hemorrhage with bipolar electrocautery, Gelfoam and thrombin, or Flo-Seal.

Wrong-level surgery can be avoided with radiographic determination of the level intraoperatively. Congenital anomalies (e.g., six non–rib-bearing vertebrae) may confuse the issue. They should be identified on the preoperative imaging studies and taken into account.

Inadequate decompression can be verified using the various probes to check the dura and nerve roots at the conclusion of the procedure. In cases in which microsurgical laminoplasty or hemilaminotomy have not allowed for adequate decompression, there should be no hesitation in converting to a more extensive procedure.

Postoperative

Postoperative infections have been reported to occur in less than 1% of all lumbar decompressions (43). All of the authors' patients receive a dose of prophylactic antibiotics before skin incision and continue these in the perioperative period for 24 to 48 hours, or until all drains and catheters have been removed.

Postoperative instability has been reported at varying rates in the literature. Patients with any radiographic sign of instability preoperatively should be strongly considered for spinal fusion at the time of decompression (46,47). It has been shown that patients with degenerative spondylolisthesis have improved clinical results from concomitant fusion (10,21–24). As noted, one study showed a 9% rate of postoperative instability after laminectomy (38), but this was not correlated with clinical symptoms. Instability may be decreased with multiple laminotomies or microsurgical laminoplasty.

CONCLUSION

Lumbar spinal stenosis is typically an acquired disease that occurs with aging and degeneration of the spine. The symptoms cause significant pain and disability for the growing numbers of elderly. The CT-myelogram and especially the MRI now allow us an unparalleled ability to pinpoint the pathology and offer a focused surgical treatment plan. With the help of the surgical microscope, the short-term morbidity can be minimized. The outcomes for standard and microscopic techniques are very successful, with all of the techniques reporting 80 to 90% patient satisfaction and improvement in functional outcomes. The risk of complications appears acceptably low. Truly, the array of lumbar decompressive techniques comprises a powerful weapon in the armamentarium of the spine surgeon.

REFERENCES

1. Turner JA, Ersek M, Herron L, et al. Surgery for lumbar spinal stenosis. Attempted meta-analysis of the literature. *Spine* 1992;17:1–8.
2. Delamarter RB. Lumbar microdiskectomy: microsurgical technique for treatment of lumbar herniated nucleus pulposus. *Instr Course Lect* 2002;51:229–232.
3. McCulloch JA, Young PH. *Essentials of spinal microsurgery*. Philadelphia: Lippincott-Raven, 1998.
4. Young S, Veerapen R, O'Laoire SA. Relief of lumbar canal stenosis using multilevel subarticular fenestrations as an alternative to wide laminectomy: preliminary report. *Neurosurgery* 1988;23:628–633.
5. Epstein JA, Epstein BS, Lavine LS. Nerve root compression associated with narrowing of the lumbar spinal canal. *J Neurol Neurosurg Psychiatry* 1962:165–172.
6. Nelson MA. Lumbar spinal stenosis. *J Bone Joint Surg Br* 1973;55:506–512.
7. Kirkaldy-Willis WH, Paine KW, Cauchoix J, et al. Lumbar spinal stenosis. *Clin Orthop* 1974;99:30–50.
8. Verbiest H. Results of surgical treatment of idiopathic developmental stenosis of the lumbar vertebral canal. A review of twenty-seven years' experience. *J Bone Joint Surg Br* 1977;59:181–188.
9. Fitzgerald JA, Newman PH. Degenerative spondylolisthesis. *J Bone Joint Surg Br* 1976;58:184–192.
10. Herkowitz HN, Kurz LT. Degenerative lumbar spondylolisthesis with spinal stenosis. A prospective study comparing decompression with decompression and intertransverse process arthrodesis. *J Bone Joint Surg Am* 1991;73:802–808.

10a. Crock HV. Normal and pathological anatomy of the lumbar spinal nerve root canals. *J Bone Joint Surg Br* 1981;63B:487–490.

11. Epstein JA, Epstein BS, Lavine LS, et al. Lumbar nerve root compression at the intervertebral foramina caused by arthritis of the posterior facets. *J Neurosurg* 1973;39:362–369.
12. Epstein JA, Epstein BS, Rosenthal AD, et al. Sciatica caused by nerve root entrapment in the lateral recess: the superior facet syndrome. *J Neurosurg* 1972;36:584–589.
13. Getty CJ, Johnson JR, Kirwan EO, et al. Partial undercutting facetectomy for bony entrapment of the lumbar nerve root. *J Bone Joint Surg Br* 1981;63-B:330–335.

13a. Hasegawa T, An HS, Haughton VM, et al. Lumbar foraminal stenosis: critical heights of the intervertebral discs and foramina. A cryomicrotome study in cadaver. *J Bone Joint Surg Am* 1995;77:32–38.

13b. Jenis LG, An HS. Spine update. Lumbar foraminal stenosis. *Spine* 2000;25:389–394.

14. Aryanpur J, Ducker T. Multilevel lumbar laminotomies: an alternative to laminectomy in the treatment of lumbar stenosis. *Neurosurgery* 1990;26:429–432; discussion 33.

14a. Lee CK, Rauschning W, Glenn W. Lateral lumbar spinal canal stenosis: classification, pathologic anatomy and surgical decompression. *Spine* 1988;13:313–320.

14b. Rauschning W. Normal and pathologic anatomy of the lumbar root canals. *Spine* 1987;12:1008–1019.

15. Rauschning W. Pathoanatomy of lumbar disc degeneration and stenosis. *Acta Orthop Scand Suppl* 1993;251:3–12.
16. Postacchini F, Cinotti G, Perugia D, et al. The surgical treatment of central lumbar stenosis. Multiple laminotomy compared with total laminectomy. *J Bone Joint Surg Br* 1993;75:386–392.

17. Weiner BK, Walker M, Brower RS, et al. Microdecompression for lumbar spinal canal stenosis. *Spine* 1999;24:2268–2272.
18. McCulloch JA, Snook D, Kruse CF. Advantages of the operating microscope in lumbar spine surgery. *Instr Course Lect* 2002;51:243–245.
19. Bookwalter JW 3rd, Busch MD, Nicely D. Ambulatory surgery is safe and effective in radicular disc disease. *Spine* 1994;19:526–530.
20. Bogduk N, Wilson AS, Tynan W. The human lumbar dorsal rami. *J Anat* 1982;134(Pt 2):383–397.
21. Booth KC, Bridwell KH, Eisenberg BA, et al. Minimum 5-year results of degenerative spondylolisthesis treated with decompression and instrumented posterior fusion. *Spine* 1999;24:1721–1727.
22. Bridwell KH, Sedgewick TA, O'Brien MF, et al. The role of fusion and instrumentation in the treatment of degenerative spondylolisthesis with spinal stenosis. *J Spinal Disord* 1993;6:461–472.
23. Fischgrund JS, Mackay M, Herkowitz HN, et al. 1997 Volvo Award winner in clinical studies. Degenerative lumbar spondylolisthesis with spinal stenosis: a prospective, randomized study comparing decompressive laminectomy and arthrodesis with and without spinal instrumentation. *Spine* 1997;22:2807–2812.
24. Vaccaro AR, Garfin SR. Degenerative lumbar spondylolisthesis with spinal stenosis, a prospective study comparing decompression with decompression and intertransverse process arthrodesis: a critical analysis. *Spine* 1997;22:368–369.
25. Abumi K, Panjabi MM, Kramer KM, et al. Biomechanical evaluation of lumbar spinal stability after graded facetectomies. *Spine* 1990;15:1142–1147.
26. Lane W. Case of spondylolisthesis associated with progressive paraplegia; laminectomy. *Lancet* 1893;1:991.
27. Verbiest H. *Sur certaines formes rares de compression de la queue de cheval hommage a clovis vincent.* Paris: Malouie 1949.
28. Verbiest H. A radicular syndrome from developmental narrowing of the lumbar vertebral canal. *J Bone Joint Surg Am* 1954;36.
29. Atlas SJ, Deyo RA, Keller RB, et al. The Maine Lumbar Spine Study, Part III. 1-year outcomes of surgical and nonsurgical management of lumbar spinal stenosis. *Spine* 1996;21:1787–1794; discussion, 94–95.
30. Atlas SJ, Keller RB, Robson D, et al. Surgical and nonsurgical management of lumbar spinal stenosis: four-year outcomes from the Maine Lumbar Spine Study. *Spine* 2000;25:556–562.
31. Cinotti G, Postacchini F, Weinstein JN. Lumbar spinal stenosis and diabetes. Outcome of surgical decompression. *J Bone Joint Surg Br* 1994;76:215–219.
32. Herno A, Airaksinen O, Saari T. Long-term results of surgical treatment of lumbar spinal stenosis. *Spine* 1993;18:1471–1474.
33. Johnsson KE. Lumbar spinal stenosis. A retrospective study of 163 cases in southern Sweden. *Acta Orthop Scand* 1995;66:403–405.
34. Katz JN, Lipson SJ, Brick GW, et al. Clinical correlates of patient satisfaction after laminectomy for degenerative lumbar spinal stenosis. *Spine* 1995;20:1155–1160.
35. Niggemeyer O, Strauss JM, Schulitz KP. Comparison of surgical procedures for degenerative lumbar spinal stenosis: a meta-analysis of the literature from 1975 to 1995. *Eur Spine J* 1997;6:423–429.
36. Postacchini F. Surgical management of lumbar spinal stenosis. *Spine* 1999;24:1043–1047.
37. Hansraj KK, Cammisa FP Jr, O'Leary PF, et al. Decompressive surgery for typical lumbar spinal stenosis. *Clin Orthop* 2001:10–17.
38. Jolles BM, Porchet F, Theumann N. Surgical treatment of lumbar spinal stenosis. Five-year follow-up. *J Bone Joint Surg Br* 2001;83:949–953.
39. Amundsen T, Weber H, Nordal HJ, et al. Lumbar spinal stenosis: conservative or surgical management?: a prospective 10-year study. *Spine* 2000;25:1424–1435; discussion 35–36.
40. Lin PM. Internal decompression for multiple levels of lumbar spinal stenosis: a technical note. *Neurosurgery* 1982;11:546–549.
41. Postacchini F, Cinotti G, Gumina S, et al. Long-term results of surgery in lumbar stenosis. 8-year review of 64 patients. *Acta Orthop Scand Suppl* 1993;251:78–80.
42. McCulloch JA. Microsurgical spinal laminotomies. In: Frymoyer JW, ed. *The adult spine*. New York: Raven Press, Ltd, 1991.
43. Deyo RA, Cherkin DC, Loeser JD, et al. Morbidity and mortality in association with operations on the lumbar spine. The influence of age, diagnosis, and procedure. *J Bone Joint Surg Am* 1992;74:536–543.
44. Wang JC, Bohlman HH, Riew KD. Dural tears secondary to operations on the lumbar spine. Management and results after a two-year-minimum follow-up of eighty-eight patients. *J Bone Joint Surg Am* 1998;80:1728–1732.
45. Cammisa FP Jr., Girardi FP, Sangani PK, et al. Incidental durotomy in spine surgery. *Spine* 2000;25:2663–2667.
46. Fox MW, Onofrio BM, Hanssen AD. Clinical outcomes and radiological instability following decompressive lumbar laminectomy for degenerative spinal stenosis: a comparison of patients undergoing concomitant arthrodesis versus decompression alone. *J Neurosurg* 1996;85:793–802.
47. Mullin BB, Rea GL, Irsik R, et al. The effect of postlaminectomy spinal instability on the outcome of lumbar spinal stenosis patients. *J Spinal Disord* 1996;9:107–116.

CHAPTER 56

Posterolateral Lumbar Fusion

John S. Kirkpatrick and Brian M. Scholl

Posterolateral lumbar arthrodesis is an integral part of the surgical management of many spinal disorders. Lumbar fusions evolved during the twentieth century from the midline interspinous and laminar techniques first described by Albee and Hibbs in early 1911 to the current technique of intertransverse fusions first described by Campbell 14 years later and popularized by Watkins in 1953 (1–4).

This utilitarian surgical procedure is indicated for the treatment of thoracolumbar and lumbar instability. It has been used successfully in acute fracture management for degenerative diseases, such as adult scoliosis and lumbar disc disease, spondylolisthesis, primary and metastatic tumors, and for pyogenic and nonpyogenic infections.

The success of the arthrodesis is dependent on attention to the biological preparation of the fusion bed. Boden et al. have demonstrated by vascular injection studies that blood flow to the fusion mass comes from the decorticated transverse processes (5). Additionally, the maximal area possible must be decorticated, as fusion rates appear to be related to the size of the exposed surface area (5). Currently, the gold standard for fusion substrate is autogenous iliac crest cancellous bone, although allograft can be used (6). Newer research has led to the identification of a variety of osteoinductive organic compounds, such as bone morphogenic proteins. Bone morphogenic protein–impregnated substrates are commercially available, and although not currently approved for posterolateral fusion, may represent the future alternatives to autogenous graft (see Chapter 51).

Despite improved techniques, nonunion occurs in 5 to 35% of noninstrumented cases—more commonly at the L-5 to S-1 level. Instrumentation has reduced this rate to 5 to 15% but is associated with increased cost, operating times, blood loss, reoperation, complication rates, and possibly increased infection (7–10). When arthrodesis is used for some degenerative conditions, a successful arthrodesis does not necessarily yield a better clinical result (7,11–13). Instrumentation, however, allows for immediate postoperative mobilization and often eliminates the need for a brace with which patients may not be entirely compliant. The higher fusion rates seen with instrumentation are directly related to the stiffness of the construct, with semirigid systems performing poorly compared to rigid constructs (14).

Although a variety of novel internal fixation devices have been used since the twentieth century, the modern era of spinal instrumentation began when Harrington introduced his distraction rod system in 1962 for the treatment of scoliosis (15). However, application of this technique in the lumbar spine resulted in flat back deformities and led to the development of other systems (16). Segmental fixation was introduced by Resina and Alves and Luque using sublaminar wires and has proved to be effective, low in cost, and particularly useful in the neuromuscular-related spinal deformities, but has the risk of neurologic injury from the passage of sublaminar wires (17,18). Second-generation segmental systems include the modular hook/rod constructs introduced by Cotrel-Dobousett (19). Pedicle screws, used with plates or rods, have significantly impacted the treatment of spinal disorders and have been incorporated into most current modular systems (20).

PATIENT SELECTION FOR ARTHRODESIS

Proper patient selection requires identification of a proper indication and consideration of medical and psychosocial factors. Well-established indications for posterolateral lumbar fusion include radiographically proven segmental instability secondary to degenerative conditions, including degenerative spondylolisthesis, degenerative scoliosis, or iatrogenic instability after spinal procedures, such as laminectomy or facetectomy, and possibly after failed disc surgery (7,9–13,21–24). Another accepted indication includes persistent back and leg pain in the adult related to isthmic spondylolisthesis (25). Additional indications include spinal stenosis with associated degenerative spondylolisthesis but without instability in patients undergoing reconstructive procedures for adult scoliosis, failed previous surgery, tumor, trauma, or infection.

Currently, no other area in lumbar spine surgery is more controversial than fusion for degenerative disc disease and discogenic back pain. Despite the difficulty of accurately and reproducibly diagnosing pain due to disc disease and the lack of long-term natural history studies, some authors are reporting successful outcomes in properly selected patients treated with isolated posterolateral fusions, posterolateral fusions with posterior instrumentation, and, more recently, circumferential fusions with anterior-interbody and posterior instrumentation (12–14,26,27). A recent randomized, prospective trial compared posterolateral fusion, posterolateral fusion with internal fixation, and posterolateral fusion with internal fixation and interbody fusion. The investigators found no clear disadvantage in clinical results from using posterolateral fusion alone (13).

Despite some well-established indications for posterolateral lumbar fusion, determination of measurable presurgical prognostic factors related to the successful posterolateral lumbar fusion is made difficult by the lack of consensus about indications, differing surgical techniques, and the lack of comparable and standardized clinical and surgical outcomes instruments. Complicating the assessment of solid arthrodesis is the fact that the interpretation of conventional radiographs or computed tomography is less reliable than surgical exploration (28–30). An additional reality is that the presence of a solid fusion does not necessarily correlate with a successful clinical outcome (7,11–13).

Factors that have been reported to have negative prognostic significance are absence of leg pain or back-dominated complaints, advancing age, previous low back surgery, increasing number of vertebral levels fused, diabetes, and tobacco abuse (14,31–36). Modifiable biologic factors should be addressed before operative intervention to maximize arthrodesis rates and minimize complications. Cessation of tobacco use and addition of pedicle screw instrumentation have been shown to increase arthrodesis rates in smokers. An often overlooked preoperatively correctable problem is malnutrition. This is particularly common in elderly patients undergoing decompression and fusion for spinal stenosis and spondylolisthesis (37). Osteopenia, although not directly associated with a poor outcome, may alter the surgeon's fixation strategy due to a higher rate of pedicle screw loosening. More commonly seen osteopenic conditions include idiopathic osteoporosis, hyperparathyroidism, malabsorption, vitamin D deficiency, calcium deficiency, immobilization [but not women with complete spinal cord injury (38)], alcoholism, and diabetes mellitus. Chronic glucocorticoid administration in conditions such as rheumatoid arthritis, sarcoidosis, lupus erythematosus, and chronic obstructive airway disease is also associated with osteopenia.

Psychosocial factors, although not always easy to investigate in clinical practice, deserve attention, because performing surgery on the wrong patient is as important as performing the wrong surgery (39). Analyses of psychosocial factors, which have proven difficult to quantify, stratify, and compare across different socioeconomic groups, have yielded inconsistent results. Studies reporting measurements of psychological well-being (Minnesota Multiphasic Personality Inventory-2, Distress and Risk Assessment Method, State Trait Anxiety Index-T, Zung) have variably implicated presurgical anxiety, depression, hypochondriasis, hysteria, and hostility as negative predictive factors of a successful posterior spinal fusion (40–42). Other negative predictive factors include the presence of disability payments, pending legal action, low level of education, and long duration of presurgical unemployment (40–42). There is also a well-documented correlation of poorer outcomes in patients receiving workers' compensation (43). The usefulness of these biopsychosocial factors lies in potentially identifying high-risk patients preoperatively, allowing practitioners to educate patients about their potential outcome and to pursue a more aggressive and monitored rehabilitation strategy preoperatively and postoperatively. Most important, these factors should alert the surgeon to those patients who need psychological intervention.

PATIENT SELECTION FOR INSTRUMENTATION

Instrumentation serves three purposes: (a) avoidance of brace wear, (b) enhancement of arthrodesis, and (c) minimizing the number of motion segments needed to be fused. There is little debate regarding the benefit of instrumentation in patients undergoing reduction and stabilization of fractures or to support anterior reconstruction in oncologic or infectious cases. Patients who have instrumentation can be started on more aggressive postoperative rehabilitation and are more easily mobilized. Addition of rigid instrumentation has also been shown in multiple studies to increase arthrodesis rates in degenerative disease at the cost of some increased risk for complications (7–10,13,14). The caveat is that increased arthrodesis rates do not necessarily equate to better clinical results, and indeed, some surgeons believe routine instrumentation is not necessary for most cases of spinal stenosis, isthmic spondylolisthesis, or degenerative spondylolisthesis. Despite this observation, some clear agreement about indications does exist.

Posterior instrumentation should be used in the tobacco abuser having lumbar fusion because of the smoking-impaired fusion rates (31,33–35). In general, patients who have spondylolisthesis or exhibit segmental instability (greater than 4 mm of translation or 10 degrees of angulation on flexion-extension films) should be instrumented (7–10,12,14,32,44). Other indications include iatrogenic instability (greater than 50% of bilateral facets or 100% of a single facet removed) and adult scoliosis. Tumors, trauma, or infection are also indicated when there is loss of the posterior elements or to supplement anterior reconstructions (45,46). Particularly in the treatment of primary and metastatic tumors, instrumentation should be used liberally, with the goal of rapid mobilization and return to function. Posterior instrumentation can also be used in failed noninstrumented fusions or a revision situation to extend construct stability or replace failed or broken hardware. As mentioned previously, routine arthrodesis and instrumentation for degenerative disc disease is controversial, although some have reported success in cases in which there is significant spondylolisthesis and angular instability or with properly selected patients undergoing posterior alone or circumferential instrumented fusions (12–14,24,26,27). Some feel relative indications include obesity and multilevel procedures.

OPERATIVE TECHNIQUE

Positioning and Exposure

In the operating room, general anesthesia is induced, any desired invasive monitoring devices are inserted, and a Foley catheter is placed. Antithrombotic stockings with or without mechanical devices for prophylaxis of deep vein thrombosis are applied to the patient. The patient is placed in a prone position with pressure relief over the abdomen to minimize distension of epidural veins and reduce bleeding. This may be accomplished to varying degrees with the knee-chest position, such as an Andrews frame or a four-point support (such as the Relton-Hall or CHOP frames), or with bolsters. All bony prominences and the face should be adequately padded or supported. A radiolucent table (i.e., Jackson table) may be desired if fluoroscopic visualization of the spine for instrumentation is desired. Hypotensive anesthesia can be used as an adjunct to minimize bleeding in the surgical field but should be used with caution in patients with known atherosclerotic vascular disease. A midline approach through skin and subcutaneous tissues is undertaken. A dermal injection of 1:500,000 epinephrine can be used to attain cutaneous vasoconstriction and minimize skin bleeding if desired before the skin incision. In general, 20 to 30 mL of this solution is sufficient for the incision to expose a one- to two-level fusion. The lumbodorsal fascia is incised the length of the skin incision, and the paraspinal muscles are subperiosteally stripped using a Cobb elevator down to the lamina, exposing the spinous processes at one or two levels. Some prefer to use monopolar cautery to elevate the paraspinals to minimize bleeding. A Kocher clamp can be placed on a spinous process and a lateral radiograph obtained to confirm the appropriate level.

Once the appropriate levels are confirmed, the remaining fascia and paraspinal muscles are subperiosteally stripped off the appropriate spinous processes and lamina down to the pars interarticularis. Caution is used to avoid damage to the facet capsules. The use of a Cobb elevator while packing with a sponge facilitates stripping of the paraspinals and obtains hemostasis. Consistently, there are small arterial feeders immediately lateral to the pars interarticularis just inferior to the facet joint. These vessels should be identified and coagulated. Self-retaining retractors, such as deep cerebellars or Beckman-Adson retractors, can be placed to expose the surgical field. Specialized lumbar retractors, such as the Karlin lumbar retractor, may be used. Once the pars is cleared of remaining tissue, the medial border of the facet capsule should be identified to prevent injury to the facet joint complex at uninvolved levels. The dissection is continued laterally by following the pars interarticularis superiorly and laterally. The facets are exposed while protecting the capsule. The dissection then proceeds laterally following the outer side of the superior facet until the transverse process is encountered. It is important to remember the transverse process of the vertebra lies superior to the facet. The paraspinals are then elevated with a Cobb or Bovie elevator off the transverse processes to the lateral tips of the transverse processes (Fig. 1). Once the transverse processes are exposed, the paraspinal muscle can be elevated from the intertransverse membrane between the levels desired. The facet capsule can be stripped, exposing the facet joint, and the articular surface denuded, if desired. If the facet capsule is removed, some believe more consideration should be given to using instrumentation (47). Once the transverse processes are exposed, the lateral gutter is developed to allow preparation for bone grafting. Hemostasis can be obtained by packing rolled sponges into the lateral gutters. If decompression is warranted, it can be performed at this time.

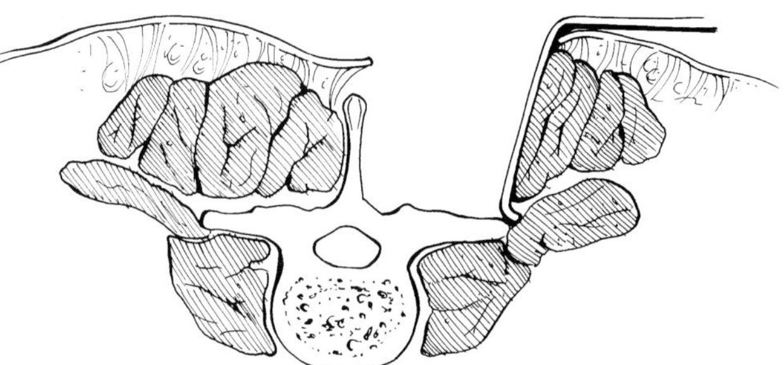

FIG. 1. Axial schematic drawing demonstrating elevation and retraction of the paraspinal muscles from one side of the spine to the tip of the transverse process.

Preparation of Lateral Gutters

The transverse processes are decorticated, exposing the largest surface area possible without removing any cancellous bone. A sharp curette can be used for this purpose. A power burr theoretically can cause thermal necrosis. In patients with osteopenic bone, a curette is generally adequate and preferred. Occasionally, a fracture of the transverse process may occur. The surgeon should use care not to remove the fractured portion but to complete decortication without further disruption of the soft-tissue attachments. These fractures heal as the fusion mass heals with no adverse effect. Patients with healthy bone often require the use of a burr to perform a corticotomy of the transverse process, which is followed by the use of a curette to complete the decortication (Fig. 2). The lateral aspect of the facet and pars interarticularis can also be decorticated if a sufficient area of the pars remains following decompression. Care must be taken to preserve the capsule of the facet joint at the next superior vertebra. If the capsule is violated, undesired fusion may occur.

Autogenous iliac crest bone grafting is then placed uniformly and directly on the decorticated transverse processes and intertransverse membrane and onto the decorticated facet joints if the capsule has been removed. The direct contact to the transverse processes is important to provide a scaffold for osteoconduction. Adequate volume of graft is needed for osteoinductive properties. Because bone quality and availability are somewhat patient-derived factors, most agree that placing as much bone as can be reasonably obtained is appropriate. Care is taken to avoid penetration of the intertransverse membrane to avoid compression of exiting nerve roots. When fusion to the sacrum is planned, the sacral ala should be exposed laterally and decorticated to receive iliac crest bone grafting as well. The sacral ala are thick enough that a cortical window can be made and reflected superiorly, exposing the cancellous bone remaining on

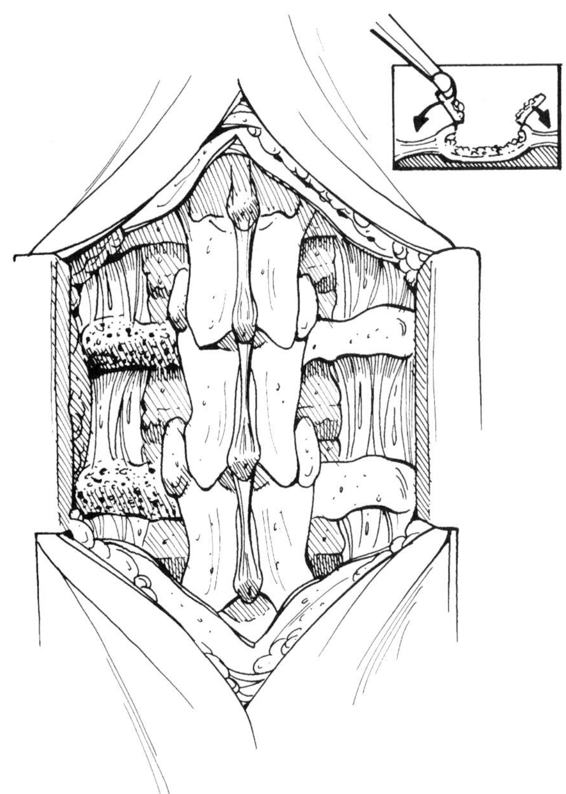

FIG. 2. Posterior view demonstrating the exposure of both sides of the spine to the tips of the transverse processes. The left transverse processes have been decorticated. Inset demonstrates a cross-section of the transverse process being decorticated with a curette. Note that the cortical bone is folded open, leaving the cancellous bone exposed.

the ala and the undersurface of the window. However, care must be taken to avoid injury to the sacroiliac joint.

Wiltse Modification

A modification of this midline approach was popularized by Wiltse and is useful for *in situ* fusions of spondylolisthesis in the pediatric population, but can also be used for far lateral disc herniations or pedicle screw placement. After the standard midline incision, a direct approach is undertaken approximately 2 cm lateral to the spinous process through the lumbodorsal fascia. The natural plane of the multifidus and longissimus muscles is developed bluntly above L-4 or sharply below this level. Retraction and dissection are carried down until the facets are found. A Cobb elevator or rongeur can then be used to remove adherent tissue and expose the lamina and transverse processes. Often, the facets and transverse processes are deeper in the operative field than expected, particularly with higher grades of spondylolisthesis. The ala of the sacrum should be exposed laterally and decorticated to receive iliac crest bone grafting as well.

Care must be taken when dissecting around the lamina of a spondylolisthesed vertebra and the transverse processes of L-5, for if dissection strays too far anterior and inferiorly, the L-5 nerve root can be injured.

INTERNAL FIXATION

Pedicle Screws

Pedicle screws and rods may be used as an adjunct to posterolateral arthrodesis to either enhance arthrodesis rates or to preserve motion segments. The screws are placed from the posterolateral aspect of the junction of the transverse process and facet, traverse the pedicle, and extend into the vertebral body. Attention to proper pedicle screw placement technique is important, particularly in patients with aberrant pedicle anatomy, which occurs in congenital or idiopathic scoliosis. Pedicle screws have been used in Europe for more than 30 years, and their complications are well understood. A survey of American Back Society members by Esses et al. demonstrated a 9.6% overall complication rate, with the following specific frequencies: 5.2% screw misplacement, 2.3% pedicle fracture, 1.9% rate dural tear with cerebrospinal leak, and 0.16% significant vessel injury (9). A larger cohort study found no significant differences for intraoperative dural tears, nerve root injuries, postoperative infection, dural leaks, or vascular injuries when pedicle screw constructs and noninstrumented fusions were done for fractures and degenerative spondylolisthesis (10). Most authors consistently report screw misplacement rates greater than 5% in degenerative conditions, but in scoliotic patients, the rates have been reported to range from a low of 0% to a high of 25% (20). Computer-assisted navigation systems present a potential alternative to minimize screw misplacement but are not widely available at present; some have questioned their benefit in routine cases (20).

The surgeon must have a three-dimensional grasp of pedicle anatomy. There are wide individual variations among patients, and there is a learning curve associated with pedicle screw placement (48). A few salient points should be emphasized to minimize intraoperative and postoperative complications. Roy-Camille initially recommended drilling the pedicle, but most surgeons use a blunt-tipped probe to minimize perforation of the pedicle wall, followed by a ball-tipped probe to directly palpate wall integrity. Return of fat droplet–laden blood has been reported to have a positive predictive value of 84% and a negative predictive value of 95% to verify nonpenetration of the pedicle wall (49).

Although advancements in pedicle screw implant design and metallurgy have lessened implant breakage, most of the stability of the pedicle screw construct occurs at the screw-bone interface (50). Screw purchase has been directly related to the fit and fill of the inner diameter of the pedicle (51), the major diameter of the screw (52), insertion depth to 80% of the vertebral body (53), insertional torque (54), and bone-marrow density (55–57). Bicortical fixation significantly increases pullout strength but has not been widely accepted due to concerns about anterior vessel injury (57,58). However, sacral bicortical fixation increases pullout strength and construct stability; it has been shown to be a safe technique (59–61). Additionally, it has been shown that triangulation and cross-linking increase the stability of constructs and pullout strength (62,63). Last, spinal column load-sharing is critical to the success of pedicle-screw constructs as described by the 4R-4bar linkage theory of Carson et al. (64) and as illustrated in concept by the load sharing classification system (65–67). It has been recommended that *in situ* contouring of the rods to correct kyphosis should be avoided, as this places stress on the pedicle screws and can decrease fixation strength. If *in situ* contouring is necessary, the addition of offset laminar hooks can decrease the stress and lower failure rates (68).

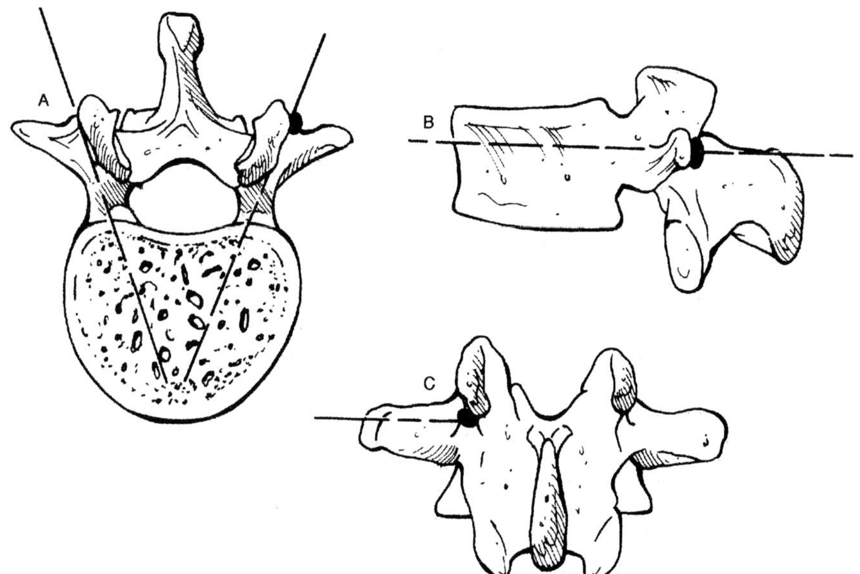

FIG. 3. Axial **(A)**, lateral **(B)**, and posterior **(C)** diagrams demonstrating the pedicle screw trajectory (*dashed lines*) and entry sites (*black dots*) on the vertebra.

Pedicle Screw Placement

Pedicle screw placement can be performed before or after the placement of the bone graft. Placement of bone graft before pedicle screw insertion may obscure landmarks for screw insertion, whereas placement of bone graft with screws present may make optimal placement of bone graft on the transverse process more difficult. Proper placement of bone graft is the more critical component.

The landmark for the entry site for the pedicle screw is at the inferior and lateral aspect of the facet complex where it intersects with the transverse process. A line running down the center of the transverse process is imagined and followed to the superior articular process of the vertebra selected for the screw (Fig. 3). A burr or rongeur is used to decorticate this area to allow for insertion of a pedicle probe. This entry site and the subsequent trajectory of the probe can be confirmed on plain film, fluoroscopy, or computer-assisted stereotaxis if desired. The pedicle probe is advanced with controlled pressure along the axis of the pedicle and small, repetitive rotations are applied. The gentle advancement of the probe in the cancellous bone of the pedicle is felt by the surgeon. A sudden ease of advancement may represent penetration of the pedicle wall, and this possibility should be checked radiographically. The difficulty of advancing the probe usually increases as the probe reaches the base of the pedicle just before entering the vertebral body. The probe is advanced until another increase in the resistance occurs, indicating that the anterior cortex has been contacted or when fluoroscopy reveals adequate length. Palpation with a smaller, straight probe confirms the integrity of the pedicle and the screw length. Special attention is used while palpating the medial and inferior aspects of the pedicle, as penetration in these directions can affect the nerve root or dura. If a decompression was done, direct examination of the pedicle in the canal and foramen can facilitate placement and confirm the absence of penetration of the pedicle walls. A tap is used to prepare the pedicle for screw insertion. Some taps are cannulated and are passed over a guide wire, which allows for fluoroscopic or radiographic confirmation of the guide wire position. Some systems use self-tapping screws, eliminating the tapping step. With the screws in place, the bone graft location is confirmed and the screws are connected by rods or plates according to the manufacturer's recommendations.

Sacral fixation requires other considerations due to larger pedicles and relatively less dense bone. Multiple techniques for fixation have been developed using screws, plates, and intramedullary devices. For relatively short (less than three levels) fusions to the sacrum, simply directing the angle of the pedicle screw more cephalad such that it crosses the superior end-plate of S-1 provides adequate fixation. The external landmark is the inferior aspect of the articular process of S-1 just cephalad and lateral to the first sacral foramen. Fluoroscopy is used to ensure proper trajectory toward the anterior portion of the superior end-plate of S-1. In some cases, the posterior aspect of the iliac wing can be prominent and make the proper trajectory difficult. This barrier can be alleviated by the removal of a small amount of soft tissue and occasionally bone from the ilium to allow the proper trajectory. A mallet is often required to aid in gaining penetration of the end-plate with the pedicle probe. For longer fusions, fixation to the pelvis and sacrum is recommended.

Sublaminar Wiring

Sublaminar wiring, a useful technique in the immature neuromuscular population, has limited use in the adult lumbar setting. The Luque technique adds rotational and translational stability over the classic Harrington technique by distributing a corrective force over multiple vertebral segments. Sublaminar wiring pullout strength appears highest in the lumbar lamina, is significantly weaker in spinous processes, and does not seem to vary among different wiring configurations or construct type (69,70).

Proper preparation of the lamina, visualization of the epidural space, and precontouring of the wire are essential to minimize potential injury. Eighteen-gauge wire should be doubled and shaped to have a gentle, semicircular curve with a radius similar to the lamina at the involved level and have a bend of less than 45 degrees at the tip. The wire is passed midline in a two-handed fashion from inferior to superior, and the tip is delivered with a blunt nerve hook and secured with a needle-driver once it is visualized at the superior border of the lamina. Pulling constant tension, the wire is pulled to create equal superior and inferior limbs. After all segments are done, the precontoured rods are placed with the wires oriented with the inferior portions lateral to the rods and the superior portions medial. The wires are cut and sequentially twisted over the rods. Cable systems are available and allow provisional tensioning of the construct. Retensioning may be necessary as more segments are secured. Experience is required to determine how much tensioning is enough before the wire breaks or cuts through the lamina, but commercially available cable tensioners are available, and the required tensions usually are specified.

Translaminar Facet Screw Fixation

Standard 4.5-mm AO screws can be used to stabilize one or two motion segments as an adjunct to anterior interbody fusion, pure dislocations (i.e., ligamentous Chance-type fractures), or standard posterolateral fusion. It is a relatively simple technique that has been reported to be superior to posterior wiring techniques and provides rigidity similar to pedicle screw fixation (71,72). Contraindications include severe osteoporosis or laminar fractures (71,73,74). Postoperative complications are uncommon and are mainly related to the bone graft donor site (73,75).

After a standard posterior midline approach, a protected 3.2-mm oscillating drill is inserted percutaneously and directed toward the base of the superior spinous process. A hole is drilled from the base of the spinous process traversing the lamina, across the facet joint, and exiting near the base of the next caudal vertebral transverse process. A tap is passed through the facet joints only if they are markedly sclerotic. Because two screws are typically placed, the entry sites must be staggered to allow the screws to cross. Aftercare is similar to routine posterolateral fusion, but as the screws act as bolts, rather than lag screws, postsurgical bracing is prudent.

Laminar or Transverse Process Hooks

Laminar or transverse process hooks can be used as a primary means of instrumentation or as an adjunct to pedicle screws. Hooks are simple and safe to use because they are placed under direct visualization. Although hooks are strongest in extension and distraction and weakest in torsion and flexion, they are useful in compression-mode with a claw-type construct. More rigid fixation can be obtained from a locked-hook construct available in some systems, which adds a locking screw that passes through the hook into the lamina.

Additionally, laminar hooks have been shown to enhance construct strength in patients with osteoporosis, as bone mineral density does not correlate with pullout strength of a laminar hook, unlike a pedicle screw (56,76–78). Flatback associated with distraction-only instrumentation is not a significant problem with newer modular systems.

AFTERCARE

Wound closure is accomplished according to the surgeon's preference. Subfascial drains are often used to help reduce the likelihood of an epidural hematoma, as the fusion bed may develop a large postoperative hematoma if they are not. The fascia is closed with large braided absorbable suture, and the subcutaneous tissues and skin are closed as desired. Postoperative intravenous analgesics (e.g., patient-controlled analgesia) and antibiotics are continued for up to 48 hours. Mechanical prophylaxis for deep vein thrombosis (e.g., sequential compression hose or pulse compression boots) is used until the patients are independently mobile, which usually ranges from 24 to 48 hours. Drains are removed when the drainage volume decreases and the color is clear. External rigid bracing (custom-molded thoracolumbosacral orthosis with thigh extension for L-5 to S-1 fusions) is used in patients without instrumentation, and nonrigid corset support may improve the early mobility of some with internal fixation.

PITFALLS AND PEARLS

Intraoperative Complications

Intraoperative complications can arise from correctly and incorrectly placed instrumentation. Identification of anatomic landmarks is essential for the placement of pedicle screws. This anatomy can often be distorted in revision situations, severe degenerative scoliosis, or congenital spinal disorders. Methods to enhance pedicle screw placement include careful attention to anatomy, technique, intraoperative radiographs, fluoroscopic visualization, or computer-assisted navigation (20,79). Anterior perforation of the vertebra is common, but vascular or visceral complications are rare even with bicortical pedicle screw fixation in the sacrum (60,61,64,80). Misplaced pedicle screws have been reported to occur in up to 25% of patients, although a large series of 4,790 patients reported a 5.1% frequency (8,9,81–84). Misplacement seems to occur at a higher rate in scoliosis and with more inexperienced surgeons (48). For pedicles missed laterally, no clear literature exists regarding whether to leave the screw as an in-out-in technique if there is a small lateral perforation of the pedicle, to redirect with the same or larger screw if there is gross malplacement, or to use unilateral fixation if the pedicle is completely split during insertion. Screws perforating the medial wall should be removed, as these have a higher risk for nerve irritation (80).

Pedicle fracture occurs rarely (0.1%) and is more common in osteoporotic bone (80). The clinical significance of a fractured pedicle is unclear, and some authors have demonstrated only an 11% decrease in pullout strength with a pedicle fracture when compared to the intact pedicle (85). It is left to the surgeon to judge stability and add an appropriate adjunct, extend the construct by an additional level, or rely on unilateral fixation. Other techniques for augmentation to pedicle screw fixation include laminar hooks, polymethylmethacrylate, or calcium-hydroxyapatite cement.

Permanent neurologic injury is the most feared complication. The risk associated with noninstrumented lumbar fusions has been reported to range from 0 to 2.7% (10) and has been variably reported with pedicle screws, ranging from a low of 0.4% to a high of 11% (8–10,20,80,86,87). Generally, it is expected to be 2 to 3% or less. Most nerve irritation comes from medial screw placement, and when present, prompt screw removal is indicated. Removal of an impinging screw even at 75 days has been associated with resolution of neurologic deficits (80). Nerve or spinal cord injury can be related to passage of sublaminar wires, although this is more common with thoracic wiring in adult scoliosis.

Dural leaks can occur in 5 to 10% of patients, mostly related to decompressive procedures performed in addition to the posterolateral arthrodesis; they occur more commonly in the patients with idiopathic or degenerative scoliosis and revision surgery. Dural leaks directly related to screw placement are uncommon and are more often related to medial wall perforation and reported at less than 1% (9,10,20,80). Dural leaks related to sublaminar wires can be avoided by correct contouring of the tip and controlled passage of the wire.

Vascular or bowel injury is exceedingly rare and occurs at a rate of 0.2% in noninstrumented fusions and a 0 to 0.3% rate in pedicle screw instrumentations (9,10,20,80). A more recent review of 4,790 pedicle screw placements revealed a 0% risk of bowel or vascular injury (80).

Considerations in Osteopenic Bone

Good biomechanical data exist regarding the pedicle and fixation techniques in the osteoporotic spine (55,56,76–78,88–90). Although trabecular bone is more affected in osteoporosis, there is also a significant decrease in the dense subcortical bone marrow density (90a) in the pedicle, accompanied by weakening of the pullout strength of a pedicle screw. Therefore, care must be taken when placing pedicle screws in osteoporotic vertebra. There is increased risk of pedicle fracture when using screws whose diameter is greater than 70% of the pedicle diameter and in a vertebra with a dual-energy x-ray absorptiometry of less than 0.7 g per cm^2 (55,88). Additionally, there is a risk incidence of pedicle screw loosening in osteoporotic vertebra and in severe osteoporosis (qCT of less than 33.3 mg/mL) (89,90). Some believe pedicle screws are contraindicated in these circumstances (90). The addition of laminar hooks has been shown to enhance construct strength in patients with osteoporosis, as bone mineral density does not correlate with pullout strength of a laminar hook, unlike a pedicle screw (56,76–78). Other adjuncts to enhance pedicle screw fixation include polymethylmethacrylate or hydroxyapatite cement (52,91,92).

Postoperative Complications

Complications typically occur in patients more than 80 years of age, patients with malignancy, or patients undergoing surgery for scoliosis or trauma. Mardjetko et al. performed a metaanalysis of the past 20 years of literature regarding degenerative spondylolisthesis. They found that complication rates were higher in instrumented patients compared to decompressive procedures or arthrodesis without instrumentation (93). In contrast, Greenfield demonstrated that expected outcomes and complications did not differ significantly in elderly patients compared to younger patients with instrumented posterolateral arthrodesis (94).

Instrumentation typically increases operating time and blood loss as well as cost (7–10). Instrumentation has also been reported to increase infection risk but typically occurs in less than 2% of patients (95–100). Infection is also higher in patients with diabetes, malignancy, steroid use, and malnutrition, but deep venous thrombosis is felt to be an uncommon complication (101).

Although rates of hardware removal are not often mentioned in reports, Lonstein reported that pain possibly associated with pedicle screw systems was the most common complication (80); screw removal was necessary in 24% of patients. Cases have been reported of late pedicle stress fracture after screw removal (102,102a), although this is not common. Reoperation rates have been reported to be similar in noninstrumented versus instrumented cases, but most reoperations in the instrumented group are for hardware removal (10).

Hardware failure usually consists of bending or breakage of the pedicle screw, which occurs in 0.5 to 25% of reported patients (80,87,103). Most authors report the risk is 5%. The risk for bending or breakage of pedicle screws has been reported to be greater in patients treated with short-segment instrumentation, particularly those with deficient anterior columns (65,66,104–106). A pseudarthrosis should be suspected when a pedicle screw fracture occurs postoperatively. Lonstein et al. reported a higher rate of screw failure with instrumentation for lumbosacral arthrodesis (15 of 20 patients or 75% with a screw fracture) and recommended exploration if the pseudarthrosis was symptomatic.

Pseudarthrosis has been reported to occur in 5 to 35% of noninstrumented cases (more commonly at L-5 to S-1), and instrumentation has reduced this rate to 5 to 15% (7–10,14). Later reoperation for pseudarthrosis typically occurs in 5 to 6% of patients.

Reoperation

Reoperation may be indicated for pseudarthrosis, degeneration or deformity at the adjacent segment, and hardware complications or symptoms. Careful dissection to avoid injury to the dura is important and is discussed in detail in Chapters 58 and 62. Scar tissue is often important to avoid injury to adjacent structures. Bovie cautery is often helpful in removing soft tissue from previously placed instruments. The pseudarthrosis usually involves a narrow fibrous union between two masses of bone. This fibrous area should be débrided with curettes or rongeurs and the adjacent bone should be decorticated. Additional bone graft, usually harvested from the iliac crest opposite the original donor site, is then placed over this newly decorticated bed. If pedicle screws are being placed, a larger diameter screw should be used if the preoperative studies indicate adequate bone. If there are no existing screws and pedicle screws are used, then fluoroscopy of the sagittal and coronal planes is used to identify entry sites and trajectory through the fusion mass to the pedicle. Treatment of pseudarthrosis of a posterior fusion may also be supplemented with anterior interbody fusion using one of the many techniques described in Chapter 57. If fusion is indicated for the adjacent segment, the fusion can be extended with a procedure similar to primary operations. If the original fusion is well healed and instrumentation was used, these implants can be removed.

CONTRAINDICATIONS

Contraindications to posterolateral fusion are variably reported and are usually patient specific. Patients must be in adequate health for general anesthesia and be able to tolerate a significant blood loss. In general, patients with limited life expectancy (less than 6 months) are not appropriate surgical candidates for fusion, although stabilization without fusion often is useful. Active infection is a relative contraindication, but posterolateral fusion may be a component of treatment for spinal infections. Multiple comorbidities yield poorer clinical results in general.

OUTCOMES

Clinical outcomes in posterolateral fusion vary with the specific indication for surgery. Radiographic fusion appears to be obtained in approximately 75% of posterolateral fusions; this increases to 90% when instrumentation is used. Clinical results are modest at best in a "worst case," in which the indication for surgery was chronic low back pain. In appropriately selected patients, reduction in visual analog pain scale of approximately one-third can be expected at 2 years. Improvement in the Oswestry Disability Index of approximately 20 to 25% (10 to 15 points) can be expected at 2 years. Somewhat better outcomes are noted in patients with more clear-cut indications, such as spondylolisthesis or traumatic instability (without spinal cord injury).

CONCLUSION

The posterolateral lumbar arthrodesis is a basic technique of spine surgery. Proper attention to biologic preparation of the transverse processes, grafting with autogenous iliac crest, or potentially newer osteoinductive substrates is critical to the biology of fusion. Supplemented by proper pedicle screw technique and rigid instrumentation, arthrodesis rates approaching 90 to 95% can be routinely expected, but successful fusion does not guarantee a successful clinical outcome. The trade-off for the use of internal fixation is an increased risk of complication.

REFERENCES

1. Albee FH. Transplantation of a portion to the tibia into the spine for Pott's disease. *JAMA* 1911;57:885.
2. Hibbs RH. An operation for progressive spinal deformities. *N Y J Med* 1911;93:1010.
3. Campbell WC. Operation for extra-articular fusion of sacroiliac joint. *Surg Gynecol Obstet* 1927;45:218–219.
4. Wilkins WB. Posterolateral fusion of the lumbar and lumbosacral spine. *J Bone Joint Surg* 1953;35(A):1014–1018.
5. Boden SD. The biology of posterolateral lumbar spinal fusion. *Orthop Clin North Am* 1998;29(4):603–619.
6. Gibson S, McLeod I, et al. Allograft versus autograft in instrumented posterolateral lumbar spinal fusion. *Spine* 2002;27:1599–1603.
7. Christensen FB, Hansen ES, Laursen M, et al. Long-term functional outcome of pedicle screw instrumentation as a support for posterolateral spinal fusion: randomized clinical study with a 5-year follow-up. *Spine* 2002;27(12):1269–1277.
8. Davne SH, Meyers DL. Complications of lumbosacral fusion for degenerative disc disease with and without instrumentation. Two-to-five year follow-up. *Spine* 1992;17:349–355.
9. Esses SI, Sachs BL, Dreyzin V. Complications associated with the technique of pedicle screw fixation. A selected survey of ABS members. *Spine* 1993;18:2231–2238.
10. Yaun HA, Garfin SR, Dickman CA, et al. A historical cohort study of pedicle screw fixation in thoracic, lumbar, and sacral fusions. *Spine* 1994;19[suppl 20]:2279S–2296S.
11. Fischgrund JS, Mackay M, Herkowitz HN, et al. Degenerative lumbar spondylolisthesis with spinal stenosis: a prospective randomized study comparing decompressive laminectomy and arthrodesis with and without spinal instrumentation. *Spine* 1997;22:2807–2818.
12. France JC, Yaszemski MJ, Lauerman WC, et al. A randomized prospective study of posterolateral lumbar fusion: outcomes with and without pedicle screw instrumentation. *Spine* 1999;24:553–560.
13. Frtizell P, Hagg O, Wessberg P, et al. Chronic low back pain and fusion: comparison of three surgical techniques: a prospective multicenter randomized study from the Swedish lumbar Spine Study Group. *Spine* 2002;27(11):1131–1141.
14. Zdbelick TA. A prospective, randomized study of lumbar fusion: preliminary results. *Spine* 1993;18:983–991.
15. Harrington PR. Treatment of scoliosis; correction and internal fixation by spinal instrumentation. *J Bone Joint Surg* 1962;44(A):591–610.
16. Aaro S, Ohlen G. The effect of Harrington instrumentation on the sagittal configuration and mobility of the spine in scoliosis. *Spine* 1983;8:570–575.
17. Luque ER, Rapp GF. A new semirigid method for intrapeduncular fixation of the spine. *Orthopaedics* 1988;11:1445–1450.
18. Resina J, Alves AF. A technique of correction and internal fixation for scoliosis. *J Bone Joint Surg* 1997;59-B(2):159–165.
19. Cotrel Y, Dubousset J, Guillaumat M. New universal instrumentation in spinal surgery. *Clin Orthop* 1988;227:10–23.
20. Gaines RW. The use of pedicle-screw internal fixation for the operative treatment of spinal disorders. *J Bone Joint Surg* 2000;82-A:1458–1476.
21. Herkowitz HN, Kurz LT. Degenerative lumbar spondylolisthesis with spinal stenosis. A prospective study comparing decompression with decompression and intertransverse process arthrodesis. *J Bone Joint Surg* 1991;73(6):802–808.
22. Lombardi JS, Wiltse LL, Reynolds J, et al. Treatment of degenerative spondylolisthesis. *Spine* 1985;10(9):821–827.
23. Grob D, Humke T, Dvorak J. Degenerative lumbar spinal stenosis: decompression with and without arthrodesis. *J Bone Joint Surg* 1995;77(A):1036–1041.
24. Bridwell KH, Sedgewick TA, O'Brien F, et al. The role of fusion and instrumentation in the treatment of degenerative spondylolisthesis with spinal stenosis. *J Spinal Disord* 1993;6:461–472.
25. Caragee EJ. Single-level posterolateral arthrodesis, with or without posterior decompression, for the treatment of isthmic spondylolisthesis in adults: a prospective randomized study. *J Bone Joint Surg* 1997;79(A):1175–1180.
26. Grubb SA, Lipscomb JH. Results of lumbosacral fusion for degenerative disc disease with and without instrumentation. Two- to five-year follow-up. *Spine* 1991;17:349–355.
27. Slosar PJ, Reynolds JB, Schofferman J, et al. Patient satisfaction after circumferential lumbar fusion. *Spine* 2000;25:722–726.
28. Blumenthal SL, Gill K. Can lumbar spine radiographs accurately determine fusion in postoperative patients? Correlation of routine radiographs with a second surgical look at lumber fusions. *Spine* 1993;18:1186–1189.
29. Kant AP, Daum WJ, Dean SM, et al. Evaluation of lumbar spine fusion: plain radiographs versus direct surgical exploration and observation. *Spine* 1995;20:2313–2317.
30. Dawson EG, Clader TJ, Bassett LW. A comparison of different methods used to diagnose pseudarthrosis following posterior spinal fusion for scoliosis. *J Bone Joint Surg* 1985;67(A):1153–1159.
31. Anderson T, Christenses FB, Laursen M, et al. Smoking as a predictor of negative outcome in lumbar spinal fusion. *Spine* 2001;26:2623–2628.
32. Deguchi M, Rapoff AJ, Zdeblick TA. Posterolateral fusion for isthmic spondylolisthesis in adults: analysis of fusion rate and clinical results. *J Spinal Disord* 1998;11:459–464.
33. Snider RK, Krumwiede NK, Snider LJ, et al. Factors affecting lumbar spinal fusion. *J Spinal Disord* 1999;12:107–114.
34. Patel TC, Erulkar JS, Grauer JN, et al. Osteogenic protein-1 overcomes the inhibitory effect of nicotine on posterolateral lumbar fusion. *Spine* 2001;26:1656–1661.
35. Glassman SD, Anagnost SC, Parker A, et al. The effect of cigarette smoking and smoking cessation on spinal fusion. *Spine* 2000;25:2608–2615.
36. Simpson JM, Silveri CP, Balderston RA, et al. The results of operations on the lumbar spine in patients who have diabetes mellitus. *J Bone Joint Surg Am* 1993;75:1823–1829.
37. Klein JD, Hey LA, Yu CS, et al. Perioperative nutrition and postoperative complications in patients undergoing spinal surgery. *Spine* 1996;21:2676–2682.
38. Garland DE, Adkins RH, Stewart CA, et al. Regional osteoporosis in women who have a complete spinal cord injury. *J Bone Joint Surg* 2001;83:1195–1200.

39. Spengler DM, Freeman C, Westbrook R, et al. Low back pain following multiple lumbar spine procedures. Failure of initial selection. *Spine* 1980;5:356–360.
40. Junge A, Frohlich M, Ahrens S, et al. Predictors of bad and good outcome of lumbar spine surgery. *Spine* 1996;21:1056–1064.
41. Trief PM, Grant W, Fredrickson B. A prospective study of psychological predictors of lumbar surgery outcome. *Spine* 2000;25:2616–2621.
42. Deberand MS, Masters KS, Colledge AL, et al. Outcomes of posterolateral lumbar fusion in Utah patients receiving workers' compensation. *Spine* 2001;26:738–747.
43. Dzioba RB, Doxey NC. A prospective investigation in the orthopaedic and psychologic predictors of outcome of first lumbar surgery following industrial injury. *Spine* 1984;9:614–623.
44. Riccairdi JE, Pflueger PC, Isaza JE, et al. Transpedicular fixation for the treatment of isthmic spondylolisthesis in adults. *Spine* 1995;20:1917–1922.
45. Guven O, Kumano L, Yalcin S, et al. A single stage posterior approach and rigid fixation for preventing kyphosis in the treatment of spinal tuberculosis. *Spine* 1994;19:1039–1043.
46. Stambough JL. Posterior instrumentation for thoracolumbar trauma. *Clin Orthop* 1997;335:73–88.
47. Kim KW, Ha KY, Moon MS, et al. Fate of the facet joints after instrumented intertransverse process fusion. *Clin Orthop Rel Res* 1999;366:110–119.
48. Gertzbein SD, Robbins SE. Accuracy of pedicular screw placement *in vivo*. *Spine* 1990;15:11–14.
49. Kosay C, Akcali O, Berk RH, et al. A new method for detecting pedicular wall perforation during pedicle screw insertion. *Spine* 2001;26:1477–1481.
50. Ashman RB, Galpin RD, Corin JD, et al. Biomechanical analysis of pedicle screw instrumentation systems in a corpectomy model. *Spine* 1989;14:1398–1405.
51. Kariakovic EE, Daubs MD, Madsen RW, et al. Morphologic characteristics of human cervical pedicles. *Spine* 1997;22:493–500.
52. Wittenberg RH, Lee KS, Shea M, et al. Effect of screw diameter, insertion technique, and bone cement augmentation of pedicular screw fixation strength. *Clin Orthop* 1993;296:278–287.
53. Krag MH, Beynnon BD, Pope MH, et al. An internal fixator for posterior application to short segments of the thoracic, lumbar, or lumbosacral spine. Design and testing. *Clin Orthop Rel Res* 1986;203:75–98.
54. Zdeblick TA, Kunz DN, Cooke ME, et al. Pedicle screw pullout strength. Correlation with insertional torque. *Spine* 1993;18:1673–1676.
55. Hirano T, Hasegawa K, Takahashi HE, et al. Structural characteristics of the pedicle and its role in screw stability. *Spine* 1997;22:2504–2510.
56. Brantley AGU, Mayfield JK, Koenman JB, et al. The effects of pedicle screw fit: an *in vitro* study. *Spine* 1994;19:1752–1758.
57. Zindrick MR, Wiltse LL, Holland WR, et al. A biomechanical study of intrapedicular screw fixation in the lumbosacral spine. *Clin Orthop Rel Res* 1986;203:99–112.
58. Weinstein JN, Rydevik BL, Rausching WR. Anatomical and technical considerations of pedicle screw fixation. *Clin Orthop* 1992;284:34–46.
59. Steffee AD, Biscup RS, Sitowske DJ. Segmental spine plates with pedicle screw fixation. A new internal fixation device for disorders of the lumbar and thoracolumbar spine. *Clin Orthop* 1986;203:45–53.
60. Mirkovic S, Abitbol JJ, Steinman J, et al. Anatomic considerations for sacral screw placement. *Spine* 1991;16(S6):S289–S294.
61. Licht NJ, Rowe DE, Ross LM. Pitfalls of pedicle screw fixation in the sacrum. A cadaver model. *Spine* 1992;17:892–896.
62. Dick JC, Zdeblick TA, Bartel BD, et al. Mechanical evaluation of cross-link designs in rigid pedicle screw systems. *Spine* 1997;22:370–375.
63. Barber JW, Boden SD, Ganey T, et al. Biomechanical study of lumbar pedicle screws: does convergence affect axial pull-out strength? *J Spinal Disord* 1998;11:215–220.
64. Carson WL, Duffield RC, Arendt M, et al. Internal forces and moments in transpedicular spine instrumentation. The effect of pedicle screw angle and transfixation–the 4R-4Bar linkage concept. *Spine* 1990;15:893–901.
65. McCormack T, Karaikovic E, Gaines RW. The load sharing classification of spine fractures. *Spine* 1994;19(15):1741–1744.
66. McLain RF, Sparling E, Benson DR. Early failure of short-segment pedicle instrumentation for thoracolumbar fractures. A preliminary report. *J Bone Joint Surg* 1993;75-A(2):162–167.
67. Parker JW, Lane JR, Gaines RW, et al. Successful short-segment instrumentation and fusion for thoracolumbar spine fractures. *Spine* 2000;25(9):1157–1169.
68. Yerby SA, Ehteshami JR, McLain RF. Offset laminar hooks decrease bending moments of pedicle screws during *in situ* contouring. *Spine* 1997;22:376–381.
69. Butler T, Asher MA, Jayarman G, et al. The strength and stability of some dorsal thoracic anchor sites in osteoporotic spines. *Proc Scoliosis Res Soc* 26th annual meeting. Minneapolis, MN, September 1991(abstr).
70. Wenger D, Miller S, Wilkerson J. Evaluation of fixation sites for segmental instrumentation of the human vertebra. *Proc Scoliosis Res Soc* 16th annual meeting. Montreal, Quebec, September 1981:101–102(abstr).
71. Lu J, Ebraheim NA, Yeasting RA. Translaminar facet screw placement: an anatomic study. *Am J Orthopaed* 1998;27(8):550–555.
72. Deguchi M, Cheng BC, Sato K, et al. Biomechanical evaluation of translaminar facet joint fixation. A comparative study of polylactide pins, screws, and pedicle fixation. *Spine* 1998;23(12):1307–1312.
73. Margulies JY, Seimon LP. Clinical efficacy of lumbar and lumbosacral fusion using the Boucher facet screw fixation technique. *Bull Hosp Jt Dis* 2000;59(1):33–39.
74. Aebi M, Thalgott JS, Webb JK. *AO ASIF principles in spine surgery*. Berlin: Springer, 1998.
75. Humke T, Grob D, Dvorak J, et al. Translaminar screw fixation of the lumbar and lumbosacral spine. A 5-year follow-up. *Spine* 1998;23(10):1180–1184.
76. Coe JD, Warden KE, Herzig M, et al. Influence of bone mineral density on the fixation of thoracolumbar implants. *Spine* 1990;15:902–907.
77. Butler TE, Asher MA, Jayarman G, et al. The strength and stiffness of thoracic implant anchors in osteoporotic spine. *Spine* 1994;19:1956–1962.
78. Hasegawa K, Takahashi H, Uchiyama S, et al. An experimental study of a combination method using pedicle screw and laminar hook for the osteoporotic spine. *Spine* 1997;22:958–962.
79. Sapkas GS, Papadakis SA, Stathakopoulos DP, et al. Evaluation of pedicle screw position in thoracic and lumbar spine fixation using plain radiographs and computed tomography a prospective study of 35 patients. *Spine* 1999;24(18):1926–1929.
80. Lonstein JE, Denis F, Perra JH, et al. Complications associated with pedicle screws. *J Bone Joint Surg* 1999;81-A;11:1519–1528.
81. Esses SI. The AO spinal internal fixture. *Spine* 1989;14:373–378.
82. Esses SI, Bednar DA. The spinal pedicle screw: techniques and systems. *Orthop Rev* 1998;18:676–682.
83. Luque ER. Complications of intrapeduncular correction and fixation. *Orthop Trans* 1988;12:238–239.
84. West JL III, Ogilvie JW, Bradford DS. Complications of the variable screw plate pedicle screw fixation. *Spine* 1992;16:576–579.
85. George DC, Krag MH, Johnson CC, et al. Hole preparation techniques for transpedicular screws. *Spine* 1991;16:181–184.
86. Louis R. Fusion of the lumbar and sacral spine by internal fixation with screw plates. *Clin Orthop* 1986;203:18–33.
87. Steffee AD, Brantigan JW. The variable screw plate spinal fixation system. Report of a prospective study of 250 patients enrolled in Food and Drug Administration clinical trials. *Spine* 1993;18:1160–1172.
88. Hirano T, Hasegawa K, Washio T, et al. Fracture risk during pedicle screw insertion in osteoporotic spine. *J Spinal Disord* 1998;11(6):493–497.
89. Wittenberg RH, Shea M, Swartz DE, et al. Importance of bone mineral density in instrumented spine fusions. *Spine* 1991;16:647–652.
90. Okuyama K, Sato K, Abe E, et al. Stability of transpedicle screwing for the osteoporotic spine: an *in vitro* study of the technical stability. *Spine* 1993;18:2240–2245.
90a. Kumano K, Hirabayashi S, Ogawa Y, et al. Pedicle screws and bone marrow density. *Spine* 1994;19:1157–1161.
91. Lotz JC, Hu SS, Chiu DFM, et al. Carbonated apatite cement augmentation of pedicle screw fixation in the lumbar spine. *Spine* 1997;22:2716–2723.
92. Hu SS, Lotz JC, Chiu DFM, et al. Pedicle screw fixation in the lumbar spine: augmentation with carbonated apatite. Presented at the

30th Annual Meeting of the Scoliosis Research Society, Washington, D.C., October 18–21, 1995.
93. Mardjetko SM, Collolly DJ, Shott S. Degenerative lumbar spondylolisthesis: a meta-analysis of literature 1970-1993. *Spine* 1994;19:2256S–2265S.
94. Greenfield III RT, Capen DA, Thomas Jr JC, et al. Pedicle screw fixation for arthrodesis of the lumbosacral spine in the elderly: an outcome study. *Spine* 1998;23:1470–1475.
95. Weinstein MA, McCabe JP, Cammisa FP. Postoperative spinal wound infection: a review of 2,391 consecutive index procedures. *J Spinal Disord* 2000;13(5):422–426.
96. Kostuik JP, Isreal J, Hall JE. Scoliosis surgery in adults. *Clin Orthop Rel Res* 1973;93:225–234.
97. Roberts FJ, Walsh A, Wing P, et al. The influence of surveillance methods on surgical wound infection rates in a tertiary care spinal surgery service. *Spine* 1998;23:366–370.
98. Capen DA, Claderons RR, Green A. Perioperative risk factors for wound infection after lower back fusions. *Orthop Clin North Am* 1996;27:83–86.
99. Massie JB, Heller JG, Abitbol JJ, et al. Postoperative posterior spinal wound infections. *Clin Orthop Rel Res* 1992;284:99–108.
100. Knapp DR, Jones ET. Use of cortical cancellous allograft for posterior spinal fusion. *Clin Orthop Rel Res* 1988;229:99–106.
101. Dearborn JT, Hu SS, Tribus CB, et al. Thromboembolic complications after major thoracolumbar spine surgery. *Spine* 1999;24:1471.
102. Macdessi SJ, Leong AK, Bentivoglio JEC. Pedicle fracture after instrumented posterolateral lumbar fusion a case report. *Spine* 2001;26:580–582.
102a. Robertson PA, Grobler LJ. Stress fracture of the pedicle: a late complication of posterolateral lumbar fusion. *Spine* 1993;18:930–932.
103. Zucherman J, Hsu K, White A, et al. Early results of spinal fusion using variable spinal plating system. *Spine* 1988;13:570–579.
104. Alanay A, Acaroglu E, Surat A, et al. Short-segment pedicle instrumentation of thoracolumbar burst fractures: does transpedicular intracorporeal grafting prevent early failure? *Spine* 2001;26(2):213–217.
105. Carl AL, Tromanhauser SG, Roger DJ. Pedicle screw instrumentation for thoracolumbar burst fractures and fracture-dislocations. *Spine* 17(8S):S317–S323.
106. Glaser JA, Estes WJ. Distal short segment fixation of thoracolumbar and lumbar injuries. *Iowa Orthop J* 1998;18:87–90.

CHAPTER 57

Interbody Fusion

Eeric Truumees and Gregory T. Brebach

Lumbar interbody fusion techniques are indicated for a variety of clinical conditions ranging from spinal trauma to infection and deformity. Most commonly, however, these fusions are performed in patients with degenerative disc disease and mechanical back pain. The vast majority of patients with mechanical low back pain (LBP) should be and are treated nonoperatively. Fusion is appropriate only when operative results have a reasonable probability to improve on the natural history of the disease.

Traditionally, posterolateral fusions without instrumentation have been the standard form of lumbar stabilization. However, posterolateral fusions have significant shortcomings, particularly in the treatment of mechanical back pain without accompanying stenosis. Reported satisfactory outcomes have varied from 16 to 95% (1,2). Pseudarthrosis rates range from 14 to 70% (2,3). Reoperation and disability rates are 24% and 25%, respectively (1).

Disadvantages of the posterolateral approach include the small surface area available for fusion and the tensile forces to which the graft is subjected. Pedicle screw instrumentation may improve fusion rates, but significant improvements in clinical outcome have not been reported (2,4,5). Finally, the wide dissection and forceful retraction of paraspinal muscles often required for posterolateral lumbar fusion (PLF) and fixation may severely jeopardize the muscles, structurally and functionally, often with a permanent decrease in fatigue characteristics (6). In one study, multifidus muscle specimens were obtained before, during, and after retraction in patients with lumbar spondylolisthesis undergoing posterolateral lumbar fusion, pedicle fixation, and laminectomy. Histopathologic and immunohistochemical analysis revealed that prolonged, continuous retraction resulted in severe muscle damage. This damage could be decreased by letting retractors down every 1.5 hours (7). This "fusion disease" may contribute to chronic LBP.

Even a solid posterolateral fusion allows residual micromotion in the disc space (8–12). Weatherly reported complete pain relief after anterior lumbar interbody fusion (ALIF) in five patients, who, despite solid posterolateral fusions, continued to suffer from disabling pain (13). In each case, discography implicated the disc as the pain source.

Historically, such interbody fusions were recommended only for salvage in patients with multiple failed posterior procedures (14,15). More recently, anterior interbody techniques have grown in popularity in degenerative disc disease as a means to completely remove the presumptive pain generator and to reduce the surgical morbidity associated with the extensor muscle stripping that accompanies a posterior approach (10–12,16–20).

Interbody fusion may also be performed to restore spinal column stability, provide anterior column support, and increase fusion rates for long posterior constructs. Interbody techniques exploit several inherent advantages of the anterior spinal column. First, wide cancellous beds are available for graft contact; second, anterior bone grafts are placed under compression; and third, the fusion mass spans the center of spinal motion. Once mature, the fused segment is more rigid construct than posterior or posterolateral fusions (21) (Table 1).

Interbody fusion may be performed from an anterior or posterior approach with a variety of techniques, grafts, and implants. This chapter explores the indications, advantages, and disadvantages of the various techniques for interbody fusion.

TABLE 1. *Indications for interbody fusion*

Clinical situations in which posterior fusion is less likely to heal
Absent posterior elements/transverse processes
Smokers
Irradiated fusion bed
Failed prior posterior fusion
Stabilization of the spine
After débridement of osteomyelitis or tumor
After hemicorpectomy in some burst fractures
Anterior column support for long posterior constructs
Degenerative disc disease
Restoration of foraminal height in some cases of foraminal stenosis
Degenerative lumbar instability
Spondylolisthesis
Isthmic but also iatrogenic and congenital
Correction of rotatory and lateral listheses
Iatrogenic spinal instability

PATHOPHYSIOLOGY

Intradiscal desiccation and degeneration are ubiquitous attributes of the aging spine. Histologically, these degenerating discs exhibit diminished proteoglycan content, nucleus pulposus volume, and cellularity. Biomechanically, disc stiffness increases (22). These changes are nearly universally noted as part of normal aging.

With disc desiccation, height is lost and facet overriding occurs. With time, bone spurs may form. These spurs or disc herniations may cause symptomatic neurologic compression, which is readily identified by radiographic imaging and easily correlated with the clinical presentation.

This degenerative process may also lead to instability in the form of degenerative spondylolisthesis or scoliosis. Kostuik and Bontiviglio found the prevalence of back pain in patients with adult scoliosis to be the same as that of the population at large, but more incapacitating pain was noted in those with curves greater than 45 degrees (23). Similarly, 10% of women older than the age of 60 years have evidence of a degenerative anterior slip, most commonly at L4-5. Such degenerative spondylolisthesis is particularly common in diabetics; women who have had an oophorectomy; and those with predisposing biomechanical factors, such as hemisacralization of the L-5 body, sagittal facet orientation, or a lowered intercrestal line (passing through L-5 instead of L-4) (4). Typically, these patients also present with neurogenic symptoms that are usually easily diagnosed by history, physical examination, and imaging studies.

In patients with mechanical pain, differentiating normal degenerative change from degenerative disease is difficult. Free nerve endings have been demonstrated in the outer half of the degenerated annulus and may contribute to the mechanical pain associated with disc degeneration (18). In some patients with a diagnosis of mechanical pain, inflammatory markers have been identified histologically within the outer annulus (19).

Degenerative disc disease is occasionally subdivided into internal disc derangement (IDD), isolated disc resorption, and lumbar segmental instability (16). Some authors prefer the single diagnosis of lumbar spondylosis for all patients with degenerative spine disorder (24,25).

IDD is a clinical syndrome of mechanical back pain due to a tear in the annulus in patients with normal plain spine radiographs and no decrease in disc height. Isolated disc resorption (or lumbar spondylosis) encompasses the most common surgically treated subgroup of degenerative disc disease. These patients exhibit mechanical spine pain with reduced intervertebral disc height, end-plate sclerosis, and osteophyte formation (4). Patients typically lose lordosis, but this finding, in isolation, has not been found to correlate with pain (26).

Lumbar segmental instability is manifested by the loss of integrity of the facets and the posterior ligaments, accompanied by advanced disc degeneration. Degenerative spondylolisthesis can lead to foraminal neural compression, but many patients present with mechanical back pain alone. Even low-grade slips are hypermobile, and the mobility increases in higher grades until the disc is completely resorbed (27).

INDICATIONS FOR INTERBODY FUSIONS

Anterior column fusions were initially described by Hodgson to stabilize the spine after anterior débridement of the tuberculous spine (28). Interbody fusion continues to be used for spinal infections, tumors, and trauma after anterior débridement and decompression (29–32). In particular, interbody techniques are advocated in patients with clinical conditions that make posterior fusion alone less likely to heal, such as a history of smoking, irradiated fusion beds, and revision fusions (17).

In patients undergoing long posterior fusions, interbody fusion may be indicated to provide anterior column support, increase fusion rates, or improve sagittal spinal balance (33). Most frequently, these issues arise in patients with spine deformities, in whom specific indications include restoration of lumbar lordosis and proper sagittal balance, lumbar curves greater than 50 degrees, rigid curves, correction of lateral and rotational listhesis, and long fusions to the sacrum (34–36). Interbody techniques are often recommended in patients with higher-grade isthmic spondylolisthesis to correct the preoperative slip angle (37–39).

Degenerative disc disease remains the most common and the most controversial indication for a lumbar interbody fusion. Much of the controversy surrounds correct identification of the pain generator. The history and physical examination, along with magnetic resonance imaging (MRI) and possibly discography all work toward identifying the source of discogenic back pain, but as of yet, there is no single or combination of examinations that definitively reveals the disc as the pain generator.

The cause of the majority of LBP is unknown. In patients with incapacitating nonradicular back pain due to disc degeneration, arthrodesis should only be considered after failure of a lengthy trial of nonoperative treatment. Initially, treatment begins with physical therapy, emphasizing core muscle strengthening and flexibility. Compliant patients eventually progress to aerobic exercise. Nonsteroidal antiinflammatory medications, muscle relaxants, and, occasionally, narcotics allow the patients to more fully participate in their rehabilitation. Smoking cessation should also be actively encouraged. If all of these measures fail, fusion may be considered. However, not all surgeons agree.

Given the frequency of similar degenerative changes in the population at large, many authors report that surgical outcomes for this vaguely defined disease do not justify the associated costs and morbidity (17,40). Other studies have shown that fusions, when performed selectively, can improve on the natural history of mechanical back pain (11,16–18,41). More than the technique used, careful patient selection predicts successful outcome.

In patients with degenerative disease and neurogenic symptoms, interbody fusions are occasionally indicated, particularly for those with spondylolisthesis and degenerative scoliosis (4,42). Although fusion is rarely indicated for primary disc herniations, it may have a role in recurrent herniations (43).

In all these patient groups, interbody fusion may be indicated to

- Increase foraminal volume in those with marked foraminal stenosis from disc height loss or in the concavity of a scoliosis
- Treat painful pseudarthrosis after attempted posterolateral fusion (17)
- Afford a suitable graft surface after laminectomy if the transverse processes have been fractured or are very small
- Stabilize isolated segments with marked lateral listhesis or focal curves causing imbalance
- Provide anterior column support in patients with long constructs extending to the sacrum

PATIENT ASSESSMENT

The determination of suitability for interbody fusion begins with a complete history and physical examination. Red flags often point to etiologies other than discogenic pain. Age older than 50 years or younger than 20 years with acute pain, night pain, nonmechanical pain, constitutional symptoms (fever, chills, malaise), and a history of cancer or immune deficiency are all potential signs and symptoms of tumor or infection. Similarly, a more detailed, multisystem evaluation is required in patients with unexplained weight loss, fever, chills, or night sweats.

The physical findings in patients with mechanical back pain are generally nonspecific. These patients do not usually exhibit point tenderness or paraspinal spasms. The vast majority of patients with acute LBP typically present with muscle spasms and identifiable painful area. Patients with discogenic back pain often report difficulty with sitting and forward lumbar flexion. Pain that increases more with extension than flexion may suggest involvement of the facet joints. Typically, however, patients display pain and difficulty with flexion and rotation maneuvers of the lumbar spine. Normal motor, sensory, and reflex findings are expected. Waddell's signs are helpful in identifying nonorganic pain syndromes in patients with significant psychosocial issues that may make them less likely to have a successful surgical outcome (Table 2).

In the absence of red flags, radiographs are recommended only if a trial of nonoperative treatment fails to relieve symptoms when indicated. When indicated, radiographic assessment begins with standing anterior-posterior and lateral views of the lumbosacral spine. The foramina and pars interarticularis are well visualized on oblique radiographs. The lateral coned down view of the lumbosacral junction affords an orthogonal view of the L-5 to S-1 interspace. These standing films identify spondylolisthesis, the extent of degenerative changes, and measurement of spinal alignment. Degenerative disc disease is frequently associated with a loss of lumbar lordosis and vertebral subluxations.

TABLE 2. *Waddell's nonorganic physical signs*

Tenderness: pain at the tip of the tailbone; pain, numbness, or giving way of the whole leg; pain to light touch

Simulation: pain with light axial loading of the head or shoulders; pain with pelvic rotation through the hips; reproduction of pain with rolling of the lumbar skin

Distraction: no pain with a sitting straight-leg raise; pain with a supine straight-leg raise

Regional: nonanatomic distributions of weakness or sensory changes (especially in stocking glove distribution)

Overreaction: moaning, trembling, collapsing, sweating, and multiple emergency admissions

From Waddell G, McCullough JA, Kummel E, et al. Nonorganic physical signs in low back pain. *Spine* 1980;5:117, with permission.

The specificity of plain radiography, however, is limited by the high prevalence of lumbar spondylosis in the general population. Signs suggestive of degenerative disc disease were present in 90% of adults in one study, of which only 53% were symptomatic (26). Frymoyer reported that traction spurs or disc space narrowing between the fourth and fifth lumbar vertebrae had a statistically significant presence in patients with severe LBP (26). These radiographic findings were also associated with lower extremity symptoms, including pain, weakness, and numbness. Flexion-extension radiographs are useful to identify occult instability and to evaluate the mobility of known spondylolisthesis. In patients with a spine deformity, standing long cassette radiographs are necessary to assess spinal balance.

MRI evidence of disc degeneration is seen as a black disc on T2-weighted images, reflecting diminished water content (44). With degeneration and subsequent dehydration, the previously discrete nuclear pulposus signal found in a T2-weighted MRI blends with the signal of the surrounding annulus. Aprill and Bogduk have described a high-intensity zone (HIZ) in the outer annulus. They concluded the HIZ represents a tear of the outer annulus and often is associated with painful, concordant discography (45). The relevance of the HIZ is not universally accepted, however (46).

TABLE 3. *Modic changes*

	Magnetic resonance image			
Stage	T1	T2	Tissue	Clinical correlation
I	D	I	Vascular fibrous tissue	Acute annular tearing; end-plate fissure
II	I	D	Fatty replacement	Chronic marrow of disuse
III	D	D	End-plate sclerosis	Chronic spondylosis

D, decreased; I, increased.

From Modic MT, Ross JS. Magnetic resonance imaging in the evaluation of low back pain. *Orthop Clin North Am* 1991;22:283, with permission.

TABLE 4. *Interbody fusion techniques*

Technique	Advantages	Disadvantages	Fusion rates	Unique complications
ALIF	Spares extensors Indirect foraminal decompression Low blood loss Better height restoration No epidural compressions Minimally invasive approach Virgin operative site if prior PSF Allows most complete disc excision	May require second surgeon No canal decompression Cannot be used alone if unstable Limited in prior abdominal surgery	16.6–97.0%	Retrograde ejaculation Ileus Lateral cage placement Iatrogenic disc herniation
PLIF	Allows direct decompression Interbody and transpedicular fix through 1 incision	Requires neural retraction Difficult if prior scar from lami May not get as much height	73–100%	Arachnoiditis Epidural bleeding Unisized cage displacement Postoperative leg pain
TLIF	Same as PLIF No significant nerve root retraction Do not remove midline ligaments anteriorly or posteriorly Maintains tension band for graft Contralateral laminar surface may be used for graft May be used higher up in lumbar spine than in PLIF Decreased risk of epidural scarring	More unusual anatomic region; difficult at L-5 to S-1 in males Long-term outcomes not available	90% (2 year)	DRG injury possible
270 degrees	Minimally invasive approach	Long-term outcomes not available Learning curve Costs for equipment	—	Implant malposition
360 degrees	Higher fusion rate	Longer procedure and higher morbidity	90% (one and two level)	Additive complication rates

ALIF, anterior lumbar interbody fusion; DRG, dorsal root ganglion; PLIF, posterior lumbar interbody fusion; PSF, posterior spinal fusion; TLIF, transforaminal lumbar interbody fusion.

Modic et al. categorized the end-plate changes seen in patients with disc degeneration (47). Type I end-plates exhibit increased T2 signal intensity, representing disruption and fissuring of the vertebral end-plates with the subsequent ingrowth of fibrous tissues. Over time, these changes evolved into type II degeneration. Here, fatty degeneration predominates, and the peridiscal bone marrow displays an increased T1 and an isointense T2 signal. Type III changes reflect sclerosis as seen on plain radiographs and are hypointense on both T1 and T2 sequences (Table 3).

Discography may have use as the sole provocative test of pain generation from the intervertebral disc (9). In discography, fluid is injected into the disc, increasing end-plate pressure. Increased end-plate pressure may elicit a pain response from the nonsedated patient.

Disc morphology can then be assessed fluoroscopically. Disruptions of normal disc morphology and dye leakage are found in up to 37% of asymptomatic patients (40). A study is positive only if the radiographic changes are accompanied by a pain response that mimics the patient's typical symptoms (8). Adjacent control levels are also injected and should be pain free. Discography is performed only as a preoperative test in psychologically normal patients with positive MRI findings. The rate of false-positive discography has been shown to be low in subjects with normal psychometric profiles and without chronic pain (10%), but false-positive painful injections were found to be very common in subjects with chronic pain (40%) or abnormal psychometric testing (83%) (48). However, discography has not been proven to improve fusion outcomes (11,40,49).

In Colhoun's study of 137 patients with positive provocative discography, 89% reported sustained benefit from fusion surgery at the painful level. In 20 additional patients fused without a positive discogram, only 52% benefited from surgery (50). Goldner noted inferior surgical outcomes when a procedure was undertaken for a positive discogram that was not related to any specific MRI abnormality (14).

OPERATIVE APPROACH AND GRAFT MATERIAL

Interbody fusion can be achieved through anterior, posterior, or circumferential approaches. Options include: ALIF; posterior interbody techniques: posterior lumbar interbody fusion (PLIF), transforaminal lumbar interbody fusion (TLIF); and anterior-posterior techniques, such as the 270-degree and 360-degree fusions. Each has inherent advantages, disadvantages, indications, risks, and benefits (11,14,16,18,51–57) (Tables 4 and 5).

These approaches are used to place a variety of interbody grafts and implants. An ideal graft is biomechanically compatible with its host tissues. When standing, 80% of spine loads are transmitted through the anterior column (58). The graft or implant must withstand these loads and provide a stable environment conducive to fusion (59).

Initially, autologous, bicortical iliac crest autograft was recommended. Often, these freestanding grafts were held in place with a screw and washer. Autologous iliac crest alone is associated with a high rate of graft collapse, loss of correction, and subsequent pseudarthrosis (60–62). To avoid graft collapse and the additional morbidity of structural versus morselized bone graft harvest, cortical allografts [e.g., femoral ring allograft (FRA), fibular strut allograft], vertical mesh cages (e.g., Harms, Pyramesh), carbon fiber cages (Brantigan), and cylindrical, threaded cages (Ray, BAK, LT) have been developed for interbody fusions (56,60,63–69). Cages are designed to prevent postoperative collapse by providing a structural support to the interspace while the cancellous graft material incorporates. The Bagby and Kuslich concept of interbody fusion was to provide stability by restoration of disc height and annular tension (70). The threads on the cage afford additional fixation strength. Many of these devices have been used in anterior and posterior approaches, but may not be U.S. Food and Drug Administration (FDA)–approved for both applications. It is important that surgeons be aware of the FDA status of the selected implant.

Similarly, in the multiple level anterior fusions performed in deformity surgery, structural grafts (e.g., rib struts) are associated with lower pseudarthrosis rates than morselized graft. However, rib struts do not maintain sagittal alignment as well as metallic implants or structural allografts (33). Overall, anterior structural allografts and fusion cages have been found to be effective in maintaining correction in deformity surgery, with pseudarthrosis rates comparable to those of autografts (36).

Allograft ring and PLIF spacers may be cut and fashioned from a segment of dense cortical, appendicular bone by the surgeon or purchased in precut and precontoured form to function as biologic cages and provide anterior column support. FRA, for example, has a compressive strength of more than 25,000 N, three times stronger than surrounding vertebral bone (62). Use of allograft bone may have some advantages over metallic implants in that progression of fusion is easier to assess than metallic cages, and the bone can easily be cut if proud or migrated.

Janssen et al. found no evidence of bone cage resorption or infectious inflammatory process in their series of allograft implants used in anterior and posterior interbody fusions (56). Butterman found that FRAs were as effective, clinically and radiographically, as tricortical iliac autografts when used as an anterior structural element in revision lumbar spine fusion for patients who have undergone multiple surgical procedures for pseudarthrosis or flatback deformity (71).

Traditionally, metallic implants have been avoided in the face of pyogenic osteomyelitis. Most authors recommend bicortical iliac crest autograft or stacked rib struts with subsequent posterior stabilization (29,72). However, others have reported success with titanium cages in the surgical treatment of vertebral osteomyelitis (73).

A typical manufactured FRA set consists of color-coded graft-sizers that correspond precisely to the size of the precut grafts. The grafts range in size from 11 to 14 mm wide and 11 to 14 mm deep and vary in height from 5 to 11 mm. The rostral and caudal faces of the grafts are corrugated, increasing resistance to migration.

Biomechanical studies have shown interlocked fibular strut allografts to be more rigid than the FRA. This added initial stability may make fibular struts preferable to ring grafts as standalone devices in ALIF surgery (60). On the other hand, although these struts or long, thin cages are convenient in higher grades of spondylolisthesis, they do not afford significant height reconstitution and foraminal decompression. Further, Janssen reported no cases of graft migration, infection, or subsidence in 100 cases using PLIF or FRA biologic cages (62). Molinari et al. reported 5-year radiographic outcomes of anterior column structural allografts in 20 patients. Of the patients, 98.5% showed incorpo-

TABLE 5. *Soft selection criteria for various means of interbody fusion*

Situation	Relative preference
Posterior decompression is necessary	PLIF[a]
Previous retroperitoneal approach	PLIF
Pedicle screw instrumentation planned	PLIF
Male patient (to avoid retrograde ejaculation)	PLIF
Previous laminectomy or discectomy	ALIF
Nerve root anomaly present (retraction more difficult)	ALIF
Loss of lumbar lordosis	ALIF
L-5 to S-1 level	ALIF
Foraminal stenosis without central or lateral stenosis	ALIF
Large cage needed for stabilization	ALIF
Multiple-level anterior support needed in deformity	ALIF
Presence of infection with psoas muscle abscess	ALIF

ALIF, anterior lumbar interbody fusion; PLIF, posterior lumbar interbody fusion.

[a]PLIF in this context means PLIF or its variant, transforaminal lumbar interbody fusion.

ration, none showed evidence of collapse, and there was no difference in sagittal plane measurements obtained immediately after surgery and those obtained at follow-up examinations (74).

Vertical titanium mesh cages are even stronger than allograft and not as brittle. These cages attach to the bone through tines of vertical cages. In one series of structural titanium mesh cages implanted into the anterior column, sagittal correction was maintained and radiographic complications were rarely observed. Seventy-eight percent of the anterior levels were judged to be fused at minimum 2-year follow-up by observers examining plain radiographs (75). Vertical cages and carbon fiber ramps are rarely indicated for stand-alone anterior placement. More typically, these devices are used as part of an anterior release and fusion procedure that precedes long posterior instrumentations or they are placed with a PLIF or TLIF approach.

BAK and similar cylindrical cage systems are also indicated for ALIF, TLIF, and PLIF. Distraction of the interspace may be maintained with these devices. In cadaveric studies, these devices increased the volume of the neuroforamen by 22.9% at L4-5 and 21.5% at L-5 to S-1. Posterior disc height increased by 37.1% at L4-5 and 45.1% at L-5 to S-1. The neuroforaminal areas significantly increased, by 29.0% at L4-5 and 33.8% at L-5 to S-1 (57).

More recently, a great deal of marketing effort has supported the idea of second-generation cylindrical cages with built-in lordosis, such as Lumbar Tapered Cage (Medtronic Sofamor Danek, Memphis, TN). The true clinical advantage of these systems remains to be proven, however. In one prospective comparative radiographic study between two geometrically varying implants used in single-level PLIF surgery, 40 patients were randomly assigned rectangular cages or wedged cages with a 4-degree inclination. Quantitative assessment of the lumbar spinal profile on standing neutral lateral radiographs was performed before surgery as well as 6 weeks and 12 months after surgery. No significant difference in the lumbar sagittal profile was noted with use of 4-degree wedged cages. The authors concluded that normal sagittal alignment after single-level lumbar fusion can be achieved with either cage design (76).

Biomechanically, ALIF cages are the weakest in flexion and rotation (57). Some reports of high failure rates with stand-alone cages have led to recommendations of supplemental posterior fixation in most, if not all cases (77). Pellise et al. performed a prospective study of L-5 to S-1 laparoscopic ALIF with twin stand-alone carbon-fiber cages in a cohort of 12 patients. An independent radiologist evaluated dynamic flexion-extension films and computed tomography (CT) scans at 6 and 12 months after surgery. Although the L-5 to S-1 mobility did not exceed 5 degrees in the dynamic study, the overall CT scan fusion rate at 2 years of follow-up was only 16.6%, an unacceptably low fusion rate (78). On the other hand, Pape and others demonstrated significant additional immobilization of the motion segment with staged ALIF after posterior transpedicular stabilization of the spondylolytic lumbosacral interspaces in 15 patients with low-grade spondylolisthesis at L-5 to S-1. They performed a two-stage open posterior and endoscopic anterior lumbar fusion using carbon fiber (Brantigan I/F) cages. At surgery, tantalum markers were implanted into the fifth lumbar (L-5) and the first sacral (S-1) vertebra. Roentgen stereophotogrammetric analysis of intervertebral motion was done after the first and second surgical procedures. The combination of ALIF and posterior transpedicular stabilization led to significant decreases in translation or angular motion (79).

The implant, whether allograft bone or a titanium cage, should be filled with autogenous, iliac crest bone graft. However, successful fusion has been reported with other strategies. Csecsei and colleagues reported a 95.7% fusion rate using local bone in PLIF constructs for isthmic slips (80). Wimmer et al. studied a group of 94 consecutive patients with painful spondylolisthesis undergoing combined anterior and posterior fusion. Pseudarthrosis occurred in seven fused levels (3%) managed with autogenic bone grafts and in seven patients (8%) managed with allogenic bone grafts. Pseudarthrosis was not significantly different between the two groups. In view of the possible complications associated with harvesting iliac crest bone, the authors concluded that the use of allogenic bone is justified (81). Hashimoto et al. reported good results with local autograft plus graft extenders, such as ceramic granules (66).

Another emerging technology involves the use of bone morphogenic protein (BMP) inside the cage. These proteins add cost but decrease graft site pain and morbidity (82). InFUSE (BMP-7) (Medtronic, Memphis, TN) bone graft has been shown to promote osteoinduction and fusion. BMP-7 is applied to an absorbable collagen sponge and is FDA approved in ALIF with threaded cortical allografts. In one recent study, all patients who received InFUSE bone graft showed radiographic evidence of bony induction and early incorporation of the cortical allografts, with fusion present at 12 and 24 months (83). A competing commercial BMP, osteogenic protein (also BMP-7), is in clinical trials for PLF and is likely to attain FDA approval in the near term.

ANTERIOR LUMBAR INTERBODY FUSION

An ALIF may be performed alone or with supporting posterior fixation. Stand-alone ALIF is best reserved for patients without significant instability. In degenerative conditions, a collapsed disc space is a better indication for ALIF than a tall disc space. The authors definitely recommend adjunctive posterior stabilization for patients with marked bone loss due to osteomyelitis, prior laminectomies, or spondylolisthesis.

The advantages of the anterior approach include wide access to the disc space, complete ligamentous release that permits interspace distraction, indirect compression of the neuroforamina, avoidance of posterior muscle stripping, avoidance of epidural scar formation, and structural support of the anterior column (21,84). Disadvantages to the stand-alone ALIF include difficulty achieving rigid fixation (especially at L-5 to S-1), the potential for graft failure or migration, and the risk of injury to the iliac veins and autonomic plexus. Relative contraindications to anterior approaches include active peritoneal or pelvic infection, previous open anterior approach to lumbar spine, previous lower abdominal surgery, pelvic inflammatory disease, atherosclerosis of vessels, obesity, and young, male patients still considering having a family.

Typically, stand-alone ALIF is not recommended in patients with significant neurogenic symptoms. However, a cadaveric CT study found that anteriorly or laterally placed interbody distraction implants provide anterior slip reduction and increases canal and foraminal volume (85). A clinical series of 56 patients with back pain, neuroclaudication, or both from degenerative spondylolisthesis and spinal stenosis underwent ALIF for reduction and fusion. Outcomes were comparable to the published outcomes of *in situ* fusion after formal laminectomy. The authors concluded that laminectomy and, hence, epidural scar may not be necessary in the treatment of degenerative spondylolisthesis with stenosis (84).

The spine may be approached anteriorly through a retroperitoneal or transperitoneal route. The retroperitoneal approach provides access to all lumbar vertebrae from L-1 to the sacrum. The transperitoneal approach is limited to intervertebral levels above L-4 because the mobilization of the great vessels and hypogastric plexus required significantly increases bleeding and genitourinary complications, particularly in males. The frequency of ileus is also reduced with the retroperitoneal approach.

Preoperative Care

For most patients undergoing anterior approaches to the lumbar spine, a bowel preparation with magnesium citrate and a pHiso-Hex (GlaxoSmithKline, Boronia, Australia) abdominal scrub are recommended the night before surgery. A nasogastric tube and Foley catheter are used to decompress the hollow viscera. In older patients with atherosclerosis, pulse oximetry attached to the great toe may detect embolic phenomena as the arteries are mobilized. All instruments for an emergency vascular repair should be available in the operating room. Somatosensory evoked potentials and electromyographic monitoring may be useful. Good lighting from headlights, overheads, or lights that attach to the retractor system greatly improves surgical visualization.

ALIF surgery is best undertaken on a radiolucent operating room table. Before preparation and draping, make sure good anterior-posterior and lateral images are possible. In tables with a central floor post, the surgeon may need to reposition head extension to the patient's feet and slide the patient down. If there are radiologic problems during surgery, such as fluoroscopic white-out, adding saline to the body cavity often improves resolution.

For surgery above L4-5, a left-sided, retroperitoneal approach is recommended, which avoids the liver and helps to protect the more fragile vena cava, lying to the right of the aorta. For procedures involving the L4-5 and L-5 to S-1 disc spaces, a lateral or anterior approach may be used. If L-5 to S-1 is the only intended fusion level, an anterior approach is undertaken in the supine position (Fig. 1).

Many spine surgeons are capable of performing retroperitoneal approaches, but a vascular surgeon should be available in case of a vessel injury. If an access surgeon performs the approach, clearly communicate the surgical goals so the right degree of exposure is achieved, and review the radiographs together preoperatively. A spine surgeon undertaking the approach must be comfortable with retroperitoneal and transperitoneal routes in case significant retroperitoneal scarring blocks access.

Once the discs are identified, the level is localized fluoroscopically. A pin should be positioned in the exact midline and well centered in the anterior-posterior view. A spinous process should appear to be equidistant to each pedicle, because small errors of rotation may lead to significant errors of malposition. Anterior osteophytes obstructing access to the disc space are removed with a rongeur, further assisting orientation.

When only a single interspace exposure is required for degenerative disease, various "mini-open" approaches yield acceptable visualization with cosmetically more appealing scars and perhaps lower procedural morbidity. These variants of the standard open retroperitoneal approach rely on the experience of the surgeon and powerful, self-contained retractor systems to minimize the incision length.

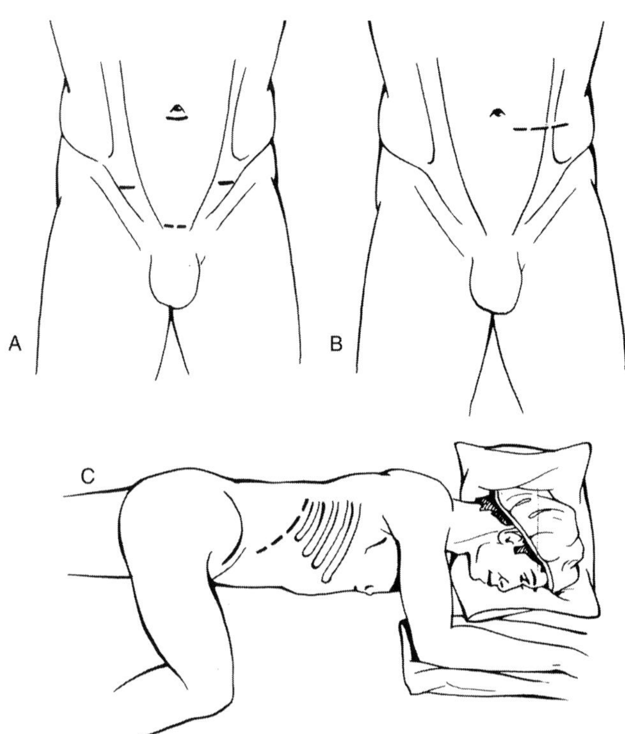

FIG. 1. Skin incisions for the anterior lumbar approach. **A:** Mini-retroperitoneal approach. The anterior rectus sheath is divided, and the rectus abdominis is protected. **B:** Laparoscopic approach allows for small skin incisions for placement of the camera (periumbilical portal, 5-mm incisions for lateral retractors, and a 15- to 20-mm incision for placement of the fusion cage. **C:** Flank approach. Position the patient laterally with the ipsilateral hip flexed to relax the psoas muscle. For L-1, the incision will be at the eleventh rib, for L2-3 access, the twelfth rib is the landmark, and an incision is made midway between the iliac crest and the inferior aspect of the twelfth rib for L3-4 disc space. (Modified from Chapman MW, Szabo RM, Marder R, et al., eds. *Chapman's orthopaedic surgery.* Philadelphia: Lippincott Williams & Wilkins, 2001:3809, with permission.)

When the endoscopic approach is used, a suprapubic incision is made in the plane of the disc space. Special working portals, usually specific to the implant system being used, are inserted through this portal and docked to the anterior spinal column once safe passage between or around the vascular structures has been confirmed.

In a 2-year follow-up retrospective review, 28 patients underwent ALIF via a 6- to 10-cm left lower quadrant transverse skin. A paramedian anterior rectus fascial Z-plasty allowed access to the retroperitoneal space for placement of a variety of implants including autogenous bone, FRAs, carbon fiber cages, and vertical mesh cages. No vascular, visceral, or urinary tract injuries occurred, but in three cases, a mild ileus was noted. The authors prefer this approach because it is safe, uses a small skin incision, avoids cutting abdominal wall musculature, allows for multiple-level anterior spinal fusions by a variety of interbody fusion techniques, and does not require transperitoneal violation or endoscopic instrumentation (86). Remember that endoscopic and open ALIF represent different approaches, not different operations, and the indications for surgery remain the same. Surgical approaches are discussed in detail in Chapters 53A and 53B.

Interbody Fusion Techniques

Regardless of when an open or "mini-open" approach has been used, once the level has been identified and surrounding soft tissues protected, the general sequence of steps for end-plate preparation and implant insertion vary with the chosen device. For most cylindrical cage systems, partial discectomies can be undertaken through various guides. First, place an alignment guide in the midline hole and make left and right pilot holes into the disc with an 8-mm drill. The authors recommend as complete a discectomy as possible regardless of the implant selected. Careful attention to the posterolateral corners of the disc space allows greater distraction and increase the area available for bone graft. Further, removing this disc material minimizes the risk of iatrogenic disc protrusion into the spinal canal when the implants are impacted into the disc space.

Incise the disc parallel to each end-plate with a long-handled 15-blade knife. Then, use a Cobb elevator to separate the disc from the end-plate. Excise as much disc material as possible with a pituitary rongeur. Completely denude the end-plates of disc and cartilage using ring curettes. Various distracters are available to improve visualization of the posterior disc space. If biologic or vertical cages are to be used, partially decorticate the end-plates with a long 4- or 5-mm power burr to enhance vascular ingrowth. Ring, vertical implants, and carbon fiber ramps are typically inserted with "all-in-one" distractor and impactor devices. Final positioning is then verified with fluoroscopy. Additional bone graft is packed around the cages.

If cylindrical cages are being used, disc space distraction is undertaken with proprietary plugs. Threaded cylindrical cages or bone dowels are easier to insert in this manner than vertical cages or femoral rings. Continuous visualization of the midline remains critical to the correct placement of these devices. Alternate pilot holes are used to gradually tap larger distractor plugs into the disc space. The plug should be recessed slightly into the annulus. Appropriate restoration of annular tension is somewhat subjective, but the plug should be difficult to pull straight out of the disc space, whereas a twisting motion will dislodge it.

Once appropriate distraction has been achieved, insert the reamer guide or sleeve over the plug. After checking the position of the iliac veins, the tines of the drill tube are tapped into the adjacent bone. Carefully check the alignment of the tube. Especially in cases of uncorrected spondylolisthesis, improper orientation will lead to asymmetric drilling of the end-plates and poor cage purchase. With the tubes in place, the implant sites are prepared with short and long reamers. Again, use a pituitary rongeur to remove disc material and bone debris from the drill hole. Insert a bone tap into the sleeve to further prepare the end-plates. Be careful not to overtap, thereby stripping the bone. If this occurs, ream up to the next-sized implant. This is not an ideal solution, as more of the stronger, cortical bone plate is lost, exposing more cancellous bone than optimal for fixation. Next, screw in the cage itself using intermittent fluoroscopic guidance by rotating the implant driver handle clockwise. Once fully seated, ensure the appropriate alignment of the cage relative to the end-plates. With the BAK device, the T-handle must be parallel to the plane of the disc space to ensure orientation of the bone ports to the end-plates (Fig. 2).

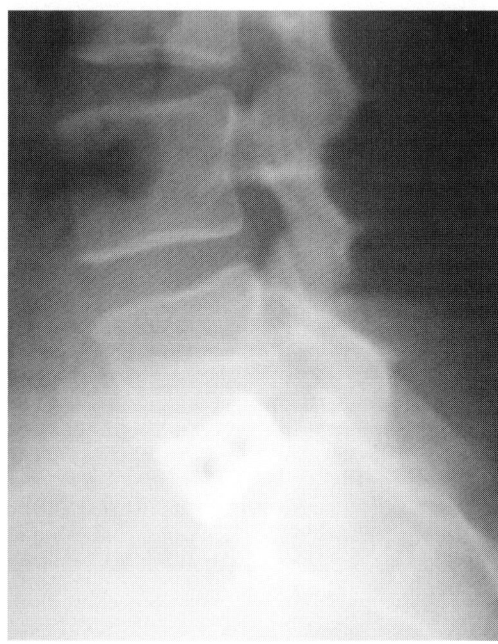

FIG. 2. Lateral radiograph taken after anterior lumbar interbody fusion, using threaded cages. Note the increase in disc height and resultant distraction of the foramina.

Sizing the implant is based on the degree of distraction achieved during surgery, and careful measurements must be made preoperatively of the end-plate dimensions on MRI or CT scan. The disc height is estimated by measuring the height of a normal lumbar disc space one level above or below the level to be fused. This height represents the goal to be achieved at the diseased level.

Many systems include templates to assist the surgeon in selecting the correct implant. Use the available trial's templates to assess ligament tension. For many systems, the appropriate trial can be countersunk 4 to 5 mm into the body and yet remain 3 to 4 mm from the posterior longitudinal ligament. Similarly, with many threaded cages, the actual implant is larger than the distraction plug (by 3 mm in the BAK system).

For metallic implants, recessed placement is ideal. The adage "ream long and cage short" emphasizes the importance of countersinking the cage and packing additional bone in front. This anterior bone graft is useful to monitor the progress of fusion (the sentinel sign) (87).

A standard closure is performed. Typically, no drains are required. If a transperitoneal approach has been used, close the anterior peritoneum to prevent bowel herniation. If an endoscopic procedure was performed, remove the fan retractor and retraction stitch and inspect the vessels for injury or thrombosis.

POSTERIOR LUMBAR INTERBODY FUSION

PLIF allows anterior column arthrodesis and posterior transpedicular stabilization through the same incision. The procedure was introduced in 1945 by Cloward to treat lumbar disc herniations (88). Initial popularity declined as high rates of pseudarthrosis and graft dislodgement became evident (89). The advent of transpedicular instrumentation and fusion cages has led to a resurgence of interest in this technique.

PLIF is especially useful in patients with LBP and symptomatic nerve root compression (88). Some surgeons have found it useful in grade I or II degenerative or isthmic spondylolisthesis with radiculopathy, reducing the percentage of the slip and increasing the posterior disc height, while achieving high 96 to 100% fusion rates (66,80). Advantages include a single, posterior approach, avoidance of injury to the hypogastric plexus and the associated risk of retrograde ejaculation, and the avoidance of a second surgery for anterior column support. Disadvantages include technical difficulty, the risk of graft displacement, potential destabilization of the anterior and posterior columns, and an increased risk of nerve root injury, dural tears, and epidural fibrosis from excessive retraction (4). Contraindications to PLIF include significant epidural scarring that prevents mobilization of roots, osteoporosis, and pathology above the midlumbar level, particularly the conus level or above. Posterior interbody fusions require adherence to the following four biomechanical principles (54,90,91):

1. Preserve the integrity of the posterior motion segment that serves to stabilize and compress the graft
2. Preserve the cortical end-plates to avoid seating the graft in the soft cancellous bone of the vertebral bodies
3. Achieve maximal removal of the disc material
4. Fill the disc space with compacted autogenous bone graft

A PLIF is performed in the prone position, using a spinal frame that allows decompression of the abdominal contents and maintenance of proper lumbar lordosis. In healthy, younger patients, hypotensive anesthesia may further decrease blood loss and improve visualization. Some authors advocate the knee-chest position, which may allow for greater thecal sac retraction, but the surgeon must restore physiologic lordosis before final instrumentation (92) (Fig. 3).

A 6- to 10-cm incision is made just cranial to the spinous process of the surgical level. Careful control of bleeding is essential at each stage, not only limiting operative blood loss, but allowing for clear and readily identifiable landmarks for dissection. Skeletonize the level to be fused, further revealing all pertinent landmarks and increasing the surface area available for fusion. Bluntly dissect over the bilateral facets with a Cobb and laparoscopic sponges. The capsules of the facets above and below the fusion level are left intact. Expose the lateral pars interarticularis and expose the transverse processes above and below the intended level, taking care not to violate the intertransverse membrane when a concomitant posterolateral intertransverse fusion is planned.

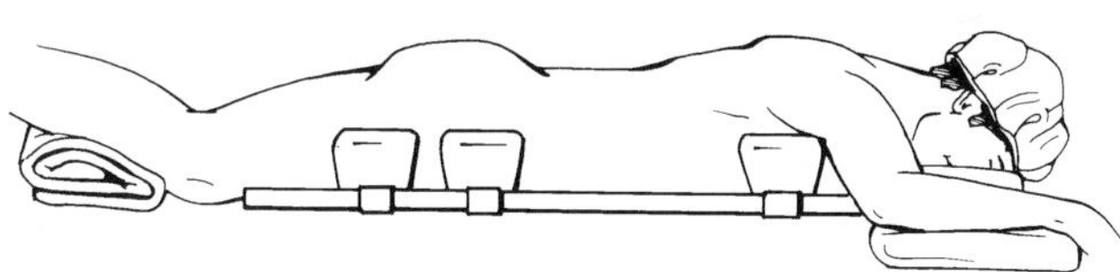

FIG. 3. Positioning for posterior lumbar interbody fusion or transforaminal lumbar interbody fusion. (Modified from Chapman MW, Szabo RM, Marder R, et al., eds. *Chapman's orthopaedic surgery*. Philadelphia: Lippincott Williams & Wilkins, 2001:3794, with permission.)

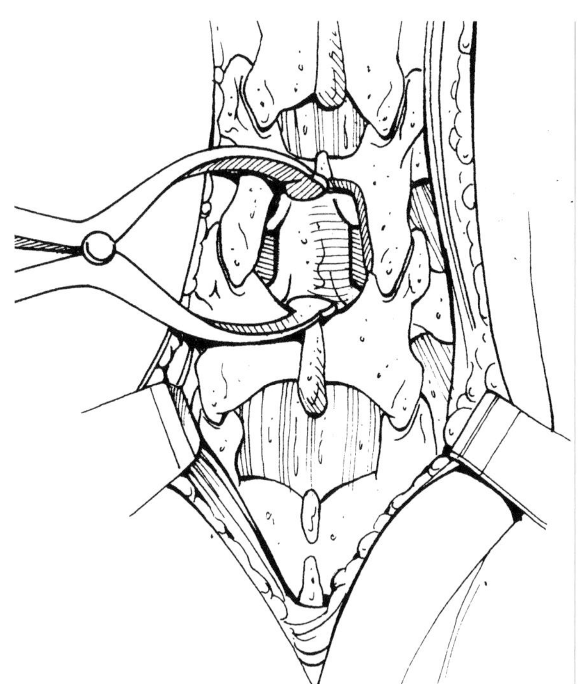

FIG. 4. Posterior lumbar interbody fusion approach midline laminectomy and partial facetectomy. A distractor is used here, but pedicle screws can also be used. (Modified from An HS, Lee RH III, eds. *An atlas of surgery of the spine*. London: William Dunitz, 1998:220, with permission.)

With the exposure completed, the three main steps of the PLIF are as follows: laminectomy, removal of the intervertebral disc, and interbody fusion. A wide laminectomy allows easy identification of the lateral border of the dura, the lateral disc space, and the exiting and traversing nerve roots. Preserve the superior portion of the superior laminae as well as the inferior portion of the inferior laminae. This adds to the stability of the construct and preserves muscle attachment sites, as well as the interspinous and supraspinous ligaments. Remove the superior one-third of the inferior facet and the medial two-thirds of the superior facet to the level of the pedicle. Often, at L-5 to S-1, less bone removal is required because of the wide canal at this level (Fig. 4).

Pedicle fixation restores posterior segmental stability after PLIF and minimizes graft retropulsion. The pedicle screws also provide a convenient way to distract the disc. A localization radiograph is taken to confirm the appropriate attitude of the pedicle in the cranial and caudal planes. In general, the L-3 pedicle is perpendicular to the floor. Superior levels incline cranially, and inferior levels decline caudally. S-1 pedicle screws are placed at the intersection of a horizontal line connecting the inferior aspect of the lumbosacral facets and a vertical line tangential to the lateral border of the superior facet (Fig. 5).

The dura and traversing nerve roots are then retracted medially and protected for appropriate visualization of the disc. Angled dural

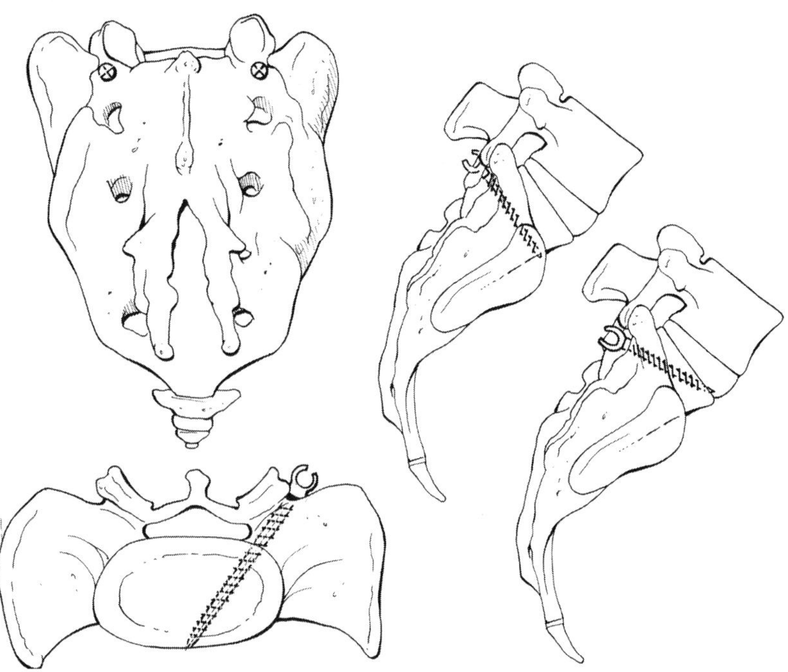

FIG. 5. Anterior-posterior and lateral view of sacral screw placement. (Modified from Chapman MW, Szabo RM, Marder R, et al., eds. *Chapman's orthopaedic surgery.* Philadelphia: Lippincott Williams & Wilkins, 2001:3798, with permission.)

retractors can be used to retract the exiting nerve root superiorly and the dura medially. It is important not to overdistract the neural structures because of the risk. This lessens the likelihood of neural fibrosis. With retractors lateral to the thecal sac, ensure that the thecal sac can be adequately mobilized to midline from either side. If the dura is immobile, gently tease the adhesions free with a Penfield 4 elevator. Meticulous cauterization of the epidural vessels with bipolar electrocautery further assists visualization. Incise the annulus with a long-handled 15-blade knife. Remove loose disc fragments with a pituitary rongeur to create a working space (Fig. 6).

A rod or working plate is placed between the previously placed pedicle screws on each side. An intervertebral distracter is used to open the disc space, and the rod is tightened to the screws to maintain distraction. If the pedicle screw purchase is tenuous, it is better to avoid distracting on the screws themselves.

With the disc space well exposed, aggressively curette the end-plates and remove the disc material and end-plate cartilage. Specialized instruments are available for disc removal. They include angled and straight disc rongeurs, osteotomes, and curettes. If these instruments are not available, curettes, pituitary rongeurs, and osteotomes can be used to prepare the disc space (Fig. 7).

Next, insert an 8-mm intradiscal shaper parallel to the end-plates. Rotate the shaper, allowing its side-cutting flutes to remove disc material and the cartilaginous end-plates. These initial steps are then repeated on the contralateral side. A pituitary rongeur is used to remove loose material, and an incrementally larger shaper is inserted. Care must be taken not to plunge the shaper, keeping in mind most lumbar vertebrae are 25 to 30 mm deep in the anterior-posterior plane. Monitor depth of penetration with lateral fluoroscopy. Leave the anterior disc and anterior longitudinal ligament intact to minimize the chance of a catastrophic vascular injury. McAfee and associates prospectively demonstrated that a complete discectomy led to higher fusion rates than partial discectomy when performed with titanium interbody cages (87). Other advantages of complete or near-complete discectomy include easier orientation to the midline, easier reduction of spondylolisthesis, and restoration of the disc space height (87) (Figs. 8–10).

Larger interbody devices should cause heightened awareness of the position of and tensioning on the dura and nerve roots. For cylindrical cages, a drill tube can be docked to the posterior disc space with an outer sleeve that conforms to the interdiscal space. Subsequent instruments can then be inserted safely. Distraction

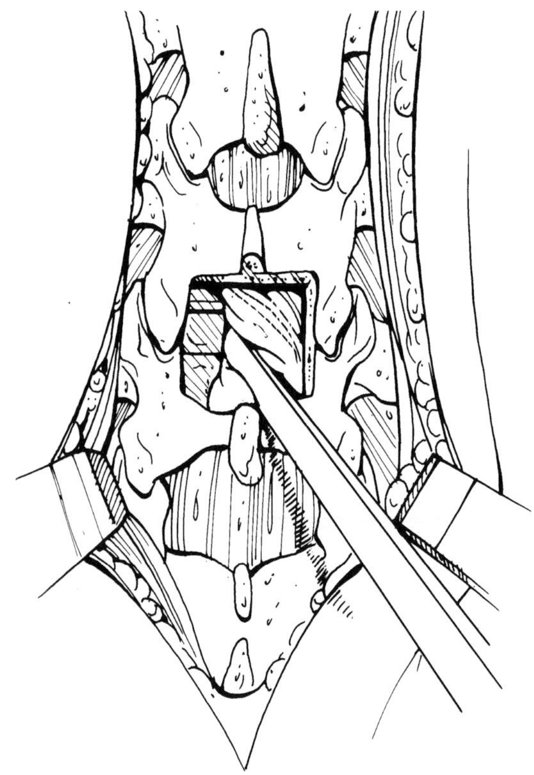

FIG. 6. Midline posterior lumbar interbody fusion exposure. (Modified from Chapman MW, Szabo RM, Marder R, et al., eds. *Chapman's orthopaedic surgery.* Philadelphia: Lippincott Williams & Wilkins, 2001:3799, with permission.)

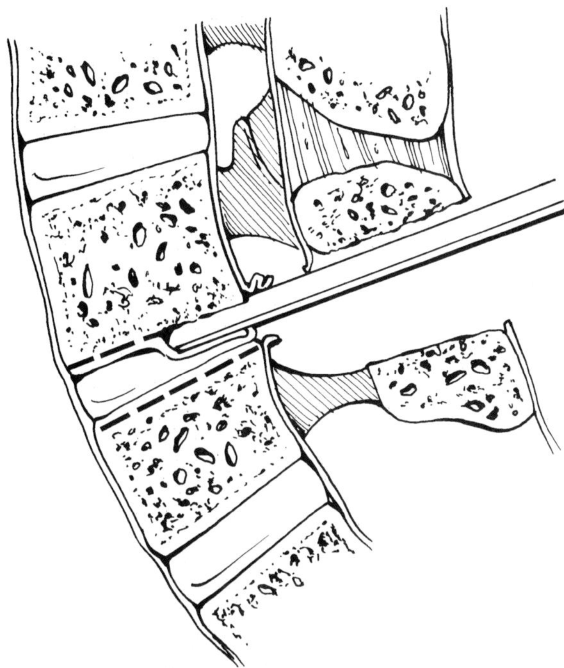

FIG. 7. In a posterior lumbar interbody fusion, an osteotome is used to remove the end-plates, followed by thorough removing of the disc. (Modified from An HS, Lee RH III, eds. *An atlas of surgery of the spine*. London: William Dunitz, 1998:221, with permission.)

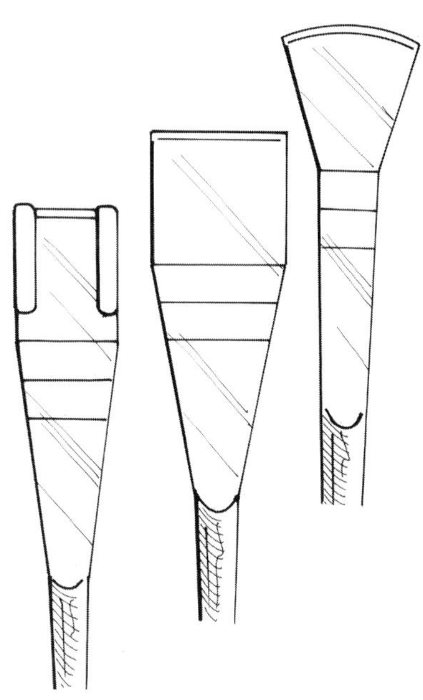

FIG. 9. Posterior lumbar interbody fusion instruments—a sampling of instruments available for completing the discectomy and disc space distraction. These instruments can also be used with transforaminal lumbar interbody fusion. (Modified from Chapman MW, Szabo RM, Marder R, et al., eds. *Chapman's orthopaedic surgery*. Philadelphia: Lippincott Williams & Wilkins, 2001:3799, with permission.)

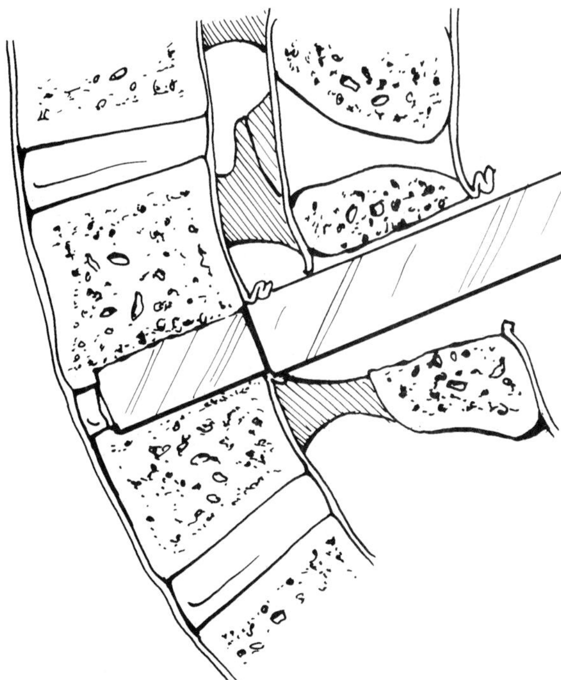

FIG. 8. Posterior lumbar interbody fusion with insertion of rectangular osteotome. These precise instruments assist with insertion of the interbody graft. (Modified from An HS, Lee RH III, eds. *An atlas of surgery of the spine*. London: William Dunitz, 1998:222, with permission.)

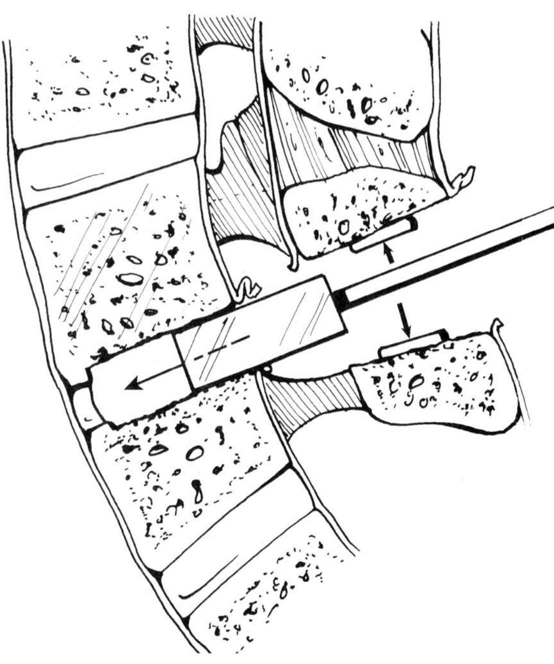

FIG. 10. Posterior lumbar interbody fusion with insertion of appropriate-sized spacer and showing posterior distraction. (Modified from An HS, Lee RH III, eds. *An atlas of surgery of the spine*. London: William Dunitz, 1998:222, with permission.)

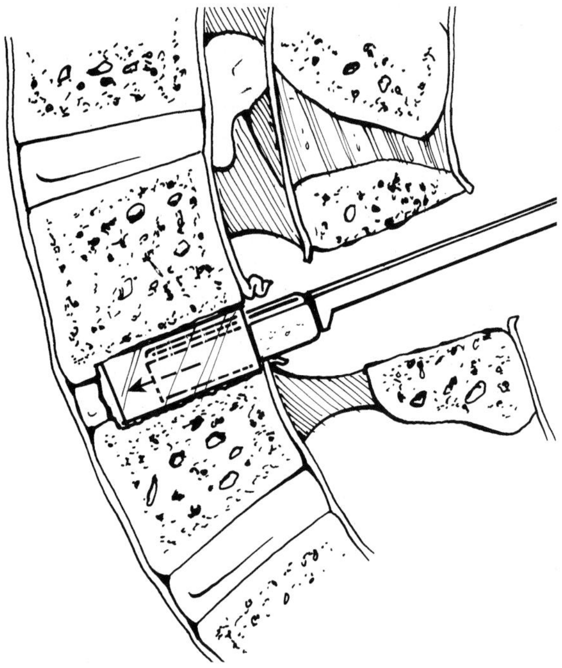

FIG. 11. Posterior lumbar interbody fusion. Placing the graft. (Modified from An HS, Lee RH III, eds. *An atlas of surgery of the spine.* London: William Dunitz, 1998:223, with permission.)

plugs are inserted with incrementally larger heights to open the disc space. Hand reamers remove any remaining end-plate tissue. Taps prepare the threaded cage path. Implant the appropriate cage using specialized cage inserters. Countersink the graft 2 to 5 mm to prevent canal encroachment. Local autograft is then added, first medially under the thecal sac, then laterally. Once the disc space has been packed, remove the distractive forces on the pedicle screws, and apply compression. Check anterior-posterior and lateral fluoroscopy to ensure implant position and sagittal spinal contour. The wound is closed in layers, creating a watertight fascial closure. A drain is left deep to the deep fascia (Figs. 11 and 12).

Similar to the "mini-open" ALIF, tubular retractor systems have been combined with microscopic dissection and fluoroscopic guidance to allow various posterior decompression and fusion techniques to be performed through smaller incisions. In one recent report, the authors performed bilateral laminotomies using a hybrid of microsurgical and microendoscopic techniques. Through this approach, the intervertebral disc spaces were distracted and prepared for interbody instrumentation. After the interbody fusion, percutaneous pedicle screws were placed. The procedure was completed in three patients in an average of 5.4 hours with an estimated blood loss of 185 cc (93).

TRANSFORAMINAL LUMBAR INTERBODY FUSION

TLIF was described by Harms as a variant to the PLIF, requiring less neural element retraction, thereby reducing risk for neural injury. There are no significant differences in blood loss, duration of hospital stay, and operative time between the PLIF and TLIF, but complications are less than those of PLIF (94). Surgical indications are the same as those for the PLIF. Because sig-

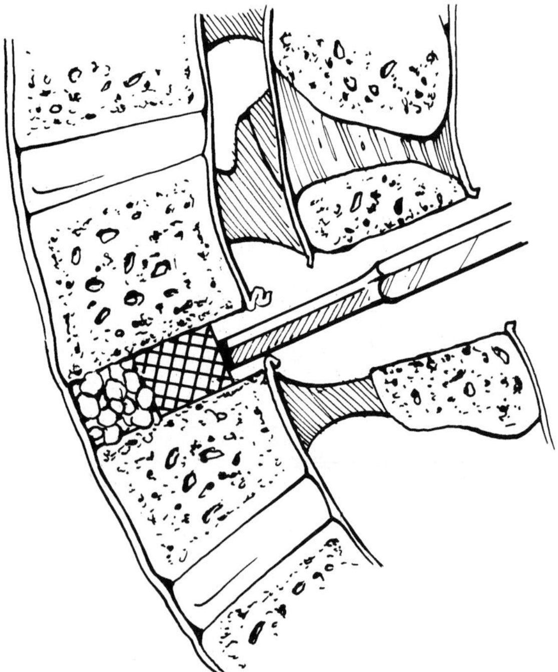

FIG. 12. Morselized autograft is placed anteriorly in the disc space; cage is inserted posteriorly. (Modified from An HS, Lee RH III, eds. *An atlas of surgery of the spine.* London: William Dunitz, 1998:224, with permission.)

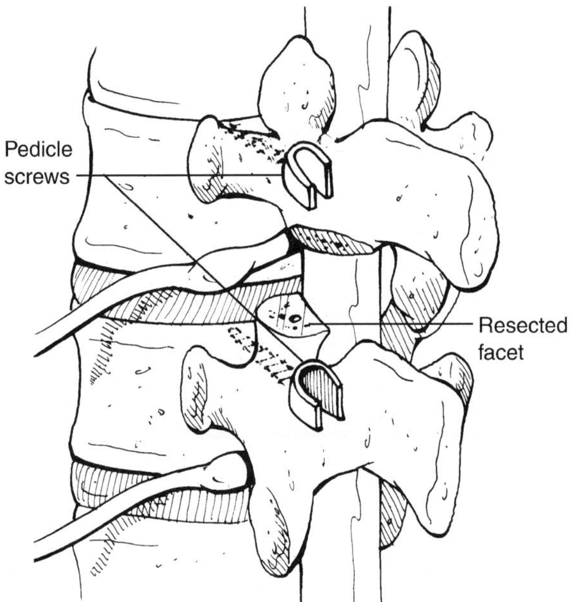

FIG. 13. Transforaminal lumbar interbody fusion: facet resection and pars removal with distraction allowing access to the disc without significant distraction of the neural elements. (Modified from Chapman MW, Szabo RM, Marder R, et al., eds. *Chapman's orthopaedic surgery.* Philadelphia: Lippincott Williams & Wilkins, 2001:3801, with permission.)

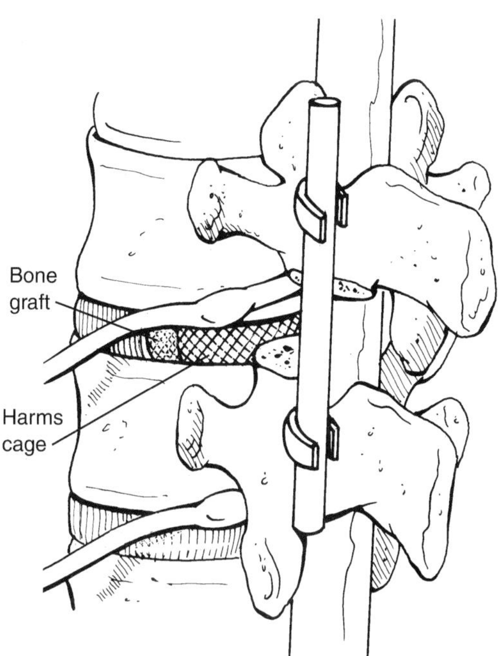

FIG. 14. After subtotal discectomy through a posterolateral annulotomy, bone graft is packed anteriorly, followed by Harms cage filled with autogenous bone graft tamped across the disc space. (Modified from Chapman MW, Szabo RM, Marder R, et al., eds. *Chapman's orthopaedic surgery.* Philadelphia: Lippincott Williams & Wilkins, 2001:3801, with permission.)

nificant thecal sac retraction is not required, TLIF can be performed at higher lumber levels.

A posterior exposure is carried out to the lateral tips of the transverse process. With an osteotome, remove the inferior facet of the superior vertebra and superior facet of the inferior vertebrae. Excise the lateral pars with a Leksel rongeur. The residual bone between the superior and inferior pedicles is removed with a Kerrison rongeur. The exiting (superior) and traversing (inferior) nerve roots are now easily identified and protected with retractors and 1-cm^3 sponges.

With the superior and inferior pedicles identified, pedicle screws are inserted bilaterally. Next, retract and protect the dural sac and nerve roots with a 90-degree angled retractor positioned in the axilla between the dura and the exiting nerve root. Remove any osteophytes from the lips of the vertebral bodies with a small rongeur. Perform an annulotomy with a 15-blade knife, creating a medially based annular flap. Begin the discectomy with angled and straight disc rongeurs and curettes. Distract the interspace with a large lamina spreader, and hold the distraction by affixing a working plate or rod to the pedicle screws. Depending on the angle of approach, both rods may be attached to both sets of screws or only the contralateral pair may be necessary (Fig. 13).

With this improved access to the interspace, use ring curette and pituitaries to remove more disc material and the cartilaginous end-plate. Harms recommends using an osteotome to remove the anterior osteophytes. Extreme care should be undertaken during this maneuver. As with the PLIF, disc spreaders are then placed into the disc space, initially with the paddle parallel to the end-plates. The spreader is then rotated 90 degrees and opened, restoring disc space height. The appropriate height is assessed with the spreader in place by fluoroscopy and feel. The corrected disc space heights usually range between 9 and 14 mm.

After the appropriate height is determined, disc shavers are inserted and rotated, removing cartilaginous material from the end-plates. Be aware of the depth of insertion of the instruments, checking insertion under fluoroscopy. Reamers and broaches are then inserted and rotated by hand. Loose, morselized, autogenous bone graft is gently tamped into the anterior disc space. The structural element, the cage, is then gently tamped into place, angling anteromedially at 45 degrees. The entry point is just lateral to the retracted dura. At this point, check fluoroscopy again, assessing the cage's position. If a

A,B

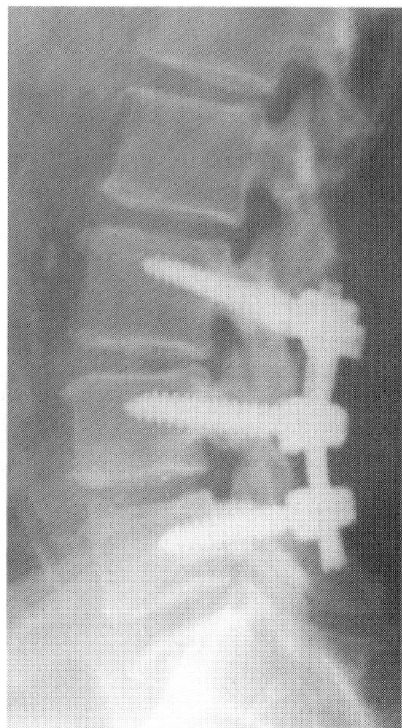

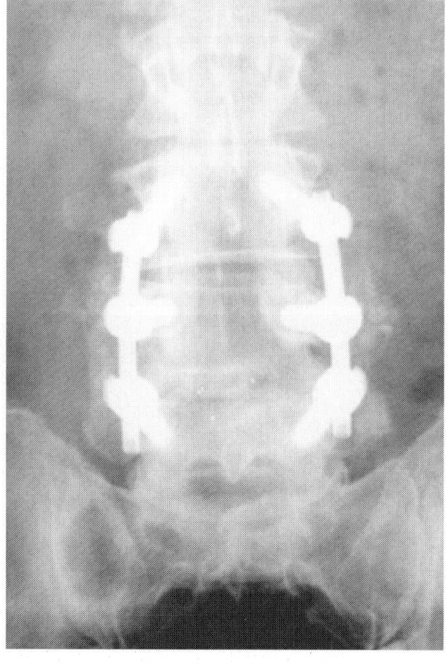

FIG. 15. Lateral **(A)** and anterior-posterior **(B)** radiographs of a 56-year-old man with a history of low back pain, L3-4 spondylolisthesis, and right L-4 radiculopathy. The patient underwent a transforaminal lumbar interbody fusion at L3-4. Note the radiographic markers (posterosuperiorly and anteroinferiorly) on the cage (Brantigan cage).

single implant is used, it should cross the midline to the contralateral side. If two cages are used, place the first graft at an angle of 40 to 45 degrees, then gently tamp the posterior aspect of the graft medially. Assess placement with fluoroscopy in both the anterior-posterior and lateral planes. A second graft is then inserted at an entry angle of 15 to 20 degrees. A cortical bone wedge, an oblong 10- to 12-mm Harms cage, two round vertical mesh cages, or one or two Brantigan cages can be inserted. Each device should have additional cancellous autograft tamped around it (Fig. 14).

Some systems require a second cage placed from the opposite side. A unilateral TLIF creates less instability because the contralateral facets are preserved. A bilateral TLIF improves access to the disc space, end-plate preparation, and an additional interbody strut but at a cost of increased operative time and blood loss.

Once the grafting is completed, compress the posterior pedicle instrumentation to regain lordosis and decrease the chance of graft migration. Closure involves watertight fascial suturing with a drain left deep to the deep fascia (Fig. 15).

CIRCUMFERENTIAL FUSION

A circumferential approach implies a separate anterior and posterior incision and approach to the spine. Traditionally, a formal 360-degree fusion includes a standard anterior retroperitoneal approach for ALIF followed by an open posterior instrumented fusion. This approach is still typically required when treating patients with deformity, tumor, or infection (Figs. 16 and 17).

In patients with degenerative disease, a number of variants on this approach have been devised. First, the anterior or posterior approach can be carried out with minimal invasion with endoscopic or percutaneous access. Second, the posterior approach may include instrumented stabilization alone, without posterolateral arthrodesis. Anterior fusion with only posterior instrumentation has been termed a *270-degree fusion.*

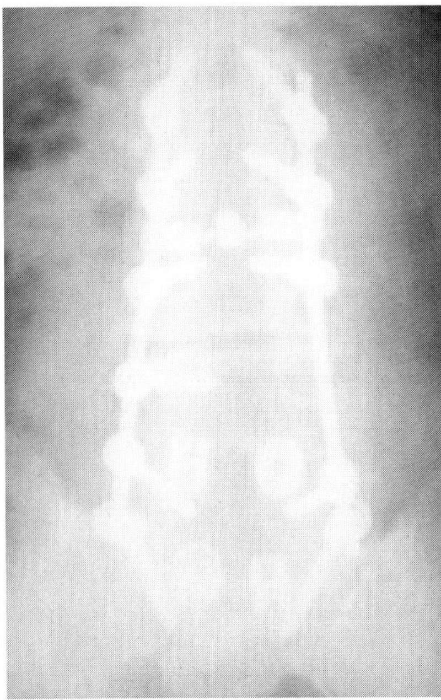

FIG. 16. Anterior-posterior view showing circumferential fusion for degenerative scoliosis.

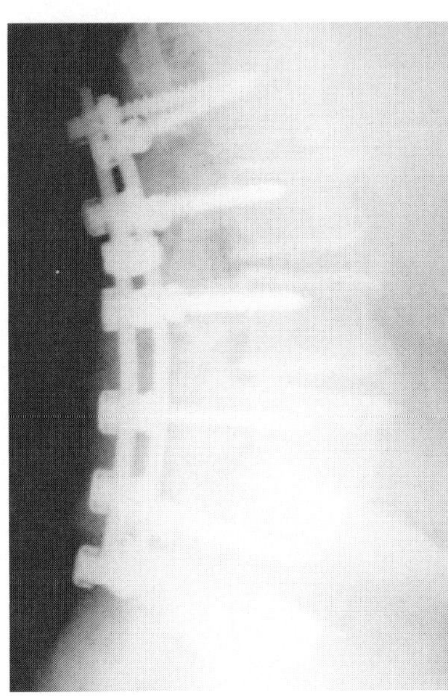

FIG. 17. Lateral radiograph of the same patient after circumferential fusion. Note the position of the anterior interbody cage: It is countersunk 3 to 4 mm.

Posterior instrumentation has been added to increase stability and fusion rates after ALIF, but the degree of stability necessary to reliably achieve a biologic union remains unclear. Formal ALIF followed by posterior pedicle screw instrumentation creates the stiffest applicable construct (11,16,18). Posterior instrumentation improves stability in extension, rotation, and compression (68).

In theory, percutaneous placement reduces the paraspinal muscle stripping necessary for open placement of posterior instrumentation, thereby limiting the morbidity of the circumferential fusion. Initially, 270-degree fusions were performed with facet screws, which provided a safe, inexpensive means to improve extension and rotation stiffness after cage ALIF (95). In one series of 18 patients, ALIF was followed by percutaneous translaminar facet fixation. Postoperative CT scanning revealed that all screws were properly placed (96). More recently, existing multiaxial lumbar pedicle screw systems have been modified to allow percutaneous placement. An extension sleeve permits remote manipulation of the polyaxial screw heads and a unique rod-insertion device [Sextant (Medtronic Sofamor Danek, Memphis, TN)] links to the screw extension sleeves and allows a precut and contoured rod to be placed through the screw tulips through a small stab wound and a muscle splitting technique. Short-term successful implantation has been reported in 12 patients (97).

Circumferential fusion is technically demanding and associated with a high rate of complications (98). This approach is most reasonable in patients with marked instability or significant anterior bone loss (e.g., osteomyelitis). In patients with degenerative disease, a circumferential approach is considered only in those with severe disability and usually previous multiple failed spinal operations. Other indications include the following (11,68,98):

- Patients at high risk for pseudarthrosis
- Multilevel involvement and marked segmental instability (infection and trauma)

- Anterior column support in patients with significant osteoporosis

POSTOPERATIVE MANAGEMENT

In most cases, interbody fusion patients start chair transfers the evening of surgery. Early physical therapy provides training, encouragement, and ambulation assistance. The majority of patients are ambulating without assistance by postoperative day three. Bracing is not routinely required, but corsets can be of use if low lumbar weakness or spasms hamper rehabilitation. The patient and the therapists are asked to limit bending and twisting and to restrict lifting to 5 lb or less. Other activities of daily living are actively encouraged.

Diet is advanced as tolerated from clear liquid for anterior and posterior surgery patients. There is higher risk for postoperative ileus following an anterior approach, particularly when the transperitoneal approach is used. Mini-open and endoscopic retroperitoneal approaches may decrease the frequency of postoperative ileus (99–101).

Patient-controlled anesthesia is begun with a basal rate of 0.5 to 1.5 mg of morphine an hour with 1 mg available every 6 minutes and a 10-mg lockout. The patient-controlled anesthesia is weaned to oral narcotics by postoperative day two or three. Nonsteroidal antiinflammatories are avoided in the postoperative period until the fusion is mature, which usually requires 6 to 8 months. The Foley catheter and operative drains are removed on postoperative day one. Intravenous perioperative antibiotics are administered, most commonly 1 mg of intravenous cefazolin for 48 hours.

Although some stand-alone ALIF patients are discharged sooner, most patients leave the hospital on postoperative day three, ambulating without assistance, tolerating a regular diet, and requiring oral pain medications. Operative time and hospital stay are both decreased in the hands of an experienced surgeon (17,21).

Return to work and sporting activities is individualized based on the patient's clinical status, radiographic assessment of union, and the nature of activities involved. An early return to work with limited or light duty is encouraged, with most patients resuming preferred activities by 6 months. Some patients, specifically those with heavy lifting and bending requirements in their occupations, may not be able to return to their previous occupations. For these individuals, occupational retraining is beneficial. Aerobic activities, spinal flexibility, and truncal strength and stability are stressed in physical therapy and as life-long aspects of the patient's personal fitness regime. Physical therapy is extended if stiffness and extensor weakness persists.

COMPLICATIONS

Complications recognized in the postoperative period can arise in the preoperative, intraoperative, or postoperative periods. However, the most common factor producing a poor outcome is improper patient selection (102).

Intraoperative complications begin with the induction of anesthesia. Interbody fusions are performed under general anesthesia and can involve significant blood loss, which can be associated with hypovolemia, fluid overload, pulmonary edema, transfusion reactions, aspiration pneumonitis, and cardiac problems.

Postoperative complications include those complications specific and nonspecific to the procedure undertaken. Nonspecific complications include wound infections, which occur in 1 to 2% of patients. This risk is lower in ALIF than in PLIF (103). Instrumentation increases the probability of postoperative infection, ranging from 1.3 to 12.0%, with a mean of 5 to 6% (104–106). Preoperative antibiotics administered 1 hour before surgery, careful soft-tissue handling, limiting muscle necrosis by relaxing paraspinal retractors at regular intervals, meticulous sterile technique, and limiting operating room traffic all decrease infection rates (107–109).

The syndrome of inappropriate antidiuretic hormone secretion is associated with spinal fusions. Excessive antidiuretic hormone secretion by the posterior pituitary gland results in a failure to excrete free water and a dilutional hyponatremia (110–112). Low urine output occurs initially, with the patient complaining of fatigue and, at times, delirium. Treatment begins with fluid restriction and continuous telemetry.

After lumbar fusion, the increased stress on the adjacent segment may accelerate its degeneration. However, in one study of 227 patients with isthmic L-5 spondylolisthesis followed for a mean 15.4 years, no significant increase in the prevalence of degeneration was observed in the adjacent disc above the fusion. Furthermore, there was no correlation between the number of degenerated discs and subjective LBP symptoms (113). Another study assessed the rate of adjacent segment degeneration in a cohort of 23 patients followed for an average of 13.3 years after ALIF for spondylolisthesis and found a 52% rate of subjacent degeneration and a 70% rate of supradjacent degeneration. Again, these changes did not correlate with long-term outcomes (61). Finally, in one series of 83 patients who underwent lumbar fusion for degenerative disc disease, a statistically significant increase in adjacent segment abnormalities was noted in patients with sagittal plane abnormalities. There was no difference in adjacent segment degeneration rates between posterior fusion alone and circumferential fusions (114).

With the advent of synthetic and metallic interbody cages, there has been a marked decrease in graft failures secondary to fracture and collapse (51,63,115). The majority of cage complications are related to the technique applied and the specific anatomic challenges of the lower lumbar spine. McAfee reported on the revision of 20 consecutive failed cages. He opined that failure was due to surgical technique rather than an intrinsic defect in cage technology (51). Factors typically implicated included failure to achieve adequate distraction of the annulus fibrosis, undersized cages (especially when placed through a PLIF approach), cerebrospinal fluid leakage or pseudomeningocele, the use of local bone graft rather than iliac crest inside the cage, anterior insertion in an excessively lateral position resulting in symptoms of a far lateral disc herniation, and failure to identify the spinal midline during an anterior approach (51). More failures were noted in patients with type 2 diabetes mellitus.

Complications specific to ALIF include retrograde ejaculation. The preaortic sympathetic autonomic plexus lies on the lateral aspect of the spine, just medial to the psoas muscle. These fibers lie close to the left iliac artery as they arch over the L-5 to S-1 disc space within the bifurcation of the aorta. Retrograde ejaculation and sterility result from disruption of this sympathetic plexus (116,117). For this reason, men still considering having children should be carefully counseled about this particular risk, and if it is possible, it may be desirable to use alternative approaches, such as TLIF or PLIF. Avoid damaging the hypogastric plexus by freeing the prevertebral plexus with blunt dissection. Do not make any transverse cuts in the annulus until the entire structure is clearly visible, and avoid electrocautery within the aortic bifurcation.

The common iliac vein is also at risk in ALIF, especially in the presence of tumor or osteomyelitis. The vein lies just posterior to the common iliac artery and is easy to confuse with soft tissue if not properly exposed. In one series, the frequency of iliac vein tear was 1 in 22 (99). Vascular complications commonly involve the iliolumbar vein, which is a branch of the vena cava or the common iliac vein. It courses right to left (from a left-sided exposure) and becomes part of the ascending lumbar venous system. Kittner dissectors or sponge sticks are used to sweep the blood vessels off of the front of the spine. Always identify, isolate, and ligate the left iliolumbar vein, especially in exposing the L4-5 interspace. A laparoscopic approach does not appear to be associated with unusual complications.

In a prospective multicenter study of 22 laparoscopic lumbar procedures, the most common complication was bone graft donor site infection (two patients). There was one case that was converted to an open procedure after a common iliac vein laceration. There were no permanent iatrogenic neurologic injuries and no deep spinal infections (99).

In PLIF and TLIF surgery, particular attention must be paid to positioning. All pressure points must be well padded. Increased ocular pressure has been reported to result in central retinal artery occlusion and resultant blindness (118,119). Failure to free the abdominal contents results in increased epidural venous pressure and increased blood loss.

PLIF procedures have been criticized for nerve root trauma resulting from the wide retraction required for placement of interbody devices. Epidural fibrosis and arachnoiditis may present as chronic radiculopathy, for which there is no treatment (120). A Japanese study of 25 consecutive patients revealed two dural tears that were repaired intraoperatively and two patients with postoperative deep venous thrombosis, with no serious complications (66). Wide decompressions and increased exposure for disc space preparation have minimized neural injury.

Complication rates associated with PLIF vary considerably. Steffee reported 104 PLIFs performed without graft dislocation, pseudarthrosis, or infection (121). On the other hand, Ma and associates reported an 11% reoperation rate, 6% for pseudarthrosis, 3% for bone graft extrusion or migration, 1% for bone graft fracture, and 1% for hematoma. Okuyama encountered a very low risk of fusion and hardware failure but noted a higher risk for neurologic impairment, with 8% of patients suffering from a temporary palsy (122).

Humphreys compared TLIF to PLIF in a recent study and determined that the transforaminal approach was similar to PLIF in all respects, other than the complication rate. In his review of 40 TLIFs and 32 PLIFs, he reported no complications with the TLIF and multiple complications with PLIF (94).

Regardless of the approach, interbody graft extrusion may have severe consequences. Anteriorly placed grafts usually displace anteriorly with a resultant loss of correction and increased kyphosis. Posterior fusion and instrumentation with compression adds stability and protection for anterior grafts and shortens time to fusion. Also, grafts that are fashioned to interlock with the superior and inferior end-plates anchor the graft in place and are less likely to extrude.

The rate of fusion is variable. Steffee reported 104 PLIF fusions performed without graft dislocation, pseudarthrosis, or infection (121). In Blumenthal's series, a single complication of graft extrusion requiring revision and associated with retrograde ejaculation was reported (9).

Circumferential fusions are not associated with unique complications, but the additional surgical time compounds the morbidity of either an anterior or posterior approach alone. But most series report complications ranging from 5 to 15% (11,18). In one series, complications included metal failure, neurologic deficit, deep infection, deep venous thrombosis, vascular injury, and fatal pulmonary embolus (98).

Pseudarthrosis results from poor surgical technique, excessive stresses across the fusion site, insufficient internal or external stabilization, and unrecognized metabolic abnormalities. Fusion rates are discussed with the individual procedures below.

OUTCOMES

Significant variability in the relief of pain and return to work after interbody fusion has been reported. Ostensibly, this variability is due to differences in surgical indications and techniques. Most of the literature includes patients with a wide variety of underlying disease states and comorbidities. Direct comparison of one technique to another, therefore, is limited.

Anterior Lumbar Interbody Fusion Outcomes

Highly variable fusion rates have been reported with stand-alone ALIF techniques, ranging from 16.6 to 97.0% (9,123,124). One outcomes study reported that 97% of 141 levels fused radiographically using the FRA spacer (64). In a series of 34 ALIFs, Blumenthal reported an overall union rate of 73%, with an average time to union of approximately 12 months (9). On the other hand, 2 years after endoscopic L-5 to S-1 ALIF using twin stand-alone carbon fiber cages, the radiographic fusion rate as measured by CT in 16 patients was only 16.6% (78). However, overall pseudarthrosis rates are lower than those reported for posterolateral fusions (5,125).

The clinical results also vary. Greenough reported a 68% clinical success rate in 150 consecutive patients, with higher success rates in noncompensation patients (20). Newman reported 86% good to excellent clinical results in a series of 36 patients treated with ALIF for internal disc disruption (126). For historic comparison, Stauffer and Coventry published only 56% good to fair results in 83 posterolateral fusions, with 44% of the patients not returning to work in spite of pain relief (15).

Fusions for multiple-level degenerative disc disease are associated with poorer outcomes (4,10,14). Knox reported that all of his multiple-level ALIF procedures had poor results, whereas 53% of his surgically treated single-level patients had good to fair results (10). Goldner followed a series of 100 patients who underwent ALIF for concordant pain on discography and reported 91% success rates with single-level fusions and 72% with multiple-level fusions (14). Of the patients, 78% reported complete to moderate pain relief. Patients with pseudarthrosis had worse clinical results.

Posterior Lumbar Interbody Fusion Outcomes

Fusion rates for PLIF range from 73 to 100% (89,90,127–129). A prospective, controlled multicentered study of a single device reported 98.9% solid union in a group of 178 patients. Multiple-level surgery did not decrease fusion rates (63).

PLIF is successful in promoting and maintaining disc space height, making it a good surgical choice for a patient with mechanical back pain and foraminal stenosis and a resultant radiculopathy. In Brantigan's series, disc space height averaged 7.9 mm before surgery, increased to 12.3 mm immediately after surgery, and was maintained at 11.7 mm at 2 years (63).

Clinical outcomes have varied from 69 to 87%, classified as good to excellent (52,80). In patients with previous failed discectomy surgery, Brantigan reported satisfactory outcomes in 86% of 92 patients (63). Other clinical studies have reported 82 to 89% good to excellent results and an 82% return to work rate (90,129). Brantigan's 2-year results of his carbon fiber cages included 83% excellent to good outcomes in 26 consecutive patients with failed back syndrome (130). Rompe reported that fair to poor outcomes are associated with prior operations, preoperative kyphosis, and preoperative motor weakness. He concluded that PLIF was no better than posterior lumbar fusion alone (131).

Transforaminal Lumbar Interbody Fusion Outcomes

There are fewer outcome reports available for TLIF. Lowe and associates reported on 40 patients treated with TLIF for degenerative diseases of the lumbar spine. At 3-year follow-up, radiographic assessment included plain and flexion-extension radiographs. Solid fusions occurred in 90%, and segmental lordosis had increased in all patients using their criteria. Clinical outcome was based on pain relief, ability to do activities of daily living, and return to work. Of the patients, 85% had excellent or good clinical outcomes (53).

Rosenberg and colleagues reported results from 22 TLIF patients treated for LBP (132). TLIF completely resolved LBP in 16 patients and moderately relieved pain in 5 patients, but the pain was unchanged in one patient. Complications included one dural tear and two postoperative wound infections. A mild, postoperative L-5 motor paresis occurred in one patient and resolved soon after surgery without further intervention.

Circumferential Fusion Outcomes

Reported outcomes for circumferential fusions have not been significantly different from those achieved with PLIF or TLIF. One report cited an overall 80% acceptable clinical result rate with combined procedures (133). O'Brien reported 90% fusion rates in one- and two-level procedures, with a 77% fusion rate in three-level procedures. He concluded that these results justify the added morbidity of the 360-degree fusion in patients with chronic disabling LBP.

Fusion rates in excess of 90% were noted in patients who had undergone one- and two-level open 360-degree fusions, whereas the fusion rate for three-level procedures dropped to 77.8% (133). Substantial pain relief was reported in 46% of all patients (133).

In another study, 150 such patients were treated with circumferential fusion; 86% of these patients were reported as improved (60% significantly) (11,18).

Comparative Outcomes

Traditional posterolateral fusions have a pseudarthrosis rate ranging between 14 and 22% (1–3). It appears that most interbody techniques are associated with significantly fewer pseudarthroses but no significant differences in clinical outcome.

Fritzell published a prospective randomized evaluation of PLF, PLF with instrumentation, and circumferential fusion with instrumentation. Eligibility included patients 25 to 65 years of age with LBP that had persisted for at least 2 years despite conservative therapy and radiologic evidence of disc degeneration (spondylosis) at L4-5, L-5 to S-1, or both (41). All surgical techniques were found to reduce pain and decrease disability substantially, but no significant differences were found between the groups. Significantly more resources were found in the two instrument groups, as measured by operator time, blood transfusions, and days in hospital. The early complication rate at 33 months was 6% in PLF, 16% in PLF with instrumentation, and 31% in the circumferential fusion. The fusion rates, as evaluated by plain radiographs, were 72%, 87%, and 91%, respectively. The study concluded that there was no obvious disadvantage in using the least-demanding surgical technique of posterolateral fusion without internal fixation (41).

Schofferman published a prospective randomized comparison of 270-degree fusion to the 360-degree fusion (134). He compared ALIF plus transpedicular instrumentation and posterolateral fusion to ALIF with transpedicular instrumentation but without posterolateral fusion. There were no significant differences in Oswestry Low Back Disability Index or percentage of solid fusions of the ALIF. Only 14% of posterolateral fusions appeared solid bilaterally. The 270-degree fusion, however, had significantly less blood loss, shorter operative times, shorter hospital stays, and lower professional fees. Both the 360- and 270-degree fusions had significant clinical improvements, with no statistical difference in outcomes between them (134).

Hee and associates recently retrospectively reviewed 164 consecutive patients treated with 360-degree fusion and TLIF (135). Fifty-three patients had same-day anterior-posterior fusion, and 111 had transforaminal interbody fusion. The investigators preferred TLIF because it was associated with shorter operating times, less blood loss, shorter hospital stays, and a lower complication rate (135).

SUMMARY

Interbody fusion is indicated to provide anterior column support and stability in a variety of spinal disorders. Although interbody fusion is commonly indicated in the surgical management of lumbar osteomyelitis and deformity, degenerative disc disease remains the most common, and the most controversial indication for a lumbar interbody fusion. As the natural history of these conditions is only partially understood, a recommendation for surgery must be carefully balanced against the surgical risks and the possibility of a poor clinical outcome. Fusion indications in adult degenerative disc disease of the lumbosacral spine include isolated disc resorption or IDD, primary and secondary instability, recurrent disc herniation, and pseudarthrosis (16). Although fusions for multiple-level degenerative disc disease typically have comparatively poorer outcomes, single-level disc disease and occasionally double-level disc disease may be considered as an indication for surgery (4,14).

In patients with neurogenic symptoms, arthrodesis is indicated as an adjunct to decompression for patients with spinal stenosis associated with degenerative spondylolisthesis, progressive degenerative lumbar scoliosis, and iatrogenic instability resulting from previous decompression (4). Interbody techniques are reserved for focal scoliosis, marked translation, foraminal stenosis, and patients with a high risk for pseudarthrosis. Isthmic spondylolisthesis may cause pain by nerve root compression, instability, or degeneration of the underlying disc (4). Interbody fusion is occasionally indicated to eradicate the painful disc, restore normal sagittal balance, and improve fusion rates.

Interbody fusion techniques include the following: standalone ALIF, PLIF, TLIF, and the circumferential fusions. The authors use stand-alone ALIF in patients with mechanical back pain and a collapsed disc but without neurogenic symptoms. The authors are more likely to offer ALIF to female rather than male patients. The authors avoid stand-alone ALIF in patients with instability and previous wide laminectomies.

PLIF is a means of achieving an anterior arthrodesis with posterior stabilization in the same approach. The authors recommend PLIF procedures for patients with marked LBP-associated nerve root compression, particularly at the L-5 to S-1 level. Disadvantages include a demanding technique, graft displacement, pseudarthrosis, potential destabilization of the anterior and posterior columns, increased risk of nerve root injury, dural tears, and epidural fibrosis from excessive retraction.

The TLIF is a PLIF variant, requiring less neural element retraction. The authors use TLIF in place of standard PLIF at L4-5 and above. The authors reserve the circumferential approach for osteomyelitis and deformity cases. Occasionally, formal 360-degree fusion is helpful in patients with multilevel involvement, osteoporosis, or marked segmental instability.

In all cases, patient selection is more important than the approach or implant selected. Less-invasive techniques refer to different approaches, not different operations; the indications remain the same.

REFERENCES

1. DeBerard MS, et al. Outcomes of posterolateral lumbar fusion in Utah patients receiving workers' compensation: a retrospective cohort study. *Spine* 2001;26(7):738–746; discussion 747.
2. Parker LM, et al. The outcome of posterolateral fusion in highly selected patients with discogenic low back pain. *Spine* 1996;21 (16):1909–1916; discussion, 1916–1917.
3. Turner JA, et al. Patient outcomes after lumbar spinal fusions. *JAMA* 1992;268(7):907–911.
4. Herkowitz HN, Sidhu KS. Lumbar spine fusion in the treatment of degenerative conditions: current indications and recommendations. *J Am Acad Orthop Surg* 1995;3(3):123–135.
5. Wood GW 2nd, et al. The effect of pedicle screw/plate fixation on lumbar/lumbosacral autogenous bone graft fusions in patients with degenerative disc disease. *Spine* 1995;20(7):819–830.
6. Zdeblick TA, et al. Indications for lumbar spinal fusion. Introduction. 1995 Focus Issue Meeting on Fusion. *Spine* 1995;20[24 Suppl]:24S–125S.
7. Lu K, et al. Oxidative stress and heat shock protein response in human paraspinal muscles during retraction. *J Neurosurg* 2002;97[1 Suppl]:75–81.
8. Park WM, et al. Fissuring of the posterior annulus fibrosus in the lumbar spine. *Br J Radiol* 1979;52(617):382–387.
9. Blumenthal SL, et al. The role of anterior lumbar fusion for internal disc disruption. *Spine* 1988;13(5):566–569.
10. Knox BD, Chapman TM. Anterior lumbar interbody fusion for discogram concordant pain. *J Spinal Disord* 1993;6(3):242–244.
11. O'Brien JP, et al. Simultaneous combined anterior and posterior fusion. A surgical solution for failed spinal surgery with a brief review of the first 150 patients. *Clin Orthop* 1986;(203):191–195.
12. Wetzel FT, LaRocca H. The failed posterior lumbar interbody fusion. *Spine* 1991;16(7):839–845.
13. Weatherley CR, Prickett CF, O'Brien JP. Discogenic pain persisting despite solid posterior fusion. *J Bone Joint Surg Br* 1986;68(1):142–143.
14. Goldner JL, Urbaniak JR, McCollum DE. Anterior disc excision and interbody spinal fusion for chronic low back pain. *Orthop Clin North Am* 1971;2(2):543–568.
15. Stauffer RN, Coventry MB. Anterior interbody lumbar spine fusion. Analysis of Mayo Clinic series. *J Bone Joint Surg Am* 1972;54(4):756–768.
16. Enker P, Steffee AD. Interbody fusion and instrumentation. *Clin Orthop* 1994;(300):90–101.
17. Nachemson A, Zdeblick TA, O'Brien JP. Lumbar disc disease with discogenic pain. What surgical treatment is most effective? *Spine* 1996;21(15):1835–1838.
18. O'Brien JP. The role of fusion for chronic low back pain. *Orthop Clin North Am* 1983;4(3):639–647.
19. Jaffray D, O'Brien JP. Isolated intervertebral disc resorption. A source of mechanical and inflammatory back pain? *Spine* 1986;11(4):397–401.
20. Greenough CG, Taylor LJ, Fraser RD. Anterior lumbar fusion. A comparison of noncompensation patients with compensation patients. *Clin Orthop* 1994;(300):30–37.
21. Zucherman JF, et al. Instrumented laparoscopic spinal fusion. Preliminary results. *Spine* 1995;20(18):2029–2034; discussion 2034–2035.
22. Norcross JP, et al. An in vivo model of degenerative disc disease. *J Orthop Res* 2003;21(1):183–188.
23. Kostuik JP, et al. Biomechanical testing of the lumbosacral spine. *Spine* 1998;23(16):1721–1728.
24. Gibson JN, Grant IC, Waddell G. The Cochrane review of surgery for lumbar disc prolapse and degenerative lumbar spondylosis. *Spine* 1999;24(17):1820–1832.
25. Gibson JN, Waddell G, Grant IC. Surgery for degenerative lumbar spondylosis. *Cochrane Database Syst Rev* 2000;(3):CD001352.
26. Frymoyer JW, et al. Spine radiographs in patients with low-back pain. An epidemiological study in men. *J Bone Joint Surg Am* 1984;66(7): 1048–1055.
27. McGregor AH, Cattermole HR, Hughes SP. Global spinal motion in subjects with lumbar spondylolysis and spondylolisthesis: does the grade or type of slip affect global spinal motion? *Spine* 2001;26(3): 282–286.
28. Hodgson AR, Wong SK. A description of a technic and evaluation of results in anterior spinal fusion for deranged intervertebral disk and spondylolisthesis. *Clin Orthop* 1968;56:133–162.
29. Arnold PM, et al. Surgical management of nontuberculous thoracic and lumbar vertebral osteomyelitis: report of 33 cases. *Surg Neurol* 1997;47(6):551–561.
30. Matsui H, Hirano N, Sakaguchi Y. Vertebral osteomyelitis: an analysis of 38 surgically treated cases. *Eur Spine J* 1998;7(1):50–54.
31. Dietze DD Jr, Fessler RG, Jacob RP. Primary reconstruction for spinal infections. *J Neurosurg* 1997;86(6):981–989.
32. Rath SA, et al. Neurosurgical management of thoracic and lumbar vertebral osteomyelitis and discitis in adults: a review of 43 consecutive surgically treated patients. *Neurosurgery* 1996;38(5):926–933.
33. Ouellet JA, Johnston CE 2nd. Effect of grafting technique on the maintenance of coronal and sagittal correction in anterior treatment of scoliosis. *Spine* 2002;27(19):2129–2135; discussion 2135–2136.
34. Emami A, et al. Outcome and complications of long fusions to the sacrum in adult spine deformity: Luque-Galveston, combined iliac and sacral screws, and sacral fixation. *Spine* 2002;27(7):776–786.
35. Buttermann GR, et al. Lumbar fusion results related to diagnosis. *Spine* 1998;23(1):116–127.
36. Buttermann GR, et al. Anterior and posterior allografts in symptomatic thoracolumbar deformity. *J Spinal Disord* 2001;14(1):54–66.
37. Smith JA, et al. Clinical outcome of trans-sacral interbody fusion after partial reduction for high-grade l5-s1 spondylolisthesis. *Spine* 2001;26(20):2227–2234.
38. Klockner C, Weber U. Correction of lumbosacral kyphosis in high grade spondylolisthesis and spondyloptosis. *Orthopade* 2001;30(12): 983–987.
39. Roca J, et al. One-stage decompression and posterolateral and interbody fusion for severe spondylolisthesis. An analysis of 14 patients. *Spine* 1999;24(7):709–714.
40. Bogduk N, Modic MT. Lumbar discography. *Spine* 1996;21 (3):402–404.

41. Fritzell P, et al. Chronic low back pain and fusion: a comparison of three surgical techniques: a prospective multicenter randomized study from the Swedish Lumbar Spine Study Group. *Spine* 2002;27(11):131–141.
42. Herkowitz H, Kurz L. Degenerative lumbar spondylolisthesis with spinal stenosis. A prospective study comparing decompression with decompression and intertransverse process arthrodesis. *J Bone Joint Surg Am* 1991;73-A:802–808.
43. Zdeblick TA. The treatment of degenerative lumbar disorders. A critical review of the literature. *Spine* 1995;20[24 Suppl]:126S–137S.
44. Modic MT, et al. Magnetic resonance imaging of intervertebral disk disease. Clinical and pulse sequence considerations. *Radiology* 1984;152(1):103–111.
45. Aprill C, Bogduk N. High-intensity zone: a diagnostic sign of painful lumbar disc on magnetic resonance imaging. *Br J Radiol* 1992;65 (773):361–369.
46. Raininko R, et al. Observer variability in the assessment of disc degeneration on magnetic resonance images of the lumbar and thoracic spine. *Spine* 1995;20(9):1029–1035.
47. Modic MT, et al. Imaging of degenerative disk disease. *Radiology* 1988;168(1):177–186.
48. Carragee EJ, et al. The rates of false-positive lumbar discography in select patients without low back symptoms. *Spine* 2000;25(11):1373–1380; discussion 1381.
49. Madan S, et al. Does provocative discography screening of discogenic back pain improve surgical outcome? *J Spinal Disord Tech* 2002;15(3):245–251.
50. Colhoun E, et al. Provocation discography as a guide to planning operations on the spine. *J Bone Joint Surg Br* 1988;70(2):267–271.
51. McAfee PC. Interbody fusion cages in reconstructive operations on the spine. *J Bone Joint Surg Am* 1999;81(6):859–880.
52. Madan S, Boeree NR. Outcome of posterior lumbar interbody fusion versus posterolateral fusion for spondylolytic spondylolisthesis. *Spine* 2002;27(14):1536–1542.
53. Lowe TG, et al. Unilateral transforaminal posterior lumbar interbody fusion (TLIF): indications, technique, and 2-year results. *J Spinal Disord Tech* 2002;15(1):31–38.
54. Lin PM. Posterior lumbar interbody fusion technique: complications and pitfalls. *Clin Orthop* 1985;(193):90–102.
55. Liljenqvist U, O'Brien JP, Renton P. Simultaneous combined anterior and posterior lumbar fusion with femoral cortical allograft. *Eur Spine J* 1998;7(2):125–131.
56. Janssen ME, Lam C, Beckham R. Outcomes of allogenic cages in anterior and posterior lumbar interbody fusion. *Eur Spine J* 2001; 10[Suppl 2]:S158–168.
57. Chen D, et al. Increasing neuroforaminal volume by anterior interbody distraction in degenerative lumbar spine. *Spine* 1995;20(1):74–79.
58. Yang K, King A. Mechanism of facet load transmission as a hypothesis for low back pain. *Spine* 1984;9:557–565.
59. Bader RJ, et al. Mechanical studies of lumbar interbody fusion implants. *Orthopade* 2002;31(5):459–465.
60. Siff TE, et al. Femoral ring versus fibular strut allografts in anterior lumbar interbody arthrodesis. A biomechanical analysis. *Spine* 1999;24(7):659–665.
61. Ishihara H, et al. Minimum 10-year follow-up study of anterior lumbar interbody fusion for isthmic spondylolisthesis. *J Spinal Disord* 2001;14(2):91–99.
62. Janssen ME, et al. Biological cages. *Eur Spine J* 2000;9[Suppl 1]:S102–109.
63. Brantigan JW, et al. Lumbar interbody fusion using the Brantigan I/F cage for posterior lumbar interbody fusion and the variable pedicle screw placement system: two-year results from a Food and Drug Administration investigational device exemption clinical trial. *Spine* 2000;25(11):1437–1446.
64. Chotivichit A, et al. Role of femoral ring allograft in anterior interbody fusion of the spine. *J Orthop Surg (Hong Kong)* 2001;9(2):1–5.
65. Hacker RJ. The Ray Threaded Fusion Cage for posterior lumbar interbody fusion. *Neurosurgery* 1998;43(4):982–983.
66. Hashimoto T, et al. Clinical results of single-level posterior lumbar interbody fusion using the Brantigan I/F carbon cage filled with a mixture of local morselized bone and bioactive ceramic granules. *Spine* 2002;27(3):258–262.
67. Onesti ST, Ashkenazi E. The Ray Threaded Fusion Cage for posterior lumbar interbody fusion. *Neurosurgery* 1998;42(1):200–204; discussion 204–205.
68. Pitzen T, Matthis D, Steudel WI. The effect of posterior instrumentation following PLIF with BAK cages is most pronounced in weak bone. *Acta Neurochir (Wien)* 2002;144(2):121–128; discussion128.
69. Tullberg T, et al. Fusion rate after posterior lumbar interbody fusion with carbon fiber implant: 1-year follow-up of 51 patients. *Eur Spine J* 1996;5(3):178–182.
70. Kuslich SD, et al. The Bagby and Kuslich method of lumbar interbody fusion. History, techniques, and 2-year follow-up results of a United States prospective, multicenter trial. *Spine* 1998;23(11):1267–1278; discussion 1279.
71. Buttermann GR, et al. Revision of failed lumbar fusions. A comparison of anterior autograft and allograft. *Spine* 1997;22(23):2748–2755.
72. Hadjipavlou AG, et al. Hematogenous pyogenic spinal infections and their surgical management. *Spine* 2000;25(13):1668–1679.
73. Hee HT, et al. Better treatment of vertebral osteomyelitis using posterior stabilization and titanium mesh cages. *J Spinal Disord Tech* 2002;15(2):149–156; discussion 156.
74. Molinari RW, et al. Minimum 5-year follow-up of anterior column structural allografts in the thoracic and lumbar spine. *Spine* 1999;24 (10):967–972.
75. Eck K, et al. Analysis of titanium mesh cages in adults with minimum two-year follow-up. *Spine* 2000;25:2407–2415.
76. Diedrich O, et al. Radiographic spinal profile changes induced by cage design after posterior lumbar interbody fusion preliminary report of a study with wedged implants. *Spine* 2001;26(12):E274–E280.
77. Barnes B, et al. Threaded cortical bone dowels for lumbar interbody fusion: over 1-year mean follow up in 28 patients. *J Neurosurg* 2001;95[1 Suppl]:1–4.
78. Pellise F, et al. Low fusion rate after L5-S1 laparoscopic anterior lumbar interbody fusion using twin stand-alone carbon fiber cages. *Spine* 2002;27(15):1665–1669.
79. Pape D, et al. Primary lumbosacral stability after open posterior and endoscopic anterior fusion with interbody implants: a roentgen stereophotogrammetric analysis. *Spine* 2000;25(19):2514–2518.
80. Csecsei GI, et al. Posterior interbody fusion using laminectomy bone and transpedicular screw fixation in the treatment of lumbar spondylolisthesis. *Surg Neurol* 2000;53(1):2–6; discussion 6–7.
81. Wimmer C, et al. Autogenic versus allogenic bone grafts in anterior lumbar interbody fusion. *Clin Orthop* 1999;(360):122–126.
82. Wozney JM. Overview of bone morphogenetic proteins. *Spine* 2002;27[16 Suppl 1]:S2–S8.
83. Burkus JK, et al. Anterior lumbar interbody fusion using rhBMP-2 with tapered interbody cages. *J Spinal Disord Tech* 2002;15(5):337–349.
84. Bednar DA. Surgical management of lumbar degenerative spinal stenosis with spondylolisthesis via posterior reduction with minimal laminectomy. *J Spinal Disord Tech* 2002;15(2):105–109.
85. Vamvanij V, et al. Quantitative changes in spinal canal dimensions using interbody distraction for spondylolisthesis. *Spine* 2001;26(3): E13–18.
86. Dewald CJ, et al. An open, minimally invasive approach to the lumbar spine. *Am Surg* 1999;65(1):61–68.
87. McAfee PC, et al. Anterior BAK instrumentation and fusion: complete versus partial discectomy. *Clin Orthop* 2002;(394):55–63.
88. Cloward RB. Posterior lumbar interbody fusion updated. *Clin Orthop* 1985;(193):16–19.
89. Brantigan JW, Steffee AD. A carbon fiber implant to aid interbody lumbar fusion. Two-year clinical results in the first 26 patients. *Spine* 1993;18(14):2106–2107.
90. Lin PM, Cautilli RA, Joyce MF. Posterior lumbar interbody fusion. *Clin Orthop* 1983;(180):154–168.
91. Stonecipher T, Wright S. Posterior lumbar interbody fusion with facet-screw fixation. *Spine* 1989;14(4):468–471.
92. Tan SB, et al. Effect of operative position on sagittal alignment of the lumbar spine. *Spine* 1994;19(3):314–318.
93. Khoo LT, et al. Minimally invasive percutaneous posterior lumbar interbody fusion. *Neurosurgery* 2002;51[5 Suppl]:166–171.
94. Humphreys SC, et al. Comparison of posterior and transforaminal approaches to lumbar interbody fusion. *Spine* 2001;26(5):567–571.
95. Frymoyer JW, Selby DK. Segmental instability. Rationale for treatment. *Spine* 1985;10(3):280–286.
96. Jang JS, Lee SH, Lim SR. Guide device for percutaneous placement of translaminar facet screws after anterior lumbar interbody fusion. Technical note. *J Neurosurg* 2003;98[1 Suppl]:100–103.

97. Foley KT, Gupta SK. Percutaneous pedicle screw fixation of the lumbar spine: preliminary clinical results. *J Neurosurg* 2002;97[1 Suppl]:7–12.
98. Gertzbein SD, et al. Semirigid instrumentation in the management of lumbar spinal conditions combined with circumferential fusion. A multicenter study. *Spine* 1996;21(16):1918–1925; discussion 1925–1926.
99. McAfee PC, et al. The incidence of complications in endoscopic anterior thoracolumbar spinal reconstructive surgery. A prospective multicenter study comprising the first 100 consecutive cases. *Spine* 1995;20(14):1624–1632.
100. Mathews HH, et al. Laparoscopic discectomy with anterior lumbar interbody fusion. A preliminary review. *Spine* 1995;20(16):797–802.
101. Kaiser MG, et al. Comparison of the mini-open versus laparoscopic approach for anterior lumbar interbody fusion: a retrospective review. *Neurosurgery* 2002;51(1):97–103; discussion 103–105.
102. Kim DH, Jaikumar S, Kam AC. Minimally invasive spine instrumentation. *Neurosurgery* 2002;51[5 Suppl]:15–25.
103. Davne SH, Myers DL. Complications of lumbar spinal fusion with transpedicular instrumentation. *Spine* 1992;17[6 Suppl]:S184–189.
104. Knapp DR Jr, Jones ET. Use of cortical cancellous allograft for posterior spinal fusion. *Clin Orthop* 1988;(229):99–106.
105. Lonstein J, et al. Wound infection with Harrington instrumentation and spine fusion for scoliosis. *Clin Orthop* 1973;96:222–233.
106. Moe JH. Complications of scoliosis treatment. *Clin Orthop* 1967;53:21–30.
107. Horwitz NH, Curtin JA. Prophylactic antibiotics and wound infections following laminectomy for lumber disc herniation. *J Neurosurg* 1975;43(6):727–731.
108. Rubinstein E, et al. Perioperative prophylactic cephazolin in spinal surgery. A double-blind placebo-controlled trial. *J Bone Joint Surg Br* 1994;76(1):99–102.
109. Whitecloud TS 3rd, et al. Complications with the variable spinal plating system. *Spine* 1989;14(4):472–476.
110. Paut O, Bissonnette B. Syndrome of inappropriate antidiuretic hormone secretion after spinal surgery in children. *Crit Care Med* 2000;28(8):3126–3127.
111. Brazel PW, McPhee IB. Inappropriate secretion of antidiuretic hormone in postoperative scoliosis patients: the role of fluid management. *Spine* 1996;21(6):724–727.
112. Callewart CC, et al. Hyponatremia and syndrome of inappropriate antidiuretic hormone secretion in adult spinal surgery. *Spine* 1994;19(15):1674–1679.
113. Seitsalo S, et al. Disc degeneration in young patients with isthmic spondylolisthesis treated operatively or conservatively: a long-term follow-up. *Eur Spine J* 1997;6(6):393–397.
114. Kumar MN, Baklanov A, Chopin D. Correlation between sagittal plane changes and adjacent segment degeneration following lumbar spine fusion. *Eur Spine J* 2001;10(4):314–319.
115. Ma GW. Posterior lumbar interbody fusion with specialized instruments. *Clin Orthop* 1985;(193):57–63.
116. Flynn JC, Price CT. Sexual complications of anterior fusion of the lumbar spine. *Spine* 1984;9(5):489–492.
117. Johnson RM, McGuire EJ. Urogenital complications of anterior approaches to the lumbar spine. *Clin Orthop* 1981;(154):114–118.
118. Stevens WR, et al. Ophthalmic complications after spinal surgery. *Spine* 1997;22(12):1319–1324.
119. Grossman W, Ward WT. Central retinal artery occlusion after scoliosis surgery with a horseshoe headrest. Case report and literature review. *Spine* 1993;18(9):1226–1228.
120. Polatin PB, et al. Psychiatric illness and chronic low-back pain. The mind and the spine—which goes first? *Spine* 1993;18(1):66–71.
121. Steffee AD, Sitkowski DJ. Posterior lumbar interbody fusion and plates. *Clin Orthop* 1988;227:99–102.
122. Okuyama K, et al. Posterior lumbar interbody fusion: a retrospective study of complications after facet joint excision and pedicle screw fixation in 148 cases. *Acta Orthop Scand* 1999;70(4):329–334.
123. Calandruccio RA, Benton BF. Anterior lumbar fusion. *Clin Orthop* 1964;35:63–68.
124. Fujimaki A, Crock HV, Bedbrook GM. The results of 150 anterior lumbar interbody fusion operations performed by two surgeons in Australia. *Clin Orthop* 1982;(165):164–167.
125. Steinmann JC, Herkowitz HN. Pseudarthrosis of the spine. *Clin Orthop* 1992;(284):80–90.
126. Newman MH, Grinstead GL. Anterior lumbar interbody fusion for internal disc disruption. *Spine* 1992;17(7):831–833.
127. Freeman BJ, Licina P, Mehdian SH. Posterior lumbar interbody fusion combined with instrumented postero-lateral fusion: 5-year results in 60 patients. *Eur Spine J* 2000;9(1):42–46.
128. Agazzi S, Reverdin A, May D. Posterior lumbar interbody fusion with cages: an independent review of 71 cases. *J Neurosurg* 1999;91[2 Suppl]:186–192.
129. Lee CK, Vessa P, Lee JK. Chronic disabling low back pain syndrome caused by internal disc derangements. The results of disc excision and posterior lumbar interbody fusion. *Spine* 1995;20(3): 356–361.
130. Brantigan JW, et al. Interbody lumbar fusion using a carbon fiber cage implant versus allograft bone. An investigational study in the Spanish goat. *Spine* 1994;19(13):1436–1444.
131. Rompe JD, Eysel P, Hopf C. Clinical efficacy of pedicle instrumentation and posterolateral fusion in the symptomatic degenerative lumbar spine. *Eur Spine J* 1995;4(4):231–237.
132. Rosenberg WS, Mummaneni PV. Transforaminal lumbar interbody fusion: technique, complications, and early results. *Neurosurgery* 2001;48(3):569–574; discussion 574–575.
133. Kozak JA, O'Brien JP. Simultaneous combined anterior and posterior fusion. An independent analysis of a treatment for the disabled low-back pain patient. *Spine* 1990;15(4):322–328.
134. Schofferman J, et al. A prospective randomized comparison of 270 degrees fusions to 360 degrees fusions (circumferential fusions). *Spine* 2001;26(10):E207–212.
135. Hee HT, et al. Anterior/posterior lumbar fusion versus transforaminal lumbar interbody fusion: analysis of complications and predictive factors. *J Spinal Disord* 2001;14(6):533–540.

CHAPTER 58

Revision Decompressive/Disc Surgery

Shawn M. Henry and Richard D. Guyer

For almost 70 years, discectomy has been used to manage lumbar disc herniations. Dependent on the population studied, the annual incidence of lumbar discectomy performed in the United States annually ranges from 50 to more than 100/100,000 (1). With significant advances in surgical technique, there has been an evolution of two different schools of thought on how much disc should be removed. Some surgeons feel that a subtotal disc excision is appropriate (2,3), whereas others advocate removal of only the offending disc fragment (4). Regardless of the surgical technique used, reported reoperation rates have been similar (5–9). In lumbar disc surgery using the conventional technique, there has been a 10 to 30% prevalence of recurrent lesions at the same level (2,8,10). The rate of recurrence is reported as 7 to 15% after the microsurgical approach (2,8,11–14), and 14 to 33% after percutaneous disc surgery (15–17). This suggests a range of 5/100,000 to 30/100,000 being treated for recurrent disc herniations each year, based on the annual incidence of surgery. Therefore, surgeons should have a clear understanding of the diagnosis and management of these patients, as well as better strategies for prevention of recurrent disc herniations.

DEFINITION OF RECURRENT LUMBAR DISC HERNIATION

Recurrent lumbar disc herniation is defined as a disc herniation occurring at the same level as a previously operated lumbar disc, regardless of whether the herniation is ipsilateral or contralateral, with a pain-free interval after the index procedure of generally greater than 6 months. In the literature, there are several conditions that have been termed "recurrent herniated disc," such as an ipsilateral herniation at the same level as the primary herniation (6,7,18–20), contralateral herniation at the same level (1,21,22), or a new herniation occurring at a different level (7,19,23,24). Because the presence of scar tissue may affect the clinical results in cases of reoperation and the annular incision performed at the primary discectomy may be a predisposing factor for recurrence, a recurrent herniation (i.e., reherniation) should be strictly defined as a herniated disc that occurs at the same level.

ETIOLOGY

In 1947, 13 years after the introduction of lumbar disc surgery, Campbell and Whitfield published the first report on the reasons for failure of lumbar disc surgery (25). They emphasized psychological factors and compensation as causes of treatment failure. Five years later, several additional papers were published on reoperation of recurrent lumbar disc herniations (26,27). Since then, numerous studies have been published regarding revision lumbar disc surgery for recurrent disc herniations. Even today, the etiology of recurrent disc herniation remains uncertain. The causes for failure in relieving radiating leg pain after lumbar discectomy include surgery performed at the wrong level, insufficient removal of herniated disc material, traumatization of a nerve root, unrecognized displaced sequestration, unrecognized second disc herniation, insufficient decompression of spinal stenosis, spondylolisthesis, tumors, extravertebral nerve compression, segmental instability, and polyneuropathy (28–31). The recurrence of back pain or sciatic leg pain after primary disc surgery may be due to a true recurrent disc herniation, a new disc herniation at a different level, epidural fibrosis, arachnoiditis, secondary spinal stenosis, iatrogenic instability, facet joint arthritis, or spondylitis or spondylodiscitis (28,32).

In patients with recurrent disc herniations, 42% related the new onset of radicular pain to an isolated injury or precipitating event (33). The onset of pain was related to trauma in 32.1% of the patients. The author felt that the annular incision performed at the time of surgery made the previously operated disc level more susceptible to sudden prolapse, particularly under conditions of mechanical overload during sports activity or heavy lifting (33). This theory may explain the higher rate of recurrent disc herniation seen in young men (6,34). The risk factors associated with recurrent disc herniation include young age, male gender, smoking, and traumatic events. There was also found to be no difference in the rate of recurrent disc herniations associated with a partial or complete discectomy (33).

Different mechanisms may be involved in the pathogenesis of contralateral versus ipsilateral recurrent disc herniations (35,36). A "complete" discectomy excises a significant amount of nuclear and annular tissue on the surgical side, whereas only a partial removal of these tissues is accomplished on the contralateral side. It is proposed the external annulus could be damaged on the opposite side, and disc material not removed at primary discectomy could extrude later through the weakened annulus and cause a recurrent contralateral herniation (37).

Although the etiology for recurrent disc herniations is unclear, biomechanical studies have shown the negative effect of discectomy on the stability of the functional spinal unit is related to the type of annular incision performed (38,39) and the amount of tissue excised (40,41). A few months after disc excision has occurred, the reparative processes that occur at the site of the disc excision may have an effect on disc biomechanics. A fibroblastic reaction is noted to fill the defect of the outer annulus, whereas the deeper layers do not heal, and progressive degenerative changes ensue (42,43). To what extent the reparative processes affect disc biomechanics is not well known. Also not well understood is to what extent the progressive degenerative changes occurring within the disc itself contribute to recurrent disc herniation. The acute biomechanical effects were studied by Ahlgren et al., who showed that up to 4 weeks after disc injury, the technique used to make the annular incision played a role in determining the mechanical strength of annular healing (38). Six weeks after the annulotomy, the biomechanical properties of the disc had returned to preinjury levels.

Patients with diabetes have a significant increase in the risk of recurrent disc herniation when compared to the general population. Mobbs et al. studied 363 patients who underwent a discectomy for herniated disc disease (44). There were 33 patients with a preoperative diagnosis of diabetes, a prevalence of 9.1%. This group of 33 patients was compared with a control group of 33 age- and sex-matched nondiabetic patients. Recurrent disc herniation occurred in 7 of 25 (28%) of the diabetic patients compared to 1 of 28 (3.5%) of the control group. Overall, good to excellent results were reported for 24 of the 28 (86%) control patients and 15 of the 25 (60%) diabetic patients. This study concluded that a diabetic patient has a greater risk for poorer surgical outcome and recurrent disc herniation after discectomy than nondiabetic patients.

It is the authors' belief that a large number of diagnosed recurrent disc herniations may in fact be retained occult disc fragments that were not removed at the time of the index procedure. Although a large disc fragment may be initially removed at the time of surgery, if particular attention is not paid to secondary disc fragments, these may cause symptoms months later and have the appearance of a recurrent disc herniation. Typically after incomplete excision of disc material, however, a pain-free interval is not seen.

HISTORY AND PHYSICAL EXAMINATION

Patients with recurrent symptoms after a prior uncomplicated lumbar disc excision constitute a diagnostic and therapeutic challenge. Differentiating between the radiculopathy of a recurrent disc herniation and epidural periradicular fibrous tissue adhesions is of utmost importance. In these cases, significant differences in outcomes can be seen after repeat surgery (45). The first step in evaluating any patient is to take a thorough history and perform a complete physical examination. It is very important to develop a time line from the time of the initial surgery to the present. Past records may reveal items the patient does not feel important enough to comment on, or that have changed with memory. It is also important to understand the symptoms, signs, and diagnostic data that led to the patient's initial surgery. Pay particular attention to the type of surgery performed, the level at which the surgery was performed, if there were any perioperative complications, and the patient's response to the surgery. If preoperative psychological screening was performed, obtaining these test results may be helpful as well.

Careful assessment of current pain complaints is an important factor in the history. First, compare the current symptoms to the pain for which the surgery was initially performed. Second, determine how much pain relief the patient experienced, if any, and for what period of time. Third, assess the present pain location if the pain is in a diffuse or well-localized pattern, and the relative magnitudes of back and leg symptoms.

If the patient failed to obtain any period of pain relief after surgery, it is likely the initial surgery failed to completely address the source of the patient's symptoms. This may be due to a missed diagnosis or failure to adequately address the problem during the surgical procedure. For example, removing a free extruded disc fragment that is compressing a nerve root while not recognizing a secondary disc fragment fails to address the pathology. If the patient experienced pain after an initial period of relief, one needs to determine the length of time before recurrent symptoms. If the time period is less than 6 months, one should suspect arachnoiditis, scarring, reflex sympathetic dystrophy, discitis, or other infection. If the patient had significant relief of pain for more than 6 months, one should suspect development of a new source of symptoms or a recurrent disc herniation, if the symptoms are similar to those initially experienced. If a patient presents with pain different from the initial symptoms, the symptoms may be caused by a newly developed pathology, such as iatrogenic instability, pathology at a different anatomic site or level (particularly those adjacent to the operated segment, including the sacroiliac joint), facet joint pathology, scarring, infection, or stenosis at a different level. Another possible but less frequent cause of pain in previously operated spine patients is related to abnormalities of the autonomic nervous system. Sachs et al. reported on a series of 11 patients (frequency, 1%) with reflex sympathetic dystrophy after lumbar spine surgery (46). All patients had burning pain, vasomotor dysfunction, and dystrophic changes in at least one of the lower extremities.

One must investigate the patient's pain location in terms of back pain versus leg pain. If significant leg pain is present and is in a well-defined pattern, then a radiculopathy is likely due to recurrent herniated disc material, scar, bony compression, arachnoiditis, or less likely reflex sympathetic dystrophy. Other anatomic sites may cause leg pain, including pain referred from the facet joints, sacroiliac joints, discs, ligaments, or other spinal structures. This type of leg pain usually is diffuse, however. If the patient's pain is primarily limited to the low back and is associated with particular motions, mechanical instability is suspect (47). This may arise after laminectomies, discectomies, or failed fusion, which cause excessive motion in the previously operated region. Hopp and Tsou reported a 17% reoperation rate for instability that followed decompressive procedures (48). The detrimental effect of surgery on spinal musculature has also been implicated as a cause of instability (49,50). Significant local denervation atrophy is identified in the paraspinal muscles after posterior lumbar surgery. In addition to denervation, the patients also are at increased risk for disuse atrophy, which supports the need for comprehensive rehabilitation after low back surgery.

It is also important to pay attention to the nature of the patient's pain. Radicular numbness may be more likely related to nerve root compression, whereas burning pain or hyperalgesia in a lower extremity may be related to postoperative reflex sympathetic dystrophy. The physician needs to assess the existence of pain at rest, night pain, pain with motion, and pain that is aggravated by coughing and sneezing. It is also important to record the consumption of analgesics as well as any disturbance of walking capacity expressed as maximal walking distance.

The purpose of the physical examination is to try to localize the area of painful pathology. Physical examination findings are more valuable when the preoperative information is available for comparison so that it can be determined if this is a new problem, a recurrent one, or one that has not resolved from the previous surgical intervention. Routine motor strength testing, sensory testing, nerve root tension signs, and deep tendon reflex testing evaluate for objective signs of radiculopathy. The interpretation of root tension signs may be more difficult in the previously operated patient, particularly when there is scar tissue or arachnoiditis.

Jönsson and Strömqvist described clinical characteristics of patients with recurrent sciatica (51). They found patients with recurrent disc herniation were more likely to have at least two of the following three characteristics present as compared to patients whose problems were associated with fibrosis: pain when coughing, pain with a straight-leg raise at less than 30 degrees, and a greatly reduced walking capacity. They also reported that patients with recurrent disc herniation tended to have a longer pain-free interval after surgery than did patients whose pain was associated with scar (51). Performing the straight-leg raising test evaluates the nerve root tension by reproducing the pain along the course of the involved nerve. The patient's response to this maneuver should be documented as pain involving the leg, the back, or both, as well as if the pain is contralateral, ipsilateral, or both. The degree at which the pain was reproduced should also be documented (e.g., ipsilateral leg pain reproduced at 30 degrees). Although reproduction of back pain with this maneuver does not signify a positive nerve root tension sign, it should still be documented. A positive contralateral straight-leg raising sign is felt to be more strongly related to the likelihood of disc herniation as a source of true sciatica (52,53).

The patient interview and physical examination may indicate psychosocial issues, a particularly important concern in patients being considered for revision lumbar surgery. Some authors suggest the routine use of a formal psychosocial evaluation (54–61). Others think these evaluations should be reserved for patients whose surgeons suspect that psychosocial issues have affected or will affect the patient's symptoms, treatment, or outcome. In the authors' practice, the use of a pain diagram and visual analog pain scale has been found to be invaluable in the screening process.

RADIOGRAPHIC EVALUATION

The interpretation of imaging studies is especially difficult in patients who have had previous surgery. Special problems encountered in this population are scarring, metallic artifact if hardware was used, and the presence of abnormalities that are unrelated to the patient's symptoms. The high rate of imaging disc abnormalities in asymptomatic individuals is well documented (62–64).

Plain Radiography

The initial radiographic workup should include standing anteroposterior and lateral lumbosacral radiographs. The anteroposterior radiograph is useful in determining the location and magnitude of a prior decompression, new degenerative changes, or some other pathology, such as tumor, metastatic lesions, or infection. The lateral x-ray shows disc height, degenerative changes, end-plate irregularities, and compression fractures, or may show potentially unstable lesions, such as spondylolisthesis or spondylolysis. In the authors' practice, flexion and extension radiographs are also obtained to evaluate instability.

Magnetic Resonance Imaging

After plain radiographs, magnetic resonance imaging (MRI) is the next diagnostic procedure (Fig. 1). In the postoperative patient, this test should be performed with and without gadolinium enhancement, to differentiate scar from recurrent disc material. The scan should be performed soon after the gadolinium injection so that the contrast can infiltrate the scar tissue, but not the denser disc tissue. Milette et al. warned that the results of postdiscectomy MRI should be used cautiously when planning future intervention (65). They reported that even though MRI was good at differentiating recurrent herniation from scar, the imaging results did not correlate with clinical outcome. In another prospective study, 36 patients with radicular pain and lumbar disc herniation underwent a single-level disc resection. One year later, clinical follow-up was combined with a gadolinium-enhanced MRI examination (66). The study concluded there was no consistent correlation between

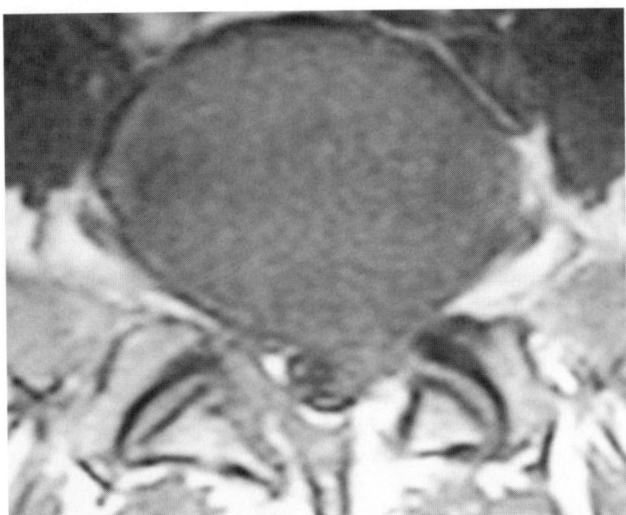

FIG. 1. Axial magnetic resonance imaging of a patient with prior laminotomy and recurrent symptoms.

postoperative back pain and/or radicular leg pain and the MRI findings. In other studies, MRI with gadolinium enhancement is reported to reliably distinguish between recurrent or residual disc herniation and scar tissue formation (67–69). Although other studies do not support that conclusion, Mullin et al. evaluated 28 patients who had surgical exploration comparing noncontrast MRI with contrast-enhanced MRI (70). They felt that the routine use of contrast-enhanced examinations in patients who have had prior lumbar surgery probably adds little diagnostic value and may be confusing. Vogelsang et al. evaluated 53 patients who underwent MRI due to recurrent pain after microdiscectomy (71). They found that the extent of peridural scarring as assessed by MRI is of minor value in the differential diagnosis of recurrent back pain after discectomy (71). In general, the criteria used to differentiate recurrent disc herniation from scar formation on contrast-enhanced MRI are that recurrent disc herniations do not enhance immediately after contrast injection, whereas scar enhances immediately (72–74). However, some authors have noted that the scar enhancement may decrease after 9 months postsurgery (75), whereas others report early epidural scar may fail to enhance at all (76). In addition, Bundschuh et al. noted that T2-weighted MRI that was unenhanced was able to correctly predict disc herniation or its absence in 13 of 14 patients (77).

Although there seems to be some controversy as to whether MRI enhancement aids in establishing a diagnosis between recurrent disc herniation and epidural fibrosis, postcontrast MRI has been established as the imaging method of choice for evaluating patients for recurrent symptoms after disc surgery (78,79). Nevertheless, one must use caution in the interpretation of gadolinium-enhanced MRI in the early postoperative period because of the normal sequence of changes that can occur (80). The degree of enhancement of scar formation is dependent on the amount of time since the operation, and decreases within the first 6 months (75,81).

Myelography

The complexity of this population of patients may require more in depth diagnostic workup. Bernard (82) evaluated a series of 45 symptomatic, previously operated patients using MRI, intrathecally enhanced computed tomography (CT), myelography, discography, and CT-discography (82). He found only 61% of patients could be accurately diagnosed using a single test (82). Among the 45 patients, 19 had more than one diagnosis confirmed at the time of surgery. A study by Byrd et al. evaluated the diagnostic use of plain films, myelography, CT, epidural venography, intravenously enhanced CT, and tomography. They concluded the plain films and enhanced CT scans were the most helpful (83). The pathologies most frequently encountered were granulation tissue, spondylosis, recurrent or residual disc herniation, and arachnoiditis.

Myelography has a role in the detection of arachnoiditis, misplaced internal fixation, and other compressive pathology such as recurrent herniated discs and epidural fibrosis, particularly when a postmyelographic CT scan is used. Arachnoiditis is difficult to identify based on clinical examination. It is generally associated with radicular pain in nonspecific patterns. In the myelogram or CT-myelogram, arachnoiditis typically appears as an irregular thecal sac that is shortened and nerve roots that are thickened or clumped together. Although the older dyes used in myelography have been found to cause arachnoiditis, this condition is not common after current nonionic water-soluble dyes.

Whereas iatrogenic instability is often identified on plain radiographs or flexion/extension views, myelography may also be helpful in making this diagnosis, particularly if the flexion/extension radiographs are taken with the myelographic contrast present. Myelography does have some shortcomings, however. Hittselberger et al. reported on myelographic imaging abnormalities in patients with no symptoms (84). It is limited wholly to identifying compressive pathology of the thecal sac or exiting nerve roots, and it is not useful in differentiating recurrent disc herniation from epidural scar tissue. Irstram reported on the use of myelography in a series of 44 patients who later underwent operation for suspected recurrent disc herniation (85). He found myelography could help identify the extent of the lesion, but it was not helpful in distinguishing scar from recurrent disc herniation. Braun et al. found that enhanced CT scan was more accurate than unenhanced CT scan in differentiating between recurrent herniated disc and epidural fibrosis (86). In another study by Benoist et al., myelography was found to be neither sensitive nor specific for differentiation of scar formation and disc herniation (87). Other authors have found CT scan with enhancement to have a 67 to 100% accuracy in assessing recurrent disc herniation versus epidural fibrosis (88–90).

Discography

Discography has been a controversial diagnostic tool since it was first introduced. It remains the only imaging study that also provides a pain provocation component. Discography may be particularly helpful in the examination of a previously operated patient in which the results of other imaging are difficult to interpret or are equivocal. Although some studies show the accuracy of combining imaging with pain provocation in discography is good (91), this evaluation may be difficult to perform in patients who have had previous surgery, scar, or a posterior fusion where the optimal placement of the needle cannot be obtained. Several investigators have reported on the use of discography in previously operated patients presenting with radicular symptoms after discectomy (92–94). They found that discography could differentiate between disc pathology and scar even in patients in whom a gadolinium-enhanced MRI yielded equivocal results.

Also, the pain provocation component of the examination can be used to determine if the visualized disc abnormality is related to the patient's presenting symptoms. Another study by Jackson et al. reported the results of comparing several diagnostic imaging methods including CT, myelography, CT-myelography, discography, and CT-discography (95). In the subgroup of patients who had previously undergone lumbar spine surgery, they found that CT-discography was the most accurate single test. It was the most sensitive at 100%, and also the most specific at 87.5% in the identification of a recurrent herniated disc.

The North American Spine Society recently published indications for lumbar discography (96). Some of the indications that may be applicable to previously operated patients include to further evaluate a disc that has been found to be abnormal, or to investigate the relationship of the imaged abnormalities to clinical symptoms (this may include recurrent disc herniation and lateral disc herniation), and patients with persistent symptoms in whom other tests have not confirmed a suspected recurrent disc herniation as a source of pain. The authors believe the provocative response to discography may be useful if it is interpreted as an extension of the physical examination.

DIAGNOSTIC AND THERAPEUTIC INJECTIONS

Injection of anesthetic or steroid agents, or both, in structures in or around the spine can be performed for therapeutic or diagnostic reasons. When the diagnosis is ambiguous, an anesthetic blockade is sometimes performed to help determine the etiology of the patient's painful condition. This becomes an important strategy in the diagnosis when the patient's history, physical examination, and imaging studies fail to clearly display the pathology that is causing the patient's pain. Anesthetizing anatomic structures within the spine can help to rule in or rule out an area in which there is a pain-provocative process. This then helps guide further treatment and may even relieve the patient's symptoms long term.

There are several sites commonly injected, including facet, nerve root, sacroiliac, epidural space, and hardware when present. Although one injection may be performed that may yield a negative response, another injection at a different anatomic site may be performed to search for the "pain generator."

Anesthetic blockade of the peripheral branches of the sciatic nerve may relieve pain in cases of radiculopathy caused by recurrent disc herniations (97,98). Selective nerve root injections are typically used in patients whose history, physical examination, imaging, and other tests are inconclusive. In cases of the multiply operated back or recurrent disc herniation, this becomes an invaluable tool to aid in the diagnosis.

PSYCHOLOGICAL EVALUATION

There is a strong tendency to rely on imaging studies in the evaluation of a surgical candidate; however, one must consider not only the visualization of pathology, but also give consideration to the patient's personality and psychological state. A study by Spengler et al. found that psychological evaluations were a better predictor of surgical outcome than were imaging studies, which were better related to operative findings (60). Their study did not specifically address previously operated patients, but it did bring recognition to the importance of psychosocial factors in surgical outcome. Block et al. developed a preoperative psychosocial screening package for spine surgery candidates (99). This package incorporates many of the factors that have been reported to be related to surgical outcome, including the hysteria and hypochondriasis scales of the Minnesota Multiphasic Personality Inventory (MMPI), coping skills, work and lifestyle stability, depression, job satisfaction, previous surgery, concomitant health conditions and other factors. Each assessment has a weighted score from which an overall evaluation is derived. The psychologist or psychiatrist can advise the surgeon of the following alternatives: (a) the patient is cleared for surgery, (b) the patient is cleared for surgery but needs psychological/psychiatric therapy, (c) the patient needs therapy before being cleared for surgery, (d) or the patient may not be a good surgical candidate. The MMPI is an effective tool in predicting surgical outcome and can be used to screen out patients who are poor surgical candidates (58,60,99).

A psychosocial problem is suspect when a patient fails to get pain relief and return to function yet the index procedure was done for well correlated clinical symptoms, signs and imaging studies, and pathology was clearly identified during the operation. The risk is greatest when patient history suggests there were major psychosocial issues before the first operation, which were never analyzed or addressed. Such patients should undergo complete psychological evaluation as well as all appropriate imaging studies before an operation is performed. A number of different tests are available for psychological assessment. Pain drawings have been shown to correlate well with the MMPI tests (22,100) and are simple and inexpensive. They found identification of life events that act as stressors can be important to predict unfavorable outcome. Crauford et al. identified the following negative predictors: childhood or sexual abuse, alcohol or drug abuse in a parent, abandonment, or emotional neglect (101). If the patient had three of five of these childhood psychological events, the likelihood of unsuccessful surgery was 85% (102).

Patient Expectations

If the patient's expectations for the proposed surgery are too great, he or she is not a good surgical candidate until he or she understands the realistic likelihood of success. Frank discussion between the surgeon and patient is particularly important in those who have already had a poor result from previous surgical intervention. The patient needs to understand an additional surgery may or may not help his or her condition, and may in fact make it worse. He or she needs to understand that total pain relief and full return to activities is unlikely. It is also important to help the patient understand a prolonged state of reduced activity requires participation in a rehabilitation program after surgery. The patient's family should be included in these discussions so their expectations also are realistic.

PATIENT SELECTION

The most important factor in achieving a good treatment result is proper patient selection. After careful consideration of the patient's history, physical examination findings, radiographic evaluation, and psychological screening results, all the important predictors of success and failure can be used to determine if further surgical intervention is warranted. A number of clinical studies have analyzed predictive risk factors. Biondi and Greenberg reported predictors of a poor outcome for surgery were workers compensation, a pain-free interval of less than 6 months, male gender, history of psychiatric illness, and primary diagnosis of perineural fibrosis (103). Finnegan et al. found that patients receiving compensation or having psychological problems tended to do more poorly after repeat surgery than patients without these factors present (104). These results are consistent with North et al., who reported the predictors of a good outcome were younger age, female gender, a history of good results from previous spine surgery, absence of epidural scar, and prevalence of radicular pain (21). However, Bernard reported that age, number of previous operations, and psychological status were unrelated to the outcome of revision surgery (82). He did find that a noncompensatable injury, return to work, a negative history of litigation, and attaining a solid fusion were significantly related to better outcomes. Quimjian and Matrka reported factors related to a good outcome after revision spine surgery were unilateral radicular pain pattern, a pain-free interval of 1 year after the initial surgery, and myelography indicative of recurrent disc herniation (105). Yaksich's study reported that the ideal patient to be accepted for a repeat spine surgery should have leg pain rather than back pain, a recurrent or residual disc herniation associated with stenosis, and be highly motivated to improve (106). Silvers et al. reported on patients with true recurrent disc herniation (herniation at the same level and same side as what was previously operated) (107). They found 64% were satisfied with the outcome of the subsequent surgery, but only 22% returned to work and 27% returned to previous activity. These figures were worse than for patients who were undergoing a subsequent discectomy for problems at different levels or on the other side.

NONOPERATIVE TREATMENT

Once a patient has been diagnosed with a recurrent disc herniation, nonoperative treatment should be implemented. If a patient has a new level or opposite-side disc herniation, they should be treated with a standard nonoperative treatment regimen for a primary disc herniation. This program includes 6 to 8 weeks of rest from vigorous activities, physical therapy, nonsteroidal antiinflammatory agents, oral steroids, and a series of epidural steroid injections. In the authors' practice, gabapentin (Neurontin) is given to the patient orally for treatment of radicular symptoms and seems to be considerably beneficial to the patient with neurogenic pain. If a patient does not improve, only then should surgical intervention be considered. In patients with true recurrent disc herniation (i.e., same level, same side), the time line from nonoperative treatment to surgical intervention may be shorter, particularly when there is muscle weakness.

If a patient fails nonoperative treatment, surgical intervention is considered. These patients generally have dominant leg pain, which is persistent and disabling. Other operative indications for recurrent disc herniation include a significant progressive neurologic deficit and cauda equina syndrome. Patients should be cleared for psychosocial contraindications, and a preoperative medical clearance should be obtained. If the patient has atypical pain patterns or other questionable findings, then a selective nerve root injection should be performed to help confirm the diagnosis before surgical intervention. The combination of anesthetic agent and steroid use can effectively provide relief of symptoms if performed at the correct root level, and may give lasting relief. It is also helpful when correlating the signs and symptoms of the suspected root level with the response obtained from the short-acting local anesthetic agent at that root level. A current MRI or CT-myelogram should also be available at the time of surgery. The patient should have informed consent carefully explaining the risks, benefits, and other alternatives, including nonoperative and operative treatment, and the risks and benefits of each of the alternatives.

OPERATIVE TREATMENT

The previous index disc surgery may have been done by percutaneous discectomy, microdiscectomy, or open laminotomy with discectomy. Nucleoplasty and chemonucleolysis may also have been used, although these techniques are no longer used in the United States. In revision disc surgery, the authors advocate a standard open laminotomy with discectomy. The goal is to decompress the nerve root that is causing the radiculopathy by removing disc material or bone, or both. Enough bone needs to be removed to allow adequate visualization so that the disc material can safely and efficiently be removed without causing later instability. In revision disc surgery, the other techniques mentioned earlier for the index operation do not adequately allow this and hence should not be used.

Fusion may be indicated in some patients, particularly those who present with a third-time disc herniation. At the authors' institution, decompression with an anterior or posterior lumbar interbody fusion is preferred for these patients. This approach allows complete removal of all disc material so that reherniation cannot occur. Also, the fusion allows the surgeon to address the already compromised disc by providing stability at this motion segment, and thus eliminates a potential cause for discogenic pain. In a study by Vishteh and Dickman, an anterior lumbar microdiscectomy and interbody fusion was performed on six patients for the treatment of recurrent disc herniation (108). These patients underwent a muscle-sparing "minilaparotomy," microscopic anterior lumbar discectomy, and fragmentectomy for recurrent lumbar disc extrusions at L-5 to S-1. Interbody fusion was then performed by placing cylindrical threaded titanium cages or threaded allograft bone dowels. With a mean follow-up of 14 months, radicular pain and neurologic deficits were resolved in all six patients. Later MRI studies showed complete resection of all herniated disc material.

A future alternative may be artificial disc replacement and/or nuclear replacement for the treatment of patients with multiple recurrent disc herniations. This procedure would potentially allow for complete removal of disc material while still maintaining motion and stability at this segment. Artificial disc replacement is currently being performed in other countries, and it is being studied at U.S. Food and Drug Administration investigational centers in the United States.

SURGICAL TECHNIQUE

Once general anesthesia is administered, the patient is placed on an Andrews table (Fig. 2). The Andrews table allows the abdomen to hang free, decreasing the intraabdominal pressure and the retrograde intravenous pressure on the epidural veins, and, therefore, decreasing bleeding. There are other special tables and devices that can also serve this purpose. The authors routinely use loop magnification and a headlamp to aid in visualization. A midline skin incision is made, typically through the incision from the previous operation, but this may need to be extended. Sharp dissection is carried through the skin and subcutaneous tissue down to the level of

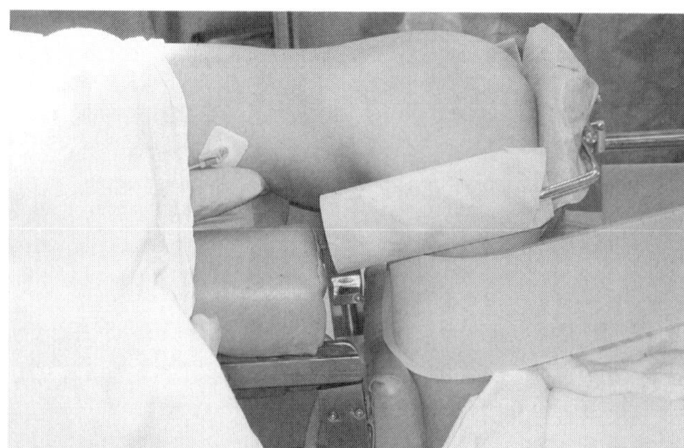

FIG. 2. Patient positioning on an Andrews table. Note the abdomen hanging free.

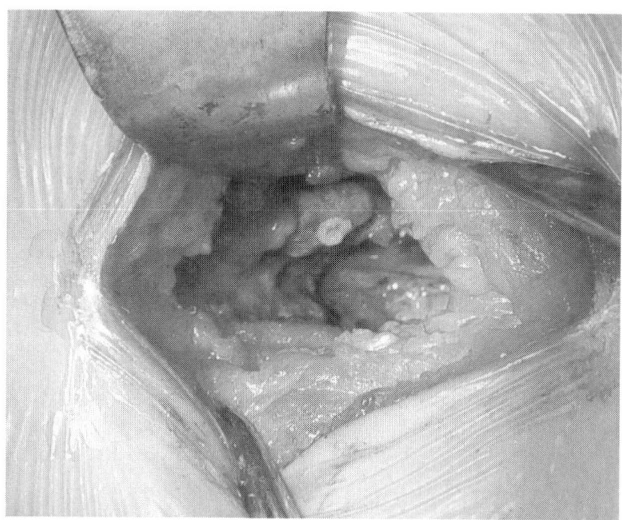

FIG. 3. The operative site.

the fascia. Care is taken to perform meticulous hemostasis throughout the surgical dissection. Next, by using electrocautery, the fascia is incised in line with the skin incision over the spinous processes and a subperiosteal dissection is carried out. The facet capsule should not be violated as dissection is taken across the lamina and out laterally. At this point, the surgical wound is packed with sponges and a localizing radiograph is taken. Once the correct level has been confirmed, the surgery is continued. A self-retaining retractor, such as a modified Taylor retractor or Crank retractor, is used. At this point, the lamina above and below the level involved should be clean and exposed and the retractor should be placed so that the interlaminar space is well visualized (Fig. 3).

Once all bony landmarks are exposed, the next step is to enter the canal. By using a sharp curette, the authors carefully detach the scar from the superior edge of the lamina below. Care is taken not to plunge with the curette. The dissection is directed medial to lateral. Next, by using a Kerrison punch or a small osteotome, a partial "thin sliver" medial facetectomy is performed. The surgeon needs to be cautious not to take more than one-third of the facet joint, which reduces the risk of iatrogenic instability. Once the osteotomized pieces of inferior medial facet joint are removed, the medial border of the superior facet will be exposed. The Kerrison punch is then used again to resect a portion of the medial border of the superior facet. One needs to be particularly careful in avoiding the nerve root because the disc herniation tends to displace the nerve root dorsally. At this point, the inferior and lateral borders of the scar should be completely free. The scar can be reflected medially to visualize the exiting nerve root, or it can be removed carefully with the Kerrison punch. The lateral border of the nerve root should then be well exposed. If the nerve root cannot be readily seen, it may be displaced by the disc material. If this occurs, a Murphy ball is used to locate the wall of the medial pedicle. It may also be necessary to extend the dissection proximally into the superior lamina until virgin dura is reached. By dissecting from the medial pedicle toward the midline and down onto the canal floor, the nerve root should eventually be visualized. Next, the nerve root needs to be mobilized to safely access the disc below. Often, the nerve root and dura may be scarred in the canal below. By using a straight curette with the blunt edge facing medially on a cottonoid patty, gentle blunt dissection can be performed until the dura and nerve root are essentially freed toward the midline. During this part of the procedure, it is very important that hemostasis be maintained. The Kerrison punch is then used to ensure that enough lamina and medial facet is removed so that the entire root is exposed as it exits from the thecal sac. A nerve root retractor is used to gently mobilize the nerve root over the offending disc fragment and provide protection during disc removal. An extruded disc fragment can be easily removed with a pituitary rongeur (Fig. 4). If the disc material has not extruded, an incision is made in the posterior annulus using a No. 11 knife blade. Next, using a pituitary rongeur the free disc material is grasped and removed. Care needs to be taken so that the pituitary rongeur is not advanced too far anteriorly in the disc space so that vascular structures are avoided. The authors tend to use a combination of different sizes, as well as up-biting and down-biting pituitary rongeurs, to ensure that all free fragments are removed from within the disc space. Once it is felt that all free disc material has been removed, a Murphy ball is then used to probe for residual disc material. There are "four checks" that specifically should be performed. These include (a) probing of the exiting foramen above, (b) the foramen below, (c) the posterior canal (above and below the disc space), and (d) the tension of the nerve. Once it is determined that all disc material is removed and that the dural sac and nerve roots have been decompressed, the decision is made as to whether a foraminotomy is necessary by probing the neural foramen. If easy passage of the nerve root is not allowed, a foraminotomy should be performed. A small Kerrison punch can be directed into the foramen to allow removal of enough bone from the lamina to provide ample space for the nerve. During the course of the surgical procedure, particular attention needs to be paid to the amount of time and the amount of retraction that are placed on nerve roots to minimize the risk of injury. Typically, nerve roots should not be retracted past midline.

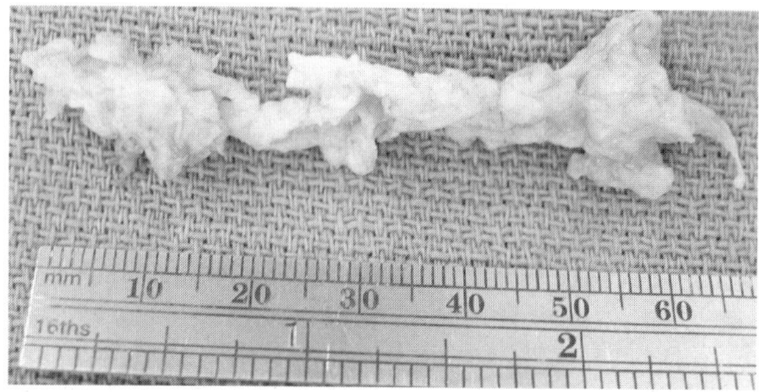

FIG. 4. Disc tissue.

If the expected pathology is not present, the level of the surgery should be reassessed using an intraoperative x-ray with a marker placed in the disc space. After the decompression has been performed, attention is paid to meticulous hemostasis. Copious irrigation is performed in the surgical wound with antibiotic irrigation solution. Next, a thin fat graft or Gelfoam is placed over the exposed dura. The lumbodorsal fascia is then closed with an absorbable suture material. A layered closure is performed in the subcutaneous tissue and skin.

In those patients in whom the disc material is intraforaminal, it may be difficult to remove the disc material through the standard surgical approach. Sometimes, removing a larger portion of the facet joint allows enough exposure to remove the disc material. It may also be necessary to perform a bilateral laminotomy to increase the exposure. This allows for better mobilization of the dura and nerve root and also allows the surgeon from the side opposite the pathology to obtain a better angle with the Kerrison punch, which can be directed toward the foramen. A portion of the lateral pars interarticularis may have to be sacrificed, however, to achieve adequate exposure. If too much of the pars is removed, it may be appropriate to fuse this segment.

Extraforaminal Herniation

Occasionally, patients present with an extraforaminal recurrent disc herniation. This lesion cannot be resolved through a standard midline approach unless the entire facet joint is taken down, which is described by some authors (109,110). An extraforaminal lateral approach has been advocated by Wiltse (111) that has a number of advantages. First, the facet joints do not have to be violated and subsequent risk of instability is avoided. Second, this approach allows the surgeon to avoid navigating through scar tissue to enter the spinal canal. Last, the nerve root can be more easily identified and the completeness of the decompression can be determined.

To perform the Wiltse approach (111,112), a 3- to 5-cm midline incision is made that is localized to the appropriate level. Dissection is carried through the subcutaneous layer down to the dorsal lumbar fascia. Next, dissection is carried through the plane between the dorsal lumbar fascia and subcutaneous tissues on the side on which the lesion is present. At this point, an incision is made through the dorsal lumbar fascia approximately 3 to 4 cm lateral to the midline, dividing the fascia over the area of the longissimus and multifidus muscles. Blunt dissection is carried through the longissimus and multifidus paraspinal muscles until the transverse processes can be palpated. The soft tissues are cleared so that the transverse process above and the transverse process below the area of pathology are clearly seen. By staying between the muscle planes of the longissimus and multifidus paraspinal muscles and without violating the muscle sheath, the amount of bleeding can be kept to a minimum. A marker is placed on the transverse process and a plain radiograph is taken to confirm the level.

Once the correct level has been confirmed, the intertransverse ligament is detached from the transverse process beginning at the caudal aspect of the lower transverse process by using a curette. Once the intertransverse ligament is removed, the nerve root can be identified approximately 2 to 4 mm deep to the intertransverse ligament. It exits at approximately a 45-degree angle. The dorsal root ganglia can also be seen as it exits under the pars interarticularis. The nerve root can then be followed medially until the disc material is visualized. The nerve root is very carefully and gently mobilized and protected with a nerve root retractor. If a free disc fragment is present, it is removed. If a free fragment is not visualized, the nerve root is protected, the annulus is incised, and pituitary rongeurs are used to remove any free disc fragments. Once it is felt that the decompression is adequate, a Murphy ball is used to probe the foramen. If the decompression still seems inadequate, then the surgeon can perform the interlaminar approach as described earlier. An alternative technique that the authors prefer is to detach the intertransverse ligament from the superior medial portion of the inferior transverse process. The disc is found in the safe "triangular zone" formed by the transverse process, superior facet, and the traversing nerve. The entry into the disc is similar to the endoscopic (arthroscopic) approaches. By working medial to the nerve root, no traction is placed on the root itself, and the disc space can be evacuated until the foramina is patent. At the time of closure, the dorsal lumbar fascia is reapproximated first. The surgeon needs to pay particular attention to closing the dead space that was made under the subcutaneous tissue layer. This layer has a tendency to collect fluid, and hence, a drain is recommended.

Cauda Equina Syndrome

In instances in which a patient presents with cauda equina syndrome, providing enough exposure is essential, and bilateral laminotomy/laminectomy is necessary. The dura is exposed by carefully removing the ligamentum flavum. When cauda equina syndrome occurs, the large offending disc fragment tends to displace the dura more dorsally under the ligament, and caution needs to be taken not to violate the dura during the midline dissection. The thecal sac then is exposed out to the lateral recesses, with removal of the superior articular facet, so that the nerve roots are adequately visualized. When cauda equina syndrome occurs after a recurrent disc herniation, dissection is more easily performed by beginning on the side that has not been previously operated. The initial goal is to provide enough exposure so that the disc can be debulked without putting excessive traction on the nerve roots. Once the large free disc fragment has been removed, steps are taken to ensure that all free fragments are removed and that all nerve roots and canals are free and patent.

Postoperative Care

Typically, the patient remains in the hospital overnight after surgery or may be discharged the same day. Pain is managed with a patient-controlled analgesia unit. Intravenous antibiotics are continued for 24 hours postoperatively. The authors often place the patients on a three-dose regimen of intravenous steroids (Decadron) administered over 24 hours if there has been a difficult dissection. Once the patient has recovered from the anesthesia, the patient is encouraged to begin ambulating immediately after surgery with physical therapy. The patient is seen for follow-up approximately 2 weeks postoperatively, and at that point, he or she is placed into a formal physical therapy rehabilitation program.

PROGNOSIS

The results of repeat spine surgery reported are not as good as those for initial procedures. The best results are obtained in carefully selected patients.

A prospective study of 26 patients who had recurrent ipsilateral radicular leg pain after a 6-month pain-free period showed an 85% satisfaction rate in the study group compared with an 88% satisfaction rate in the control group (i.e., no radicular leg pain) (33). A study by Cinotti et al. investigated the surgical outcomes of patients who underwent discectomy for contralateral recurrent disc herniation and compared these with results from a group of patients who had a primary discectomy performed for herniated nucleus pulposus (35). This prospective evaluation found that 14 of 16 patients with recurrent disc herniations were satisfied at 2 years after surgery compared with 45 of 50 patients who were satisfied at 2 years who had a primary discectomy performed. They concluded that the clinical results showed that patients who were reoperated on for contralateral recurrent disc herniation compared favorably to those who had a primary discectomy performed (35).

There are some studies in the literature suggesting that repeat discectomy performed on patients with recurrent disc herniations tend to have poorer results. In a study by Silvers et al., a retrospective analysis was performed on 82 patients who underwent a microdiscectomy for treatment of recurrent back and leg pain (107). Although 73% of the patients were satisfied with their results, the authors concluded that workers' compensation patients presenting within 1 year after discectomy with recurrent complaints and a same-side recurrence are at risk for poor outcomes. In another retrospective study of 211 patients, a comparison was made between the results of a primary discectomy and a discectomy for recurrent disc herniation. The reoperated group had significantly worse results (114). In a study by Fritsch et al., a retrospective study was performed on 182 revision surgeries for recurrent disc (115). There were 44 patients in this study who had multiple procedures. They concluded a laminectomy performed at the time of primary surgery was a factor leading to a high rate of recurrence, which the authors attributed to late instability and epidural fibrosis. Although their definitions of instability and postdiscotomy syndrome were ill-defined, the study suggests subsequent surgery is most successful when there is pure recurrent disc herniation with isolated radicular syndromes. Herron et al. reported on 46 patients who were treated for recurrent disc herniation. They noted that 28 (69%) of these patients had good results, whereas only three patients (7%) had poor results. They concluded (in the absence of instability) that recurrent disc herniation may be treated by repeat discectomy (54). In another retrospective evaluation of 28 patients with recurrent lumbar disc herniations, the outcomes correlated with a number of covariant risk factors (36). Age, gender, smoking, profession, traumatic events, level and degree of herniation, and pain-free interval did not appear to affect clinical outcomes. Conventional open discectomy as a revision procedure for recurrent disc herniation yielded satisfactory results comparable to those of primary discectomy. Ozgen et al. analyzed 114 patients who underwent re-exploration for intractable back and leg pain (116). At the time of reoperation, they found 78% disc herniations, 12.2% epidural fibrosis, 3.5% adhesive arachnoiditis, 2.6% isolated spinal stenosis, and 3.5% iatrogenic instability. Fifty-six of the one hundred fourteen patients (50%) were found to have a true recurrent disc herniation. There were several conclusions derived from this study: recurrent disc disease and particularly extruded disc fragments were the most important cause for re-exploration. The most favorable outcomes were achieved in patients in whom disc herniations occurred at the same level. The presence of epidural fibrosis and arachnoiditis was associated with a poor result.

Another significant issue is low back pain after discectomy. Hanley and Shapiro evaluated 87 patients with 120 primary discectomies (113). Of these patients, 14% reported poor results secondary to disabling low back pain and 7% were found to have recurrent disc herniation. Other studies suggested the risk for significant chronic low back pain after discectomy is 15% (6,52,86,113). In a study by Finnegan et al., patients were noted to have an 80% satisfactory outcome with revision surgery (104). This occurred when a pain-free interval followed the previous operation, and when mechanical compression or instability was seen.

SUMMARY

The best treatment for recurrent disc herniations is prevention. By having a thorough understanding of the factors that are predisposed to recurrent disc herniations, one can hopefully minimize the number of recurrences in the surgeon's practice. However, a recurrent disc herniation should not be considered a surgical complication. The approach is to carefully assess the patient's condition and determine an appropriate course of treatment. The decision to subject the patient to additional surgery should not be undertaken lightly. Unless there are indications for surgery, a clinical history and physical examination findings that correlate with radiographic findings, and clearance by a psychologist, additional surgery should be avoided. On the other hand, if a patient does present with well-defined indications for surgery, one should not be overly hesitant to pursue this course simply because the patient has had prior surgery.

Ultimately, the keys for successful treatment are to obtain an accurate diagnosis, practice good surgical technique, and most importantly, for the surgeon, the patient, and their family, to have realistic expectations about the outcome.

REFERENCES

1. Davis H. Increasing rates of cervical and lumbar spine surgery in the United States 1979–1990. *Spine* 1994;19:1117–1124.
2. Casper W, Campbell B, Barbier DD, et al. The Casper microsurgical discectomy and comparison with a conventional standard lumbar disc procedure. *Neurosurgery* 1991;28:78–86.
3. Wilson DH, Harbaugh R. Microsurgical and standard removal of the protruded lumbar disc: a comparative study. *Neurosurgery* 1981;8:422–427.
4. Williams RW. Microlumbar discectomy: a conservative surgical approach to the virgin herniated lumbar disc. *Spine* 1978;3:175–182.
5. Burton CV, Kirkaldy-Willis WH, Yong-Hing K, et al. Causes of failure of surgery on the lumbar spine. *Clin Orthop* 1981;157:191–199.
6. Ebeling U, Kalbarcyk H, Reulen HJ. Microsurgical reoperation following lumbar disc surgery. *J Neurosurg* 1989;70:397–404.
7. Law JD, Lehman RAW, Kirsch WM. Reoperation after lumbar intervertebral disc surgery. *J Neurosurg* 1978;48:259–263.
8. Silvers HR. Microsurgical versus standard lumbar discectomy. *Neurosurgery* 1988;22:837–841.
9. Weir BKA, Jacobs GA. Reoperation rate following lumbar discectomy. *Spine* 1980;5:366–370.
10. Tullberg T, Isacson J, Weidenhielm L. Does microscopic removal of lumbar disc herniation lead to better results than the standard procedure? Results of a one-year randomized study. *Spine* 1993;18:24–27.
11. Barrios C, Ahmed M, Arrotegui J, et al. Microsurgery versus standard removal of the herniated lumbar disc: a 3-year comparison in 150 cases. *Acta Orthop Scand* 1990;61:399–403.
12. Ebeling U, Reichenberg W, Reulen HJ. Results of microsurgical lumbar discectomy: review of 485 patients. *Acta Neurochir* 1986; 81:45–52.

13. Nyström B. Experience of microsurgical compared with conventional technique in lumbar disc operations. *Acta Neurol Scand* 1987; 76:129–144.
14. Pappas CTE, Harrington T, Sonntag VKH. Outcome analysis of 654 surgically treated lumbar disc herniations. *Neurosurgery* 1992;30:862–866.
15. Hoppenfeld S. Percutaneous removal of herniated lumbar discs: 50 cases with ten-year follow-up periods. *Clin Orthop* 1989;238:92–97.
16. Onik G, Mooney V, Maroon JC, et al. Automated percutaneous discectomy: a prospective multi-institutional study. *Neurosurgery* 1990;26:228–232.
17. Revel M, Payan C, Vallee C, et al. Automated percutaneous lumbar discectomy versus chemonucleolysis in the treatment of sciatica: a randomized multicenter trial. *Spine* 1993;18:1–7.
18. Fandino J, Botana C, Viladrich A, et al. Reoperation after lumbar disc surgery: results in 130 cases. *Acta Neurochir Wien* 1993;122:102–104.
19. O'Sullivan MG, Connolly AE, Buckley TF. Recurrent lumbar disc protrusion. *Br J Neurosurg* 1990;4:319–325.
20. Pheasant HC. Sources of failure in laminectomies. *Orthop Clin North Am* 1975;6:319–329.
21. North RB, Campbell JN, James CS, et al. Failed back surgery syndrome: 5-year follow-up in 102 patients undergoing repeat operation. *Neurosurgery* 1991;28:685–690.
22. Ransford AO, Cairns D, Mooney V. The pain drawing as an aid to the psychological evaluation of patients with low back pain. *Spine* 1976;1:127–135.
23. Connolly ES. Surgery for recurrent lumbar disc herniation. *Clin Neurosurg* 1992;39:211–216.
24. Epstein JA, Lavine LS, Epstein BS. Recurrent herniation of the lumbar intervertebral disk. *Clin Orthop* 1967;52:169–178.
25. Campbell E, Whitfield RD. Certain reasons for failure following disc operations. *N Y State J Med* 1947;47:2569–2572.
26. Greenwood J Jr, McGuire TH, Kimbell F. A study of the causes of failure in the herniated intervertebral disc operation. An analysis of sixty-seven reoperated cases. *J Neurosurg* 1952;9:15–20.
27. Kelly JH, Vordis DC, Svien HJ, et al. Multiple operations for protruded intervertebral disk. *Proc Staff Meet Mayo Clin* 1954;29:546–550.
28. Dahmen G. Editorial. Rezidivoperationen nacnNucleotomie. Bericht uber ein Kolloquium. In: Schollner D, ed. *Rezidive nach lumbalen Bandscheibenoperationen: Ursachen, Diagnostik, Behandlung*. Uelzen, Germany: Medizinisch Literarische Verlags Gesellschaft, 1980.
29. Keyl W, Wirth C-J. Indikation, Technik und Ergebnisse der Operationen bei Nucleusrezidiven. In: Schollner D, ed. *Rezidive nach lumbalen Bandscheibenoperationen: Ursachen, Diagnostik, Behandlung*. Uelzen, Germany: Medizinisch Literarische Verlags Gesellschaft, 1980.
30. Kramer J. *Bandscheibenbedingte Erkrankungen. Ursachen, Diagnose, Behandlung, Vorbeugung, Begutachtung*, 2nd ed. New York: Thieme, 1986.
31. Martin G. Recurrent disc prolapse as a cause of recurrent pain after laminectomy for lumbar disc lesions. *N Z Med J* 1980;91:206–208.
32. Crock HV. Observation on the management of failed spinal operations. *J Bone Joint Surg [Br]* 1976;58:193–199.
33. Cinotti G, Roysam GS, Eisenstein SM, et al. Ipsilateral recurrent lumbar disc herniation. *J Bone Joint Surg [Br]* 1998;80:825–832.
34. Reith C, Lausberg G. Risk factors of recurrent disc herniation. *Neurosurg Rev* 1989;12:147–150.
35. Cinotti G, Gumina S, Giannicola G, et al. Contralateral recurrent lumbar disc herniation. Results of discectomy compared with those in primary herniation. *Spine* 1999;24:800–806.
36. Suk KS, Lee HM, Moon SH, et al. Recurrent lumbar disc herniation. Results of operative management. *Spine* 2001;26:672–676.
37. Jacchia GE, Bardelli M, Barile L, et al. Casistica, risultati e cause di insuccessi di ernie discali operate. *Ital J Orthop Traumatol* 1980;6 [Suppl]:5–23.
38. Ahlgren BD, Vasavada A, Brower RS, et al. Annular incision technique on the strength and multidirectional flexibility of the healing intervertebral disc. *Spine* 1994;19:948–954.
39. Ethier DB, Cain JC, Yaszemski MJ, et al. The influence of annulotomy section on disc competence. A radiographic, biomechanical, and histologic analysis. *Spine* 1994;19:2071–2076.
40. Brinckmann P, Grootenboer H. Change of the disc height, radial bulge, and intradiscal pressure from discectomy. An in vitro investigation on human lumbar discs. *Spine* 1991;16:641–646.
41. Goel VK, Nishiyama K, Weinstein JN, et al. Mechanical properties of lumbar spinal motion segments as affected by partial disc removal. *Spine* 1986;11:1008–1012.
42. Hampton D, Laros G, McCarron R, et al. Healing potential of the anulus fibrosus. *Spine* 1989;14:398–401.
43. Osti OL, Vernon-Roberts B, Fraser RD. Anulus tear and intervertebral disc degeneration. An experimental study using an animal model. *Spine* 1990;15:762–767.
44. Mobbs R, Newcombe R, Chandran K. Lumbar discectomy and the diabetic patient: incidence and outcome. *J Clin Neurosci* 2001;8:10–13.
45. Jönsson B, Strömqvist B. Repeat decompression of lumbar nerve roots: prospective two-year evaluation. *J Bone Joint Surg [Br]* 1993;75:894–897.
46. Sachs BL, Zindrick MR, Beasley RD. Reflex sympathetic dystrophy after operative procedures on the lumbar spine. *J Bone Joint Surg [Am]* 1993;75:721–731.
47. Lauerman WC, Wiesel SW. The failed back: an algorithm. *Semin Spine Surg* 1996;8:208–220.
48. Hopp E, Tsou PM. Postdecompression lumbar instability. *Clin Orthop* 1988; 227:143–151.
49. Kawaguchi Y, Matsui H, Tsuji H. Back muscle injury after posterior lumbar spine surgery. Part 2: Histologic and histochemical analysis in humans. *Spine* 1994;19:2598–2602.
50. Sihvonen T, Herno A, Paljarvi L, et al. Local denervation atrophy of paraspinal muscles in postoperative failed back syndrome. *Spine* 1993;18:575–581.
51. Jönsson B, Strömqvist B. Clinical characteristics of recurrent sciatica after lumbar discectomy. *Spine* 1996;21:500–505.
52. Garvey TA. Surgical decision making in lumbar disc herniation. *Phys Ther Pract* 1992;1:10–19.
53. Stambough JL. Recurrent same-level, ipsilateral lumbar disc herniation. *Orthop Rev* 1994;23:810–816.
54. Herron L. Recurrent lumbar disc herniation: results of repeat laminectomy and discectomy. *J Spinal Disord* 1994;7:161–166.
55. Herron LD, Turner J. Patient selection for lumbar laminectomy and discectomy with a revised objective rating system. *Clin Orthop* 1985;199:145–152.
56. Herron LD, Turner J, Clancy S, et al. The differential utility of the Minnesota Multiphasic Personality Inventory: a predictor of outcome in lumbar laminectomy for disc herniation versus spinal stenosis. *Spine* 1986;11:847–850.
57. Pheasant HC, Gilbert D, Goldfarb J, et al. The MMPI as a predictor of outcome in low-back surgery. *Spine* 1979;4:78–84.
58. Spengler DM, Freeman CW. Patient selection for lumbar discectomy. *Spine* 1979;4:129–134.
59. Spengler D. Lumbar discectomy results with limited excision and selective foraminectomy. *Spine* 1982;7:604–607.
60. Spengler DM, Ouellette E, Battie M, et al. Elective discectomy for herniation of a lumbar disc. *J Bone Joint Surg [Am]* 1990;72:230–237.
61. Wiltse LL. Psychologic testing in predicting the success of low back surgery. *Orthop Clin North Am* 1975;6:317–318.
62. Boden SD, Davis DO, Dina TS, et al. Abnormal magnetic resonance scans of the lumbar spine in asymptomatic subjects. *J Bone Joint Surg [Am]* 1990;72:403–408.
63. Boos N, Reider R, Schnade V, et al. The diagnostic accuracy of MRI, work perception and psychological factors in identifying symptomatic disc herniations. *Spine* 1995;20:2613–2625.
64. Jenson MC, Brant-Zawadzki MN, Obuchowski N, et al. Magnetic resonance imaging of the lumbar spine in people without back pain. *New Engl J Med* 1994;331:69–73.
65. Milette PC, Fontaine S, Lepanto L, et al. Clinical impact of contrast-enhanced MR imaging reports in patients with previous lumbar disc surgery. *AJR Am J Roentgenol* 1996;167:217–223.
66. Tullberg T, Grane P, Isacson J. Gadolinium-enhanced magnetic resonance imaging of 36 patients one year after lumbar disc resection. *Spine* 1994;19:176–182.
67. Hirabayashi S, Kumano K, Ogawa Y, et al. Microdiscectomy and second operation for lumbar disc herniation. *Spine* 1993;18:2206–2211.
68. Hu RW, Jaglal S, Axcell T, et al. A population-based study of reoperations after back surgery. *Spine* 1997;22:2265–2271.

69. Salmela R, Koistinen V. Is the discharge register of general hospitals complete and reliable? (Published in Finnish.) *Sairaala* 1987;49: 480–482.
70. Mullin W, Heithoff K, Gilbert T, et al. Magnetic resonance evaluation of recurrent disc herniation. Is gadolinium necessary? *Spine* 2000;25:1493–1499.
71. Vogelsang J, Finkenstaedt M, Vogelsang M, et al. Recurrent pain after lumbar discectomy: the diagnostic value of peridural scar on MRI. *Eur Spine J* 1999;8:475–479.
72. Cavanagh S, Stevens J, Johnson JR. High-resolution MRI in the investigation of recurrent pain after lumbar discectomy. *J Bone Joint Surg [Br]* 1993;75:524–528.
73. Hueftle MG, Modic MT, Ros JS, et al. Lumbar spine: postoperative MR imaging with GD-DTPA. *Radiology* 1988;167:817–824.
74. Ross JS, Masaryk TJ, Schrader M, et al. MR imaging of the postoperative lumbar spine: assessment with gadopentetate dimeglumine. *AJR Am J Roentgenol* 1990;155:8670–8672.
75. Glickstein MF, Sussman SK. Time-dependent enhancement in magnetic resonance imaging of the postoperative lumbar spine. *Skeletal Radiol* 1991;20:333–337.
76. Dina TS, Boden SD, Davis DO. Lumbar spine after surgery for herniated disk; imaging findings in the early postoperative period. *AJR Am J Roentgenol* 1995;164:665–671.
77. Bundschuh CV, Modic MT, Ross JS, et al. Epidural fibrosis and recurrent disk herniation in the lumbar spine: MR imaging assessment. *AJR Am J Roentgenol* 1988;150:923–932.
78. Grane P. The postoperative lumbar spine. A radiological investigation of the lumbar spine after discectomy using MR imaging and CT. *Acta Radiol* 1998;414[Suppl]:1–23.
79. Hamm B, Haring B, Traupe H, et al. The diagnostic role of contrast medium-enhanced MR tomography in the diagnosis of the post-diskectomy syndrome. A prospective study of 109 patients. *Röfo Fortschr Geb Röntgenstr Neuen Bildgeb Verfahr* 1993;159:269–277.
80. Van de Kelft EJ, Van Goethem JW, de la Porte C, et al. Early postoperative gadolinium-DTPA-enhanced MR imaging after successful lumbar discectomy. *Br J Neurosurg* 1996;10:41–49.
81. Van Goethem JW, Van de Kelft E, Van Hasselt BA, et al. MRI after successful lumbar discectomy. *Neuroradiology* 1996;38[Suppl]:90–96.
82. Bernard TN Jr. Repeat lumbar spine surgery: factors influencing outcome. *Spine* 1993;18:2196–2200.
83. Byrd SE, Cohn ML, Biggers SL, et al. The radiographic evaluation of the symptomatic postoperative lumbar spine patient. *Spine* 1985;10:652–661.
84. Hiltselberger WE, Witten RM. Abnormal myelograms in asymptomatic patients. *J Neurosurg* 1968;28:204–208.
85. Irstam L. Differential diagnosis of recurrent lumbar disc herniation and postoperative deformation by myelography. An impossible task. *Spine* 1984;9:759–763.
86. Braun IF, Hoffman JC, Davis PC, et al. Contrast enhancement in CT differentiation between recurrent disk herniation and postoperative scar; prospective study. *AJNR Am J Neuroradiol* 1985;6:607–612.
87. Benoist M, Ficat C, Baraf P, et al. Postoperative lumbar epiduroarachnoiditis. *Spine* 1980;5:432–436.
88. Weiss T, Treisch J, Kazner E, et al. CT of the postoperative spine: the value of intravenous contrast. *Neuroradiology* 1986;28:241–245.
89. Modic MT, Masaryk T, Boumphrey F, et al. Lumbar herniated disc disease and canal stenosis: prospective evaluation by surface coil MR, CT and myelography. *Neuroradiology* 1987;7:709–717.
90. Modic MT, Ross JS. Magnetic resonance imaging in the evaluation of low back pain. *Orthop Clin North Am* 1991;22:283–301.
91. Walsh TR, Weinstein JN, Spratt KF, et al. Lumbar discography in normal subjects: a controlled, prospective study. *J Bone Joint Surg [Am]* 1990;72:1081–1088.
92. Bernard TN Jr. Using computed tomography/discography and enhanced magnetic resonance imaging to distinguish between scar tissue and recurrent lumbar disc herniation. *Spine* 1994;19:2826–2832.
93. Guyer RD, Ohnmeiss DD, Hochschuler SH, et al. The use of CT/discography to identify recurrent herniation not visualized by gadolinium enhanced MRI. Presented to the Federation of Spine Associations. Anaheim, CA: March 1991.
94. Rappoport LH, Pravda J, Leipzig JM, et al. The role of discogram/CT in assessing postoperative disc herniations. Presented to the International Society for the Study of the Lumbar Spine. Chicago, IL: May 1992.
95. Jackson RP, Cain JE Jr, Jacobs RR, et al. The neuroradiographic diagnosis of lumbar herniated nucleus pulposus: a comparison of CT, myelography, CT-myelography, discography, and CT-discography. *Spine* 1989;14:1356–1361.
96. Guyer RD, Ohnmeiss DD. Contemporary concepts in spine care: lumbar discography. Position statement from the North American Spine Society Diagnostic and Therapeutic Committee. *Spine* 1995; 20:2048–2059.
97. Kibler RF, Nathan PW. Relief of pain and paraesthesias by nerve block distal to a lesion. *J Neurol Neurosurg Psychiatry* 1960;23:91–98.
98. Xavier AV, McDanal J, Kissin I. Relief of sciatic radicular pain by sciatic nerve block. *Anesth Analg* 1988;67:1177–1180.
99. Block AR, Ohnmeiss DD, Guyer RD, et al. The use of presurgical psychological screening to predict the outcome of spine surgery. *Spine Journal* 2001;1:274–282.
100. Spengler DM. *Low back pain*. New York: Grune & Stratton, 1982.
101. Crauford DI, Creed F, Jayson MI. Life events and psychological disturbance in patients with low-back pain. *Spine* 1990;15:490–494.
102. Schofferman J, Anderson D, Hines R, et al. Childhood psychological trauma correlates with unsuccessful lumbar spine surgery. *Spine* 1992;17:S138–S144.
103. Biondi J, Greenberg BJ. Redecompression and fusion in failed back syndrome patients. *J Spinal Disord* 1990;3:362–369.
104. Finnegan WJ, Fenlin JM, Marvel JP, et al. Result of surgical intervention in the symptomatic multiply operated back patient: analysis of 67 cases followed three to seven years. *J Bone Joint Surg [Am]* 1979;61:1077–1082.
105. Quimjian JD, Matrla PJ. Decompression laminectomy and lateral spinal fusion in patients with previously failed lumbar spine surgery. *Orthopedics* 1988;11:563–569.
106. Yaksich I. Failed back surgery syndrome: problems, pitfalls, and prevention. *Ann Acad Med Singapore* 1993;22[3 Suppl]:414–417.
107. Silvers HR, Lewis PJ, Asch HL, et al. Lumbar diskectomy for recurrent disk herniation. *J Spinal Disord* 1994;7:408–419.
108. Vishteh AG, Dickman CA. Anterior lumbar microdiscectomy and interbody fusion for the treatment of recurrent disc herniation. *Neurosurg* 2001;48:334–338.
109. Epstein JA. Discussion on extreme lateral lumbar disc herniation. *J Spinal Disord* 1989;2:138.
110. Tarlov ET. Discussion on extreme lateral lumbar disc herniation. *J Spinal Disord* 1989;2:137–138.
111. Wiltse LL. Discussion on extreme lateral lumbar disc herniation. *J Spinal Disord* 1989;2:134–137.
112. Wiltse LL. The intervertebral foramina. In: Watkins RG, Collis JC, eds. *Lumbar discectomy and laminectomy*. Rockville, MD: Aspen Publishers, Inc., 1987:203–213.
113. Hanley EN, Shapiro DE. The development of low back pain after excision of a lumbar disc. *J Bone Joint Surg [Am]* 1989;71:719–721.
114. Vik A, Zwart JA, Hulleberg G, et al. Eight year outcome after surgery for lumbar disc herniation: a comparison of reoperated and not reoperated patients. *Acta Neurochir (Wien)* 2001;143:607–611.
115. Fritsch EW, Heisel J, Rupp S. The failed back syndrome: reasons, intraoperative findings, and long-term results: a report of 182 operative treatments. *Spine* 1996;21:626–633.
116. Ozgen S, Naderi S, Ozek MM, et al. Findings and outcome of revision lumbar disc surgery. *J Spinal Disord* 1999;12:287–292.

CHAPTER 59

Failure of Lumbar Fusion

A. Failures Other Than Pseudarthrosis

John W. Frymoyer

In 1911, Albee (1) and Hibbs (2) described two different methods for posterior lumbar spinal arthrodesis. Since their publications, the indications for lumbar fusion have progressively broadened, particularly as a treatment alternative for patients with chronic low back complaints. In the past two decades, population growth and advances in perioperative care, combined with the development of more reliable fixation devices, have led to a very rapid increase in the number of spinal fusions performed annually. There are also data that suggest a direct relationship exists between the rate of spinal surgery and the number of available specially trained spine surgeons (3). Because many of the indications remain controversial, it is not surprising there also are significant differences between the annual rate of spinal fusion performed in different countries, as well as between geographic areas of the United States (4).

What constitutes success and failure for a spinal fusion is often measured as a function of the investigator's preference and the specific condition being treated. Common outcome measures include the patient's symptom relief, return to work, correction of deformity, and successful biologic fusion. The type of outcome measure used significantly affect the apparent rate of success. For example, the authors (5) compared 13 published outcome measurements used to assess the success of lumbar disc excision with and without fusion. There were significant differences, with results ranging from 55 to 95% successful simply as a function of the outcome measure used. Furthermore, some of the failures occur early, but others are late, and thus the shorter the term of the follow-up, the more optimistic the outcomes appear. Long-term surveillance is required to give a true representation of success rate.

The most complete evaluation of the literature was performed by Turner et al. (6), who did a Medline search of all published reports of lumbar spinal fusion from 1966 to 1991. Selection criteria included a minimum 1 year of follow-up data that could permit the classification of outcome as satisfactory or unsatisfactory, and the report must have included a cohort of at least 30 patients. They identified 47 articles that met their criteria; none were randomized trials. The range of satisfactory results ranged from 16 to 19%, with an average of 68%. Table 1 gives the characteristic of the patient populations from the 47 studies. Table 2 displays the probability of a satisfactory outcome by diagnosis, and Table 3 demonstrates the probability of satisfactory outcome by type of fusion performed. The overall rates for a variety of complications are given in Table 4. Pseudarthrosis was the most common complication and was identified in 14%. That figure is different than Slipman (7) who reported stenosis and internal disc disruption were the most common sources of failure.

TABLE 1. *Preoperative clinical features of 47 patient cohorts taken from the literature[a]*

Characteristics	Mean	Range	Number of articles reporting variables
Mean age (yr)	43.4	33.0–61.0	33
Men (%)	52.9	33.3–92.9	38
Mean symptom duration (mo)	76.2	27.0–123.0	12
Symptoms/findings (%)			
Low back pain	96.4	82.5–100.0	25
Leg pain	75.9	46.6–100.0	20
Sensory deficit	52.9	28.0–75.0	4
Objective weakness	44.0	16.0–83.3	6
Bowel/bladder dysfunction	12.0	4.1–20.0	2
Normal neurologic findings	33.5	0.0–72.7	8
Previous back surgery	33.5	0.0–100.0	34
Diagnosis (%)			
Disc herniation	46.0	0.0–100.0	19
Degenerative disc disease/internal disc derangement	45.8	0.0–100.0	27
Degenerative scoliosis	7.1	0.0–22.4	5
Segmental instability	28.7	0.0–100.0	10
Pseudarthrosis	14.7	0.0–60.2	20
Postlaminectomy pain/ instability; failed back surgery syndrome	24.9	0.0–100.0	25
Spondylolisthesis	39.9	0.0–100.0	37
Spinal stenosis	30.8	0.0–100.0	8

[a]Sample size mean, 98.4; range, 33–492.

From Turner JA, Ersek M, Herron L, et al. Patient outcomes after lumbar spinal fusions. *JAMA* 1992;268:907–911, with permission.

However, an exacting analysis of the selection criterion used to determine a patient's suitability for the index fusion is absent in both Turner and Slipman's studies. If there is a single critical determinant to predict the chance for success or failure, it is the criteria by which a patient is selected for the original operation.

When low back pain is the predominant complaint, the causation is attributed to some causative event. Particularly when it occurs at work, the patient has been disabled more than 6 months, and if there is any evidence of substance abuse or psychologic dysfunction, the operation is most likely doomed to fail irrespective of the operative techniques used. Often, it is difficult to cull this subpopulation out of the published outcomes of spinal fusion, particularly if return to work, quality of life, and functional status are not measured. However, there are a number of studies that explicitly have measured outcomes in this type of patient cohort.

Franklin et al. (8) assessed the outcomes in all patients who had a lumbar spine fusion in the state of Washington in 1986.

TABLE 2. *Probability of a satisfactory outcome after surgery as a function of diagnosis*

Diagnosis	Satisfactory clinical outcomes (%)	
	Mean	Range
Herniated disc	70.1	52.6–85.3
Spondylolisthesis[a]	82.1	60.0–95.0
Isthmic spondylolisthesis	76.6	60.0–92.5
Degenerative spondylolisthesis	90.1	85.2–95.0
All studies	68.0	16.2–95.0

[a]Any type.

From Turner JA, Ersek M, Herron L, et al. Patient outcomes after lumbar spinal fusions. *JAMA* 1992;268:907–911, with permission.

All patients attributed their back symptoms to a work-related event and were covered by workers' compensation. Most patients (67%) reported no improvement or worsened back pain, and 56% rated their quality of life worse than their preoperative status. These abysmal results were independent of the type of instrumentation used, although the later rate of reoperation was greater in those who had an implant as part of the procedure. Similarly, Hanley (9) evaluated the results of fusion for ischemic spondylolisthesis in two cohorts, one with workers' compensation, the other without. The success rate was 65% in the former and 95% in the latter. Hanley's study is particularly relevant because the condition being treated, spondylolisthesis, is easily identifiable, and the indications for its treatment are well established. In comparison, many of the initial indications for spinal fusion are far more debatable. For example, Slipman (7) noted that 54% of patients in whom the original diagnosis was internal disc disruption were considered failures after fusion for that condition. Dhar and Porter (10) studied the outcomes in 160 patients who underwent lumbar spinal fusion. Twenty factors that might influence the result were used in a predictive risk model. Of these 20 variables, the most common cause of a poor surgical outcome was failure to recognize abnormal pain behaviors before surgery. The other major predictor was the number of previous operations.

This chapter gives an overview of the common complications after spinal fusion. Because pseudarthrosis is the most common longer-term failure and involves complex biologic issues, that topic is covered in an accompanying chapter. Also, there are certain complications highly specific to the condition that originally was being treated. For example, the crankshaft phenomenon and flatback deformity typically follow fusions performed for scoliosis and kyphosis (see Chapters 22 and 23). Similarly, the failures of treating high-grade spondylolisthesis are detailed in Chapter 24.

CAUSES OF FAILURE AFTER FUSION

In the earlier editions of *The Adult Spine*, the authors (11,12) developed a classification scheme based on two factors. The first was the time between the index operation and the appearance of symptoms connoting a failure; this period was

TABLE 3. *Probability of a satisfactory outcome as a function of the type of fusion performed*

	Satisfactory clinical outcomes[a]			Solid arthrodesis[a]		
Type of fusion	Mean (%)[b]	SD (%)	Number	Mean (%)	SD (%)	Number
Posterior	65.8	21.7	9	87.8	10.3	5
Posterolateral	67.7	18.5	19	89.0[c]	7.6	15
Anterior interbody	67.0	22.6	5	73.1[c,d]	14.5	7
Posterior lumbar interbody fusion	74.5	25.6	5	94.5[d]	4.1	4

SD, standard deviation.

[a]Number indicates number of studies in which 100% of patients had the indicated type of fusion.

[b]Differences not statistically significant.

[c]The posterolateral and anterior interbody means for solid arthrodesis were significantly different (p <.05) in pairwise comparisons using Scheffe's method.

[d]The anterior interbody and posterior lumbar interbody fusion means for solid arthrodesis were significantly different (p <.05) in pairwise comparisons using Scheffe's method.

From Turner JA, Ersek M, Herron L, et al. Patient outcomes after lumbar spinal fusions. *JAMA* 1992;268:907–911, with permission.

subdivided into early (weeks), midterm (months), and long-term (years). The reason for such a temporal division was based on the authors' studies (13) of the long-term outcomes of lumbar disc excision compared to disc excision with spinal fusion. These studies showed three relatively distinct time intervals for failure after lumbar disc surgery (Fig. 1). The second factor in the classification scheme was whether the predominant symptom was back or radicular pain. If radicular pain was not part of the symptom before the index operation and is part of the new symptom complex, this is an extremely important observation in establishing a diagnosis (Table 5). The authors also differentiated failures of fusion from a myriad of other complications that followed lumbar spinal surgery. As seen in Table 6, some of these complications are specific to the surgical approach used and fusion technique, whereas others are generic.

TABLE 4. *Reported rates of complications for lumbar spinal fusion*

Complication	Mean (%)	Range (%)	Number of articles reporting variables
In-hospital mortality	0.2	0.0–2.3	27
Deep infection	1.5	0.0–5.2	17
Superficial infection	1.6	0.0–4.0	17
Deep vein thrombosis/ thrombophlebitis	3.7	0.0–11.2	20
Pulmonary embolus	2.2	0.0–6.1	14
Neural injury	2.8	0.0–16.5	21
Any donor site complication	10.8	1.1–37.1	11
Donor site infection	1.5	0.0–5.2	17
Donor site chronic pain	8.7	0.0–37.1	10
Donor site pelvic instability	1.9	1.1–2.6	2
Graft extrusion	2.0	0.0–9.8	6
Instrumentation failure[a]	7.3	0.0–24.7	13
Other	8.7	1.0–42.6	29

[a]Percent of total instrumentation cases.

From Turner JA, Ersek M, Herron L, et al. Patient outcomes after lumbar spinal fusions. *JAMA* 1992;268:907–911, with permission.

DIAGNOSTIC EVALUATION

History

A complete history details the symptoms and impairments preceding each of the previous surgical interventions. Did the patient obtain relief of symptoms initially? Was the symptom relief complete after the surgery within a reasonable time frame? What level of function did the patient regain compared with the functional level before the original onset of symptoms? Was the patient able to work before the index operation? How long did it take to return to work after the procedure and to what type of work? What is the history of medication use preopera-

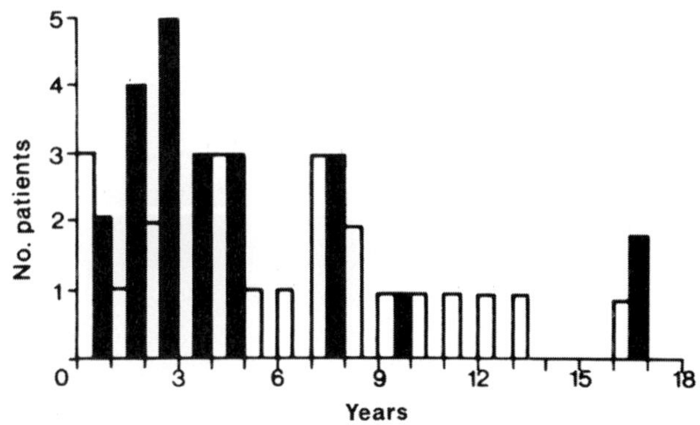

FIG. 1. Failure of spinal surgery as a function of years after the index procedure. (From Frymoyer JW, et al. Failed lumbar disc surgery requiring second operation. A long-term follow-up study. *Spine* 1978;3:7–118, with permission.)

TABLE 5. *Other complications after spinal fusion*

Local	General
Posterior	
Early:	
Hemorrhage	Blood transfusion reactions
Ecchymoses	Hemolysis
Wound dehiscence	Anemia
Neurologic	Urinary retention
Laminal fracture	Sepsis
Pedicle fracture	Metabolic disorders
Sepsis	Psychosis
Vascular (anterior)	Drug overdose
Iliac crest	Hypotension
Anterior	
Early:	
Hemorrhage	Cholecystitis
Vascular (vessel)	Pancreatitis
Ureteric damage	+ All listed from Posterior
Renal damage	
Splenic damage	
Bowel damage	
Sympathetic disruption	
Iliac crest hemorrhage	
Iliac crest fracture	
Wound dehiscence	
Sepsis	
Graft extrusion	
Anterior and posterior	
Intermediate:	
Wound sepsis	
Fracture at fixation points	
Instrumentation failure	
Vascular aneurysm (anterior only)	
Retroperitoneal fractures	
Ureteric obstruction (anterior only)	
Hydronephrosis	
Incisional hernia	
Iliac crest fracture	
Nerve irritation secondary to donor site	
Late:	
Late sepsis	
Instrumentation failure	
Donor site problems	
Retroperitoneal fibrosis	
Ureteric obstruction (anterior only)	
Hydronephrosis (anterior only)	
Vascular aneurysm (anterior only)	
Incisional hernia	

TABLE 6. *Causes of failure after spinal fusion*

Time	Back pain predominant	Leg symptoms
Early (wk)	Infection Wrong level fused Insufficient levels fused Psychosocial distress	Nerve impingement by fixation device or cement
Midterm (mo)	Pseudarthrosis Disc disruption Early adjacent disc degeneration Inadequate reconditioning Graft donor site	Fixation loose Early adjacent disc degeneration Graft donor site
Long-term (yr)	Late pseudarthrosis Adjacent level instability Acquired spondylolysis Abutment syndrome Compression fracture above fusion	Disc with pseudarthrosis Adjacent level stenosis Adjacent level disc Stenosis above fusion

tively, postoperatively, and at present? If there has been more than one operation, this information must be obtained for each previous procedure.

It is vital to obtain all previous medical records, which, ideally, should give additional data about the patient's original presenting complaints, physical findings, imaging studies, and operative findings, as well as greater detail about the intraoperative events, including any untoward complications. These data are particularly helpful if a patient has a well-documented history of absent neurologic complaints and findings before the index procedure and now is presenting with radicular pain and associated neurologic abnormalities. One of the more difficult problems is to distinguish spinal pain from pain attributed to the graft donor site. In general, graft donor pain tends to be part of a constellation of symptoms referable to the spine rather than due to local mechanical or other disturbances in the pelvis and sacroiliac joint (14).

Because psychosocial issues can be a significant part of a failure of spine fusion, it is important to elicit information about the patient's self assessment of his or her psychologic state. Are depression or anxiety issues of concern? What medications are being taken, including psychotropic drugs and pain relievers? If married, what is the marital relationship? If there is workers' compensation, are those issues resolving? The profile of a patient at particular risk would be an individual whose original preoperative symptoms were attributable to a work-related event, whose preoperative studies did not reveal unequivocal pathology, who never had significant pain relief after surgery, and who has not returned to work. There are no hard and fast rules about who should have additional standard psychologic testing, such as a Minnesota Multiphasic Personality Inventory or Beck Depression Inventory, or who should be referred to a psychiatrist or psychologist for additional formal evaluation. There rarely is any adverse effect for such evaluation, however, and therefore, it is suggested as part of the routine evaluation, particularly in patients who have had more than two failed back operations.

Physical Examination

Most of the physical findings are quite nonspecific and include a limited range of spinal motion and usually some degree of local tenderness to palpation. Specific findings of importance are fairly obvious and include swelling (e.g., infection, meningocele), sinuses or any other drainage, prominent hardware, particularly if there is an overlying tender bursa, as well as postural abnormalities, such as a flat back. The neurologic examination often is negative other than for hamstring tightness, which can be misinterpreted as a positive nerve root tension sign. If there are positive finding, such as altered reflex, sensation, or strength, the critical issue is: Is this a new finding or was this finding present before the previous operation? The other observation of particular interest is the Waddell signs (15), which, if present, serve as a warning there are major psychosocial issues that must be addressed.

Imaging

Plain radiographs are taken, including anteroposterior, lateral, and oblique films. Again, the important findings are often based on a comparison of the preoperative and postoperative films. Many of the so-called abnormalities are nonspecific and include disc space narrowing, the presence of osteophytes, and most of the minor congenital abnormalities such as translational vertebrae (16). The more specific findings are the presence of a pseudarthrosis and the type of implants present as well as their structural integrity and positioning. If there was a deformity present, such as scoliosis or spondylolisthesis, it is important to determine if there has been any loss of correction or progression of deformity (Fig. 2). Often, a flexion-extension lateral is obtained to assess for pseudarthrosis or a new level of instability above or below a fusion. The sensitivity and specificity of these dynamic radiographs for the diagnosis of pseudarthrosis is discussed in Chapter 59B. Bone scans have limited value, even in the diagnosis of pseudarthrosis (Chapter 59B).

A computed tomography scan is particularly useful in defining pseudarthrosis, and Kostuik (12) in particular lauded the use of three-dimensional reconstructions, as have others (17). The other particular indications are to assess the spinal canal, fusion, and instrumentation in patients who have had ferrous metal implants. If intraspinal pathology is suggested by the history or physical examination, a myelogram should be performed, followed by computed tomography enhancement. In the absence of ferrous metal implants, magnetic resonance imaging (MRI) is the favored alternative and has benefit of giving additional information about disc degeneration under, above, and below the fusion mass.

Other studies, including the use of diagnostic injections such as facet blocks and selective nerve root injections, are detailed in Chapter 6B. As noted in that chapter, preoperative facet blocks correlated poorly with the later results of a primary fusion in Esse and Moro's analysis of 126 patients (18). A somewhat different perspective was a study by Markwalder and Battaglia (19). Their analysis of 171 patients with failed back surgery suggested facet blocks could be predictive of later surgical success. Hasue (20) has advocated local nerve root injections, and radiculograms are indicated when there are discrepancies between the physical examination and imaging studies in patients with radicular pain.

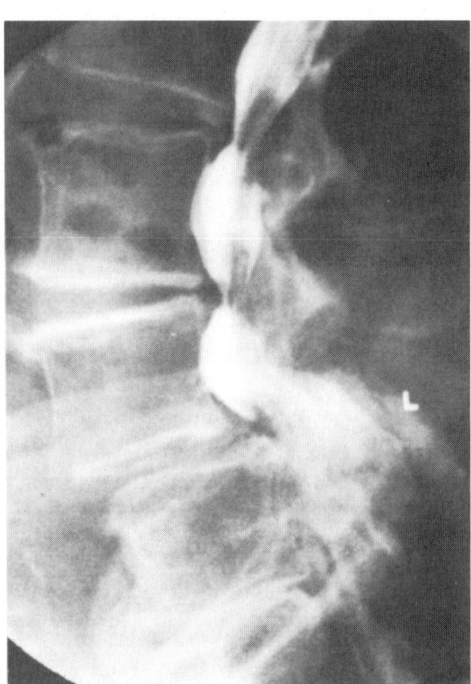

FIG. 2. This patient had an L-5 to S-1 fusion performed 2 years previously. Recurrent back and leg pain was confirmed to be secondary to a degenerative spondylolisthesis above the level of the prior fusion.

Perhaps the most controversial diagnostic study is discography. The advocates cite three general indications in a patient with a previous failed fusion: (a) the assessment of junctional interspaces, particularly when there is evidence of significant degeneration identified either on plain film or MRI—the production of concordant pain would identify this level as the likely site of symptoms and would suggest the benefit of extension of the fusion; (b) a patient with pain unrelieved by a posterior or posterolateral fusion in whom no abnormalities are identified other than evidence of disc degeneration at an intervertebral level under the fusion—this set of findings suggests the presence of disc disruption syndrome as described by Crock (21) and should be relieved by an interbody fusion; or (c) discography at the level affected by a pseudarthrosis, as MacNab advocated (22). He concluded that the production of concordant pain was a sensitive and specific confirmation that this level was the source of symptoms.

EARLY FAILURES (BACK PAIN PREDOMINANT)

Infection

The published rate of infections after spinal fusion varies as a function of the era in which the surgery was performed, possibly the type of fusion, the presence or absence of metal implants, the age of the patient, and the existence of comorbidities, and probably the use of prophylactic antibiotics. Older publications gave a somewhat higher rate of infection than contemporary series. The type of fusion may or not have an influence; Kostuik and

Hall (23) thought but did not prove that anterior fusions had a lower infection risk than posterior fusions. Implants are typically associated with high infection rates, which may be as great as 13%. The older the patient, the higher the risk of infection, particularly when there are comorbidities such as diabetes (24). Finally, preoperative and postoperative antibiotics are routinely administered, but evidence favoring their efficacy is debatable. What has become clear over the past two decades is that prolonged antibiotic use has no apparent benefits and has significant and growing risks for complications such as intestinal superinfections with *Clostridia difficile*.

The presentation of infection typically occurs 5 to 7 days postoperatively and is manifested by variable levels of fever, local wound symptoms (particularly pain), and sometimes by localized erythema. There are wide variations, however, ranging from acute severe presentations to indolent presentations in which the presence of infection is only suggested by progressive loosening of an implant. Similarly, the treatment is somewhat variable. An essential element of treatment is to obtain deep cultures. If the infection is superficial, the wound should be relieved of local tension and drained, cultures obtained, and appropriate antibiotic therapy initiated. If the infection is deeper, the strategy for treatment usually includes open drainage, débridement of necrotic tissues, and antibiotics. A significant issue is what to do with the bone graft and fixation devices. In acute infections presenting soon after the operation, a reasonable strategy is to débride the wound, wash off the grafts with antibiotic solution and replace them, and leave the fixation intact. Significant preoperative instability increases the desirability of maintaining instrumentation, whereas gram-negative organisms make retention of these devices less likely. If the infection is more indolent, the fixation devices commonly have become loose and are removed. Based on the patient's condition, the local condition of the fusion, and the organism, the surgeon's judgment determines if the instrumentation should be reimplanted or if a second stage procedure should be done such as an anterior interbody fusion in the face of failed, infected posterior fusion.

Wrong Level Surgery or Inadequate Number of Levels

Performance of the operation at the wrong level or failure to include all affected vertebral levels is significantly more of a problem in decompressive surgery, particularly in patients with multilevel spinal stenosis, than it is with spinal fusion. The situation in which inadequate fusion length is a problem that is likely to occur is when fusion was performed for a deformity (see Chapters 22 and 23). Extension of the fusion is the appropriate solution. A second and more controversial issue is the extent of fusion required in patients with multilevel degenerative disease, no associated deformity, and no evidence of stenosis. The decision to perform a multilevel fusion is based on chronic back pain combined with degenerative disc disease identified by MRI and often discographic replication of pain. The extent of the fusion in these instances is uncertain. Kostuik (12) recommended discography be performed at all levels until a normal level was encountered, and all discographically abnormal levels be incorporated in the fusion. If a patient has persistent symptoms and solid fusion is identified, it is difficult to determine if the symptoms relate to failure to include sufficient levels, a symptomatic disc under a solid posterior fusion, or if the indications were inappropriate in the first place. If one is convinced the symptoms are related to insufficient levels, extension of the fusion is a solution, whereas identification of a painful disc with a solid posterior fusion indicates the need for anterior fusion.

EARLY FAILURES (LEG PAIN PREDOMINANT)

If a patient had preoperative radicular symptoms and these persist postoperatively, this usually indicates the affected nerve root was inadequately decompressed. This situation most commonly arises in spinal stenosis. The common site for continued compression is in the lateral recesses. Another potential cause is the so-called battered root. The most catastrophic situation is a postoperative cauda equina syndrome, which may result from displacement of a graft or interbody device, an extradural hematoma, or in patients treated for high-grade spondylolisthesis, with or without reduction. Far more common after instrumented fusion is nerve root impingement from a pedicle screw or displacement of an interbody implant (Fig. 3). If methylmethacrylate has been used in an osteoporotic patient to provide better screw anchorage, extravasation of the cement is another potential cause, producing thermal injury or direct compression on the nerve. How commonly these events occur is unknown and varies particularly as a function of the experience of the surgeon. Weinstein (25) simulated pedicle screw placements in the lumbar spine and compared experienced to inexperienced surgeons. Screw misplacement occurred in 21% of the specimens. It is difficult to obtain an accurate assessment of how commonly screw impingement on nerve roots occurs sufficient to cause radicular symptoms.

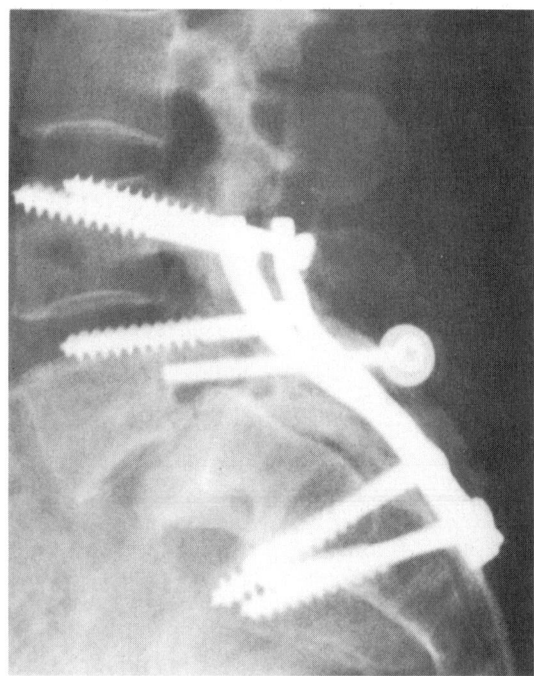

FIG. 3. This patient underwent a two-level fusion for spondylolisthesis. She had postoperative leg pain. The lateral radiograph demonstrates one screw has missed the L-4 pedicle, and screws were in the disc space of L4-5. The screws were removed and replaced, with relief of symptoms.

The evaluation of patients with unresolving postoperative leg pain is similar to that given in Chapter 47. The treatment usually entails decompression of the affected nerve root(s) or removal of a displaced or misplaced device.

MIDTERM FAILURES

Back Pain Predominant

Pseudarthrosis is the most common cause of midterm failure and is discussed in detail in Chapter 59B.

Inadequate Reconditioning

Intuitively, it makes sense that patients who have had significant low back pain and then have undergone a major operation would, in general, be physically deconditioned. Furthermore, a well-established consequence of posterior lumbar spinal fusion is denervation of the paraspinal muscles. Despite the logic, it is surprising how deconditioning often is not included in a differential diagnosis, nor is a carefully planned reconditioning program considered as treatment. Despite an absence of much data, a physical therapy program, combined with aerobic exercise conditioning, makes sense as a first line of treatment before any further surgery is considered. If a patient has had multiple operations, a comprehensive rehabilitation program should be considered as described in Chapter 14.

Leg Pain Predominant

Historically, spinal fusions commonly were performed in association with disc excisions based on the premise that the affected level was mechanically unstable. A common cause of failure, affecting as many as 20% of patients, was a new disc herniation above the level of the fusion, particularly if the fusion had been performed only at L-5 to S-1 (13) (Fig. 4). Another, less common cause of leg pain was a new or recurrent disc herniation underneath a fusion with pseudarthrosis. Today, these complications are rarer. However, recurrent leg pain can occur when a decompression was performed for spinal stenosis, and in the presence of a pseudarthrosis, the radicular complaints reoccur. A rare event is fracture of a facet joint that impinges on the nerve root in the lateral recess. Other causes of leg pain include arachnoiditis, a meningocele, and reflex sympathetic dystrophy.

Treatment is dependent on the cause of pain. Disc herniation and spinal stenosis are treated by decompression, and usually the fusion mass is reinforced if there is any evidence of pseudarthrosis. Arachnoiditis is not amenable to direct surgical intervention, although a variety of pain-relieving strategies, including implanting nerve stimulators, are options. A meningocele is treated by closure.

LONG-TERM FAILURES

Back Pain Predominant

The most common cause of back pain in the years after an apparently successful spinal fusion is degeneration at adjacent motion segments. Whether this should be considered a failure or simply the progression of a disease process can be debated. Moreover, radiographic degeneration is not synonymous with symptoms. The spectrum of radiologic degenerative signs above or below a fusion includes disc space narrowing, osteophytic overgrowth, segmental instability, and spinal stenosis, which may be identified in as many as 50% of patients years after the index operation (16,26). When back pain is the predominant symptom, it is far more difficult to determine the cause than when radicular symptoms are predominant. If there are rapidly developing and clear signs of degeneration, the likelihood is greater that level is the source of symptoms (Fig. 5). Other rarer causes of predominant back pain were more common when midline fusions were performed and included abutment syndromes (where the fusion abuts against the next adjacent spinous process, producing a local pseudojoint) and acquired spondylolysis and spondylolisthesis (27,28). Other later complications, such as flatback deformity, are discussed in Chapters 22, 23, and 25.

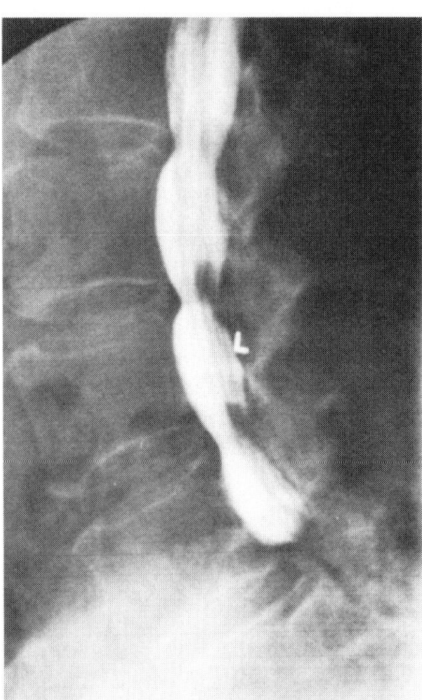

FIG. 4. Myelogram demonstrating disc herniation with complete block above an L-5 to S-1 fusion.

If one is assured the source of symptoms comes from an adjacent level(s), the appropriate treatment is extension of the fusion. Normally, this can be done from a posterior approach.

Leg Pain Predominant

When leg pain is present, the most common cause is degenerative spinal stenosis above or below the fusion. The usual symptoms are neurologic claudication, occasionally with more focal radiculopathy. A rarer cause is frank lumbar disc herniation, usually affecting the L3-4 disc above a previous spinal fusion. When midline fusions were common, spinal stenosis also occurred in some patients secondary to overgrowth of the fusion mass (29).

A,B

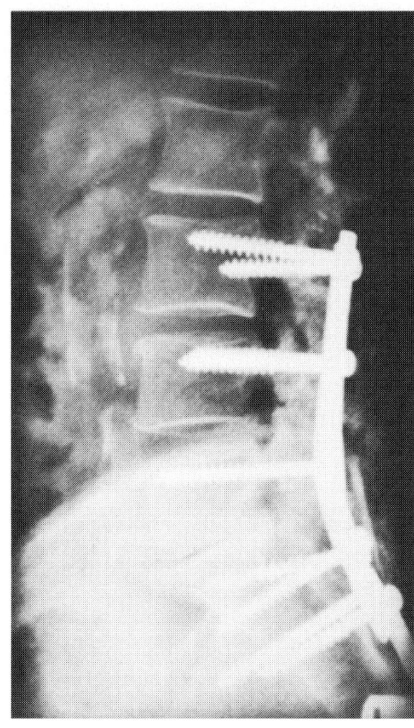

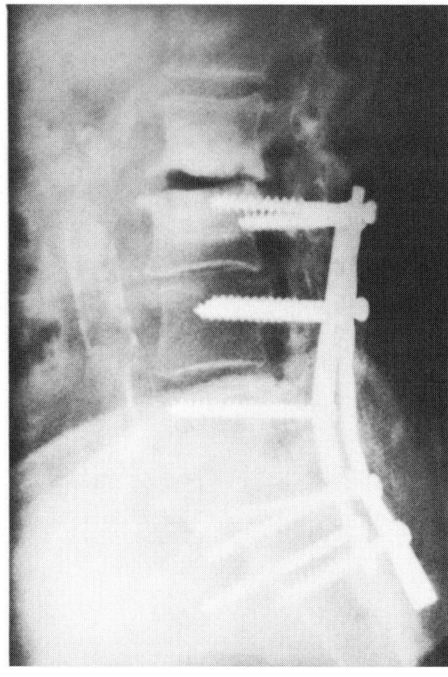

FIG. 5. This patient had a previous L-3 to S-1 instrumented fusion with relief of symptoms **(A)**. Three years later, she developed recurrent severe back pain. Radiographs demonstrated a vacuum sign, significant osteophytic overgrowth, and end-plate irregularity indicative of severe degenerative changes **(B)**.

Treatment of the patients is decompression of the affected level(s). Typically, this is done in conjunction with extension of the fusion.

REFERENCES

1. Albee FH. Transplantation of a portion of the tibia into the spine for Pott's disease. *JAMA* 1911;57:885.
2. Hibbs RA. An operation for progressive spinal deformities *N Y Med J* 1911;93:1013.
3. Cherkin DC, Deyo RA, Loeser JD, et al. An international comparison of back surgery rates. *Spine* 1994;19:1201–1206.
4. Volinn E, Mayer J, Diehr P, et al. Small area analysis of surgery for low-back pain. *Spine* 1992;17:575–579.
5. Howe J, Frymoyer JW. The effects of questionnaire design on the determination of end results in lumbar spine surgery. *Spine* 1985; 10:804–805.
6. Turner JA, Ersek M, Herron L, et al. Patient outcomes after lumbar spine fusions. *JAMA* 1992;268:907–911.
7. Slipman CW, Shin CH, Patel RK, et al. Etiologies of failed back surgery syndrome. *Pain Med* 2002;3:200–214.
8. Franklin GM, Haug J, Heyer NJ, et al. Outcome of lumbar fusion in Washington state worker's compensation. *Spine* 1994;19:1897–1903.
9. Hanley EN Jr, Levy JA. Surgical treatment of isthmic lumbosacral spondylolisthesis. Analysis of variables influencing results. *Spine* 1989;14:48–50.
10. Dhar S, Porter RW. Failed lumbar surgery. *Int Orthop* 1992;16(2): 152–156.
11. KostuiK JP, Frymoyer JW. Failures after spinal fusion: causes and surgical treatment results. In: Frymoyer JW, ed. *The adult spine*. New York: Raven Press, 1991.
12. Kostuik JP. Failures after spinal fusion. In: Frymoyer JW, ed. *The adult spine,* 2nd ed. Philadelphia: Lippincott–Raven, 1997.
13. Frymoyer JW, Matteri RE, Hanley EN, et al. Failed lumbar disc surgery requiring second operation. A long-term follow-up study. *Spine* 1976;3:7–11.
14. Frymoyer JW, Howe J, Kuhlmann D. The long-term effects of spinal fusion on the sacroiliac joints and ilium. *Clin Orthop* 1978;134:196–201.
15. Waddell G, McCullough JA, Kummel, ED, et al. Nonorganic physical signs in low back pain. *Spine* 1980;5:117–125.
16. Frymoyer JW, Hanley EN Jr, Howe J, et al. A comparison of radiographic findings in fusion and nonfusion patients ten or more years following lumbar disc surgery. *Spine* 1979;4:435–440.
17. Zinreich SJ, Long DM, Davis R, et al. Three-dimensional CT imaging in postsurgical "failed back" syndrome. *J Comput Assist Tomogr* 1990;14:574–580.
18. Esses SI, Moro JK. The value of facet joint blocks in patient selection for lumbar fusion. *Spine* 1993;18:185–190.
19. Markwalder T, Battaglia M. Failed back surgery syndrome. Part I: analysis of the clinical presentation and results of testing procedures for instability of the lumbar spine in 171 patients. *Acta Neurochir (Wien)* 1993;123:46–51.
20. Hasue M, Kikuchi S. Nerve root injections. In: Frymoyer JW, ed. *The adult spine*, 2nd ed. Philadelphia: Lippincott–Raven, 1997.
21. Crock HV. Internal disc disruption. In: Frymoyer JW, ed. *The adult spine*. New York: Raven Press, 1991.
22. Macnab I, Dali D. The blood supply of the lumbar spine and its application to the technique of intertransverse lumbar fusion. *J Bone Joint Surg (Br)* 1971;53:628–638.
23. Kostuik JP, Halkl BB. Spinal fusions to the sacrum in adults with scoliosis. *Spine* 1982;8:489–500.
24. Deyo RA, Ciol MA, Cherkin DC, et al. Lumbar spinal fusion. A cohort study of complications, repoerations and resource use in the Medicare population. *Spine* 1993;18:1463–1470.
25. Weinstein JN, Spratt KF, Spengler D, et al. Spinal pedical fixation: reliability and validity of roentgenogram-based assessment and surgical factors on successful screw placement. *Spine* 1988;13:1412–1418.
26. Lehmann TR, Spratt KF, Tozzi JE. Long-term follow-up of lower lumbar fusion patients. *Spine* 1987;12:97–114.
27. Rumbold C. Spondylolysis: a complication of spinal fusion. *J Bone Joint Surg (Am)* 1965;51:1237–1242.
28. Cleveland M, Bosworth DM, Thompson FR. Pseudoarthrosis in the lumbosacral spine. *J Bone Joint Surg (Am)* 1948;30:302–312.
29. Brodsky AI. Post-laminectomy and post-fusion stenosis of the lumbar spine. *Clin Orthop* 1976;115:130.

CHAPTER 59

Failure of Lumbar Fusion

B. Pseudarthrosis

Mark B. Dekutoski

More than 200,000 spinal fusions are performed each year in the United States, the goal of which is to permanently stabilize the involved motion segment. Success of fusion procedures has evolved each decade since the 1960s, when facet grafting techniques were developed. Subsequent departure from posterior midline to posterolateral fusion, and then to anterior interbody techniques was believed to improve the rates of bone unions. Spine instrumentation evolved in the 1970s and 1980s from hook-rod techniques to segmental fixation. Each decade has provided new optimism about the reduction of the 20 to 50% risk of pseudarthrosis noted with historic *in situ* midline technique. In the 1990s, the promise of osteoinductive materials was first reported for demineralized bone matrixes and, subsequently, bone morphogenic proteins (BMPs). Despite the development of BMPs and the hope for gene therapy in the first decade of the twenty-first century, pseudarthrosis remains an important cause of clinical failure after attempted spinal fusion.

A daunting task for the clinician is to discern which of these evolving techniques is fad and which is fundamental to the contemporary treatment of the spinal fusion patient.

BIOLOGY AND NATURAL HISTORY OF FUSION MATURATION

Bone formation in the adult human is a complex and closely regulated process involving inflammatory, reparative, and remodeling phases. A cascade of cellular processes occurs, triggered by growth factors and external stimuli that are pertinent to the formation of bony union or pseudarthrosis (Fig. 1) (1–3).

The basis of fracture or fusion healing is the proliferation and differentiation of precursor stromal cells into osteoblasts and osteoclasts. These stromal cells are stimulated by local growth factors and undergo differentiation from mesenchymal stem cells to preosteoblasts, subsequent osteocytes, and lining cells. The osteoblasts are responsible for production of bone matrix constituents and collagen and noncollagen proteins, and do not function individually but in clusters through interaction with the surrounding matrix and cells. Bony extracellular matrix of collagen and noncollagen proteins is produced by the osteoblasts. Resorption is induced by the osteoclast function.

Noncollagenous proteins include the proteoglycans, biglycan, decortin, glycoproteins such as osteonectin, enzymes such

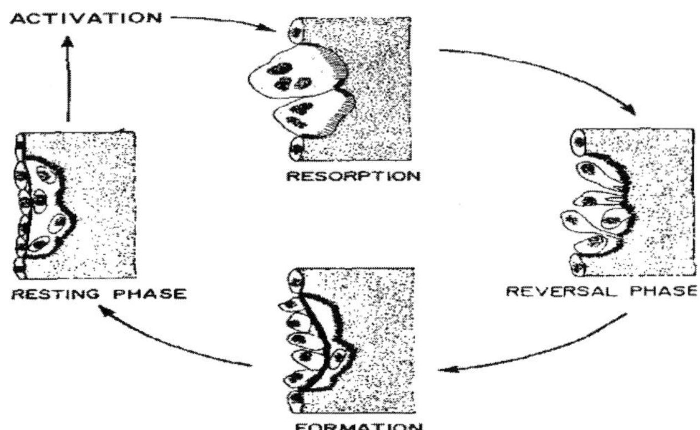

FIG. 1. Cellular events in the formation of bone.

as alkaline phosphatase, and cell attachment proteins such as osteopontin, fibronectin, thrombospondin, and sialoprotein and γ-carboxyglutamic acid protein, osteocalcin and matrix protein Growth factors, such as transforming growth factor-β, immunoglobulin A platelet-derived growth factor, α– and β–fibroblast growth factor, and BMPs are also active in the stimulation of and inducement of cell maturation. The BMPs have been classified in the transforming growth factor-β subfamily and in animal and clinical studies appear to induce bone formation (1,4).

Bone forms by endochondral and intramembranous ossification. Endochondral ossification is characterized by the development of an epiphyseal growth plate from cartilage precursor, which then secondarily calcifies at the zone of calcified cartilage. Intramembranous bone formation occurs by osteoblastic differentiation of mesenchymal tissues and direct formation of woven bone characteristic of the cranial bulb and clavicle. Fracture healing and fusion maturation is a contiguous cascade of cellular and molecular events wherein there is complete remodeling with absence of fibrous tissue.

Fracture healing has three phases. The inflammatory phase involves the formation of a hematoma and cellular necrosis, which causes an acute inflammatory response. Platelet factors, platelet-derived growth factor, and transforming growth factor-β are activated. Periosteum and local bone stimulate cell differentiation, which heralds the reparative phase in which immature callus is formed. This appears several weeks after an acute fracture or a surgical attempt to cause fusion. In this phase, bone mineral is produced and osteoid forms, creating an internal or medullary callus and some external callus. This medullary callus is characteristic of the intramembranous bone formation wherein a narrow endosteal cleft of mesenchymal cells proliferate and there is primary osteonal healing only where there is bone-to-bone interface. In external callus intramembranous subperiosteal bone formation occurs as well as enchondral bone formation with chondrogenesis, vascular ingrowth, and formation of woven bone. Motion and low oxygen tension in this phase of bone healing induce cartilage formation in favor of bone formation.

Finally, in the ensuing months to up to 2 years after a fracture or fusion, the remodeling phase occurs. Bone is reorganized in accordance with Wolff's law to optimize strength in relationship to imposed load. This process involves bone growth factors and the effects of activation, resorption and reformation of bone in the activation, resorption, and formation cycle (2). The time course of bone remodeling is characterized by the maturation of osteoblasts and subsequent proliferation over a period of 6 months (3,4). When bone grafting has been performed, creeping substitution occurs with progressive resorption of the graft material and replacement osteoid. This process lines the cancellous graft with osteoid and induces osteoblastic formation by the rules of determined osteogenic precursor cells and inducible osteogenic progenitor cells. This process is affected by the graft composition, local factors, and hypoxia as well as systemic factors, such as malnutrition, lack of thyroid hormone, and insulin growth factors.

The healing sequence of intertransverse autogenous spinal fusion has been described and consists of the rabbit model, the early inflammatory phase occurs in weeks 1 through 3, the middle reparative phase in weeks 4 and 5, and the late remodeling phase in weeks 6 to 10 (5a,5b,6).

During the early phase of healing there is disruption of local blood supply. The transverse process decortication results in early hematoma formation, within which inflammatory cells are present. Fibroblast-like cells transform the hematoma into a fibrovascular stroma. Earlier vascular buds are seen, which grow into the fusion site. Primary membranous bone formation develops near the decorticated transverse processes. There is very minimal cartilage and endochondral ossification at this phase, and limited osteoid is seen in new trabecular bone forming near the decorticated transverse processes. Likewise, there is little osteoid formation on the transplanted bone grafts.

In the reparative phase, there is remodeling of the cancellous bone especially near the vascularized transverse processes. The inflammatory process abates with initiation of revascularization and resorption of necrotic debris. Early differentiation of osteoblastic and chondroblastic cells is observed with the extension of newborn bone toward the central zone of the fusion mass, which is the area between the transverse processes. In the central zone, the pleuri potential cells are differentiated in the less vascularized area with formation of cartilage rather than direct membranous bone formation. This may be critical to later development in these more "ischemic" areas of pseudarthrosis. This evolves to an interface zone, which is initially cartilage, followed by endochondral ossification from the end points toward the center.

During the late remodeling phase of the rabbit model, there is an increase in trabecular osteoid bone, a dramatic remodeling evident by formation of a peripheral cortical rim, an increased formation of secondary spongiosa bone, and an increase in marrow volume.

The newly formed trabecular process extends from this periphery centrally in concert with the neovascularization of this fusion mass.

After 10 weeks, there is a variable maturation of the fusion mass, which is most advanced near the transverse processes and diminishes centrally. It appears that decortication of the transverse processes is a critical source of ingrowing vascular tissue. Osteoprogenitor cells have an important role in this process. Throughout bone healing, the cancellous graft bone undergoes resorption and remodeling at a higher rate than the cortical bone. In many areas, it is completely resorbed.

The biologic properties of bone grafts vary significantly. Bone grafts have osteogenic, osteoconductive, and osteoinductive characteristics. Osteogenesis is the new bone formation that is the result of transplantation of viable cells in the harvested iliac crest bone graft. Viable cells are transplanted in approximately 20% (1). Osteoconduction is the ability of graft material to present a three-dimensional matrix or framework to support bony ingrowth;

allograft and autograft have this property. Osteoinduction is the ability to stimulate mesenchymal cells to differentiate into bone-forming elements.

Potential graft materials include cancellous and cortical autografts and allografts, which may be fresh-frozen, freeze-dried, or demineralized bone matrix as well as newer recombinant bone graft materials (1,7). Cancellous graft allows for progressive appositional bone replacement, and there is some autograft reestablishing of blood supply within 24 to 48 hours after transplantation where some vascular ingrowth may be observed. Normal revascularization occurs within 2 weeks into the fusion bed. Although as few as 20% of graft cells survive, the osteoinductive properties of cancellous autogenous bone make it the ideal graft. Cortical grafts have an initial strength greater than cancellous bone, but they also have fewer osteogenic cell precursors. Cortical autograft undergoes osteoclastic resorption, which results in a delay in bone deposition strength compared to autograft fusion. However, at 2 years the mechanical strengths are equivalent. Vascularized autograft, such as rib and fibula, maintain a blood supply and are ideal in a challenging host environment, such as an infection or tumor. Fresh-frozen allograft has decreased immunogenicity and a minimal reduction in strength and is osteoinductive, but it can be associated with the risk of disease transmission. Less than optimal procurement and storage can increase these risks significantly. Allograft can be sterilized with ethylene oxide, which reduces the immunogenicity and has no effect on the biomechanical strain. Ethylene oxide–treated allograft is minimally osteoinductive, however, and has had limited clinical success owing to its reduced proinflammatory potential. Radiation can also affect graft strength. At greater than 3 mrad, this reduced axial loading strength is found. Radiation also reduces the osteoinductive and conductive properties of graft.

Studies of the rat femur fracture model (8) have demonstrated a delay in mineralization and subsequent development of pseudarthrosis when motion persists at the fracture site. Interfragmentary motion characteristically retards the cartilaginous phase of bone healing; type II collagen production is extended and results in an interposing membrane, which differentiates into matrix tissue with a low propensity to mineralize. Typically, type II collagen secretion is substituted for by type I collagen in normal fracture healing (8–10).

ADJUNCTS FOR ENHANCEMENT OF FUSION MATURATION THROUGH ELECTRICAL STIMULATION

The use of electrical stimulation as an adjunct to stimulation of spinal fusion was evaluated in a canine posterior lumbar fusion model by Dwyer in 1975 and Nerubay et al. in 1986 (11,12). Two months after fusion the animals with the bone-grown stimulator demonstrated an enhanced fusion mass. Electrical stimulation involves direct current (DC) stimulation via an implantable back stimulator. Implanted anodes and cathodes deliver the current to the arthrodesis site (13–15). External pulsed electromagnetic field therapy (PEMF) has also been reported to enhance the rate and quality of lumbar spinal fusion (16–18).

Limitations of these devices have been the need for removal of the DC implant. Poor patient compliance and intermittent usage during the postoperative period have been identified as problems with the external PEMF intervention.

Clinical investigations have analyzed the efficacy of implantable DC stimulation on instrumented and uninstrumented fusions. Tejano et al. (13) reported their results in multilevel noninstrumented fusions and found the results comparable to the increased fusion rate caused by instrumentation alone. Kane (14) reported a successful lumbar fusion rate of 91% with and 81% without the electrical stimulator. In this same study, a subset of more difficult fusion situations (i.e., those with previous failed fusion, multilevel surgery with grade 2 or greater spondylolisthesis, or obesity) were evaluated. Fusion was noted in 81% of patients treated with electrical stimulation compared to 54% of those treated without.

PEMF has also been studied in posterolateral lumbar fusions in animal models and in humans. Animal studies by Kahanovitz found that PEMF had no effect on healing rate or quality of spinal fusions (16).

Later open-trial clinical studies by Simmons (19) evaluated PEMF. Successful intertransverse fusion occurred in 71% of patients treated with this adjunct.

Jenis (17) compared PEMF, no adjunct, and implanted DC stimulator treatment in instrumented spinal fusions and could demonstrate no difference in fusion rate in over 60 patients randomized between the three treatment modalities. There was a significant increase in fusion mass bone density, however. An interesting finding in the PEMF and DC-stimulator patients was a significant increase in fusion mass bone density of 24% in PEMF and 36% in DC-stimulated patients, compared to the nonaugmented control group.

Currently, the use of DC current electrical stimulation or PEMF is not indicated for primary instrumented spinal fusion. There may be a benefit in an uninstrumented spinal fusion and/or in the high-risk patient (20,21).

EXTRACORPOREAL SHOCK WAVE THERAPY

Delayed and nonunion of fractures and osteotomies of the long bones have been treated experimentally and clinically with the application of extracorporeal shock waves. A high-energy extracorporeal shock wave has shown a method to enhance spinal fusion (17,18) and induce calcification of pseudarthrotic tissue and neogenesis of bone in experimental models (22–24). Acceleration of long-bone fracture healing has been found in sheep, rat, and dogs by Haupt (22) and Johannes (25).

The efficacy in long-bone fractures with delayed union in humans 6 months after initial injury has been 60%. More recently, application of this technique to the spine has been conducted in select cases by Valchanou (24) and Haupt (22), but its role is not yet established (26). A drawback of this technique is the requirement for anesthesia due to the discomfort induced by the therapy.

HISTORY AND PHYSICAL EXAMINATION IN THE EVALUATION OF PSEUDARTHROSIS

Patients with cervicothoracic thoracolumbar and lumbar fusion most typically have an interval of postoperative pain followed by gradual resolution, accompanied by the ability to increase their activities. Very characteristic of the pseudarthrosis patient is an interval of improvement followed by an early plateau during the pre–fusion consolidation phase owing to early loosening of implants or later when the bone implant fails. Pain patterns with pseudarthrosis are often confusing due to the physical deconditioning and chronic pain syndromes often preceding a fusion. A mechanical component to the patient's pain (i.e., positional or a direct activity-related component) can be helpful.

It is important in interviewing the patient with suspected pseudarthrosis to identify a previous history of significant postoperative wound drainage and/or treatment for suspected or proven infection.

PLAIN RADIOGRAPH COMPONENTS

Evaluation of the patient with residual symptoms after spinal fusion should always include plain radiographs (i.e., anteroposterior, lateral, and flexion-extension laterals). A confluent trabecularized fusion mass is believed to rule out pseudarthrosis. The sensitivity of this finding is suspect. Direct exploration of a fusion mass previously thought to be intact radiographically often reveals a pseudarthrosis (27). A 70% correlation is found between confluent trabeculation and the appearance of fusion mass during surgical exploration (28,29). Radiographic evidence suggestive of fusion failure may indicate progressive resorption of bone graft, development of fissure, failure of spinal implants, or progression of deformity.

Use of flexion-extension lateral radiographs has become standard. Historically, a difference of 1 or 2 degrees of motion has been cited as evidence of pseudarthrosis, but is within the intraobserver measurement error and therefore not diagnostic. A more reliable figure is motion greater than 5 degrees, as well as increased separation of the spinous process in flexion, particularly in the cervical spine (28,30).

NUCLEAR IMAGING

Technetium scintigraphy and single-photon emission computed tomography (SPECT) imaging initially were felt to have great promise for the noninvasive evaluation and diagnosis of pseudarthrosis. Several prospective studies compared these modalities to exploration and direct inspection of the fusion mass and found a very poor predictive value of scintigraphy in the diagnosis of pseudarthrosis. Albert and colleagues (31) evaluated SPECT scanning in 38 patients, in whom SPECT correctly identified 7 of the 14 pseudarthroses and 14 of 24 solid fusions, with a sensitivity of 0.50 and specificity of 0.58. Similarly, Bohnsack et al. (32) reported a specificity of 50% and a positive predictive value for technetium bone scintigraphy of 40% in their study of 42 patients and concluded the technique was inadequate to assess the integrity of spinal fusion. Other studies have compared plain flexion-extension radiographs, computed tomography findings, and bone scintigraphy, and found scintigraphy least sensitive (33). Likewise, McMasters and Merrick found the predictive value of technetium scans was negligible in fused scoliosis patients 6 months after surgery (34).

DETECTION OF LOW-GRADE INFECTION

Infection is a significant retardant to arthrodesis. The rate of infection after *in situ* fusion ranges to 5%, but some believe occult infections may be more common. When a wound infection is evident, management includes wound irrigation, débridement, and intravenous antibiotics as outlined by Glassman (35). He treated 19 acute postoperative infections with this regimen. One year later, 5 out of 19 (24%) patients had clear evidence of pseudarthrosis. Not all infections are obvious, however. Schofferman and colleagues (36) found a positive culture for diphtheroids in several pseudarthrosis patients; two out of the seven had a normal erythrocyte sedimentation rate.

Similarly, at 5-year follow-up Aydinli et al. (37) found that eight patients out of 174 had later evidence of recurrent infection and pseudarthrosis after an initial acute postoperative infection. The late culture in the patients was low-virulence *Staphylococcus epidermis.*

The contemporary use of white count energy testing, C-reactive proteins, erythrocyte sedimentation rate, and the importance of the history of wound drainage cannot be emphasized enough. Patients who are leukopenic with absolute lymphocyte counts less than 1,200 are at greater risk for an occult infection. Because of their malnourished or relatively anergic state, they also are at greater risk for an infection when pseudarthrosis repair is undertaken.

Indium-labeled bone scans have not been effective in discerning acute or chronic infections. Gratz et al. (38) and Merkle et al. (39) have reported SPECT imaging in combination with technetium or gallium enhances the sensitivity and is preferred over indium-labeled white blood cell studies.

INTERVENTION FOR PSEUDARTHROSIS

The rate of pseudarthrosis varies widely depending on pathology and the patient's age. The risk may be as low as 1 to 2% in the adolescent idiopathic scoliosis population, whereas in the adult population, a risk of 25 to 30% has been reported with instrumented posterolumbar fusion, and it may be as high as 45% when a thoracolumbar fusion is extended to the sacrum (40). The decision of when to intervene is a complex one and varies according to the original indication of fusion and presence or absence of symptoms.

CONCOMITANT DEFORMITY

Local tissue factors, alignment, and methods of stabilization all affect the risk of pseudarthrosis in the spinal deformity patient. Residual sagittal imbalance contributes to the development of early hardware failure and lumbosacral pseudarthrosis. Likewise, fixation across segments with changing contours or rigidity, such as the thoracolumbar junction or the thoracic apex, are sites at greater risk.

Although surgical intervention typically relies on débridement of the pseudarthrosis and regrafting, osteotomies to rebalance the spine have been recommended based on a small clinical series.

ANTERIOR COLUMN DEFICIT

Anterior column deficit, especially at the junctional segments, significantly increases the likelihood of hardware failure and pseudarthrosis.

The use of anterior structural grafts aids in restoration of sagittal alignment and creates load sharing between the anterior and posterior implants, and contributes significantly to the successful treatment of pseudarthrosis. Indeed, there are settings wherein there is evidence of radiographic clef where intact instrumentation in the scoliotic curve with some loss of overall sagittal line may connote pseudarthrosis. In these settings, anterior interbody fusion may forestall hardware failure and allow for arthrodesis to be accomplished.

OLIGOTROPHIC VERSUS HYPERTROPHIC PSEUDARTHROSIS

Studies of hypertrophic pseudarthroses in long-bone fractures indicate that a lack of mechanical stability and continued motion are causative. Often the bony cleft is associated with a synovial pocket on magnetic resonance imaging. These large, often-mobile pseudarthroses occur in the spine and can be associated with Charcot arthropathy. In the spinal cord injury patient, these findings suggest an increased risk of low-grade infection or excessive mechanical demands through these segments.

In the thoracic spinal cord injury patient, thoracolumbar or lumbar pseudarthrosis can be a significant challenge due to the mechanical demands of activities of daily living, wheelchair transfer, and/or sports such as wheelchair marathon racing. Extending the length of a fusion may impair a patient's ability to transfer or sporting activities. The challenge is to achieve a structural vascularized graft bridging any anterior defects and rigid immobilization in osteopenic bone.

An oligotrophic pseudarthrosis should raise additional red flags regarding the potential for an ongoing inflammatory process that disrupted the early phases of bone healing. This situation is seen in patients who have had an early postoperative wound infection. It is also seen in patients who have been on high doses of corticosteroids or receiving chemotherapy that has disrupted the fusion's biology.

TECHNIQUES OF PSEUDARTHROSIS REPAIR

Early loss of bone implant interface mechanics and severe disabling pain can certainly push a surgical decision so as to reduce patient discomfort. After initial spinal fusions by Albe and Hibs, infection of nonunion of the posterior spinal fusions was reported in the early era of spinal fusion *in situ* after reduction for the idiopathic scoliosis patient; the principles of fusion reexploration were initiated through this time. The second-look operations for decortication, débridement, and pseudarthrosis were quite common and were practiced routinely in large scoliosis centers.

In the late 1950s after the introduction of instrumentation for reduction of scoliosis, the advent of the Moe technique of pseudarthrosis became widely touted. In this technique, as the pseudarthrosis cleft was débrided, this was bone grafted with autogenous bone graft and then compressed via application of the early generation Harrington compression hooks and other wiring or clawing techniques. With these techniques, generally external immobilization was used.

In the contemporary practice, pseudarthrosis repair is generally attempted with operative means that serve to enhance fusion mass area and affect rigid immobilization of the spinal segments.

After addressing the issues of infection and nutrition, techniques that affect pseudarthrosis repair must take into account the patient's overall sagittal balance and functional capacity.

In pseudarthrosis repair, there are several considerations as to the role of osteotomy and sagittal balance, the role of anterior column deficit, and the adjunctive role of free-tissue transfer or local vascularized osseous transfer flaps and the reconstruction of these patients.

LOCAL VASCULARIZED OSSEOUS TRANSFER FLAPS

Pseudarthrosis repair has often involved use of local bone graft to create local osseous flaps, which hopefully preserved an endogenous blood supply. Local turndown flaps from the transverse process facets with débridement of facet cartilage were typical of the technique.

FREE VASCULAR TRANSFER FLAPS

Free vascular transfer flaps have been used in the form of vascularized ribs. In larger structural defects, free vascularized tissue transfers in the form of vascularized fibula can be used but require microsurgical techniques and intervention, which result in increased operating room time and potential for donor site deficiencies, such as foot drop, ankle weakness, and compartment syndrome.

STRUCTURAL BONE GRAFTING

Structural bone graft is the mainstay of anterior column support and has been used in the form of cages and structural allograft bone.

The delayed ossification can result in resorption and pseudarthrosis development; nevertheless, this allows for the greatest potential for ingrowth.

REFERENCES

1. Friedlander GE, Curtin SL, Huo MH. Bone grafts and bone graft substitutes. In: Frymoyer JW, ed. *The adult spine*, 2nd ed. Philadelphia: Lippincott Williams & Wilkins, 1997:719–732.
2. Baron R, Vignery A, Horowitz M. Lymphocytes, macrophages, and bone remodeling. *J Bone Miner Res* 1984;2:175–273.
3. Burchardt H. Biology of bone transformation. *Orthop Clin North Am* 1987;18:187–196.
4. Baylink DJ, Finkelman RD, Mohan S. Growth factors to stimulate bone formation. *J Bone Miner Res* 1993;8:5565–5572.

5a. Boden SD, Schimandle JH, Hutton WC. An experimental lumbar transverse process spinal fusion model: radiographic, histologic, and biomechanical healing characteristics. Spine 1995;20:412–420.

5b. Boden SD, Schimandle JH, Hutton WC, et al. The 1995 Volvo Aware in Basic Sciences. The use of an osteoinductive growth factor for lumbar spinal fusion. Part I: the biology of spinal fusion. Spine 1995;20:2626–2632.

6. Chen MI, Boden SD, Ugbo JL, et al. A new semi-automated method for histologic quantitation of lumbar spine fusion process. Neuro-orthop 1998;24:43–57.
7. An H, Lynch K, Toth J. Prospective comparison of autograft vs. allograft for adult posterolateral lumbar spine fusion: differences among freeze-dried, frozen, and mixed grafts. *J Spinal Disord* 1995;8:131–135.

8. McKibbin B. The biology of fracture healing in long bones. *J Bone Joint Surg* 1978;60B(2):150–162.
9. Hietaniemi K. Retarded mineralization cascade in an experimental nonunion—a sequential polyfluorochrome labeling study in rats. *Ann Chir Gynaecol* 1998;87(3):236–239.
10. Perren SM. Physical and biological aspects of fracture healing with special reference to internal fixation. *CORR* 1979;138:175–196.
11. Dwyer A. The use of electrical current stimulation in spinal fusion. *Orthop Clin North Am* 1975;6:265–279.
12. Nerubay J, Margarit B, Bubis J, et al. Stimulation of bone formation by electrical current on spinal fusion. *Spine* 1986;11:167–169.
13. Tejano N, Puno R, Ignacio J. The use of implantable direct current stimulation in multilevel spinal fusion without instrumentation. *Spine* 1996;21:1904–1908.
14. Kane W. Direct current electrical bone growth stimulation for spinal fusion. *Spine* 1988;24:363–365.
15. Kahanovitz N, Aroczny S, Hulse D, et al. The effect of postoperative electromagnetic pulsing on canine posterior spinal fusions. *Spine* 1984;9:273–279.
16. Kahanovitz N, Aroczny S, Nemzek J, et al. The effect of electromagnetic pulsing on posterior lumbar spinal fusions in dogs. *Spine* 1994;19:705–709.
17. Jenis LG, An HS, Stein R, et al. Prospective comparison of the effect of direct current electrical stimulation and pulsed electromagnetic fields on instrumented posterolateral lumbar arthrodesis. *J Spinal Disord* 2000;13(4):290–296.
18. Mooney V. A randomized double-blind prospective study of the efficacy of pulsed electromagnetic fields for interbody lumbar fusions. *Spine* 1990;15:708–712.
19. Simmons J. Treatment of failed posterior lumbar interbody fusion (PLIF) of the spine with pulsing electromagnetic fields. *Clin Orthop* 1985;183:127–132.
20. Rogozinski A, Rogozinski C. Efficacy of implanted bone growth stimulation in instrumented lumbosacral spinal fusion. *Spine* 1996; 21:2479–483.
21. Meril A. Direct current (DC) stimulation of allograft in anterior and posterior lumbar interbody fusions. *Spine* 1994;19:2393–2397.
22. Haupt G, Haupt A, Ekkernkamp A, et al. Influence of shock waves on fracture healing. *Urology* 1992;39(6):529–532.
23. Schleberger R, Senge T. Non-invasive treatment of long-bone pseudarthrosis by shock waves (ESWL). *Arch Orthop Trauma Surg* 1992;111(4):224–227.
24. Valchanou VD, Michailov P. High energy shock waves in the treatment of delayed and nonunion of fractures. *Int Orthop* 1991;15 (3):181-184.
25. Johannes EJ, Kaulesar Sukul DM, Matura E. High-energy shock waves for the treatment of nonunions: an experiment on dogs. *J Surg Res* 1994;57(2):246–252.
26. Vogel J, Hopf C, Eysel P, et al. Application of extracorporeal shock-waves in the treatment of pseudarthrosis of the lower extremity. Preliminary results. *Arch Orthop Trauma Surg* 1997; 116(8):480–483.
27. Turner JA, Ersek M, Herron L, et al. Patient outcomes after lumbar spinal fusions. *JAMA* 1992;268(7):907–911.
28. Kant AP, Daum WJ, Dean SM, et al. Evaluation of lumbar spine fusion: plain radiographs versus direct surgical exploration and observation. *Spine* 1995;20(21):2313–2317.
29. Lauerman WC, Bradford DS, Transfeldt EE, et al. Management of pseudarthrosis after arthrodesis of the spine for idiopathic scoliosis. *J Bone Joint Surg* 1992;73(2):222–236.
30. Herzog RJ, Marcotte PJ. Assessment of spinal fusion. Critical evaluation of imaging techniques. *Spine* 1996;21(9):1114–1118.
31. Albert TJ, Pinto M, Smith MD, et al. Accuracy of SPECDT scanning in diagnosing pseudoarthrosis: a prospective study. *J Spinal Disord* 1998;11(3):197–199.
32. Bohnsack M, Gosse F, Ruhmann O, et al. The value of scintigraphy in the diagnosis of pseudarthrosis after spinal fusion surgery. *J Spinal Disord* 1999;12(6):482–484.
33. Larsen JM, Rimoldi RL, Capen DA, et al. Assessment of pseudarthrosis in pedicle screw fusion: a prospective study comparing plain radiographs, flexion/extension radiographs, CT scanning, and bone scintigraphy with operative findings. *J Spinal Disord* 1996;9(2): 117–120.
34. McMaster MJ, Merrick MV. The scintigraphic assessment of the scoliotic spine after fusion. *J Bone Joint Surg* 1980;62B(1):65–72.
35. Glassman SD, Dimar JR, Puno RM, et al. Salvage of instrumental lumbar fusions complicated by surgical wound infection. *Spine* 1996;21(18):2163–2169.
36. Schofferman L, Zucherman J, Schofferman J, et al. Diphtheroids and associated infections as a cause of failed instrument stabilization procedures in the lumbar spine. *Spine* 1991;16(3):356–358.
37. Aydinli U, Karaeminogullari O, Tiskaya K. Postoperative deep wound infection in instrumented spinal surgery. *Acta Orthop Belg* 1999;65(2):182–187.
38. Gratz S, Dorner J, Ostermann WJ, et al. ^{67}Ga-citrate and ^{99}Tcm-MDP for estimating the severity of vertebral osteomyelitis. *Nuclear Med* 2000;21(1):111–120.
39. Merkel KD, Brown ML, Dewanjee MK, et al. Comparison of indium-labeled-leukocyte imaging with sequential technetium-gallium scanning in the diagnosis of low-grade musculoskeletal sepsis. *J Bone Joint Surg* 1985;67:465–476.
40. Bernhardt M, Schwartz D, Clotiaux P, et al. Posterolateral lumbar and lumbosacral fusion with and without pedicle screw fixation. *Clin Orthop* 1992;284:109–115.

CHAPTER 60

Reconstruction of the Osteoporotic Spine

Sigurd H. Berven and Serena S. Hu

Vertebral compression fractures are the most common clinical presentation of osteoporosis. These fractures may often be managed by percutaneous techniques of vertebral augmentation, including vertebroplasty and kyphoplasty, as discussed in Chapter 27. The patient with osteoporosis and progressive spinal deformity, instability, or insufficiency fractures with neurologic deficits cannot be managed effectively by techniques of percutaneous vertebral augmentation and may present a difficult challenge for reconstruction.

Instrumentation and internal fixation of the osteoporotic spine is measurably compromised by bone stock insufficiency. Strategies for management of deformity in the osteoporotic spine are now available and expand the ability of the surgeon to provide a stable and effective reconstruction. The purpose of this chapter is to identify osteoporosis as a significant comorbidity in the evaluation and treatment of patients who require spinal reconstruction, and to describe biomechanical and surgical problems associated with internal fixation of the osteoporotic spine. The information in this chapter is intended to guide decision making regarding preoperative evaluation and intraoperative management of the patient with osteoporosis requiring spinal reconstruction.

EPIDEMIOLOGY OF OSTEOPOROSIS

Osteoporosis is a skeletal disorder characterized by compromised bone strength leading to an increased risk of fracture (1). The pathophysiology of osteoporosis involves an uncoupling of the processes of bone resorption and bone formation, resulting in a microarchitectural deterioration of bony trabeculae and cortices (2–4). The definition of Albright and Reifenstein is descriptive, defining *osteoporosis* as the condition of having too little bone, but what bone there is, is normal (5). Osteoporosis is a systemic disease that is recognized as one of the major public health problems facing postmenopausal women and aging individuals of both genders (6). The World Health Organization has established diagnostic criteria for osteoporosis based on the results of dual x-ray absorptiometry (DEXA) scanning (7). Patients with a bone mineral density (BMD) between 1.0 and 2.5 standard deviations below peak BMD for gender are classified as having low bone mass. Patients with DEXA measurements less than 2.5 standard deviations below peak density for gender are classified as having osteoporosis (Fig. 1). Fractures and spinal deformity are important consequences of osteoporosis, and the lifetime prevalence of an insufficiency fracture is 40 to 75% in white women and 13% in white men (8). The prevalence of vertebral compression fractures may vary significantly depending on the criteria used to define a vertebral fracture; it also has been observed that less than one-third of vertebral compression fractures noted on radiographs come to medical attention (9). Osteoporosis of the spine is characterized by a high rate of nontraumatic vertebral fractures, disproportionate loss of trabecular bone within the vertebral bodies, and an association with spinal deformity and unstable scoliosis (10–12).

OSTEOPOROSIS AND SPINAL DEFORMITY

Osteoporosis has a significant impact on the etiology and clinical presentation of disorders of the spine. The association between BMD and spinal pathology is complex. Degenerative conditions of the spine, including facet arthropathy and intervertebral disc

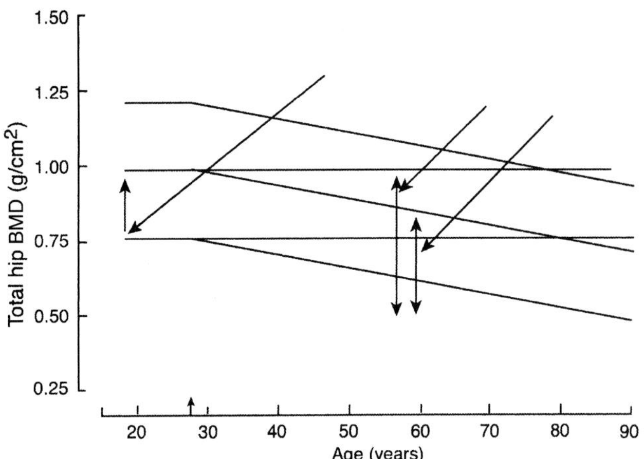

FIG. 1. Bone mineral density (BMD) changes with age, based on dual x-ray absorptiometry values.

degeneration, appear to be associated with increased BMD in the axial and appendicular skeleton (13–16). In patients with more severe osteoporosis, however, facet arthropathy and disc degeneration may be correspondingly more severe (17). Spinal deformity with scoliosis and kyphosis is a characteristic feature of osteogenesis imperfecta, with most patients being affected (18). Deformity of the spine is influenced importantly by BMD, and the spectrum of deformity associated with osteoporosis is broad.

Sagittal plane deformity resulting from vertebral compression fractures is the most characteristic manifestation of osteoporosis of the spine (19). The European Vertebral Osteoporosis Study Group described three types of vertebral deformity associated with osteoporotic compression fractures: crush, wedge, and biconcave (20). Crush and wedge fractures were most prevalent at the thoracic and thoracolumbar spine, whereas biconcave fractures were predominant at the lumbar spine. The prevalence of all types of osteoporotic compression fractures is higher in women than in men, and increases with age. A parallel epidemiologic pattern has also been demonstrated in a Japanese population (21). Prior back pain, loss of body height, and kyphotic deformity are the characteristic clinical presentation for vertebral compression fractures. The impact of compression fractures and progressive kyphosis on quality of life and on mortality has been well documented (22–28). BMD has a direct effect on the incidence of vertebral compression fractures (29–32). Patients with two or more vertebral compression fractures have a lower BMD than age-matched patients without fractures, and more severe fractures are observed in patients with lower bone density (33). When the incidence of vertebral fractures is adjusted for BMD, the gender differences observed in epidemiologic studies are eliminated, which denotes the primary importance of vertebral body strength rather than gender in determining fracture risk (34). In the child and adolescent, low BMD is directly associated with the development of kyphotic deformity. Children with idiopathic juvenile osteoporosis are characterized by kyphosis in all cases (35). Bradford has also demonstrated that osteoporosis is a significant factor in the development of Scheuermann's kyphosis, further emphasizing a clear relationship between osteoporosis and sagittal plane deformity (36).

The relationship between other spinal deformities and osteoporosis has not been well defined. Adult scoliosis, rotatory subluxation of the spine, and spondylolisthesis are spinal deformities for which the causative relationship is not as well defined as it is with sagittal deformities. Several reviews of scoliosis have concluded there is no causal relationship between scoliosis and osteoporosis in the elderly population (37–42). However, others have identified an association between osteoporosis and deformity in the adult spine (43–47). Healey and Lane estimated a prevalence of structural scoliosis in osteoporotic women of nearly 50%, with a predominance of lumbar and thoracolumbar curves (48). Curves were generally small, with only 10% measuring greater than 30 degrees. They also observed a high percentage of osteoporotic patients with lateral subluxation and anterolisthesis. Fractures occurred within the curve patterns, but did not contribute to the coronal plane deformity. Healy and Lane concluded that scoliosis in elderly women may be a sensitive marker for osteoporosis.

The presence of rotatory subluxation has been identified as a predictor of scoliosis morbidity, and it is a feature of unstable scoliosis and accelerated rate of deformity progression (10). Velis et al. identified osteoporosis as a distinct characteristic of patients with unstable scoliosis but found no association with stable scoliosis. Patients with unstable scoliosis had femoral neck density determined by dual-photon absorptiometry techniques averaging 26 to 48% lower than age-matched controls, whereas patients with stable scoliosis had a similar BMD at the femoral neck. These studies indicate a direct relationship between osteoporosis and rotatory subluxation of lumbar vertebra and unstable scoliosis, with a less reliable relationship between osteoporosis and stable scoliosis.

Healey and Lane also observed a higher prevalence of spondylolisthesis within the lumbar spine in patients with osteoporosis. The Study of Osteoporotic Fractures demonstrates that lumbar olisthesis is associated with higher BMD at L4-5, and lower BMD at L-5 to S-1 (49,50). Tabrizi reported a case of acquired spondylolisthesis related to *de novo* elongation of the L-5 pars interarticularis reportedly owing to osteoporosis, and this is consistent with one pathologic mechanism of spondylolisthesis (51,52). Spondylolisthesis occurring during childhood and adolescence is unrelated to osteoporosis, however (53,54).

Osteoporosis appears to be a characteristic of adolescents with scoliosis, and the association between scoliosis and osteoporosis in adults may be a long-term result of a compromised peak BMD in affected adolescents. Peak skeletal mass in young adulthood is a major determinant of adult bone density (10). Adolescents with scoliosis have lower BMD than age-adjusted controls (10,55–59). This difference is not a simple effect of bracing (60). In a longitudinal follow-up study, Cheng et al. demonstrated that compromised BMD in adolescents persists over time, and may lead to low peak bone mass in adulthood (61). These data suggest the association of spinal deformity, and osteoporosis may be an effect of compromised peak BMD during adolescence. In addition, osteoporosis in adulthood may predispose to collapsing of the spine, progressive kyphotic deformity, and unstable scoliosis, as well as rotatory subluxation of the spine (10).

A final category of deformity associated with osteoporosis involves postsurgical deformity. The patient with osteoporosis may be susceptible to significant and progressive deformity after surgery on limited segments of the spine. Natelson identified the potential hazards of laminectomy and facetectomy in a small group of patients with osteoporosis and compression fractures in the area treated, demonstrating progressive instability, deformity, and "disastrous results" (62). Progressive deformity after decompression without internal fixation or adjacent to fused segments of the spine is an important contemporary cause of deformity in the cervical, thoracic, and lumbar spine, and common indication for surgical revision (63–70). Osteoporosis is a comorbidity in these cases that presents a difficult challenge for effective reconstruction.

PREOPERATIVE EVALUATION

The prevalence of osteoporosis in postmenopausal white women is estimated to be 16 to 30% (71–73). Prevalence in African-American men and women is lower but remains an important consideration in preoperative evaluation of patients. The measurement of osteoporosis requires a quantitative radiographic system. DEXA scanning is the standardized test based on the definitions of the World Health Organization. Other techniques for quantifying BMD include quantitative computed tomography (CT), nuclear scanning, radiographic absorptiometry, and ultrasonography (74). Plain radiographs or CT scans without quantification have poor sensitivity and specificity for the evaluation of osteoporosis (75). Although osteoporosis is a systemic condition, DEXA scan results may vary significantly depending on the anatomic site of measurement. DEXA measurements may be made centrally at the spine or hip, or peripherally at the calcaneus or distal or proximal radius. Measurement of BMD in the spine is limited by concurrent conditions, including calcification of the aorta, sclerosis of the vertebral end-plates, calcification of the intervertebral discs, osteophyte formation, and facet hypertrophy (76–79). Similarly, the accuracy of DEXA measurements on the lateral view of the spine is compromised by the superimposition of ribs, iliac crest, and, in scoliosis, overlap of vertebral bodies (80). Measurement at the spine and hip increases the accuracy and the precision of the DEXA measurement (74). The use of bone densitometry is significantly limited in children and adolescents who have not reached peak BMD (81). Anticipation of compromised BMD in chronically ill children and in children with compromised mobility and activity is important in planning surgical intervention.

It is also important to determine if osteoporosis is primary or secondary. Some risk factors may be modified and others cannot (3). Idiopathic, or primary osteoporosis, accounts for more than 95% of the cases of osteoporosis in the elderly population (2,4,82). The Study of Osteoporotic Fractures identified important risk factors for osteoporotic insufficiency fractures including postmenopausal white women older than 50 years; history of a fracture after age 40 years; history of a fracture of the hip, wrist, or spine in a first-degree relative; and current cigarette smoking (83).

Primary osteoporosis also is clearly related to a genetic predisposition and factors that are not modifiable, including white race, poor health, and comorbidities (84). Secondary osteoporosis is caused by pathologies that may be modifiable, including endocrine disturbances (e.g., hyperparathyroidism, hyperthyroidism, hypercortisolism, estrogen withdrawal); renal failure; and drug use, including heparin, prednisone, alcohol, cigarette smoking, and excessive vitamin A. Patients with secondary osteoporosis may have a measurable improvement in BMD with treatment (85–88.) Because their condition may be improved, the identification of secondary osteoporosis is of value in the preoperative evaluation and treatment of the patient who is being considered for spinal reconstruction.

The value of preoperative treatment of the patient with osteoporosis with antiresorptive agents has not been demonstrated to reduce rates of hardware failure or improve rates of arthrodesis. Antiresorptive agents approved for the treatment of osteoporosis include bisphosphonates, calcitonin, estrogen, and selective estrogen receptor modulators. Bae et al. demonstrated that alendronate positively affects the process of spinal fusion at low doses in a rabbit model, although this effect is inhibitory at higher doses (89). In fracture healing models, bisphosphonates have been shown to have an inhibitory effect on callus remodeling and the process of healing (90). However, these effects may not compromise the overall strength and mechanical properties of the healed bone (91–93). In a clinical trial of clodronate of Colles' fractures, Adolphson et al. demonstrated increased BMD in patients treated compared with placebo (94). Intermittent parathyroid hormone has a potent anabolic effect in the treatment of osteoporosis (95). Animal studies have demonstrated that intermittent parathyroid hormone may have a positive effect on fracture healing by enhancing callus formation, increasing production of bone matrix proteins, and enhancing osteoclastogenesis during the phase of callus remodeling (96,97). The resultant effect is an increase in callus mechanical strength. In a study of screw fixation strength and intermittent parathyroid hormone administration in rats, Skripitz et al. demonstrated enhanced strength of the bone-implant interface with the treated group (98). Despite these data, the role of pharmacologic therapies in the perioperative management of patients with osteoporosis remains to be established.

SURGICAL STRATEGIES: INTERNAL FIXATION AND THE OSTEOPOROTIC SPINE

Fractures in patients with osteoporosis most commonly involve the spine. Other areas commonly affected by insufficiency fractures include the peritrochanteric region, pelvis, and distal radius (9). Osteoporosis is recognized as an important risk factor for the etiology of these fractures, and a significant factor in compromising the stability of internal fixation of the skeleton (99–107). In a study of hip fractures, osteoporosis was identified as an independent predictor of nonunion and implant failure, regardless of the implant used (108). Similarly, osteoporosis is a predictor of implant failure in the spine. Complications of internal fixation of the osteoporotic spine are well known, and include implant pull-out and failure, adjacent segment fractures, nonunion with secondary implant fracture, and progressive deformity (109–111). Therefore, establishing stable internal fixation in osteoporotic bone is a challenge in many areas of skeletal reconstruction.

In the spine, implants serve to provide stability where there is a fracture, deformity, or intrinsically unstable biologic environment. The use of implants in the spine for the correction and maintenance of correction of spinal deformity was introduced by Paul Harrington. He studied the anatomy of the spine and the pathology of scoliosis in approximately 3,000 patients with poliomyelitis and began using an implantable device in 1949 (112). The original Harrington device included a prestressed distraction rod using a ratchet system and hooks, a threaded compression rod with hooks, and a sacral bar for pelvic fixation. The device was designed to achieve correction through distraction of the concavity and compression of the convexity of the curve. He proposed using the device with or without a Hibbs midline fusion to supplement the instrumentation. Harrington recognized that different

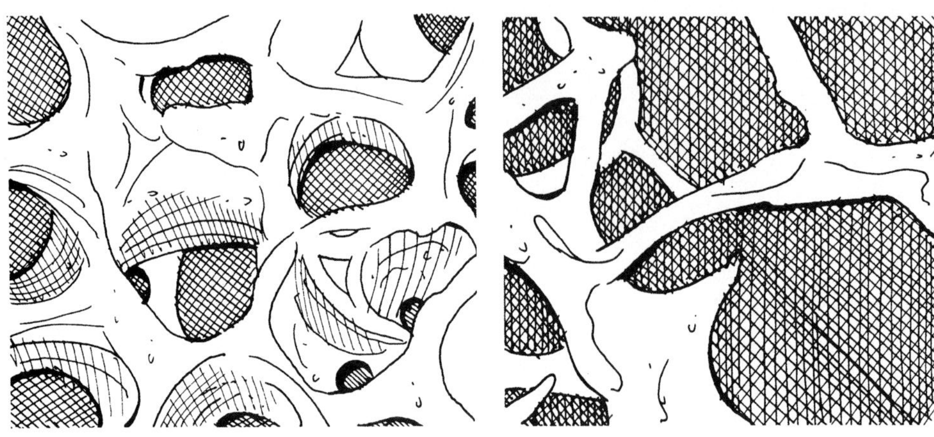

FIG. 2. Depiction of a photomicrograph of bone mineral density in normal and osteoporotic bone.

portions of the vertebra had variable strength as points of fixation for distraction and compression hooks, varying from 5 lb of force application before fracture at the tip of the transverse process to 300 lb or greater at the sublaminar region and pars interarticularis. He reported instrument failure in 58% of his early cases, and instrument dislocation in up to 10% of cases. In 1973, Eduardo Luque recognized an unacceptably high rate of complications using Harrington spinal instrumentation in "soft, young, postpoliomyelitic bone" (113). This concern led him to introduce a method of spinal segmental instrumentation using sublaminar wires in addition to hook fixation, recognizing that "the more points utilized to apply corrective forces, the less corrective force was required at a given point." The Luque method of segmental instrumentation provides a transverse force at every vertebra by applying a moment arm of correction in a plane that is perpendicular to the plane of the Harrington distraction/compression system (114). A direct comparison of the two methods demonstrated a failure pattern at the metal-bone interface in the Harrington system, and this did not occur with segmental fixation (115).

The use of transpedicular fixation in the spine was first reported by Boucher in 1959 (116). He described the use of long screws through the facet joints and into the pedicles as a technique to avoid an unacceptably high incidence of failure in lumbar spine fusion. Roy-Camille introduced the use of metal plates with transpedicular fixation to gain segmental fixation in spinal fusions (117). The screw and plate construct extended the use of segmental fixation to applications including treatment of fractures, malunions, and tumors, as well as deformity (118).

Contemporary instrumentation systems for the management of spinal deformity may involve combinations of fixation strategies, using devices to maximize strength of fixation at the bone-metal interface, and to maximize corrective power of the implant on the spine. A clear benefit for the use of transpedicular segmental fixation compared with wires and hooks remains to be demonstrated in clinical outcomes (119). McAfee et al. demonstrated that successful arthrodesis of the spine is enhanced by rigid internal fixation. However, they also observed that rigid internal fixation of the spine also led to device-related osteoporosis (i.e., stress shielding) of the vertebra. They concluded the improved mechanical properties of spinal instrumentation on spinal arthrodesis more than compensates for the occurrence of device-related osteoporosis in the spine. The mechanical properties of fixation in the osteoporotic spine depend impcrtantly on the relationship between the bone and the implant.

OSTEOPOROSIS AND THE BONE-IMPLANT INTERFACE

In the osteoporotic spine, it is particularly important to recognize the relationship between implant position and performance relative to BMD. BMD is directly related to the mechanical properties of the surgical construct, and it has measurable effects on insertional torque and pullout strength of the implant (120). The relationship between load to failure of a bone-implant construct and BMD has been studied for thoracolumbar implants by Coe et al., and this work lends important insight into the use of various implants in fixation of the osteoporotic spine (121). Those authors demonstrated transpedicular screws and spinous process wires had a load to failure when subjected to posteriorly directed tensile forces that correlated with BMD. In contrast, laminar hooks demonstrated a load to failure that was significantly higher than pedicle screws or spinous process wires, and this load to failure was not compromised by diminished BMD. The authors concluded that the relative strength of laminar fixation compared with pedicle screw fixation in the osteoporotic spine is related to the reduced rate of bone turnover in cortical bone compared with cancellous bone.

In addition to BMD, trabecular orientation is an important factor in the strength of the bone-implant construct (122). The structural characteristics of the osteoporotic spine differ significantly from those of the normal spine, accounting for important difference in properties of internal fixation. The overall strength and stiffness of an individual vertebral body is defined mainly by trabecular bone. Osteoporosis greatly affects trabecular bone, as the large surface area exposed leads to increased bone turnover (84). With a decrease in bone mass comes a decrease in the size and the number of trabeculae (Fig. 2). In addition, osteoporosis causes a decreased connectivity of the trabecular bone. Connectivity refers to the number of connections between individual trabeculae, which creates a lattice-like structure. In normal bone, the microstructure resembles a plate, whereas osteoporotic bone resembles a collection of narrow, unconnected bars. These unconnected bars are much weaker in axial compression and shear, resulting in a decrease in vertebral body strength in compression (123).

The apparent density of bone is defined as mass per bulk volume and is an indicator of the porosity of a structure. Carter and

Hayes modeled bone as a two-phase porous structure, and they determined that in normal and osteoporotic bone, the compressive strength of bone (trabecular or cortical) is proportional to the square of the apparent density, and the compressive modulus of elasticity is proportional to the cube of the apparent density (124). Hirano et al. examined the regional BMD of the pedicle measured by peripheral quantitative CT in normal and osteoporotic cadaveric specimens (125). They found that the BMD increased from the inner core of trabecular bone to the outer cortical shell in all specimens. The osteoporotic specimens had decreased BMD in all layers, and their cortices were significantly thinner. Those investigators also found that the pedicle rather than the vertebral body is responsible for 80% of the bone-screw interface stiffness, and 60% of the pullout strength of 6.25-mm diameter pedicle screws.

Characteristics of the implant may have an important effect on the bone-screw interface in a spinal construct. The integrity of the bone-screw interface is key to the maintenance of rigidity in spinal instrumentation systems. Factors that influence the bone-screw interface include the geometry of the screw, the elastic modulus of the bone, and the "quality of fit" of the screw. The interface is compromised in the osteoporotic patient, leading to micromotion and subsequent loss of fixation. The mechanism of screw failure is usually a combination of toggling in the sagittal plane and axial pullout (126–129). Zindrick et al. showed that when screws fail in the osteoporotic spine, they do so by toggling in the sagittal plane. This toggling can be minimized by contact with the cortical bone of the pedicle. The BMD at the tip of the screw within the vertebral body was found to affect the toggling less than the pedicle contact, owing to the fact that the motion occurs about the isthmus of the pedicle. The same study also noted that toggling was minimized by purchase of the anterior cortex of the vertebral body, mainly because the fulcrum then moves anteriorly. The associated risks to the anterior vascular and visceral structures are significant, however, and this technique is not recommended except at the sacrum below the vascular bifurcation.

The geometry of the screw has an important influence on the strength of the bone-screw interface. Pedicle screws have been designed to optimize the bone-screw interface. Factors such as length of threaded portion, ratio of inner to outer diameter (i.e., thread depth), and pitch greatly affect the pullout strength. DeCoster et al. looked at various screw design parameters and their effects on pullout strength (130). They found that pullout strength was linearly related to major diameter; it was also related to the ratio of major to minor diameter, although the increase was not as great. An increase in pitch also increased pullout strength, in some cases to a greater extent than an increase in major diameter. To maximize pullout strength and minimize the risk of cutout and pedicle fracture, pedicle screw major diameter should be 70 to 80% of the pedicle diameter (131). However, screws larger than 80% of the outer diameter (medial/lateral) of the pedicle may increase the risk of pedicle fracture (131,132). Cook et al. compared the pullout strengths of self-tapping pedicle screws with an expansile type of pedicle screw. The latter has a fin on the anterior tip that increases the screw diameter by 2 mm, much like drywall bolts. Pullout strengths in normal and low BMD groups were increased significantly, by 30% and 50%, respectively.

Pullout strength of pedicle screws has been found to be inversely proportional to BMD by a number of authors (126,132–135). Augmentation of osteoporotic bone with polymethylmethacrylate (PMMA) enhances the effective modulus of elasticity of bone and the apparent density of the bone surrounding the screw. PMMA augmentation has been shown to increase pullout strength of pedicle screws between 49% and 162% compared with nonaugmented pedicle screws. Zindrick et al. reported that pressurization of cement increases the pullout strength by 96%, compared with nonpressurized cement, which restored mechanical pullout to levels for normal bone (129).

The use of PMMA in the spine does have significant potential drawbacks. PMMA polymerization is an exothermic reaction, which can lead to local necrosis; it gives off toxic monomers on polymerization; it is not resorbed, leading to potential problems with further bone loss in revision spinal surgery; and extravasation into the spinal canal and the vascular system has been reported (136a–136c). Hydroxyapatite composite resin cements and bioresorbable polymers may be a substitute for PMMA in the spine. Although most of the materials investigated have mechanical properties that are inferior to those of PMMA, the material properties are certainly superior to those of osteoporotic bone. These substances have, in general, enhanced the bone-screw interface as manifested by pullout strength, albeit not as much as PMMA. However, they have the advantage of not causing local toxicity by heat or chemicals, and they are resorbed with time, avoiding the problems caused by cement removal. The property of bioresorbability also introduces the potential complication of late loosening of fixation. *In vivo* studies are in progress with some of these materials in animal and human models. For example, Lotz et al. examined screws augmented with carbonated apatite *in vitro* in a human cadaveric model (128). They found an increase in pullout strength of 68%, and the peak pullout strength was linearly related to BMD. They then looked at a rigid beam on elastic foundation analysis, and found that the cement increased stiffness by 30% within the vertebral body and 74% within the pedicle. Goodman et al. used Norian Skeletal Repair System (SRS) to augment screws in the femur and found higher load to failure and less screw sliding when cement was used (137). Heini et al. performed vertebroplasty in a cadaveric model with PMMA and brushite ($CaPO_4$) cement (138). The PMMA significantly increased stiffness in osteoporotics only, whereas the brushite increased stiffness in all specimens by 120%. Both substances significantly increased the loads to failure. They did caution that overstiffening may lead to adjacent segment fracture and did note cement leakage with high volumes. Eriksson et al. tested PMMA versus Norian SRS in foam blocks of different densities (139). Femoral neck implants were pulled out of the augmented blocks. They found that PMMA significantly increased pullout strength for all densities; the SRS increase was less pronounced and most obvious in the low-density blocks. They also noted that the PMMA failed at the cement-bone interface, whereas the SRS failed at the screw-cement interface. Ignatius et al. compared a bioabsorbable polymer versus PMMA in bovine vertebral bodies and human femur (140). They found that both substances significantly increased pullout strength as well as insertion torque and found that polymer augmentation was most effective in low-density specimens. They also demonstrated a linear correlation between pullout strength and BMD, but only in the nonaugmented specimens, indicating that augmentation decreased the adverse effects of osteoporosis. Moore et al. compared PMMA

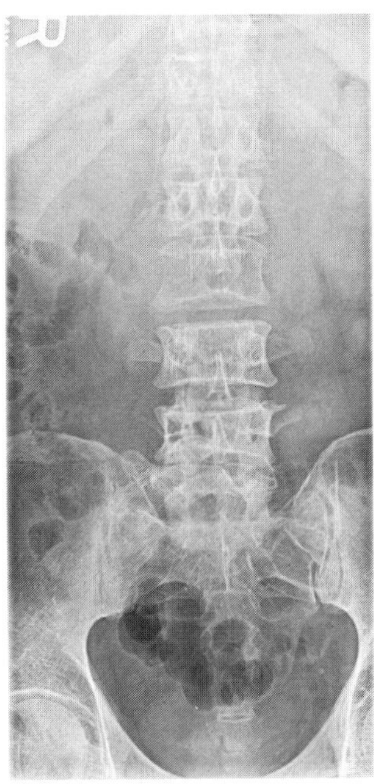
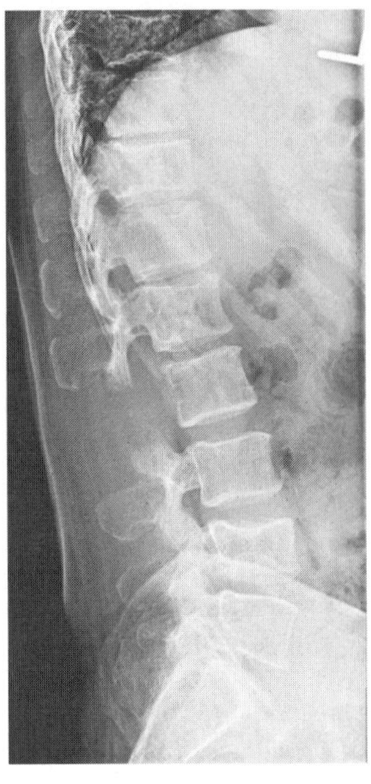
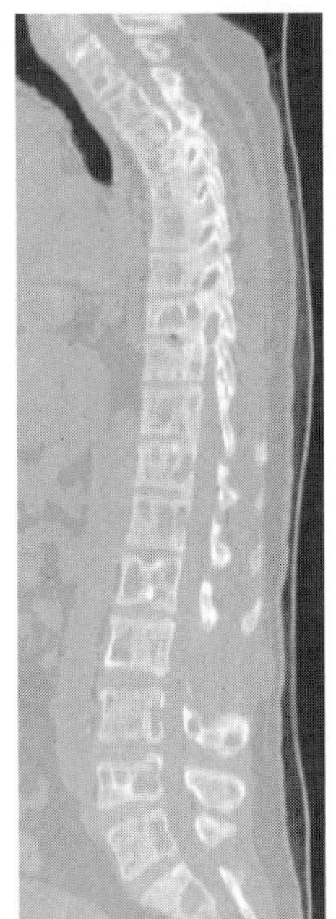
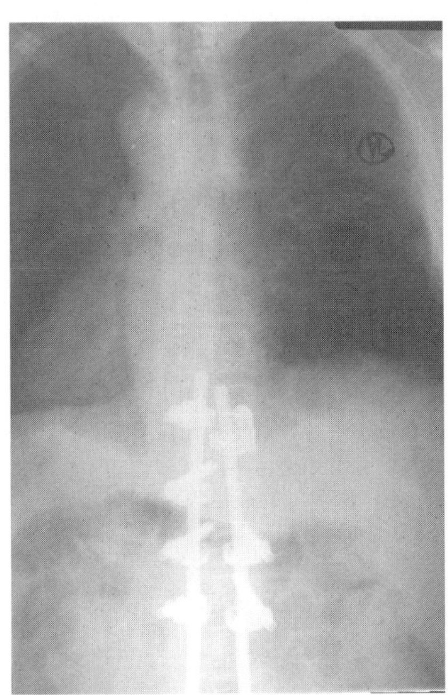
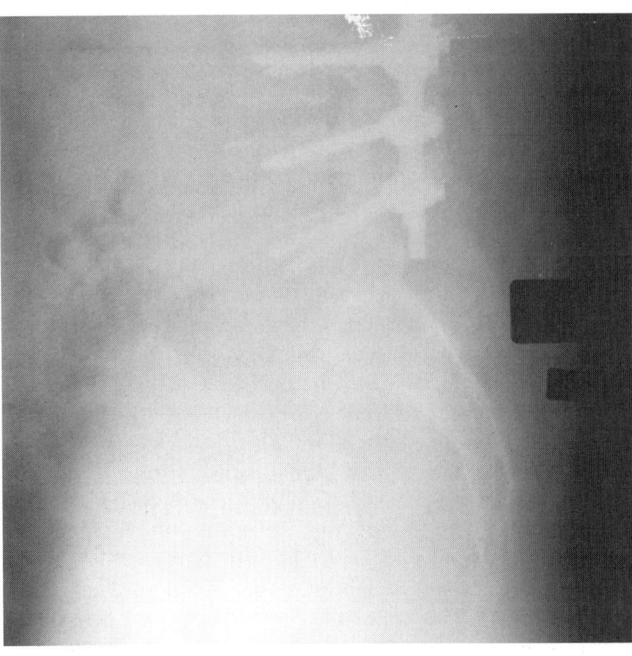

FIG. 3. Thirty-eight-year-old man with multiple myeloma and vertebral column insufficiency. Reconstruction of the spine involved posterior segmental fixation with vertebral augmentation using polymethylmethacrylate at each level of the fusion.

to $CaPO_4$ cement augmentation in human cadaveric vertebrae (141). Both substances significantly increased pullout strengths of various screw types (147% for PMMA, 102% for $CaPO_4$). Wittenberg et al. compared PMMA and polyglycol fumarate augmentation in human and bovine vertebra (128). They found that both substances increased pullout strength significantly, but that only PMMA significantly increased transverse bending stiffness. Yerby et al. used hydroxyapatite cement to rescue failed pedicle screws in human lumbar vertebrae (142). They found that augmentation of 6.0-mm and 7.0-mm failed screws increased pullout strength more than 300%. In a clinical review of experience using calcium apatite cement to augment anteriorly-placed vertebral screws and posteriorly placed pedicle screws, Wuisman et al. reported cement leakage in four of forty-eight augmented dorsal screws, with no complications reported (143). Jang et al. demonstrated stronger stabilization and facilitation of short segment instrumentation using PMMA augmentation for fixation in metastatic disease (144). Metastatic involvement of the vertebral column presents challenges that are similar to osteoporosis (Fig. 3) Overall, augmentation of osteoporotic bone with a bone filler material significantly increases the rigidity of the bone-screw interface, and improves the efficacy of instrumentation in the osteoporotic spine. The long-term effect of implant loosening between PMMA and a resorbable material remains to be demonstrated in clinical study.

The "quality of fit" is a final important consideration in optimization of the bone-screw interface. The "strength" of a pedicle screw lies in its ability to transfer stresses to the bony

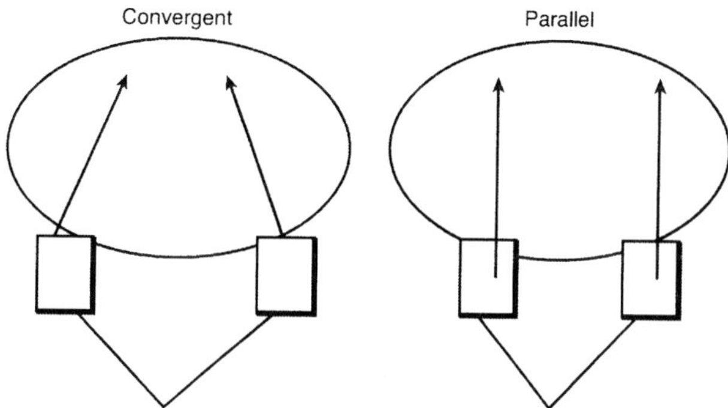

FIG. 4. Drawing of convergent versus parallel pedicle screws.

shell of the pedicle, which is cortical bone and able to bear higher loads than trabecular bone. Therefore, a large-diameter pedicle screw should increase the stability of the bone-screw interface. Fatigue failure (cycles to failure) of an individual pedicle screw is related to the ratio of the screw diameter to the pedicle diameter, again implicating the importance of the "quality of fit" (131). In the osteoporotic patient, the pedicle is affected as well as the trabecular bone of the vertebral body, although to a lesser degree (84,127). The BMD of the entire pedicle (i.e., cortical and subcortical bone) is decreased, increasing the risk of pedicle fracture or screw cutout during track preparation and screw insertion. Modified methods of screw track preparation and screw insertion may be useful in the osteoporotic spine. Untapped and undertapped tracks have been shown to enhance pullout strengths *in vitro* (132, 139,145). Halvorson et al. looked at different insertion techniques as well as supplemental fixation techniques in a human cadaveric model, and found that in osteoporotic specimens, not tapping and undertapping increased the pullout strength for 6.5-mm diameter screws. It is interesting that no significant difference was noted with these techniques in spines with normal BMD. Enhancing the amount of bone between the screws by triangulating has also been shown to be effective in stabilizing the bone-screw interface. Barber and colleagues tested screw configurations of varying degrees of convergence and found that 30 degrees of convergence resulted in significantly increased resistance to pullout and sustained higher loads than parallel screws (146) (Fig. 4). Rudland et al. compared the pullout strengths of a variety of instrumentation configurations: laminar hooks, single screws, and triangulated screws connected via a transverse plate (147). They found that the pullout strengths of the triangulated screws were significantly higher than any other group, and postulated that the mass of bone between the screws was more important than the amount of bone in contact with the screw threads.

OTHER STRATEGIES

The use of laminar hooks or interbody cages in combination with transpedicular fixation may significantly improve construct rigidity. Halvorson et al. demonstrated that the addition of two laminar hooks, one at the level of and one above the pedicle screw, serves to stabilize the construct and minimize micromotion at the bone-screw interface (132). Hasegawa and colleagues examined the fixation of a screw alone, and one coupled with a same-level laminar hook in a nondestructive manner (148). They found that the hook significantly increased the stiffness of the bone-screw interface. In addition, they found similar improvements in the normal BMD and low BMD groups, indicating that supplemental fixation should be beneficial in all patients. At the cephalad extent of a long fusion, the upper thoracic spine presents a challenge for adequate fixation. Hooks, wires, pedicle screws, or combinations may be used effectively. Butler et al. demonstrated that a pedicle hook claw is superior to sublaminar wires alone in strength to failure using osteoporotic spine (149). Hilibrand et al. demonstrated that a supralaminar hook may restore the fixation strength when added to a compromised pedicle screw (150). Figure 5 demonstrates the case of a 69-year-old woman with hook failure at the cephalad portion of a long fusion. The patient was revised with a combination construct using pedicle screws and wires with good result.

The relationship between osteoporosis and pseudarthrosis has not been defined, and osteoporosis is not identified as an independent risk factor for pseudarthrosis (151,152). Osteoprogenitor cells from osteoporotic bone marrow are less in number, however, and function with a reduced capacity compared with cells derived from normal bone marrow (153–157). Rodriguez et al. demonstrated that mesenchymal stem cells from osteoporotic women have a lower growth rate than control marrow stem cells, respond to growth signals less potently, and have a compromised capacity to differentiate into an osteoblastic lineage (158). These data may provide a physiologic basis for compromised bone formation in the osteoporotic spine.

Stable arthrodesis is more reliable with the use of combined anterior and posterior surgery (159–161). Hasegawa et al. studied the biomechanics of anterior interbody devices in a cadaveric model (148). The authors demonstrated that larger cages transferred load borne by the body to the cortical shell, sparing the weaker cancellous bone, and resulting in higher maximum loads before fracture. Jost and colleagues examined the compressive strengths and load/displacement curves of a variety of interbody fusion cages, and noted that low BMD specimens failed at lower loads and exhibited less resistance to compressive loading compared with normal BMD specimens (162).

The addition of anterior column support clearly contributes to the overall stability of a spinal reconstruction instrumentation strategy. Circumferential fusion of the spine is also useful in improving the stability of fixation in the osteoporotic spine in the perioperative period and in the late postoperative period by reducing the rate of pseudarthrosis. Anterior column support also introduces risk of significant morbidity as discussed later, and this risk must be balanced against the benefits in determining an optimal surgical strategy. Osteoporosis has a measurable effect on the efficacy of implants in the anterior and posterior columns of the spine. The addition of laminar and anterior interbody fixation improves the overall rigidity of the construct in osteoporotic bone.

In summary, internal fixation of the osteoporotic spine is a difficult surgical challenge. Techniques for optimizing construct rigidity include implant combinations with multiple sites of fixation, screw augmentation, and circumferential arthrodesis. Sublaminar hooks and wires have mechanical characteristics, including pullout strength, that are relatively preserved even in the presence of osteo-

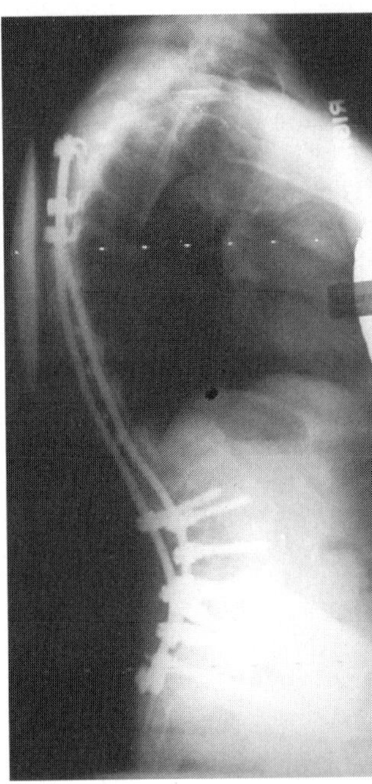

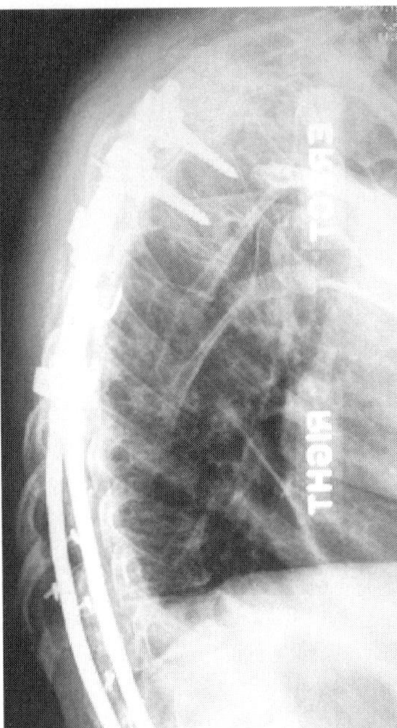

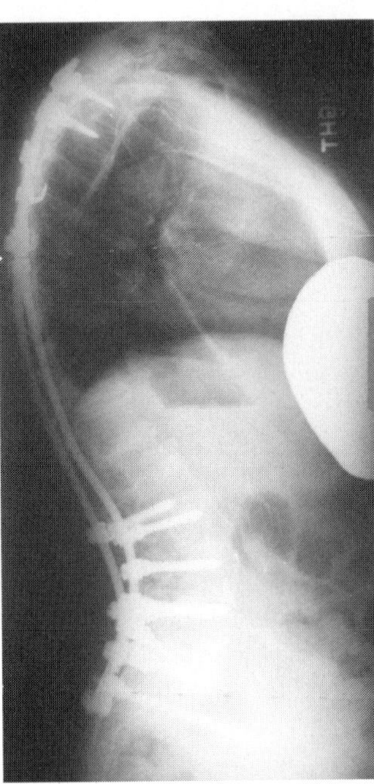

FIG. 5. Failure of fixation at the cephalad end of the construct. Revision with transpedicular fixation and sublaminar wiring.

porosis. However, in the patient with previous laminectomy and in the lumbar spine, pedicle screws with augmentation may provide more reliable fixation. The goals of deformity correction in the osteoporotic spine may be less than those in a patient with normal BMD, as compromise of the bone-implant interface may prevent the safe use of some corrective maneuvers.

OUTCOMES AND COMPLICATIONS OF SURGERY ON THE OSTEOPOROTIC SPINE

Surgical strategies in the spinal reconstructive surgery require attention to the physiologic status and comorbidities of the patient as well as to the biomechanics of internal fixation. Implant failure, adjacent segment decompensation, and complications related to medical comorbidities in the elderly or functionally compromised patient population are of particular concern in treating patients with osteoporosis. Implant failure may be avoided by optimization of the rigidity of internal fixation, as outlined previously. Progressive kyphosis above or below a region of fixation is an important consideration in the osteoporotic spine, and attention to fusion of the spine above the area of maximal kyphosis in the thoracic spine or into the area of lordosis in the lumbar spine protects the spine from progressive deformity in the adjacent segments. Termination of the implant construct with a rigid claw construct or screw fixation rather than wires prevents settling of the end vertebrae and progressive kyphosis. The addition of anterior column reconstruction clearly contributes to the stability of a spinal column reconstruction. However, complication rates for combined anterior and posterior surgery are clearly higher than posterior-only surgery (163–166).

The rate of complications in surgery on the spine is age dependent, and this further contributes to complex considerations in choosing a strategy for reconstruction of the osteoporotic spine. In an age-related assessment of outcome in spinal deformity surgery, Takahashi et al. reported significantly less correction of deformity and inadequate restoration of lumbar lordosis in patients older than 50 years (167). The overall complication rate was 29%, and was unrelated to age. The authors identified factors that contribute to potential complications and surgical difficulty in elderly patients, including curve rigidity, osteoporosis, and comorbidities. In a study of perioperative complications after anterior spine surgery for deformity, McDonnell et al. reported that patients between 61 and 80 years of age had a significantly higher rate of perioperative complications than younger cohorts, with pulmonary complications identified as the most common (168). There also is an increased risk in the elderly for cardiac morbidity and pancreatitis in the postoperative period (169,170). Age and comorbidities were identified as independent predictors of hospital stay, operative time, and intraoperative blood loss in patients undergoing lumbar decompression with segmental instrumentation (171). Kostuik et al. identified age and preoperative American Society of Anesthesiologists score as important predictors of minor and major complications in adult spinal deformity surgery, reporting an overall complication rate of 57% and major complications in 27% of patients. They concluded that age is an important preoperative consideration for surgical planning and avoidance of complications (172).

Given all of the surgical challenges of complex rigid deformities, osteoporosis, and an increased risk for intraoperative and perioperative complications, the surgeon may consider options including decompression alone or *in situ* arthrodesis. Nonoperative options, including activity modification and physical therapy to improve endurance, may be shared with the patient as alternatives to reconstruction of the spine. Sharing knowledge of complication rates and risks of surgical intervention empowers the patient to participate in an informed choice regarding his or her care, and contributes to the patient's overall satisfaction with management.

When a patient presents with deformity, vertebral body fracture, pain, or neurologic involvement, the physician must decide if there are any risk factors for osteoporosis. If yes, the condition should be confirmed by DEXA and secondary causes evaluated by the appropriate laboratory tests. If a secondary cause is confirmed, it should probably be treated radically.

Once the basic spine problem is evaluated (e.g., deformity, fracture, pain), nonoperative treatment should first be attempted. If symptoms continue, surgical assessment should proceed including an assessment of comorbidities.

If surgery is felt to be possible, and instrumentation is necessary, several strategies should be followed. For pedicle screws, 70 to 80% of the pedicle should be filled by the screw—"best fit." The vertebral body should be penetrated without going through the anterior cortex, and the screws should not be tapped. If secure fixation cannot be obtained, cement should be considered.

CONCLUSION

Spinal reconstruction in the setting of osteoporosis is an important and contemporary topic for the spinal deformity physician. The mean age of the population is increasing in nearly all industrialized countries. In the year 2000, 12.6% of the U.S. population was older than 65 years (173). By 2030, 20% of the U.S. population will be older than 65 years. In correlation with the increase in life expectancy and increased population age, the activity level and health care expectations of older people may increase (174,175). The mission of health care providers in contributing to the health of the population includes consideration of physical, mental, and social well being (176). Reconstruction of the spine is an important intervention for the population of patients with spinal instability, progressive deformity, and pain related to vertebral column insufficiency. The development of safe and effective techniques for reconstruction of the osteoporotic spine offers the spinal deformity physician the opportunity to contribute to health in this growing patient population.

REFERENCES

1. NIH Consensus Development Conference, March 27, 2000.
2. Mankin HJ. Metabolic bone disease. *Instr Course Lect* 1995;44(3).
3. Lane JM, Russell L, Khan SN. Osteoporosis. *Clin Orthop* 2000; 372:139–150.
4. Lindsay R, Cosman F. Primary osteoporosis. In: Coe FL, Favus MJ, eds. *Disorders of bone and mineral metabolism*. New York: Raven Press, 1992:831–888.
5. Albright F, Reifenstein EC Jr, eds. Metabolic bone disease: osteoporosis. In: *The parathyroid glands and metabolic bone disease*. Baltimore: Williams & Wilkins, 1948:145–204.
6. Riggs BL, Melton LJ. The worldwide problem of osteoporosis: insights afforded by epidemiology. *Bone* 1995;17(5):505S–511S.
7. Assessment of fracture risk and its applications to screening for postmenopausal osteoporosis. Report of a World Health Organization Study Group. *World Health Organ Tech Rep Ser* 1994;843:1–129.
8. Melton LJ III, Chrischilles EA, Cooper C, et al. How many women have osteoporosis? *J Bone Miner Res* 1992;7:1005–1010.
9. Cummings SR, Melton LJ. Osteoporosis I: epidemiology and outcomes of osteoporotic fractures. *Lancet* 2002;359(9319):1761–1767.
10. Velis KP, Healey JH, Schneider R. Osteoporosis in unstable adult scoliosis. *Clin Orthop* 1988;(237):132–141.
11. Riggs BL, Wahner WL, Dunn RB, et al. Differential changes in bone mineral density of the appendicular and axial skeleton with aging. *J Clin Invest* 1981;67:328.
12. Bell GH, Dunbar O, Beck JS, et al. Variation in strength of vertebrae with age and their relation to osteoporosis. *Calcif Tissue Res* 1967;1:75.
13. Dequeker J. The relationship between osteoporosis and osteoarthritis. *Clin Rheum Dis* 1985;11:271–296.
14. Harada A, Okuizumi H, Miyagi N, et al. Correlation between bone mineral density and intervertebral disc degeneration. *Spine* 1998;23: 857–862.
15. Dai L. The relationship between vertebral body deformity and disc degeneration in the lumbar spine of the senile. *Eur Spine J* 1998;7: 40–44.
16. Knight SM, Ring EFJ, Bhalla AK. Bone mineral density and osteoarthritis. *Ann Rheum Dis* 1992;1:1025–1026.
17. Marguiles JY, Payzer A, Nyska M, et al. The relationship between degenerative changes and osteoporosis in the lumbar spine. *Clin Orthop* 1996;324:146–152.
18. Cristofaro RL, Hoek KJ, Bonnett CA, et al. Operative treatment of spine deformity in osteogenesis imperfecta. *Clin Orthop* 1979;139: 40–48.
19. Cortet B, Roches E, Logier R, et al. Evaluation of spinal curvatures after a recent osteoporotic vertebral fracture. *J Bone Spine* 2002; 69(2):201–208.
20. Ismail AA, Cooper C, Felsenberg D, et al. EVOS Group. Number and type of vertebral deformities: epidemiological characteristics and relation to back pain and height loss. *Osteoporosis Int* 1999;9:206–213.
21. Jinbayashi H, Aoyagi K, Ross PD, et al. Prevalence of vertebral deformity and its associations with physical impairment among Japanese women: The Hizen-Oshima Study. *Osteoporosis Int* 2002; 13(9):723–730.
22. Matthis C, Weber U, O'Neill WO, et al., and the European Vertebral Osteoporosis Study Group. *Osteoporosis Int* 1998;8:364–372.
23. Ettinger B, Black DM, Nevitt MC, et al. Contribution of vertebral deformities to chronic back pain and disability. The study of osteoporotic fractures research group. *J Bone Miner Res* 1992;7(4):449–456.
24. Badia X, Diez-Perez A, Alvarez-Sanz C, et al. The Spanish GRECO Study Group. *Qual Life Res* 2001;10(4):307–317.
25. Silverman SL. The clinical consequences of vertebral compression fractures. *Bone* 1992;13S:S27–S31.
26. Cooper C, Kinson EJ, Atkinson J, et al. Population based study of survival after osteoporotic fractures. *Am J Epidemiol* 1993;137: 1001–1005.
27. Schlaich C, Minne HW, Bruckner T, et al. Reduced pulmonary function in patients with spinal osteoporotic fractures. *Osteoporos Int* 1998;8:261–267.
28. Gold JW. The clinical impact of vertebral fractures: quality of life in women with osteoporosis. *Bone* 1996;18(3S):185S–189S.
29. Edmondston SJ, Singer KP, Day RE, et al. *Ex vivo* estimation of thoracolumbar vertebral body compressive strength: the relative contributions of bone densitometry and vertebral morphometry. *Osteoporosis Int* 1997;7L:142–148.
30. Marshall D, Johnell O, Wedel H. Meta-analysis of how well measures of bone mineral density predict occurrence of osteoporotic fractures. *BMJ* 1996;312:1254–1259.
31. Jones G, White C, Bguyen T, et al. Prevalent vertebral deformities: relationship to bone mineral density and spinal osteophytosis in elderly men and women. *Osteoporos Int* 1996;6(3):233–239.
32. Myers ER, Wilson SE. Biomechanics of osteoporosis and vertebral fracture. *Spine* 1997;22(24S):25S–31S.
33. Antoniou J, Nguyen C, Lander P, et al. Osteoporosis of the spine: correlation between vertebral deformity and bone mineral density in postmenopausal women. *Am J Orthop* 2000;29(1):956–959.
34. The European Vertebral Osteoporosis Study Group. The relationship between bone density and incident vertebral fracture in men and women. *J Bone Miner Res* 2002;17(12):2214–2221.
35. Jones ET, Hensinger RN. Spinal deformity in idiopathic juvenile osteoporosis. *Spine* 1981;6(1):1–4.
36. Bradford DS, Brown DM, Moe JH, et al. Scheuermann's kyphosis: a form of osteoporosis? *Clin Orthop* 1976;118:10–14.
37. Robin D, Span Y, Steinberg R, et al. Scoliosis in the elderly: a follow-up study. *Spine* 1982;7:355–361.

38. Robin G, Span Y, Makin M, et al. Scoliosis in the elderly: idiopathic or osteoporotic? In: Zorab PA, ed. *Scoliosis. Proceedings of the fifth symposium*. London: Academic Press, 1977:215–219.
39. Leichter I, Hazan G, Weinren A, et al. The effect of age and sex on bone density, bone mineral content and cortical index. *Clin Orthop* 1981;156:232–238.
40. Hans D, Biot B, Schott AM, et al. No diffuse osteoporosis in lumbar scoliosis but lower femoral bone density on the convexity. *Bone* 18(1):15–17.
41. Korovessis P, Piperos G, Sidiropoulos P, et al. Adult idiopathic lumbar scoliosis: a formula for prediction of progression and review of the literature. *Spine* 1994;19(17):1926–1932.
42. Grubb SA, Lipscomb HJ. Diagnostic findings in painful adult scoliosis. *Spine* 1992;17(5).
43. Vanderpool DW, James JIP, Wynne-Davis R. Scoliosis in the elderly. *J Bone Joint Surg* 1969;51A:446–451.
44. Thevenon A, Pollez B, Cantegrit F, et al. Relationship between kyphosis, scoliosis and osteoporosis in the elderly population. *Spine* 1987;12:744–745.
45. Shands AR, Eisberg HB. The incidence of scoliosis in the state of Delaware. A study of 50,000 minifilms of the chest made during a survey for tuberculosis. *J Bone Joint Surg* 1955;37A:1243.
46. Carter OD, Haynes SG. Prevalence rates for scoliosis in US adults: results from the first National Health and Nutrition Examination Survey. *Int J Epidemiol* 1987;16(4):537–544.
47. Gillespy T III, Gillespy T Jr, Revak CS. Progressive senile scoliosis: seven cases of increasing spinal curves in elderly patients. *Skel Radiol* 1985;13(4):280–286.
48. Healey JH, Lane JM. Structural scoliosis in osteoporotic women. *Clin Orthop* 1985;195:216–223.
49. Vogt MT, Rubin DA, SanValentin R, et al. Degenerative lumbar listhesis and bone mineral density in elderly women. The study of osteoporotic fractures. *Spine* 1999;24(23):2536–2541.
50. Vogt MT, Rubin DA, SanValentin R, et al. Lumbar olisthesis and low back symptoms in elderly white women. The study of osteoporotic fractures. *Spine* 1998;23(23):2640–2647.
51. Tabrizi P, Bouchard JA. Osteoporotic spondylolisthesis: a case report. *Spine* 2001;26(13):1482–1485.
52. Newman PH. The etiology of spondylolisthesis. *J Bone Joint Surg* 1963;45B:39–59.
53. Wiltse LL. The etiology of spondylolisthesis. *J Bone Joint Surg* 1962;44A:539–560.
54. Wiltse LL, Widell EH, Jackson DW. Fatigue fracture: the basic lesion in isthmic spondylolisthesis. *J Bone Joint Surg* 1975;57A: 17–22.
55. Courtois I, Collet P, Mouilleseaux B, et al. Bone mineral density at the femur and lumbar spine in a population of young women treated for scoliosis in adolescence. *Rev Rheum Engl Ed* 1999;66(12):705–710.
56. Burber WL, Badger VM, et al. Osteoporosis and acquired back deformities. *J Pediatr Orthop* 1982;118:10–15.
57. Cheng JCY, Guo X. Osteopenia in adolescent idiopathic scoliosis, a primary problem or secondary to spinal deformity? *Spine* 1997;22:1716–1721.
58. Thomas KA, Cook SD, Skalley TC, et al. Lumbar spine and femoral neck bone mineral density in idiopathic scoliosis: a follow-up study. *J Pediatr Orthop* 1992;12(2):235–240.
59. Cook SD, Harding AF, Morgan EL, et al. Trabecular bone density in idiopathic scoliosis. *J Pediatr Orthop* 1987;7(2):168–174.
60. Snyder BD, Zaltz I, Breitenbach MA, et al. Does bracing affect bone density in adolescent scoliosis? *Spine* 1995;20(14):1554–1560.
61. Cheng JCY, Guo X, Sher AHL. Persistent osteopenia in adolescent idiopathic scoliosis. A longitudinal follow-up study. *Spine* 1999;24(12):1218–1222.
62. Natelson SE. The injudicious laminectomy. *Spine* 1986;11(9):966–969.
63. Azuma S, Seichi A, Ohnishi I, et al. Long-term results of operative treatment for cervical spondylotic myelopathy in patients with athetoid cerebral palsy: an over 10-year follow-up study. *Spine* 2002;27(9):943–948.
64. Guigui P, Benoist M, Deburge A. Spinal deformity and instability after multilevel cervical laminectomy for spondylotic myelopathy. *Spine* 1998;23(4):440–447.
65. Saito T, Yamamuro T, Shikata J, et al. Analysis and prevention of spinal column deformity following cervical laminectomy. I. Pathogenetic analysis of postlaminectomy deformities. *Spine* 1991;16(5): 494–502.
66. Lonstein JE. Post-laminectomy kyphosis. *Clin Orthop* 1977;(128): 93–100.
67. Benner B, Ehni G. Degenerative lumbar scoliosis. *Spine* 1979;4(6): 548–552.
68. Papagelopoulos PJ, Peterson HA, Ebersold MJ, et al. Spinal column deformity and instability after lumbar or thoracolumbar laminectomy for intraspinal tumors in children and young adults. *Spine* 1997;22(4):442–451.
69. Kostuik JP, Errico TJ, Gleason TF. Techniques of internal fixation for degenerative conditions of the lumbar spine. *Clin Orthop* 1986;(203):219–231.
70. Sano S, Yokokura S, Nagata Y, et al. Unstable lumbar spine without hypermobility in postlaminectomy cases. Mechanism of symptoms and effect of spinal fusion with and without spinal instrumentation. *Spine* 1990;15(11):1190–1197.
71. Melton LJ III. Epidemiology of spinal osteoporosis. *Spine* 1997;22(24S):2S–11S.
72. Melton LJ III. How many women have osteoporosis now? *J Bone Miner Res* 1993;10:175–177.
73. Looker AC, Johnston CC Jr, Wahner HW, et al. Prevalence of low femoral bone density in older US women from NHANES III. *J Bone Miner Res* 1995;10:796–802.
74. Seeger LL. Bone density determination. *Spine* 1997;22(24S):49S–57S.
75. Koot VCM, Kesselaer SMMJ, Clevers GJ, et al. Evaluation of the Singh index for measuring osteoporosis. *J Bone Joint Surg* 1996;78B:831–834.
76. Smith JA, Vento JA, Spencer RP, et al. Aortic calcification contributing to bone densitometry measurement. *J Clin Densitom* 1999;2(2): 181–183.
77. Guglielmi G, Grimston SK, Fischer KC, et al. Osteoporosis: diagnosis with lateral and posteroanterior dual x-ray absorptiometry compared with quantitative CT. *Radiology* 1994;192:845–850.
78. Antonnaci MD, Hanson DS, LeBlanc A, et al. Regional variation in vertebral bone density and trabecular architecture are influenced by osteoarthritic change and osteoporosis. *Spine* 1997;22(20):2393–2401, discussion, 2401–2402.
79. Rand T, Seidl G, Kainberger F, et al. Impact of spinal degenerative changes on the evaluation of bone mineral density with dual energy X-ray absorptiometry (DXA). *Calcif Tissue Int* 1997;60(5):430–433.
80. Rupich RC, Griffin MG, Pacifici R, et al. Lateral dual-energy radiography: artifact error from rib and pelvic bone. *J Bone Miner Res* 1992;7:97–101.
81. van Rijn RR, Van der Sluis IM, Link TM, et al. Bone densitometry in children: a critical appraisal. *Eur Radiol* 2003;13:700–710.
82. Riggs BL, Melton LJ III. Involutional osteoporosis. *N Engl J Med* 1986;314:1676–1686.
83. Cummings SR, Nevitt MC, Browner WC, et al. Risk factors for hip fracture in white women. *N Engl J Med* 1995;332:767–773.
84. Lane JM, Riley EH, Wirganowicz PZ. Osteoporosis: diagnosis and treatment. *J Bone Joint Surg* 1996;78A:618–632.
85. Marcus R. Secondary forms of osteoporosis. In: Coe FL, Flavus MJ, eds. *Disorders of bone and mineral metabolism*. New York: Raven Press, 1992:889–904.
86. Saville PD, Kharmosh O. Osteoporosis of rheumatoid arthritis: influence of age, sex, and corticosteroids. *Arthritis Rheum* 1967;10:423–430.
87. Aloia JF, Roginsky M, Ellis K, et al. Skeletal metabolism and body composition in Cushing's Syndrome. *J Clin Endocrinol Metab* 1974;39:981–985.
88. Fraser SA, Anderson JB, Smith DA, et al. Osteoporosis and fractures following thyrotoxicosis. *Lancet* 1971;1:981–983.
89. Bae H, Yee A, Friess D, et al. Alendronate influences bone volume in rabbit posterolateral spine fusion. *Spine J* 2002;2(5S):98S–99S.
90. Li C, Mori S, Li J, et al. Long-term effect of incadronate disodium (YM-175) on fracture healing of femoral shaft in growing rats. *J Bone Miner Res* 2001;16(3):429–436.
91. Li J, Mori S, Kaji Y, et al. Concentration of bisphosphonate (incadronate) in callus area and its effects on fracture healing in rats. *J Bone Miner Res* 2000;15(10):2042–2051.
92. Koivukangas A, Tuukkanen J, Kippo K, et al. Long-term administration of clodronate does not prevent fracture healing in rats. *Clin Orthop* 2003;(408):268–278.

93. Peter CP, Cook WO, Nunamaker DM, et al. Effect of alendronate on fracture healing and bone remodeling in dogs. *J Orthop Res* 1996;14(1):74–79.
94. Adolphson P, Abbaszadegan H, Boden H, et al. Clodronate increases mineralization of callus after Colles' fracture: a randomized, double-blind, placebo-controlled, prospective trial in 32 patients. *Acta Orthop Scand* 2000;71(2):195–200.
95. Morley P, Whitfield JF, Willick GE. Parathyroid hormone: an anabolic treatment for osteoporosis. *Curr Pharm Des* 2001;7(8):671–687. Review.
96. Nakajima A, Shimoji N, Shiomi K, et al. Mechanisms for the enhancement of fracture healing in rats treated with intermittent low-dose human parathyroid hormone (1-34). *J Bone Miner Res* 2002;17(11):2038–2047.
97. Andreassen TT, Fledelius C, Ejersted C, et al. Increases in callus formation and mechanical strength of healing fractures in old rats treated with parathyroid hormone. *Acta Orthop Scand* 2001;72(3): 304–307.
98. Skripitz R, Aspenberg P. Implant fixation enhanced by intermittent treatment with parathyroid hormone. *J Bone Joint Surg Br* 2001; 83(3):437–440.
99. Laros GS. Intertrochanteric fractures. The role of complications of fixation. *Arch Surg* 1975;110(1):37–40.
100. Kim WY, Han CH, Park JI, et al. Failure of intertrochanteric fracture fixation with a dynamic hip screw in relation to pre-operative fracture stability and osteoporosis. *Int Orthop* 2001;25(6):360–362.
101. Handoll HH, Madhok R. Surgical interventions for treating distal radial fractures in adults. *Cochrane Database Syst Rev* 2001;(3):CD003209. Review.
102. Kuokkanen H, Raty S, Korkala O, et al. Osteosynthesis and allogeneic bone grafting in complex osteoporotic fractures. *Orthopedics* 2001;24(3):249–252.
103. Spangler L, Cummings P, Tencer AF, et al. Biomechanical factors and failure of transcervical hip fracture repair. *Injury* 2001;32(3): 223–228.
104. Chmell MC, Moran MA, Scott RD. Periarticular fractures after total knee replacement. *J Am Acad Orthop Surg* 1996;4(2):109–116.
105. Kitajima I, Tachibana S, Mikami Y, et al. Insufficiency fracture of the femoral neck after intramedullary nailing. *J Orthop Sci* 1999;4(4):304–306.
106. Matsuda M, Kiyoshige M, Takagi M, et al. Intramedullary bone-cement fixation for proximal humeral fracture in elderly patients. A report of 5 cases. *Acta Orthop Scand* 1999;70(3):283–285.
107. Kawaguchi S, Sawado K, Nabeta Y. Cutting-out of the lag screw after internal fixation with the Asiatic gamma nail. *Injury* 1998;29(1):47–53.
108. Barrios C, Brostrom LA, Stark A, et al. Healing complications after internal fixation of trochanteric hip fractures: the prognostic value of osteoporosis. *J Orthop Trauma* 1993;7(5):438–442.
109. Andersson S, Rodrigues M, Olerud C. Odontoid fractures: high complication rate associated with anterior screw fixation in the elderly. *Eur Spine J* 2000;9(1):56–59, discussion, 60.
110. Swank M. Adjacent segment failure above lumbosacral fusions instrumented to L1 or L2. *Spine J* 2(5S):48S.
111. Bayley JC, Yuan HA, Fredrickson BE. The Syracuse I-plate. *Spine* 1991;16[3 Suppl]:S120–S124.
112. Harrington PR. Treatment of scoliosis. Correction and internal fixation by spine instrumentation. *J Bone Joint Surg* 44(4):591–610.
113. Luque ER. The anatomic basis and development of segmental spinal instrumentation. *Spine* 1982;7(3):256–259.
114. Wenger DR, Carollo JJ, Wilkerson JA. Biomechanics of scoliosis correction by segmental spinal instrumentation. *Spine* 7(3):260–264.
115. Wenger DR, Carollo JJ, Wilkerson JA, et al. Laboratory testing of segmental spinal instrumentation versus traditional Harrington Instrumentation for scoliosis treatment. *Spine* 1982;7(3):265–269.
116. Boucher HH. A method of spinal fusion. *J Bone Joint Surg* 1959;41B:248–259.
117. Roy-Camille R, Saillant G, Berteaux D, et al. Osteosynthesis of thoracolumbar spine fractures with metal plates screwed through the vertebral pedicles. *Reconstr Surg Traumatol* 1976;15:2–16.
118. Roy-Camille R, Saillant G, Mazel C. Internal fixation of the lumbar spine with pedicle screw plating. *Clin Orthop* 1986;203:7–17.
119. Bridwell KH, Hanson DS, Rhee JM, et al. Correction of thoracic adolescent idiopathic scoliosis with segmental hooks, rods, and Wisconsin wires posteriorly. It's bad and obsolete, correct? *Spine* 2002;27(18):2059–2066.
120. Okuyama K, Sato K, Abe E, et al. Stability of transpedicular screwing for the osteoporotic spine. An *in vitro* study of the mechanical stability. *Spine* 1993;18(15):2240–2245.
121. Coe JD, Warden KE, Herzig MA, et al. Influence of bone mineral density on the fixation of thoracolumbar implants. A comparative study of transpedicular screws, laminar hooks, and spinous process wires. *Spine* 1990;15(9):902–907.
122. Turner IG, Rice GN. Comparison of bone screw holding strength in healthy bovine and osteoporotic human cancellous bone. *Clin Mater* 1992;9(2):105–107.
123. Parisien M, Cosman F, Mellish RW, et al. Bone structure in postmenopausal hyperparathyroid, osteoporotic, and normal women. *J Bone Miner Res* 1995;10(9):1393–1399.
124. Carter DR, Hayes WC. The compressive behavior of bone as two-phase porous structure. *J Bone Joint Surg* 1977;59A(7):954–962.
125. Hirano T, Hasegawa K, Takahashi HE, et al. Structural characteristics of the pedicle and its role in screw stability. *Spine* 1997;22(21):2504–2509, discussion 2510.
126. Lotz JC, Hu SS, Chiu DFM, et al. Carbonated apatite cement augmentation of pedicle screw fixation in the lumbar spine. *Spine* 1997;22(23):2716–2723.
127. Turner AWL, Gillies RM, Svehla MJ, et al. Hydroxyapatite composite resin cement augmentation of pedicle screw fixation. *CORR* 2003;406:253–261.
128. Wittenberg RH, Lee KS, Shea M, et al. Effect of screw diameter, insertion technique, and bone cement augmentation of pedicular screw strength. *CORR* 1993;296:278–297.
129. Zindrick MR, Wiltse LL, Widell EH, et al. A biomechanical study of intrapedicular screw fixation in the lumbosacral spine. *CORR* 1986;203:99–112.
130. DeCoster TA, Heetderks DB, Downey DJ, et al. Optimizing bone screw pullout force. *J Orthop Trauma* 1990;4(2):169–174.
131. Misenhimer GR, Peek RD, Wiltse LL, et al. Anatomic analysis of pedicle cortical and cancellous diameter as related to screw size. *Spine* 1989;14(4):367–372.
132. Pitzen T, Barbier D, Tintinger F, et al. Screw fixation to the posterior cortical shell does not influence peak torque and pullout in anterior cervical plating. *Eur Spine J* 2002;11:494–499.
133. Halvorson TL, Kelley LA, Thomas KA, et al. Effects of bone mineral density on pedicle screw fixation. *Spine* 1994;19(21):2415–2420.
134. Hitchon PW, Brenton MD, Coppes JK, et al. Factors affecting the pullout strength of self-drilling and self-tapping anterior cervical screws. *Spine* 2003;28(1):9–13.
135. Hackenberg L, Link T, Liljenqvist U. Axial and tangential fixation strength of pedicle screws versus hooks in the thoracic spine in relation to bone mineral density. *Spine* 2002;27(9):937–942.
136a. Yeom JS, Kim WJ, Choy WS, et al. Leakage of cement in percutaneous transpedicular vertebroplasty for painful osteoporotic compression fractures. *J Bone Joint Surg* 2003;85B:83–89.
136b. Peters KR, Guiot BH, Martin PA, et al. Vertebroplasty for osteoporotic compression fractures: current practice and evolving techniques. *Neurosurgery* 2002;51[5 Suppl]:96–103.
136c. Phillips FM, Todd Wetzel F, Lieberman I, et al. An *in vivo* comparison of the potential for extravertebral cement leak after vertebroplasty and kyphoplasty. *Spine* 2002;27(19):2173–2178; discussion 2178–2179.
137. Goodman SB, Bauer TW, Carter D, et al. Norian SRS cement augmentation in hip fracture treatment. *CORR* 1998;348:42–50.
138. Heini PF, Berlemann U, Kaufmann M, et al. Augmentation of mechanical properties in osteoporotic vertebral bones—a biomechanical investigation of vertebroplasty efficacy with different bone cements. *Eur Spine J* 2001;10:164–171.
139. Eriksson F, Mattson P, Larsson S. The effect of augmentation with resorbable or conventional bone cement on the holding strength for femoral neck fixation devices. *J Orthop Trauma* 2002;16(5):302–310.
140. Ignatius AA, Augat P, Ohnmacht M, et al. A new bioresorbable polymer for screw augmentation in the osteosynthesis of osteoporotic cancellous bone: a biomechanical evaluation. *J Biomed Mater Res* 2001;58:254–260.
141. Moore DC, Maitra RS, Farjo LA, et al. Restoration of pedicle screw fixation with an in situ setting calcium phosphate cement. *Spine* 1997;22(15):1696–1705.

142. Yerby SA, Toh E, McLain RF. Revision of failed pedicle screws using hydroxyapatite cement. *Spine* 1998;23(15):1657–1661.
143. Wuisman PIJ, Van Dijk M, Staal H, et al. Augmentation of pedicle screws with calcium apatite cement in patients with severe progressive osteoporotic spinal deformities: an innovative technique. *Eur Spine J* 2000;9:528–533.
144. Jang JS, Lee SH, Rhee CH, et al. Polymethylmethacrylate-augmented screw fixation for stabilization in metastatic spine tumors. *J Neurosurg* 2002;96:131–134.
145. Oktenoglu BT, Ferrara LA, Andalkar N, et al. Effects of hole preparation on screw pullout resistance and insertional torque: a biomechanical study. *J Neurosurg* 2001;94[1 Suppl]:91–96.
146. Barber JW, Boden SD, Ganey T, et al. Biomechanical study of lumbar pedicle screws: does convergence affect axial pullout strength? *J Spinal Disord* 1998;11(3):215–220.
147. Rudland CM, McAfee PC, Warden KE, et al. Triangulation of pedicular instrumentation. A biomechanical analysis. *Spine* 1991;16(6):S270–S276.
148. Hasegawa K, Takahashi HE, Uchiyama S, et al. An experimental study of a combination method using a pedicle screw and laminar hook for the osteoporotic spine. *Spine* 1997;22(9):958–962, discussion, 963.
149. Butler TE, Asher MA, Jayaraman G, et al. The strength and stiffness of thoracic implant anchors in osteoporotic spines. *Spine* 1994;19(17):1956–1962.
150. Hilibrand AS, Moore DC, Graziano GP. The role of pediculolaminar fixation in compromised pedicle bone. *Spine* 1996;21(4):445–451.
151. Simmons E, Kuhele J, Lee J, et al. Evaluation of metabolic bone disease as a risk factor for lumbar fusion. *Spine J* 2002;2:98S.
152. Schofferman J, Schofferman L, Zucherman J, et al. Metabolic bone disease in lumbar pseudarthrosis. *Spine* 1990;15(7):687–689.
153. Oreffo RO, Bord S, Triffitt JT. Skeletal progenitor cells and ageing human populations. *Clin Sci (Lond)* 1998;94(5):549–555.
154. Muschler GF, Nitto H, Boehm CA, et al. Age- and gender-related changes in the cellularity of human bone marrow and the prevalence of osteoblastic progenitors. *J Orthop Res* 2001;19(1):117–125.
155. Bergman RJ, Gazit D, Kahn AJ, et al. Age-related changes in osteogenic stem cells in mice. *J Bone Miner Res* 1996;11(5):568–577.
156. D'Ippolito G, Schiller PC, Ricordi C, et al. Age-related osteogenic potential of mesenchymal stromal stem cells from human vertebral bone marrow. *J Bone Miner Res* 1999;14(7):1115–1122.
157. Rodriguez JP, Montecinos L, Rios S, et al. Mesenchymal stem cells from osteoporotic patients produce a type I collagen-deficient extracellular matrix favoring adipogenic differentiation. *J Cell Biochem* 2000;79(4):557–565.
158. Rodriguez JP, Garat S, Gajardo H, et al. Abnormal osteogenesis in osteoporotic patients is reflected by altered mesenchymal stem cells dynamics. *J Cell Biochem* 1999;75(3):414–423.
159. Saer EH III, Winter RB, Lonstein JE. Long scoliosis fusion to the sacrum in adults with nonparalytic scoliosis: an improved method. *Spine* 1990;15:650–653.
160. O'Brien JP, Dawson MH, Heard CW, et al. Simultaneous combined anterior and posterior fusion. A surgical solution for failed spinal surgery with a brief review of the first 150 patients. *Clin Orthop* 1986;(203):191–195.
161. Albert TJ, Pinto M, Denis F. Management of symptomatic lumbar pseudarthrosis with anteroposterior fusion. *Spine* 2000;25:123–129.
162. Jost B, Cripton PA, Lund T, et al. Compressive strength of interbody cages in the lumbar spine: the effect of cage shape, posterior instrumentation and bone density. *Eur Spine J* 1998;7(2):132–141.
163. Byrd JA III, Scoles PV, Winter RB, et al. Adult idiopathic scoliosis treated by anterior and posterior spinal fusion. *J Bone Joint Surg Am* 1987;69:843–850.
164. Floman Y, Micheli LJ, Penny JN, et al. Combined anterior and posterior fusion in seventy-three spinally deformed patients: Indications, results and complications. *Clin Orthop* 1982;164:110–122.
165. Winter RB. Combined Dwyer and Harrington instrumentation and fusion in the treatment of selected patients with painful adult idiopathic scoliosis. *Spine* 1978;3:135–141.
166. Berven S, Deviren V, Smith JA, et al. Management of fixed sagittal plane deformity: outcome of combined anterior and posterior surgery. *Spine (in press)*.
167. Takahashi S, Delecrin J, Passuti N. Surgical treatment of idiopathic scoliosis in adults: an age-related analysis of outcome. *Spine* 2002;27(16):1742–1748.
168. McDonnell MF, Glassman SD, Dimar JR 2nd, et al. Perioperative complications of anterior procedures on the spine. *J Bone Joint Surg Am* 1996;78(6):839–847.
169. Shapiro G, Green DW, Fatica NS, et al. Medical complications in scoliosis surgery. *Curr Opin Pediatr* 2001;13:36–41.
170. Laplaza FJ, Widmann RF, Fealy S, et al. Pancreatitis after surgery in adolescent idiopathic scoliosis: incidence and risk factors. *J Pediatr Orthop* 2002;22(1):80–83.
171. Zheng F, Cammisa FP Jr, Sandhu HS, et al. Factors predicting hospital stay, operative time, blood loss, and transfusion in patients undergoing revision posterior lumbar spine decompression, fusion, and segmental instrumentation. *Spine* 2002;27(8):818–824.
172. Kostuik JP, Chang JY, Sieber AN, et al. Complications of spinal fusion in treatment of adult spinal deformity. Poster #308, American Academy of Orthopedic Surgeons, New Orleans, 2003.
173. U.S. Bureau of Census, Current Population Reports, Series P25–1130, 1996.
174. Reference deleted.
175. Sarkisian CA, Hays RD, Mangione CM. Do older adults expect to age successfully? The association between expectations regarding aging and beliefs regarding healthcare seeking among older adults. *J Am Geriatr Soc* 2002;50(11):1837–1843.
176. WHO definition of health, 1948.

CHAPTER 61

Bone Grafting: Techniques and Complications

Kirkham B. Wood

Currently, more than 200,000 spine fusions are performed annually in the United States (1,2). The most common indications are instability (e.g., fracture, degeneration) or deformity (e.g., scoliosis, kyphosis, spondylolisthesis). Posterolateral intertransverse process fusions remain the most commonly used technique. However, the rate of pseudarthrosis can rise as high as 40% primarily as a function of the number of vertebral levels spanned (3–6). Today, autologous iliac crest bone grafts remain the biologic and biomechanical standard for spinal fusions. The most common donor site is the posterior iliac crest because of the quantity and the quality of the graft material obtained. The anterior ilium is the second most common site, especially applicable for cervical fusions because the bi- or tricortical graph is mechanically well suited for the interbody position (1,7–10). As technology has evolved and the problems associated with harvesting bone from the patient's own ilium have been clarified, human allograft and bone graft substitutes have become more popular.

BIOPHYSIOLOGY

Autograft bone carries the three fundamental factors needed for a successful fusion: osteogenicity, osteoinductivity, and osteoconductivity (11). Other bone fusion materials (e.g., allograft, ceramics, coral, etc.) also have these characteristics to varying degrees, but autologous bone remains the gold standard. Osteogenic cells in the form of viable osteoblasts and stem cells initiate the fusion process. Appropriate decortication of the fusion site's bony surfaces is important to provide bone marrow, vascularization, and osteoprogenitor cells to the fusion area. Other osteoinductive factors, such as bone morphogenetic proteins, also stimulate neovascularization and the migration of other bone-forming cells to the site. The rigid mechanical osteoconductive lattice provided by the hydroxyapatite and collagen provides a scaffold for the new blood vessels.

The majority of autograft used is cancellous bone. Because of its great trabecular area, it offers great osteoconductivity. It lacks mechanical strength, however, and initially needs protection by instrumentation or external bracing. With time, the fusion mass remodels and increases in strength (i.e., osteointegration). Cortical bone in the form of struts or long-bone "rings" offers early stability, but cortical bone can lose up to one-third of its initial strength during incorporation and may take up to 2 years to complete the fusion process by integrating with the host bone. This long time interval is because cortical grafts have fewer marrow spaces for osteogenetic cells, with less surface area onto which new bone can form.

ANATOMY OF GRAFT DONOR SITES

The ilium is composed of an irregular posterosuperior surface and a concave anterosuperior surface (Fig. 1). The ilium is thickest from 2 to 3 cm posterior to the anterior superior iliac spine and the posteroinferior ilium. The anterior ilium in normal subjects measures approximately 10.6 to 11.7 cm in width and

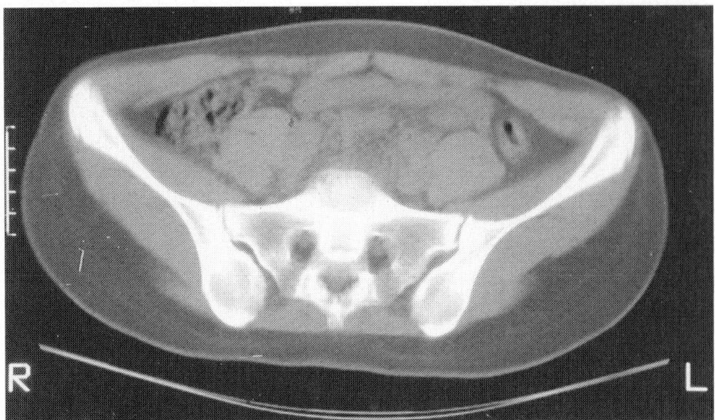

FIG. 1. Axial computed tomographic scan through pelvis demonstrating the curvilinear surfaces of the anterior and posterior ilium.

almost 17 mm in width at the iliac tubercle and posteriorly (12,13). The medial-superior cortex of the iliac crest at the level of the iliac tubercle facilitates the harvesting of ample amounts of cancellous bone, while preserving the contour of the iliac crest. Posteriorly, the average thickness of the crest ranges from 14.2 to 17.1 cm, but some crests can have much more than 2 cm of cancellous bone for harvesting.

Important neurovascular structures include the ilioinguinal, iliohypogastric, and lateral femoral cutaneous nerves anteriorly and the superior cluneal and gluteal nerves posteriorly (Fig. 2). Special attention should be paid to the location of these structures, including their anatomic variations, before embarking on open harvesting of bone from the ilium.

The lateral femoral cutaneous nerve is a sensory branch of the lumbar plexus and supplies sensation to the anterolateral thigh (Fig. 3). It typically courses just under the inguinal ligament into the thigh, medial to the anterior superior iliac spine. It can, on occasion, pass over the crest laterally and thus come under some risk during exposure to the lateral anterior ilium (12).

Posteriorly, the cluneal nerves originate as branches of the L-1, L-2, and L-3 dorsal rami and supply sensation to the posterior buttocks. They pass over the iliac crest posteriorly approximately 7 to 8 cm from the posterior iliac spine and can be injured during aggressive harvesting of bone from the posterior ilium (Fig. 4).

The superior gluteal artery is a branch of the internal iliac artery (Fig. 5) and presents potential danger as it exits the pelvis through the sciatic notch to enter the gluteal region.

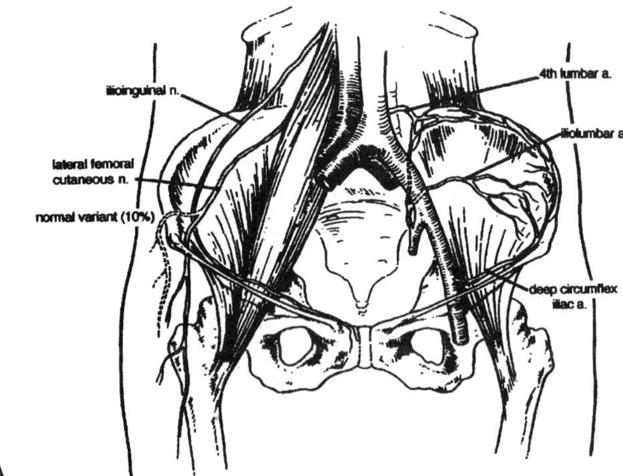

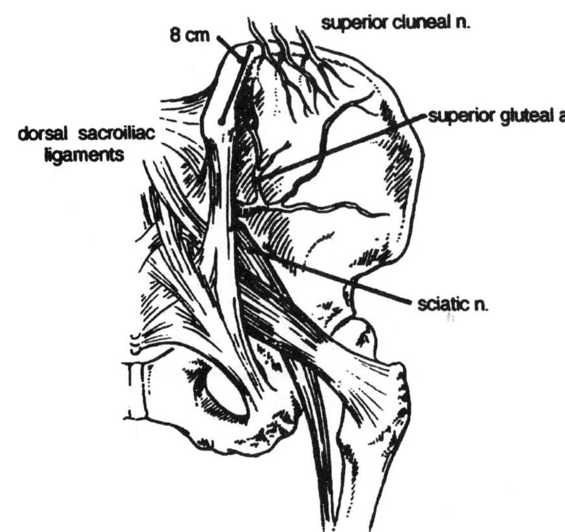

FIG. 2. A: Important neural and vascular structures in relation to the anterior ilium. **B:** Important anterior structures in relation to the posterior ilium. a, artery; n, nerve. (From Fowler BL, Dall BE, Rowe DE. Complications associated with harvesting autogenous iliac bone graft. *Am J Orthop* 1995;24:895–903, with permission.)

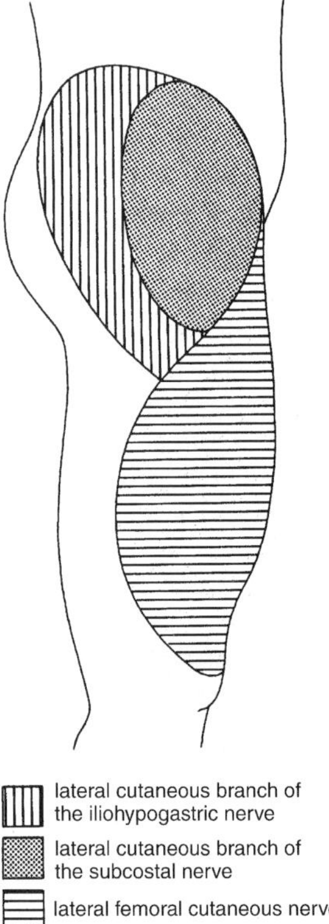

FIG. 3. Sensory distribution of nerves at risk during bone harvesting from the anterior ilium. (From Kalk W, et al. Morbidity from iliac crest bone harvesting. *J Oral Maxillofac Surg* 1996;54:1424–1429, with permission.)

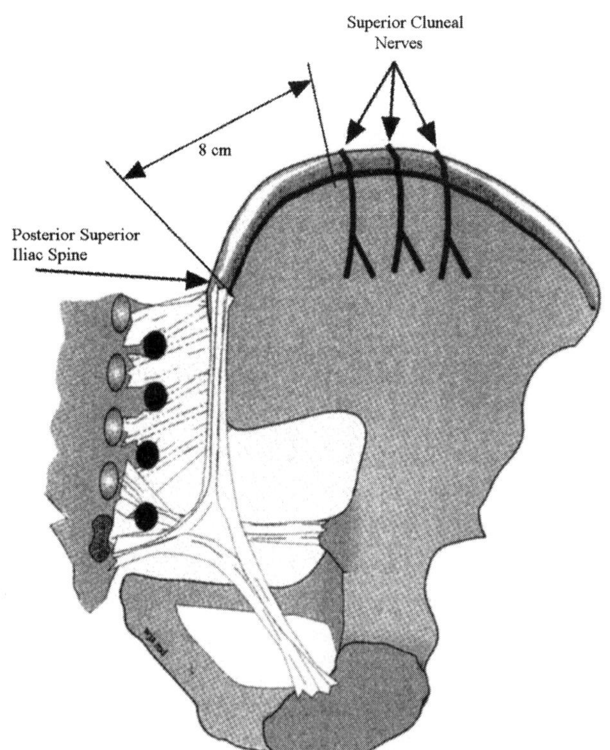

FIG. 4. Distribution of the cluneal nerves over the posterior ilium. Surgeons should take care to limit their exposure to within 8 cm of the posterior superior iliac spine.

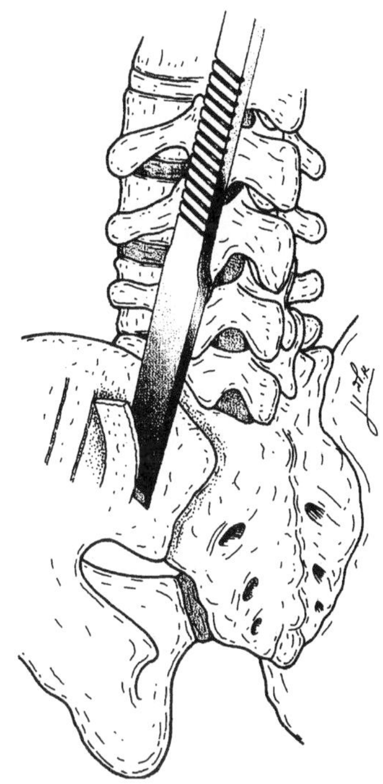

FIG. 6. Harvesting corticocancellous strips from the posterior ilium. [From Mirovsky Y, et al. Comparison between the outer table and intracortical methods of obtaining autogenous bone graft from the iliac crest. *Spine* 2000;25(13):1722–1725, with permission.]

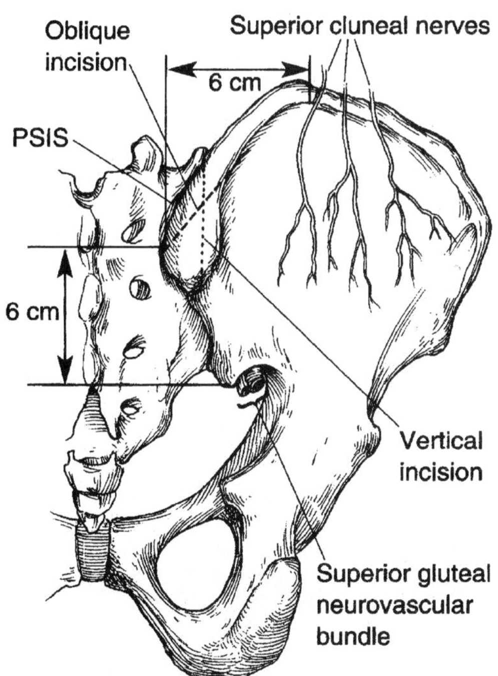

FIG. 5. Description of the superior gluteal artery (along with nerve) as it exits the pelvis through the sciatic notch. PSIS, posterior superior iliac spine. [© 2001 American Academy of Orthopaedic Surgeons. From Ebraheim NA, Hossein E, Xu R. Bone-graft harvesting from iliac and fibular donor sites: techniques and complications. *J Am Acad Orthop Surg* 2001;9(3):210–218, with permission.]

Harvesting from the Posterior Ilium

Five harvesting techniques are used to obtain graft from the posterior ilium. These include the most commonly used removal of corticocancellous strips from the outer table using osteotomes and gouges, trephine curettage, a trap door (14), Wolfe's (15), and the subcrestal techniques.

The traditional harvesting of corticocancellous strips begins by making one or several longitudinal cuts in the outer cortical ilium with an osteotome, the number depending on the amount of bone needed (Fig. 6). Additional cancellous bone down to, but not penetrating the inner table, is removed with a gouge or curette.

The posterior ilium is approached via a vertical or lateral oblique incision (Fig. 5). It should be kept within an 8-cm distance from the posterior superior iliac spine so as to avoid the superior cluneal nerves. The working area should also be kept within 4 cm of the crest to avoid injury to the sacroiliac joint. Full-thickness grafts, such as those taken commonly from the anterior ilium, are ill advised in the posterior ileum because of the risk of injury to the sacroiliac ligaments (13,16).

The "trap-door" technique involves hinging a section of the iliac crest on its periosteal and muscular attachments, removing the cancellous bone from within using curettes or gouges, then closing the crest back down to maintain the crest's normal contour (Fig. 7). Wolfe and Kawamoto described a technique wherein the crest is split longitudinally, the cancellous bone removed from within, then closing the crest with the use of wire or suture (Fig. 8) (15).

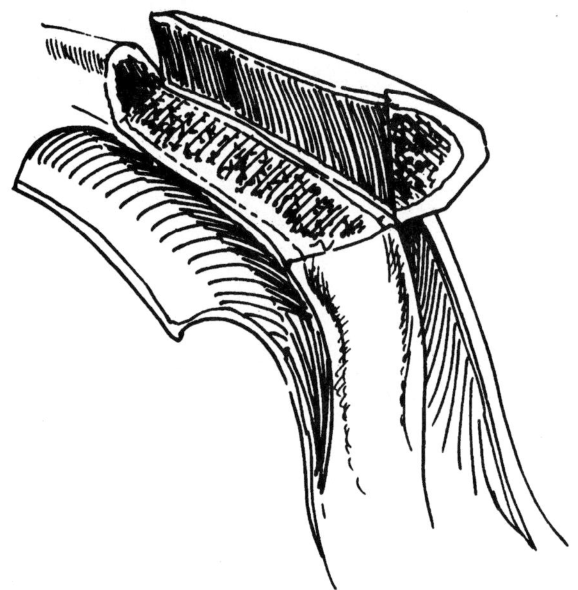

FIG. 7. Diagram depicting the iliac crest reflected to expose cancellous bone for harvesting. (© 1999 The Cleft Palate-Craniofacial Journal, by De La Torre JI, et al. Reprinted with permission of Alliance Communications Group, a division of Allen Press, Inc.)

In the subcrestal window technique, graft, including full-thickness harvesting, can be removed from inferior to the crest itself again preserving the contour (Fig. 9B). One alternative method for harvesting bone is a trephine technique, which uses a serrated cylinder, standard curettes, or even a Craig bone biopsy instrument that can be manually driven between the tables of the ilium so as to remove cancellous bone in a less invasive manner (Fig. 10) (17–22). The skin incision can be as short as 1 to 2 cm or through the same spine incision, if appropriate (22). Local anesthetic can be injected, and often no drains are required. The postoperative pain and risks of cosmetic deformity and fracture are considerably less than with open techniques, although the amount of bone harvested may be less.

Another novel technique for harvesting bone involves trephining bone from within a vertebral body adjacent to the fusion level. This obviously is principally applicable during an anterior approach. The defect thus created can be filled with a ceramic or allograft plug (20).

Harvested cancellous bone can and does regenerate within the iliac crest, although it takes approximately 24 months to do so (11,23), and the amount is less than available from a normal iliac crest. The greatest amount of graft follows a trap-door technique. If use of a previously used graft site is contemplated, computed tomography (CT) scanning is recommended preoperatively for a precise description of the available graft and anatomy.

Harvesting from the Anterior Ilium

When making the approach to the anterior ilium, it is best to mobilize the skin craniomedially before incision so that the scar is located somewhat caudolateral to the crest. This has a better cosmetic appearance and avoids possible scar irritation from clothing. Bone commonly is removed from the medial rather than lateral cortex, which preserves muscular attachments, particularly the abductors.

The anterior ilium is an excellent source of bicortical or tricortical grafts for use in cervical fusions. Tricortical grafts are procured by parallel cuts through the inner and outer tables using an oscillating saw (Fig. 9A) (12,24,25). It is particularly important to harvest the bone at least 3 cm posterior to the anterior superior iliac spine and to assure the cut is directed away from the spine. Bicortical or corticocancellous strip grafts may be taken from below the iliac crest, using the subcrestal window technique.

Large structural autografts for thoracic and thoracolumbar vertebrectomy can sometimes be taken from the anterior crest. However, at least 4 to 6 cm should remain from the graft donor

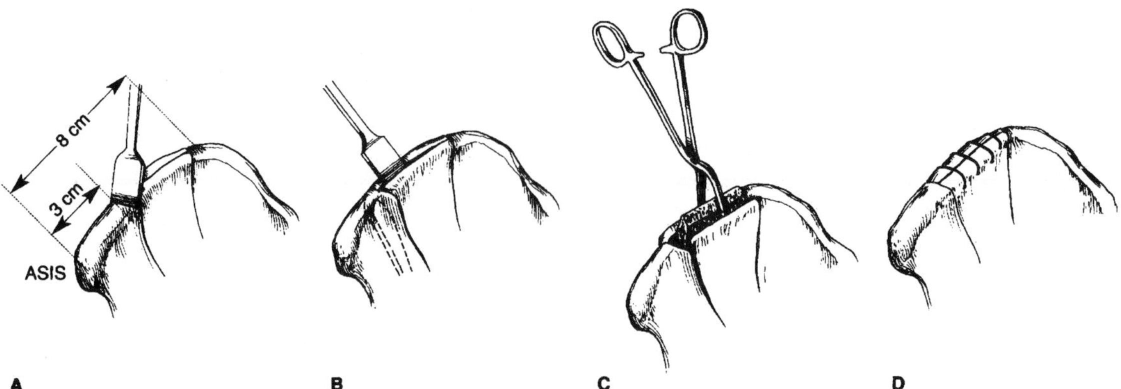

FIG. 8. Wolfe technique. A: Parallel cuts though the iliac crest. B: A longitudinal cut splits the crest. C: Cancellous bone removed. D: Inner and outer tables reapproximated with suture or wire. ASIS, anterior superior iliac spine. [© 2001 American Academy of Orthopaedic Surgeons. From Ebraheim NA, Hossein E, Xu R. Bone-graft harvesting from iliac and fibular donor sites: techniques and complications. *J Am Acad Orthop Surg* 2001;9(3):210–218, with permission.]

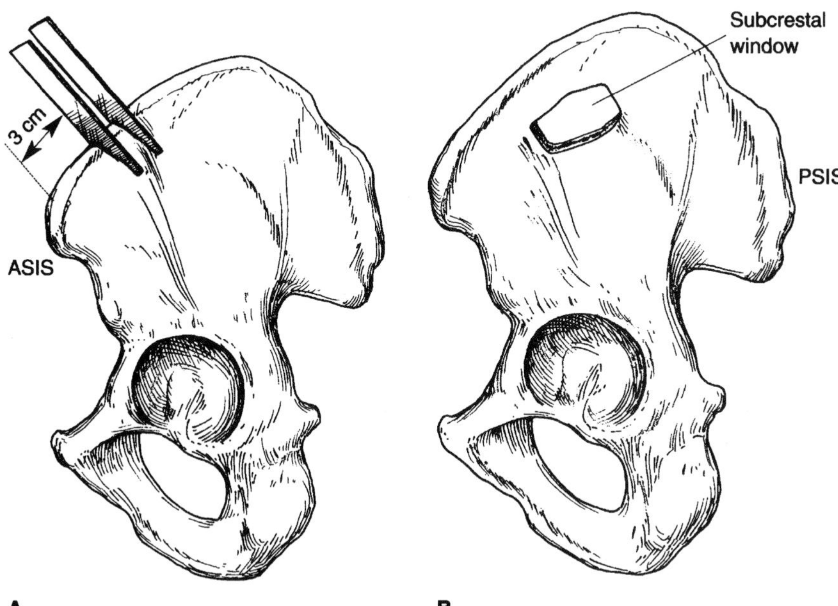

FIG. 9. A: Harvesting of tricortical graft from the anterior ilium, taking care to remain at least 3 cm from the anterior superior iliac spine (ASIS) crest. **B:** Subcrestal window technique harvesting bicortical bone. PSIS, posterior superior iliac spine. [© 2001 American Academy of Orthopaedic Surgeons. From Ebraheim NA, Hossein E, Xu R. Bone-graft harvesting from iliac and fibular donor sites: techniques and complications. *J Am Acad Orthop Surg* 2001; 9(3):210–218, with permission.]

site to the anterior superior iliac spine. To preserve the mechanical strength of the autograft, it is important to use an oscillating saw. Finally, if large defects in the bone are created, for cosmetic reasons, reconstruction of the crest contour with methylmethacrylate should be considered.

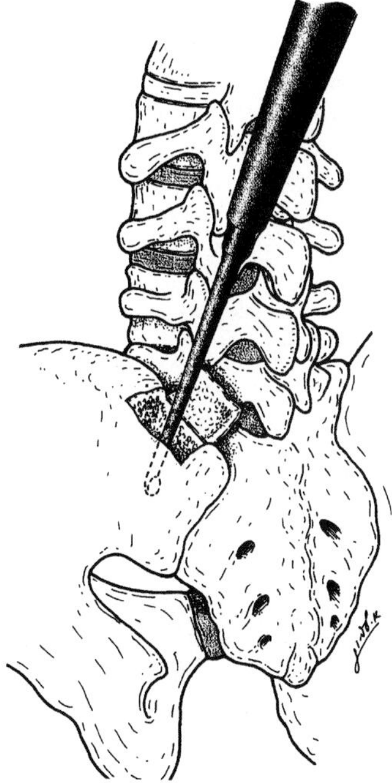

FIG. 10. Trephine technique using curettes to harvest cancellous bone from within the tables of the ilium. [From Mirovsky Y, et al. Comparison between the outer table and intracortical methods of obtaining autogenous bone graft from the iliac crest. *Spine* 2000;25(13):1722–1725, with permission.]

ALLOGRAFT

Allograft is an alternative to autograft and its use has increased dramatically over the past two decades as preparation and storage methods have improved (26). It is available in cancellous cubes, crushed particles, long bone shafts, or machined dowels for use in interbody fusions. Allograft is only weakly osteoinductive, and that property depends on the method of preparation. Advantages of allograft include its availability, ease of use, initial strength, and avoidance of the problems with autograft donor sites. Drawbacks include slower rates of incorporation, greater resorption, and the potential for an increased rate of local infection, as well as the risk of disease transmission, such as acquired immunodeficiency syndrome, hepatitis B and C, and so forth. However, no new cases of human immunodeficiency virus (HIV) transmission in bone allograft have been reported since 1992 (26). Modern preparatory methods, including sonication, tumbling, high-pressure hosing, and soaking, are used to remove all blood and blood products, which dramatically reduces the possibility of disease transmission to almost nothing. Additionally, bone bank donors are routinely tested for HIV-1, HIV-2, and hepatitis C and hepatitis B surface antigens.

Autograft is basically nonimmunogenic. Depending on the method of preparation, different allograft types produce different immune responses. The magnitude of the response depends on the degree of enzymatic degradation of allograft proteins during processing (27). For example, minimally prepared fresh allograft produces an intense immune response and has little application in spine surgery. Freeze-dried allograft, processed by vacuum removal of water, has substantially lower immunogenicity, yet has a diminished compressive strength. Fresh-frozen bone has intermediate immunogenicity but greater biomechanical strength.

The success of allograft significantly depends on revascularization and the mechanical stresses to which it is subjected. If it does not successfully incorporate into the host bone, the graft is not subjected to physiologic stresses of Wolff's law (28) and eventually fatigues and fractures. When placed under compression in a large vascularized surface area, such as the anterior interbody spaces, the fusion rates can be high. In comparison, an allograft subjected to low loads or tension, such as posteriorly on the laminae, has lower rates of fusion (29,30). Large cortical bone dowels, because of their density, are less easily revascularized, and incorporate less successfully than cancellous bone. Smaller segments, such as cortical struts, are more easily revascularized than whole segments of long bones. Cancellous cubes, on the other hand, because of their anatomy and surface area, incorporate significantly more quickly and completely because they are easily vascularized and have a large surface area for accretion of new bone.

BONE GRAFTING ALTERNATIVES

Donor site morbidity; less than perfect rates of fusion; increased operative time, hospital stay, and recovery; and the limited and variable supply of autogenous bone has led to the search for a variety of bone graft substitutes.

Bone Graft Biosubstitutes

Demineralized bone matrix is a frequently used alternative to autologous bone graft. Although lacking some of the fundamental properties of autograft (i.e., osteogenicity, osteoinductivity, and osteoconductivity), it has nonetheless been useful principally as a fusion extender. It is made from allograft cortical bone and decalcified by acid extraction, leaving behind collagen, some growth factors, and some noncollagenous proteins. Similar to freeze-dried allograft, this extensive processing makes demineralized bone matrix the least immunogenic of all bone substitutes. When used in stabilized constructs, such as anterior interbody grafts, it has shown excellent graft incorporation in animal models (31), but the cost of augmenting a one-level fusion can be as high as $1,100 (30).

Other bone graft substitutes include ceramics and coralline implants. These are osteoconductive substitutes that function as a scaffold to deliver the bone growth elements, but do not contain growth factors to attract bone precursor cells or initiate osteoblastic differentiation. Ceramics are comprised of hydroxyapatite and are somewhat porous, but lack the high surface area anatomy of trabecular bone (2). Because they contain no proteins, they do not incite an inflammatory response, although seromas have been reported with their use (32). Because no human tissue is used, there is no real risk of disease transmission. Coralline implants may be used as a filler or graft extender, but their success rates have been varied. In general, corals are brittle and provide little compressive resistance or tensile strength; hence, they behave poorly as stand-alone devices and must be shielded from loading until incorporation occurs.

Bone Morphogenic Proteins

It has been long understood that devitalized bone, when implanted, still induces a cellular response leading to new bone formation. Newer techniques have allowed large quantities of osteoinductive proteins to be produced, such as bone morphogenic proteins (BMPs) and their recombinant forms, including human BMP-2 and BMP-7 (Osteogenic Protein-1, OP-1). BMPs are dimeric cytokines belonging to the transforming growth factor-β (TGF-β) superfamily that have strong osteoinductive properties and play a primary role in the remodeling of bone and fracture healing (33). Their many important osteoinductive functions occur during embryogenesis, mesenchymal cell infiltration, skeletal morphogenesis, and angiogenesis. They function principally by promoting the differentiation of mesenchymal stem cells into osteochondrogenic cells and regulating the proliferation and matrix synthesis of such cells, including osteoblasts, chondrocytes, and endothelial cells.

Research has clearly shown the applicability and use of BMPs in animal fusion models (34–41). Schimandle et al., using a posterolateral rabbit fusion model, reported 100% fusion success at 4 weeks with BMPs compared to a 42% fusion using autograft controls (41). Patel et al. then studied the ability of OP-1 to overcome the inhibitory effects of nicotine in the same rabbit posterolateral intertransverse process fusion model, reporting all sites were solid with BMP versus only 25% of the autograft controls (42). Paramore et al. studied OP-1 in a dog laminectomy and fusion model and also showed superior fusion success with OP-1 compared to autograft controls (40).

Current research is now focusing on the optimum application and carrier for BMPs, as well as safety issues, such as the potential for unwanted neurologic compression. Current systemic safety and toxicity profiles of BMPs have been established through numerous tests analyzing their distribution, carcinogenicity, and systemic toxicity. To date, there have been no clinically significant adverse events (2,43). A study of biodistribution in rabbits has shown that OP-1 remains well within the fusion site. By 5 days, 20 to 27% of the BMP remains, whereas by day 28, only 0.02% can be detected (44). Although BMPs and their receptors have been identified within certain tumors, to date there remains no evidence that they are actually carcinogenic, and what is seen probably represents up-regulated proteins within these cell types (45).

Some technical points have emerged as the surgical use of BMPs has expanded. Commercial BMP is combined with bone collagen (carrier) and then reconstituted with saline to form a paste for implantation. BMP and its carrier must be carefully placed, because leakage of BMP outside the intended fusion area may lead to an adjacent-level fusion. Once the BMP has been placed, irrigation of the surgical site should be withheld and suction drains should not be placed in contact with the material. Because of its strong interaction with the host's bone-forming cellular environment, new bone formation has been shown to occur experimentally if BMP comes in direct contact with fresh laminectomy/laminotomy sites or decompressed foramina (45). In experimental laminectomy sites, BMP has failed to produce significant bony regrowth (46–48). Nonetheless, the placement of BMP on freshly laminectomized bone probably should be avoided.

Placement of BMP on the intact dura can result in extradural bone formation and dural compression (43). On the other hand, the application of BMP on nerve tissue has not demonstrated any adverse effects in animal models (43,49).

The early experience with human clinical trials has been encouraging as well. A safety and efficacy study compared autograft alone to autograft augmented with OP-1 for posterolateral fusions (50). At 6 months, nine of 12 autograft plus BMP sites were fused, versus two of four autograft-alone sites. No adverse effects were reported. Similarly, a study of patients with degenerative spondylolisthesis compared uninstrumented posterolateral fusions with autograft on one side and OP-1 putty on the other. CT scans at 6 months showed equal or greater bone formation on the BMP side than controls.

COMPLICATIONS OF GRAFT HARVEST

Complications reported after harvesting of bone from the posterior or anterior iliac crest include chronic pain, neurovascular injury, infection, cosmetic deformity, sacroiliac disruption, fracture of the iliac wing or the anterior iliac spine, and herniation of abdominal contents. The frequency of reported major and minor complications has ranged from 3 to 49% (7,11,51–54). In their review of 180 patients, Banwart et al. reported 88 of 180 patients (49%) and 90 of 195 donor sites (47%) as having complications (54). Major complications (10%) included seroma, unsightly scar requiring revision, and chronic pain. Minor complications included scar or buttock dysesthesia, prolonged wound drainage, superficial infection and a broken drain, and scar unsightliness. Russell and Block reviewed the literature and found major complications (3 to 39%) and minor complications (10 to 40%) (11). Examples of the former included neurologic injuries, vascular injuries, infection, hematoma, bowel herniation, fracture, pelvic instability, and chronic pain. Minor complications included superficial infection, seroma, dissatisfaction with cosmesis, temporary hypesthesia, and mild pain (20). Throughout the literature, certain factors appear to be associated with an increased risk of adverse occurrence: older age, obesity, female gender, comorbidities, and large reconstructive spine surgery (7,11,55–59).

Donor Site Pain

Donor site pain is probably the most common reported complaint after surgical bone harvesting. Its reported prevalence has ranged from 3 to 50% (7,53,55,60–63). The figures may be imprecise, however, as most reports are retrospective chart reviews. Heary et al. prospectively followed 105 patients, of whom 87 had anterior and 33 had posterior donor sites (60). Structural corticocancellous grafts were used in 79 cases and morselized cancellous bone in 41 obtained by a variety of techniques. Assessment by an independent examiner 4 years later revealed acceptable, but nonetheless present pain in 31% of individuals, and unacceptable pain in 3%. Schnee et al. reviewed 184 anterior iliac crest bone grafts for cervical fusions and reported 4% prevalence of protracted pain lasting beyond 3 months. In their series, they found a risk of increased pain in women and obese patients (7).

Most pain from bone graft harvesting is reported at the time of hospital discharge and tends to clear by 3 months (64). Pain persisting beyond 3 months is termed chronic and has been reported by many authors. In their review of 60 individuals with bone harvested from the posterior ilium, however, Mirovsky and Neuwirth found significant pain persisting beyond 2 years in 20% of their patients (65). Frymoyer et al. found persistent graft donor pain even 10 years after surgery (66). The complaint of donor site pain was significantly greater in patients with continuing back pain. The pain may be related to injury to the nerves in proximity (e.g., cluneal nerves), owing to a great deal of muscle stripping to gain exposure (13,56,60), or perhaps is part of a more generalized pain syndrome in some patients (66). Suggested means of minimizing graft site pain include local anesthetics, vertical or oblique incisions to avoid cutaneous nerves, incisions inferior to the crest prominence to reduce chafing from clothes and belts, harvesting from the medial cortex, and subcrestal or unicortical (crest splitting) techniques (7,15,16,65,67,68).

Vascular Injury

A rare but serious injury is laceration or puncture of the superior gluteal artery as it exits the pelvis through the greater sciatic notch. Harvesting bone from too close to the sciatic notch, or improper placement of retractors or elevators, places the vessel at risk (16,51). Primary ligation of a lacerated vessel sometimes cannot be accomplished, because the artery retracts into the pelvis. Exposure then may require osteotomy of the pelvis or an urgent transpelvic intraabdominal approach. On occasion, arteriography may be useful to study the source of an expanding buttock hematoma, or unexplained anemia postoperatively, to exclude injury to the gluteal vessel (51). Besides laceration, other reported injuries to the gluteal vasculature have included pseudoaneurysm and arteriovenous fistulas (69,70).

Anteriorly, the fourth lumbar, iliolumbar, and deep iliac circumflex arteries (Fig. 2A) are at some potential risk when the anterior crest is approached.

Neurologic Injury

Nerves are in close proximity to the iliac wings and thus at risk for injury. These structures include the lateral femoral cutaneous, ilioinguinal, and iliohypogastric nerves anteriorly, and the superior gluteal, sciatic, and cluneal nerves posteriorly. There is considerable variability in the anatomic placement of these nerves, however: In an anatomic study, Murata et al. showed that more than 10% of the time, the lateral femoral cutaneous nerve can be found coursing laterally over the iliac crest more than 3 cm from the anterior spine (71).

Because the nerves at risk are primarily sensory, symptoms after injury or laceration include dysesthetic pain, numbness, and paresthesias (i.e., meralgia paresthetica) that can be localized or radiate to the buttocks or thighs. The degree of discomfort may increase with belts or tight-fitting clothes over the harvest site. Ten percent of individuals may require local anesthetics or surgical exploration to excise painful neuromas (16,51). Excessive traction on the nerves during exposure is probably the most common cause of injury. Scar dysesthesias and cluneal nerve pain may actually be related to the direction of the scar at the time of graft harvesting. A recent study compared an incision directed superolaterally to inferomedially with one superomedial to inferolateral and found less numbness, tenderness, and pain with the second incision (62). It is theorized this direction spares the cluneal nerves rather than potentially dividing them.

The femoral, ilioinguinal, superior gluteal, and sciatic nerves all exit the pelvis and thus are theoretically at some risk for injury; however, actual reports of their disruption are exceedingly rare (72).

Iliac Fractures

After the harvesting of large amounts of bone, the ilium can suffer fracture posteriorly or anteriorly. The former is typically

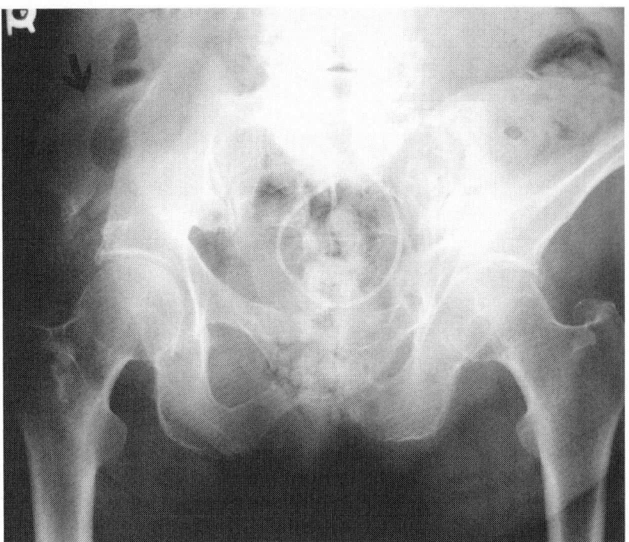

FIG. 11. Radiograph of a 62-year-old woman who suffered a fracture of the right anterior ilium after tricortical graft harvest for cervical fusion (*arrow*).

associated with excessive bone removal down to and through the inner table of the posterior ilium (73,74). Coventry and Tapper reported stress fractures of the posterior ilium and subsequent sacroiliac instability in six patients after aggressive posterior bone harvesting (75). Anteriorly, avulsion of the anterior iliac spine is associated with the harvesting of tricortical or bicortical grafts, typically for anterior cervical fusions (76). When graft is taken too close [less than 3 cm (77)] to the anterior superior iliac spine, a stress riser is created and forces generated by hip flexors can avulse the bone (Fig. 11), especially in older, more osteopenic women (77,78). Hu and Bohlman reported 10 patients with avulsion type fractures of the anterior ilium associated with anterior cervical decompression and fusion (77). According to the authors, the diagnosis was made easily in patients with sudden onset of moderate to severe pain in the region of the bone graft harvest site. Taking care to remove bone at least 3 cm posterior to the iliac spine has been shown to dramatically increase the force required to produce an avulsion fracture. In a concomitant study, Jones et al. showed significant differences in the bone graft compressive strength when anterior iliac bone grafts were harvested using an oscillating saw or an osteotome (25). The authors suggested that use of an osteotome not only produces a weaker iliac graft, but it may also leave occult fracture lines in the pelvis that propagate later (25,76). The treatment for a stress fracture is largely nonsurgical, with bed rest for pain control followed by gradual mobilization.

Sacroiliac Disruption

Coventry and Tapper reported six cases of what they called an unstable sacroiliac joint after excessive removal of bone from the posterior ilium with violation of the sacroiliac ligaments or the joint itself, or both (75). Typically, the injury was not obvious clinically but was evident in radiographs. Injection may be helpful for making the diagnosis, and if the pain and disability is resistant to other treatments, a fusion may be indicated. Lichtblau also reported a case of sacroiliac joint disruption after aggressive posterior iliac crest graft harvesting (79).

Infection

The rate of donor site infection has been reported to range from 1 to 5% (7,16,51,53). Suggested risk factors for deep wound infection or fascial dehiscence include obesity, female gender, immunocompromised host, nutritional depletion, improper surgical techniques, and the presence of medical comorbidities (7,51). Treatment follows the standard orthopedic principles of careful cultures, débridement, irrigation, and antibiotic therapy. Taking care to limit hematoma formation is probably one of the most important measures for reducing the risk of postoperative infection. Suggested methods include careful subperiosteal dissection, the use of bone wax or other clotting agents to control exposed cancellous bleeding, and postoperative Hemovac drainage.

Cosmetic Deformity

The harvesting of large segments of tricortical bone, especially from the anterior ilium, can sometimes result in an unsightly and painful cosmetic deformity (16). In Schnee et al.'s work, a poor cosmetic result after graft harvest was reported in five patients, all of whom were women (p = .04) (7). Rish et al. reported "unsightly scarring" in 25% of autograft donor sites, although the methods of how this information was obtained were not given (80). A significant soft-tissue defect can result from a detached gluteus maximus origin, or in certain cases, subcutaneous fat atrophy (53). Methods used to avoid a poor cosmetic result have included cement reconstruction of the crest, ceramic spacers, and biologic substitutes (78), as well as careful reconstruction of the fascial attachments.

Herniation

Muscle or bowel herniation can occur after the removal of large portions of bicortical ilium along with their muscular attachments (13,51,77). Presenting from 2 weeks to years postoperatively, symptoms can range from vague lower abdominal pain to a mass with bowel sounds. Herniation can become a surgical emergency, as incarceration, volvulus, and strangulation of small bowel have all been reported sometimes, associated with hypotension and shock (11,51,81,82). This complication is rare, however, with fewer than 20 cases reported in the literature, but at least one presented 15 years after the initial surgery (82).

HETEROTOPIC BONE FORMATION

Heterotopic bone formation is an unusual case of recurrent iliac crest donor site pain (83,84). The etiology may be some factor that encourages mesenchymal cells to undergo differentiation, or possibly the presence of residual bony fragments within the wound (84). Patients who seem most to be at risk for developing this complication include males, those with hypertrophic osteoarthropathy, and those who have previously developed heterotopic bone. It may be difficult to visualize on standard radiography; hence, a certain index of suspicion must be maintained. CT has been recommended as the imaging study of choice to confirm the diagnosis.

SUMMARY

Bone autographs are commonly used for spinal fusion and still remain the gold standard. Their use is associated with significant morbidity at the donor site, which can be minimized by careful surgical technique. In the future, further development of human allografts, BMPs, and synthetic or artificial graft materials will allow the surgeon greater latitude. These materials are of particular use when performing salvage fusions in troublesome situations, such as pseudarthrosis, revision surgery in which there is limited bone supply, or when there is compromised vasculature in the graft bed. Currently, these bone graft substitutes and stimulators are expensive, but many of the historic risks of transmitted infection virtually have been eliminated. Newer, somewhat less-invasive techniques for obtaining autographs appear to lessen the risk of complications, such as chronic donor site pain, fracture, hernia, and nerve injury. However, the key to successful fusion is the biologic viability of the harvested bones; its capacity for osteoinduction, conduction, and osteogenesis; the area of decorticated bone onto which the graft is placed; and the vascularity of the adjacent graft site tissues.

REFERENCES

1. Clements DH, O'Leary PF. Anterior cervical discectomy and fusion. *Spine* 1990;15:1023–1025.
2. Vaccaro AR, Chiba K, Heller JG, et al. Bone grafting alternatives in spinal surgery. *Spine J* 2002;2:206–215.
3. Bridwell KH, Sedgewick TA, O'Brien MF. The role of fusion and instrumentation in the treatment of degenerative spondylolisthesis with spinal stenosis. *J Spinal Disord* 1993;6:461–472.
4. France JC, Yaszemski MJ, Lauerman WC. A randomized prospective study of posterolateral lumbar fusion: outcomes with and without pedicle screw instrumentation. *Spine* 1999;24:553–560.
5. Steinmann JC, Herkowitz HN. Pseudarthrosis of the spine. *Clin Orthop* 1992;284:80–90.
6. Cotler JM, Star AM. Complications of spinal fusion. In: Cotler JM, Cotler HB, eds. *Spine fusions: science and technique.* New York: Springer-Verlag, 1990:361–387.
7. Schnee CL, Freese A, Weil RJ, et al. Analysis of harvest morbidity and radiographic outcome using autograft for anterior cervical fusion. *Spine* 1997;22(19):2222–2227.
8. An HS, Simpson JM, Glover JM, et al. Comparison between allograft plus demineralized bone matrix versus autograft in anterior cervical fusion: a prospective multicenter study. *Spine* 1995;20:2211–2216.
9. Bohlman HH, Emery SE, Goodfellow DB, et al. Robinson anterior cervical discectomy and arthrodesis for cervical radiculopathy. *J Bone Joint Surg [Am]* 1993;75:1298–1307.
10. Lane JM, Muschler GF, Kurz LT. Spinal fusion. In: Rothman RH, Simeone FA, eds. *The spine.* Philadelphia: WB Saunders, 1992:1739–1773.
11. Russell JL, Block JE. Surgical harvesting of bone graft from the ilium: point of view. *Med Hypothesis* 2000;55(6):474–479.
12. Ebraheim NA, Yang H, Lu J, et al. Anterior iliac crest bone graft. Anatomic considerations. *Spine* 1997;22(8):847–849.
13. Fowler BL, Dall BE, Rowe DE. Complications associated with harvesting autogenous iliac bone graft. *Am J Orthop* 1995;24(12):895–903.
14. de la Torre JI, Tenehaus M, Gallagher PM, et al. Harvesting iliac bone graft: decreasing the morbidity. *Cleft Palate Craniofac J* 1999;36(5): 388–390.
15. Wolfe SA, Kawamoto HK. Taking the iliac-bone graft: a new technique. *J Bone Joint Surg [Am]* 1978;60:411.
16. Kurz LT, Garfin SR, Booth RE. Harvesting autogenous iliac bone grafts: a review of complications and techniques. *Spine* 1989;14(12): 1324–1331.
17. Lamb DR. A minimally invasive method of harvesting iliac cancellous bone. *Plast Reconstr Surg* 1999;103(3):1090–1091.
18. Boustred AM, Fernandes D, van Zyl AE. Minimally invasive iliac cancellous bone graft harvesting. *Plast Reconstr Surg* 1997;99(6):1760–1764.
19. Caddy CM, Reid CD. An atraumatic technique for harvesting cancellous bone for secondary alveolar bone grafting in cleft palate. *Br J Plast Surg* 1985;38:540–543.
20. Steffen T, Downer P, Steiner B, et al. Minimally invasive bone harvesting tools. *Eur Spine J* 2000;9[Suppl 1]:S114–118.
21. Burnstein FD, Simms C, Cohen SR, et al. Iliac crest bone graft harvesting techniques: a comparison. *Plast Reconstr Surg* 2000;105(1):34–39.
22. Eufinger H, Leppanen H. Iliac crest donor site morbidity following open and closed methods of bone harvesting for alveolar cleft osteoplasty. *J Craniomaxillofac Surg* 2000;28:31–38.
23. Moed BR, Thorderson N, Linden MD. Reharvest of iliac crest donor site cancellous bone. *Clin Orthop Rel Res* 1998;346:223–227.
24. Behairy YM, Al-Sebai W. A modified technique for harvesting full-thickness iliac crest bone graft. *Spine* 2001;26(6):695–697.
25. Jones AA, Dougherty PJ, Sharkey NA, et al. Iliac crest bone graft. Osteotome versus saw. *Spine* 1993;18:2048–2052.
26. Tomford WW, Mankin HJ. Bone banking: update on methods and materials. *Orthop Clin North Am* 1999;30(4):565–570.
27. Gazdag AR, Lane JM, Glaser D, et al. Alternatives to autologous bone graft. Efficacy and indications. *J Am Acad Orthop Surg* 1995;3:1–8.
28. Wolff J. *Des gesetz der transformation der knochen.* Berlin: A Hirschwald,1892.
29. Boden SD, Schimandle JH. Fusion. Biology of lumbar spine fusion and bone graft materials. In: International Society for Study of the Lumbar Spine Editorial Committee, ed. *The lumbar spine*, 2nd ed. Philadelphia: WB Saunders, 1996:1284–1306.
30. Boden SD. Overview of the biology of lumbar spine fusion and principles for selecting a bone graft substitute. *Spine* 2002;27(16S):S26–S31.
31. Oikarinen J. Experimental spinal fusion with decalcified bone matrix and deep frozen allogenic bone in rabbits. *Clin Orthop Rel Res* 1982;162:210–218.
32. Buckholz RW, Carlton A. Interporous hydroxyapatite as a bone graft substitute in tibial plateau fractures. *Clin Orthop Rel Res* 1989;240:53–62.
33. Nakase T, Nomura S, Yoshikawa H. Transient and localized expression of bone morphogenic protein 4 messenger RNA during fracture healing. *J Bone Miner Res* 1994;1994(9).
34. Sandhu HS, Kanim LE, Toth JM. Experimental spinal fusion with recombinant human bone morphogenic protein-2 without decortication of osseous elements. *Spine* 1997;22:1171–1180.
35. Zdeblick TA, Ghanayem AJ, Rapoff AJ. Cervical interbody fusion cages: an animal model with and without bone morphogenetic protein. *Spine* 1998;23:758–765.
36. Boden SD, Schimandle JH, Hutton WC. Lumbar intertransverse-process spinal arthrodesis with use of a bovine bone-derived osteoinductive protein. A preliminary report. *J Bone Joint Surg [Am]* 1995;77:1404–1417.
37. Cunningham BW, Shimanoto N, Sefter JC. Posterolateral spinal arthrodesis using osteogenic protein-1: an *in vivo* time course study using a canine model. In: 15th Annual Meeting of the North American Spine Society. New Orleans, 2000.
38. Sandhu HS, Toth JM, Diwan AD. Histologic evaluation of the efficacy of rhBMP-2 compared with autograft bone in sheep spinal anterior interbody fusion. *Spine* 2002;27:567–575.
39. Takahashi T, Tominaga T, Watanabe N. Use of porous hydroxyapatite graft containing recombinant human bone morphogenetic protein-2 for cervical fusion in a caprine model. *J Neurosurg* 1999;90[4Suppl]:224–230.
40. Paramore CG, Lauryssen C, Rauzzino J. The safety of OP-1 for lumbar fusion with decompression: a canine study. *Neurosurgery* 1999;44:1151–1156.
41. Schimandle JH, Boden SD, Hutton WC. Experimental spinal fusion with recombinant human bone morphogenic protein-2. *Spine* 1995;20:1326–1337.
42. Patel TC, Erulkar JS, Grauner JS. OP-1 overcomes the inhibitory effects of nicotine on lumbar fusion. In: 15th Annual Meeting of the North American Spine Society. New Orleans, 2000.
43. Sandhu HS, Anderson DG, Andersson GBJ, et al. Summary statement: safety of bone morphogenic proteins for spine fusion. *Spine* 2002;27(16S):S39.

44. Vaccaro AR, Anderson DG, Toth CA. Recombinant human osteogenic protein-1 (bone morphogenic protein-7) as an osteoinductive agent in spinal fusion. *Spine* 2002;40(16S):S59–S65.
45. Poynton AR, Lane JM. Safety profile for the clinical use of bone morphogenetic proteins in the spine. *Spine* 2002;27(16S):S40–S48.
46. Boden SD, Martin GJ, Monroe MA. Posterolateral lumbar intertransverse process spine arthrodesis with recombinant human bone morphogenetic protein-2/hydroxyapatite-tricalcium phosphate after laminectomy in the nonhuman primate. *Spine* 1999;24:1179–1186.
47. David SM, Murakami T, Tabor OB. Lumbar spinal fusion using recombinant human bone morphogenetic protein-2 (rhBMP-2): a randomized, blinded and controlled study. *Trans Int Soc Study Lumbar Spine* 1995;22:14.
48. Martin GJ, Boden SD, Morone MA. Posterolateral intertransverse process spinal arthrodesis with rhBMP-2 in a nonhuman primate: important lessons learned regarding dose, carrier, and safety. *J Spinal Disord* 1999;12:179–189.
49. Meyer RAJ, Gruber HE, Howard BA. Safety of recombinant human bone morphogenetic protein-2 after spinal laminectomy in the dog. *Spine* 1999;24:747–754.
50. Patel TC, Vaccaro AR, Truumees E. A safety and efficacy study of Op-1 (Rhbmp-7) as an adjunct to posterolateral lumbar fusion. In: North American Spine Society, Seattle, 2001.
51. Arrington ED, Smith WJ, Chambers HG, et al. Complications of iliac crest bone graft harvesting. *Clin Orthop Rel Res* 1996;329: 300–309.
52. Laurie SW, Kaban LB, Mulliken JB, et al. Donor-site morbidity after harvesting rib and iliac bone. *Plast Reconstr Surg* 1984;73:933.
53. Robertson PA, Wray AC. Natural history of posterior iliac crest bone graft donation for spinal surgery. *Spine* 2001;26(13):1473–1476.
54. Banwart JC, Asher MA, Hassanein RS. Iliac crest bone graft harvest donor site morbidity. A statistical evaluation. *Spine* 1995;20(9): 1055–1060.
55. Sawin PD, Traynelis VC, Menezes AH. A comparative analysis of fusion rates and donor-site morbidity for autogenetic rib and iliac crest bone grafts in posterior cervical fusions. *J Neurosurg* 1998;88: 255–265.
56. Fernyhough JC, Schimandle JJ, Weigel MC, et al. Chronic donor site pain complicating bone graft harvesting from the posterior iliac crest for spinal fusion. *Spine* 1992;17:1474–1480.
57. Younger EM, Chapman MW. Morbidity at bone graft donor sites. *J Orthop Trauma* 1989;3:192–195.
58. Chapman MW, Buckholz RW, Cornell C. Treatment of acute fractures with a collagen-calcium phosphate graft material. A randomized clinical trial. *J Bone Joint Surg [Am]* 1997;79:495–502.
59. Summers BN, Eisenstein SM. Donor site pain from the ilium. A complication of lumbar spine fusion. *J Bone Joint Surg [Br]* 1989; 71:677–680.
60. Heary RF, Schlenk RP, Sacchieri TA, et al. Persistent iliac crest donor site pain: independent outcome assessment. *Neurosurgery* 2002;50(3):510–516.
61. Turner JA, Ersek M, Herron L. Patient outcomes after lumbar spinal fusions. *JAMA* 1992;268:907–911.
62. Colterjohn NR, Bedner DA. Procurement of bone graft from the iliac crest: an operative approach with decreased morbidity. *J Bone Joint Surg [Am]* 1997;79:756–759.
63. Goulet JA, Senunas LE, DeSilva GL, et al. Autogenous iliac crest bone graft: complications and functional assessment. *Clin Orthop* 1997;339:76–81.
64. Polly DW, Kuklo TR. Bone graft donor site pain. In: 37th annual meeting of the Scoliosis Research Society, Seattle, 2002:178.
65. Mirovsky Y, Neuwirth MG. Comparison between the outer table and intracortical methods of obtaining autogenous bone graft from the iliac crest. *Spine* 2000;25(13):1722–1725.
66. Frymoyer JW, Hanley E, Howe J, et al. Disc excision and spine fusion in the management of lumbar disc disease: a minimum ten-year follow-up. *Spine* 1978;3:1–6.
67. Nicholson MW. Technique for obtaining iliac bone graft for anterior cervical fusion. *J Neurosurg* 1974;41:260–261.
68. Wacaser LE. A nearly painless method of obtaining Cloward bone plugs. *J Neurosurg* 1972;37:619.
69. Escalas F, De Wald RL. Combined traumatic arteriovenous fistula and ureteral injury. A complication of iliac bone-grafting. *J Bone Joint Surg [Am]* 1977;59:270–271.
70. Catinella FP, Delaria GA, De Wald RL. False aneurysm of the superior gluteal artery. *Spine* 1990;15:1360–1362.
71. Murata Y, Takahashi K, Yamagata M, et al. The anatomy of the lateral femoral cutaneous nerve, with special reference to the harvesting of iliac bone graft. *J Bone Joint Surg [Am]* 2000;82(5):746–747.
72. Weikel AM, Habal MB. Meralgia paresthetica: a complication of iliac bone procurement. *Plast Reconstr Surg* 1977;60:572–574.
73. Reynolds AFJ, Turner PT, Loeser JD. Fracture of the anterior superior iliac spine following anterior cervical fusion using iliac crest. *J Neurosurg* 1978;48:809–810.
74. Ubhi CS, Morris DL. Fracture and herniation of bowel at bone graft donor site in the iliac crest. *J Trauma* 1984;16:202–203.
75. Coventry MT, Tapper EM. Pelvic instability, a consequence of removing iliac bone for grafting. *J Bone Joint Surg [Am]* 1972;54: 83–101.
76. Porchet F, Jaques B. Unusual complications at iliac crest bone graft donor site: experience with two cases. *Neurosurgery* 1996;39(4): 856–859.
77. Hu R, Hearn T, Yang J. Bone graft harvest site as a determinant of iliac crest strength. *Clin Orthop Rel Res* 1995;310:252–256.
78. Ebraheim NA, Hossein E, Xu R. Bone-graft harvesting from iliac and fibular donor sites: techniques and complications. *J Am Acad Orthop Surg* 2001;9(3):210–218.
79. Lichtblau S. Dislocation of the sacroiliac joint: a complication of bone grafting. *J Bone Joint Surg [Am]* 1962;44:193–198.
80. Rish BL, McFadden JT, Penix JO. Anterior cervical fusion using homologous bone grafts. A comparative study. *Surg Neurol* 1976;5: 119–121.
81. Challis JH, Lyttle JA, Stuart AE. Strangulated lumbar hernia and volvulus following removal of iliac crest bone grafts. *Acta Orthop Scand* 1975;46:230–233.
82. Cowley SP, Anderson LD. Hernias through donor sites for iliac bone grafts. *J Bone Joint Surg [Am]* 1983;65:1032–1035.
83. Hutchinson MR, Dall BE. Midline fascial splitting approach to the iliac crest for bone graft. *Spine* 1994;19:62–66.
84. Ross N, Tacconi L, Miles JB. Heterotopic bone formation causing recurrent donor site pain following iliac crest bone harvesting. *Br J Neuro Surg* 2000;14(5):476–479.

CHAPTER 62

Complications of Lumbar Laminectomy and Discectomy

Peter J. Lennarson, Vincent C. Traynelis, and Alexandre Marinho

Laminectomies and discectomies are the most common spinal procedures performed in the United States (1). Although many prospective patients recount anecdotal "horror stories" related to lumbar surgery, the success rates are quite high, ranging from 88.0 to 98.5% for simple one-level discectomy (1). Despite these success rates, lumbar laminectomy and discectomy are not without associated complications (2). Even a careful and knowledgeable spine surgeon encounters a variety of complications during and after lumbar decompressive surgery. Awareness of the risks, use of meticulous operative technique, and close attention to perioperative details limit the occurrence of these potentially irreversible and sometimes dramatic injuries.

ANATOMY OF THE COMPLICATIONS

A brief review of the anatomy relevant to surgical complications includes neural and adjacent vascular structures. Knowledge of the pertinent neural anatomy is essential to minimizing direct neural injuries. In the adult, the conus medullaris most frequently ends at the inferior border of L-1. Occasionally, it may only reach the level of T-12, or it may extend to L-2. Although nerve roots generally tolerate transient traction or compression, minimal manipulation of the spinal cord or conus may cause profound neurologic disturbances.

Spinal nerve roots, although more tolerant of mechanical deformation than the spinal cord, are less forgiving than the peripheral nerves. A thin membranous root sheath covers the intradural nerve rootlets, and its permeability to cerebrospinal fluid (CSF) is essential for nutrition. In contrast, peripheral nerves are protected by an epineurium and a perineurium, making them much less susceptible to injury.

The lumbar nerve roots exit below their corresponding pedicle and tend to hug its inferior and medial aspect. In the rostrocaudal dimension, the lumbar nerve roots tend to fill the rostral third of the keyhole-shaped foramina. This makes inferior or medial pedicle breach much more likely than a superior or lateral breakout to cause nerve injury, for example, when cannulating a pedicle for screw placement. Nerve root anomalies, such as conjoined roots, are well described and predispose to misdiagnosis as well as intraoperative nerve injury (3–6). The prevalence of nerve root anomalies may be as high as 14%; L-5 to S-1 is the most commonly involved level (6).

Lumbar laminectomy for discectomy usually involves minimal blood loss, but substantial bleeding can occur from the extradural vertebral venous plexus within the spinal canal overlying the posterior vertebral bodies. Although hemodynamically significant blood losses are rare, bleeding can obscure the surgeon's vision leading to inadvertent nerve injury during efforts to cauterize or tamponade the source of hemorrhage. Bleeding from the dilated venous channels tends to abate after disc removal because of external decompression of the thecal sac and nerve roots. Conversely, bleeding may increase with deflation of the thecal sac, as occurs in the case of a dural tear and CSF leakage.

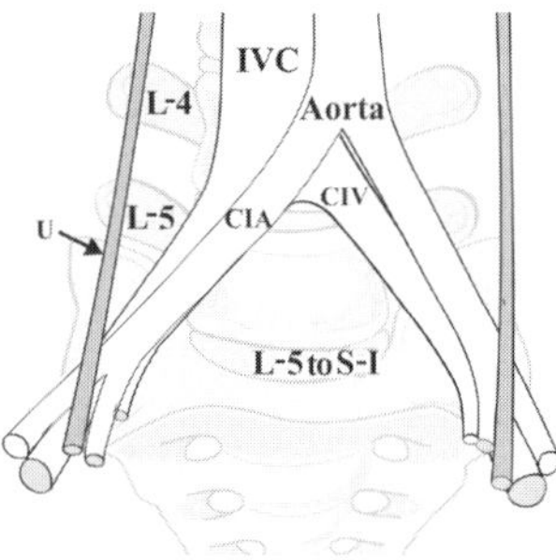

FIG. 1. Drawing showing the relationship between the ureters, vascular structures, and the lumbar spine. CIA, common iliac artery; CIV, common iliac vein; IVC, inferior vena cava; U, ureter.

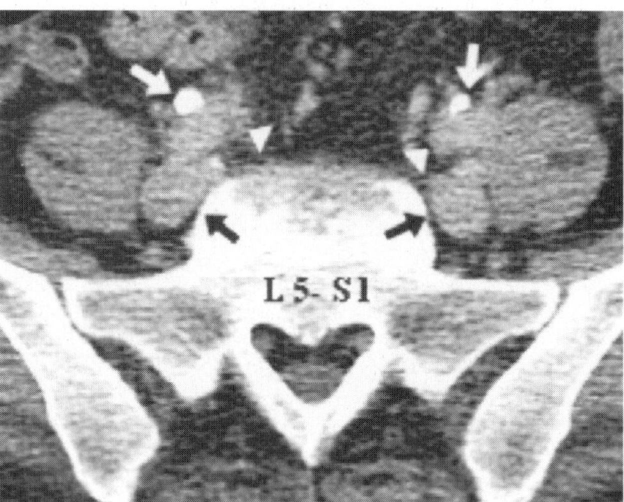

FIG. 3. Computed tomography image through the L-5 to S-1 disc space. The ureters (*white arrows*), common iliac veins (*black arrows*), and common iliac arteries (*white arrowheads*) are identified.

Structures anterior to the spine are not directly visualized during surgery; however, knowledge of their anatomy is essential in preventing and/or diagnosing complications associated with their injury (Figs. 1–3). The common iliac veins join anterior and eccentric to the right of the fourth lumbar vertebra to form the inferior vena cava (IVC). The aorta lies just anterior and to the left of the IVC and bifurcates into the common iliac arteries more proximally, over the upper part of L-4. These relationships explain why these vessels are occasionally damaged if the anterior longitudinal ligament (ALL) is perforated during lumbar disc surgery.

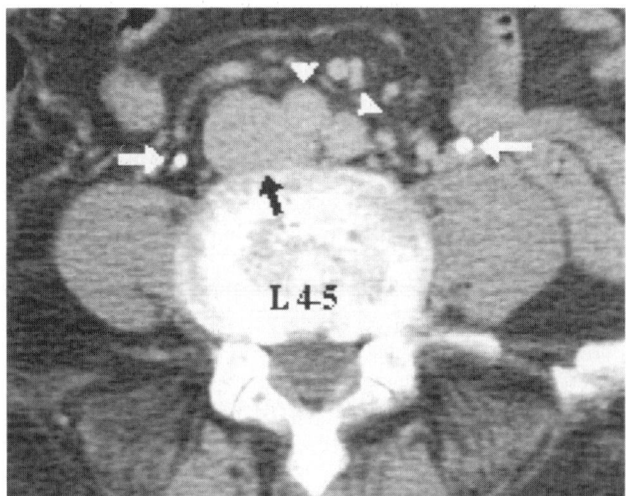

FIG. 2. Computed tomography image through the L4-5 disc space. The ureters (*white arrows*), inferior vena cava (*black arrow*), and common iliac arteries (*white arrowheads*) are identified.

The aorta, the vena cava, and collateral vessels are prevertebral and in close proximity to the hypogastric nerve plexus. The hypogastric nerve plexus is approximately 6 to 8 cm in length and runs along the surface of the aorta, extending from the cephalad aspect of L-4 (as the superior hypogastric plexus) to the first sacral vertebra. These fibers innervate the seminal vesicles and vas deferens in men, and operative injury can lead to retrograde ejaculation. Injury to the sympathetic chain, which lies along the ventrolateral curve of the lumbar vertebrae, can also occur.

The abdominal portion of the ureter runs in the retroperitoneal connective tissue anterior to the psoas muscle until it crosses the bifurcation of the common iliac arteries and descends into the pelvis (Figs. 1–3).

VASCULAR AND VISCERAL INJURIES: RISK FACTORS

The prevalence of symptomatic injury involving vascular and visceral prevertebral structures is estimated to range from 1.6 to 17.0 per 10,000 operations. Although vascular injuries are rare, they have been more commonly reported than visceral injuries. For these injuries to occur, inadvertent perforation of the anterior annulus fibrosis and ALL must take place. Preexisting defects in the annulus and ALL, such as an anterior disc rupture or a previous discectomy, may be predisposing factors. The surgeon should always be cognizant of the depth of the tip of the rongeurs within the disc space. Various other factors have been thought to increase the risk of intraabdominal injury. Body habitus, patient positioning, use of certain instruments, use of the operating microscope, history of previous intraabdominal surgery, and experience of the surgeon have all been discussed in the literature (7,8). None of these variables alone has been found to be a consistent risk factor.

If the injury is inflicted with a biting instrument, such as a pituitary rongeur, the first clue of an injury may be the presence of unusual material in the specimen, such as mucosa, vessel wall, or fat. Although not all surgeons send specimen to pathology on "routine" discectomies, gross inspection of material collected during a procedure may facilitate early diagnosis and treatment of this potentially lethal complication. In Smith and Hanigan's review of 29 visceral injuries, all three cases diagnosed intraoperatively were identified by abnormal tissue within the surgical specimen (8). Although injuries to the various structures are discussed separately, perforation of the anterior annulus with incursion into the prevertebral space may result in more than one injury. In one series, 16% of visceral injuries had an associated vascular injury as well (8). As Smith and Debord note, if preoperative studies did not include an evaluation of the bowel, blood vessels, and ureters, surgical exploration to fix the suspected problem should include careful examination of each of these structures (9).

Vascular Injuries

Vascular insults associated with lumbar discectomy have included injury to the aorta, iliac arteries, superior rectal artery, IVC, and iliac veins and their branches. Of these vessels, the left iliac artery appears to be the most vulnerable.

Vascular injuries have been associated with discectomies at L3-4, L4-5, and L-5 to S-1. Vascular injury usually results in immediate hemorrhage; however, pseudoaneurysms and arteriovenous fistulas (AVF) involving various combinations of the aforementioned vessels have also been reported. Fistulas between the common iliac artery and IVC are purportedly the most common (10) and have generally been associated with discectomy at L4-5. In a review of iatrogenic AVF, Rossi et al. found discectomy to be the most common surgical cause (11).

Vascular wounds generally result from perforation of the anterior annulus and ALL with a curette or rongeur. Brisk bleeding from the disc space may suggest a problem; however, this is seen in less than 50% of patients (7). In a review of 73 cases of AVF, bleeding from the disc space was reported in only 28% (12). Unexplained hypotension intra- or postoperatively may also herald vascular injury. Other presenting signs and symptoms have included abdominal distention or discomfort, nausea, vomiting, and a pale, cool, or pulseless extremity.

AVF or pseudoaneurysm usually presents later. Delays in diagnosis average 17 months, but may be as long as 9 years (13). The presentation may be a pulsating abdominal mass; ruptures have been reported. AVF may also present with high-output cardiac failure and cardiomegaly. Additional signs and symptoms are swelling of the legs, a continuous murmur in the lower part of the abdomen, and intermittent claudication (14).

Treatment of vascular injury depends in part on what the injury is and when it presents. If brisk hemorrhage from the disc space is apparent intraoperatively and/or the patient becomes hemodynamically unstable, the wound should be closed and emergent laparotomy undertaken. If the patient can be stabilized with blood transfusion and other appropriate hemodynamic support, diagnostic studies including ultrasonography, computed tomography (CT), and angiography may establish the diagnosis. In one case of left iliac artery and vein perforation, the authors were able to stabilize the patient in the recovery room using blood and fluid resuscitation in addition to medical antishock trousers. This intervention enabled temporization for 2 hours until the vascular surgeon was ready. In reporting this, the authors stressed the patient's need for anesthesia and mechanical ventilation to avoid the pulmonary effects of compression. The medical antishock trousers must be deflated cautiously before laparotomy to avoid circulatory collapse (15).

Although treatment of vascular injury usually entails urgent or emergent surgical repair, one report documents successful treatment of active bleeding from the superior rectal artery using coil embolization (16). If such an approach is attempted, it is recommended that a backup operating team be standing by in case surgical repair becomes necessary (16). Additionally, the patient's hypotension must be manageable with volume resuscitation to justify the potential delay in treatment required to obtain the angiographic and CT studies needed.

Multiple case reports of vascular injury document "favorable," "uneventful," and "good" outcomes after treatment (14–16). Goodkin and Laska presented 18 patients with vascular injury and pending litigation. The mortality rate was 39%. Six of nine surviving patients experienced new problems postoperatively, including leg, back, and abdominal pain; numbness and paralysis of the legs; claudication; bladder and bowel dysfunction; and impotency (7). The reported mortality has varied widely. The overall mortality in several older reports ranged from 15 to 61% (17), whereas more recent series cite rates from 12.9 to 22.2% (7).

Visceral Injuries

Visceral complications including injury to the bowel, pancreas, ureters, and bladder have been reported with an estimated frequency of 3.8 per 10,000 cases (7–9). Unlike vascular injuries, mortality as a direct result of a visceral injury has seldom been reported (8). Persistent flank pain, ileus, or fever in the postoperative period that cannot otherwise be explained should raise the concern of possible intraabdominal injury (7).

Bowel Injuries

At least 15 cases of isolated bowel injury during posterior lumbar discectomy have been described in the literature (9). The majority of bowel injuries reported have been associated with discectomies performed at L-5 to S-1, while the remainder has been associated with surgery at L4-5. Most injuries have involved the small bowel, usually the ileum, whereas fewer have involved the sigmoid colon (7,8). Vascular injuries may be identified intraoperatively because of visible hemorrhage or associated hypotension; however, injuries to the bowel may present more insidiously. Signs and symptoms of an acute abdomen may present while the patient is in the recovery room, or several days may elapse. Radiographic studies may show free air in the peritoneal cavity. Other cases have presented later, with chronic wound infections at the discectomy site growing intestinal organisms. Abdominal/pelvic abscesses and enterocutaneous fistulas also have been observed (9).

Treatment entails laparotomy and repair of the injured viscus. The majority of patients recover uneventfully.

Ureteral Injuries

Reports of ureteral injuries from lumbar disk surgery are rare. Seventeen cases have been reported in the literature (8,18). As with other prevertebral injuries, ureteral injury is associated with inadvertent perforation of the anterior annulus fibrosis and ALL. Frequently, the injured ureter is contralateral to the side of the laminotomy because of the tangential angle of passage of the instrument (18). The majority of these injuries have occurred in association with a discectomy at L4-5.

Ureteral injuries are rarely diagnosed intraoperatively, and delay in diagnosis has ranged from 3 to 60 days postoperatively. Initial signs and symptoms may include abdominal or flank pain, hematuria, and fever. Urinalysis is abnormal in only one-third of patients and reveals biochemical or cytological abnormalities (8). Over time, a urinoma, or mass of encapsulated urine holding as much as 2 L of fluid may develop. Urinomas may present with varying degrees of abdominal distention and occasionally are palpable as a tender, fluctuant mass. Abdominal radiographs may reveal a soft-tissue mass that obliterates the normal retroperitoneal structures. Ultrasonography, CT, and intravenous pyelogram should demonstrate the mass as well as displacement of the kidney and hydronephrosis.

Once identified, a ureteral injury is initially treated with an indwelling stent. In most cases, end-to-end ureteral anastomosis can be performed after mobilization of the kidney. However, in some patients nephrectomy becomes necessary (18). Approximately 80% of patients in Smith and Hanigan's review retained function of their injured kidney (8).

Adynamic Ileus

A well-known complication of spinal disease and trauma is adynamic ileus, or cessation of normal intestinal motility, which may cause intestinal pseudoobstruction (19). It has also been reported after otherwise uncomplicated lumbar laminectomy and/or discectomy (19–22). Reported cases have involved small and large bowel ileus together, or have involved only the colon (also known as *Ogilvie's syndrome*). Of the ten cases with Ogilvie's syndrome described in the literature, nine had a disc herniation affecting the L4-5 level, whereas the remaining case had pathology at L-5 to S-1.

Adynamic ileus is thought to result from temporary inhibition of the extrinsic control of motility, but why uncomplicated posterior lumbar surgery should affect this control remains unclear (19). The well-known signs and symptoms of an ileus include abdominal pain and distention, nausea, vomiting, and failure to pass flatus or have a bowel movement postoperatively. Bowel sounds are typically absent or hypoactive.

The diagnosis of suspected ileus is usually confirmed by plain abdominal radiographs, which demonstrate distended loops of bowel. Most patients are effectively treated with several days of nasogastric decompression, intravenous fluids, and withdrawal or minimization of narcotic medication. Early postoperative mobilization, although beneficial for other reasons, has not been shown to prevent or shorten the length of ileus (23). Use of prokinetic agents, such as metoclopramide, is controversial. Metoclopramide has commonly been used for treatment of postoperative ileus; however, multiple studies have shown it to have no effect on the duration of the ileus (24). Intravenous administration of neostigmine has been reported to help in patients with Ogilvie's syndrome (21). If colonic (cecal) dilatation continues despite these conservative measures, colonoscopy for immediate decompression may be necessary to prevent bowel perforation.

Other precursors for adynamic ileus include electrolyte disturbances (hypokalemia), hypothyroidism, uremia, sympathectomy and retroperitoneal hematomas.

Unintended Durotomy

Dural tears are one of the most frequent complications associated with surgery of the lumbar spine. Although the name *dural tear* is commonly used, another term, *unintended, incidental durotomy* has been suggested as an alternative out of concern that the word "tear" implies a degree of carelessness (25). The incidence of breach of the dura during spinal surgery has been estimated to range from 0.3 to 13.0% (25,26) for primary operations and as high as 17% for reoperations (25–28). In a prospective study of 412 primary and 69 reoperations, Stolke et al. reported perforation of the dura in 1.8% of microdiscectomies, 5.3% of macrodiscectomies, and 17.4% of reoperations (27). Although the majority of dural injuries are recognized intraoperatively, 6.8% of these injuries went unnoticed at the time of surgery.

The dura is vulnerable to injury throughout much of the exposure involved in decompressive surgery. During the initial soft-tissue dissection to expose the spine, the dura can be violated inadvertently if instruments such as a Bovie or periosteal elevator pass through the interlaminar space. Particular caution must be exercised when defects such as spina bifida occulta are present or a prior laminectomy was performed. Dural tears may also occur during removal of the lamina or ligamentum flavum. Stripping away any dural adhesions with an instrument such as a Woodson dissector or separating the dura from the posterior elements with temporary placement of a cottonoid may afford some protection. The epidural cottonoid may increase extradural compression, however, which can be a potential risk in a patient with severe spinal stenosis.

The choice of instrument used for decompression may influence the risk of dural injury. Although a 45-degree angled footplate rongeur is helpful when biting bone or ligament in a caudal to rostral direction, it is more likely to include redundant dura in its jaws when used in a rostral to caudal direction (29). When working on the inferior lamina or in the rostral to caudal direction, a 90-degree punch is recommended. This is particularly important in cases of severe spinal stenosis.

Dissection through scar tissue during reoperation also makes dural perforation more likely. Beginning dissection in a virgin area, if possible, allows the correct tissue plane to be identified and developed, thereby minimizing the risk. Care should also be taken to avoid leaving sharp bony edges or spicules, which may later perforate the dura.

Finally, an increased incidence of spinal fluid leaks associated with the use of ADCON-L, an anti-adhesion barrier gel, has been reported by Hieb and Sevens (30). In their series, five of 27 patients on whom ADCON-L was used developed CSF leaks postoperatively, despite the fact that dural tears were not seen intraoperatively (30).

Although intraoperative identification of a spinal fluid leak is generally straightforward, small leaks or "potential leaks" sometimes go unnoticed. Potential leaks arise when the dura is only partially torn or when the arachnoid is still intact, preventing overt extravasation of CSF. Incidental increases in cerebrospinal pressure almost inevitably lead to rupture and a fluid leak postoperatively. A Valsalva maneuver may be performed intraoperatively to raise the intraspinal pressure and may help demonstrate a leak that would otherwise be overlooked.

Postoperative CSF leaks may present in various ways. The most common presentation is a spinal or postural headache relieved by recumbency. Accompanying symptoms may include nausea, vomiting, and photophobia. The patient may complain of increasing back or radicular pain. A fluctuant subcutaneous mass consistent with a pseudomeningocele may be observed (31). Patients with a dural-cutaneous fistula may present with signs and symptoms of meningitis, in addition to drainage from the wound. When the nature of the wound drainage is unclear (liquefied hematoma, seroma, or abscess might be other possibilities), a laboratory test identifying beta-2-transferrin, a substance specific to CSF, confirms the diagnosis.

Myelography, CT, post-myelography CT, and magnetic resonance imaging (MRI) can all be useful imaging modalities to confirm a CSF leak. CT obtained after intrathecal administration of water-soluble contrast may confirm the presence of a pseudomeningocele as well as demonstrate its connection to the thecal sac. However, injection of contrast intrathecally may confuse the diagnosis. If a post-myelogram headache develops, it may further confound the issue, particularly if it remains after the repair of the original site of CSF leakage. A persistent spinal headache may be interpreted as failure of the surgical procedure to stop the CSF leak, when in fact it was a result of the myelogram. MRI can also demonstrate a fluid collection consistent with a pseudomeningocele and may help localize the source of the leak (Figs. 4 and 5). In the early postoperative period, normal postsurgical changes observed on MRI can be confusing. Additionally, obtaining a good quality, motion-free MRI can be difficult in the patient with pain. The authors believe that CT provides all the necessary information, is easily obtained, and is well tolerated.

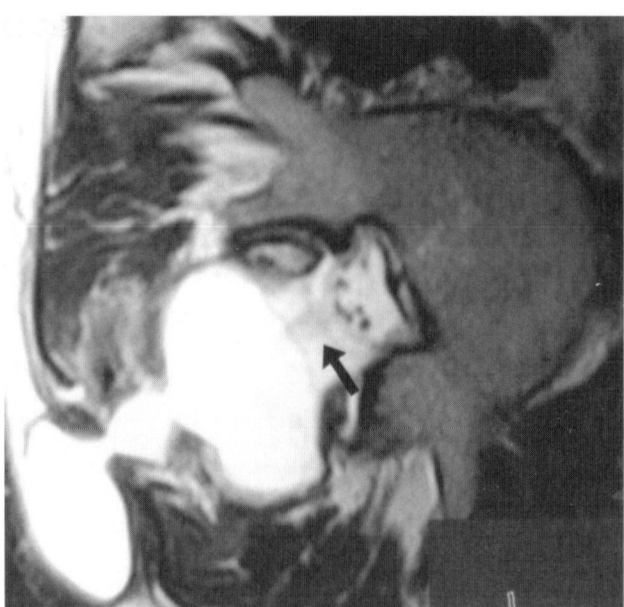

FIG. 5. Axial T2-weighted magnetic resonance image of the lumbar spine revealing a postoperative pseudomeningocele. The slightly hypointense signal extending posteriorly from the thecal sac (*arrow*) may represent flow through the dural opening into the pseudomeningocele.

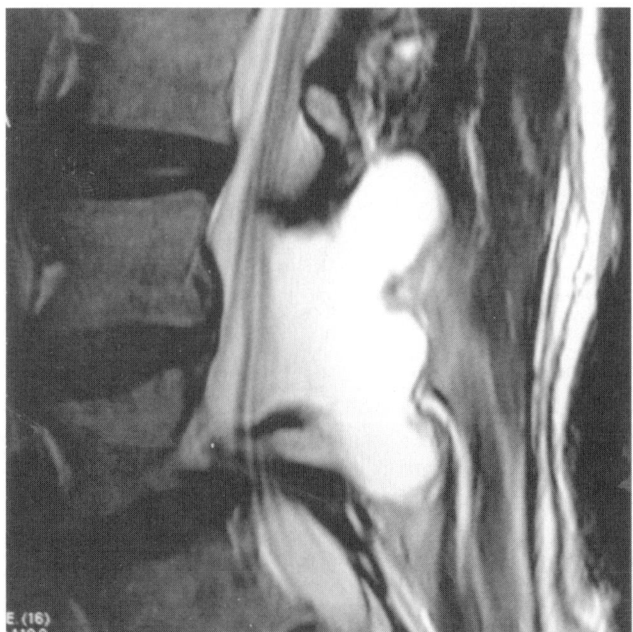

FIG. 4. Sagittal T2-weighted magnetic resonance image of the lumbar spine revealing a postoperative pseudomeningocele behind the L-4 and L-5 vertebral bodies.

Durotomy recognized intraoperatively should be closed primarily with a permanent suture, such as 4-0, 5-0, or 6-0 Prolene, Neurelan, or silk. Despite a "watertight" suture line, fragile dura occasionally leaks from the holes created by passage of the needle or suture. Therefore, the smallest manageable suture and needle should be selected. Adequate exposure of the tear and surrounding normal dura is essential and may necessitate additional bone removal. Good lighting and magnification with loupes or a microscope are also recommended.

When a watertight closure is achieved with suture, no additional treatments are required. A subfascial drain is not contraindicated in those at risk for hematoma (26). No period of bed rest is necessary, and the patient is allowed to ambulate immediately (32).

When watertight closure is not attainable with suture alone, patching or plugging with locally harvested muscle or fascia is useful. The defect may additionally be covered with blood or thrombin-soaked Gelfoam and/or fibrin glue. Watertight fascial and skin closures help prevent leakage from the skin and reduce the risk of subsequent meningitis in the event that the repair is unsuccessful. At the conclusion of the procedure, a smooth reversal of anesthesia is critical so that coughing and retching on the endotracheal tube is kept to an absolute minimum. When repair has required some or all of these adjuvant treatments for leak control, it is the authors' practice to leave the patient at bed rest for 3 days postoperatively. A urinary catheter is often left in place to facilitate the bed rest. Laxatives are indicated, and narcotic usage should be minimized to decrease the chance of constipation that requires straining by the patient.

Some leaks, when located relatively ventrally or at the nerve root axilla, for example, are not directly repairable with suture. In this instance, the tear may be covered with thrombin-soaked Gelfoam or fibrin glue if feasible, and watertight fascial and skin closures are performed. Postoperatively, a lumbar drain is placed percutaneously several segments from the operative site. Drainage of approximately 10 cc per hour is allowed for 5 days. It has been the authors' practice to allow patients to ambulate with the drain in place. Care has to be taken to prevent overdrainage by adjusting the level of the drain as the patient's activity and position dictate. Others prefer to keep patients on strict bed rest while lumbar drains are being used (33,34). During the period of drainage, a prophylactic antibiotic such as nafcillin is administered and samples of CSF are withdrawn every 2 to 3 days for analysis. On the sixth day the drain is withdrawn, and a skin suture is placed at the drain exit site.

Although management of durotomy recognized intraoperatively is somewhat standardized, treatment of CSF leaks that appear postoperatively remains controversial. Various nonoperative methods of treatment have been described (34–38). Kitchell et al. advocated lumbar drainage for 4 days in the supine position followed by an additional day of bed rest (34). Fifteen of nineteen (79%) of their patients healed, while two patients developed meningitis. Prophylactic antibiotics were not used.

Waisman and Schweppe advocated a technique of resuturing the skin under local anesthesia to achieve a watertight skin closure, bed rest in the Trendelenburg position, antibiotic coverage, and daily puncture and drainage of the subcutaneous fluid (35). All eight patients in their series recovered within 10 to 28 days, none required reoperation, no infections were reported, and no patients developed long-term complications in 8 years of surveillance.

CT-guided aspiration of CSF followed by a blood or fibrin glue patch has also been described (37,38). A single case report described resolution of a large lumbar pseudomeningocele after 4 weeks of mechanical compression obtained by a wide belt (36).

Despite varying success with conservative treatments, the authors recommend direct surgical repair of postoperative spinal fluid leaks and pseudomeningocele using the previously described methods. Cultures are obtained intraoperatively.

Unintended durotomy does not increase perioperative morbidity or adversely affect the long-term results of operations on the lumbar spine, provided it is diagnosed early and treated effectively (26,34,39,40). In Wang et al.'s series of 88 patients who incurred a dural tear, the repair added 20 to 30 minutes to the length of the operation, but it did not result in increased blood loss, neurologic deficit, or pain when compared to patients without durotomy (26). Although extra bone removal often was required for exposure of the leak, there were no cases of spinal instability or unplanned arthrodesis (26).

Not all reports are that optimistic. Goodkin and Laska note a dural tear may allow herniation of nerve roots and subsequent nerve injury, at the time of the initial operation or later if nerve roots herniate into a pseudomeningocele cavity. Additionally, a CSF leak may be a contributing factor to infection, arachnoiditis, and/or chronic pain. The associated complications and sequelae rather than the dural tear itself are the stimuli for malpractice lawsuits (25). It is therefore recommended that incidental durotomy and its potential associated complications be discussed during the informed consent process.

Neural Injury

Although direct neural injury during lumbar spinal surgery is known to happen, it is rarely discussed in the literature, making estimates of the frequency uncertain. In a prospective study of 412 primary and 69 reoperations, two cases of nerve root injury were reported in the primary surgery group (0.5%), and one case occurred in the reoperation group (1.4%) (27). The severity of the injuries went unreported. Blaauw et al. detailed the 1-year outcome of 443 patients who underwent low-back surgery for disc herniation and/or stenosis (41). Of 320 patients without preoperative weakness who underwent low-back surgery for disc herniation or stenosis, nine had a motor deficit at 1 year postoperatively (3%) as identified by the surgeon. However, 5% of patients reported significant weakness (21 of 389). Of patients with preoperative motor weakness, 4% (5 of 123) deteriorated, and 10% (13 of 123) failed to improve after surgery. On the other hand, 85% (105 of 123) of patients with preoperative weakness regained normal strength (75%) or had improved strength compared to their preoperative status (10%).

In the same study, 30 of 242 (12%) patients with normal sensation on admission showed some sensory loss 1 year after surgery (41). Thirty of 210 (15%) patients who denied paresthesias before surgery reported them 1 year postoperatively. On the other hand, paresthesias in 161 of 233 patients resolved, and sensory examination had normalized in 138 of 201.

With regard to reflexes, 3% of patients with normal knee jerks and 10% of patients with normal ankle jerks preoperatively were found to have diminished or absent reflexes after surgery (41). On the other hand, 60% of patients with reflex abnormalities before surgery had regained normal reflexes at 1-year follow-up.

Nerve roots may be injured by a variety of mechanisms including excessive retraction, laceration, and crushing or thermal injury (2,3,42). Nerve roots may also be injured in association with dural tears, as a result of the trauma that caused the tear as well as the repair itself. When closing a durotomy, one must be extremely careful not to injure rootlets with suction or incorporate a rootlet into the closure. Such injuries are more likely to occur in a reoperation where epidural scar is adherent to the root. Individual nerve roots can also be injured if allowed to herniate through a dural opening. Such nerve root strangulation can be prevented by closing all durotomies primarily, even those that fail to leak intraoperatively because of an intact arachnoid layer (43).

Medial nerve root retraction is best tolerated when gentle and intermittent. Less retraction is required if there is adequate lateral exposure (42). Occasionally, a large medial disc herniation precludes retraction without undue tension. In these instances, partial decompression can be attempted lateral to the nerve root, or through the nerve root axilla to facilitate later atraumatic retraction. When there is a massive central herniation with cauda equina syndrome (CES), it may be necessary to perform bilateral laminectomies and decompress the disc through the side, which requires less nerve root tension.

Laceration or avulsion of a root generally results from poor visualization of the nerve root or failure to recognize a flattened nerve root over an extruded disc and nerve root abnormality (2). The annulus or presumed disc herniation should not be incised until the nerve root is identified. Use of a microscope providing light and magnification, and obtaining adequate exposure and hemostasis minimizes the risk of inadvertent nerve injury. Nerve root anomalies when present alter the "normal" anatomy and also predispose to neural injury (6). The best treatment lies in prevention, as the damage is generally not amenable to surgical repair.

Contusion of a nerve root may result from contact with a high-speed burr or the footplate of a Kerrison rongeur. Shielding the nerve root with a retractor while burring may prevent nerve contact should the burr skip off the bone. Using a rongeur with a thin footplate lessens the risk of nerve injury, particularly when the instrument is introduced into an already tight canal or foramen.

Thermal injury can be minimized by setting the current level on the bipolar electrocautery as low as possible and by preventing contact between the bipolar and the nerve root. Immediate irrigation after cauterization also helps avoid injury. Temporary placement of hemostatic agents, such as thrombin-soaked Gelfoam, Surgicel, or cottonoid (with or without thrombin), often obviates or minimizes the need for electrocautery.

CLINICAL CONSEQUENCES OF NERVE ROOT INJURY

Often nerve root injury is not discovered until the patient is examined postoperatively. Symptoms of a "battered" root may comprise pain, often described as a constant burning, ice-cold, or aching pain that is exacerbated by certain postures or movements (42). Alternatively, nerve root injury may be evidenced by failure of preoperative symptoms to resolve despite adequate decompression. In some instances, new signs or symptoms of nerve injury that were not present on admission are apparent after surgery (41).

There is no specific treatment for the battered root, but this condition should be differentiated from a persistent compressive lesion or a root entrapped through a dural opening. Postoperative imaging with MRI, CT, or CT-myelography may give useful information, but it frequently is difficult to interpret. The authors have reexplored the operative site when a new deficit or severe pain presents in the immediate postoperative period. This approach has not resulted in further deficit, and occasionally, pathology has been identified and treated with a satisfactory outcome.

Recovery from root injury may take weeks to months and is often incomplete.

Cauda Equina Syndrome

CES, caused by neuropathy of multiple lumbar and sacral nerve roots, is the most significant form of neural injury associated with lumbar spine surgery. The frequency of CES as a result of lumbar surgery is approximately 0.2% (25,44). Although rare, CES is the most commonly cited complication of lumbar spine surgery that leads to malpractice suits (25).

Mechanical trauma, postoperative hematoma, and vascular/ischemic injury have all been proposed as precipitating factors in the development of CES (2,44). McLaren and Bailey presented six cases of 2,842 lumbar discectomies. Spinal stenosis was identified at the level of the disc protrusion but was not decompressed. These authors postulated the etiology was a trauma or compressive ischemia (44). In five patients, the discectomy was done through an interlaminar approach without a laminotomy or laminectomy. In the sixth patient, a vascular insult was hypothesized as the mechanism leading to the injury. In a series of 244 patients with spinal stenosis, two patients suffered postoperative epidural hematomas, one of whom had CES before hematoma evacuation (40). Placement of free epidural fat grafts after laminectomy has also been blamed for postoperative CES (45). Kothbauer and Seiler reported a case of CES in which multiple nerve roots herniated through a small ventral dural rent, filling the available space in the intervertebral disc and becoming incarcerated "in much the same manner that bowel loops are incarcerated in an abdominal wall hernia" (43).

CES usually presents in the immediate postoperative period, but it can occasionally develop days to weeks later (43,44,46). Patients present with a complex of back pain, saddle anesthesia, variable sensory deficits in the lower extremities, bilateral leg weakness, and bladder and/or bowel dysfunction (retention or incontinence). In some patients, not all findings are present, but all develop if the condition goes untreated.

Although the diagnosis of CES can be made clinically, emergent imaging, if available, may help clarify the etiology. Modalities used for confirmation include MRI, CT, CT-myelography, and myelography.

Treatment of CES, in most cases, entails emergency decompression of the neural elements. If the cause of compression is an epidural hematoma, meticulous hemostasis on reoperation must be attained. If hemostasis is not reliably obtained, an epidural drain should be placed. Rarely, CES involves a vascular/ischemic event without neural compression. In such cases, operative intervention may cause further neurologic deterioration (44).

Recovery after CES is variable and only partial recovery is often seen (40). The best outcomes, including full recovery, have followed early diagnosis and decompression (43,44). In McLaren and Bailey's series, patients with mild to moderate motor deficits recovered, whereas patients with severe paraparesis before decompression made only incomplete recoveries (44). Sensory deficits improved universally, with only minimal subjective complaints persisting. Functional bladder and bowel recovery occurred in two-thirds of cases.

Infection

Postoperative wound infection after lumbar laminectomy and/or discectomy has been well described but is uncommon. Infection may be superficial, such as in a local cellulitis, or may involve deeper structures, causing an epidural empyema. Involvement of the disc space defines discitis. The reported frequency of postoperative infection after operations on the lumbar spine ranges from 0.4 to 2.9% (3,47).

Superficial wound infections after lumbar surgery present with pain or tenderness. Signs may include fever, wound erythema, swelling, local wound discharge, and dehiscence. Diagnosis is frequently evident on physical examination and often does not require additional imaging studies. Treatment consists of wound débridement, wound culture, and a short course of empiric antibiotics aimed at *Staphylococcus* and *Streptococcus* species until the organism is identified. Wounds with superficial dehiscence may be allowed to heal by secondary intention or may be closed secondarily in a delayed fashion.

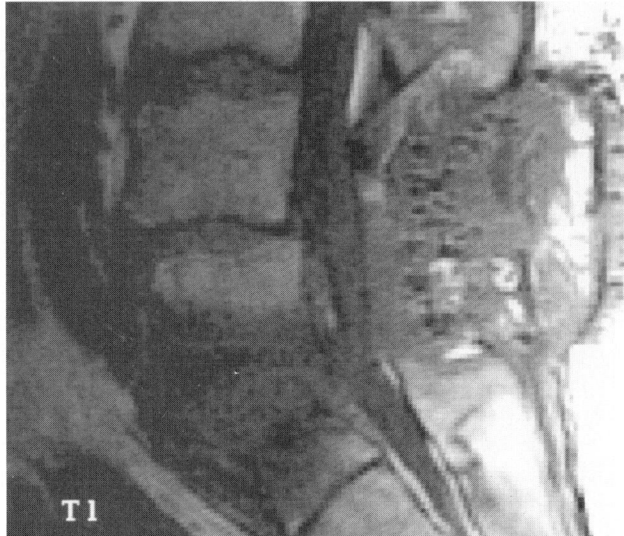

FIG. 6. Sagittal T1-weighted magnetic resonance image of the lumbar spine in a patient with postoperative discitis at L-5 to S-1. Note the hypointense signal in the disc and adjacent vertebral bodies.

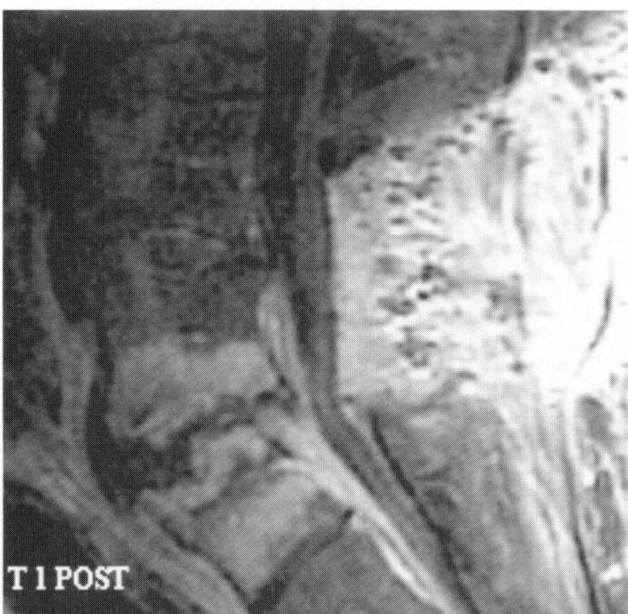

FIG. 8. Sagittal T1-weighted, post-contrast magnetic resonance image of the lumbar spine in a patient with postoperative discitis at L-5 to S-1. Note the adjacent vertebral marrow, the disc space, and the annulus fibrosus enhancement.

Deep wound infections, including epidural empyema, are more problematic. In Spiegelmann et al.'s series of 589 lumbar discectomies, the frequency of epidural empyema was 0.67% (48). In some patients, symptoms and signs similar to those of superficial infections may be present; in other patients, the clinical features are "surprisingly vague and misleading" (48). For example, in one report of four patients with epidural empyema, fever was present in only two patients, neurologic deficit attributable to infection was present in one, and leukocytosis was absent in all four (48). Pain and tenderness about the wound were present in all four patients.

An elevated white blood cell count, erythrocyte sedimentation rate (ESR), and C-reactive protein (CRP) are consistent with the diagnosis of postoperative infection but are not always

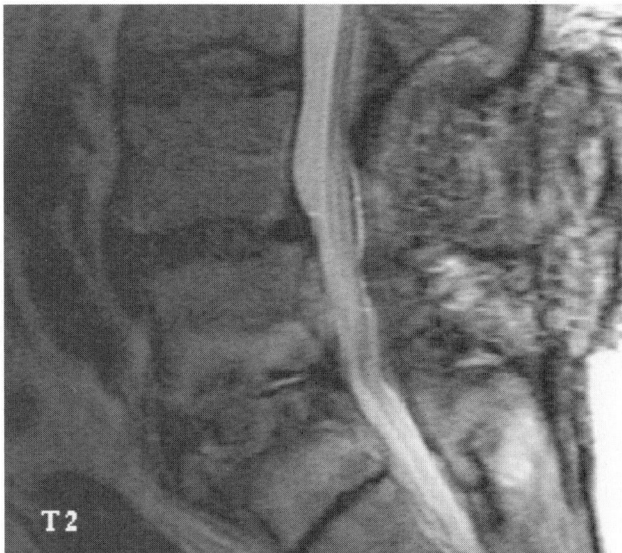

FIG. 7. Sagittal T2-weighted magnetic resonance image of the lumbar spine in a patient with postoperative discitis at L-5 to S-1. Note the hyperintense signal in the disc and adjacent vertebral bodies.

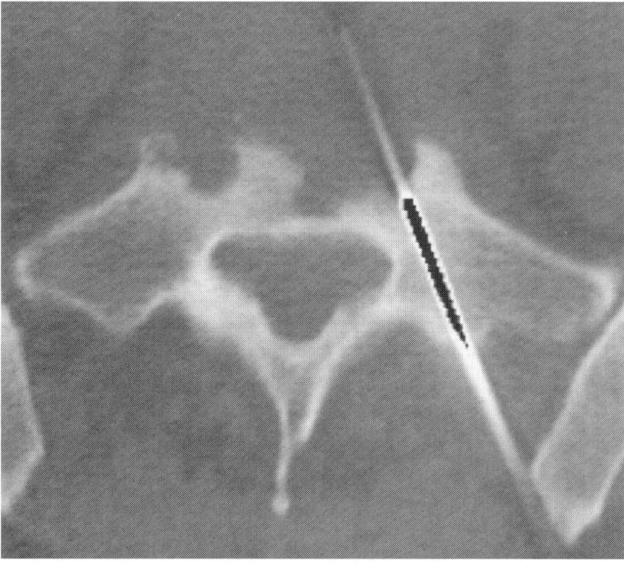

FIG. 9. Computed tomography image at the level of the S-1 pedicles obtained during needle biopsy through the left S-1 pedicle. Note the fragmentation of the anterior vertebral body and end-plate.

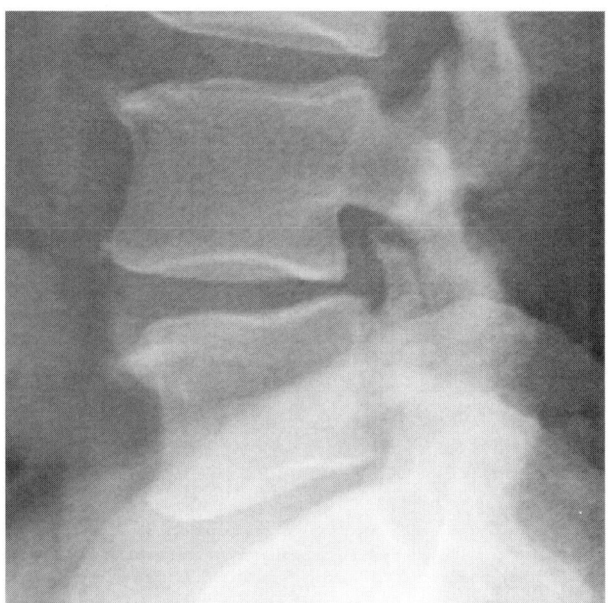

FIG. 10. Preoperative lumbar radiograph in a patient who developed discitis postoperatively.

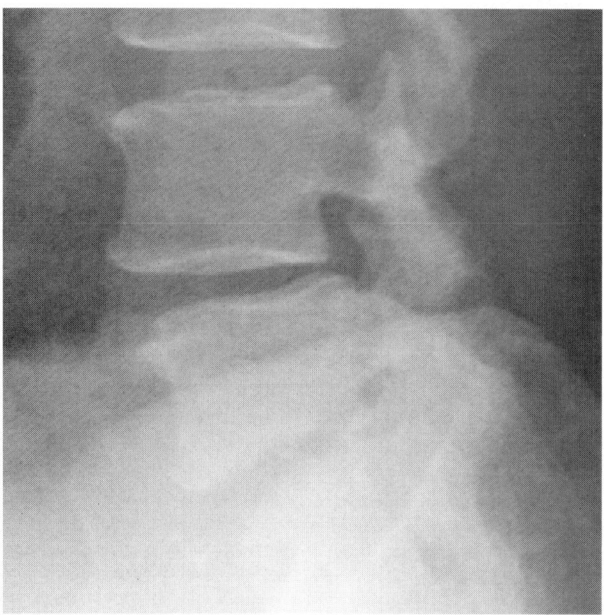

FIG. 11. Postoperative lumbar radiograph obtained 3 months after surgery, at which time the patient was found to have discitis. Note the fragmentation of the anterior S-1 vertebral body and end-plate.

present. CT and MRI scans typically show fluid collections. Peripheral enhancement often takes 1 to 2 weeks to develop, and scans performed in the early stages of infection may be not enhanced at all. If diagnosis is uncertain, needle aspiration with ultrasonography or CT guidance as needed may be helpful.

Treatment of deep wound infections, including epidural empyema, involves irrigation and drainage of pus, as well as débridement of the surrounding devitalized soft tissues. Primary wound closure is usually achievable but must be tension free. In some cases, this may necessitate mobilization of the paraspinal muscles by freeing the muscle from the facets bilaterally. Other cases may require a more extensive rotational muscle flap (49). Some authors advocate closure of the wound over drains or irrigation systems (49,50). In addition to surgical treatment, antibiotic therapy is important. The reported duration of antibiotic treatment ranges from 10 days to 6 weeks (48,50).

Postoperative discitis has been reported to occur with a frequency of 0.75 to 1.00% (27,51). Aseptic or chemical discitis must be separated from the septic form (52). The most likely mechanism of the septic form is direct inoculation of the disc space at the time of surgery.

Moderate to severe back pain aggravated by any spinal motion and associated paravertebral muscle spasms are the most common presenting symptoms. Pain may radiate to the abdomen, perineum, hips, or legs, but true radicular pain is uncommon. Fever is present in up to one-half of the patients. The interval from surgery to the development of symptoms can range from several days to 8 months, but the majority of cases present between 1 and 4 weeks after surgery (53).

The white blood cell count may be mildly elevated. The ESR is almost universally elevated in discitis. The ESR remains elevated for up to 6 weeks after uncomplicated surgery, making that test relatively nonspecific. However, an ESR that fails to normalize or increases after surgery is suggestive of discitis in patients with symptoms. CRP, an acute phase reactant, may be more helpful in making the diagnosis. In the absence of discitis, the CRP peaks 2 to 3 days postoperatively and should return to normal levels within 5 to 14 days after uncomplicated discectomy (54).

MRI, CT, nuclear medicine scans, and plain radiographs all may show characteristic findings, but MRI appears to be the most sensitive and specific test available (Figs. 6–11). Characteristic MRI findings may be present within 3 days of symptom onset and include hypointense signal in the disc and adjacent vertebral bodies on T1-weighted images and hyperintense signal from these structures on T2-weighted images (Figs. 6 and 7). The adjacent vertebral marrow, the disc space, and the annulus fibrosus all enhance after gadolinium administration (Fig. 8) (55). MRI may also delineate an associated abscess formation. CT findings include vertebral end-plate fragmentation and obliteration of paravertebral fat planes (Fig. 9). Technetium and gallium scans may show increased uptake in the adjacent vertebral end-plates within 7 and 14 days, respectively. Plain radiographic findings include narrowing of the disc space and loss of end-plate definition followed by end-plate sclerosis and eventual fusion of the disc space (Figs. 10 and 11).

If imaging studies demonstrate discitis, needle biopsy for culture may be attempted to help guide therapy (Fig. 9). Blood cultures should also be drawn. If cultures are unrevealing, empiric therapy with antistaphylococcal agents is recommended. Duration of antibiotic therapy ranges from 6 to 12 weeks and may include intravenous and oral regimens. Additional symptomatic treatments for discitis include analgesics, muscle relaxants, and bed rest. Back braces or corsets may also be helpful.

REFERENCES

1. Koebbe CJ, Maroon JC, Abla A, et al. Lumbar microdiscectomy: a historical perspective and current technical considerations. *Neurosurg Focus* 2002;13:1–6.

2. Wiesel SW. Neurologic complications and lumbar laminectomy: a standardized approach to the multiply operated lumbar spine. In: Garfin SR, ed. *Complications of spine surgery.* Baltimore: Williams & Wilkins, 1989:64–74.
3. An HS, Booth RE, Rothman RH. Complications in lumbar disc disease and spinal stenosis surgery. In: Balderston RA, An HS, eds. *Complications in spinal surgery*. Philadelphia: WB Saunders, 1991:61–78.
4. Bernini PM, Wiesel SW, Rothman RH. Metrizamide myelography and the identification of anomalous lumbosacral nerve roots. *J Bone Joint Surg* 1980;62-A:1203–1208.
5. Cannon BW, Hunter SE, Picaza JA. Nerve root anomalies in lumbar disc surgery. *J Neurosurg* 1961;19:208–214.
6. Kadish LJ, Simmons EH. Anomalies of the lumbosacral nerve roots an anatomical investigation and myelographic study. *J Bone Joint Surg* 1984;66-B:411–416.
7. Goodkin R, Laska LL. Vascular and visceral injuries associated with lumbar disc surgery: medicolegal implications. *Surg Neurol* 1998;49:358–372.
8. Smith EB, Hanigan WC. Injuries to the intra-abdominal viscera associated with lumbar disk excision. In: Tarlov EC, ed. *Neurosurgical topics: complications of spinal surgery*. Park Ridge, IL: American Association of Neurological Surgeons, 1991:41–49.
9. Smith EB, DeBord JR. Intestinal injury after lumbar discectomy. *Surg Gynecol Obstet* 1991;173:22–24.
10. Hildreth DH, Trucke DA. Post laminectomy arteriovenous fistula. *Surgery* 1977;81:512–520.
11. Rossi P, Carillo FJ, Alfidi RJ, et al. Iatrogenic arteriovenous fistulas. *Radiology* 1971;111:47–51.
12. Jarstfer BS, Rich NM. The challenge of arteriovenous fistula formation following disk surgery: a collective review. *J Trauma* 1976;16:726–733.
13. Boyd DP, Farha GJ. Arteriovenous fistula and isolated vascular injuries secondary to intervertebral disk surgery. Report of four cases and review of the literature. *Ann Surg* 1965;161:524–531.
14. Santos E, Peral V, Aroca M, et al. Arteriovenous fistula as a complication of lumbar disc surgery: case report. *Neuroradiology* 1998;40:459–461.
15. Hanouz JL, Bessodes A, Samba D, et al. Delayed diagnosis of vascular injuries during lumbar discectomy. *J Clin Anesth* 2000;12:64–66.
16. Tsai Y, Yu P, Lee T, et al. Superior rectal artery injury following lumbar disc surgery. *J Neurosurg* 2001;95:108–110.
17. Harbison SP. Major vascular complications of intervertebral disc surgery. *Ann Surg* 1954;40:342–348.
18. Trinchieri A, Montanari E, Salvini P, et al. Renal autotransplantation for complete ureteral avulsion following lumbar disk surgery. *J Urol* 2001;165:1210–1211.
19. Price SJ, Buxton N. Adynamic ileus complicating lumbar laminectomy: a report of two cases. *Br J Neurosurg* 1998;12:162–164.
20. Haimovic IC, Arbit E, Posner JB. Colonic ileus complicating laminectomy. *Neurosurgery* 1978;3:369–372.
21. Caner H, Bavbek M, Albayrak A, et al. Ogilvie's syndrome as a rare complication of lumbar disc surgery. *Can J Neurol Sci* 2000;27:77–78.
22. Melamed M, Rabushka SE, Melamed JL. Colon ileus associated with low spine disease. *Clin Radiol* 1969;20:47–51.
23. Waldhausen JH, Schirmer BD. The effect of ambulation on recovery from postoperative ileus. *Ann Surg* 1990;212:671–677.
24. Bungard TJ, Kale-Pradhan PB. Prokinetic agents for the treatment of postoperative ileus in adults: a review of the literature. *Pharmacotherapy* 1999;19:416–423.
25. Goodkin R, Laska LL. Unintended "incidental" durotomy during surgery of the lumbar spine: medicolegal implications. *Surg Neurol* 1995;43:4–14.
26. Wang JC, Bohlman HH, Riew KD. Dural tears secondary to operations on the lumbar spine. *J Bone Joint Surg* 1998;80-A:1728–1732.
27. Stolke D, Sollmann WP, Seifert V. Intra- and postoperative complication in lumber disc surgery. *Spine* 1989;14:56–59.
28. Le AX, Rogers DE, Dawson EG, et al. Unrecognized durotomy after lumbar discectomy. *Spine* 2001;26:115–118.
29. Finneson BE, Schmidek HH. Lumbar disk excision. In: Schmidek HH, ed. *Operative neurosurgical techniques. Indications, methods and results,* 4th ed. Philadelphia: WB Saunders, 2000:2219–2231.
30. Hieb LD, Stevens DL. Spontaneous postoperative cerebrospinal fluid leaks following application of anti-adhesion barrier gel: case report and review of the literature. *Spine* 2001;26:748–751.
31. Lee KS, Hardy IM. Postlaminectomy lumbar pseudomeningocele: report of four cases. *Neurosurgery* 1992;30:111–114.
32. Hodges SD, Humphreys SC, Eck JC, et al. Management of incidental durotomy without mandatory bedrest: a retrospective review of 20 cases. *Spine* 1999;24:2062–2068.
33. Shapiro SA, Scully T. Closed continuous drainage of cerebrospinal fluid via a lumbar subarachnoid catheter for treatment or prevention of cranial/spinal cerebrospinal fluid fistula. *Neurosurgery* 1992;30:241–245.
34. Kitchell SH, Eismont FJ, Green BA. Closed subarachnoid drainage for management of cerebrospinal fluid leakage after an operation on the spine. *J Bone Joint Surg* 1989;71-A:984–987.
35. Waisman M, Schweppe Y. Postoperative cerebrospinal fluid leakage after lumbar spine operations. Conservative treatment. *Spine* 1991;16:52–53.
36. Leis AA, Leis JM, Leis JR. Pseudomeningoceles: a role for mechanical compression in the treatment of dural tears. *Neurology* 2001;56:1116–1117.
37. Patel MR, Louie W, Rachlin J. Postoperative cerebrospinal fluid leaks of the lumbosacral spine: management with percutaneous fibrin glue. *AJNR Am J Neuroradiol* 1996;17:495–500.
38. Elbiaadi-Aziz N, Benzon HT, Russell EJ, et al. Cerebrospinal fluid leak treated by aspiration and epidural blood patch under computed tomography guidance. *Reg Anesth Pain Med* 2001;26:363–367.
39. Jones AAM, Stambough JL, Balderston RA, et al. Long-term results of lumbar spine surgery complicated by unintended incidental durotomy. *Spine* 1989;14:443–446.
40. Silvers HR, Lewis PJ, Asch HL. Decompressive lumbar laminectomy for spinal stenosis. *J Neurosurg* 1993;78:695–701.
41. Blaauw G, Braakman R, Gelpke GJ, et al. Changes in radicular function following low-back surgery. *J Neurosurg* 1988;69:649–652.
42. Bertrand G. The "battered" root problem. *Orthop Clin North Am* 1975;6:305–310.
43. Kothbauer KF, Seiler RW. Transdural cauda equina incarceration after microsurgical lumbar discectomy: case report. *Neurosurgery* 2000;47:1449.
44. McLaren AC, Bailey SI. Cauda equina syndrome: a complication of lumbar discectomy. *Clin Orthop Rel Res*1986;204:143–149.
45. Prusick VR, Lint DS, Bruder WJ. Cauda equina syndrome as a complication of free epidural fat-grafting. A report of two cases and a review of the literature. *J Bone Joint Surg* 1988;70:1256–1258.
46. Spanier DE, Stambough JL. Delayed postoperative epidural hematoma formation after heparinization in lumbar spinal surgery. *J Spinal Disord* 2000;13:46–49.
47. Deyo RA, Cherkin DC, Loeser JD, et al. Morbidity and mortality in association with operations on the lumbar spine. *J Bone Joint Surg* 1992;74-A:536–543.
48. Spiegelmann R, Findler G, Faibel M, et al. Postoperative spinal epidural empyema. Clinical and computed tomography features. *Spine* 1991;16:1146–1149.
49. Shektman A, Granick M, Solomon MP, et al. Management of infected laminectomy wounds case report. *Neurosurgery* 1994;35:307–309.
50. Dernbach PD, Gomez H, Hahn J. Primary closure of infected spinal wounds. *Neurosurgery* 1990;26:707–709.
51. Lindholm TS, Pylkanen P. Discitis following removal of intervertebral disc. *Spine* 1982;7:618–622.
52. Fouquet B, Goupille P, Jattiot F, et al. Discitis after lumbar disc surgery. Features of "aseptic" and "septic" forms. *Spine* 1992;17:356–358.
53. Rawlings CE, Wilkins RH, Gallis HA, et al. Postoperative intervertebral disc space infection. *Neurosurgery* 1983;13:371–376.
54. Thelander U, Larsson S. Quantitation of c-reactive protein levels and erythrocyte sedimentation rate after spinal surgery. *Spine* 1992;17:400–404.
55. Boden SD, Davis DO, Dina TS, et al. Postoperative diskitis: distinguishing early MR imaging findings from normal postoperative disk space changes. *Radiology* 1992;184:765–771.

Index

Note: Page numbers followed by *f* refer to figures; page numbers followed by *t* refer to tables.

C

E

F

G

J

K